The Comparative Guide to American Hospitals

Volume 4

Second Edition

The Comparative Guide to American Hospitals

Volume 4: Western Region

4,383 Hospitals with Key Personnel and
24 Quality Measures in Treating Heart Attack, Heart Failure,
Pneumonia, Pregnancy and Surgical Infection Prevention

A SEDGWICK PRESS Book

Grey House Publishing

PUBLISHER . . . . Leslie Mackenzie
EDITOR. . . . . David Garoogian
EDITORIAL DIRECTOR. . . . . Laura Mars-Proietti
PRODUCTION MANAGER . . . . Karen Stevens
MARKETING DIRECTOR . . . . Jessica Moody

A Sedgewick Press Book
Grey House Publishing, Inc.
185 Millerton Road
Millerton, NY 12546
518.789.8700
FAX 518.789.0545
www.greyhouse.com
e-mail: books @greyhouse.com

Second Edition

Printed in the USA

10 9 8 7 6 5 4 3 2

Comparative guide to American hospitals. Vol. 1, Eastern region; [ed. David Garoogian]. -- 2nd ed. (2007)

v. ; cm.

Includes index.
"4,383 hospitals with key personnel and 24 quality measures in treating heart attack, heart failure, pneumonia, pregnancy and surgical infection prevention."

1. Hospitals--United States--Directories. 2. Hospitals--United States--Periodicals. 3. Hospitals--Ratings--United States--Statistics--Periodicals. 4. Myocardial infarction--Hospitals--United States--Directories. 5. Heart failure--Hospitals--United States--Directories. 6. Pneumonia--Hospitals--United States--Directories. I. Garoogian, David.

RA977 .C66
610/.025

4-Volume Set ISBN: 978-1-59237-182-2
Volume 1 ISBN: 978-1-59237-280-5
Volume 2 ISBN: 978-1-59237-281-2
Volume 3 ISBN: 978-1-59237-282-9
Volume 4 ISBN: 978-1-59237-283-6

Table of Contents

Introduction

Welcome to the second edition of *The Comparative Guide to American Hospitals*. It reports on how 4,383 hospitals in America measure up when caring for patients with a number of specific conditions. The first edition reported on **Heart Attacks, Heart Failure** and **Pneumonia**. In this second edition, each hospital profile includes additional data on **Pregnancy Care** and **Surgical Infection Prevention.** Also new are two Appendixes - **30-Day Mortality Data** and **Glossary of Terms**.

The content of this work is based on a Federal study (Hospital Compare) in which short-term acute care and critical access hospitals around the country voluntarily reported on quality measures in order to receive an incentive payment established by the Medicare Prescription Drug, Improvement and Modernization Act of 2003. Each hospital is rated on 24 recognized quality measures - **Seven More Than Last Edition** -- and is compared to both state and national averages, and to the top hospitals in the country (best practices).

Due to the increased data, and the regional use of such data, this edition is comprised of four regional volumes - **Eastern, Southern, Central** and **Western**. In addition to comprehensive hospital profiles for all states in the region, each volume includes a **State-by-State Statistical Summary**.

Each hospital profile in *The Comparative Guide to American Hospitals* is comprised of data from Hospital Compare (the Medicare sponsored web site) and The Joint Commission plus value-added data from Grey House's *Directory of Hospital Personnel*. You will find **20,700 key contact names** managing the care at 4,383 hospitals - that's 5,509 more names at 180 more hospitals than last edition. In addition, each state chapter includes **State Rankings**.

Section One: Hospital Rankings & State Profiles

The first section of each regional volume of *The Comparative Guide to American Hospitals* is arranged alphabetically by state. Each state starts with a ranking section that rates hospitals in that state on how often they meet the accepted quality protocols. Following the ranking section, hospital profiles are listed first by city, then alpha within city. Profiles include name, address, phone, fax, web site and number of licensed beds. Further, each profile includes an average of 10 key medical contacts -- **Five More Than Last Edition** -- including hospital administration, patients, and those who provide products and services to the industry -- representing not only the facility's top administration but also the physicians specifically responsible for the care of heart, pneumonia, and pregnant patients, as well as surgical infection prevention.

The first section of *The Comparative Guide to American Hospitals*:

- **Evaluates 24 Quality Measures:** The quality measures rated in *The Comparative Guide to American Hospitals* are based on accepted, effective treatments supported by the Centers for Medicare & Medical Services of the US Department of Health & Human Services and the Hospital Quality Alliance (HQA) - a public/private collaboration established to promote on hospital quality of care. HQA represents consumers, hospitals, doctors, employers, accrediting organizations and Federal agencies.
- **Examines Critical Conditions: Heart Attack Care** measures include aspirin at arrival and discharge, beta blockers at arrival and discharge, use of ACE/ARB inhibitors, and PCI administration and fibrinolytic medication timing. **Heart Failure Care** measures include LVF assessment, use of ACE/ARB inhibitors, discharge instructions and smoking cessation advice. **Pneumonia Care** measures include use of initial antibiotics and pneumococcal vaccine, use of oxygenation and blood culture results, smoking cessation advice, and administration of influenza vaccine. **Surgical Infection Prevention** measures ***(NEW)*** include use of prophylactic antibiotics. **Pregnancy Care** measures ***(NEW)*** include inpatient neonatal mortality, and degree of vaginal lacerations.

Section Two: Statistical Summary, Appendixes & Index

The second section of *The Comparative Guide to American Hospitals includes:*

- **Regional State-by-State Statistical Summary Tables** show at a glance how hospitals in the same state score and compare with each other. They are arranged alphabetically by state in easy-to-read landscape format.

- **Appendix A: 30-Day Mortality Chart** *(NEW)* lists hospitals nationwide that are "better" or "worse" than the national average, plus a State Summary of Hospital Mortality.

- **Appendix B: Glossary of Terms** *(NEW)* provides a list of 60 medical terms to make the best use possible of the data in this edition.

- **Regional Hospital Profile Index** lists hospitals alphabetically, including city and state.

This completely revised second edition of *The Comparative Guide to American Hospitals,* **now in four regional volumes**, is a valuable guide for the entire medical community, with more hospitals, more criteria measures and more key executives than the first edition. It offers an indispensable snapshot of how hospitals measure up, not only to established "best practices," but also to each other.

We welcome your comments to this edition.

User's Guide

Shown below is a fictitious listing illustrating the kind of information that is or might be included in a Hospital Profile. Each numbered item of information is described in the paragraphs following the example.

❶ Bowling Green Medical Center

250 Park Street — Phone: 270-745-1255
Bowling Green, KY 42101 — Fax: 270-745-1253
E-mail: SKWebb@mcbg.org
URL: www.mcbg.org
Ownership: Voluntary non-profit - Private — Accredited: Yes
Emergency Services: Yes — Licensed Beds: 330

❷ **Key Personnel:**

CEO/President. . . . . Wayne Bush, MD
Emergency Room Director. . . . . Pliois Prerost
Director Medical/Surgical Nursing . . . . Kathleen Riley, RN
Chief OB/GYN . . . . Joseph Gass, MD
Surgery Chair. . . . . James Bergin, MD
Chief Radiology . . . . Ken Bartholomew, MD

	Measure	Cases	This Hospital	State Average	U.S. Average	Top Hospital
❸						
❹	**Heart Attack Care**					
	ACE Inhibitor or ARB for LVSD	63	73%	75%	82%	100%
	Aspirin at Arrival	191	95%	89%	92%	100%
	Aspirin at Discharge	243	96%	86%	90%	100%
	Beta Blocker at Arrival	140	91%	82%	87%	100%
	Beta Blocker at Discharge	274	97%	86%	90%	100%
	Fibrinolytic Medication Timing[1]	10	10%	31%	31%	100%
	PCI Within 90 Minutes of Arrival[1]	6	17%	44%	54%	95%
	Smoking Cessation Advice	147	100%	84%	88%	100%
❺	**Heart Failure Care**					
	ACE Inhibitor or ARB for LVSD	162	84%	78%	82%	100%
	Discharge Instructions	394	50%	59%	61%	93%
	Evaluation of LVS Function	466	90%	79%	83%	99%
	Smoking Cessation Advice	123	100%	82%	82%	100%
❻	**Pneumonia Care**					
	Appropriate Initial Antibiotic	277	84%	82%	83%	94%
	Blood Culture Timing	225	92%	89%	90%	100%
	Influenza Vaccine	87	84%	76%	70%	100%
	Initial Antibiotic Timing	382	69%	82%	80%	93%
	Oxygenation Assessment	483	100%	99%	99%	100%
	Pneumococcal Vaccine	284	87%	75%	69%	94%
	Smoking Cessation Advice	170	100%	84%	80%	100%
❼	**Surgical Infection Prevention**					
	Prophylactic Antibiotic Given[3]	427	89%	74%	77%	95%
	Prophylactic Antibiotic Selection	245	87%	85%	90%	100%
	Prophylactic Antibiotic Stopped[3]	424	91%	69%	72%	95%
❽	**Pregnancy Care**					
	Inpatient Neonatal Mortality	1,979	0.25%	-	-	-
	Third or Fourth Degree Laceration	1,283	4.36%	3.25%	3.63%	3.27%

➊ **Hospital Name and Record Header:** hospital name; alternate name (if applicable); street address; phone; fax; e-mail; URL; ownership; accredited (Yes/No); emergency services (Yes/No); and number of licensed beds. *Source: Directory of Hospital Personnel, 2007, Grey House Publishing; www.hospitalcompare.hhs.gov, Centers for Medicare & Medicaid Services (CMS), an agency of the U.S. Department of Health and Human Services (DHHS) along with the Hospital Quality Alliance (HQA).*

➋ **Key Personnel:** includes the names of key personnel primarily related to the five conditions covered in this publication. *Source: Directory of Hospital Personnel, 2007, Grey House Publishing*

➌ **Hospital Compare Data:** each table contains data covering the five conditions and twenty-four associated measures contained in the Hospital Compare database. There are six columns:

Measure: the twenty-four quality measures reported.

There are five possible footnotes:

1. *The number of cases is too small (n<25) for purposes of reliably predicting hospital performance.*
   For each measure, the rate is displayed as a percent of the number of patients for whom the measured treatment is appropriate. For hospitals with small numbers of patients for whom the measured treatment is appropriate during the reporting period (fewer than 25 patients), the calculated rate may not be predictive of the hospital's future performance. As the quality data base is expanded to a full rolling four quarters of data for each measure, the number of cases used to determine hospitals' rates will likely increase, thereby increasing the reliability and stability of the rates. Note: This footnote does not necessarily reflect hospital size or overall patient volume.

2. *Measure reflects the hospital's indication that its submission was based upon a sample of its relevant discharges.*
   Rates are based on the cases reported by hospitals. A rate may be based upon the total number of cases treated by a hospital, or for a facility with a large caseload, a rate may be based on a random sample of the cases the hospital treated. This footnote indicates that a hospital chose to submit data for a sample of its total cases (following specific rules for how to the select the cases).

3. *Rate reflects fewer than the maximum possible quarters of data for the measure.*
   Each rate reflects the care provided over a specific time period, up to a maximum of four quarters. The number of quarters of data available is determined by when hospitals first began to report data using a specific measure. For example, for the ten measures in the "Starter Set", the maximum number of quarters for which a hospital could have provided data is four quarters. For measures added more recently, the maximum will be fewer than four quarters. This footnote indicates that the hospital's rate was based on data from fewer than the maximum possible number of quarters that the measure was generally collected.

4. *Inaccurate information submitted and suppressed for one or more quarters.*
   Hospitals are required to submit accurate, reportable data to the Centers for Medicare and Medicaid Services (CMS). The rates for these measures were calculated by excluding data that had been suppressed for one or more quarters because they were identified as inaccurate.

5. *No data is available from the hospital for this measure.*
   Hospitals volunteer to provide data for reporting on Hospital Compare. This footnote is applied when the hospital did not submit any cases for a measure.

Cases: the size of the data sample (number of patients) for each hospital and quality measure. In addition, the notation "0" is applied when a hospital provided care to patients with a condition, such as pneumonia, but the cases that the hospital submitted did not meet the specific criteria for being included in the calculation of the measure.

This Hospital: the performance rate that the hospital achieved for each quality measure. This value is expressed as a percentage of the sample size that was measured.

State Average: the average rate for all hospitals reporting data in the state the hospital is located in.

U.S. Average: the average rate for all hospitals reporting nationwide.

Top Hospital: the average rate for the 90th percentile (or top 10%) of hospitals reporting data.

Note: A two-step process was used to calculate the national and state comparison group rates. The national and state comparison rates for each measure were calculated using all of the data submitted to the QIO Clinical Data Warehouse for hospitals with at least one case that met the measure's inclusion criteria (that is, for which the denominator was greater than zero).

First, the individual hospital performance rates were calculated using the method described above for all hospitals. Next, hospitals with "0 patients" were excluded from the calculation. For the determination of the 90th percentile (or top 10%) of hospitals on a national basis, the individual rates were then rank ordered and the top 10th percentile score identified. For the national and state averages, a simple average was constructed where the numerator was the sum of all non-excluded hospitals' scores and the denominator was the total number of hospitals, each calculated at either the national or individual state level.

❹ Heart Attack Care

Every year, about one million people suffer a heart attack (acute myocardial infarction or AMI). AMI is among the leading causes of hospital admission for Medicare beneficiaries, age 65 and older.

Scientific evidence indicates that the following process of care measures represent the best practices for the treatment of AMI. Higher scores are better.

- **ACE Inhibitor or ARB for LVSD** - AMI patients with left ventricular systolic dysfunction (LVSD) and without angiotensin converting enzyme inhibitor (ACE inhibitor) contraindications or angiotensin receptor blocker (ARB) contraindications who are prescribed an ACE inhibitor or an ARB at hospital discharge.
- **Aspirin at Arrival** - Acute myocardial infarction (AMI) patients without aspirin contraindications who received aspirin within 24 hours before or after hospital arrival.
- **Aspirin at Discharge** - AMI patients without aspirin contraindications who were prescribed aspirin at hospital discharge.
- **Beta Blocker at Arrival** - AMI patients without beta-blocker contraindications who received a beta-blocker within 24 hours after hospital arrival.
- **Beta Blocker at Discharge** - AMI patients without beta-blocker contraindications who were prescribed a beta-blocker at hospital discharge.
- **Fibrinolytic Medication Timing** - AMI patients receiving fibrinolytic therapy during the hospital stay and having a time from hospital arrival to fibrinolysis of 30 minutes or less.
- **PCI Within 90 Minutes of Arrival** - AMI patients receiving Percutaneous Coronary Intervention (PCI) during the hospital stay with a time from hospital arrival to PCI of 90 minutes or less.
- **Smoking Cessation Advice** - AMI patients with a history of smoking cigarettes, who are given smoking cessation advice or counseling during a hospital stay.

❺ Heart Failure Care

Heart failure is the most common hospital admission diagnosis in patients age 65 or older, accounting for more than 700,000 hospitalizations among Medicare beneficiaries every year. It is associated with severe functional impairments and high rates of mortality and morbidity.

Substantial scientific evidence indicates that the following process of care measures represent the best practices for the treatment of heart failure. Higher scores are better.

- **ACE Inhibitor or ARB for LVSD** - Heart failure patients with left ventricular systolic dysfunction (LVSD) and without angiotensin converting enzyme inhibitor (ACE inhibitor) contraindications or angiotensin receptor blocker (ARB) contraindications who are prescribed an ACE inhibitor or an ARB at hospital discharge.
- **Discharge Instructions** - Heart failure patients discharged home with written instructions or educational material given to patient or care giver at discharge or during the hospital stay addressing all of the following: activity level, diet, discharge medications, follow-up appointment, weight monitoring, and what to do if symptoms worsen.
- **Evaluation of LVS Function** - Heart failure patients with documentation in the hospital record that an evaluation of the left ventricular systolic (LVS) function was performed before arrival, during hospitalization, or is planned for after discharge.
- **Smoking Cessation Advice** - Heart failure patients with a history of smoking cigarettes, who are given smoking cessation advice or counseling during a hospital stay.

❻ Pneumonia Care

Community acquired pneumonia is a major contributor to illness and mortality in the United States, causing four million episodes of illness and nearly one million hospital admissions each year.

Scientific evidence indicates that the following process of care measures represent the best practices for the treatment of community-acquired pneumonia. Higher scores are better.

- **Appropriate Initial Antibiotic** - Immunocompetent patients with pneumonia who receive an initial antibiotic regimen that is consistent with current guidelines.
- **Blood Culture Timing** - Pneumonia patients whose initial emergency room blood culture specimen was collected prior to first hospital dose of antibiotics.
- **Influenza Vaccination** - Pneumonia patients age 50 years and older, hospitalized during October, November, December, January, or February who were screened for influenza vaccine status and were vaccinated prior to discharge, if indicated.
- **Initial Antibiotic Timing** - Pneumonia inpatients who receive antibiotics within 4 hours of hospital arrival. Evidence shows better outcomes for administration times less than four hours.
- **Oxygenation Assessment** - Pneumonia inpatients who receive an oxygenation assessment, arterial blood gas (ABG), or pulse oximetry within 24 hours of hospital arrival.
- **Pneumococcal Vaccination** - Pneumonia inpatients age 65 and older who were screened for pneumococcal vaccine status and were administered the vaccine prior to discharge, if indicated.
- **Smoking Cessation Advice** - Pneumonia patients with a history of smoking cigarettes, who are given smoking cessation advice or counseling during a hospital stay.

❼ Surgical Infection Prevention

Hospitals can reduce the risk of wound infection after surgery by providing the right medicines at the right time on the day of surgery. Studies show a strong association of reduced incidence of post-operative infection with administration of antibiotics within the one hour prior to surgery. After the incision is closed, however, studies show that prolonged administration of prophylaxis with antibiotics may increase the risk of certain other infections at no additional benefit to the surgical patient.

Scientific evidence indicates that the following process of care measures represent the best practices for the prevention of infections after selected surgeries (colon surgery, hip and knee arthroplasty, abdominal and vaginal hysterectomy, cardiac surgery (including coronary artery bypass grafts (CABG)) and vascular surgery). Higher scores are better.

- **Prophylactic Antibiotic Given** - Surgical patients who received prophylactic antibiotics within 1 hour prior to surgical incision.
- **Prophylactic Antibiotic Selection** - Surgical patients who received the recommended antibiotics for their particular type of surgery.
- **Prophylactic Antibiotic Stopped** - Surgical patients whose prophylactic antibiotics were discontinued within 24 hours after surgery end time.

❽ Pregnancy Care

- **Inpatient Neonatal Mortality** - This measure reports how often infants died before 28 days of birth; it is adjusted to reflect the fact that some babies are sicker than others at or shortly after birth.
- **Third or Fourth Degree Laceration** - This measure reports how often patients have significant tears between the vagina and anus while having a baby. These types of tears can lead to other medical complications.

Information about Hospital Performance

Hospital performance rates tell you the proportion of cases where a hospital provided the recommended process of care. Only patients meeting the inclusion criteria for a measure are included in the calculation of the rate for a measure. A rate of 88% means that the hospital provided the recommended process of care 88% of the time. For example, the rates for initial antibiotic timing tell you the percentage of patients who received their first dose of antibiotics within four hours of arrival to the hospital. The ultimate goal for all measures listed (except Pregnancy Care) is 100%. With the two measures under Pregnancy Care, lower numbers are preferable. Hospitals with effective quality improvement programs are continually working toward this goal.

Confidence Intervals

The table below enables the user to calculate confidence intervals for each reported measure.

Confidence intervals can be used to estimate the precision of the calculated rates for an individual hospital. A confidence interval is the range of values, within which an estimated value or rate is likely to fall. A confidence interval is a statistical determination of the degree of certainty associated with an estimated value. As can be seen in the table of estimated values (below), large differences between individual hospitals' rates may be significant, and small differences between hospitals are usually not significant.

The smaller the sample size, the greater the difference in rates must be order for that difference to be statistically meaningful. Also, as sample size varies between hospitals, it is difficult to precisely compare their rates, without considering the confidence intervals.

Over time, as the quality data base is expanded, a full four quarters of data will ultimately be available, so the number of cases used to determine hospitals' rates will likely increase, thereby increasing the reliability and stability of the rates.

Estimating Confidence Intervals for the Quality Measures: Estimated Values for Proportion Data

Sample Size	Observed Rate								
	10%	20%	30%	40%	50%	60%	70%	80%	90%
< 25	*	*	24.9	26.6	27.2	26.6	24.9	*	*
25 - 75	8.3	11.1	12.7	13.6	13.9	13.6	12.7	11.1	8.3
76 - 125	5.9	7.8	9.0	9.6	9.8	9.6	9.0	7.8	5.9
126 - 175	4.8	6.4	7.3	7.8	8.0	7.8	7.3	6.4	4.8
176 - 225	4.2	5.5	6.4	6.8	6.9	6.8	6.4	5.5	4.2
226 -275	3.7	5.0	5.7	6.1	6.2	6.1	5.7	5.0	3.7
276+	2.9	3.9	4.5	4.8	4.9	4.8	4.5	3.9	2.9

Source: CMS/OCSQ/QIG. The values in the table are the approximate amount to add and subtract from the observed rate to estimate a 95 percent confidence interval for the given sample size. (Interpolation between the values in the table is appropriate.)
** Estimates of an interval in these cells exceed the natural limits for proportions.*

Source of Data

The information in this book comes from the quality data submitted by hospitals to the QIO Clinical Data Warehouse for inpatient discharges. Heart Attack Care, Heart Failure Care, Pneumonia Care, Pregnancy Care and Surgical Infection Prevention data is from www.hospitalcompare.hhs.gov, a website tool developed by the Centers for Medicare & Medicaid Services (CMS). Data covers October 2005 through September 2006. Hospital Mortality data is also from www.hospitalcompare.hhs.gov. Data covers July 2005 through June 2006.

Pregnancy Care data is from www.qualitycheck.org, a service of The Joint Commission. The Joint Commission (formerly the Joint Commission on Accreditation of Healthcare Organizations (JCAHO)), is a US-based non-profit organization formed in 1951 with a mission to maintain and elevate the standards of healthcare delivery through evaluation and accreditation of healthcare organizations. Data covers January 2006 through December 2006.

Heart Attack Care

1. ACE Inhibitor or ARB for LVSD

Hospital Name	City	Rate	Cases
Providence Alaska Medical Center	Anchorage	85%	82

2. Aspirin at Arrival

Hospital Name	City	Rate	Cases
Alaska Regional Hospital	Anchorage	100%	67
Valley Hospital	Palmer	100%	37
Providence Alaska Medical Center	Anchorage	98%	191

3. Aspirin at Discharge

Hospital Name	City	Rate	Cases
Alaska Regional Hospital	Anchorage	100%	117
Providence Alaska Medical Center	Anchorage	95%	362

4. Beta Blocker at Arrival

Hospital Name	City	Rate	Cases
Alaska Regional Hospital	Anchorage	96%	69
Providence Alaska Medical Center	Anchorage	95%	150
Valley Hospital	Palmer	91%	32

5. Beta Blocker at Discharge

Hospital Name	City	Rate	Cases
Alaska Regional Hospital	Anchorage	97%	115
Providence Alaska Medical Center	Anchorage	97%	354

8. Smoking Cessation Advice

Hospital Name	City	Rate	Cases
Alaska Regional Hospital	Anchorage	92%	49
Providence Alaska Medical Center	Anchorage	90%	137

Heart Failure Care

9. ACE Inhibitor or ARB for LVSD

Hospital Name	City	Rate	Cases
Alaska Native Medical Center	Anchorage	100%	42
Alaska Regional Hospital	Anchorage	92%	36
Fairbanks Memorial Hospital	Fairbanks	90%	39
Providence Alaska Medical Center	Anchorage	90%	183

10. Discharge Instructions

Hospital Name	City	Rate	Cases
Central Peninsula Hospital	Soldotna	83%	35
Valley Hospital	Palmer	68%	56
Fairbanks Memorial Hospital	Fairbanks	66%	85
Bartlett Regional Hospital	Juneau	51%	41
Alaska Regional Hospital	Anchorage	49%	75
Providence Alaska Medical Center	Anchorage	43%	289
Alaska Native Medical Center	Anchorage	5%	65

11. Evaluation of LVS Function

Hospital Name	City	Rate	Cases
Fairbanks Memorial Hospital	Fairbanks	99%	86
Alaska Native Medical Center	Anchorage	97%	66
Alaska Regional Hospital	Anchorage	97%	78
Central Peninsula Hospital	Soldotna	97%	38
Providence Alaska Medical Center	Anchorage	96%	305
Valley Hospital	Palmer	91%	57
Bartlett Regional Hospital	Juneau	89%	45

12. Smoking Cessation Advice

Hospital Name	City	Rate	Cases
Providence Alaska Medical Center	Anchorage	55%	80

Pneumonia Care

13. Appropriate Initial Antibiotic

Hospital Name	City	Rate	Cases
Alaska Native Medical Center	Anchorage	91%	64
Alaska Regional Hospital	Anchorage	91%	34
Central Peninsula Hospital	Soldotna	89%	35
Valley Hospital	Palmer	83%	75
Fairbanks Memorial Hospital	Fairbanks	80%	89
Ketchikan General Hospital	Ketchikan	77%	31
Providence Alaska Medical Center	Anchorage	76%	165
Bartlett Regional Hospital	Juneau	70%	50

14. Blood Culture Timing

Hospital Name	City	Rate	Cases
Central Peninsula Hospital	Soldotna	100%	30
Fairbanks Memorial Hospital	Fairbanks	97%	62
Bartlett Regional Hospital	Juneau	96%	26
Valley Hospital	Palmer	96%	48
Alaska Native Medical Center	Anchorage	90%	59
Ketchikan General Hospital	Ketchikan	89%	27
Providence Alaska Medical Center	Anchorage	89%	135

15. Influenza Vaccine

Hospital Name	City	Rate	Cases
Providence Alaska Medical Center	Anchorage	63%	30

16. Initial Antibiotic Timing

Hospital Name	City	Rate	Cases
Alaska Regional Hospital	Anchorage	84%	37
Bartlett Regional Hospital	Juneau	83%	42
Valley Hospital	Palmer	82%	80
Fairbanks Memorial Hospital	Fairbanks	80%	109
Alaska Native Medical Center	Anchorage	77%	79
Central Peninsula Hospital	Soldotna	77%	39
Ketchikan General Hospital	Ketchikan	72%	36
Providence Alaska Medical Center	Anchorage	72%	166
Yukon-Kuskokwim Delta Regional Hospital	Bethel	64%	58

17. Oxygenation Assessment

Hospital Name	City	Rate	Cases
Alaska Regional Hospital	Anchorage	100%	50
Bartlett Regional Hospital	Juneau	100%	58
Central Peninsula Hospital	Soldotna	100%	52
Fairbanks Memorial Hospital	Fairbanks	100%	136
Ketchikan General Hospital	Ketchikan	100%	48
Providence Alaska Medical Center	Anchorage	100%	227
Valley Hospital	Palmer	100%	91
Yukon-Kuskokwim Delta Regional Hospital	Bethel	100%	83
Alaska Native Medical Center	Anchorage	99%	96
South Peninsula Hospital	Homer	96%	25

18. Pneumococcal Vaccine

Hospital Name	City	Rate	Cases
Alaska Native Medical Center	Anchorage	94%	36
Fairbanks Memorial Hospital	Fairbanks	88%	69
Valley Hospital	Palmer	83%	54
Central Peninsula Hospital	Soldotna	81%	32
Ketchikan General Hospital	Ketchikan	76%	25
Yukon-Kuskokwim Delta Regional Hospital	Bethel	63%	54
Providence Alaska Medical Center	Anchorage	48%	103
Bartlett Regional Hospital	Juneau	47%	34

19. Smoking Cessation Advice

Hospital Name	City	Rate	Cases
Fairbanks Memorial Hospital	Fairbanks	95%	38
Providence Alaska Medical Center	Anchorage	66%	61
Alaska Native Medical Center	Anchorage	65%	48

Surgical Infection Prevention

20. Prophylactic Antibiotic Given

Hospital Name	City	Rate	Cases
Providence Alaska Medical Center	Anchorage	87%	228
Alaska Native Medical Center	Anchorage	84%	198
Ketchikan General Hospital	Ketchikan	84%	37
Valley Hospital	Palmer	84%	141
Central Peninsula Hospital	Soldotna	81%	75
Fairbanks Memorial Hospital	Fairbanks	71%	132
Alaska Regional Hospital	Anchorage	63%	273
Bartlett Regional Hospital	Juneau	37%	57

21. Prophylactic Antibiotic Selection

Hospital Name	City	Rate	Cases
Alaska Regional Hospital	Anchorage	95%	133
Providence Alaska Medical Center	Anchorage	95%	75
Alaska Native Medical Center	Anchorage	93%	60
Valley Hospital	Palmer	87%	38
Fairbanks Memorial Hospital	Fairbanks	85%	52
Bartlett Regional Hospital	Juneau	56%	27

NOTE: Hospital profiles are in alphabetical order by state, then city, then hospital within the city; Rankings are sorted by rate in descending order and exclude hospitals with less than 25 cases; (1) The number of cases is too small (n<25) for purposes of reliably predicting hospital performance; (2) Measure reflects the hospital's indication that its submission was based upon a sample of its relevant discharges; (3) Rate reflects fewer than the maximum possible quarters of data for the measure; (4) Inaccurate information submitted and suppressed for one or more quarters; (5) No data is available from the hospital for this measure; Please refer to the User's Guide for a full explanation of data

22. Prophylactic Antibiotic Stopped

Hospital Name	City	Rate	Cases
Central Peninsula Hospital	Soldotna	94%	78
Fairbanks Memorial Hospital	Fairbanks	82%	128
Valley Hospital	Palmer	82%	136
Alaska Native Medical Center	Anchorage	81%	195
Alaska Regional Hospital	Anchorage	76%	271
Ketchikan General Hospital	Ketchikan	76%	37
Providence Alaska Medical Center	Anchorage	71%	222
Bartlett Regional Hospital	Juneau	63%	52

Pregnancy Care

23. Inpatient Neonatal Mortality

Hospital Name	City	Rate	Cases
Alaska Native Medical Center	Anchorage	0.40%	1501

24. Third or Fourth Degree Laceration

Hospital Name	City	Rate	Cases
Alaska Native Medical Center	Anchorage	3.07%	1207

NOTE: Hospital profiles are in alphabetical order by state, then city, then hospital within the city; Rankings are sorted by rate in descending order and exclude hospitals with less than 25 cases; (1) The number of cases is too small (n<25) for purposes of reliably predicting hospital performance; (2) Measure reflects the hospital's indication that its submission was based upon a sample of its relevant discharges; (3) Rate reflects fewer than the maximum possible quarters of data for the measure; (4) Inaccurate information submitted and suppressed for one or more quarters; (5) No data is available from the hospital for this measure; Please refer to the User's Guide for a full explanation of data

Alaska Native Medical Center

4315 Diplomacy Drive
Anchorage, AK 99508
URL: www.anmc.org
Ownership: Government - Federal
Emergency Services: Yes
Phone: 907-563-2662
Fax: 907-729-1984
Accredited: Yes

Key Personnel:

Hospital Administrator . . . . Dee Hutchison, RN
Chief Medical Staff. . . . . David Snyder, MD
Cardiac Lab . . . . Matt Schenellbacher
Emergency Room . . . . Richard Brodsky
Infection Control. . . . . Carol Bromley
ICU . . . . Phyllis Goodwin
Medical Surgical Nurse . . . . Julie Palm
OB/GYN Womens Health. . . . . Kristen Cady

Measure	Cases	This Hospital	State Average	U.S. Average	Top Hospital
Heart Attack Care					
ACE Inhibitor or ARB for LVSD[1]	6	100%	84%	82%	100%
Aspirin at Arrival[1]	3	100%	95%	92%	100%
Aspirin at Discharge[1]	11	91%	98%	90%	100%
Beta Blocker at Arrival[1]	3	100%	86%	87%	100%
Beta Blocker at Discharge[1]	12	92%	87%	90%	100%
Fibrinolytic Medication Timing	0	-	17%	31%	100%
PCI Within 90 Minutes of Arrival	0	-	63%	54%	95%
Smoking Cessation Advice[1]	7	57%	75%	88%	100%
Heart Failure Care					
ACE Inhibitor or ARB for LVSD	42	100%	88%	82%	100%
Discharge Instructions	65	5%	40%	61%	93%
Evaluation of LVS Function	66	97%	83%	83%	99%
Smoking Cessation Advice[1]	23	57%	80%	82%	100%
Pneumonia Care					
Appropriate Initial Antibiotic	64	91%	86%	83%	94%
Blood Culture Timing	59	90%	94%	90%	100%
Influenza Vaccine[1]	13	54%	64%	70%	100%
Initial Antibiotic Timing	79	77%	78%	80%	93%
Oxygenation Assessment	96	99%	100%	99%	100%
Pneumococcal Vaccine	36	94%	69%	69%	94%
Smoking Cessation Advice	48	65%	79%	80%	100%
Surgical Infection Prevention					
Prophylactic Antibiotic Given[2,3]	198	84%	78%	77%	95%
Prophylactic Antibiotic Selection[2]	60	93%	90%	90%	100%
Prophylactic Antibiotic Stopped[2,3]	195	81%	72%	72%	95%
Pregnancy Care					
Inpatient Neonatal Mortality	1,501	0.40%	-	-	-
Third or Fourth Degree Laceration	1,207	3.07%	-	3.63%	3.27%

Alaska Regional Hospital

Alternate Name: Humana Hospital-Alaska
2801 DeBarr Road
Anchorage, AK 99508
URL: www.alaskaregional.com
Ownership: Proprietary
Emergency Services: Yes
Phone: 907-276-1131
Fax: 907-264-1143
Accredited: Yes
Licensed Beds: 238

Key Personnel:

CEO. . . . . Ed Lamb
Chief Medical Staff. . . . . Richard Chung, MD
Director Radiology . . . . Dennis Cherry
Emergency Room . . . . Hilliard Pettus, RN
Director Medical/Surgical Nursing . . . . Paula Fair
Director Medical/Surgical Nursing . . . . Norman Wilder, MD
OB/GYN Womens Health. . . . . Rhene Merkouts, MD
Chief Radiology . . . . Bradley Cruz, MD
Director Respiratory Therapy . . . . Connie Spahn

Measure	Cases	This Hospital	State Average	U.S. Average	Top Hospital
Heart Attack Care					
ACE Inhibitor or ARB for LVSD[1]	21	100%	84%	82%	100%
Aspirin at Arrival	67	100%	95%	92%	100%
Aspirin at Discharge	117	100%	98%	90%	100%
Beta Blocker at Arrival	69	96%	86%	87%	100%
Beta Blocker at Discharge	115	97%	87%	90%	100%
Fibrinolytic Medication Timing	0	-	17%	31%	100%
PCI Within 90 Minutes of Arrival[1]	7	71%	63%	54%	95%
Smoking Cessation Advice	49	92%	75%	88%	100%
Heart Failure Care					
ACE Inhibitor or ARB for LVSD	36	92%	88%	82%	100%
Discharge Instructions	75	49%	40%	61%	93%
Evaluation of LVS Function	78	97%	83%	83%	99%
Smoking Cessation Advice[1]	16	81%	80%	82%	100%
Pneumonia Care					
Appropriate Initial Antibiotic	34	91%	86%	83%	94%
Blood Culture Timing[1]	20	85%	94%	90%	100%
Influenza Vaccine[1]	5	60%	64%	70%	100%
Initial Antibiotic Timing	37	84%	78%	80%	93%
Oxygenation Assessment	50	100%	100%	99%	100%
Pneumococcal Vaccine[1]	22	55%	69%	69%	94%
Smoking Cessation Advice[1]	18	78%	79%	80%	100%
Surgical Infection Prevention					
Prophylactic Antibiotic Given[2,3]	273	63%	78%	77%	95%
Prophylactic Antibiotic Selection[2]	133	95%	90%	90%	100%
Prophylactic Antibiotic Stopped[2,3]	271	76%	72%	72%	95%
Pregnancy Care					
Inpatient Neonatal Mortality	-	-	-	-	-
Third or Fourth Degree Laceration	-	-	-	3.63%	3.27%

Providence Alaska Medical Center

Alternate Name: Providence Hospital
3200 Providence Drive
Anchorage, AK 99508
URL: www.providence.org
Ownership: Voluntary non-profit - Church
Emergency Services: Yes
Phone: 907-562-2211
Fax: 907-261-3041
Accredited: Yes
Licensed Beds: 293

Key Personnel:

CEO. . . . . Douglas A Bruce
OB/GYN Womens Health. . . . . Maicylyn Pique
Chief Radiology . . . . Denise Farleigh, MD
Director Respiratory Therapy . . . . LuAnn Moss

Measure	Cases	This Hospital	State Average	U.S. Average	Top Hospital
Heart Attack Care					
ACE Inhibitor or ARB for LVSD	82	85%	84%	82%	100%
Aspirin at Arrival	191	98%	95%	92%	100%
Aspirin at Discharge	362	95%	98%	90%	100%
Beta Blocker at Arrival	150	95%	86%	87%	100%
Beta Blocker at Discharge	354	97%	87%	90%	100%
Fibrinolytic Medication Timing	0	-	17%	31%	100%
PCI Within 90 Minutes of Arrival[1]	13	54%	63%	54%	95%
Smoking Cessation Advice	137	90%	75%	88%	100%
Heart Failure Care					
ACE Inhibitor or ARB for LVSD	183	90%	88%	82%	100%
Discharge Instructions	289	43%	40%	61%	93%
Evaluation of LVS Function	305	96%	83%	83%	99%
Smoking Cessation Advice	80	55%	80%	82%	100%
Pneumonia Care					
Appropriate Initial Antibiotic	165	76%	86%	83%	94%
Blood Culture Timing	135	89%	94%	90%	100%
Influenza Vaccine	30	63%	64%	70%	100%
Initial Antibiotic Timing	166	72%	78%	80%	93%
Oxygenation Assessment	227	100%	100%	99%	100%
Pneumococcal Vaccine	103	48%	69%	69%	94%
Smoking Cessation Advice	61	66%	79%	80%	100%
Surgical Infection Prevention					
Prophylactic Antibiotic Given[2,3]	228	87%	78%	77%	95%
Prophylactic Antibiotic Selection[2]	75	95%	90%	90%	100%
Prophylactic Antibiotic Stopped[2,3]	222	71%	72%	72%	95%
Pregnancy Care					
Inpatient Neonatal Mortality	-	-	-	-	-
Third or Fourth Degree Laceration	-	-	-	3.63%	3.27%

Samuel Simmonds Memorial Hospital

Alternate Name: PHS Alaska Native Hospital

NOTE: Hospital profiles are in alphabetical order by state, then city, then hospital within the city; Rankings are sorted by rate in descending order and exclude hospitals with less than 25 cases; (1) The number of cases is too small (n<25) for purposes of reliably predicting hospital performance; (2) Measure reflects the hospital's indication that its submission was based upon a sample of its relevant discharges; (3) Rate reflects fewer than the maximum possible quarters of data for the measure; (4) Inaccurate information submitted and suppressed for one or more quarters; (5) No data is available from the hospital for this measure; Please refer to the User's Guide for a full explanation of data

1296 Agvik Street
Barrow, AK 99723
Ownership: Government - Federal
Emergency Services: No

Phone: 907-852-4611
Fax: 907-852-6408
Accredited: Yes
Licensed Beds: 14

Key Personnel:
Administrator/CEO . . . . Mike Herring
Chief Medical Staff . . . . Dina Villauera
Infection Control . . . . Drew Komensky

Measure	Cases	This Hospital	State Average	U.S. Average	Top Hospital
Heart Attack Care					
ACE Inhibitor or ARB for LVSD[5]	-	-	84%	82%	100%
Aspirin at Arrival[5]	-	-	95%	92%	100%
Aspirin at Discharge[5]	-	-	98%	90%	100%
Beta Blocker at Arrival[5]	-	-	86%	87%	100%
Beta Blocker at Discharge[5]	-	-	87%	90%	100%
Fibrinolytic Medication Timing[5]	-	-	17%	31%	100%
PCI Within 90 Minutes of Arrival[5]	-	-	63%	54%	95%
Smoking Cessation Advice[5]	-	-	75%	88%	100%
Heart Failure Care					
ACE Inhibitor or ARB for LVSD[3]	0	-	88%	82%	100%
Discharge Instructions[1,3]	1	0%	40%	61%	93%
Evaluation of LVS Function[1,3]	2	50%	83%	83%	99%
Smoking Cessation Advice[3]	0	-	80%	82%	100%
Pneumonia Care					
Appropriate Initial Antibiotic[5]	-	-	86%	83%	94%
Blood Culture Timing[5]	-	-	94%	90%	100%
Influenza Vaccine[5]	-	-	64%	70%	100%
Initial Antibiotic Timing[1,3]	5	80%	78%	80%	93%
Oxygenation Assessment[1,3]	5	100%	100%	99%	100%
Pneumococcal Vaccine[1,3]	2	100%	69%	69%	94%
Smoking Cessation Advice[5]	-	-	79%	80%	100%
Surgical Infection Prevention					
Prophylactic Antibiotic Given[5]	-	-	78%	77%	95%
Prophylactic Antibiotic Selection[5]	-	-	90%	90%	100%
Prophylactic Antibiotic Stopped[5]	-	-	72%	72%	95%
Pregnancy Care					
Inpatient Neonatal Mortality	-	-	-	-	-
Third or Fourth Degree Laceration	-	-	-	3.63%	3.27%

Yukon-Kuskokwim Delta Regional Hospital

PO Box 528
Bethel, AK 99559
E-mail: info@ykhc.org
URL: www.ykhc.org
Ownership: Government - Federal
Emergency Services: Yes

Phone: 907-543-6000
Fax: 907-543-6366
Accredited: Yes
Licensed Beds: 50

Measure	Cases	This Hospital	State Average	U.S. Average	Top Hospital
Heart Attack Care					
ACE Inhibitor or ARB for LVSD[3]	0	-	84%	82%	100%
Aspirin at Arrival[1,3]	1	100%	95%	92%	100%
Aspirin at Discharge[1,3]	1	100%	98%	90%	100%
Beta Blocker at Arrival[1,3]	1	100%	86%	87%	100%
Beta Blocker at Discharge[1,3]	1	100%	87%	90%	100%
Fibrinolytic Medication Timing[5]	-	-	17%	31%	100%
PCI Within 90 Minutes of Arrival[5]	-	-	63%	54%	95%
Smoking Cessation Advice[5]	-	-	75%	88%	100%
Heart Failure Care					
ACE Inhibitor or ARB for LVSD[1]	1	100%	88%	82%	100%
Discharge Instructions[1,3]	5	0%	40%	61%	93%
Evaluation of LVS Function[1]	15	40%	83%	83%	99%
Smoking Cessation Advice[1,3]	1	100%	80%	82%	100%
Pneumonia Care					
Appropriate Initial Antibiotic[1,3]	15	100%	86%	83%	94%
Blood Culture Timing[1,3]	18	89%	94%	90%	100%
Influenza Vaccine[5]	-	-	64%	70%	100%
Initial Antibiotic Timing	58	64%	78%	80%	93%
Oxygenation Assessment	83	100%	100%	99%	100%
Pneumococcal Vaccine	54	63%	69%	69%	94%
Smoking Cessation Advice[1,3]	3	67%	79%	80%	100%
Surgical Infection Prevention					
Prophylactic Antibiotic Given[5]	-	-	78%	77%	95%
Prophylactic Antibiotic Selection[5]	-	-	90%	90%	100%
Prophylactic Antibiotic Stopped[5]	-	-	72%	72%	95%
Pregnancy Care					
Inpatient Neonatal Mortality	-	-	-	-	-
Third or Fourth Degree Laceration	-	-	-	3.63%	3.27%

Fairbanks Memorial Hospital

1650 Cowles Street
Fairbanks, AK 99701
E-mail: lsmith@bannerhealth.com
URL: www.bannerhealth.com
Ownership: Voluntary non-profit - Private
Emergency Services: Yes

Phone: 907-452-8181
Fax: 907-458-5151
Accredited: Yes
Licensed Beds: 162

Key Personnel:
Chief Medical Staff . . . . Elizabeth Kohnen, MD
Emergency Room . . . . Carol Meyer
Director Medical/Surgical Nursing . . . . Karl Sanford
OB/GYN Womens Health . . . . Nigel Wappett, MD
Manager Radiology . . . . Jim Button
Director Respiratory Therapy . . . . Charles Holyfield

Measure	Cases	This Hospital	State Average	U.S. Average	Top Hospital
Heart Attack Care					
ACE Inhibitor or ARB for LVSD[1]	4	75%	84%	82%	100%
Aspirin at Arrival[1]	20	90%	95%	92%	100%
Aspirin at Discharge[1]	12	100%	98%	90%	100%
Beta Blocker at Arrival[1]	16	94%	86%	87%	100%
Beta Blocker at Discharge[1]	10	100%	87%	90%	100%
Fibrinolytic Medication Timing[1]	6	50%	17%	31%	100%
PCI Within 90 Minutes of Arrival	0	-	63%	54%	95%
Smoking Cessation Advice[1]	2	100%	75%	88%	100%
Heart Failure Care					
ACE Inhibitor or ARB for LVSD	39	90%	88%	82%	100%
Discharge Instructions	85	66%	40%	61%	93%
Evaluation of LVS Function	86	99%	83%	83%	99%
Smoking Cessation Advice[1]	22	95%	80%	82%	100%
Pneumonia Care					
Appropriate Initial Antibiotic	89	80%	86%	83%	94%
Blood Culture Timing	62	97%	94%	90%	100%
Influenza Vaccine[1]	22	95%	64%	70%	100%
Initial Antibiotic Timing	109	80%	78%	80%	93%
Oxygenation Assessment	136	100%	100%	99%	100%
Pneumococcal Vaccine	69	88%	69%	69%	94%
Smoking Cessation Advice	38	95%	79%	80%	100%
Surgical Infection Prevention					
Prophylactic Antibiotic Given[3]	132	71%	78%	77%	95%
Prophylactic Antibiotic Selection	52	85%	90%	90%	100%
Prophylactic Antibiotic Stopped[3]	128	82%	72%	72%	95%
Pregnancy Care					
Inpatient Neonatal Mortality	-	-	-	-	-
Third or Fourth Degree Laceration	-	-	-	3.63%	3.27%

South Peninsula Hospital

4300 Bartlett Street
Homer, AK 99603
URL: www.sphosp.com
Ownership: Voluntary non-profit - Other
Emergency Services: Yes

Phone: 907-235-8101
Fax: 907-235-0253
Accredited: No
Licensed Beds: 40

Key Personnel:
CEO . . . . Charles Franv
Chief Medical Staff . . . . Paul Eneboe, MD
Emergency Room . . . . Sharon Merchant
Emergency Room . . . . Yal Smith, MD
Infection Control . . . . Donna Libal, RN
Medical/Surgical Nursing . . . . Sharon Merchant

Measure	Cases	This Hospital	State Average	U.S. Average	Top Hospital
Heart Attack Care					
ACE Inhibitor or ARB for LVSD[3]	0	-	84%	82%	100%
Aspirin at Arrival[1,3]	2	50%	95%	92%	100%
Aspirin at Discharge[1,3]	2	100%	98%	90%	100%
Beta Blocker at Arrival[1,3]	1	0%	86%	87%	100%

NOTE: Hospital profiles are in alphabetical order by state, then city, then hospital within the city; Rankings are sorted by rate in descending order and exclude hospitals with less than 25 cases; (1) The number of cases is too small (n<25) for purposes of reliably predicting hospital performance; (2) Measure reflects the hospital's indication that its submission was based upon a sample of its relevant discharges; (3) Rate reflects fewer than the maximum possible quarters of data for the measure; (4) Inaccurate information submitted and suppressed for one or more quarters; (5) No data is available from the hospital for this measure; Please refer to the User's Guide for a full explanation of data

Beta Blocker at Discharge[1,3]	1	0%	87%	90%	100%
Fibrinolytic Medication Timing[3]	0	-	17%	31%	100%
PCI Within 90 Minutes of Arrival	0	-	63%	54%	95%
Smoking Cessation Advice[1,3]	1	100%	75%	88%	100%
Heart Failure Care					
ACE Inhibitor or ARB for LVSD[1,3]	3	67%	88%	82%	100%
Discharge Instructions[1,3]	15	93%	40%	61%	93%
Evaluation of LVS Function[1,3]	16	62%	83%	83%	99%
Smoking Cessation Advice[1,3]	2	50%	80%	82%	100%
Pneumonia Care					
Appropriate Initial Antibiotic[1,3]	22	73%	86%	83%	94%
Blood Culture Timing[1,3]	7	100%	94%	90%	100%
Influenza Vaccine[5]	-	-	64%	70%	100%
Initial Antibiotic Timing[1,3]	17	59%	78%	80%	93%
Oxygenation Assessment[3]	25	96%	100%	99%	100%
Pneumococcal Vaccine[1,3]	19	42%	69%	69%	94%
Smoking Cessation Advice[1,3]	3	67%	79%	80%	100%
Surgical Infection Prevention					
Prophylactic Antibiotic Given[1,3]	6	83%	78%	77%	95%
Prophylactic Antibiotic Selection[1]	4	100%	90%	90%	100%
Prophylactic Antibiotic Stopped[1,3]	5	20%	72%	72%	95%
Pregnancy Care					
Inpatient Neonatal Mortality	-	-	-	-	-
Third or Fourth Degree Laceration	-	-	-	3.63%	3.27%

Bartlett Regional Hospital

3260 Hospital Drive
Juneau, AK 99801
URL: www.bartletthospital.org
Ownership: Proprietary
Emergency Services: Yes

Phone: 907-796-8900
Fax: 907-796-8909
Accredited: Yes
Licensed Beds: 55

Key Personnel:
CEO. . . . . Robert F Valliant
Chief Medical Staff. . . . . Greg Dostal

Measure	Cases	This Hospital	State Average	U.S. Average	Top Hospital
Heart Attack Care					
ACE Inhibitor or ARB for LVSD[1]	2	100%	84%	82%	100%
Aspirin at Arrival[1]	12	100%	95%	92%	100%
Aspirin at Discharge[1]	12	100%	98%	90%	100%
Beta Blocker at Arrival[1]	15	93%	86%	87%	100%
Beta Blocker at Discharge[1]	12	100%	87%	90%	100%
Fibrinolytic Medication Timing[1]	7	14%	17%	31%	100%
PCI Within 90 Minutes of Arrival	0	-	63%	54%	95%
Smoking Cessation Advice[1]	3	33%	75%	88%	100%
Heart Failure Care					
ACE Inhibitor or ARB for LVSD[1]	13	85%	88%	82%	100%
Discharge Instructions	41	51%	40%	61%	93%
Evaluation of LVS Function	45	89%	83%	83%	99%
Smoking Cessation Advice[1]	6	50%	80%	82%	100%
Pneumonia Care					
Appropriate Initial Antibiotic	50	70%	86%	83%	94%
Blood Culture Timing	26	96%	94%	90%	100%
Influenza Vaccine[1]	4	75%	64%	70%	100%
Initial Antibiotic Timing	42	83%	78%	80%	93%
Oxygenation Assessment	58	100%	100%	99%	100%
Pneumococcal Vaccine	34	47%	69%	69%	94%
Smoking Cessation Advice[1]	9	78%	79%	80%	100%
Surgical Infection Prevention					
Prophylactic Antibiotic Given[3]	57	37%	78%	77%	95%
Prophylactic Antibiotic Selection	27	56%	90%	90%	100%
Prophylactic Antibiotic Stopped[3]	52	63%	72%	72%	95%
Pregnancy Care					
Inpatient Neonatal Mortality	-	-	-	-	-
Third or Fourth Degree Laceration	-	-	-	3.63%	3.27%

Ketchikan General Hospital

3100 Tongass Avenue
Ketchikan, AK 99901
Ownership: Voluntary non-profit - Church
Emergency Services: Yes

Phone: 907-225-5171
Fax: 907-228-8322
Accredited: No
Licensed Beds: 85

Key Personnel:
CEO. . . . . Patrick J Branco
Chief Medical Staff. . . . . Stacy Schultz, MD
Emergency Manager . . . . Ben Crum
ICU . . . . Kathy Smith
Manager Medical/Surgical Nursing. . . . . Kendall Sawa

Measure	Cases	This Hospital	State Average	U.S. Average	Top Hospital
Heart Attack Care					
ACE Inhibitor or ARB for LVSD[1,3]	1	100%	84%	82%	100%
Aspirin at Arrival[1,3]	3	100%	95%	92%	100%
Aspirin at Discharge[1,3]	2	100%	98%	90%	100%
Beta Blocker at Arrival[1,3]	3	67%	86%	87%	100%
Beta Blocker at Discharge[1,3]	2	100%	87%	90%	100%
Fibrinolytic Medication Timing[1,3]	1	0%	17%	31%	100%
PCI Within 90 Minutes of Arrival	0	-	63%	54%	95%
Smoking Cessation Advice[1,3]	2	100%	75%	88%	100%
Heart Failure Care					
ACE Inhibitor or ARB for LVSD[1]	3	100%	88%	82%	100%
Discharge Instructions[1]	15	33%	40%	61%	93%
Evaluation of LVS Function[1]	16	81%	83%	83%	99%
Smoking Cessation Advice[1]	3	100%	80%	82%	100%
Pneumonia Care					
Appropriate Initial Antibiotic	31	77%	86%	83%	94%
Blood Culture Timing	27	89%	94%	90%	100%
Influenza Vaccine[1]	7	57%	64%	70%	100%
Initial Antibiotic Timing	36	72%	78%	80%	93%
Oxygenation Assessment	48	100%	100%	99%	100%
Pneumococcal Vaccine	25	76%	69%	69%	94%
Smoking Cessation Advice[1]	14	100%	79%	80%	100%
Surgical Infection Prevention					
Prophylactic Antibiotic Given[3]	37	84%	78%	77%	95%
Prophylactic Antibiotic Selection[1]	11	100%	90%	90%	100%
Prophylactic Antibiotic Stopped[3]	37	76%	72%	72%	95%
Pregnancy Care					
Inpatient Neonatal Mortality	-	-	-	-	-
Third or Fourth Degree Laceration	-	-	-	3.63%	3.27%

Valley Hospital

Alternate Name: Mat-Su Regional Medical Center
515 East Dahlia Street
Palmer, AK 99645
URL: www.valley-hosp.com
Ownership: Voluntary non-profit - Private
Emergency Services: Yes

Phone: 907-746-8600
Fax: 907-861-6578
Accredited: Yes
Licensed Beds: 36

Key Personnel:
President/CEO. . . . . George Larson
Chief Medical Staff. . . . . Tom Leigh, MD
Emergency Room . . . . Shiela La Mar
Infection Control. . . . . Pat Ball, RN
ICU . . . . Greta Banning, RN
Intensive/Coronary Care . . . . Greta Banning, RN
Medical/Surgical Nursing . . . . Bev Miles, RN
OB/GYN Womens Health. . . . . Pat Smith
Respiratory/Cardiopulmonary. . . . . Greta Banning, RN

Measure	Cases	This Hospital	State Average	U.S. Average	Top Hospital
Heart Attack Care					
ACE Inhibitor or ARB for LVSD[1]	3	100%	84%	82%	100%
Aspirin at Arrival	37	100%	95%	92%	100%
Aspirin at Discharge[1]	23	96%	98%	90%	100%
Beta Blocker at Arrival	32	91%	86%	87%	100%
Beta Blocker at Discharge[1]	22	95%	87%	90%	100%
Fibrinolytic Medication Timing[1]	5	20%	17%	31%	100%
PCI Within 90 Minutes of Arrival	0	-	63%	54%	95%
Smoking Cessation Advice[1]	11	100%	75%	88%	100%
Heart Failure Care					
ACE Inhibitor or ARB for LVSD[1]	20	90%	88%	82%	100%

NOTE: Hospital profiles are in alphabetical order by state, then city, then hospital within the city; Rankings are sorted by rate in descending order and exclude hospitals with less than 25 cases; (1) The number of cases is too small (n<25) for purposes of reliably predicting hospital performance; (2) Measure reflects the hospital's indication that its submission was based upon a sample of its relevant discharges; (3) Rate reflects fewer than the maximum possible quarters of data for the measure; (4) Inaccurate information submitted and suppressed for one or more quarters; (5) No data is available from the hospital for this measure; Please refer to the User's Guide for a full explanation of data

Measure	Cases	This Hospital	State Average	U.S. Average	Top Hospital
Discharge Instructions	56	68%	40%	61%	93%
Evaluation of LVS Function	57	91%	83%	83%	99%
Smoking Cessation Advice[1]	14	100%	80%	82%	100%
Pneumonia Care					
Appropriate Initial Antibiotic	75	83%	86%	83%	94%
Blood Culture Timing	48	96%	94%	90%	100%
Influenza Vaccine[1]	9	78%	64%	70%	100%
Initial Antibiotic Timing	80	82%	78%	80%	93%
Oxygenation Assessment	91	100%	100%	99%	100%
Pneumococcal Vaccine	54	83%	69%	69%	94%
Smoking Cessation Advice[1]	24	96%	79%	80%	100%
Surgical Infection Prevention					
Prophylactic Antibiotic Given	141	84%	78%	77%	95%
Prophylactic Antibiotic Selection	38	87%	90%	90%	100%
Prophylactic Antibiotic Stopped	136	82%	72%	72%	95%
Pregnancy Care					
Inpatient Neonatal Mortality	-	-	-	-	-
Third or Fourth Degree Laceration	-	-	-	3.63%	3.27%

Mount Edgecumbe Hospital

Alternate Name: Searhc, Mount Edgecumbe Hospital
222 Tongass Drive
Sitka, AK 99835
Phone: 907-966-2411
Fax: 907-966-8300
URL: www.searhc.org
Ownership: Voluntary non-profit - Other
Accredited: Yes
Emergency Services: No
Licensed Beds: 78

Key Personnel:

CEO. . . . . Frank Sutton
Chief Medical Staff. . . . . Susan Carlson, MD
Emergency Room . . . . Robert Carlson
Chief Radiology . . . . Emory Gonzales
Director Respiratory Therapy . . . . Julene Logue

Measure	Cases	This Hospital	State Average	U.S. Average	Top Hospital
Heart Attack Care					
ACE Inhibitor or ARB for LVSD[3]	0	-	84%	82%	100%
Aspirin at Arrival[1,3]	2	100%	95%	92%	100%
Aspirin at Discharge[1,3]	2	100%	98%	90%	100%
Beta Blocker at Arrival[1,3]	2	100%	86%	87%	100%
Beta Blocker at Discharge[1,3]	2	100%	87%	90%	100%
Fibrinolytic Medication Timing[3]	0	-	17%	31%	100%
PCI Within 90 Minutes of Arrival[5]	-	-	63%	54%	95%
Smoking Cessation Advice[3]	0	-	75%	88%	100%
Heart Failure Care					
ACE Inhibitor or ARB for LVSD[1,3]	5	100%	88%	82%	100%
Discharge Instructions[1,3]	9	33%	40%	61%	93%
Evaluation of LVS Function[1,3]	9	100%	83%	83%	99%
Smoking Cessation Advice[1,3]	1	100%	80%	82%	100%
Pneumonia Care					
Appropriate Initial Antibiotic[1]	15	100%	86%	83%	94%
Blood Culture Timing[1]	12	100%	94%	90%	100%
Influenza Vaccine[1]	3	100%	64%	70%	100%
Initial Antibiotic Timing[1]	14	79%	78%	80%	93%
Oxygenation Assessment[1]	23	100%	100%	99%	100%
Pneumococcal Vaccine[1]	12	100%	69%	69%	94%
Smoking Cessation Advice[1]	11	73%	79%	80%	100%
Surgical Infection Prevention					
Prophylactic Antibiotic Given[1,3]	10	80%	78%	77%	95%
Prophylactic Antibiotic Selection[1]	2	100%	90%	90%	100%
Prophylactic Antibiotic Stopped[1,3]	8	50%	72%	72%	95%
Pregnancy Care					
Inpatient Neonatal Mortality	-	-	-	-	-
Third or Fourth Degree Laceration	-	-	-	3.63%	3.27%

Sitka Community Hospital

209 Moller Avenue
Sitka, AK 99835
Phone: 907-747-3241
Fax: 907-747-1794
Ownership: Government - Local
Accredited: No
Emergency Services: Yes
Licensed Beds: 27

Key Personnel:

Chief Medical Staff. . . . . Robert Hunter, MD
OB/GYN Womens Health. . . . . Robert Klem, MD
Chief Radiology . . . . Rebecca MacGregor, MD

Measure	Cases	This Hospital	State Average	U.S. Average	Top Hospital
Heart Attack Care					
ACE Inhibitor or ARB for LVSD[1,3]	1	0%	84%	82%	100%
Aspirin at Arrival[1,3]	4	100%	95%	92%	100%
Aspirin at Discharge[1,3]	3	100%	98%	90%	100%
Beta Blocker at Arrival[1,3]	4	100%	86%	87%	100%
Beta Blocker at Discharge[1,3]	3	67%	87%	90%	100%
Fibrinolytic Medication Timing[3]	0	-	17%	31%	100%
PCI Within 90 Minutes of Arrival	0	-	63%	54%	95%
Smoking Cessation Advice[1,3]	1	0%	75%	88%	100%
Heart Failure Care					
ACE Inhibitor or ARB for LVSD[1,3]	6	50%	88%	82%	100%
Discharge Instructions[1,3]	7	0%	40%	61%	93%
Evaluation of LVS Function[1,3]	11	73%	83%	83%	99%
Smoking Cessation Advice[1,3]	1	100%	80%	82%	100%
Pneumonia Care					
Appropriate Initial Antibiotic[1,3]	3	100%	86%	83%	94%
Blood Culture Timing[1,3]	1	100%	94%	90%	100%
Influenza Vaccine[1]	2	0%	64%	70%	100%
Initial Antibiotic Timing[1,3]	2	100%	78%	80%	93%
Oxygenation Assessment[1,3]	4	100%	100%	99%	100%
Pneumococcal Vaccine[1,3]	4	25%	69%	69%	94%
Smoking Cessation Advice[3]	0	-	79%	80%	100%
Surgical Infection Prevention					
Prophylactic Antibiotic Given[1,3]	1	100%	78%	77%	95%
Prophylactic Antibiotic Selection	0	-	90%	90%	100%
Prophylactic Antibiotic Stopped[1,3]	1	100%	72%	72%	95%
Pregnancy Care					
Inpatient Neonatal Mortality	-	-	-	-	-
Third or Fourth Degree Laceration	-	-	-	3.63%	3.27%

Central Peninsula Hospital

250 Hospital Place
Soldotna, AK 99669
Phone: 907-714-4404
Fax: 907-714-4669
E-mail: bnichols@cpgh.org
URL: www.cpgh.org
Ownership: Voluntary non-profit - Other
Accredited: Yes
Emergency Services: Yes
Licensed Beds: 62

Key Personnel:

President . . . . Loretta Flanders
CEO. . . . . Ryan Smith
Chief Medical Staff. . . . . Nets Anderson, MD
Infection Control. . . . . Ken Simmons, RN
Director, Medical Surgical . . . . Gypsy Jolly, RN
Director Radiology . . . . Mark McVee, MD
Director Respiratory Care. . . . . Paul Drake, RT

Measure	Cases	This Hospital	State Average	U.S. Average	Top Hospital
Heart Attack Care					
ACE Inhibitor or ARB for LVSD[1]	1	100%	84%	82%	100%
Aspirin at Arrival[1]	3	100%	95%	92%	100%
Aspirin at Discharge[1]	1	100%	98%	90%	100%
Beta Blocker at Arrival[1]	3	100%	86%	87%	100%
Beta Blocker at Discharge[1]	1	100%	87%	90%	100%
Fibrinolytic Medication Timing[1]	1	0%	17%	31%	100%
PCI Within 90 Minutes of Arrival	0	-	63%	54%	95%
Smoking Cessation Advice	0	-	75%	88%	100%
Heart Failure Care					
ACE Inhibitor or ARB for LVSD[1]	10	90%	88%	82%	100%
Discharge Instructions	35	83%	40%	61%	93%
Evaluation of LVS Function	38	97%	83%	83%	99%
Smoking Cessation Advice[1]	7	71%	80%	82%	100%
Pneumonia Care					
Appropriate Initial Antibiotic	35	89%	86%	83%	94%
Blood Culture Timing	30	100%	94%	90%	100%
Influenza Vaccine[1]	5	60%	64%	70%	100%
Initial Antibiotic Timing	39	77%	78%	80%	93%
Oxygenation Assessment	52	100%	100%	99%	100%
Pneumococcal Vaccine	32	81%	69%	69%	94%
Smoking Cessation Advice[1]	10	90%	79%	80%	100%
Surgical Infection Prevention					
Prophylactic Antibiotic Given[2,3]	75	81%	78%	77%	95%

NOTE: Hospital profiles are in alphabetical order by state, then city, then hospital within the city; Rankings are sorted by rate in descending order and exclude hospitals with less than 25 cases; (1) The number of cases is too small (n<25) for purposes of reliably predicting hospital performance; (2) Measure reflects the hospital's indication that its submission was based upon a sample of its relevant discharges; (3) Rate reflects fewer than the maximum possible quarters of data for the measure; (4) Inaccurate information submitted and suppressed for one or more quarters; (5) No data is available from the hospital for this measure; Please refer to the User's Guide for a full explanation of data

Prophylactic Antibiotic Selection[1,2]	21	90%	90%	90%	100%
Prophylactic Antibiotic Stopped[2,3]	78	94%	72%	72%	95%
Pregnancy Care					
Inpatient Neonatal Mortality	-	-	-	-	-
Third or Fourth Degree Laceration	-	-	-	3.63%	3.27%

NOTE: Hospital profiles are in alphabetical order by state, then city, then hospital within the city; Rankings are sorted by rate in descending order and exclude hospitals with less than 25 cases; (1) The number of cases is too small (n<25) for purposes of reliably predicting hospital performance; (2) Measure reflects the hospital's indication that its submission was based upon a sample of its relevant discharges; (3) Rate reflects fewer than the maximum possible quarters of data for the measure; (4) Inaccurate information submitted and suppressed for one or more quarters; (5) No data is available from the hospital for this measure; Please refer to the User's Guide for a full explanation of data

Heart Attack Care

1. ACE Inhibitor or ARB for LVSD

Hospital Name	City	Rate	Cases
Saint Joseph's Hospital & Medical Center	Phoenix	100%	29
Tucson Heart Hospital	Tucson	100%	45
University Medical Center	Tucson	99%	70
Carondelet Saint Mary's Hospital	Tucson	97%	66
Verde Valley Medical Center	Cottonwood	95%	41
Northwest Medical Center	Tucson	93%	44
Phoenix Baptist Hospital and Medical Center	Phoenix	93%	29
John C Lincoln Hospital-Deer Valley	Phoenix	90%	52
Carondelet Saint Joseph's Hospital	Tucson	89%	35
Arizona Heart Hospital	Phoenix	88%	82
Chandler Regional Hospital	Chandler	88%	73
Mayo Clinic Hospital	Phoenix	88%	33
Banner Baywood Heart Hospital	Mesa	85%	60
Desert Samaritan Medical Center	Mesa	85%	62
Tucson Medical Center	Tucson	85%	66
John C Lincoln Hospital-North Mountain	Phoenix	84%	44
Mesa General Hospital	Mesa	84%	25
Banner Estrella Medical Center	Phoenix	83%	30
Phoenix Memorial Health System	Phoenix	82%	33
Banner Thunderbird Medical Center	Glendale	81%	63
Scottsdale Healthcare-Osborn	Scottsdale	81%	47
West Valley Hospital	Goodyear	81%	27
Flagstaff Medical Center	Flagstaff	79%	29
Yuma Regional Medical Center	Yuma	79%	68
Scottsdale Healthcare	Scottsdale	78%	51
Banner Good Samaritan Medical Center	Phoenix	77%	75
Sun Health Boswell Hospital	Sun City	64%	66

2. Aspirin at Arrival

Hospital Name	City	Rate	Cases
Arizona Heart Hospital	Phoenix	100%	83
Maricopa Integrated Health	Phoenix	100%	69
Tucson Heart Hospital	Tucson	100%	140
Maryvale Hospital Medical Center	Phoenix	99%	148
Phoenix Baptist Hospital and Medical Center	Phoenix	99%	88
Verde Valley Medical Center	Cottonwood	99%	133
Banner Estrella Medical Center	Phoenix	98%	143
Banner Good Samaritan Medical Center	Phoenix	98%	110
Carondelet Saint Joseph's Hospital	Tucson	98%	174
Del E Webb Memorial Hospital	Sun City West	98%	227
Flagstaff Medical Center	Flagstaff	98%	96
John C Lincoln Hospital-Deer Valley	Phoenix	98%	172
Mayo Clinic Hospital	Phoenix	98%	162
Northwest Medical Center	Tucson	98%	174
Northwest Medical Center Oro Valley	Oro Valley	98%	83
Phoenix Memorial Health System	Phoenix	98%	96
West Valley Hospital	Goodyear	98%	132
Western Arizona Regional Medical Center	Bullhead City	98%	140
Arrowhead Community Hospital	Glendale	97%	101
Chandler Regional Hospital	Chandler	97%	313
Mesa General Hospital	Mesa	97%	59
Saint Joseph's Hospital & Medical Center	Phoenix	97%	112
Scottsdale Healthcare	Scottsdale	97%	245
Tempe Saint Luke's Hospital	Tempe	97%	33
UPH Hospital at Kino campus	Tucson	97%	30
Yavapai Regional Medical Center	Prescott	97%	122
Carondelet Saint Mary's Hospital	Tucson	96%	311
Desert Samaritan Medical Center	Mesa	96%	227
Paradise Valley Hospital	Phoenix	96%	80
Tucson Medical Center	Tucson	96%	224
Yuma Regional Medical Center	Yuma	96%	277
Navapache Regional Medical Center	Show Low	95%	41
Scottsdale Healthcare-Osborn	Scottsdale	95%	243
University Medical Center	Tucson	95%	192
Banner Thunderbird Medical Center	Glendale	94%	260
Casa Grande Regional Medical Center	Casa Grande	94%	80
John C Lincoln Hospital-North Mountain	Phoenix	94%	177
Sierra Vista Regional Health Center	Sierra Vista	94%	77
Sun Health Boswell Hospital	Sun City	94%	193
Saint Luke's Medical Center	Phoenix	89%	44
Kingman Regional Medical Center	Kingman	88%	168
Havasu Regional Medical Center	Lake Havasu City	85%	119
Banner Baywood Medical Center	Mesa	76%	51

3. Aspirin at Discharge

Hospital Name	City	Rate	Cases
Navapache Regional Medical Center	Show Low	100%	34
Saint Joseph's Hospital & Medical Center	Phoenix	100%	142
University Medical Center	Tucson	100%	267
Arizona Heart Hospital	Phoenix	99%	319
Arrowhead Community Hospital	Glendale	99%	78
John C Lincoln Hospital-Deer Valley	Phoenix	99%	153
John C Lincoln Hospital-North Mountain	Phoenix	99%	151
Northwest Medical Center	Tucson	99%	202
Northwest Medical Center Oro Valley	Oro Valley	99%	70
Phoenix Baptist Hospital and Medical Center	Phoenix	99%	88
Verde Valley Medical Center	Cottonwood	99%	186
Western Arizona Regional Medical Center	Bullhead City	99%	144
Banner Baywood Heart Hospital	Mesa	98%	248
Banner Good Samaritan Medical Center	Phoenix	98%	211
Carondelet Saint Joseph's Hospital	Tucson	98%	167
Chandler Regional Hospital	Chandler	98%	306
Mayo Clinic Hospital	Phoenix	98%	129
Scottsdale Healthcare-Osborn	Scottsdale	98%	218
Tucson Heart Hospital	Tucson	98%	261
Banner Estrella Medical Center	Phoenix	97%	116
Flagstaff Medical Center	Flagstaff	97%	127
Mesa General Hospital	Mesa	97%	73
Paradise Valley Hospital	Phoenix	97%	59
Scottsdale Healthcare	Scottsdale	97%	233
Carondelet Saint Mary's Hospital	Tucson	96%	280
Del E Webb Memorial Hospital	Sun City West	96%	175
Desert Samaritan Medical Center	Mesa	96%	221
Saint Luke's Medical Center	Phoenix	96%	48
UPH Hospital at Kino campus	Tucson	96%	26
Banner Thunderbird Medical Center	Glendale	95%	245
Sun Health Boswell Hospital	Sun City	95%	201
Tucson Medical Center	Tucson	95%	270
West Valley Hospital	Goodyear	95%	126
Yavapai Regional Medical Center	Prescott	95%	93
Yuma Regional Medical Center	Yuma	94%	236
Maryvale Hospital Medical Center	Phoenix	93%	121
Phoenix Memorial Health System	Phoenix	91%	128
Maricopa Integrated Health	Phoenix	84%	68
Havasu Regional Medical Center	Lake Havasu City	83%	101
Casa Grande Regional Medical Center	Casa Grande	82%	28
Kingman Regional Medical Center	Kingman	82%	144
Banner Baywood Medical Center	Mesa	76%	25
Sierra Vista Regional Health Center	Sierra Vista	66%	29

4. Beta Blocker at Arrival

Hospital Name	City	Rate	Cases
Arizona Heart Hospital	Phoenix	100%	67
Tucson Heart Hospital	Tucson	100%	132
Verde Valley Medical Center	Cottonwood	99%	113
Del E Webb Memorial Hospital	Sun City West	98%	167
Mayo Clinic Hospital	Phoenix	98%	138
Western Arizona Regional Medical Center	Bullhead City	98%	112
Chandler Regional Hospital	Chandler	97%	190
Saint Joseph's Hospital & Medical Center	Phoenix	97%	96
Arrowhead Community Hospital	Glendale	96%	81
Carondelet Saint Joseph's Hospital	Tucson	96%	135
Mesa General Hospital	Mesa	96%	45
Northwest Medical Center	Tucson	96%	120
West Valley Hospital	Goodyear	95%	116
Banner Good Samaritan Medical Center	Phoenix	94%	81
Phoenix Memorial Health System	Phoenix	94%	87
Banner Estrella Medical Center	Phoenix	93%	122
John C Lincoln Hospital-North Mountain	Phoenix	93%	112
Scottsdale Healthcare-Osborn	Scottsdale	93%	165
Saint Luke's Medical Center	Phoenix	92%	26
Scottsdale Healthcare	Scottsdale	92%	171
University Medical Center	Tucson	92%	169
Yavapai Regional Medical Center	Prescott	92%	106
Flagstaff Medical Center	Flagstaff	91%	76
Phoenix Baptist Hospital and Medical Center	Phoenix	91%	70
UPH Hospital at Kino campus	Tucson	91%	32
Carondelet Saint Mary's Hospital	Tucson	90%	253
John C Lincoln Hospital-Deer Valley	Phoenix	90%	129
Northwest Medical Center Oro Valley	Oro Valley	90%	60
Tucson Medical Center	Tucson	90%	202
Maricopa Integrated Health	Phoenix	89%	66
Maryvale Hospital Medical Center	Phoenix	89%	143
Yuma Regional Medical Center	Yuma	89%	227
Desert Samaritan Medical Center	Mesa	88%	146
Paradise Valley Hospital	Phoenix	88%	57
Sierra Vista Regional Health Center	Sierra Vista	88%	74
Sun Health Boswell Hospital	Sun City	88%	121
Casa Grande Regional Medical Center	Casa Grande	84%	67
Kingman Regional Medical Center	Kingman	82%	152
Banner Thunderbird Medical Center	Glendale	81%	238
Havasu Regional Medical Center	Lake Havasu City	78%	113
Tempe Saint Luke's Hospital	Tempe	75%	32

NOTE: Hospital profiles are in alphabetical order by state, then city, then hospital within the city; Rankings are sorted by rate in descending order and exclude hospitals with less than 25 cases; (1) The number of cases is too small (n<25) for purposes of reliably predicting hospital performance; (2) Measure reflects the hospital's indication that its submission was based upon a sample of its relevant discharges; (3) Rate reflects fewer than the maximum possible quarters of data for the measure; (4) Inaccurate information submitted and suppressed for one or more quarters; (5) No data is available from the hospital for this measure; Please refer to the User's Guide for a full explanation of data

Hospital Name	City	Rate	Cases
Banner Baywood Medical Center	Mesa	72%	43

5. Beta Blocker at Discharge

Hospital Name	City	Rate	Cases
Arrowhead Community Hospital	Glendale	100%	82
Saint Joseph's Hospital & Medical Center	Phoenix	100%	143
Tucson Heart Hospital	Tucson	100%	243
John C Lincoln Hospital-Deer Valley	Phoenix	99%	160
Mayo Clinic Hospital	Phoenix	99%	150
University Medical Center	Tucson	99%	260
Carondelet Saint Joseph's Hospital	Tucson	98%	160
Carondelet Saint Mary's Hospital	Tucson	98%	291
Del E Webb Memorial Hospital	Sun City West	98%	168
Northwest Medical Center	Tucson	98%	199
Scottsdale Healthcare	Scottsdale	98%	238
Scottsdale Healthcare-Osborn	Scottsdale	98%	226
Western Arizona Regional Medical Center	Bullhead City	98%	139
Arizona Heart Hospital	Phoenix	97%	304
Banner Baywood Heart Hospital	Mesa	97%	247
Banner Estrella Medical Center	Phoenix	97%	121
Desert Samaritan Medical Center	Mesa	97%	237
John C Lincoln Hospital-North Mountain	Phoenix	97%	151
Banner Thunderbird Medical Center	Glendale	96%	253
Chandler Regional Hospital	Chandler	96%	263
Mesa General Hospital	Mesa	96%	76
Phoenix Baptist Hospital and Medical Center	Phoenix	96%	100
Saint Luke's Medical Center	Phoenix	96%	52
Sun Health Boswell Hospital	Sun City	96%	229
Verde Valley Medical Center	Cottonwood	96%	167
Banner Good Samaritan Medical Center	Phoenix	95%	199
West Valley Hospital	Goodyear	95%	119
Maryvale Hospital Medical Center	Phoenix	94%	123
Paradise Valley Hospital	Phoenix	94%	71
Tucson Medical Center	Tucson	94%	271
Flagstaff Medical Center	Flagstaff	93%	109
Navapache Regional Medical Center	Show Low	93%	30
Northwest Medical Center Oro Valley	Oro Valley	93%	70
Phoenix Memorial Health System	Phoenix	93%	124
Banner Baywood Medical Center	Mesa	91%	34
Havasu Regional Medical Center	Lake Havasu City	87%	103
Kingman Regional Medical Center	Kingman	86%	147
Yavapai Regional Medical Center	Prescott	86%	102
UPH Hospital at Kino campus	Tucson	85%	26
Yuma Regional Medical Center	Yuma	85%	275
Maricopa Integrated Health	Phoenix	81%	68
Sierra Vista Regional Health Center	Sierra Vista	79%	33
Casa Grande Regional Medical Center	Casa Grande	77%	30

6. Fibrinolytic Medication Timing

Hospital Name	City	Rate	Cases
Yuma Regional Medical Center	Yuma	13%	30

8. Smoking Cessation Advice

Hospital Name	City	Rate	Cases
Banner Baywood Heart Hospital	Mesa	100%	99
Carondelet Saint Joseph's Hospital	Tucson	100%	66
Carondelet Saint Mary's Hospital	Tucson	100%	76
Chandler Regional Hospital	Chandler	100%	106
John C Lincoln Hospital-Deer Valley	Phoenix	100%	72
Paradise Valley Hospital	Phoenix	100%	32
Phoenix Baptist Hospital and Medical Center	Phoenix	100%	46
Saint Joseph's Hospital & Medical Center	Phoenix	100%	66
Scottsdale Healthcare	Scottsdale	100%	53
Scottsdale Healthcare-Osborn	Scottsdale	100%	79
Tucson Heart Hospital	Tucson	100%	70
Tucson Medical Center	Tucson	100%	85
University Medical Center	Tucson	100%	91
Western Arizona Regional Medical Center	Bullhead City	100%	72
Desert Samaritan Medical Center	Mesa	98%	98
Del E Webb Memorial Hospital	Sun City West	97%	30
Flagstaff Medical Center	Flagstaff	97%	37
John C Lincoln Hospital-North Mountain	Phoenix	97%	58
Northwest Medical Center	Tucson	97%	70
Arizona Heart Hospital	Phoenix	96%	116
Verde Valley Medical Center	Cottonwood	96%	55
Yavapai Regional Medical Center	Prescott	96%	27
Banner Good Samaritan Medical Center	Phoenix	95%	98
Maryvale Hospital Medical Center	Phoenix	95%	59
Banner Estrella Medical Center	Phoenix	94%	53
Yuma Regional Medical Center	Yuma	92%	74
Banner Thunderbird Medical Center	Glendale	90%	81
Sun Health Boswell Hospital	Sun City	89%	45
Kingman Regional Medical Center	Kingman	88%	69
Saint Luke's Medical Center	Phoenix	88%	26
West Valley Hospital	Goodyear	86%	50
Phoenix Memorial Health System	Phoenix	81%	64
Havasu Regional Medical Center	Lake Havasu City	74%	27
Mesa General Hospital	Mesa	72%	36
Maricopa Integrated Health	Phoenix	50%	32

Heart Failure Care

9. ACE Inhibitor or ARB for LVSD

Hospital Name	City	Rate	Cases
Mesa General Hospital	Mesa	100%	61
Tucson Heart Hospital	Tucson	100%	98
Arrowhead Community Hospital	Glendale	98%	51
Flagstaff Medical Center	Flagstaff	97%	38
Mayo Clinic Hospital	Phoenix	97%	120
Saint Joseph's Hospital & Medical Center	Phoenix	96%	139
Carondelet Saint Mary's Hospital	Tucson	95%	133
Phoenix Memorial Health System	Phoenix	95%	59
University Medical Center	Tucson	95%	183
Phoenix Baptist Hospital and Medical Center	Phoenix	94%	85
John C Lincoln Hospital-Deer Valley	Phoenix	91%	109
Arizona Heart Hospital	Phoenix	90%	170
Carondelet Saint Joseph's Hospital	Tucson	88%	102
John C Lincoln Hospital-North Mountain	Phoenix	88%	112
West Valley Hospital	Goodyear	88%	57
Tucson Medical Center	Tucson	87%	95
Banner Baywood Heart Hospital	Mesa	86%	145
Banner Baywood Medical Center	Mesa	86%	76
Maricopa Integrated Health	Phoenix	86%	102
Banner Estrella Medical Center	Phoenix	85%	112
Desert Samaritan Medical Center	Mesa	85%	130
Havasu Regional Medical Center	Lake Havasu City	85%	55
Yavapai Regional Medical Center	Prescott	84%	97
Northwest Medical Center	Tucson	83%	117
Scottsdale Healthcare-Osborn	Scottsdale	82%	173
Kingman Regional Medical Center	Kingman	81%	104
Paradise Valley Hospital	Phoenix	81%	43
Yuma Regional Medical Center	Yuma	81%	221
Chandler Regional Hospital	Chandler	80%	130
Western Arizona Regional Medical Center	Bullhead City	80%	123
Verde Valley Medical Center	Cottonwood	79%	34
Banner Thunderbird Medical Center	Glendale	78%	148
Banner Mesa Medical Center	Mesa	77%	26
Maryvale Hospital Medical Center	Phoenix	77%	83
Northwest Medical Center Oro Valley	Oro Valley	76%	41
Banner Good Samaritan Medical Center	Phoenix	75%	142
Sierra Vista Regional Health Center	Sierra Vista	75%	28
Tempe Saint Luke's Hospital	Tempe	75%	32
Tuba City Indian Medical Center	Tuba City	75%	28
Saint Luke's Medical Center	Phoenix	72%	69
Del E Webb Memorial Hospital	Sun City West	69%	120
Scottsdale Healthcare	Scottsdale	69%	189
Sun Health Boswell Hospital	Sun City	65%	129
Casa Grande Regional Medical Center	Casa Grande	63%	54

10. Discharge Instructions

Hospital Name	City	Rate	Cases
Carondelet Saint Mary's Hospital	Tucson	100%	350
Carondelet Saint Joseph's Hospital	Tucson	94%	233
Tucson Heart Hospital	Tucson	92%	262
Arizona Heart Hospital	Phoenix	85%	245
Flagstaff Medical Center	Flagstaff	85%	111
Arrowhead Community Hospital	Glendale	83%	101
Mayo Clinic Hospital	Phoenix	81%	265
Saint Joseph's Hospital & Medical Center	Phoenix	81%	244
Banner Baywood Heart Hospital	Mesa	78%	260
University Medical Center	Tucson	76%	295
UPH Hospital at Kino campus	Tucson	73%	91
Banner Estrella Medical Center	Phoenix	70%	241
Tucson Medical Center	Tucson	70%	197
Banner Baywood Medical Center	Mesa	68%	206
Banner Mesa Medical Center	Mesa	67%	83
Chandler Regional Hospital	Chandler	67%	298
Western Arizona Regional Medical Center	Bullhead City	67%	276
John C Lincoln Hospital-North Mountain	Phoenix	66%	215
Casa Grande Regional Medical Center	Casa Grande	65%	163
Northwest Medical Center	Tucson	64%	286
Payson Regional Medical Center	Payson	61%	33
Scottsdale Healthcare	Scottsdale	61%	347
Yavapai Regional Medical Center	Prescott	61%	239
Verde Valley Medical Center	Cottonwood	60%	86
West Valley Hospital	Goodyear	60%	157
Desert Samaritan Medical Center	Mesa	59%	234

NOTE: Hospital profiles are in alphabetical order by state, then city, then hospital within the city; Rankings are sorted by rate in descending order and exclude hospitals with less than 25 cases; (1) The number of cases is too small (n<25) for purposes of reliably predicting hospital performance; (2) Measure reflects the hospital's indication that its submission was based upon a sample of its relevant discharges; (3) Rate reflects fewer than the maximum possible quarters of data for the measure; (4) Inaccurate information submitted and suppressed for one or more quarters; (5) No data is available from the hospital for this measure; Please refer to the User's Guide for a full explanation of data

Hospital Name	City	Rate	Cases
Havasu Regional Medical Center	Lake Havasu City	58%	125
John C Lincoln Hospital-Deer Valley	Phoenix	57%	212
Scottsdale Healthcare-Osborn	Scottsdale	55%	363
Yuma Regional Medical Center	Yuma	55%	425
Banner Good Samaritan Medical Center	Phoenix	54%	249
Northwest Medical Center Oro Valley	Oro Valley	51%	79
Banner Thunderbird Medical Center	Glendale	49%	241
Mesa General Hospital	Mesa	48%	112
Phoenix Baptist Hospital and Medical Center	Phoenix	48%	183
Chinle Comprehensive Health Care Facility	Chinle	42%	33
Kingman Regional Medical Center	Kingman	41%	260
La Paz Regional Hospital	Parker	37%	30
Paradise Valley Hospital	Phoenix	34%	108
Maryvale Hospital Medical Center	Phoenix	33%	170
Saint Luke's Medical Center	Phoenix	31%	113
Phoenix Memorial Health System	Phoenix	28%	109
Sun Health Boswell Hospital	Sun City	24%	231
Del E Webb Memorial Hospital	Sun City West	23%	209
Sierra Vista Regional Health Center	Sierra Vista	16%	80
Navapache Regional Medical Center	Show Low	13%	68
Tempe Saint Luke's Hospital	Tempe	12%	112
Maricopa Integrated Health	Phoenix	9%	154
Tuba City Indian Medical Center	Tuba City	0%	36

11. Evaluation of LVS Function

Hospital Name	City	Rate	Cases
Mayo Clinic Hospital	Phoenix	100%	274
Banner Baywood Heart Hospital	Mesa	99%	283
Saint Joseph's Hospital & Medical Center	Phoenix	99%	272
University Medical Center	Tucson	99%	318
John C Lincoln Hospital-North Mountain	Phoenix	98%	246
Arizona Heart Hospital	Phoenix	97%	278
Arrowhead Community Hospital	Glendale	97%	124
Banner Good Samaritan Medical Center	Phoenix	97%	282
John C Lincoln Hospital-Deer Valley	Phoenix	97%	236
Mesa General Hospital	Mesa	97%	144
Northwest Medical Center	Tucson	97%	352
Phoenix Memorial Health System	Phoenix	97%	120
Tuba City Indian Medical Center	Tuba City	97%	36
Banner Thunderbird Medical Center	Glendale	96%	292
Carondelet Saint Joseph's Hospital	Tucson	96%	281
Paradise Valley Hospital	Phoenix	96%	139
Tucson Medical Center	Tucson	96%	256
Chandler Regional Hospital	Chandler	95%	361
Scottsdale Healthcare-Osborn	Scottsdale	95%	432
Tucson Heart Hospital	Tucson	95%	283
Maricopa Integrated Health	Phoenix	94%	188
Maryvale Hospital Medical Center	Phoenix	94%	190
Saint Luke's Medical Center	Phoenix	94%	129
Western Arizona Regional Medical Center	Bullhead City	94%	302
Banner Baywood Medical Center	Mesa	93%	264
Carondelet Saint Mary's Hospital	Tucson	93%	382
Scottsdale Healthcare	Scottsdale	93%	418
Banner Estrella Medical Center	Phoenix	92%	260
Desert Samaritan Medical Center	Mesa	92%	273
Sun Health Boswell Hospital	Sun City	92%	294
UPH Hospital at Kino campus	Tucson	92%	95
Verde Valley Medical Center	Cottonwood	92%	84
Flagstaff Medical Center	Flagstaff	91%	130
Northwest Medical Center Oro Valley	Oro Valley	91%	90
Phoenix Baptist Hospital and Medical Center	Phoenix	91%	209
Banner Mesa Medical Center	Mesa	90%	105
Casa Grande Regional Medical Center	Casa Grande	90%	182
West Valley Hospital	Goodyear	90%	174
Del E Webb Memorial Hospital	Sun City West	88%	268
Payson Regional Medical Center	Payson	87%	38
Yavapai Regional Medical Center	Prescott	87%	290
Valley View Medical Center	Fort Mohave	86%	28
Navapache Regional Medical Center	Show Low	85%	73
Sierra Vista Regional Health Center	Sierra Vista	85%	106
Tempe Saint Luke's Hospital	Tempe	82%	127
Yuma Regional Medical Center	Yuma	81%	488
Havasu Regional Medical Center	Lake Havasu City	80%	139
White Mountain Regional Medical Center	Springerville	71%	28
Kingman Regional Medical Center	Kingman	70%	285
La Paz Regional Hospital	Parker	61%	31
Chinle Comprehensive Health Care Facility	Chinle	51%	37

12. Smoking Cessation Advice

Hospital Name	City	Rate	Cases
Carondelet Saint Mary's Hospital	Tucson	100%	58
Chandler Regional Hospital	Chandler	100%	55
John C Lincoln Hospital-Deer Valley	Phoenix	100%	61
Mayo Clinic Hospital	Phoenix	100%	25
Scottsdale Healthcare-Osborn	Scottsdale	100%	74
Tucson Medical Center	Tucson	100%	42
University Medical Center	Tucson	100%	59
Banner Baywood Heart Hospital	Mesa	98%	44
Saint Joseph's Hospital & Medical Center	Phoenix	98%	66
Scottsdale Healthcare	Scottsdale	95%	43
Maryvale Hospital Medical Center	Phoenix	94%	71
Western Arizona Regional Medical Center	Bullhead City	94%	94
Arizona Heart Hospital	Phoenix	93%	81
Carondelet Saint Joseph's Hospital	Tucson	92%	36
John C Lincoln Hospital-North Mountain	Phoenix	92%	53
Northwest Medical Center	Tucson	92%	48
Paradise Valley Hospital	Phoenix	92%	26
Phoenix Baptist Hospital and Medical Center	Phoenix	91%	46
West Valley Hospital	Goodyear	91%	32
Yuma Regional Medical Center	Yuma	90%	78
Banner Good Samaritan Medical Center	Phoenix	89%	63
Banner Estrella Medical Center	Phoenix	87%	54
Desert Samaritan Medical Center	Mesa	87%	52
Phoenix Memorial Health System	Phoenix	87%	52
Yavapai Regional Medical Center	Prescott	85%	52
Havasu Regional Medical Center	Lake Havasu City	82%	39
Casa Grande Regional Medical Center	Casa Grande	76%	33
Mesa General Hospital	Mesa	73%	33
Saint Luke's Medical Center	Phoenix	73%	41
Kingman Regional Medical Center	Kingman	67%	81
Sun Health Boswell Hospital	Sun City	66%	29
Banner Thunderbird Medical Center	Glendale	63%	68
Maricopa Integrated Health	Phoenix	56%	68
Tempe Saint Luke's Hospital	Tempe	33%	30
UPH Hospital at Kino campus	Tucson	32%	47

Pneumonia Care

13. Appropriate Initial Antibiotic

Hospital Name	City	Rate	Cases
Northern Cochise Community Hospital	Willcox	98%	42
Banner Mesa Medical Center	Mesa	97%	98
Fort Defiance Indian Hospital	Fort Defiance	97%	39
La Paz Regional Hospital	Parker	96%	72
Mayo Clinic Hospital	Phoenix	96%	202
Tucson Heart Hospital	Tucson	96%	52
Banner Baywood Medical Center	Mesa	95%	118
Carondelet Holy Cross Hospital	Nogales	94%	36
Saint Joseph's Hospital & Medical Center	Phoenix	94%	142
Sun Health Boswell Hospital	Sun City	94%	88
Navapache Regional Medical Center	Show Low	93%	128
University Medical Center	Tucson	93%	73
Northwest Medical Center	Tucson	92%	358
Payson Regional Medical Center	Payson	92%	100
Tucson Medical Center	Tucson	92%	72
Benson Hospital	Benson	91%	35
Chandler Regional Hospital	Chandler	91%	356
Northwest Medical Center Oro Valley	Oro Valley	91%	117
Scottsdale Healthcare	Scottsdale	91%	289
Carondelet Saint Mary's Hospital	Tucson	90%	319
Del E Webb Memorial Hospital	Sun City West	90%	96
Desert Samaritan Medical Center	Mesa	90%	139
Havasu Regional Medical Center	Lake Havasu City	90%	202
John C Lincoln Hospital-Deer Valley	Phoenix	90%	122
Kingman Regional Medical Center	Kingman	90%	167
Paradise Valley Hospital	Phoenix	90%	151
Banner Thunderbird Medical Center	Glendale	89%	101
Carondelet Saint Joseph's Hospital	Tucson	89%	317
Flagstaff Medical Center	Flagstaff	89%	151
Scottsdale Healthcare-Osborn	Scottsdale	89%	253
UPH Hospital at Kino campus	Tucson	89%	107
Arrowhead Community Hospital	Glendale	88%	312
PHS Indian Hospital-San Carlos	San Carlos	88%	41
John C Lincoln Hospital-North Mountain	Phoenix	87%	103
Saint Luke's Medical Center	Phoenix	87%	90
Banner Estrella Medical Center	Phoenix	86%	241
Banner Good Samaritan Medical Center	Phoenix	86%	99
Sierra Vista Regional Health Center	Sierra Vista	86%	131
Yavapai Regional Medical Center	Prescott	86%	146
Phoenix Memorial Health System	Phoenix	85%	151
Verde Valley Medical Center	Cottonwood	85%	158
Wickenburg Regional Hospital	Wickenburg	85%	33
Yavapai Regional Medical Center-East	Prescott Valley	85%	26
Arizona Heart Hospital	Phoenix	84%	49
Casa Grande Regional Medical Center	Casa Grande	84%	334
Phoenix Indian Medical Center	Phoenix	84%	38
Maricopa Integrated Health	Phoenix	83%	157
Maryvale Hospital Medical Center	Phoenix	82%	176

NOTE: Hospital profiles are in alphabetical order by state, then city, then hospital within the city; Rankings are sorted by rate in descending order and exclude hospitals with less than 25 cases; (1) The number of cases is too small (n<25) for purposes of reliably predicting hospital performance; (2) Measure reflects the hospital's indication that its submission was based upon a sample of its relevant discharges; (3) Rate reflects fewer than the maximum possible quarters of data for the measure; (4) Inaccurate information submitted and suppressed for one or more quarters; (5) No data is available from the hospital for this measure; Please refer to the User's Guide for a full explanation of data

Hospital Name	City	Rate	Cases
Mesa General Hospital	Mesa	82%	85
West Valley Hospital	Goodyear	82%	159
Phoenix Baptist Hospital and Medical Center	Phoenix	81%	186
Yuma Regional Medical Center	Yuma	81%	354
Whiteriver Indian Hospital	Whiteriver	79%	57
Tuba City Indian Medical Center	Tuba City	77%	79
Chinle Comprehensive Health Care Facility	Chinle	76%	34
Tempe Saint Luke's Hospital	Tempe	76%	149
Western Arizona Regional Medical Center	Bullhead City	76%	119
Southeast Arizona Medical Center	Douglas	73%	41
Mount Graham Regional Medical Center	Safford	67%	92
Hopi Health Care Center	Polacca	45%	31
Sage Memorial Hospital	Ganado	33%	33

14. Blood Culture Timing

Hospital Name	City	Rate	Cases
Sun Health Boswell Hospital	Sun City	97%	88
Desert Samaritan Medical Center	Mesa	96%	119
Casa Grande Regional Medical Center	Casa Grande	95%	187
Flagstaff Medical Center	Flagstaff	95%	105
John C Lincoln Hospital-Deer Valley	Phoenix	95%	111
Del E Webb Memorial Hospital	Sun City West	94%	81
Mayo Clinic Hospital	Phoenix	94%	249
Northwest Medical Center Oro Valley	Oro Valley	94%	107
Verde Valley Medical Center	Cottonwood	94%	127
Banner Good Samaritan Medical Center	Phoenix	93%	86
John C Lincoln Hospital-North Mountain	Phoenix	92%	77
Navapache Regional Medical Center	Show Low	92%	83
Saint Luke's Medical Center	Phoenix	92%	79
Banner Thunderbird Medical Center	Glendale	91%	96
Northwest Medical Center	Tucson	91%	331
Sierra Vista Regional Health Center	Sierra Vista	91%	70
Tuba City Indian Medical Center	Tuba City	91%	54
Paradise Valley Hospital	Phoenix	90%	164
Scottsdale Healthcare-Osborn	Scottsdale	90%	258
Yavapai Regional Medical Center	Prescott	90%	83
Arizona Heart Hospital	Phoenix	89%	38
University Medical Center	Tucson	89%	45
Banner Baywood Medical Center	Mesa	88%	82
Payson Regional Medical Center	Payson	88%	83
Saint Joseph's Hospital & Medical Center	Phoenix	88%	119
Scottsdale Healthcare	Scottsdale	88%	271
Tucson Heart Hospital	Tucson	88%	65
Western Arizona Regional Medical Center	Bullhead City	88%	89
Banner Mesa Medical Center	Mesa	87%	89
Chandler Regional Hospital	Chandler	87%	298
Carondelet Saint Mary's Hospital	Tucson	86%	288
Tucson Medical Center	Tucson	86%	74
Arrowhead Community Hospital	Glendale	85%	170
Havasu Regional Medical Center	Lake Havasu City	85%	137
Phoenix Baptist Hospital and Medical Center	Phoenix	85%	95
Maryvale Hospital Medical Center	Phoenix	84%	121
Yuma Regional Medical Center	Yuma	84%	370
Carondelet Saint Joseph's Hospital	Tucson	82%	308
Kingman Regional Medical Center	Kingman	81%	128
Phoenix Memorial Health System	Phoenix	80%	104
Maricopa Integrated Health	Phoenix	79%	113
Whiteriver Indian Hospital	Whiteriver	79%	52
Tempe Saint Luke's Hospital	Tempe	77%	47
UPH Hospital at Kino campus	Tucson	77%	62
Mount Graham Regional Medical Center	Safford	76%	38
West Valley Hospital	Goodyear	76%	90
Mesa General Hospital	Mesa	72%	60
Banner Estrella Medical Center	Phoenix	57%	163

15. Influenza Vaccine

Hospital Name	City	Rate	Cases
Tucson Heart Hospital	Tucson	100%	26
John C Lincoln Hospital-North Mountain	Phoenix	96%	26
Tuba City Indian Medical Center	Tuba City	93%	27
Mayo Clinic Hospital	Phoenix	91%	99
John C Lincoln Hospital-Deer Valley	Phoenix	84%	25
Saint Joseph's Hospital & Medical Center	Phoenix	82%	34
Payson Regional Medical Center	Payson	78%	32
Havasu Regional Medical Center	Lake Havasu City	75%	67
Northwest Medical Center	Tucson	74%	119
Verde Valley Medical Center	Cottonwood	72%	50
Sierra Vista Regional Health Center	Sierra Vista	70%	27
Yavapai Regional Medical Center	Prescott	70%	30
Western Arizona Regional Medical Center	Bullhead City	65%	26
Scottsdale Healthcare	Scottsdale	64%	107
Northwest Medical Center Oro Valley	Oro Valley	58%	40
West Valley Hospital	Goodyear	58%	36
Scottsdale Healthcare-Osborn	Scottsdale	57%	110
Flagstaff Medical Center	Flagstaff	56%	43
Yuma Regional Medical Center	Yuma	51%	172
Carondelet Saint Mary's Hospital	Tucson	50%	114
Sun Health Boswell Hospital	Sun City	48%	25
Arrowhead Community Hospital	Glendale	46%	80
Banner Estrella Medical Center	Phoenix	44%	87
Maryvale Hospital Medical Center	Phoenix	41%	41
Paradise Valley Hospital	Phoenix	41%	37
Banner Thunderbird Medical Center	Glendale	40%	25
Casa Grande Regional Medical Center	Casa Grande	29%	112
Maricopa Integrated Health	Phoenix	23%	48

16. Initial Antibiotic Timing

Hospital Name	City	Rate	Cases
Fort Defiance Indian Hospital	Fort Defiance	95%	42
Hopi Health Care Center	Polacca	94%	32
Wickenburg Regional Hospital	Wickenburg	91%	33
Payson Regional Medical Center	Payson	89%	132
Verde Valley Medical Center	Cottonwood	89%	183
Mayo Clinic Hospital	Phoenix	87%	284
Paradise Valley Hospital	Phoenix	86%	206
Yavapai Regional Medical Center-East	Prescott Valley	86%	28
PHS Indian Hospital-San Carlos	San Carlos	85%	41
Tucson Heart Hospital	Tucson	85%	72
Western Arizona Regional Medical Center	Bullhead City	85%	142
Kingman Regional Medical Center	Kingman	84%	187
La Paz Regional Hospital	Parker	84%	73
Saint Joseph's Hospital & Medical Center	Phoenix	84%	168
Scottsdale Healthcare	Scottsdale	84%	353
Scottsdale Healthcare-Osborn	Scottsdale	84%	346
Whiteriver Indian Hospital	Whiteriver	83%	59
Maryvale Hospital Medical Center	Phoenix	82%	196
Tuba City Indian Medical Center	Tuba City	82%	85
Arrowhead Community Hospital	Glendale	81%	342
Carondelet Saint Mary's Hospital	Tucson	81%	396
Winslow Memorial Hospital	Winslow	81%	27
Carondelet Saint Joseph's Hospital	Tucson	80%	388
Northwest Medical Center Oro Valley	Oro Valley	79%	150
White Mountain Regional Medical Center	Springerville	79%	33
Chandler Regional Hospital	Chandler	78%	418
Phoenix Indian Medical Center	Phoenix	78%	46
Southeast Arizona Medical Center	Douglas	78%	37
Benson Hospital	Benson	77%	39
Del E Webb Memorial Hospital	Sun City West	77%	140
John C Lincoln Hospital-North Mountain	Phoenix	77%	141
Northern Cochise Community Hospital	Willcox	77%	53
Banner Mesa Medical Center	Mesa	76%	136
Phoenix Baptist Hospital and Medical Center	Phoenix	76%	238
Yavapai Regional Medical Center	Prescott	76%	186
Banner Estrella Medical Center	Phoenix	75%	288
Navapache Regional Medical Center	Show Low	75%	152
West Valley Hospital	Goodyear	75%	168
Arizona Heart Hospital	Phoenix	74%	61
Chinle Comprehensive Health Care Facility	Chinle	72%	43
Phoenix Memorial Health System	Phoenix	72%	184
Northwest Medical Center	Tucson	71%	479
Flagstaff Medical Center	Flagstaff	70%	172
Sierra Vista Regional Health Center	Sierra Vista	70%	141
Banner Good Samaritan Medical Center	Phoenix	67%	133
Maricopa Integrated Health	Phoenix	67%	212
Valley View Medical Center	Fort Mohave	66%	29
Sun Health Boswell Hospital	Sun City	65%	141
Casa Grande Regional Medical Center	Casa Grande	63%	400
Tempe Saint Luke's Hospital	Tempe	63%	148
Tucson Medical Center	Tucson	62%	108
Saint Luke's Medical Center	Phoenix	61%	117
Carondelet Holy Cross Hospital	Nogales	59%	29
John C Lincoln Hospital-Deer Valley	Phoenix	59%	141
Banner Baywood Medical Center	Mesa	58%	134
Desert Samaritan Medical Center	Mesa	58%	154
Sage Memorial Hospital	Ganado	58%	36
Banner Thunderbird Medical Center	Glendale	57%	130
Mesa General Hospital	Mesa	57%	109
University Medical Center	Tucson	57%	142
Mount Graham Regional Medical Center	Safford	55%	94
UPH Hospital at Kino campus	Tucson	55%	147
Havasu Regional Medical Center	Lake Havasu City	50%	250
Yuma Regional Medical Center	Yuma	46%	721

17. Oxygenation Assessment

Hospital Name	City	Rate	Cases
Arizona Heart Hospital	Phoenix	100%	76
Arrowhead Community Hospital	Glendale	100%	382
Banner Baywood Medical Center	Mesa	100%	163

NOTE: Hospital profiles are in alphabetical order by state, then city, then hospital within the city; Rankings are sorted by rate in descending order and exclude hospitals with less than 25 cases; (1) The number of cases is too small (n<25) for purposes of reliably predicting hospital performance; (2) Measure reflects the hospital's indication that its submission was based upon a sample of its relevant discharges; (3) Rate reflects fewer than the maximum possible quarters of data for the measure; (4) Inaccurate information submitted and suppressed for one or more quarters; (5) No data is available from the hospital for this measure; Please refer to the User's Guide for a full explanation of data

Banner Estrella Medical Center	Phoenix	100%	356
Banner Good Samaritan Medical Center	Phoenix	100%	164
Banner Mesa Medical Center	Mesa	100%	165
Banner Thunderbird Medical Center	Glendale	100%	181
Benson Hospital	Benson	100%	47
Carondelet Holy Cross Hospital	Nogales	100%	51
Carondelet Saint Joseph's Hospital	Tucson	100%	499
Carondelet Saint Mary's Hospital	Tucson	100%	483
Casa Grande Regional Medical Center	Casa Grande	100%	449
Chandler Regional Hospital	Chandler	100%	549
Chinle Comprehensive Health Care Facility	Chinle	100%	47
Del E Webb Memorial Hospital	Sun City West	100%	167
Desert Samaritan Medical Center	Mesa	100%	198
Flagstaff Medical Center	Flagstaff	100%	217
Fort Defiance Indian Hospital	Fort Defiance	100%	45
Hopi Health Care Center	Polacca	100%	33
John C Lincoln Hospital-Deer Valley	Phoenix	100%	186
John C Lincoln Hospital-North Mountain	Phoenix	100%	176
Kingman Regional Medical Center	Kingman	100%	214
Maricopa Integrated Health	Phoenix	100%	257
Maryvale Hospital Medical Center	Phoenix	100%	229
Mayo Clinic Hospital	Phoenix	100%	403
Mesa General Hospital	Mesa	100%	123
Mount Graham Regional Medical Center	Safford	100%	125
Navapache Regional Medical Center	Show Low	100%	168
Northern Cochise Community Hospital	Willcox	100%	57
Northwest Medical Center	Tucson	100%	604
Northwest Medical Center Oro Valley	Oro Valley	100%	167
PHS Indian Hospital-San Carlos	San Carlos	100%	44
Paradise Valley Hospital	Phoenix	100%	257
Payson Regional Medical Center	Payson	100%	139
Phoenix Baptist Hospital and Medical Center	Phoenix	100%	283
Phoenix Indian Medical Center	Phoenix	100%	47
Phoenix Memorial Health System	Phoenix	100%	195
Saint Joseph's Hospital & Medical Center	Phoenix	100%	219
Saint Luke's Medical Center	Phoenix	100%	139
Scottsdale Healthcare	Scottsdale	100%	465
Scottsdale Healthcare-Osborn	Scottsdale	100%	457
Sells Indian Hospital	Sells	100%	32
Sun Health Boswell Hospital	Sun City	100%	172
Tuba City Indian Medical Center	Tuba City	100%	98
Tucson Heart Hospital	Tucson	100%	84
Tucson Medical Center	Tucson	100%	151
University Medical Center	Tucson	100%	188
Valley View Medical Center	Fort Mohave	100%	31
Verde Valley Medical Center	Cottonwood	100%	216
West Valley Hospital	Goodyear	100%	198
Western Arizona Regional Medical Center	Bullhead City	100%	162
White Mountain Regional Medical Center	Springerville	100%	38
Winslow Memorial Hospital	Winslow	100%	30
Yavapai Regional Medical Center	Prescott	100%	213
Yavapai Regional Medical Center-East	Prescott Valley	100%	33
Yuma Regional Medical Center	Yuma	100%	848
Havasu Regional Medical Center	Lake Havasu City	99%	279
La Paz Regional Hospital	Parker	99%	79
Sierra Vista Regional Health Center	Sierra Vista	99%	168
Tempe Saint Luke's Hospital	Tempe	99%	163
UPH Hospital at Kino campus	Tucson	99%	161
Whiteriver Indian Hospital	Whiteriver	99%	81
Sage Memorial Hospital	Ganado	98%	47
Southeast Arizona Medical Center	Douglas	96%	47
Wickenburg Regional Hospital	Wickenburg	88%	33

18. Pneumococcal Vaccine

Hospital Name	City	Rate	Cases
Tucson Heart Hospital	Tucson	97%	64
Whiteriver Indian Hospital	Whiteriver	97%	37
Carondelet Saint Mary's Hospital	Tucson	96%	249
Mayo Clinic Hospital	Phoenix	96%	324
Carondelet Saint Joseph's Hospital	Tucson	92%	305
Verde Valley Medical Center	Cottonwood	88%	164
Tuba City Indian Medical Center	Tuba City	85%	71
Fort Defiance Indian Hospital	Fort Defiance	83%	29
Kingman Regional Medical Center	Kingman	83%	96
Chandler Regional Hospital	Chandler	82%	310
Payson Regional Medical Center	Payson	82%	92
Northwest Medical Center Oro Valley	Oro Valley	81%	109
John C Lincoln Hospital-North Mountain	Phoenix	80%	103
La Paz Regional Hospital	Parker	80%	46
Saint Joseph's Hospital & Medical Center	Phoenix	80%	101
Arrowhead Community Hospital	Glendale	79%	210
Scottsdale Healthcare-Osborn	Scottsdale	79%	310
John C Lincoln Hospital-Deer Valley	Phoenix	78%	95
Scottsdale Healthcare	Scottsdale	78%	301
University Medical Center	Tucson	78%	74
Yavapai Regional Medical Center	Prescott	78%	138
Southeast Arizona Medical Center	Douglas	74%	31
Northwest Medical Center	Tucson	73%	361
Benson Hospital	Benson	71%	28
Northern Cochise Community Hospital	Willcox	70%	33
Havasu Regional Medical Center	Lake Havasu City	69%	199
Mount Graham Regional Medical Center	Safford	69%	77
Desert Samaritan Medical Center	Mesa	68%	87
Navapache Regional Medical Center	Show Low	68%	78
Banner Baywood Medical Center	Mesa	67%	99
Phoenix Baptist Hospital and Medical Center	Phoenix	66%	164
Western Arizona Regional Medical Center	Bullhead City	66%	80
Sierra Vista Regional Health Center	Sierra Vista	65%	99
Arizona Heart Hospital	Phoenix	62%	52
Del E Webb Memorial Hospital	Sun City West	60%	124
Banner Mesa Medical Center	Mesa	59%	81
Flagstaff Medical Center	Flagstaff	58%	115
Sun Health Boswell Hospital	Sun City	58%	138
Tucson Medical Center	Tucson	58%	86
Paradise Valley Hospital	Phoenix	56%	124
Banner Estrella Medical Center	Phoenix	55%	150
Yuma Regional Medical Center	Yuma	50%	545
Banner Good Samaritan Medical Center	Phoenix	49%	74
Saint Luke's Medical Center	Phoenix	49%	70
Mesa General Hospital	Mesa	48%	66
Maryvale Hospital Medical Center	Phoenix	45%	87
West Valley Hospital	Goodyear	44%	86
Carondelet Holy Cross Hospital	Nogales	43%	30
Tempe Saint Luke's Hospital	Tempe	41%	69
Sage Memorial Hospital	Ganado	40%	40
UPH Hospital at Kino campus	Tucson	40%	58
Banner Thunderbird Medical Center	Glendale	39%	98
Casa Grande Regional Medical Center	Casa Grande	27%	254
Phoenix Memorial Health System	Phoenix	27%	73
Wickenburg Regional Hospital	Wickenburg	24%	25
Chinle Comprehensive Health Care Facility	Chinle	21%	47
Maricopa Integrated Health	Phoenix	21%	81

19. Smoking Cessation Advice

Hospital Name	City	Rate	Cases
Carondelet Saint Mary's Hospital	Tucson	100%	145
Mayo Clinic Hospital	Phoenix	100%	39
Tucson Medical Center	Tucson	100%	32
University Medical Center	Tucson	100%	48
John C Lincoln Hospital-Deer Valley	Phoenix	98%	62
Scottsdale Healthcare-Osborn	Scottsdale	98%	85
Arrowhead Community Hospital	Glendale	97%	86
Carondelet Saint Joseph's Hospital	Tucson	97%	102
Scottsdale Healthcare	Scottsdale	95%	66
Chandler Regional Hospital	Chandler	94%	89
Paradise Valley Hospital	Phoenix	91%	66
Northwest Medical Center Oro Valley	Oro Valley	90%	30
Navapache Regional Medical Center	Show Low	88%	33
Payson Regional Medical Center	Payson	88%	32
John C Lincoln Hospital-North Mountain	Phoenix	87%	38
Yavapai Regional Medical Center	Prescott	87%	46
Phoenix Memorial Health System	Phoenix	86%	84
Verde Valley Medical Center	Cottonwood	86%	51
Northwest Medical Center	Tucson	85%	119
Western Arizona Regional Medical Center	Bullhead City	85%	72
Phoenix Baptist Hospital and Medical Center	Phoenix	82%	89
Maryvale Hospital Medical Center	Phoenix	80%	82
Arizona Heart Hospital	Phoenix	79%	29
Yuma Regional Medical Center	Yuma	78%	131
Havasu Regional Medical Center	Lake Havasu City	77%	64
West Valley Hospital	Goodyear	77%	52
Del E Webb Memorial Hospital	Sun City West	76%	25
Flagstaff Medical Center	Flagstaff	76%	45
Mount Graham Regional Medical Center	Safford	73%	26
Banner Estrella Medical Center	Phoenix	72%	83
Mesa General Hospital	Mesa	72%	36
Desert Samaritan Medical Center	Mesa	71%	56
Sierra Vista Regional Health Center	Sierra Vista	71%	42
Saint Joseph's Hospital & Medical Center	Phoenix	68%	62
Saint Luke's Medical Center	Phoenix	68%	47
Kingman Regional Medical Center	Kingman	66%	86
Maricopa Integrated Health	Phoenix	63%	98
Casa Grande Regional Medical Center	Casa Grande	61%	108
Banner Baywood Medical Center	Mesa	60%	30
Banner Thunderbird Medical Center	Glendale	57%	54
Banner Mesa Medical Center	Mesa	51%	35
UPH Hospital at Kino campus	Tucson	47%	76
Tempe Saint Luke's Hospital	Tempe	44%	48

NOTE: Hospital profiles are in alphabetical order by state, then city, then hospital within the city; Rankings are sorted by rate in descending order and exclude hospitals with less than 25 cases; (1) The number of cases is too small (n<25) for purposes of reliably predicting hospital performance; (2) Measure reflects the hospital's indication that its submission was based upon a sample of its relevant discharges; (3) Rate reflects fewer than the maximum possible quarters of data for the measure; (4) Inaccurate information submitted and suppressed for one or more quarters; (5) No data is available from the hospital for this measure; Please refer to the User's Guide for a full explanation of data

Banner Good Samaritan Medical Center	Phoenix	40%	45

Surgical Infection Prevention

20. Prophylactic Antibiotic Given

Hospital Name	City	Rate	Cases
Tucson Heart Hospital	Tucson	99%	107
UPH Hospital at Kino campus	Tucson	98%	56
Arizona Spine and Joint Hospital	Mesa	94%	71
Chandler Regional Hospital	Chandler	94%	208
Mayo Clinic Hospital	Phoenix	92%	695
Northwest Medical Center Oro Valley	Oro Valley	91%	491
Yavapai Regional Medical Center	Prescott	91%	246
Flagstaff Medical Center	Flagstaff	89%	222
Scottsdale Healthcare-Osborn	Scottsdale	89%	73
Phoenix Baptist Hospital and Medical Center	Phoenix	86%	541
Sun Health Boswell Hospital	Sun City	86%	280
John C Lincoln Hospital-North Mountain	Phoenix	85%	252
Banner Baywood Heart Hospital	Mesa	84%	182
John C Lincoln Hospital-Deer Valley	Phoenix	84%	190
Paradise Valley Hospital	Phoenix	84%	354
Banner Mesa Medical Center	Mesa	83%	151
Northwest Medical Center	Tucson	83%	1638
Carondelet Saint Mary's Hospital	Tucson	82%	144
Sierra Vista Regional Health Center	Sierra Vista	82%	347
Arizona Heart Hospital	Phoenix	81%	365
Yuma Regional Medical Center	Yuma	80%	898
Casa Grande Regional Medical Center	Casa Grande	79%	224
Del E Webb Memorial Hospital	Sun City West	79%	168
Tucson Medical Center	Tucson	79%	266
Arrowhead Community Hospital	Glendale	77%	485
Desert Samaritan Medical Center	Mesa	77%	233
University Medical Center	Tucson	76%	66
Navapache Regional Medical Center	Show Low	75%	159
Banner Estrella Medical Center	Phoenix	74%	209
Mesa General Hospital	Mesa	74%	121
Banner Thunderbird Medical Center	Glendale	73%	201
Maryvale Hospital Medical Center	Phoenix	72%	76
Payson Regional Medical Center	Payson	72%	127
Phoenix Indian Medical Center	Phoenix	72%	46
Banner Good Samaritan Medical Center	Phoenix	71%	241
Mount Graham Regional Medical Center	Safford	71%	114
Carondelet Holy Cross Hospital	Nogales	70%	54
Saint Joseph's Hospital & Medical Center	Phoenix	70%	149
Verde Valley Medical Center	Cottonwood	69%	90
West Valley Hospital	Goodyear	69%	287
Phoenix Memorial Health System	Phoenix	63%	76
Carondelet Saint Joseph's Hospital	Tucson	61%	183
Valley View Medical Center	Fort Mohave	60%	40
Kingman Regional Medical Center	Kingman	59%	190
Scottsdale Healthcare	Scottsdale	59%	87
Arizona Orthopedic Surgical Hospital	Chandler	52%	25
Banner Baywood Medical Center	Mesa	50%	121
Havasu Regional Medical Center	Lake Havasu City	50%	464
Saint Luke's Medical Center	Phoenix	47%	145
Western Arizona Regional Medical Center	Bullhead City	44%	317
Tempe Saint Luke's Hospital	Tempe	7%	30

21. Prophylactic Antibiotic Selection

Hospital Name	City	Rate	Cases
Arizona Spine and Joint Hospital	Mesa	100%	71
Tucson Heart Hospital	Tucson	100%	37
Banner Baywood Heart Hospital	Mesa	98%	61
Navapache Regional Medical Center	Show Low	98%	41
Yavapai Regional Medical Center	Prescott	98%	58
Arizona Heart Hospital	Phoenix	97%	98
John C Lincoln Hospital-Deer Valley	Phoenix	97%	61
Mayo Clinic Hospital	Phoenix	97%	211
West Valley Hospital	Goodyear	97%	98
Chandler Regional Hospital	Chandler	96%	68
Maryvale Hospital Medical Center	Phoenix	96%	26
Northwest Medical Center	Tucson	96%	382
Northwest Medical Center Oro Valley	Oro Valley	96%	127
Tucson Medical Center	Tucson	96%	96
Sierra Vista Regional Health Center	Sierra Vista	95%	74
Verde Valley Medical Center	Cottonwood	95%	64
Arrowhead Community Hospital	Glendale	94%	155
Banner Mesa Medical Center	Mesa	94%	150
Paradise Valley Hospital	Phoenix	94%	109
Carondelet Saint Joseph's Hospital	Tucson	93%	60
Mesa General Hospital	Mesa	93%	29
Yuma Regional Medical Center	Yuma	93%	182
Banner Good Samaritan Medical Center	Phoenix	92%	80
Flagstaff Medical Center	Flagstaff	92%	76
Saint Joseph's Hospital & Medical Center	Phoenix	92%	53
Kingman Regional Medical Center	Kingman	91%	46
Banner Estrella Medical Center	Phoenix	89%	61
Casa Grande Regional Medical Center	Casa Grande	88%	73
Del E Webb Memorial Hospital	Sun City West	88%	48
John C Lincoln Hospital-North Mountain	Phoenix	87%	75
Payson Regional Medical Center	Payson	84%	38
Carondelet Saint Mary's Hospital	Tucson	83%	48
Banner Baywood Medical Center	Mesa	82%	39
Banner Thunderbird Medical Center	Glendale	80%	76
Phoenix Baptist Hospital and Medical Center	Phoenix	79%	149
Scottsdale Healthcare	Scottsdale	79%	84
Havasu Regional Medical Center	Lake Havasu City	78%	103
Desert Samaritan Medical Center	Mesa	76%	83
Scottsdale Healthcare-Osborn	Scottsdale	75%	75
Saint Luke's Medical Center	Phoenix	72%	50
Western Arizona Regional Medical Center	Bullhead City	68%	77
University Medical Center	Tucson	60%	72

22. Prophylactic Antibiotic Stopped

Hospital Name	City	Rate	Cases
Phoenix Baptist Hospital and Medical Center	Phoenix	100%	511
Tucson Heart Hospital	Tucson	100%	107
Western Arizona Regional Medical Center	Bullhead City	98%	291
Carondelet Holy Cross Hospital	Nogales	96%	49
UPH Hospital at Kino campus	Tucson	96%	56
Verde Valley Medical Center	Cottonwood	96%	69
Phoenix Indian Medical Center	Phoenix	95%	38
Mount Graham Regional Medical Center	Safford	94%	112
Mesa General Hospital	Mesa	92%	108
Mayo Clinic Hospital	Phoenix	90%	670
Banner Estrella Medical Center	Phoenix	87%	195
Yuma Regional Medical Center	Yuma	74%	886
Arrowhead Community Hospital	Glendale	73%	496
Banner Baywood Heart Hospital	Mesa	72%	161
Tucson Medical Center	Tucson	72%	249
Casa Grande Regional Medical Center	Casa Grande	71%	220
Payson Regional Medical Center	Payson	70%	115
Banner Mesa Medical Center	Mesa	69%	146
Yavapai Regional Medical Center	Prescott	69%	226
Arizona Heart Hospital	Phoenix	67%	356
Arizona Spine and Joint Hospital	Mesa	66%	71
Saint Joseph's Hospital & Medical Center	Phoenix	66%	143
Scottsdale Healthcare	Scottsdale	66%	82
West Valley Hospital	Goodyear	66%	268
Northwest Medical Center	Tucson	65%	1523
Valley View Medical Center	Fort Mohave	65%	37
Arizona Orthopedic Surgical Hospital	Chandler	64%	25
Banner Good Samaritan Medical Center	Phoenix	64%	226
John C Lincoln Hospital-Deer Valley	Phoenix	64%	174
Banner Thunderbird Medical Center	Glendale	63%	186
Paradise Valley Hospital	Phoenix	63%	347
Flagstaff Medical Center	Flagstaff	61%	213
Sierra Vista Regional Health Center	Sierra Vista	61%	332
Carondelet Saint Joseph's Hospital	Tucson	60%	167
John C Lincoln Hospital-North Mountain	Phoenix	60%	247
Maryvale Hospital Medical Center	Phoenix	60%	72
Chandler Regional Hospital	Chandler	59%	194
University Medical Center	Tucson	58%	65
Phoenix Memorial Health System	Phoenix	57%	72
Desert Samaritan Medical Center	Mesa	55%	223
Carondelet Saint Mary's Hospital	Tucson	50%	145
Banner Baywood Medical Center	Mesa	49%	109
Kingman Regional Medical Center	Kingman	48%	183
Northwest Medical Center Oro Valley	Oro Valley	47%	480
Havasu Regional Medical Center	Lake Havasu City	46%	450
Sun Health Boswell Hospital	Sun City	46%	272
Del E Webb Memorial Hospital	Sun City West	42%	158
Scottsdale Healthcare-Osborn	Scottsdale	41%	69
Navapache Regional Medical Center	Show Low	34%	158
Saint Luke's Medical Center	Phoenix	34%	139

Pregnancy Care

23. Inpatient Neonatal Mortality

Hospital Name	City	Rate	Cases
Mesa General Hospital	Mesa	0.00%	1312
Tuba City Indian Medical Center	Tuba City	0.00%	498
Del E Webb Memorial Hospital	Sun City West	0.10%	1951
Carondelet Saint Joseph's Hospital	Tucson	0.11%	2631
Chandler Regional Hospital	Chandler	0.11%	5238
Yavapai Regional Medical Center	Prescott	0.22%	1378
Yuma Regional Medical Center	Yuma	0.24%	3712
Desert Samaritan Medical Center	Mesa	0.56%	9031

NOTE: Hospital profiles are in alphabetical order by state, then city, then hospital within the city; Rankings are sorted by rate in descending order and exclude hospitals with less than 25 cases; (1) The number of cases is too small (n<25) for purposes of reliably predicting hospital performance; (2) Measure reflects the hospital's indication that its submission was based upon a sample of its relevant discharges; (3) Rate reflects fewer than the maximum possible quarters of data for the measure; (4) Inaccurate information submitted and suppressed for one or more quarters; (5) No data is available from the hospital for this measure; Please refer to the User's Guide for a full explanation of data

Saint Joseph's Hospital & Medical Center	Phoenix	1.01%	6028

24. Third or Fourth Degree Laceration

Hospital Name	City	Rate	Cases
Tuba City Indian Medical Center	Tuba City	1.50%	399
Saint Joseph's Hospital & Medical Center	Phoenix	2.11%	4116
Del E Webb Memorial Hospital	Sun City West	2.20%	1409
Yuma Regional Medical Center	Yuma	3.02%	2580
Desert Samaritan Medical Center	Mesa	3.84%	5599
Chandler Regional Hospital	Chandler	3.93%	3434
Yavapai Regional Medical Center	Prescott	5.47%	896
Carondelet Saint Joseph's Hospital	Tucson	6.07%	1795
Mesa General Hospital	Mesa	8.76%	993

NOTE: Hospital profiles are in alphabetical order by state, then city, then hospital within the city; Rankings are sorted by rate in descending order and exclude hospitals with less than 25 cases; (1) The number of cases is too small (n<25) for purposes of reliably predicting hospital performance; (2) Measure reflects the hospital's indication that its submission was based upon a sample of its relevant discharges; (3) Rate reflects fewer than the maximum possible quarters of data for the measure; (4) Inaccurate information submitted and suppressed for one or more quarters; (5) No data is available from the hospital for this measure; Please refer to the User's Guide for a full explanation of data

Benson Hospital

450 S Ocotillo Street Phone: 520-586-2261
Benson, AZ 85602 Fax: 520-586-2265
URL: www.personal.riverusers.com/~bensonhospital
Ownership: Voluntary non-profit - Other Accredited: No
Emergency Services: Yes Licensed Beds: 22

Key Personnel:

CEO . . . . . Ronald McKinnon
Chief Medical Staff . . . . . Barbara Haftley
Emergency Room . . . . . Jefferey Beeley, MD
Director Medical/Surgical Nursing . . . . . Beverly Hazelton
Chief Radiology . . . . . Brian Kirkwood

Measure	Cases	This Hospital	State Average	U.S. Average	Top Hospital
Heart Attack Care					
ACE Inhibitor or ARB for LVSD[3]	0	-	83%	82%	100%
Aspirin at Arrival[3]	0	-	96%	92%	100%
Aspirin at Discharge[3]	0	-	91%	90%	100%
Beta Blocker at Arrival[3]	0	-	88%	87%	100%
Beta Blocker at Discharge[3]	0	-	93%	90%	100%
Fibrinolytic Medication Timing[3]	0	-	10%	31%	100%
PCI Within 90 Minutes of Arrival[5]	-	-	47%	54%	95%
Smoking Cessation Advice[3]	0	-	89%	88%	100%
Heart Failure Care					
ACE Inhibitor or ARB for LVSD[1]	4	50%	81%	82%	100%
Discharge Instructions[1]	14	21%	48%	61%	93%
Evaluation of LVS Function[1]	18	39%	84%	83%	99%
Smoking Cessation Advice[1]	3	100%	76%	82%	100%
Pneumonia Care					
Appropriate Initial Antibiotic	35	91%	84%	83%	94%
Blood Culture Timing[1]	22	91%	87%	90%	100%
Influenza Vaccine[1]	4	100%	61%	70%	100%
Initial Antibiotic Timing	39	77%	73%	80%	93%
Oxygenation Assessment	47	100%	100%	99%	100%
Pneumococcal Vaccine	28	71%	64%	69%	94%
Smoking Cessation Advice[1]	16	75%	69%	80%	100%
Surgical Infection Prevention					
Prophylactic Antibiotic Given[5]	-	-	74%	77%	95%
Prophylactic Antibiotic Selection[5]	-	-	88%	90%	100%
Prophylactic Antibiotic Stopped[5]	-	-	68%	72%	95%
Pregnancy Care					
Inpatient Neonatal Mortality	-	-	-	-	-
Third or Fourth Degree Laceration	-	-	3.70%	3.63%	3.27%

Copper Queen Community Hospital

101 Cole Avenue Phone: 520-432-5383
Bisbee, AZ 85603 Fax: 520-432-8018
URL: www.cqch.org
Ownership: Voluntary non-profit - Other Accredited: No
Emergency Services: No Licensed Beds: 28

Key Personnel:

CEO . . . . . James Dickson
Chief Medical Staff . . . . . Stephen Lindstrom, MD
Infection Control . . . . . Elizabeth Mitchell, RN
Respiratory/Cardiopulmonary . . . . . Ben Vavila

Measure	Cases	This Hospital	State Average	U.S. Average	Top Hospital
Heart Attack Care					
ACE Inhibitor or ARB for LVSD[5]	-	-	83%	82%	100%
Aspirin at Arrival[5]	-	-	96%	92%	100%
Aspirin at Discharge[5]	-	-	91%	90%	100%
Beta Blocker at Arrival[5]	-	-	88%	87%	100%
Beta Blocker at Discharge[5]	-	-	93%	90%	100%
Fibrinolytic Medication Timing[5]	-	-	10%	31%	100%
PCI Within 90 Minutes of Arrival[5]	-	-	47%	54%	95%
Smoking Cessation Advice[5]	-	-	89%	88%	100%
Heart Failure Care					
ACE Inhibitor or ARB for LVSD[3]	0	-	81%	82%	100%
Discharge Instructions[1,3]	4	0%	48%	61%	93%
Evaluation of LVS Function[1,3]	3	0%	84%	83%	99%
Smoking Cessation Advice[1,3]	1	0%	76%	82%	100%
Pneumonia Care					
Appropriate Initial Antibiotic[1,3]	6	0%	84%	83%	94%
Blood Culture Timing[1,3]	6	100%	87%	90%	100%
Influenza Vaccine[5]	-	-	61%	70%	100%
Initial Antibiotic Timing[1,3]	4	75%	73%	80%	93%
Oxygenation Assessment[1,3]	8	100%	100%	99%	100%
Pneumococcal Vaccine[1,3]	3	100%	64%	69%	94%
Smoking Cessation Advice[1,3]	3	33%	69%	80%	100%
Surgical Infection Prevention					
Prophylactic Antibiotic Given[5]	-	-	74%	77%	95%
Prophylactic Antibiotic Selection[5]	-	-	88%	90%	100%
Prophylactic Antibiotic Stopped[5]	-	-	68%	72%	95%
Pregnancy Care					
Inpatient Neonatal Mortality	-	-	-	-	-
Third or Fourth Degree Laceration	-	-	3.70%	3.63%	3.27%

Western Arizona Regional Medical Center

Alternate Name: Bullhead Community Hospital
2735 Silver Creek Road Phone: 928-763-2273
Bullhead City, AZ 86442 Fax: 928-704-6734
URL: www.warmc.com
Ownership: Proprietary Accredited: Yes
Emergency Services: Yes Licensed Beds: 123

Key Personnel:

CEO . . . . . Lee Christenson
Director Medical/Surgical Nursing . . . . . Dona Osborn
Director Respiratory Therapy . . . . . Jim Berryman

Measure	Cases	This Hospital	State Average	U.S. Average	Top Hospital
Heart Attack Care					
ACE Inhibitor or ARB for LVSD[1]	21	95%	83%	82%	100%
Aspirin at Arrival	140	98%	96%	92%	100%
Aspirin at Discharge	144	99%	91%	90%	100%
Beta Blocker at Arrival	112	98%	88%	87%	100%
Beta Blocker at Discharge	139	98%	93%	90%	100%
Fibrinolytic Medication Timing[1]	19	26%	10%	31%	100%
PCI Within 90 Minutes of Arrival[1]	2	50%	47%	54%	95%
Smoking Cessation Advice	72	100%	89%	88%	100%
Heart Failure Care					
ACE Inhibitor or ARB for LVSD	123	80%	81%	82%	100%
Discharge Instructions	276	67%	48%	61%	93%
Evaluation of LVS Function	302	94%	84%	83%	99%
Smoking Cessation Advice	94	94%	76%	82%	100%
Pneumonia Care					
Appropriate Initial Antibiotic[2]	119	76%	84%	83%	94%
Blood Culture Timing[2]	89	88%	87%	90%	100%
Influenza Vaccine[2]	26	65%	61%	70%	100%
Initial Antibiotic Timing[2]	142	85%	73%	80%	93%
Oxygenation Assessment[2]	162	100%	100%	99%	100%
Pneumococcal Vaccine[2]	80	66%	64%	69%	94%
Smoking Cessation Advice[2]	72	85%	69%	80%	100%
Surgical Infection Prevention					
Prophylactic Antibiotic Given[2,3]	317	44%	74%	77%	95%
Prophylactic Antibiotic Selection[2]	77	68%	88%	90%	100%
Prophylactic Antibiotic Stopped[2,3]	291	98%	68%	72%	95%
Pregnancy Care					
Inpatient Neonatal Mortality	-	-	-	-	-
Third or Fourth Degree Laceration	-	-	3.70%	3.63%	3.27%

Casa Grande Regional Medical Center

1800 E Florence Boulevard Phone: 520-381-6300
Casa Grande, AZ 85222 Fax: 520-381-6435
URL: www.casagrandehospital.com
Ownership: Voluntary non-profit - Other Accredited: Yes
Emergency Services: Yes Licensed Beds: 201

Key Personnel:

President/CEO . . . . . J Marty Dernier
CEO . . . . . Marty Dernier
Chief Medical Staff . . . . . Gilda Eakin
Emergency Room Director . . . . . Nancy Hicks-Arsenal
Director Infection/Disease Control . . . . . Mary Kay Johnson
Chief OB/GYN . . . . . Eleanor Clark, MD
Chief Radiology . . . . . John James, MD
Director Respiratory Therapy . . . . . Mark Nunley

NOTE: Hospital profiles are in alphabetical order by state, then city, then hospital within the city; Rankings are sorted by rate in descending order and exclude hospitals with less than 25 cases; (1) The number of cases is too small (n<25) for purposes of reliably predicting hospital performance; (2) Measure reflects the hospital's indication that its submission was based upon a sample of its relevant discharges; (3) Rate reflects fewer than the maximum possible quarters of data for the measure; (4) Inaccurate information submitted and suppressed for one or more quarters; (5) No data is available from the hospital for this measure; Please refer to the User's Guide for a full explanation of data

Measure	Cases	This Hospital	State Average	U.S. Average	Top Hospital
Heart Attack Care					
ACE Inhibitor or ARB for LVSD[1]	14	50%	83%	82%	100%
Aspirin at Arrival	80	94%	96%	92%	100%
Aspirin at Discharge	28	82%	91%	90%	100%
Beta Blocker at Arrival	67	84%	88%	87%	100%
Beta Blocker at Discharge	30	77%	93%	90%	100%
Fibrinolytic Medication Timing[1]	1	0%	10%	31%	100%
PCI Within 90 Minutes of Arrival	0	-	47%	54%	95%
Smoking Cessation Advice[1]	6	67%	89%	88%	100%
Heart Failure Care					
ACE Inhibitor or ARB for LVSD	54	63%	81%	82%	100%
Discharge Instructions	163	65%	48%	61%	93%
Evaluation of LVS Function	182	90%	84%	83%	99%
Smoking Cessation Advice	33	76%	76%	82%	100%
Pneumonia Care					
Appropriate Initial Antibiotic	334	84%	84%	83%	94%
Blood Culture Timing	187	95%	87%	90%	100%
Influenza Vaccine	112	29%	61%	70%	100%
Initial Antibiotic Timing	400	63%	73%	80%	93%
Oxygenation Assessment	449	100%	100%	99%	100%
Pneumococcal Vaccine	254	27%	64%	69%	94%
Smoking Cessation Advice	108	61%	69%	80%	100%
Surgical Infection Prevention					
Prophylactic Antibiotic Given[3]	224	79%	74%	77%	95%
Prophylactic Antibiotic Selection	73	88%	88%	90%	100%
Prophylactic Antibiotic Stopped[3]	220	71%	68%	72%	95%
Pregnancy Care					
Inpatient Neonatal Mortality	-	-	-	-	-
Third or Fourth Degree Laceration	-	-	3.70%	3.63%	3.27%

Arizona Orthopedic Surgical Hospital

2905 West Warne Road
Chandler, AZ 85225
Phone: 480-603-9000
Ownership: Proprietary
Accredited: No
Emergency Services: No

Measure	Cases	This Hospital	State Average	U.S. Average	Top Hospital
Heart Attack Care					
ACE Inhibitor or ARB for LVSD[5]	-	-	83%	82%	100%
Aspirin at Arrival[5]	-	-	96%	92%	100%
Aspirin at Discharge[5]	-	-	91%	90%	100%
Beta Blocker at Arrival[5]	-	-	88%	87%	100%
Beta Blocker at Discharge[5]	-	-	93%	90%	100%
Fibrinolytic Medication Timing[5]	-	-	10%	31%	100%
PCI Within 90 Minutes of Arrival[5]	-	-	47%	54%	95%
Smoking Cessation Advice[5]	-	-	89%	88%	100%
Heart Failure Care					
ACE Inhibitor or ARB for LVSD[5]	-	-	81%	82%	100%
Discharge Instructions[5]	-	-	48%	61%	93%
Evaluation of LVS Function[5]	-	-	84%	83%	99%
Smoking Cessation Advice[5]	-	-	76%	82%	100%
Pneumonia Care					
Appropriate Initial Antibiotic[5]	-	-	84%	83%	94%
Blood Culture Timing[5]	-	-	87%	90%	100%
Influenza Vaccine[5]	-	-	61%	70%	100%
Initial Antibiotic Timing[5]	-	-	73%	80%	93%
Oxygenation Assessment[5]	-	-	100%	99%	100%
Pneumococcal Vaccine[5]	-	-	64%	69%	94%
Smoking Cessation Advice[5]	-	-	69%	80%	100%
Surgical Infection Prevention					
Prophylactic Antibiotic Given[2,3]	25	52%	74%	77%	95%
Prophylactic Antibiotic Selection[5]	-	-	88%	90%	100%
Prophylactic Antibiotic Stopped[2,3]	25	64%	68%	72%	95%
Pregnancy Care					
Inpatient Neonatal Mortality	-	-	-	-	-
Third or Fourth Degree Laceration	-	-	3.70%	3.63%	3.27%

Chandler Regional Hospital

475 S Dobson Road
Phone: 480-728-3000
Chandler, AZ 85224
Fax: 480-899-5548
URL: www.chandlerregional.com
Ownership: Voluntary non-profit - Other
Accredited: Yes
Emergency Services: Yes
Licensed Beds: 210

Key Personnel:

President/CEO. . . . . David G Covert
Chief Medical Staff. . . . . Dr. Terry Happle
Emergency Room . . . . Timothy Johns, MD
ICU . . . . Nancy Wood, RN
Intensive/Coronary Care . . . . Nancy Wood, RN
OB/GYN Womens Health. . . . . Steven Eddy, DO
Respiratory/Cardiopulmonary. . . . . Ghaleb Okla

Measure	Cases	This Hospital	State Average	U.S. Average	Top Hospital
Heart Attack Care					
ACE Inhibitor or ARB for LVSD	73	88%	83%	82%	100%
Aspirin at Arrival	313	97%	96%	92%	100%
Aspirin at Discharge	306	98%	91%	90%	100%
Beta Blocker at Arrival	190	97%	88%	87%	100%
Beta Blocker at Discharge	263	96%	93%	90%	100%
Fibrinolytic Medication Timing	0	-	10%	31%	100%
PCI Within 90 Minutes of Arrival[1]	17	41%	47%	54%	95%
Smoking Cessation Advice	106	100%	89%	88%	100%
Heart Failure Care					
ACE Inhibitor or ARB for LVSD	130	80%	81%	82%	100%
Discharge Instructions	298	67%	48%	61%	93%
Evaluation of LVS Function	361	95%	84%	83%	99%
Smoking Cessation Advice	55	100%	76%	82%	100%
Pneumonia Care					
Appropriate Initial Antibiotic	356	91%	84%	83%	94%
Blood Culture Timing	298	87%	87%	90%	100%
Influenza Vaccine[4,5]	-	-	61%	70%	100%
Initial Antibiotic Timing	418	78%	73%	80%	93%
Oxygenation Assessment	549	100%	100%	99%	100%
Pneumococcal Vaccine	310	82%	64%	69%	94%
Smoking Cessation Advice	89	94%	69%	80%	100%
Surgical Infection Prevention					
Prophylactic Antibiotic Given[2,3]	208	94%	74%	77%	95%
Prophylactic Antibiotic Selection[2]	68	96%	88%	90%	100%
Prophylactic Antibiotic Stopped[2,3]	194	59%	68%	72%	95%
Pregnancy Care					
Inpatient Neonatal Mortality	5,238	0.11%	-	-	-
Third or Fourth Degree Laceration	3,434	3.93%	3.70%	3.63%	3.27%

Chinle Comprehensive Health Care Facility

Alternate Name: PHS Indian Hospital
N US Highway 191
Phone: 928-674-7001
PO Box PH
Fax: 928-674-7372
Chinle, AZ 86503
Ownership: Government - Federal
Accredited: Yes
Emergency Services: Yes
Licensed Beds: 60

Key Personnel:

CEO. . . . . Ronald Tso
Chief Medical Director . . . . Christian Thompson
Emergency Room . . . . Deborah Levitt, MD
OB/GYN Womens Health. . . . . Jean Howe, MD
Chief Radiology . . . . Don Yellow
Director Respiratory Therapy . . . . Sean M Ward

Measure	Cases	This Hospital	State Average	U.S. Average	Top Hospital
Heart Attack Care					
ACE Inhibitor or ARB for LVSD[1,3]	1	100%	83%	82%	100%
Aspirin at Arrival[1,3]	2	100%	96%	92%	100%
Aspirin at Discharge[1,3]	3	100%	91%	90%	100%
Beta Blocker at Arrival[1,3]	1	100%	88%	87%	100%
Beta Blocker at Discharge[1,3]	3	100%	93%	90%	100%
Fibrinolytic Medication Timing[3]	0	-	10%	31%	100%
PCI Within 90 Minutes of Arrival	0	-	47%	54%	95%
Smoking Cessation Advice[3]	0	-	89%	88%	100%
Heart Failure Care					
ACE Inhibitor or ARB for LVSD[1,3]	11	82%	81%	82%	100%

NOTE: Hospital profiles are in alphabetical order by state, then city, then hospital within the city; Rankings are sorted by rate in descending order and exclude hospitals with less than 25 cases; (1) The number of cases is too small (n<25) for purposes of reliably predicting hospital performance; (2) Measure reflects the hospital's indication that its submission was based upon a sample of its relevant discharges; (3) Rate reflects fewer than the maximum possible quarters of data for the measure; (4) Inaccurate information submitted and suppressed for one or more quarters; (5) No data is available from the hospital for this measure; Please refer to the User's Guide for a full explanation of data

Measure	Cases	This Hospital	State Average	U.S. Average	Top Hospital
Discharge Instructions[3]	33	42%	48%	61%	93%
Evaluation of LVS Function[3]	37	51%	84%	83%	99%
Smoking Cessation Advice[3]	0	-	76%	82%	100%
Pneumonia Care					
Appropriate Initial Antibiotic[3]	34	76%	84%	83%	94%
Blood Culture Timing[1]	12	75%	87%	90%	100%
Influenza Vaccine[1]	14	14%	61%	70%	100%
Initial Antibiotic Timing[3]	43	72%	73%	80%	93%
Oxygenation Assessment[3]	47	100%	100%	99%	100%
Pneumococcal Vaccine[3]	47	21%	64%	69%	94%
Smoking Cessation Advice[1,3]	1	0%	69%	80%	100%
Surgical Infection Prevention					
Prophylactic Antibiotic Given[3]	0	-	74%	77%	95%
Prophylactic Antibiotic Selection	0	-	88%	90%	100%
Prophylactic Antibiotic Stopped[3]	0	-	68%	72%	95%
Pregnancy Care					
Inpatient Neonatal Mortality	-	-	-	-	-
Third or Fourth Degree Laceration	-	-	3.70%	3.63%	3.27%

Verde Valley Medical Center

Alternate Name: Marcus J Lawrence Medical Center
269 S Candy Lane Phone: 928-634-2251
Cottonwood, AZ 86326 Fax: 928-639-6070
URL: www.nahealth.com/pp_vvmc/vvmc_about.htm
Ownership: Government - Federal Accredited: No
Emergency Services: Yes Licensed Beds: 110

Key Personnel:

CEO. . . . . Craig Owens
Director Medical/Surgical Nursing . . . . Mary Jewett
Director Respiratory Therapy . . . . Maggie Mansfield

Measure	Cases	This Hospital	State Average	U.S. Average	Top Hospital
Heart Attack Care					
ACE Inhibitor or ARB for LVSD	41	95%	83%	82%	100%
Aspirin at Arrival	133	99%	96%	92%	100%
Aspirin at Discharge	186	99%	91%	90%	100%
Beta Blocker at Arrival	113	99%	88%	87%	100%
Beta Blocker at Discharge	167	96%	93%	90%	100%
Fibrinolytic Medication Timing	0	-	10%	31%	100%
PCI Within 90 Minutes of Arrival[1]	14	79%	47%	54%	95%
Smoking Cessation Advice	55	96%	89%	88%	100%
Heart Failure Care					
ACE Inhibitor or ARB for LVSD	34	79%	81%	82%	100%
Discharge Instructions	86	60%	48%	61%	93%
Evaluation of LVS Function	84	92%	84%	83%	99%
Smoking Cessation Advice[1]	19	89%	76%	82%	100%
Pneumonia Care					
Appropriate Initial Antibiotic	158	85%	84%	83%	94%
Blood Culture Timing	127	94%	87%	90%	100%
Influenza Vaccine	50	72%	61%	70%	100%
Initial Antibiotic Timing	183	89%	73%	80%	93%
Oxygenation Assessment	216	100%	100%	99%	100%
Pneumococcal Vaccine	164	88%	64%	69%	94%
Smoking Cessation Advice	51	86%	69%	80%	100%
Surgical Infection Prevention					
Prophylactic Antibiotic Given[3]	90	69%	74%	77%	95%
Prophylactic Antibiotic Selection	64	95%	88%	90%	100%
Prophylactic Antibiotic Stopped[3]	69	96%	68%	72%	95%
Pregnancy Care					
Inpatient Neonatal Mortality	-	-	-	-	-
Third or Fourth Degree Laceration	-	-	3.70%	3.63%	3.27%

Southeast Arizona Medical Center

2174 W Oak Ave Phone: 520-364-7931
Douglas, AZ 85607 Fax: 520-364-2551
URL: samcdouglas.org
Ownership: Voluntary non-profit - Private Accredited: Yes
Emergency Services: No Licensed Beds: 25

Key Personnel:

President/CEO. . . . . Michael Carter
Chief of Medical Staff. . . . . Rajesh Pillai, MD
Emergency Room . . . . Debbie Thornby
Infection Control. . . . . Ann Benson
Surgical Services . . . . Mike Morales
Respiratory/Cardiopulmonary. . . . . George Gomez

Measure	Cases	This Hospital	State Average	U.S. Average	Top Hospital
Heart Attack Care					
ACE Inhibitor or ARB for LVSD[3]	0	-	83%	82%	100%
Aspirin at Arrival[1,3]	1	100%	96%	92%	100%
Aspirin at Discharge[3]	0	-	91%	90%	100%
Beta Blocker at Arrival[1,3]	1	100%	88%	87%	100%
Beta Blocker at Discharge[3]	0	-	93%	90%	100%
Fibrinolytic Medication Timing[1,3]	2	0%	10%	31%	100%
PCI Within 90 Minutes of Arrival[5]	-	-	47%	54%	95%
Smoking Cessation Advice[3]	0	-	89%	88%	100%
Heart Failure Care					
ACE Inhibitor or ARB for LVSD[1,2,3]	2	100%	81%	82%	100%
Discharge Instructions[1,2,3]	10	30%	48%	61%	93%
Evaluation of LVS Function[1,2,3]	11	55%	84%	83%	99%
Smoking Cessation Advice[1,2,3]	3	100%	76%	82%	100%
Pneumonia Care					
Appropriate Initial Antibiotic[2]	41	73%	84%	83%	94%
Blood Culture Timing[1,2]	6	100%	87%	90%	100%
Influenza Vaccine[1]	6	83%	61%	70%	100%
Initial Antibiotic Timing[2]	37	78%	73%	80%	93%
Oxygenation Assessment[2]	47	96%	100%	99%	100%
Pneumococcal Vaccine[2]	31	74%	64%	69%	94%
Smoking Cessation Advice[1,2]	9	56%	69%	80%	100%
Surgical Infection Prevention					
Prophylactic Antibiotic Given[5]	-	-	74%	77%	95%
Prophylactic Antibiotic Selection[5]	-	-	88%	90%	100%
Prophylactic Antibiotic Stopped[5]	-	-	68%	72%	95%
Pregnancy Care					
Inpatient Neonatal Mortality	-	-	-	-	-
Third or Fourth Degree Laceration	-	-	3.70%	3.63%	3.27%

Flagstaff Medical Center

1200 North Beaver Street Phone: 928-779-3366
Flagstaff, AZ 86001 Fax: 928-773-2579
URL: www.nahealth.com
Ownership: Proprietary Accredited: Yes
Emergency Services: Yes Licensed Beds: 238

Key Personnel:

CEO. . . . . Stephen G Carlson
Chief Medical Staff. . . . . Thomas Gaughan, MD
Emergency Room Director. . . . . Sheila' O Connor
Director Medical/Surgical Nursing . . . . Randy McKusick

Measure	Cases	This Hospital	State Average	U.S. Average	Top Hospital
Heart Attack Care					
ACE Inhibitor or ARB for LVSD	29	79%	83%	82%	100%
Aspirin at Arrival	96	98%	96%	92%	100%
Aspirin at Discharge	127	97%	91%	90%	100%
Beta Blocker at Arrival	76	91%	88%	87%	100%
Beta Blocker at Discharge	109	93%	93%	90%	100%
Fibrinolytic Medication Timing	0	-	10%	31%	100%
PCI Within 90 Minutes of Arrival[1]	9	33%	47%	54%	95%
Smoking Cessation Advice	37	97%	89%	88%	100%
Heart Failure Care					
ACE Inhibitor or ARB for LVSD	38	97%	81%	82%	100%
Discharge Instructions	111	85%	48%	61%	93%
Evaluation of LVS Function	130	91%	84%	83%	99%
Smoking Cessation Advice[1]	22	86%	76%	82%	100%
Pneumonia Care					
Appropriate Initial Antibiotic	151	89%	84%	83%	94%
Blood Culture Timing	105	95%	87%	90%	100%
Influenza Vaccine	43	56%	61%	70%	100%
Initial Antibiotic Timing	172	70%	73%	80%	93%
Oxygenation Assessment	217	100%	100%	99%	100%
Pneumococcal Vaccine	115	58%	64%	69%	94%
Smoking Cessation Advice	45	76%	69%	80%	100%
Surgical Infection Prevention					
Prophylactic Antibiotic Given[2,3]	222	89%	74%	77%	95%
Prophylactic Antibiotic Selection[2]	76	92%	88%	90%	100%

NOTE: Hospital profiles are in alphabetical order by state, then city, then hospital within the city; Rankings are sorted by rate in descending order and exclude hospitals with less than 25 cases; (1) The number of cases is too small (n<25) for purposes of reliably predicting hospital performance; (2) Measure reflects the hospital's indication that its submission was based upon a sample of its relevant discharges; (3) Rate reflects fewer than the maximum possible quarters of data for the measure; (4) Inaccurate information submitted and suppressed for one or more quarters; (5) No data is available from the hospital for this measure; Please refer to the User's Guide for a full explanation of data

Prophylactic Antibiotic Stopped[2,3]	213	61%	68%	72%	95%
Pregnancy Care					
Inpatient Neonatal Mortality	-	-	-	-	-
Third or Fourth Degree Laceration	-	-	3.70%	3.63%	3.27%

Fort Defiance Indian Hospital

Alternate Name: PHS Indian Hospital
PO Box 649 — Phone: 928-729-3356
Fort Defiance, AZ 86504 — Fax: 928-871-7850
E-mail: cecelia.yazzie@fdih.his.gov
URL: www.home.navajo.his.gov
Ownership: Government - Federal — Accredited: No
Emergency Services: Yes — Licensed Beds: 76

Key Personnel:
CEO. . . . . Franklin R Freeland
Director Cardiology . . . . . David Downing
Emergency Room . . . . . Cathey Arviso
Emergency Room . . . . . Sherry Killingsworth, RN
OB/GYN Womens Health. . . . . W Perry Killam, MD
Chief Radiology . . . . . Virginia Barker
Director Respiratory Therapy . . . . . Yvette Cayeito

Measure	Cases	This Hospital	State Average	U.S. Average	Top Hospital
Heart Attack Care					
ACE Inhibitor or ARB for LVSD[3]	0	-	83%	82%	100%
Aspirin at Arrival[1,3]	1	100%	96%	92%	100%
Aspirin at Discharge[1,3]	1	100%	91%	90%	100%
Beta Blocker at Arrival[1,3]	1	100%	88%	87%	100%
Beta Blocker at Discharge[1,3]	1	100%	93%	90%	100%
Fibrinolytic Medication Timing[3]	0	-	10%	31%	100%
PCI Within 90 Minutes of Arrival	0	-	47%	54%	95%
Smoking Cessation Advice[3]	0	-	89%	88%	100%
Heart Failure Care					
ACE Inhibitor or ARB for LVSD[1]	3	100%	81%	82%	100%
Discharge Instructions[1]	10	10%	48%	61%	93%
Evaluation of LVS Function[1]	10	60%	84%	83%	99%
Smoking Cessation Advice	0	-	76%	82%	100%
Pneumonia Care					
Appropriate Initial Antibiotic	39	97%	84%	83%	94%
Blood Culture Timing[1]	22	82%	87%	90%	100%
Influenza Vaccine[1]	8	50%	61%	70%	100%
Initial Antibiotic Timing	42	95%	73%	80%	93%
Oxygenation Assessment	45	100%	100%	99%	100%
Pneumococcal Vaccine	29	83%	64%	69%	94%
Smoking Cessation Advice[1]	3	0%	69%	80%	100%
Surgical Infection Prevention					
Prophylactic Antibiotic Given[5]	-	-	74%	77%	95%
Prophylactic Antibiotic Selection[5]	-	-	88%	90%	100%
Prophylactic Antibiotic Stopped[5]	-	-	68%	72%	95%
Pregnancy Care					
Inpatient Neonatal Mortality	-	-	-	-	-
Third or Fourth Degree Laceration	-	-	3.70%	3.63%	3.27%

Valley View Medical Center

5330 South Highway 95 — Phone: 928-788-2273
Fort Mohave, AZ 86426
Ownership: Proprietary — Accredited: No
Emergency Services: Yes

Measure	Cases	This Hospital	State Average	U.S. Average	Top Hospital
Heart Attack Care					
ACE Inhibitor or ARB for LVSD[3]	0	-	83%	82%	100%
Aspirin at Arrival[1,3]	7	100%	96%	92%	100%
Aspirin at Discharge[3]	0	-	91%	90%	100%
Beta Blocker at Arrival[1,3]	6	100%	88%	87%	100%
Beta Blocker at Discharge[3]	0	-	93%	90%	100%
Fibrinolytic Medication Timing[3]	0	-	10%	31%	100%
PCI Within 90 Minutes of Arrival	0	-	47%	54%	95%
Smoking Cessation Advice[3]	0	-	89%	88%	100%
Heart Failure Care					
ACE Inhibitor or ARB for LVSD[1,3]	12	75%	81%	82%	100%
Discharge Instructions[1,3]	15	53%	48%	61%	93%
Evaluation of LVS Function[3]	28	86%	84%	83%	99%
Smoking Cessation Advice[1,3]	5	80%	76%	82%	100%
Pneumonia Care					
Appropriate Initial Antibiotic[1,3]	8	62%	84%	83%	94%
Blood Culture Timing[1,3]	5	100%	87%	90%	100%
Influenza Vaccine[5]	-	-	61%	70%	100%
Initial Antibiotic Timing[3]	29	66%	73%	80%	93%
Oxygenation Assessment[3]	31	100%	100%	99%	100%
Pneumococcal Vaccine[1,3]	17	71%	64%	69%	94%
Smoking Cessation Advice[1,3]	5	60%	69%	80%	100%
Surgical Infection Prevention					
Prophylactic Antibiotic Given[3]	40	60%	74%	77%	95%
Prophylactic Antibiotic Selection[5]	-	-	88%	90%	100%
Prophylactic Antibiotic Stopped[3]	37	65%	68%	72%	95%
Pregnancy Care					
Inpatient Neonatal Mortality	-	-	-	-	-
Third or Fourth Degree Laceration	-	-	3.70%	3.63%	3.27%

Sage Memorial Hospital

Highway 264 & US 191 — Phone: 928-755-4500
PO Box 457 — Fax: 928-755-4659
Ganado, AZ 86505
URL: www.navajosage.org
Ownership: Voluntary non-profit - Private — Accredited: Yes
Emergency Services: Yes — Licensed Beds: 45

Key Personnel:
CEO. . . . . Taylor McKenzie
Chief of Medical Staff. . . . . Mohammed Illias
Emergency Room . . . . . Wanda Begay
Supervisor of Respiratory Therapy. . . . . Hector Bermudas

Measure	Cases	This Hospital	State Average	U.S. Average	Top Hospital
Heart Attack Care					
ACE Inhibitor or ARB for LVSD[5]	-	-	83%	82%	100%
Aspirin at Arrival[5]	-	-	96%	92%	100%
Aspirin at Discharge[5]	-	-	91%	90%	100%
Beta Blocker at Arrival[5]	-	-	88%	87%	100%
Beta Blocker at Discharge[5]	-	-	93%	90%	100%
Fibrinolytic Medication Timing[5]	-	-	10%	31%	100%
PCI Within 90 Minutes of Arrival[5]	-	-	47%	54%	95%
Smoking Cessation Advice[5]	-	-	89%	88%	100%
Heart Failure Care					
ACE Inhibitor or ARB for LVSD[3]	0	-	81%	82%	100%
Discharge Instructions[1,3]	8	0%	48%	61%	93%
Evaluation of LVS Function[1,3]	9	33%	84%	83%	99%
Smoking Cessation Advice[3]	0	-	76%	82%	100%
Pneumonia Care					
Appropriate Initial Antibiotic[3]	33	33%	84%	83%	94%
Blood Culture Timing[1,3]	13	92%	87%	90%	100%
Influenza Vaccine[1]	19	53%	61%	70%	100%
Initial Antibiotic Timing[3]	36	58%	73%	80%	93%
Oxygenation Assessment[3]	47	98%	100%	99%	100%
Pneumococcal Vaccine[3]	40	40%	64%	69%	94%
Smoking Cessation Advice[1,3]	2	0%	69%	80%	100%
Surgical Infection Prevention					
Prophylactic Antibiotic Given[5]	-	-	74%	77%	95%
Prophylactic Antibiotic Selection[5]	-	-	88%	90%	100%
Prophylactic Antibiotic Stopped[5]	-	-	68%	72%	95%
Pregnancy Care					
Inpatient Neonatal Mortality	-	-	-	-	-
Third or Fourth Degree Laceration	-	-	3.70%	3.63%	3.27%

Mercy Gilbert Medical Center

3555 S Val Vista Drive — Phone: 480-728-8327
Gilbert, AZ 85296
Ownership: Voluntary non-profit - Church — Accredited: Yes
Emergency Services: Yes

Measure	Cases	This Hospital	State Average	U.S. Average	Top Hospital
Heart Attack Care					
ACE Inhibitor or ARB for LVSD[5]	-	-	83%	82%	100%
Aspirin at Arrival[5]	-	-	96%	92%	100%

NOTE: Hospital profiles are in alphabetical order by state, then city, then hospital within the city; Rankings are sorted by rate in descending order and exclude hospitals with less than 25 cases; (1) The number of cases is too small (n<25) for purposes of reliably predicting hospital performance; (2) Measure reflects the hospital's indication that its submission was based upon a sample of its relevant discharges; (3) Rate reflects fewer than the maximum possible quarters of data for the measure; (4) Inaccurate information submitted and suppressed for one or more quarters; (5) No data is available from the hospital for this measure; Please refer to the User's Guide for a full explanation of data

Measure	Cases	This Hospital	State Average	U.S. Average	Top Hospital
Aspirin at Discharge[5]	-	-	91%	90%	100%
Beta Blocker at Arrival[5]	-	-	88%	87%	100%
Beta Blocker at Discharge[5]	-	-	93%	90%	100%
Fibrinolytic Medication Timing[5]	-	-	10%	31%	100%
PCI Within 90 Minutes of Arrival[5]	-	-	47%	54%	95%
Smoking Cessation Advice[5]	-	-	89%	88%	100%
Heart Failure Care					
ACE Inhibitor or ARB for LVSD[5]	-	-	81%	82%	100%
Discharge Instructions[5]	-	-	48%	61%	93%
Evaluation of LVS Function[5]	-	-	84%	83%	99%
Smoking Cessation Advice[5]	-	-	76%	82%	100%
Pneumonia Care					
Appropriate Initial Antibiotic[5]	-	-	84%	83%	94%
Blood Culture Timing[5]	-	-	87%	90%	100%
Influenza Vaccine[5]	-	-	61%	70%	100%
Initial Antibiotic Timing[5]	-	-	73%	80%	93%
Oxygenation Assessment[5]	-	-	100%	99%	100%
Pneumococcal Vaccine[5]	-	-	64%	69%	94%
Smoking Cessation Advice[5]	-	-	69%	80%	100%
Surgical Infection Prevention					
Prophylactic Antibiotic Given[5]	-	-	74%	77%	95%
Prophylactic Antibiotic Selection[5]	-	-	88%	90%	100%
Prophylactic Antibiotic Stopped[5]	-	-	68%	72%	95%
Pregnancy Care					
Inpatient Neonatal Mortality[5]	0	0.00%	-	-	-
Third or Fourth Degree Laceration[5]	0	0.00%	3.70%	3.63%	3.27%

Arrowhead Community Hospital

18701 N 67th Avenue
Glendale, AZ 85308
Phone: 623-561-1000
Fax: 623-561-7142
URL: www.arrowheadhospital.com
Ownership: Proprietary
Emergency Services: Yes
Accredited: Yes
Licensed Beds: 115

Measure	Cases	This Hospital	State Average	U.S. Average	Top Hospital
Heart Attack Care					
ACE Inhibitor or ARB for LVSD[1]	14	100%	83%	82%	100%
Aspirin at Arrival	101	97%	96%	92%	100%
Aspirin at Discharge	78	99%	91%	90%	100%
Beta Blocker at Arrival	81	96%	88%	87%	100%
Beta Blocker at Discharge	82	100%	93%	90%	100%
Fibrinolytic Medication Timing	0	-	10%	31%	100%
PCI Within 90 Minutes of Arrival[1]	3	67%	47%	54%	95%
Smoking Cessation Advice[1]	22	100%	89%	88%	100%
Heart Failure Care					
ACE Inhibitor or ARB for LVSD	51	98%	81%	82%	100%
Discharge Instructions	101	83%	48%	61%	93%
Evaluation of LVS Function	124	97%	84%	83%	99%
Smoking Cessation Advice[1]	20	90%	76%	82%	100%
Pneumonia Care					
Appropriate Initial Antibiotic	312	88%	84%	83%	94%
Blood Culture Timing	170	85%	87%	90%	100%
Influenza Vaccine	80	46%	61%	70%	100%
Initial Antibiotic Timing	342	81%	73%	80%	93%
Oxygenation Assessment	382	100%	100%	99%	100%
Pneumococcal Vaccine	210	79%	64%	69%	94%
Smoking Cessation Advice	86	97%	69%	80%	100%
Surgical Infection Prevention					
Prophylactic Antibiotic Given[3]	485	77%	74%	77%	95%
Prophylactic Antibiotic Selection	155	94%	88%	90%	100%
Prophylactic Antibiotic Stopped[3]	496	73%	68%	72%	95%
Pregnancy Care					
Inpatient Neonatal Mortality	-	-	-	-	-
Third or Fourth Degree Laceration	-	-	3.70%	3.63%	3.27%

Banner Thunderbird Medical Center

5555 W Thunderbird Road
Glendale, AZ 85306
Phone: 602-865-5555
Fax: 602-865-5930
URL: www.bannerhealth.com
Ownership: Govt - Hospital District or Authority
Emergency Services: Yes
Accredited: Yes
Licensed Beds: 397

Key Personnel:

CEO. . . . . Tom Dickinson, FACHE
CEO. . . . . Vicki Noyes, MBA
Chief Medical Officer . . . . Ted Laughlin
Emergency Room . . . . Linda Lindquist
Director of Pulmonary/Respiratory Care. . . . . . . Cathy Garcia

Measure	Cases	This Hospital	State Average	U.S. Average	Top Hospital
Heart Attack Care					
ACE Inhibitor or ARB for LVSD[2]	63	81%	83%	82%	100%
Aspirin at Arrival[2]	260	94%	96%	92%	100%
Aspirin at Discharge[2]	245	95%	91%	90%	100%
Beta Blocker at Arrival[2]	238	81%	88%	87%	100%
Beta Blocker at Discharge[2]	253	96%	93%	90%	100%
Fibrinolytic Medication Timing[2]	0	-	10%	31%	100%
PCI Within 90 Minutes of Arrival[1,2]	8	50%	47%	54%	95%
Smoking Cessation Advice[2]	81	90%	89%	88%	100%
Heart Failure Care					
ACE Inhibitor or ARB for LVSD[2]	148	78%	81%	82%	100%
Discharge Instructions[2]	241	49%	48%	61%	93%
Evaluation of LVS Function[2]	292	96%	84%	83%	99%
Smoking Cessation Advice[2]	68	63%	76%	82%	100%
Pneumonia Care					
Appropriate Initial Antibiotic[2]	101	89%	84%	83%	94%
Blood Culture Timing[2]	96	91%	87%	90%	100%
Influenza Vaccine	25	40%	61%	70%	100%
Initial Antibiotic Timing[2]	130	57%	73%	80%	93%
Oxygenation Assessment[2]	181	100%	100%	99%	100%
Pneumococcal Vaccine[2]	98	39%	64%	69%	94%
Smoking Cessation Advice[2]	54	57%	69%	80%	100%
Surgical Infection Prevention					
Prophylactic Antibiotic Given[3]	201	73%	74%	77%	95%
Prophylactic Antibiotic Selection	76	80%	88%	90%	100%
Prophylactic Antibiotic Stopped[3]	186	63%	68%	72%	95%
Pregnancy Care					
Inpatient Neonatal Mortality	-	-	-	-	-
Third or Fourth Degree Laceration	-	-	3.70%	3.63%	3.27%

West Valley Hospital

13677 W McDowell Road
Goodyear, AZ 85338
Phone: 623-882-1500
Fax: 623-848-5959
URL: www.wvhospital.com
Ownership: Government - State
Emergency Services: Yes
Accredited: Yes
Licensed Beds: 74

Key Personnel:

CEO. . . . . Jim Resendez

Measure	Cases	This Hospital	State Average	U.S. Average	Top Hospital
Heart Attack Care					
ACE Inhibitor or ARB for LVSD	27	81%	83%	82%	100%
Aspirin at Arrival	132	98%	96%	92%	100%
Aspirin at Discharge	126	95%	91%	90%	100%
Beta Blocker at Arrival	116	95%	88%	87%	100%
Beta Blocker at Discharge	119	95%	93%	90%	100%
Fibrinolytic Medication Timing	0	-	10%	31%	100%
PCI Within 90 Minutes of Arrival[1]	10	10%	47%	54%	95%
Smoking Cessation Advice	50	86%	89%	88%	100%
Heart Failure Care					
ACE Inhibitor or ARB for LVSD	57	88%	81%	82%	100%
Discharge Instructions	157	60%	48%	61%	93%
Evaluation of LVS Function	174	90%	84%	83%	99%
Smoking Cessation Advice	32	91%	76%	82%	100%
Pneumonia Care					
Appropriate Initial Antibiotic	159	82%	84%	83%	94%
Blood Culture Timing	90	76%	87%	90%	100%
Influenza Vaccine	36	58%	61%	70%	100%
Initial Antibiotic Timing	168	75%	73%	80%	93%

NOTE: Hospital profiles are in alphabetical order by state, then city, then hospital within the city; Rankings are sorted by rate in descending order and exclude hospitals with less than 25 cases; (1) The number of cases is too small (n<25) for purposes of reliably predicting hospital performance; (2) Measure reflects the hospital's indication that its submission was based upon a sample of its relevant discharges; (3) Rate reflects fewer than the maximum possible quarters of data for the measure; (4) Inaccurate information submitted and suppressed for one or more quarters; (5) No data is available from the hospital for this measure; Please refer to the User's Guide for a full explanation of data

Oxygenation Assessment	198	100%	100%	99%	100%
Pneumococcal Vaccine	86	44%	64%	69%	94%
Smoking Cessation Advice	52	77%	69%	80%	100%
Surgical Infection Prevention					
Prophylactic Antibiotic Given[3]	287	69%	74%	77%	95%
Prophylactic Antibiotic Selection	98	97%	88%	90%	100%
Prophylactic Antibiotic Stopped[3]	268	66%	68%	72%	95%
Pregnancy Care					
Inpatient Neonatal Mortality	-	-	-	-	-
Third or Fourth Degree Laceration	-	-	3.70%	3.63%	3.27%

Gilbert Hospital

5656 South Power Road
Higley, AZ 85236
Phone: 480-279-5835
Ownership: Proprietary
Accredited: No
Emergency Services: Yes

Measure	Cases	This Hospital	State Average	U.S. Average	Top Hospital
Heart Attack Care					
ACE Inhibitor or ARB for LVSD[5]	-	-	83%	82%	100%
Aspirin at Arrival[5]	-	-	96%	92%	100%
Aspirin at Discharge[5]	-	-	91%	90%	100%
Beta Blocker at Arrival[5]	-	-	88%	87%	100%
Beta Blocker at Discharge[5]	-	-	93%	90%	100%
Fibrinolytic Medication Timing[5]	-	-	10%	31%	100%
PCI Within 90 Minutes of Arrival[5]	-	-	47%	54%	95%
Smoking Cessation Advice[5]	-	-	89%	88%	100%
Heart Failure Care					
ACE Inhibitor or ARB for LVSD[5]	-	-	81%	82%	100%
Discharge Instructions[5]	-	-	48%	61%	93%
Evaluation of LVS Function[5]	-	-	84%	83%	99%
Smoking Cessation Advice[5]	-	-	76%	82%	100%
Pneumonia Care					
Appropriate Initial Antibiotic[5]	-	-	84%	83%	94%
Blood Culture Timing[5]	-	-	87%	90%	100%
Influenza Vaccine[5]	-	-	61%	70%	100%
Initial Antibiotic Timing[5]	-	-	73%	80%	93%
Oxygenation Assessment[5]	-	-	100%	99%	100%
Pneumococcal Vaccine[5]	-	-	64%	69%	94%
Smoking Cessation Advice[5]	-	-	69%	80%	100%
Surgical Infection Prevention					
Prophylactic Antibiotic Given[5]	-	-	74%	77%	95%
Prophylactic Antibiotic Selection[5]	-	-	88%	90%	100%
Prophylactic Antibiotic Stopped[5]	-	-	68%	72%	95%
Pregnancy Care					
Inpatient Neonatal Mortality	-	-	-	-	-
Third or Fourth Degree Laceration	-	-	3.70%	3.63%	3.27%

Kingman Regional Medical Center

3269 Stockton Hill Road
Kingman, AZ 86409
Toll-Free: 877-757-2101
Phone: 928-757-2101
Fax: 928-692-4110
URL: www.azkrmc.com
Ownership: Govt - Hospital District or Authority
Accredited: Yes
Emergency Services: Yes
Licensed Beds: 124

Key Personnel:

CEO. . . . . Brian Turney
Chief Medical Staff. . . . . SI Bokhari
Emergency Room . . . . Janet Godi
OB/GYN Womens Health. . . . . Joseph Tedesco, DO
Chief Radiology . . . . Mansour Tafazol, MD
Director Respiratory Therapy . . . . Fred Knarr

Measure	Cases	This Hospital	State Average	U.S. Average	Top Hospital
Heart Attack Care					
ACE Inhibitor or ARB for LVSD[1]	22	73%	83%	82%	100%
Aspirin at Arrival	168	88%	96%	92%	100%
Aspirin at Discharge	144	82%	91%	90%	100%
Beta Blocker at Arrival	152	82%	88%	87%	100%
Beta Blocker at Discharge	147	86%	93%	90%	100%
Fibrinolytic Medication Timing	0	-	10%	31%	100%
PCI Within 90 Minutes of Arrival[1]	7	14%	47%	54%	95%
Smoking Cessation Advice	69	88%	89%	88%	100%
Heart Failure Care					
ACE Inhibitor or ARB for LVSD[2]	104	81%	81%	82%	100%
Discharge Instructions[2]	260	41%	48%	61%	93%
Evaluation of LVS Function[2]	285	70%	84%	83%	99%
Smoking Cessation Advice[2]	81	67%	76%	82%	100%
Pneumonia Care					
Appropriate Initial Antibiotic[2]	167	90%	84%	83%	94%
Blood Culture Timing[2]	128	81%	87%	90%	100%
Influenza Vaccine[4,5]	-	-	61%	70%	100%
Initial Antibiotic Timing[2]	187	84%	73%	80%	93%
Oxygenation Assessment[2]	214	100%	100%	99%	100%
Pneumococcal Vaccine[2]	96	83%	64%	69%	94%
Smoking Cessation Advice[2]	86	66%	69%	80%	100%
Surgical Infection Prevention					
Prophylactic Antibiotic Given[2,3]	190	59%	74%	77%	95%
Prophylactic Antibiotic Selection[2]	46	91%	88%	90%	100%
Prophylactic Antibiotic Stopped[2,3]	183	48%	68%	72%	95%
Pregnancy Care					
Inpatient Neonatal Mortality	-	-	-	-	-
Third or Fourth Degree Laceration	-	-	3.70%	3.63%	3.27%

Havasu Regional Medical Center

Alternate Name: Havasu Samaritan Regional Hospital
101 Civic Center Lane
Lake Havasu City, AZ 86403
Phone: 928-855-8185
Fax: 928-505-5744
URL: www.havasuregional.com
Ownership: Proprietary
Accredited: Yes
Emergency Services: Yes
Licensed Beds: 138

Key Personnel:

CEO. . . . . Dorothy Sawyer
Chief of Medical Staff. . . . . Douglas Hade
Chief of Pulmonary Department. . . . . Paul Aiken

Measure	Cases	This Hospital	State Average	U.S. Average	Top Hospital
Heart Attack Care					
ACE Inhibitor or ARB for LVSD[1]	18	89%	83%	82%	100%
Aspirin at Arrival	119	85%	96%	92%	100%
Aspirin at Discharge	101	83%	91%	90%	100%
Beta Blocker at Arrival	113	78%	88%	87%	100%
Beta Blocker at Discharge	103	87%	93%	90%	100%
Fibrinolytic Medication Timing[1]	1	0%	10%	31%	100%
PCI Within 90 Minutes of Arrival[1]	4	50%	47%	54%	95%
Smoking Cessation Advice	27	74%	89%	88%	100%
Heart Failure Care					
ACE Inhibitor or ARB for LVSD	55	85%	81%	82%	100%
Discharge Instructions	125	58%	48%	61%	93%
Evaluation of LVS Function	139	80%	84%	83%	99%
Smoking Cessation Advice	39	82%	76%	82%	100%
Pneumonia Care					
Appropriate Initial Antibiotic	202	90%	84%	83%	94%
Blood Culture Timing	137	85%	87%	90%	100%
Influenza Vaccine	67	75%	61%	70%	100%
Initial Antibiotic Timing	250	50%	73%	80%	93%
Oxygenation Assessment	279	99%	100%	99%	100%
Pneumococcal Vaccine	199	69%	64%	69%	94%
Smoking Cessation Advice	64	77%	69%	80%	100%
Surgical Infection Prevention					
Prophylactic Antibiotic Given	464	50%	74%	77%	95%
Prophylactic Antibiotic Selection	103	78%	88%	90%	100%
Prophylactic Antibiotic Stopped	450	46%	68%	72%	95%
Pregnancy Care					
Inpatient Neonatal Mortality	-	-	-	-	-
Third or Fourth Degree Laceration	-	-	3.70%	3.63%	3.27%

Arizona Spine and Joint Hospital

4620 East Baseline Road
Mesa, AZ 85206
Phone: 480-832-4770
Ownership: Proprietary
Accredited: Yes
Emergency Services: No

Measure	Cases	This Hospital	State Average	U.S. Average	Top Hospital

NOTE: Hospital profiles are in alphabetical order by state, then city, then hospital within the city; Rankings are sorted by rate in descending order and exclude hospitals with less than 25 cases; (1) The number of cases is too small (n<25) for purposes of reliably predicting hospital performance; (2) Measure reflects the hospital's indication that its submission was based upon a sample of its relevant discharges; (3) Rate reflects fewer than the maximum possible quarters of data for the measure; (4) Inaccurate information submitted and suppressed for one or more quarters; (5) No data is available from the hospital for this measure; Please refer to the User's Guide for a full explanation of data

Measure	Cases	This Hospital	State Average	U.S. Average	Top Hospital
Heart Attack Care					
ACE Inhibitor or ARB for LVSD[5]	-	-	83%	82%	100%
Aspirin at Arrival[5]	-	-	96%	92%	100%
Aspirin at Discharge[5]	-	-	91%	90%	100%
Beta Blocker at Arrival[5]	-	-	88%	87%	100%
Beta Blocker at Discharge[5]	-	-	93%	90%	100%
Fibrinolytic Medication Timing[5]	-	-	10%	31%	100%
PCI Within 90 Minutes of Arrival[5]	-	-	47%	54%	95%
Smoking Cessation Advice[5]	-	-	89%	88%	100%
Heart Failure Care					
ACE Inhibitor or ARB for LVSD[5]	-	-	81%	82%	100%
Discharge Instructions[5]	-	-	48%	61%	93%
Evaluation of LVS Function[5]	-	-	84%	83%	99%
Smoking Cessation Advice[5]	-	-	76%	82%	100%
Pneumonia Care					
Appropriate Initial Antibiotic[5]	-	-	84%	83%	94%
Blood Culture Timing[5]	-	-	87%	90%	100%
Influenza Vaccine[5]	-	-	61%	70%	100%
Initial Antibiotic Timing[5]	-	-	73%	80%	93%
Oxygenation Assessment[5]	-	-	100%	99%	100%
Pneumococcal Vaccine[5]	-	-	64%	69%	94%
Smoking Cessation Advice[5]	-	-	69%	80%	100%
Surgical Infection Prevention					
Prophylactic Antibiotic Given[2,3]	71	94%	74%	77%	95%
Prophylactic Antibiotic Selection[2]	71	100%	88%	90%	100%
Prophylactic Antibiotic Stopped[2,3]	71	66%	68%	72%	95%
Pregnancy Care					
Inpatient Neonatal Mortality	-	-	-	-	-
Third or Fourth Degree Laceration	-	-	3.70%	3.63%	3.27%

Banner Baywood Heart Hospital

6750 East Baywood Avenue
Mesa, AZ 85206
Phone: 480-854-5050
Ownership: Government - Local
Accredited: Yes
Emergency Services: Yes

Measure	Cases	This Hospital	State Average	U.S. Average	Top Hospital
Heart Attack Care					
ACE Inhibitor or ARB for LVSD[2]	60	85%	83%	82%	100%
Aspirin at Arrival[1,2]	7	100%	96%	92%	100%
Aspirin at Discharge[2]	248	98%	91%	90%	100%
Beta Blocker at Arrival[1,2]	4	50%	88%	87%	100%
Beta Blocker at Discharge[2]	247	97%	93%	90%	100%
Fibrinolytic Medication Timing[2]	0	-	10%	31%	100%
PCI Within 90 Minutes of Arrival[2]	0	-	47%	54%	95%
Smoking Cessation Advice[2]	99	100%	89%	88%	100%
Heart Failure Care					
ACE Inhibitor or ARB for LVSD[2]	145	86%	81%	82%	100%
Discharge Instructions[2]	260	78%	48%	61%	93%
Evaluation of LVS Function[2]	283	99%	84%	83%	99%
Smoking Cessation Advice[2]	44	98%	76%	82%	100%
Pneumonia Care					
Appropriate Initial Antibiotic[1,2]	1	100%	84%	83%	94%
Blood Culture Timing[2]	0	-	87%	90%	100%
Influenza Vaccine[1]	14	57%	61%	70%	100%
Initial Antibiotic Timing[1,2]	1	0%	73%	80%	93%
Oxygenation Assessment[1,2]	2	100%	100%	99%	100%
Pneumococcal Vaccine[1,2]	20	60%	64%	69%	94%
Smoking Cessation Advice[1,2]	4	100%	69%	80%	100%
Surgical Infection Prevention					
Prophylactic Antibiotic Given[2,3]	182	84%	74%	77%	95%
Prophylactic Antibiotic Selection[2]	61	98%	88%	90%	100%
Prophylactic Antibiotic Stopped[2,3]	161	72%	68%	72%	95%
Pregnancy Care					
Inpatient Neonatal Mortality	-	-	-	-	-
Third or Fourth Degree Laceration	-	-	3.70%	3.63%	3.27%

Banner Baywood Medical Center

6644 E Baywood Avenue
Mesa, AZ 85206
Phone: 480-981-2000
Fax: 480-981-4198
URL: www.bannerhealth.com
Ownership: Govt - Hospital District or Authority
Accredited: Yes
Emergency Services: Yes
Licensed Beds: 239

Key Personnel:

CEO. . . . . Don Evans
Chief of Medical Staff . . . . Larry Stratling
Director Respiratory Therapy . . . . Bruce Lawrey

Measure	Cases	This Hospital	State Average	U.S. Average	Top Hospital
Heart Attack Care					
ACE Inhibitor or ARB for LVSD[1]	11	73%	83%	82%	100%
Aspirin at Arrival	51	76%	96%	92%	100%
Aspirin at Discharge	25	76%	91%	90%	100%
Beta Blocker at Arrival	43	72%	88%	87%	100%
Beta Blocker at Discharge	34	91%	93%	90%	100%
Fibrinolytic Medication Timing	0	-	10%	31%	100%
PCI Within 90 Minutes of Arrival	0	-	47%	54%	95%
Smoking Cessation Advice[1]	4	50%	89%	88%	100%
Heart Failure Care					
ACE Inhibitor or ARB for LVSD[2]	76	86%	81%	82%	100%
Discharge Instructions[2]	206	68%	48%	61%	93%
Evaluation of LVS Function[2]	264	93%	84%	83%	99%
Smoking Cessation Advice[1,2]	24	58%	76%	82%	100%
Pneumonia Care					
Appropriate Initial Antibiotic[2]	118	95%	84%	83%	94%
Blood Culture Timing[2]	82	88%	87%	90%	100%
Influenza Vaccine[1,2]	23	74%	61%	70%	100%
Initial Antibiotic Timing[2]	134	58%	73%	80%	93%
Oxygenation Assessment[2]	163	100%	100%	99%	100%
Pneumococcal Vaccine[2]	99	67%	64%	69%	94%
Smoking Cessation Advice[2]	30	60%	69%	80%	100%
Surgical Infection Prevention					
Prophylactic Antibiotic Given[2,3]	121	50%	74%	77%	95%
Prophylactic Antibiotic Selection[2]	39	82%	88%	90%	100%
Prophylactic Antibiotic Stopped[2,3]	109	49%	68%	72%	95%
Pregnancy Care					
Inpatient Neonatal Mortality	-	-	-	-	-
Third or Fourth Degree Laceration	-	-	3.70%	3.63%	3.27%

Banner Mesa Medical Center

1010 N Country Club Drive
Mesa, AZ 85201
Phone: 480-834-1211
Fax: 480-461-2939
URL: www.bannerhealth.com
Ownership: Govt - Hospital District or Authority
Accredited: Yes
Emergency Services: Yes

Key Personnel:

CEO. . . . . Becky Kuhn

Measure	Cases	This Hospital	State Average	U.S. Average	Top Hospital
Heart Attack Care					
ACE Inhibitor or ARB for LVSD[1]	2	50%	83%	82%	100%
Aspirin at Arrival[1]	20	95%	96%	92%	100%
Aspirin at Discharge[1]	5	80%	91%	90%	100%
Beta Blocker at Arrival[1]	20	80%	88%	87%	100%
Beta Blocker at Discharge[1]	6	100%	93%	90%	100%
Fibrinolytic Medication Timing	0	-	10%	31%	100%
PCI Within 90 Minutes of Arrival	0	-	47%	54%	95%
Smoking Cessation Advice	0	-	89%	88%	100%
Heart Failure Care					
ACE Inhibitor or ARB for LVSD	26	77%	81%	82%	100%
Discharge Instructions	83	67%	48%	61%	93%
Evaluation of LVS Function	105	90%	84%	83%	99%
Smoking Cessation Advice[1]	19	89%	76%	82%	100%
Pneumonia Care					
Appropriate Initial Antibiotic[2]	98	97%	84%	83%	94%
Blood Culture Timing[2]	89	87%	87%	90%	100%
Influenza Vaccine[1,2]	24	38%	61%	70%	100%
Initial Antibiotic Timing[2]	136	76%	73%	80%	93%
Oxygenation Assessment[2]	165	100%	100%	99%	100%

NOTE: Hospital profiles are in alphabetical order by state, then city, then hospital within the city; Rankings are sorted by rate in descending order and exclude hospitals with less than 25 cases; (1) The number of cases is too small (n<25) for purposes of reliably predicting hospital performance; (2) Measure reflects the hospital's indication that its submission was based upon a sample of its relevant discharges; (3) Rate reflects fewer than the maximum possible quarters of data for the measure; (4) Inaccurate information submitted and suppressed for one or more quarters; (5) No data is available from the hospital for this measure; Please refer to the User's Guide for a full explanation of data

Pneumococcal Vaccine[2]	81	59%	64%	69%	94%
Smoking Cessation Advice[2]	35	51%	69%	80%	100%
Surgical Infection Prevention					
Prophylactic Antibiotic Given[3]	151	83%	74%	77%	95%
Prophylactic Antibiotic Selection	150	94%	88%	90%	100%
Prophylactic Antibiotic Stopped[3]	146	69%	68%	72%	95%
Pregnancy Care					
Inpatient Neonatal Mortality	-	-	-	-	-
Third or Fourth Degree Laceration	-	-	3.70%	3.63%	3.27%

Desert Samaritan Medical Center

Alternate Name: Banner Desert Medical Center
1400 South Dobson Road — Phone: 480-512-2000
Mesa, AZ 85202 — Fax: 480-835-8711
URL: www.bannerhealth.com/channels
Ownership: Voluntary non-profit - Private — Accredited: Yes
Emergency Services: Yes — Licensed Beds: 414

Key Personnel:
Chief Medical Staff . . . . Joseph Gutman, MD
Director Infection/Disease Control . . . . Patt Madson
Chief Radiology . . . . M Kornreich, MD

Measure	Cases	This Hospital	State Average	U.S. Average	Top Hospital
Heart Attack Care					
ACE Inhibitor or ARB for LVSD[2]	62	85%	83%	82%	100%
Aspirin at Arrival[2]	227	96%	96%	92%	100%
Aspirin at Discharge[2]	221	96%	91%	90%	100%
Beta Blocker at Arrival[2]	146	88%	88%	87%	100%
Beta Blocker at Discharge[2]	237	97%	93%	90%	100%
Fibrinolytic Medication Timing[2]	0	-	10%	31%	100%
PCI Within 90 Minutes of Arrival[1,2]	15	60%	47%	54%	95%
Smoking Cessation Advice[2]	98	98%	89%	88%	100%
Heart Failure Care					
ACE Inhibitor or ARB for LVSD[2]	130	85%	81%	82%	100%
Discharge Instructions[2]	234	59%	48%	61%	93%
Evaluation of LVS Function[2]	273	92%	84%	83%	99%
Smoking Cessation Advice[2]	52	87%	76%	82%	100%
Pneumonia Care					
Appropriate Initial Antibiotic[2]	139	90%	84%	83%	94%
Blood Culture Timing[2]	119	96%	87%	90%	100%
Influenza Vaccine[1,2]	20	45%	61%	70%	100%
Initial Antibiotic Timing[2]	154	58%	73%	80%	93%
Oxygenation Assessment[2]	198	100%	100%	99%	100%
Pneumococcal Vaccine[2]	87	68%	64%	69%	94%
Smoking Cessation Advice[2]	56	71%	69%	80%	100%
Surgical Infection Prevention					
Prophylactic Antibiotic Given[3]	233	77%	74%	77%	95%
Prophylactic Antibiotic Selection	83	76%	88%	90%	100%
Prophylactic Antibiotic Stopped[3]	223	55%	68%	72%	95%
Pregnancy Care					
Inpatient Neonatal Mortality	9,031	0.56%	-	-	-
Third or Fourth Degree Laceration	5,599	3.84%	3.70%	3.63%	3.27%

Mesa General Hospital

515 N Mesa Drive — Phone: 480-969-9111
Mesa, AZ 85201 — Fax: 480-969-0095
URL: www.mesageneralhospital.com
Ownership: Government - State — Accredited: Yes
Emergency Services: Yes — Licensed Beds: 126

Key Personnel:
President/CEO . . . . Brent A Cope
Catheterization Lab . . . . Scott Nelson, RN
Emergency Room . . . . Cundi Smith
Infection Control . . . . Betty Burnham
ICU . . . . Scott Nelson
Intensive/Coronary Care . . . . Scott Nelson
Medical/Surgical Nursing . . . . Kathy Davis, RN
OB/GYN Womens Health . . . . Maria Hayes, RN
Respiratory/Cardiopulmonary . . . . Geeta Joshi

Measure	Cases	This Hospital	State Average	U.S. Average	Top Hospital
Heart Attack Care					
ACE Inhibitor or ARB for LVSD	25	84%	83%	82%	100%
Aspirin at Arrival	59	97%	96%	92%	100%
Aspirin at Discharge	73	97%	91%	90%	100%
Beta Blocker at Arrival	45	96%	88%	87%	100%
Beta Blocker at Discharge	76	96%	93%	90%	100%
Fibrinolytic Medication Timing	0	-	10%	31%	100%
PCI Within 90 Minutes of Arrival[1]	2	50%	47%	54%	95%
Smoking Cessation Advice	36	72%	89%	88%	100%
Heart Failure Care					
ACE Inhibitor or ARB for LVSD	61	100%	81%	82%	100%
Discharge Instructions	112	48%	48%	61%	93%
Evaluation of LVS Function	144	97%	84%	83%	99%
Smoking Cessation Advice	33	73%	76%	82%	100%
Pneumonia Care					
Appropriate Initial Antibiotic	85	82%	84%	83%	94%
Blood Culture Timing	60	72%	87%	90%	100%
Influenza Vaccine[4,5]	-	-	61%	70%	100%
Initial Antibiotic Timing	109	57%	73%	80%	93%
Oxygenation Assessment	123	100%	100%	99%	100%
Pneumococcal Vaccine	66	48%	64%	69%	94%
Smoking Cessation Advice	36	72%	69%	80%	100%
Surgical Infection Prevention					
Prophylactic Antibiotic Given[3]	121	74%	74%	77%	95%
Prophylactic Antibiotic Selection	29	93%	88%	90%	100%
Prophylactic Antibiotic Stopped[3]	108	92%	68%	72%	95%
Pregnancy Care					
Inpatient Neonatal Mortality	1,312	0.00%	-	-	-
Third or Fourth Degree Laceration	993	8.76%	3.70%	3.63%	3.27%

Carondelet Holy Cross Hospital

Alternate Name: Holy Cross Hospital & Health Center
1171 W Target Range Road — Phone: 520-285-3000
Nogales, AZ 85621 — Fax: 520-285-8015
URL: www.carondelet.org
Ownership: Voluntary non-profit - Private — Accredited: No
Emergency Services: No — Licensed Beds: 80

Key Personnel:
SVP/CEO . . . . Richard Polheber
CNO . . . . Marlene Wade
Chief Medical Staff . . . . Maria Pina
Emergency Room . . . . Dan Luther, MD
Medical Staff Services . . . . Karla Bregen
Respiratory Care . . . . Johnette Addy

Measure	Cases	This Hospital	State Average	U.S. Average	Top Hospital
Heart Attack Care					
ACE Inhibitor or ARB for LVSD[3]	0	-	83%	82%	100%
Aspirin at Arrival[1,3]	1	100%	96%	92%	100%
Aspirin at Discharge[1,3]	1	100%	91%	90%	100%
Beta Blocker at Arrival[1,3]	1	100%	88%	87%	100%
Beta Blocker at Discharge[1,3]	1	100%	93%	90%	100%
Fibrinolytic Medication Timing[3]	0	-	10%	31%	100%
PCI Within 90 Minutes of Arrival	0	-	47%	54%	95%
Smoking Cessation Advice[3]	0	-	89%	88%	100%
Heart Failure Care					
ACE Inhibitor or ARB for LVSD[1]	3	67%	81%	82%	100%
Discharge Instructions[1]	12	67%	48%	61%	93%
Evaluation of LVS Function[1]	10	60%	84%	83%	99%
Smoking Cessation Advice	0	-	76%	82%	100%
Pneumonia Care					
Appropriate Initial Antibiotic[2]	36	94%	84%	83%	94%
Blood Culture Timing[1,2]	17	82%	87%	90%	100%
Influenza Vaccine[1]	12	50%	61%	70%	100%
Initial Antibiotic Timing[2]	29	59%	73%	80%	93%
Oxygenation Assessment[2]	51	100%	100%	99%	100%
Pneumococcal Vaccine[2]	30	43%	64%	69%	94%
Smoking Cessation Advice[1,2]	9	56%	69%	80%	100%
Surgical Infection Prevention					
Prophylactic Antibiotic Given[2,3]	54	70%	74%	77%	95%
Prophylactic Antibiotic Selection[1,2]	13	100%	88%	90%	100%
Prophylactic Antibiotic Stopped[2,3]	49	96%	68%	72%	95%
Pregnancy Care					
Inpatient Neonatal Mortality	-	-	-	-	-

NOTE: Hospital profiles are in alphabetical order by state, then city, then hospital within the city; Rankings are sorted by rate in descending order and exclude hospitals with less than 25 cases; (1) The number of cases is too small (n<25) for purposes of reliably predicting hospital performance; (2) Measure reflects the hospital's indication that its submission was based upon a sample of its relevant discharges; (3) Rate reflects fewer than the maximum possible quarters of data for the measure; (4) Inaccurate information submitted and suppressed for one or more quarters; (5) No data is available from the hospital for this measure; Please refer to the User's Guide for a full explanation of data

Third or Fourth Degree Laceration	-	-	3.70%	3.63%	3.27%

Page Hospital

501 N Navajo Drive
PO Box 1447
Page, AZ 86040
Phone: 928-645-2424
Fax: 928-645-3549
Ownership: Govt - Hospital District or Authority
Accredited: Yes
Emergency Services: Yes
Licensed Beds: 25

Key Personnel:
CEO. . . . . Sandy Haryasz
Chief Medical Staff. . . . . Barbara Zimmerman
Director Respiratory Therapy . . . . Patty Cantrell

Measure	Cases	This Hospital	State Average	U.S. Average	Top Hospital
Heart Attack Care					
ACE Inhibitor or ARB for LVSD[5]	-	-	83%	82%	100%
Aspirin at Arrival[5]	-	-	96%	92%	100%
Aspirin at Discharge[5]	-	-	91%	90%	100%
Beta Blocker at Arrival[5]	-	-	88%	87%	100%
Beta Blocker at Discharge[5]	-	-	93%	90%	100%
Fibrinolytic Medication Timing[5]	-	-	10%	31%	100%
PCI Within 90 Minutes of Arrival[5]	-	-	47%	54%	95%
Smoking Cessation Advice[5]	-	-	89%	88%	100%
Heart Failure Care					
ACE Inhibitor or ARB for LVSD[1]	5	100%	81%	82%	100%
Discharge Instructions[1]	11	91%	48%	61%	93%
Evaluation of LVS Function[1]	11	100%	84%	83%	99%
Smoking Cessation Advice[1]	2	100%	76%	82%	100%
Pneumonia Care					
Appropriate Initial Antibiotic[1]	16	100%	84%	83%	94%
Blood Culture Timing[1]	9	67%	87%	90%	100%
Influenza Vaccine[1]	3	100%	61%	70%	100%
Initial Antibiotic Timing[1]	14	93%	73%	80%	93%
Oxygenation Assessment[1]	17	100%	100%	99%	100%
Pneumococcal Vaccine[1]	14	100%	64%	69%	94%
Smoking Cessation Advice[1]	2	50%	69%	80%	100%
Surgical Infection Prevention					
Prophylactic Antibiotic Given[1,3]	3	100%	74%	77%	95%
Prophylactic Antibiotic Selection[1]	3	100%	88%	90%	100%
Prophylactic Antibiotic Stopped[1,3]	3	100%	68%	72%	95%
Pregnancy Care					
Inpatient Neonatal Mortality	-	-	-	-	-
Third or Fourth Degree Laceration	-	-	3.70%	3.63%	3.27%

La Paz Regional Hospital

1200 Mohave Road
Parker, AZ 85344
Phone: 928-669-9201
Fax: 928-669-7417
E-mail: hr@LaPazHospital.org
URL: www.lapazhospital.org
Ownership: Voluntary non-profit - Other
Accredited: Yes
Emergency Services: Yes
Licensed Beds: 39

Key Personnel:
CEO. . . . . M Victoria Clark
Chief Medical Staff. . . . . Edward Fuller, MD
Emergency Room . . . . Kathleen Shrewsburg, RN
Infection Control. . . . . Barbara Heeringa, RN
ICU . . . . Bonnie Viloria, RN, CNO
Medical/Surgical Nursing . . . . Bonnie Viloria, RN
Surgical Services . . . . Teri Forbis
Respiratory/Cardiopulmonary. . . . . Angela Young

Measure	Cases	This Hospital	State Average	U.S. Average	Top Hospital
Heart Attack Care					
ACE Inhibitor or ARB for LVSD[3]	0	-	83%	82%	100%
Aspirin at Arrival[1,3]	2	100%	96%	92%	100%
Aspirin at Discharge[1,3]	2	100%	91%	90%	100%
Beta Blocker at Arrival[1,3]	2	100%	88%	87%	100%
Beta Blocker at Discharge[1,3]	2	100%	93%	90%	100%
Fibrinolytic Medication Timing[3]	0	-	10%	31%	100%
PCI Within 90 Minutes of Arrival[5]	-	-	47%	54%	95%
Smoking Cessation Advice[3]	0	-	89%	88%	100%
Heart Failure Care					
ACE Inhibitor or ARB for LVSD[1]	1	100%	81%	82%	100%
Discharge Instructions	30	37%	48%	61%	93%
Evaluation of LVS Function	31	61%	84%	83%	99%
Smoking Cessation Advice[1]	7	86%	76%	82%	100%
Pneumonia Care					
Appropriate Initial Antibiotic	72	96%	84%	83%	94%
Blood Culture Timing[1]	22	68%	87%	90%	100%
Influenza Vaccine[1]	19	79%	61%	70%	100%
Initial Antibiotic Timing	73	84%	73%	80%	93%
Oxygenation Assessment	79	99%	100%	99%	100%
Pneumococcal Vaccine	46	80%	64%	69%	94%
Smoking Cessation Advice[1]	14	64%	69%	80%	100%
Surgical Infection Prevention					
Prophylactic Antibiotic Given[1]	12	67%	74%	77%	95%
Prophylactic Antibiotic Selection[1]	2	0%	88%	90%	100%
Prophylactic Antibiotic Stopped[1]	11	9%	68%	72%	95%
Pregnancy Care					
Inpatient Neonatal Mortality	-	-	-	-	-
Third or Fourth Degree Laceration	-	-	3.70%	3.63%	3.27%

Payson Regional Medical Center

Alternate Name: Lewis R Pyle Memorial Hospital
807 S Ponderosa
Payson, AZ 85541
Phone: 928-474-3222
Fax: 928-472-1295
URL: www.paysonhospital.com
Ownership: Voluntary non-profit - Other
Accredited: Yes
Emergency Services: Yes
Licensed Beds: 66

Key Personnel:
CEO. . . . . Chris Wolf
Chief Medical Staff. . . . . Charlie Caulkins
Director of Cardiology/Cardiac Lab. . . . . David Alexander
Emergency Room . . . . Richard Moreno
Chief Radiology . . . . David Plone, DO
Director Respiratory Therapy . . . . Tim Sillin

Measure	Cases	This Hospital	State Average	U.S. Average	Top Hospital
Heart Attack Care					
ACE Inhibitor or ARB for LVSD	0	-	83%	82%	100%
Aspirin at Arrival[1]	3	67%	96%	92%	100%
Aspirin at Discharge[1]	2	50%	91%	90%	100%
Beta Blocker at Arrival[1]	7	57%	88%	87%	100%
Beta Blocker at Discharge[1]	3	100%	93%	90%	100%
Fibrinolytic Medication Timing	0	-	10%	31%	100%
PCI Within 90 Minutes of Arrival	0	-	47%	54%	95%
Smoking Cessation Advice	0	-	89%	88%	100%
Heart Failure Care					
ACE Inhibitor or ARB for LVSD[1]	14	71%	81%	82%	100%
Discharge Instructions	33	61%	48%	61%	93%
Evaluation of LVS Function	38	87%	84%	83%	99%
Smoking Cessation Advice[1]	7	71%	76%	82%	100%
Pneumonia Care					
Appropriate Initial Antibiotic	100	92%	84%	83%	94%
Blood Culture Timing	83	88%	87%	90%	100%
Influenza Vaccine	32	78%	61%	70%	100%
Initial Antibiotic Timing	132	89%	73%	80%	93%
Oxygenation Assessment	139	100%	100%	99%	100%
Pneumococcal Vaccine	92	82%	64%	69%	94%
Smoking Cessation Advice	32	88%	69%	80%	100%
Surgical Infection Prevention					
Prophylactic Antibiotic Given[2,3]	127	72%	74%	77%	95%
Prophylactic Antibiotic Selection[2]	38	84%	88%	90%	100%
Prophylactic Antibiotic Stopped[2,3]	115	70%	68%	72%	95%
Pregnancy Care					
Inpatient Neonatal Mortality	-	-	-	-	-
Third or Fourth Degree Laceration	-	-	3.70%	3.63%	3.27%

Arizona Heart Hospital

1930 East Thomas Road
Phoenix, AZ 85016
Phone: 602-532-1000
Fax: 602-532-2000
URL: www.azhearthospital.com
Ownership: Proprietary
Accredited: Yes
Emergency Services: Yes

Key Personnel:
President . . . . Ken Howell

NOTE: Hospital profiles are in alphabetical order by state, then city, then hospital within the city; Rankings are sorted by rate in descending order and exclude hospitals with less than 25 cases; (1) The number of cases is too small (n<25) for purposes of reliably predicting hospital performance; (2) Measure reflects the hospital's indication that its submission was based upon a sample of its relevant discharges; (3) Rate reflects fewer than the maximum possible quarters of data for the measure; (4) Inaccurate information submitted and suppressed for one or more quarters; (5) No data is available from the hospital for this measure; Please refer to the User's Guide for a full explanation of data

Measure	Cases	This Hospital	State Average	U.S. Average	Top Hospital
Heart Attack Care					
ACE Inhibitor or ARB for LVSD	82	88%	83%	82%	100%
Aspirin at Arrival	83	100%	96%	92%	100%
Aspirin at Discharge	319	99%	91%	90%	100%
Beta Blocker at Arrival	67	100%	88%	87%	100%
Beta Blocker at Discharge	304	97%	93%	90%	100%
Fibrinolytic Medication Timing	0	-	10%	31%	100%
PCI Within 90 Minutes of Arrival[1]	5	80%	47%	54%	95%
Smoking Cessation Advice	116	96%	89%	88%	100%
Heart Failure Care					
ACE Inhibitor or ARB for LVSD	170	90%	81%	82%	100%
Discharge Instructions	245	85%	48%	61%	93%
Evaluation of LVS Function	278	97%	84%	83%	99%
Smoking Cessation Advice	81	93%	76%	82%	100%
Pneumonia Care					
Appropriate Initial Antibiotic	49	84%	84%	83%	94%
Blood Culture Timing	38	89%	87%	90%	100%
Influenza Vaccine[1]	19	42%	61%	70%	100%
Initial Antibiotic Timing	61	74%	73%	80%	93%
Oxygenation Assessment	76	100%	100%	99%	100%
Pneumococcal Vaccine	52	62%	64%	69%	94%
Smoking Cessation Advice	29	79%	69%	80%	100%
Surgical Infection Prevention					
Prophylactic Antibiotic Given[3]	365	81%	74%	77%	95%
Prophylactic Antibiotic Selection	98	97%	88%	90%	100%
Prophylactic Antibiotic Stopped[3]	356	67%	68%	72%	95%
Pregnancy Care					
Inpatient Neonatal Mortality	-	-	-	-	-
Third or Fourth Degree Laceration	-	-	3.70%	3.63%	3.27%

Arizona Surgical Hospital

Alternate Name: Community Hospital Medical Center
6501 N 19th Avenue Phone: 602-795-6020
Phoenix, AZ 85015 Fax: 602-795-6021
Ownership: Voluntary non-profit - Private Accredited: Yes
Emergency Services: No

Key Personnel:

CEO. . . . . Beverly Carpenter
Chief Medical Staff. . . . . Marky Siegel, DO
Infection Control. . . . . Colleen Clarke, RN
Medical Surgical Nursing . . . . Deborah Roberts

Measure	Cases	This Hospital	State Average	U.S. Average	Top Hospital
Heart Attack Care					
ACE Inhibitor or ARB for LVSD[5]	-	-	83%	82%	100%
Aspirin at Arrival[5]	-	-	96%	92%	100%
Aspirin at Discharge[5]	-	-	91%	90%	100%
Beta Blocker at Arrival[5]	-	-	88%	87%	100%
Beta Blocker at Discharge[5]	-	-	93%	90%	100%
Fibrinolytic Medication Timing[5]	-	-	10%	31%	100%
PCI Within 90 Minutes of Arrival[5]	-	-	47%	54%	95%
Smoking Cessation Advice[5]	-	-	89%	88%	100%
Heart Failure Care					
ACE Inhibitor or ARB for LVSD[5]	-	-	81%	82%	100%
Discharge Instructions[5]	-	-	48%	61%	93%
Evaluation of LVS Function[5]	-	-	84%	83%	99%
Smoking Cessation Advice[5]	-	-	76%	82%	100%
Pneumonia Care					
Appropriate Initial Antibiotic[5]	-	-	84%	83%	94%
Blood Culture Timing[5]	-	-	87%	90%	100%
Influenza Vaccine[5]	-	-	61%	70%	100%
Initial Antibiotic Timing[5]	-	-	73%	80%	93%
Oxygenation Assessment[5]	-	-	100%	99%	100%
Pneumococcal Vaccine[5]	-	-	64%	69%	94%
Smoking Cessation Advice[5]	-	-	69%	80%	100%
Surgical Infection Prevention					
Prophylactic Antibiotic Given[2,3]	0	-	74%	77%	95%
Prophylactic Antibiotic Selection[5]	-	-	88%	90%	100%
Prophylactic Antibiotic Stopped[2,3]	0	-	68%	72%	95%
Pregnancy Care					
Inpatient Neonatal Mortality	-	-	-	-	-
Third or Fourth Degree Laceration	-	-	3.70%	3.63%	3.27%

Banner Estrella Medical Center

9201 West Thomas Road Phone: 623-327-5003
Phoenix, AZ 85037
Ownership: Voluntary non-profit - Other Accredited: Yes
Emergency Services: Yes

Measure	Cases	This Hospital	State Average	U.S. Average	Top Hospital
Heart Attack Care					
ACE Inhibitor or ARB for LVSD	30	83%	83%	82%	100%
Aspirin at Arrival	143	98%	96%	92%	100%
Aspirin at Discharge	116	97%	91%	90%	100%
Beta Blocker at Arrival	122	93%	88%	87%	100%
Beta Blocker at Discharge	121	97%	93%	90%	100%
Fibrinolytic Medication Timing	0	-	10%	31%	100%
PCI Within 90 Minutes of Arrival[1]	8	12%	47%	54%	95%
Smoking Cessation Advice	53	94%	89%	88%	100%
Heart Failure Care					
ACE Inhibitor or ARB for LVSD[2]	112	85%	81%	82%	100%
Discharge Instructions[2]	241	70%	48%	61%	93%
Evaluation of LVS Function[2]	260	92%	84%	83%	99%
Smoking Cessation Advice[2]	54	87%	76%	82%	100%
Pneumonia Care					
Appropriate Initial Antibiotic[2]	241	86%	84%	83%	94%
Blood Culture Timing[2]	163	57%	87%	90%	100%
Influenza Vaccine[2]	87	44%	61%	70%	100%
Initial Antibiotic Timing[2]	288	75%	73%	80%	93%
Oxygenation Assessment[2]	356	100%	100%	99%	100%
Pneumococcal Vaccine[2]	150	55%	64%	69%	94%
Smoking Cessation Advice[2]	83	72%	69%	80%	100%
Surgical Infection Prevention					
Prophylactic Antibiotic Given[3]	209	74%	74%	77%	95%
Prophylactic Antibiotic Selection	61	89%	88%	90%	100%
Prophylactic Antibiotic Stopped[3]	195	87%	68%	72%	95%
Pregnancy Care					
Inpatient Neonatal Mortality	-	-	-	-	-
Third or Fourth Degree Laceration	-	-	3.70%	3.63%	3.27%

Banner Good Samaritan Medical Center

1111 East McDowell Road Phone: 602-239-2000
Phoenix, AZ 85006 Fax: 602-239-3749
URL: www.bannerhealth.com
Ownership: Govt - Hospital District or Authority Accredited: Yes
Emergency Services: Yes Licensed Beds: 659

Key Personnel:

CEO. . . . . Paul Mullings
Chief Medical Staff. . . . . John Harlend, MD
Director Infection/Disease Control . . . . Beth Urndinski
OB/GYN Womens Health. . . . . William Clewell, MD
Director Respiratory Therapy . . . . Glen Davis

Measure	Cases	This Hospital	State Average	U.S. Average	Top Hospital
Heart Attack Care					
ACE Inhibitor or ARB for LVSD[2]	75	77%	83%	82%	100%
Aspirin at Arrival[2]	110	98%	96%	92%	100%
Aspirin at Discharge[2]	211	98%	91%	90%	100%
Beta Blocker at Arrival[2]	81	94%	88%	87%	100%
Beta Blocker at Discharge[2]	199	95%	93%	90%	100%
Fibrinolytic Medication Timing[2]	0	-	10%	31%	100%
PCI Within 90 Minutes of Arrival[1,2]	7	14%	47%	54%	95%
Smoking Cessation Advice[2]	98	95%	89%	88%	100%
Heart Failure Care					
ACE Inhibitor or ARB for LVSD[2]	142	75%	81%	82%	100%
Discharge Instructions[2]	249	54%	48%	61%	93%
Evaluation of LVS Function[2]	282	97%	84%	83%	99%
Smoking Cessation Advice[2]	63	89%	76%	82%	100%
Pneumonia Care					
Appropriate Initial Antibiotic[2]	99	86%	84%	83%	94%
Blood Culture Timing[2]	86	93%	87%	90%	100%
Influenza Vaccine[1,2]	19	37%	61%	70%	100%

NOTE: Hospital profiles are in alphabetical order by state, then city, then hospital within the city; Rankings are sorted by rate in descending order and exclude hospitals with less than 25 cases; (1) The number of cases is too small (n<25) for purposes of reliably predicting hospital performance; (2) Measure reflects the hospital's indication that its submission was based upon a sample of its relevant discharges; (3) Rate reflects fewer than the maximum possible quarters of data for the measure; (4) Inaccurate information submitted and suppressed for one or more quarters; (5) No data is available from the hospital for this measure; Please refer to the User's Guide for a full explanation of data

Measure	Cases	This Hospital	State Average	U.S. Average	Top Hospital
Initial Antibiotic Timing[2]	133	67%	73%	80%	93%
Oxygenation Assessment[2]	164	100%	100%	99%	100%
Pneumococcal Vaccine[2]	74	49%	64%	69%	94%
Smoking Cessation Advice[2]	45	40%	69%	80%	100%
Surgical Infection Prevention					
Prophylactic Antibiotic Given[2,3]	241	71%	74%	77%	95%
Prophylactic Antibiotic Selection[2]	80	92%	88%	90%	100%
Prophylactic Antibiotic Stopped[2,3]	226	64%	68%	72%	95%
Pregnancy Care					
Inpatient Neonatal Mortality	-	-	-	-	-
Third or Fourth Degree Laceration	-	-	3.70%	3.63%	3.27%

John C Lincoln Hospital-Deer Valley

19829 N 27th Avenue Phone: 623-879-6100
Phoenix, AZ 85027 Fax: 623-879-5400
URL: www.jcl.com
Ownership: Voluntary non-profit - Private Accredited: Yes
Emergency Services: Yes Licensed Beds: 149
Key Personnel:
President/CEO. . . . . Dan C Coleman
Chief Medical Staff. . . . . Clark York, DO

Measure	Cases	This Hospital	State Average	U.S. Average	Top Hospital
Heart Attack Care					
ACE Inhibitor or ARB for LVSD	52	90%	83%	82%	100%
Aspirin at Arrival	172	98%	96%	92%	100%
Aspirin at Discharge	153	99%	91%	90%	100%
Beta Blocker at Arrival	129	90%	88%	87%	100%
Beta Blocker at Discharge	160	99%	93%	90%	100%
Fibrinolytic Medication Timing	0	-	10%	31%	100%
PCI Within 90 Minutes of Arrival[1]	6	17%	47%	54%	95%
Smoking Cessation Advice	72	100%	89%	88%	100%
Heart Failure Care					
ACE Inhibitor or ARB for LVSD[2]	109	91%	81%	82%	100%
Discharge Instructions[2]	212	57%	48%	61%	93%
Evaluation of LVS Function[2]	236	97%	84%	83%	99%
Smoking Cessation Advice[2]	61	100%	76%	82%	100%
Pneumonia Care					
Appropriate Initial Antibiotic[2]	122	90%	84%	83%	94%
Blood Culture Timing[2]	111	95%	87%	90%	100%
Influenza Vaccine	25	84%	61%	70%	100%
Initial Antibiotic Timing[2]	141	59%	73%	80%	93%
Oxygenation Assessment[2]	186	100%	100%	99%	100%
Pneumococcal Vaccine[2]	95	78%	64%	69%	94%
Smoking Cessation Advice[2]	62	98%	69%	80%	100%
Surgical Infection Prevention					
Prophylactic Antibiotic Given[2,3]	190	84%	74%	77%	95%
Prophylactic Antibiotic Selection[2]	61	97%	88%	90%	100%
Prophylactic Antibiotic Stopped[2,3]	174	64%	68%	72%	95%
Pregnancy Care					
Inpatient Neonatal Mortality	-	-	-	-	-
Third or Fourth Degree Laceration	-	-	3.70%	3.63%	3.27%

John C Lincoln Hospital-North Mountain

250 E Dunlap Road Phone: 602-943-2381
Phoenix, AZ 85020 Fax: 602-944-9610
URL: www.jcl.com
Ownership: Voluntary non-profit - Private Accredited: No
Emergency Services: Yes Licensed Beds: 262
Key Personnel:
CEO. . . . . Dan C Coleman
Chief Medical Staff. . . . . Tim Tracy

Measure	Cases	This Hospital	State Average	U.S. Average	Top Hospital
Heart Attack Care					
ACE Inhibitor or ARB for LVSD	44	84%	83%	82%	100%
Aspirin at Arrival	177	94%	96%	92%	100%
Aspirin at Discharge	151	99%	91%	90%	100%
Beta Blocker at Arrival	112	93%	88%	87%	100%
Beta Blocker at Discharge	151	97%	93%	90%	100%
Fibrinolytic Medication Timing	0	-	10%	31%	100%
PCI Within 90 Minutes of Arrival[1]	10	30%	47%	54%	95%
Smoking Cessation Advice	58	97%	89%	88%	100%
Heart Failure Care					
ACE Inhibitor or ARB for LVSD[2]	112	88%	81%	82%	100%
Discharge Instructions[2]	215	66%	48%	61%	93%
Evaluation of LVS Function[2]	246	98%	84%	83%	99%
Smoking Cessation Advice[2]	53	92%	76%	82%	100%
Pneumonia Care					
Appropriate Initial Antibiotic[2]	103	87%	84%	83%	94%
Blood Culture Timing[2]	77	92%	87%	90%	100%
Influenza Vaccine	26	96%	61%	70%	100%
Initial Antibiotic Timing[2]	141	77%	73%	80%	93%
Oxygenation Assessment[2]	176	100%	100%	99%	100%
Pneumococcal Vaccine[2]	103	80%	64%	69%	94%
Smoking Cessation Advice[2]	38	87%	69%	80%	100%
Surgical Infection Prevention					
Prophylactic Antibiotic Given[2,3]	252	85%	74%	77%	95%
Prophylactic Antibiotic Selection[2]	75	87%	88%	90%	100%
Prophylactic Antibiotic Stopped[2,3]	247	60%	68%	72%	95%
Pregnancy Care					
Inpatient Neonatal Mortality	-	-	-	-	-
Third or Fourth Degree Laceration	-	-	3.70%	3.63%	3.27%

Maricopa Integrated Health

2601 East Roosevelt Street Phone: 602-344-5011
Phoenix, AZ 85008 Fax: 602-344-1132
E-mail: copanet@hcs.maricopa.gov
URL: www.mihs.org
Ownership: Government - Local Accredited: Yes
Emergency Services: Yes Licensed Beds: 449
Key Personnel:
CEO. . . . . James Kennedy
Chief Medical Staff. . . . . James Campbell Davis
Emergency Room . . . . Charles Pollack, MD
Director Infection/Disease Control . . . . Rita Neibauer
Director of Respiratory . . . . Lora McKay

Measure	Cases	This Hospital	State Average	U.S. Average	Top Hospital
Heart Attack Care					
ACE Inhibitor or ARB for LVSD[1]	13	69%	83%	82%	100%
Aspirin at Arrival	69	100%	96%	92%	100%
Aspirin at Discharge	68	84%	91%	90%	100%
Beta Blocker at Arrival	66	89%	88%	87%	100%
Beta Blocker at Discharge	68	81%	93%	90%	100%
Fibrinolytic Medication Timing[1]	1	0%	10%	31%	100%
PCI Within 90 Minutes of Arrival[1]	2	50%	47%	54%	95%
Smoking Cessation Advice	32	50%	89%	88%	100%
Heart Failure Care					
ACE Inhibitor or ARB for LVSD	102	86%	81%	82%	100%
Discharge Instructions	154	9%	48%	61%	93%
Evaluation of LVS Function	188	94%	84%	83%	99%
Smoking Cessation Advice	68	56%	76%	82%	100%
Pneumonia Care					
Appropriate Initial Antibiotic	157	83%	84%	83%	94%
Blood Culture Timing	113	79%	87%	90%	100%
Influenza Vaccine	48	23%	61%	70%	100%
Initial Antibiotic Timing	212	67%	73%	80%	93%
Oxygenation Assessment	257	100%	100%	99%	100%
Pneumococcal Vaccine	81	21%	64%	69%	94%
Smoking Cessation Advice	98	63%	69%	80%	100%
Surgical Infection Prevention					
Prophylactic Antibiotic Given[1,3]	14	50%	74%	77%	95%
Prophylactic Antibiotic Selection[1]	9	89%	88%	90%	100%
Prophylactic Antibiotic Stopped[1,3]	12	100%	68%	72%	95%
Pregnancy Care					
Inpatient Neonatal Mortality	-	-	-	-	-
Third or Fourth Degree Laceration	-	-	3.70%	3.63%	3.27%

NOTE: Hospital profiles are in alphabetical order by state, then city, then hospital within the city; Rankings are sorted by rate in descending order and exclude hospitals with less than 25 cases; (1) The number of cases is too small (n<25) for purposes of reliably predicting hospital performance; (2) Measure reflects the hospital's indication that its submission was based upon a sample of its relevant discharges; (3) Rate reflects fewer than the maximum possible quarters of data for the measure; (4) Inaccurate information submitted and suppressed for one or more quarters; (5) No data is available from the hospital for this measure; Please refer to the User's Guide for a full explanation of data

Maryvale Hospital Medical Center

5102 W Campbell Avenue
Phoenix, AZ 85031
Phone: 623-848-5000
Fax: 623-848-5553
URL: www.maryvalehospital.com
Ownership: Proprietary
Accredited: Yes
Emergency Services: Yes
Licensed Beds: 239

Key Personnel:

CEO. . . . . Gregory Pizilla
Chief of Medical Staff. . . . . Frederick Scott
Emergency Room . . . . Stacy Aragon
Director Medical/Surgical Nursing . . . . Caroline Rosen

Measure	Cases	This Hospital	State Average	U.S. Average	Top Hospital
Heart Attack Care					
ACE Inhibitor or ARB for LVSD[1]	24	75%	83%	82%	100%
Aspirin at Arrival	148	99%	96%	92%	100%
Aspirin at Discharge	121	93%	91%	90%	100%
Beta Blocker at Arrival	143	89%	88%	87%	100%
Beta Blocker at Discharge	123	94%	93%	90%	100%
Fibrinolytic Medication Timing	0	-	10%	31%	100%
PCI Within 90 Minutes of Arrival[1]	10	30%	47%	54%	95%
Smoking Cessation Advice	59	95%	89%	88%	100%
Heart Failure Care					
ACE Inhibitor or ARB for LVSD	83	77%	81%	82%	100%
Discharge Instructions	170	33%	48%	61%	93%
Evaluation of LVS Function	190	94%	84%	83%	99%
Smoking Cessation Advice	71	94%	76%	82%	100%
Pneumonia Care					
Appropriate Initial Antibiotic	176	82%	84%	83%	94%
Blood Culture Timing	121	84%	87%	90%	100%
Influenza Vaccine	41	41%	61%	70%	100%
Initial Antibiotic Timing	196	82%	73%	80%	93%
Oxygenation Assessment	229	100%	100%	99%	100%
Pneumococcal Vaccine	87	45%	64%	69%	94%
Smoking Cessation Advice	82	80%	69%	80%	100%
Surgical Infection Prevention					
Prophylactic Antibiotic Given[3]	76	72%	74%	77%	95%
Prophylactic Antibiotic Selection	26	96%	88%	90%	100%
Prophylactic Antibiotic Stopped[3]	72	60%	68%	72%	95%
Pregnancy Care					
Inpatient Neonatal Mortality	-	-	-	-	-
Third or Fourth Degree Laceration	-	-	3.70%	3.63%	3.27%

Mayo Clinic Hospital

5777 East Mayo Boulevard
Phoenix, AZ 85054
Phone: 480-515-6296
Fax: 480-342-3523
URL: www.mayoclinic.org
Ownership: Voluntary non-profit - Private
Accredited: Yes
Emergency Services: Yes
Licensed Beds: 208

Key Personnel:

Administrator . . . . Thomas C Bour

Measure	Cases	This Hospital	State Average	U.S. Average	Top Hospital
Heart Attack Care					
ACE Inhibitor or ARB for LVSD	33	88%	83%	82%	100%
Aspirin at Arrival	162	98%	96%	92%	100%
Aspirin at Discharge	129	98%	91%	90%	100%
Beta Blocker at Arrival	138	98%	88%	87%	100%
Beta Blocker at Discharge	150	99%	93%	90%	100%
Fibrinolytic Medication Timing	0	-	10%	31%	100%
PCI Within 90 Minutes of Arrival[1]	9	78%	47%	54%	95%
Smoking Cessation Advice[1]	23	100%	89%	88%	100%
Heart Failure Care					
ACE Inhibitor or ARB for LVSD	120	97%	81%	82%	100%
Discharge Instructions	265	81%	48%	61%	93%
Evaluation of LVS Function	274	100%	84%	83%	99%
Smoking Cessation Advice	25	100%	76%	82%	100%
Pneumonia Care					
Appropriate Initial Antibiotic	202	96%	84%	83%	94%
Blood Culture Timing	249	94%	87%	90%	100%
Influenza Vaccine	99	91%	61%	70%	100%
Initial Antibiotic Timing	284	87%	73%	80%	93%
Oxygenation Assessment	403	100%	100%	99%	100%
Pneumococcal Vaccine	324	96%	64%	69%	94%
Smoking Cessation Advice	39	100%	69%	80%	100%
Surgical Infection Prevention					
Prophylactic Antibiotic Given[2,3]	695	92%	74%	77%	95%
Prophylactic Antibiotic Selection[2]	211	97%	88%	90%	100%
Prophylactic Antibiotic Stopped[2,3]	670	90%	68%	72%	95%
Pregnancy Care					
Inpatient Neonatal Mortality	-	-	-	-	-
Third or Fourth Degree Laceration	-	-	3.70%	3.63%	3.27%

Paradise Valley Hospital

3929 E Bell Road
Phoenix, AZ 85032
Phone: 602-867-1881
Fax: 602-923-5657
URL: www.paradisevalleyhospital.com
Ownership: Proprietary
Accredited: Yes
Emergency Services: Yes
Licensed Beds: 140

Key Personnel:

CEO. . . . . John Harrington
Head Surgeon . . . . Rick Low
Emergency Room . . . . Brian Helender
Director of Respiratory Therapy . . . . Karan Jasinski

Measure	Cases	This Hospital	State Average	U.S. Average	Top Hospital
Heart Attack Care					
ACE Inhibitor or ARB for LVSD[1]	15	80%	83%	82%	100%
Aspirin at Arrival	80	96%	96%	92%	100%
Aspirin at Discharge	59	97%	91%	90%	100%
Beta Blocker at Arrival	57	88%	88%	87%	100%
Beta Blocker at Discharge	71	94%	93%	90%	100%
Fibrinolytic Medication Timing	0	-	10%	31%	100%
PCI Within 90 Minutes of Arrival[1]	5	40%	47%	54%	95%
Smoking Cessation Advice	32	100%	89%	88%	100%
Heart Failure Care					
ACE Inhibitor or ARB for LVSD	43	81%	81%	82%	100%
Discharge Instructions	108	34%	48%	61%	93%
Evaluation of LVS Function	139	96%	84%	83%	99%
Smoking Cessation Advice	26	92%	76%	82%	100%
Pneumonia Care					
Appropriate Initial Antibiotic	151	90%	84%	83%	94%
Blood Culture Timing	164	90%	87%	90%	100%
Influenza Vaccine	37	41%	61%	70%	100%
Initial Antibiotic Timing	206	86%	73%	80%	93%
Oxygenation Assessment	257	100%	100%	99%	100%
Pneumococcal Vaccine	124	56%	64%	69%	94%
Smoking Cessation Advice	66	91%	69%	80%	100%
Surgical Infection Prevention					
Prophylactic Antibiotic Given[3]	354	84%	74%	77%	95%
Prophylactic Antibiotic Selection	109	94%	88%	90%	100%
Prophylactic Antibiotic Stopped[3]	347	63%	68%	72%	95%
Pregnancy Care					
Inpatient Neonatal Mortality	-	-	-	-	-
Third or Fourth Degree Laceration	-	-	3.70%	3.63%	3.27%

Phoenix Baptist Hospital and Medical Center

2000 W Bethany Home Road
Phoenix, AZ 85015
Phone: 602-249-0212
Fax: 602-246-5849
URL: www.phoenixbaptisthospital.com
Ownership: Proprietary
Accredited: Yes
Emergency Services: Yes
Licensed Beds: 202

Key Personnel:

CEO. . . . . Dennis Knox
Chief Medical Staff. . . . . James Kennedy, MD
Emergency Room . . . . Christiene Sinon
OB/GYN Womens Health. . . . . Rodney Smith
Chief Radiology . . . . Robert Lewis, MD
Director Respiratory Therapy . . . . Steve Brown

Measure	Cases	This Hospital	State Average	U.S. Average	Top Hospital
Heart Attack Care					
ACE Inhibitor or ARB for LVSD	29	93%	83%	82%	100%
Aspirin at Arrival	88	99%	96%	92%	100%

NOTE: Hospital profiles are in alphabetical order by state, then city, then hospital within the city; Rankings are sorted by rate in descending order and exclude hospitals with less than 25 cases; (1) The number of cases is too small (n<25) for purposes of reliably predicting hospital performance; (2) Measure reflects the hospital's indication that its submission was based upon a sample of its relevant discharges; (3) Rate reflects fewer than the maximum possible quarters of data for the measure; (4) Inaccurate information submitted and suppressed for one or more quarters; (5) No data is available from the hospital for this measure; Please refer to the User's Guide for a full explanation of data

Measure	Cases	This Hospital	State Average	U.S. Average	Top Hospital
Aspirin at Discharge	88	99%	91%	90%	100%
Beta Blocker at Arrival	70	91%	88%	87%	100%
Beta Blocker at Discharge	100	96%	93%	90%	100%
Fibrinolytic Medication Timing	0	-	10%	31%	100%
PCI Within 90 Minutes of Arrival[1]	6	33%	47%	54%	95%
Smoking Cessation Advice	46	100%	89%	88%	100%
Heart Failure Care					
ACE Inhibitor or ARB for LVSD	85	94%	81%	82%	100%
Discharge Instructions	183	48%	48%	61%	93%
Evaluation of LVS Function	209	91%	84%	83%	99%
Smoking Cessation Advice	46	91%	76%	82%	100%
Pneumonia Care					
Appropriate Initial Antibiotic	186	81%	84%	83%	94%
Blood Culture Timing	95	85%	87%	90%	100%
Influenza Vaccine[4,5]	-	-	61%	70%	100%
Initial Antibiotic Timing	238	76%	73%	80%	93%
Oxygenation Assessment	283	100%	100%	99%	100%
Pneumococcal Vaccine	164	66%	64%	69%	94%
Smoking Cessation Advice	89	82%	69%	80%	100%
Surgical Infection Prevention					
Prophylactic Antibiotic Given[3]	541	86%	74%	77%	95%
Prophylactic Antibiotic Selection	149	79%	88%	90%	100%
Prophylactic Antibiotic Stopped[3]	511	100%	68%	72%	95%
Pregnancy Care					
Inpatient Neonatal Mortality	-	-	-	-	-
Third or Fourth Degree Laceration	-	-	3.70%	3.63%	3.27%

Phoenix Indian Medical Center

4212 N 16th Street
Phoenix, AZ 85016
URL: www.ihs.gov
Phone: 602-263-1200
Fax: 602-263-1631
Ownership: Government - Federal
Accredited: Yes
Emergency Services: Yes
Licensed Beds: 199

Key Personnel:

OB/GYN Womens Health. . . . . Richard Hays, MD
Chief Radiology . . . . Terence Hamel, MD
Director Respiratory Therapy . . . . Leo Hernandez

Measure	Cases	This Hospital	State Average	U.S. Average	Top Hospital
Heart Attack Care					
ACE Inhibitor or ARB for LVSD[5]	-	-	83%	82%	100%
Aspirin at Arrival[5]	-	-	96%	92%	100%
Aspirin at Discharge[5]	-	-	91%	90%	100%
Beta Blocker at Arrival[5]	-	-	88%	87%	100%
Beta Blocker at Discharge[5]	-	-	93%	90%	100%
Fibrinolytic Medication Timing[5]	-	-	10%	31%	100%
PCI Within 90 Minutes of Arrival[5]	-	-	47%	54%	95%
Smoking Cessation Advice[5]	-	-	89%	88%	100%
Heart Failure Care					
ACE Inhibitor or ARB for LVSD[1,3]	3	67%	81%	82%	100%
Discharge Instructions[1,3]	6	83%	48%	61%	93%
Evaluation of LVS Function[1,3]	6	100%	84%	83%	99%
Smoking Cessation Advice[1,3]	3	100%	76%	82%	100%
Pneumonia Care					
Appropriate Initial Antibiotic	38	84%	84%	83%	94%
Blood Culture Timing[1]	10	90%	87%	90%	100%
Influenza Vaccine[1]	4	50%	61%	70%	100%
Initial Antibiotic Timing	46	78%	73%	80%	93%
Oxygenation Assessment	47	100%	100%	99%	100%
Pneumococcal Vaccine[1]	4	75%	64%	69%	94%
Smoking Cessation Advice[1]	17	41%	69%	80%	100%
Surgical Infection Prevention					
Prophylactic Antibiotic Given	46	72%	74%	77%	95%
Prophylactic Antibiotic Selection[1]	11	64%	88%	90%	100%
Prophylactic Antibiotic Stopped	38	95%	68%	72%	95%
Pregnancy Care					
Inpatient Neonatal Mortality	-	-	-	-	-
Third or Fourth Degree Laceration	-	-	3.70%	3.63%	3.27%

Phoenix Memorial Health System

1201 S 7th Avenue
Phoenix, AZ 85007
E-mail: info@phxmemorialhospital.com
URL: www.phxmemorialhospital.com
Phone: 602-258-5111
Fax: 602-824-3383
Ownership: Proprietary
Accredited: Yes
Emergency Services: Yes
Licensed Beds: 203

Key Personnel:

CEO. . . . . Thomas Keller
Emergency Room . . . . Joyce Hughes
Director Medical/Surgical Nursing . . . . Joyce Hughes
OB/GYN Womens Health. . . . . Farshad Agahi, MD
Director Respiratory Therapy . . . . Howard Jones

Measure	Cases	This Hospital	State Average	U.S. Average	Top Hospital
Heart Attack Care					
ACE Inhibitor or ARB for LVSD	33	82%	83%	82%	100%
Aspirin at Arrival	96	98%	96%	92%	100%
Aspirin at Discharge	128	91%	91%	90%	100%
Beta Blocker at Arrival	87	94%	88%	87%	100%
Beta Blocker at Discharge	124	93%	93%	90%	100%
Fibrinolytic Medication Timing[1]	1	0%	10%	31%	100%
PCI Within 90 Minutes of Arrival[1]	6	50%	47%	54%	95%
Smoking Cessation Advice	64	81%	89%	88%	100%
Heart Failure Care					
ACE Inhibitor or ARB for LVSD	59	95%	81%	82%	100%
Discharge Instructions	109	28%	48%	61%	93%
Evaluation of LVS Function	120	97%	84%	83%	99%
Smoking Cessation Advice	52	87%	76%	82%	100%
Pneumonia Care					
Appropriate Initial Antibiotic	151	85%	84%	83%	94%
Blood Culture Timing	104	80%	87%	90%	100%
Influenza Vaccine[4,5]	-	-	61%	70%	100%
Initial Antibiotic Timing	184	72%	73%	80%	93%
Oxygenation Assessment	195	100%	100%	99%	100%
Pneumococcal Vaccine	73	27%	64%	69%	94%
Smoking Cessation Advice	84	86%	69%	80%	100%
Surgical Infection Prevention					
Prophylactic Antibiotic Given[3]	76	63%	74%	77%	95%
Prophylactic Antibiotic Selection[1]	14	100%	88%	90%	100%
Prophylactic Antibiotic Stopped[3]	72	57%	68%	72%	95%
Pregnancy Care					
Inpatient Neonatal Mortality	-	-	-	-	-
Third or Fourth Degree Laceration	-	-	3.70%	3.63%	3.27%

Saint Joseph's Hospital & Medical Center

Alternate Name: Select Specialty Hospital
350 W Thomas Road
Phoenix, AZ 85013
URL: www.stjosephs-phx.org
Phone: 602-406-3000
Fax: 602-406-7143
Ownership: Voluntary non-profit - Church
Accredited: Yes
Emergency Services: Yes
Licensed Beds: 535

Key Personnel:

President/CEO. . . . . Linda Hunt
Head of Emergency Room. . . . . Kim Flannders
Director Emergency Department . . . . Julie Ward

Measure	Cases	This Hospital	State Average	U.S. Average	Top Hospital
Heart Attack Care					
ACE Inhibitor or ARB for LVSD	29	100%	83%	82%	100%
Aspirin at Arrival	112	97%	96%	92%	100%
Aspirin at Discharge	142	100%	91%	90%	100%
Beta Blocker at Arrival	96	97%	88%	87%	100%
Beta Blocker at Discharge	143	100%	93%	90%	100%
Fibrinolytic Medication Timing	0	-	10%	31%	100%
PCI Within 90 Minutes of Arrival[1]	7	71%	47%	54%	95%
Smoking Cessation Advice	66	100%	89%	88%	100%
Heart Failure Care					
ACE Inhibitor or ARB for LVSD	139	96%	81%	82%	100%
Discharge Instructions	244	81%	48%	61%	93%
Evaluation of LVS Function	272	99%	84%	83%	99%
Smoking Cessation Advice	66	98%	76%	82%	100%
Pneumonia Care					

NOTE: Hospital profiles are in alphabetical order by state, then city, then hospital within the city; Rankings are sorted by rate in descending order and exclude hospitals with less than 25 cases; (1) The number of cases is too small (n<25) for purposes of reliably predicting hospital performance; (2) Measure reflects the hospital's indication that its submission was based upon a sample of its relevant discharges; (3) Rate reflects fewer than the maximum possible quarters of data for the measure; (4) Inaccurate information submitted and suppressed for one or more quarters; (5) No data is available from the hospital for this measure; Please refer to the User's Guide for a full explanation of data

Measure	Cases	This Hospital	State Average	U.S. Average	Top Hospital
Appropriate Initial Antibiotic	142	94%	84%	83%	94%
Blood Culture Timing	119	88%	87%	90%	100%
Influenza Vaccine	34	82%	61%	70%	100%
Initial Antibiotic Timing	168	84%	73%	80%	93%
Oxygenation Assessment	219	100%	100%	99%	100%
Pneumococcal Vaccine	101	80%	64%	69%	94%
Smoking Cessation Advice	62	68%	69%	80%	100%
Surgical Infection Prevention					
Prophylactic Antibiotic Given[2,3]	149	70%	74%	77%	95%
Prophylactic Antibiotic Selection[2]	53	92%	88%	90%	100%
Prophylactic Antibiotic Stopped[2,3]	143	66%	68%	72%	95%
Pregnancy Care					
Inpatient Neonatal Mortality	6,028	1.01%	-	-	-
Third or Fourth Degree Laceration	4,116	2.11%	3.70%	3.63%	3.27%

Saint Luke's Medical Center

1800 E Van Buren
Phoenix, AZ 85006
URL: www.stlukesmedcenter.com
Ownership: Government - State
Emergency Services: No

Phone: 602-251-8100
Fax: 602-251-8761

Accredited: Yes
Licensed Beds: 235

Key Personnel:

CEO. . . . . J Neil Basset
Chief Medical Staff. . . . . Robert Kearl, MD
Chief Surgery. . . . . Darwin Zahn, MD
Emergency Room . . . . . David Leinen Veber
Infection Control. . . . . Tery Thuoite
ICU . . . . . Joesph Lotsko
Medical & Surgical Nursing . . . . . Colleen Wlookouiski

Measure	Cases	This Hospital	State Average	U.S. Average	Top Hospital
Heart Attack Care					
ACE Inhibitor or ARB for LVSD[1]	17	82%	83%	82%	100%
Aspirin at Arrival	44	89%	96%	92%	100%
Aspirin at Discharge	48	96%	91%	90%	100%
Beta Blocker at Arrival	26	92%	88%	87%	100%
Beta Blocker at Discharge	52	96%	93%	90%	100%
Fibrinolytic Medication Timing	0	-	10%	31%	100%
PCI Within 90 Minutes of Arrival[1]	1	0%	47%	54%	95%
Smoking Cessation Advice	26	88%	89%	88%	100%
Heart Failure Care					
ACE Inhibitor or ARB for LVSD	69	72%	81%	82%	100%
Discharge Instructions	113	31%	48%	61%	93%
Evaluation of LVS Function	129	94%	84%	83%	99%
Smoking Cessation Advice	41	73%	76%	82%	100%
Pneumonia Care					
Appropriate Initial Antibiotic	90	87%	84%	83%	94%
Blood Culture Timing	79	92%	87%	90%	100%
Influenza Vaccine[1]	19	58%	61%	70%	100%
Initial Antibiotic Timing	117	61%	73%	80%	93%
Oxygenation Assessment	139	100%	100%	99%	100%
Pneumococcal Vaccine	70	49%	64%	69%	94%
Smoking Cessation Advice	47	68%	69%	80%	100%
Surgical Infection Prevention					
Prophylactic Antibiotic Given[3]	145	47%	74%	77%	95%
Prophylactic Antibiotic Selection	50	72%	88%	90%	100%
Prophylactic Antibiotic Stopped[3]	139	34%	68%	72%	95%
Pregnancy Care					
Inpatient Neonatal Mortality	-	-	-	-	-
Third or Fourth Degree Laceration	-	-	3.70%	3.63%	3.27%

Hopi Health Care Center

PO Box 6000
Polacca, AZ 86042
Ownership: Government - Federal
Emergency Services: Yes

Phone: 928-737-6000

Accredited: Yes

Measure	Cases	This Hospital	State Average	U.S. Average	Top Hospital
Heart Attack Care					
ACE Inhibitor or ARB for LVSD[5]	-	-	83%	82%	100%
Aspirin at Arrival[5]	-	-	96%	92%	100%
Aspirin at Discharge[5]	-	-	91%	90%	100%
Beta Blocker at Arrival[5]	-	-	88%	87%	100%
Beta Blocker at Discharge[5]	-	-	93%	90%	100%
Fibrinolytic Medication Timing[5]	-	-	10%	31%	100%
PCI Within 90 Minutes of Arrival[5]	-	-	47%	54%	95%
Smoking Cessation Advice[5]	-	-	89%	88%	100%
Heart Failure Care					
ACE Inhibitor or ARB for LVSD[1]	4	100%	81%	82%	100%
Discharge Instructions[1]	6	0%	48%	61%	93%
Evaluation of LVS Function[1]	8	88%	84%	83%	99%
Smoking Cessation Advice[1]	1	100%	76%	82%	100%
Pneumonia Care					
Appropriate Initial Antibiotic	31	45%	84%	83%	94%
Blood Culture Timing[1]	16	94%	87%	90%	100%
Influenza Vaccine[1]	6	83%	61%	70%	100%
Initial Antibiotic Timing	32	94%	73%	80%	93%
Oxygenation Assessment	33	100%	100%	99%	100%
Pneumococcal Vaccine[1]	20	60%	64%	69%	94%
Smoking Cessation Advice[1]	2	0%	69%	80%	100%
Surgical Infection Prevention					
Prophylactic Antibiotic Given[5]	-	-	74%	77%	95%
Prophylactic Antibiotic Selection[5]	-	-	88%	90%	100%
Prophylactic Antibiotic Stopped[5]	-	-	68%	72%	95%
Pregnancy Care					
Inpatient Neonatal Mortality	-	-	-	-	-
Third or Fourth Degree Laceration	-	-	3.70%	3.63%	3.27%

Yavapai Regional Medical Center

1003 Willow Creek Road
Prescott, AZ 86301

Toll-Free: 877-843-9762
Phone: 928-445-2700
Fax: 928-771-5755

E-mail: webmaster@yrmc.org
URL: www.yrmc.org
Ownership: Voluntary non-profit - Other
Emergency Services: Yes

Accredited: Yes
Licensed Beds: 127

Key Personnel:

CEO. . . . . Timothy Barnett
Chief Medical Staff. . . . . DJ Patel, MD
Emergency Room . . . . . Judy Denton
Director Medical/Surgical Nursing . . . . . Donna Kennedy, RN
OB/GYN Womens Health. . . . . Wade Kartchner, MD
Chief Radiology . . . . . Warren Goodman, MD
Director Respiratory Therapy. . . . . Mike Martin

Measure	Cases	This Hospital	State Average	U.S. Average	Top Hospital
Heart Attack Care					
ACE Inhibitor or ARB for LVSD[1]	12	83%	83%	82%	100%
Aspirin at Arrival	122	97%	96%	92%	100%
Aspirin at Discharge	93	95%	91%	90%	100%
Beta Blocker at Arrival	106	92%	88%	87%	100%
Beta Blocker at Discharge	102	86%	93%	90%	100%
Fibrinolytic Medication Timing	0	-	10%	31%	100%
PCI Within 90 Minutes of Arrival[1]	3	67%	47%	54%	95%
Smoking Cessation Advice	27	96%	89%	88%	100%
Heart Failure Care					
ACE Inhibitor or ARB for LVSD[2]	97	84%	81%	82%	100%
Discharge Instructions[2]	239	61%	48%	61%	93%
Evaluation of LVS Function[2]	290	87%	84%	83%	99%
Smoking Cessation Advice[2]	52	85%	76%	82%	100%
Pneumonia Care					
Appropriate Initial Antibiotic[2]	146	86%	84%	83%	94%
Blood Culture Timing[2]	83	90%	87%	90%	100%
Influenza Vaccine[2]	30	70%	61%	70%	100%
Initial Antibiotic Timing[2]	186	76%	73%	80%	93%
Oxygenation Assessment[2]	213	100%	100%	99%	100%
Pneumococcal Vaccine[2]	138	78%	64%	69%	94%
Smoking Cessation Advice[2]	46	87%	69%	80%	100%
Surgical Infection Prevention					
Prophylactic Antibiotic Given[2,3]	246	91%	74%	77%	95%
Prophylactic Antibiotic Selection[2]	58	98%	88%	90%	100%
Prophylactic Antibiotic Stopped[2,3]	226	69%	68%	72%	95%
Pregnancy Care					
Inpatient Neonatal Mortality	1,378	0.22%	-	-	-
Third or Fourth Degree Laceration	896	5.47%	3.70%	3.63%	3.27%

NOTE: Hospital profiles are in alphabetical order by state, then city, then hospital within the city; Rankings are sorted by rate in descending order and exclude hospitals with less than 25 cases; (1) The number of cases is too small (n<25) for purposes of reliably predicting hospital performance; (2) Measure reflects the hospital's indication that its submission was based upon a sample of its relevant discharges; (3) Rate reflects fewer than the maximum possible quarters of data for the measure; (4) Inaccurate information submitted and suppressed for one or more quarters; (5) No data is available from the hospital for this measure; Please refer to the User's Guide for a full explanation of data

Yavapai Regional Medical Center-East

7700 East Florentine Road
Prescott Valley, AZ 86314
Phone: 928-442-8165
Ownership: Voluntary non-profit - Private
Accredited: No
Emergency Services: Yes

Measure	Cases	This Hospital	State Average	U.S. Average	Top Hospital
Heart Attack Care					
ACE Inhibitor or ARB for LVSD[3]	0	-	83%	82%	100%
Aspirin at Arrival[3]	0	-	96%	92%	100%
Aspirin at Discharge[3]	0	-	91%	90%	100%
Beta Blocker at Arrival[3]	0	-	88%	87%	100%
Beta Blocker at Discharge[1,3]	1	100%	93%	90%	100%
Fibrinolytic Medication Timing[3]	0	-	10%	31%	100%
PCI Within 90 Minutes of Arrival	0	-	47%	54%	95%
Smoking Cessation Advice[3]	0	-	89%	88%	100%
Heart Failure Care					
ACE Inhibitor or ARB for LVSD[1,3]	4	25%	81%	82%	100%
Discharge Instructions[1,3]	10	40%	48%	61%	93%
Evaluation of LVS Function[1,3]	11	91%	84%	83%	99%
Smoking Cessation Advice[1,3]	1	0%	76%	82%	100%
Pneumonia Care					
Appropriate Initial Antibiotic[3]	26	85%	84%	83%	94%
Blood Culture Timing[1,3]	17	94%	87%	90%	100%
Influenza Vaccine[5]	-	-	61%	70%	100%
Initial Antibiotic Timing[3]	28	86%	73%	80%	93%
Oxygenation Assessment[3]	33	100%	100%	99%	100%
Pneumococcal Vaccine[1,3]	22	77%	64%	69%	94%
Smoking Cessation Advice[1,3]	7	71%	69%	80%	100%
Surgical Infection Prevention					
Prophylactic Antibiotic Given[1,2,3]	23	70%	74%	77%	95%
Prophylactic Antibiotic Selection[5]	-	-	88%	90%	100%
Prophylactic Antibiotic Stopped[1,2,3]	23	26%	68%	72%	95%
Pregnancy Care					
Inpatient Neonatal Mortality	-	-	-	-	-
Third or Fourth Degree Laceration	-	-	3.70%	3.63%	3.27%

Mount Graham Regional Medical Center

1600 20th Avenue
Safford, AZ 85546
Phone: 928-348-4000
Fax: 928-348-5701
URL: www.mtgraham.org
Ownership: Govt - Hospital District or Authority
Accredited: No
Emergency Services: No
Licensed Beds: 59

Key Personnel:

CEO. . . . . Pat O'Brien
Chief Medical Staff. . . . . Drew Christensen, MD
Emergency Room . . . . Debbie Cherry, RN
Director Medical/Surgical Nursing . . . . Katrina Pearsson
Chief Radiology . . . . Zane Kartchner, MD
Director Respiratory Therapy . . . . Eric Gibbons

Measure	Cases	This Hospital	State Average	U.S. Average	Top Hospital
Heart Attack Care					
ACE Inhibitor or ARB for LVSD[3]	0	-	83%	82%	100%
Aspirin at Arrival[1,3]	1	100%	96%	92%	100%
Aspirin at Discharge[3]	0	-	91%	90%	100%
Beta Blocker at Arrival[3]	0	-	88%	87%	100%
Beta Blocker at Discharge[3]	0	-	93%	90%	100%
Fibrinolytic Medication Timing[3]	0	-	10%	31%	100%
PCI Within 90 Minutes of Arrival	0	-	47%	54%	95%
Smoking Cessation Advice[3]	0	-	89%	88%	100%
Heart Failure Care					
ACE Inhibitor or ARB for LVSD[1]	7	29%	81%	82%	100%
Discharge Instructions[1]	24	4%	48%	61%	93%
Evaluation of LVS Function[1]	24	67%	84%	83%	99%
Smoking Cessation Advice[1]	3	100%	76%	82%	100%
Pneumonia Care					
Appropriate Initial Antibiotic	92	67%	84%	83%	94%
Blood Culture Timing	38	76%	87%	90%	100%
Influenza Vaccine[4,5]	-	-	61%	70%	100%
Initial Antibiotic Timing	94	55%	73%	80%	93%
Oxygenation Assessment	125	100%	100%	99%	100%
Pneumococcal Vaccine	77	69%	64%	69%	94%
Smoking Cessation Advice	26	73%	69%	80%	100%
Surgical Infection Prevention					
Prophylactic Antibiotic Given	114	71%	74%	77%	95%
Prophylactic Antibiotic Selection[1]	21	100%	88%	90%	100%
Prophylactic Antibiotic Stopped	112	94%	68%	72%	95%
Pregnancy Care					
Inpatient Neonatal Mortality	-	-	-	-	-
Third or Fourth Degree Laceration	-	-	3.70%	3.63%	3.27%

PHS Indian Hospital-San Carlos

PO Box 208
San Carlos, AZ 85550
Phone: 928-475-2371
Ownership: Government - Federal
Accredited: Yes
Emergency Services: Yes

Measure	Cases	This Hospital	State Average	U.S. Average	Top Hospital
Heart Attack Care					
ACE Inhibitor or ARB for LVSD[5]	-	-	83%	82%	100%
Aspirin at Arrival[5]	-	-	96%	92%	100%
Aspirin at Discharge[5]	-	-	91%	90%	100%
Beta Blocker at Arrival[5]	-	-	88%	87%	100%
Beta Blocker at Discharge[5]	-	-	93%	90%	100%
Fibrinolytic Medication Timing[5]	-	-	10%	31%	100%
PCI Within 90 Minutes of Arrival[5]	-	-	47%	54%	95%
Smoking Cessation Advice[5]	-	-	89%	88%	100%
Heart Failure Care					
ACE Inhibitor or ARB for LVSD[3]	0	-	81%	82%	100%
Discharge Instructions[1,3]	1	0%	48%	61%	93%
Evaluation of LVS Function[1,3]	1	100%	84%	83%	99%
Smoking Cessation Advice[3]	0	-	76%	82%	100%
Pneumonia Care					
Appropriate Initial Antibiotic	41	88%	84%	83%	94%
Blood Culture Timing[1]	20	70%	87%	90%	100%
Influenza Vaccine[4,5]	-	-	61%	70%	100%
Initial Antibiotic Timing	41	85%	73%	80%	93%
Oxygenation Assessment	44	100%	100%	99%	100%
Pneumococcal Vaccine[1]	15	87%	64%	69%	94%
Smoking Cessation Advice[1]	4	0%	69%	80%	100%
Surgical Infection Prevention					
Prophylactic Antibiotic Given[5]	-	-	74%	77%	95%
Prophylactic Antibiotic Selection[5]	-	-	88%	90%	100%
Prophylactic Antibiotic Stopped[5]	-	-	68%	72%	95%
Pregnancy Care					
Inpatient Neonatal Mortality	-	-	-	-	-
Third or Fourth Degree Laceration	-	-	3.70%	3.63%	3.27%

Scottsdale Healthcare

Alternate Name: Scottsdale Memorial Hospital-North
9003 E Shea Boulevard
Scottsdale, AZ 85260
Phone: 480-860-3000
Fax: 480-860-3510
URL: www.shc.org
Ownership: Proprietary
Accredited: Yes
Emergency Services: Yes
Licensed Beds: 343

Key Personnel:

Chief Medical Staff. . . . . James Burke, MD
Emergency Room . . . . Mary Kopp, RN
OB/GYN Womens Health. . . . . Ken Welch, MD
Director Radiology . . . . Julie Hughes
Manager Respiratory Therapy . . . . Henry Fronczak

Measure	Cases	This Hospital	State Average	U.S. Average	Top Hospital
Heart Attack Care					
ACE Inhibitor or ARB for LVSD	51	78%	83%	82%	100%
Aspirin at Arrival	245	97%	96%	92%	100%
Aspirin at Discharge	233	97%	91%	90%	100%
Beta Blocker at Arrival	171	92%	88%	87%	100%
Beta Blocker at Discharge	238	98%	93%	90%	100%
Fibrinolytic Medication Timing	0	-	10%	31%	100%
PCI Within 90 Minutes of Arrival[1]	6	83%	47%	54%	95%
Smoking Cessation Advice	53	100%	89%	88%	100%
Heart Failure Care					

NOTE: Hospital profiles are in alphabetical order by state, then city, then hospital within the city; Rankings are sorted by rate in descending order and exclude hospitals with less than 25 cases; (1) The number of cases is too small (n<25) for purposes of reliably predicting hospital performance; (2) Measure reflects the hospital's indication that its submission was based upon a sample of its relevant discharges; (3) Rate reflects fewer than the maximum possible quarters of data for the measure; (4) Inaccurate information submitted and suppressed for one or more quarters; (5) No data is available from the hospital for this measure; Please refer to the User's Guide for a full explanation of data

ACE Inhibitor or ARB for LVSD[2]	189	69%	81%	82%	100%
Discharge Instructions[2]	347	61%	48%	61%	93%
Evaluation of LVS Function[2]	418	93%	84%	83%	99%
Smoking Cessation Advice[2]	43	95%	76%	82%	100%
Pneumonia Care					
Appropriate Initial Antibiotic[2]	289	91%	84%	83%	94%
Blood Culture Timing[2]	271	88%	87%	90%	100%
Influenza Vaccine	107	64%	61%	70%	100%
Initial Antibiotic Timing[2]	353	84%	73%	80%	93%
Oxygenation Assessment[2]	465	100%	100%	99%	100%
Pneumococcal Vaccine[2]	301	78%	64%	69%	94%
Smoking Cessation Advice[2]	66	95%	69%	80%	100%
Surgical Infection Prevention					
Prophylactic Antibiotic Given[2,3]	87	59%	74%	77%	95%
Prophylactic Antibiotic Selection[2]	84	79%	88%	90%	100%
Prophylactic Antibiotic Stopped[2,3]	82	66%	68%	72%	95%
Pregnancy Care					
Inpatient Neonatal Mortality	-	-	-	-	-
Third or Fourth Degree Laceration	-	-	3.70%	3.63%	3.27%

Scottsdale Healthcare-Osborn

7400 E Osborn Road
Scottsdale, AZ 85251
URL: www.shc.org
Ownership: Proprietary
Emergency Services: Yes

Phone: 480-882-4000
Fax: 480-882-4989

Accredited: Yes
Licensed Beds: 337

Key Personnel:

President/CEO. . . . . Thomas J Sadvary
Emergency Room . . . . Linda Ott, RN
Chief Medical Officer . . . . Jeff Burke
Supervisor of Respiratory. . . . . Nancy Hibbert

Measure	Cases	This Hospital	State Average	U.S. Average	Top Hospital
Heart Attack Care					
ACE Inhibitor or ARB for LVSD	47	81%	83%	82%	100%
Aspirin at Arrival	243	95%	96%	92%	100%
Aspirin at Discharge	218	98%	91%	90%	100%
Beta Blocker at Arrival	165	93%	88%	87%	100%
Beta Blocker at Discharge	226	98%	93%	90%	100%
Fibrinolytic Medication Timing	0	-	10%	31%	100%
PCI Within 90 Minutes of Arrival[1]	8	25%	47%	54%	95%
Smoking Cessation Advice	79	100%	89%	88%	100%
Heart Failure Care					
ACE Inhibitor or ARB for LVSD[2]	173	82%	81%	82%	100%
Discharge Instructions[2]	363	55%	48%	61%	93%
Evaluation of LVS Function[2]	432	95%	84%	83%	99%
Smoking Cessation Advice[2]	74	100%	76%	82%	100%
Pneumonia Care					
Appropriate Initial Antibiotic[2]	253	89%	84%	83%	94%
Blood Culture Timing[2]	258	90%	87%	90%	100%
Influenza Vaccine	110	57%	61%	70%	100%
Initial Antibiotic Timing[2]	346	84%	73%	80%	93%
Oxygenation Assessment[2]	457	100%	100%	99%	100%
Pneumococcal Vaccine[2]	310	79%	64%	69%	94%
Smoking Cessation Advice[2]	85	98%	69%	80%	100%
Surgical Infection Prevention					
Prophylactic Antibiotic Given[2,3]	73	89%	74%	77%	95%
Prophylactic Antibiotic Selection[2]	75	75%	88%	90%	100%
Prophylactic Antibiotic Stopped[2,3]	69	41%	68%	72%	95%
Pregnancy Care					
Inpatient Neonatal Mortality	-	-	-	-	-
Third or Fourth Degree Laceration	-	-	3.70%	3.63%	3.27%

Sells Indian Hospital

Alternate Name: PHS Indian Hospital
Highway 86 and Taopwa Road
Sells, AZ 85634
Ownership: Government - Federal
Emergency Services: Yes

Phone: 520-383-7251
Fax: 520-383-7216
Accredited: Yes
Licensed Beds: 34

Key Personnel:

CEO. . . . . Priscilla Whitethorne
Chief Medical Staff. . . . . Lois Steele
Chief of Medical Staff . . . . Peter Zigler
Head of Emergency Room. . . . . Ernie Reyes
Emergency Room . . . . Cantace Chapirl

Measure	Cases	This Hospital	State Average	U.S. Average	Top Hospital
Heart Attack Care					
ACE Inhibitor or ARB for LVSD[5]	-	-	83%	82%	100%
Aspirin at Arrival[5]	-	-	96%	92%	100%
Aspirin at Discharge[5]	-	-	91%	90%	100%
Beta Blocker at Arrival[5]	-	-	88%	87%	100%
Beta Blocker at Discharge[5]	-	-	93%	90%	100%
Fibrinolytic Medication Timing[5]	-	-	10%	31%	100%
PCI Within 90 Minutes of Arrival[5]	-	-	47%	54%	95%
Smoking Cessation Advice[5]	-	-	89%	88%	100%
Heart Failure Care					
ACE Inhibitor or ARB for LVSD[3]	0	-	81%	82%	100%
Discharge Instructions[3]	0	-	48%	61%	93%
Evaluation of LVS Function[1,3]	7	0%	84%	83%	99%
Smoking Cessation Advice[3]	0	-	76%	82%	100%
Pneumonia Care					
Appropriate Initial Antibiotic[1,3]	4	50%	84%	83%	94%
Blood Culture Timing[1,3]	4	100%	87%	90%	100%
Influenza Vaccine[5]	-	-	61%	70%	100%
Initial Antibiotic Timing[1]	22	82%	73%	80%	93%
Oxygenation Assessment	32	100%	100%	99%	100%
Pneumococcal Vaccine[1]	11	0%	64%	69%	94%
Smoking Cessation Advice[3]	0	-	69%	80%	100%
Surgical Infection Prevention					
Prophylactic Antibiotic Given[5]	-	-	74%	77%	95%
Prophylactic Antibiotic Selection[5]	-	-	88%	90%	100%
Prophylactic Antibiotic Stopped[5]	-	-	68%	72%	95%
Pregnancy Care					
Inpatient Neonatal Mortality	-	-	-	-	-
Third or Fourth Degree Laceration	-	-	3.70%	3.63%	3.27%

Navapache Regional Medical Center

2200 Show Low Lake Road
Show Low, AZ 85901
URL: www.nrmc.org
Ownership: Voluntary non-profit - Private
Emergency Services: Yes

Phone: 928-537-4375
Fax: 928-537-8839

Accredited: No

Key Personnel:

CEO. . . . . Leigh Cox
Director of Obstetrics . . . . Shelly Lanagan, RN
Surgery Department. . . . . Thia Ebert

Measure	Cases	This Hospital	State Average	U.S. Average	Top Hospital
Heart Attack Care					
ACE Inhibitor or ARB for LVSD[1]	4	100%	83%	82%	100%
Aspirin at Arrival	41	95%	96%	92%	100%
Aspirin at Discharge	34	100%	91%	90%	100%
Beta Blocker at Arrival[1]	20	90%	88%	87%	100%
Beta Blocker at Discharge	30	93%	93%	90%	100%
Fibrinolytic Medication Timing[1]	6	0%	10%	31%	100%
PCI Within 90 Minutes of Arrival[1]	1	0%	47%	54%	95%
Smoking Cessation Advice[1]	18	83%	89%	88%	100%
Heart Failure Care					
ACE Inhibitor or ARB for LVSD[1]	18	89%	81%	82%	100%
Discharge Instructions	68	13%	48%	61%	93%
Evaluation of LVS Function	73	85%	84%	83%	99%
Smoking Cessation Advice[1]	14	71%	76%	82%	100%
Pneumonia Care					
Appropriate Initial Antibiotic	128	93%	84%	83%	94%
Blood Culture Timing	83	92%	87%	90%	100%
Influenza Vaccine[1]	23	57%	61%	70%	100%
Initial Antibiotic Timing	152	75%	73%	80%	93%
Oxygenation Assessment	168	100%	100%	99%	100%
Pneumococcal Vaccine	78	68%	64%	69%	94%
Smoking Cessation Advice	33	88%	69%	80%	100%
Surgical Infection Prevention					
Prophylactic Antibiotic Given	159	75%	74%	77%	95%
Prophylactic Antibiotic Selection	41	98%	88%	90%	100%
Prophylactic Antibiotic Stopped	158	34%	68%	72%	95%

NOTE: Hospital profiles are in alphabetical order by state, then city, then hospital within the city; Rankings are sorted by rate in descending order and exclude hospitals with less than 25 cases; (1) The number of cases is too small (n<25) for purposes of reliably predicting hospital performance; (2) Measure reflects the hospital's indication that its submission was based upon a sample of its relevant discharges; (3) Rate reflects fewer than the maximum possible quarters of data for the measure; (4) Inaccurate information submitted and suppressed for one or more quarters; (5) No data is available from the hospital for this measure; Please refer to the User's Guide for a full explanation of data

Pregnancy Care					
Inpatient Neonatal Mortality	-	-	-	-	-
Third or Fourth Degree Laceration	-	-	3.70%	3.63%	3.27%

Sierra Vista Regional Health Center

300 El Camino Real
Sierra Vista, AZ 85635

Toll-Free: 800-880-0088
Phone: 520-458-4641
Fax: 520-458-2268

E-mail: admin@szch.com
URL: www.svch.com
Ownership: Voluntary non-profit - Other
Emergency Services: Yes
Accredited: Yes
Licensed Beds: 86

Key Personnel:
President/CEO. . . . . Margaret Hepburn
Department Chair Surgery . . . . Raul Monzon
Director of Pulmonary/Respiratory Care. . . . . . . Craig Haris

Measure	Cases	This Hospital	State Average	U.S. Average	Top Hospital
Heart Attack Care					
ACE Inhibitor or ARB for LVSD[1]	6	83%	83%	82%	100%
Aspirin at Arrival	77	94%	96%	92%	100%
Aspirin at Discharge	29	66%	91%	90%	100%
Beta Blocker at Arrival	74	88%	88%	87%	100%
Beta Blocker at Discharge	33	79%	93%	90%	100%
Fibrinolytic Medication Timing[1]	2	50%	10%	31%	100%
PCI Within 90 Minutes of Arrival	0	-	47%	54%	95%
Smoking Cessation Advice[1]	9	56%	89%	88%	100%
Heart Failure Care					
ACE Inhibitor or ARB for LVSD	28	75%	81%	82%	100%
Discharge Instructions	80	16%	48%	61%	93%
Evaluation of LVS Function	106	85%	84%	83%	99%
Smoking Cessation Advice[1]	17	71%	76%	82%	100%
Pneumonia Care					
Appropriate Initial Antibiotic	131	86%	84%	83%	94%
Blood Culture Timing	70	91%	87%	90%	100%
Influenza Vaccine	27	70%	61%	70%	100%
Initial Antibiotic Timing	141	70%	73%	80%	93%
Oxygenation Assessment	168	99%	100%	99%	100%
Pneumococcal Vaccine	99	65%	64%	69%	94%
Smoking Cessation Advice	42	71%	69%	80%	100%
Surgical Infection Prevention					
Prophylactic Antibiotic Given[2]	347	82%	74%	77%	95%
Prophylactic Antibiotic Selection[2]	74	95%	88%	90%	100%
Prophylactic Antibiotic Stopped[2]	332	61%	68%	72%	95%
Pregnancy Care					
Inpatient Neonatal Mortality	-	-	-	-	-
Third or Fourth Degree Laceration	-	-	3.70%	3.63%	3.27%

White Mountain Regional Medical Center

Alternate Name: White Mountain Communities Hospital
118 South Mountain Avenue
Springerville, AZ 85938

Phone: 928-333-4368
Fax: 928-333-4369

E-mail: info@wmrmc.com
URL: www.wmrmc.com
Ownership: Voluntary non-profit - Private
Emergency Services: Yes
Accredited: No
Licensed Beds: 16

Key Personnel:
President . . . . Darlene West
CEO. . . . . Ann Coleman-Hall
Chief Medical Staff. . . . . Scott Hamblin, MD
Infection Control. . . . . Jennifer Belisle
Director Respiratory Therapy . . . . Rogenia Dunn

Measure	Cases	This Hospital	State Average	U.S. Average	Top Hospital
Heart Attack Care					
ACE Inhibitor or ARB for LVSD[3]	0	-	83%	82%	100%
Aspirin at Arrival[1,3]	2	100%	96%	92%	100%
Aspirin at Discharge[1,3]	2	50%	91%	90%	100%
Beta Blocker at Arrival[1,3]	3	67%	88%	87%	100%
Beta Blocker at Discharge[1,3]	2	100%	93%	90%	100%
Fibrinolytic Medication Timing[5]	-	-	10%	31%	100%
PCI Within 90 Minutes of Arrival[5]	-	-	47%	54%	95%
Smoking Cessation Advice[5]	-	-	89%	88%	100%
Heart Failure Care					
ACE Inhibitor or ARB for LVSD[1]	3	100%	81%	82%	100%
Discharge Instructions[1,3]	4	25%	48%	61%	93%
Evaluation of LVS Function	28	71%	84%	83%	99%
Smoking Cessation Advice[1,3]	2	0%	76%	82%	100%
Pneumonia Care					
Appropriate Initial Antibiotic[1,3]	5	80%	84%	83%	94%
Blood Culture Timing[1,3]	2	100%	87%	90%	100%
Influenza Vaccine[5]	-	-	61%	70%	100%
Initial Antibiotic Timing	33	79%	73%	80%	93%
Oxygenation Assessment	38	100%	100%	99%	100%
Pneumococcal Vaccine[1]	22	36%	64%	69%	94%
Smoking Cessation Advice[1,3]	2	50%	69%	80%	100%
Surgical Infection Prevention					
Prophylactic Antibiotic Given[5]	-	-	74%	77%	95%
Prophylactic Antibiotic Selection[5]	-	-	88%	90%	100%
Prophylactic Antibiotic Stopped[5]	-	-	68%	72%	95%
Pregnancy Care					
Inpatient Neonatal Mortality	-	-	-	-	-
Third or Fourth Degree Laceration	-	-	3.70%	3.63%	3.27%

Sun Health Boswell Hospital

10401 W Thunderbird Blvd
Sun City, AZ 85351

Toll-Free: 800-815-0115
Phone: 623-977-7211
Fax: 623-876-5795

URL: www.sunhealth.org
Ownership: Voluntary non-profit - Private
Emergency Services: Yes
Accredited: Yes
Licensed Beds: 323

Key Personnel:
CEO. . . . . George Perez
Chief Radiology . . . . Robert Charney
Director Respiratory Therapy . . . . Penny Schmiege

Measure	Cases	This Hospital	State Average	U.S. Average	Top Hospital
Heart Attack Care					
ACE Inhibitor or ARB for LVSD[2]	66	64%	83%	82%	100%
Aspirin at Arrival[2]	193	94%	96%	92%	100%
Aspirin at Discharge[2]	201	95%	91%	90%	100%
Beta Blocker at Arrival[2]	121	88%	88%	87%	100%
Beta Blocker at Discharge[2]	229	96%	93%	90%	100%
Fibrinolytic Medication Timing[1,2]	2	50%	10%	31%	100%
PCI Within 90 Minutes of Arrival[1,2]	5	20%	47%	54%	95%
Smoking Cessation Advice[2]	45	89%	89%	88%	100%
Heart Failure Care					
ACE Inhibitor or ARB for LVSD[2]	129	65%	81%	82%	100%
Discharge Instructions[2]	231	24%	48%	61%	93%
Evaluation of LVS Function[2]	294	92%	84%	83%	99%
Smoking Cessation Advice[2]	29	66%	76%	82%	100%
Pneumonia Care					
Appropriate Initial Antibiotic[2]	88	94%	84%	83%	94%
Blood Culture Timing[2]	88	97%	87%	90%	100%
Influenza Vaccine[2]	25	48%	61%	70%	100%
Initial Antibiotic Timing[2]	141	65%	73%	80%	93%
Oxygenation Assessment[2]	172	100%	100%	99%	100%
Pneumococcal Vaccine[2]	138	58%	64%	69%	94%
Smoking Cessation Advice[1,2]	19	74%	69%	80%	100%
Surgical Infection Prevention					
Prophylactic Antibiotic Given[2]	280	86%	74%	77%	95%
Prophylactic Antibiotic Selection[5]	-	-	88%	90%	100%
Prophylactic Antibiotic Stopped[2]	272	46%	68%	72%	95%
Pregnancy Care					
Inpatient Neonatal Mortality	-	-	-	-	-
Third or Fourth Degree Laceration	-	-	3.70%	3.63%	3.27%

Del E Webb Memorial Hospital

Alternate Name: Webb Memorial Hospital
14502 W Meeker Boulevard
Sun City West, AZ 85375

Phone: 623-214-4000
Fax: 623-214-4105

URL: www.sunhealth.org
Ownership: Voluntary non-profit - Private
Emergency Services: Yes
Accredited: Yes
Licensed Beds: 235

Key Personnel:
CEO. . . . . Thomas Dickson

NOTE: Hospital profiles are in alphabetical order by state, then city, then hospital within the city; Rankings are sorted by rate in descending order and exclude hospitals with less than 25 cases; (1) The number of cases is too small (n<25) for purposes of reliably predicting hospital performance; (2) Measure reflects the hospital's indication that its submission was based upon a sample of its relevant discharges; (3) Rate reflects fewer than the maximum possible quarters of data for the measure; (4) Inaccurate information submitted and suppressed for one or more quarters; (5) No data is available from the hospital for this measure; Please refer to the User's Guide for a full explanation of data

Chief Medical Staff. . . . . Steven Charney, MD
Emergency Room . . . . Corlean Kuhl

Measure	Cases	This Hospital	State Average	U.S. Average	Top Hospital
Heart Attack Care					
ACE Inhibitor or ARB for LVSD[1,2]	14	86%	83%	82%	100%
Aspirin at Arrival[2]	227	98%	96%	92%	100%
Aspirin at Discharge[2]	175	96%	91%	90%	100%
Beta Blocker at Arrival[2]	167	98%	88%	87%	100%
Beta Blocker at Discharge[2]	168	98%	93%	90%	100%
Fibrinolytic Medication Timing[2]	0	-	10%	31%	100%
PCI Within 90 Minutes of Arrival[1,2]	5	100%	47%	54%	95%
Smoking Cessation Advice[2]	30	97%	89%	88%	100%
Heart Failure Care					
ACE Inhibitor or ARB for LVSD[2]	120	69%	81%	82%	100%
Discharge Instructions[2]	209	23%	48%	61%	93%
Evaluation of LVS Function[2]	268	88%	84%	83%	99%
Smoking Cessation Advice[1,2]	20	70%	76%	82%	100%
Pneumonia Care					
Appropriate Initial Antibiotic[2]	96	90%	84%	83%	94%
Blood Culture Timing[2]	81	94%	87%	90%	100%
Influenza Vaccine[1,2]	23	43%	61%	70%	100%
Initial Antibiotic Timing[2]	140	77%	73%	80%	93%
Oxygenation Assessment[2]	167	100%	100%	99%	100%
Pneumococcal Vaccine[2]	124	60%	64%	69%	94%
Smoking Cessation Advice[2]	25	76%	69%	80%	100%
Surgical Infection Prevention					
Prophylactic Antibiotic Given[2]	168	79%	74%	77%	95%
Prophylactic Antibiotic Selection[2]	48	88%	88%	90%	100%
Prophylactic Antibiotic Stopped[2]	158	42%	68%	72%	95%
Pregnancy Care					
Inpatient Neonatal Mortality	1,951	0.10%	-	-	-
Third or Fourth Degree Laceration	1,409	2.20%	3.70%	3.63%	3.27%

Tempe Saint Luke's Hospital

1500 S Mill Avenue
Tempe, AZ 85281
Phone: 480-784-5500
Fax: 480-784-5539
URL: www.tempestlukeshospital.com
Ownership: Proprietary
Accredited: Yes
Emergency Services: Yes
Licensed Beds: 110

Key Personnel:

CEO. . . . . Kevin Stockton
Chief Medical Staff. . . . . James E Gerace, MD
Emergency Room . . . . Debra Wagner, RN
ICU . . . . Jamie McFarland
OB/GYN Womens Health. . . . . Farshad Agahi, MD
Chief Radiology . . . . Ron Christianson, MD
Director Respiratory Therapy . . . . Nancy Henderson, RN

Measure	Cases	This Hospital	State Average	U.S. Average	Top Hospital
Heart Attack Care					
ACE Inhibitor or ARB for LVSD[1]	4	50%	83%	82%	100%
Aspirin at Arrival	33	97%	96%	92%	100%
Aspirin at Discharge[1]	12	67%	91%	90%	100%
Beta Blocker at Arrival	32	75%	88%	87%	100%
Beta Blocker at Discharge[1]	12	83%	93%	90%	100%
Fibrinolytic Medication Timing[1]	1	0%	10%	31%	100%
PCI Within 90 Minutes of Arrival	0	-	47%	54%	95%
Smoking Cessation Advice[1]	3	33%	89%	88%	100%
Heart Failure Care					
ACE Inhibitor or ARB for LVSD	32	75%	81%	82%	100%
Discharge Instructions	112	12%	48%	61%	93%
Evaluation of LVS Function	127	82%	84%	83%	99%
Smoking Cessation Advice	30	33%	76%	82%	100%
Pneumonia Care					
Appropriate Initial Antibiotic	149	76%	84%	83%	94%
Blood Culture Timing	47	77%	87%	90%	100%
Influenza Vaccine[1]	19	53%	61%	70%	100%
Initial Antibiotic Timing	148	63%	73%	80%	93%
Oxygenation Assessment	163	99%	100%	99%	100%
Pneumococcal Vaccine	69	41%	64%	69%	94%
Smoking Cessation Advice	48	44%	69%	80%	100%
Surgical Infection Prevention					
Prophylactic Antibiotic Given[3]	30	7%	74%	77%	95%
Prophylactic Antibiotic Selection[1]	9	78%	88%	90%	100%
Prophylactic Antibiotic Stopped[1,3]	24	92%	68%	72%	95%
Pregnancy Care					
Inpatient Neonatal Mortality	-	-	-	-	-
Third or Fourth Degree Laceration	-	-	3.70%	3.63%	3.27%

Tuba City Indian Medical Center

167 North Main Street
PO Box 610
Tuba City, AZ 86045
Phone: 928-283-2501
Fax: 928-283-2516
E-mail: contacat@tcrhcc.org/
URL: www.tcrhcc.org
Ownership: Government - Federal
Accredited: Yes
Emergency Services: Yes
Licensed Beds: 65

Key Personnel:

CEO. . . . . Joseph T Engelken
Chief of Medical Staff. . . . . Steve Xolve
OB/GYN Womens Health. . . . . Holly Van Dyke, MD
Respiratory Care . . . . David Errikson

Measure	Cases	This Hospital	State Average	U.S. Average	Top Hospital
Heart Attack Care					
ACE Inhibitor or ARB for LVSD[3]	0	-	83%	82%	100%
Aspirin at Arrival[3]	0	-	96%	92%	100%
Aspirin at Discharge[1,3]	1	0%	91%	90%	100%
Beta Blocker at Arrival[3]	0	-	88%	87%	100%
Beta Blocker at Discharge[1,3]	1	0%	93%	90%	100%
Fibrinolytic Medication Timing[3]	0	-	10%	31%	100%
PCI Within 90 Minutes of Arrival	0	-	47%	54%	95%
Smoking Cessation Advice[3]	0	-	89%	88%	100%
Heart Failure Care					
ACE Inhibitor or ARB for LVSD	28	75%	81%	82%	100%
Discharge Instructions	36	0%	48%	61%	93%
Evaluation of LVS Function	36	97%	84%	83%	99%
Smoking Cessation Advice[1]	2	0%	76%	82%	100%
Pneumonia Care					
Appropriate Initial Antibiotic	79	77%	84%	83%	94%
Blood Culture Timing	54	91%	87%	90%	100%
Influenza Vaccine	27	93%	61%	70%	100%
Initial Antibiotic Timing	85	82%	73%	80%	93%
Oxygenation Assessment	98	100%	100%	99%	100%
Pneumococcal Vaccine	71	85%	64%	69%	94%
Smoking Cessation Advice	0	-	69%	80%	100%
Surgical Infection Prevention					
Prophylactic Antibiotic Given[1,3]	9	67%	74%	77%	95%
Prophylactic Antibiotic Selection[1]	3	100%	88%	90%	100%
Prophylactic Antibiotic Stopped[1,3]	8	100%	68%	72%	95%
Pregnancy Care					
Inpatient Neonatal Mortality[2]	498	0.00%	-	-	-
Third or Fourth Degree Laceration[2]	399	1.50%	3.70%	3.63%	3.27%

Carondelet Saint Joseph's Hospital

350 N Wilmot Road
Tucson, AZ 85711
Phone: 520-873-3000
Fax: 520-873-3921
URL: www.carondelet.org
Ownership: Voluntary non-profit - Church
Accredited: Yes
Emergency Services: Yes
Licensed Beds: 309

Key Personnel:

CEO. . . . . Greg Angle
Director Emergency Services. . . . . Maggie McClellan
Manager Emergency Room . . . . Karri Mcglone, RN
Chief Medical Officer . . . . Jose Santiago
DirectorOB/GYN Womens Health . . . . Diann Neal
Director Radiology . . . . Fred Swiderski
Manager Respiratory Therapy . . . . Greg Hermann

Measure	Cases	This Hospital	State Average	U.S. Average	Top Hospital
Heart Attack Care					
ACE Inhibitor or ARB for LVSD	35	89%	83%	82%	100%
Aspirin at Arrival	174	98%	96%	92%	100%

NOTE: Hospital profiles are in alphabetical order by state, then city, then hospital within the city; Rankings are sorted by rate in descending order and exclude hospitals with less than 25 cases; (1) The number of cases is too small (n<25) for purposes of reliably predicting hospital performance; (2) Measure reflects the hospital's indication that its submission was based upon a sample of its relevant discharges; (3) Rate reflects fewer than the maximum possible quarters of data for the measure; (4) Inaccurate information submitted and suppressed for one or more quarters; (5) No data is available from the hospital for this measure; Please refer to the User's Guide for a full explanation of data

Aspirin at Discharge	167	98%	91%	90%	100%
Beta Blocker at Arrival	135	96%	88%	87%	100%
Beta Blocker at Discharge	160	98%	93%	90%	100%
Fibrinolytic Medication Timing[1]	2	0%	10%	31%	100%
PCI Within 90 Minutes of Arrival[1]	13	77%	47%	54%	95%
Smoking Cessation Advice	66	100%	89%	88%	100%
Heart Failure Care					
ACE Inhibitor or ARB for LVSD	102	88%	81%	82%	100%
Discharge Instructions	233	94%	48%	61%	93%
Evaluation of LVS Function	281	96%	84%	83%	99%
Smoking Cessation Advice	36	92%	76%	82%	100%
Pneumonia Care					
Appropriate Initial Antibiotic	317	89%	84%	83%	94%
Blood Culture Timing	308	82%	87%	90%	100%
Influenza Vaccine[4,5]	-	-	61%	70%	100%
Initial Antibiotic Timing	388	80%	73%	80%	93%
Oxygenation Assessment	499	100%	100%	99%	100%
Pneumococcal Vaccine	305	92%	64%	69%	94%
Smoking Cessation Advice	102	97%	69%	80%	100%
Surgical Infection Prevention					
Prophylactic Antibiotic Given[2,3]	183	61%	74%	77%	95%
Prophylactic Antibiotic Selection[2]	60	93%	88%	90%	100%
Prophylactic Antibiotic Stopped[2,3]	167	60%	68%	72%	95%
Pregnancy Care					
Inpatient Neonatal Mortality	2,631	0.11%	-	-	-
Third or Fourth Degree Laceration	1,795	6.07%	3.70%	3.63%	3.27%

Carondelet Saint Mary's Hospital

1601 W Street Mary's Road
Tucson, AZ 85745
URL: www.carondelet.org
Ownership: Proprietary
Emergency Services: Yes

Phone: 520-872-3000
Fax: 520-872-6066
Accredited: Yes
Licensed Beds: 393

Key Personnel:

President/CEO. . . . . Sallly Jeffcoat
Chief Medical Staff . . . . D Bowman
Director of Emergency . . . . D McReynolds, MD
Director Pulmonary . . . . Caroline Schalger

Measure	Cases	This Hospital	State Average	U.S. Average	Top Hospital
Heart Attack Care					
ACE Inhibitor or ARB for LVSD	66	97%	83%	82%	100%
Aspirin at Arrival	311	96%	96%	92%	100%
Aspirin at Discharge	280	96%	91%	90%	100%
Beta Blocker at Arrival	253	90%	88%	87%	100%
Beta Blocker at Discharge	291	98%	93%	90%	100%
Fibrinolytic Medication Timing	0	-	10%	31%	100%
PCI Within 90 Minutes of Arrival[1]	7	57%	47%	54%	95%
Smoking Cessation Advice	76	100%	89%	88%	100%
Heart Failure Care					
ACE Inhibitor or ARB for LVSD	133	95%	81%	82%	100%
Discharge Instructions	350	100%	48%	61%	93%
Evaluation of LVS Function	382	93%	84%	83%	99%
Smoking Cessation Advice	58	100%	76%	82%	100%
Pneumonia Care					
Appropriate Initial Antibiotic	319	90%	84%	83%	94%
Blood Culture Timing	288	86%	87%	90%	100%
Influenza Vaccine	114	50%	61%	70%	100%
Initial Antibiotic Timing	396	81%	73%	80%	93%
Oxygenation Assessment	483	100%	100%	99%	100%
Pneumococcal Vaccine	249	96%	64%	69%	94%
Smoking Cessation Advice	145	100%	69%	80%	100%
Surgical Infection Prevention					
Prophylactic Antibiotic Given[2,3]	144	82%	74%	77%	95%
Prophylactic Antibiotic Selection[2]	48	83%	88%	90%	100%
Prophylactic Antibiotic Stopped[2,3]	145	50%	68%	72%	95%
Pregnancy Care					
Inpatient Neonatal Mortality	-	-	-	-	-
Third or Fourth Degree Laceration	-	-	3.70%	3.63%	3.27%

Northwest Medical Center

Alternate Name: Northwest Hospital

6200 N La Cholla Boulevard
Tucson, AZ 85741
URL: www.northwestmedicalcenter.com
Ownership: Proprietary
Emergency Services: Yes

Phone: 520-742-9000
Fax: 520-469-8101
Accredited: Yes
Licensed Beds: 278

Key Personnel:

CEO. . . . . Jeff Comer
Chief Medical Staff. . . . . Mitzi Barmatz, MD
Catheterization Lab . . . . Robin Athey
Emergency Room . . . . Katie Gleason
Infection Control. . . . . Melvin Morrow
OB/GYN Womens Health. . . . . Dale Reimer

Measure	Cases	This Hospital	State Average	U.S. Average	Top Hospital
Heart Attack Care					
ACE Inhibitor or ARB for LVSD	44	93%	83%	82%	100%
Aspirin at Arrival	174	98%	96%	92%	100%
Aspirin at Discharge	202	99%	91%	90%	100%
Beta Blocker at Arrival	120	96%	88%	87%	100%
Beta Blocker at Discharge	199	98%	93%	90%	100%
Fibrinolytic Medication Timing[1]	1	0%	10%	31%	100%
PCI Within 90 Minutes of Arrival[1]	10	90%	47%	54%	95%
Smoking Cessation Advice	70	97%	89%	88%	100%
Heart Failure Care					
ACE Inhibitor or ARB for LVSD	117	83%	81%	82%	100%
Discharge Instructions	286	64%	48%	61%	93%
Evaluation of LVS Function	352	97%	84%	83%	99%
Smoking Cessation Advice	48	92%	76%	82%	100%
Pneumonia Care					
Appropriate Initial Antibiotic	358	92%	84%	83%	94%
Blood Culture Timing	331	91%	87%	90%	100%
Influenza Vaccine	119	74%	61%	70%	100%
Initial Antibiotic Timing	479	71%	73%	80%	93%
Oxygenation Assessment	604	100%	100%	99%	100%
Pneumococcal Vaccine	361	73%	64%	69%	94%
Smoking Cessation Advice	119	85%	69%	80%	100%
Surgical Infection Prevention					
Prophylactic Antibiotic Given	1,638	83%	74%	77%	95%
Prophylactic Antibiotic Selection	382	96%	88%	90%	100%
Prophylactic Antibiotic Stopped	1,523	65%	68%	72%	95%
Pregnancy Care					
Inpatient Neonatal Mortality	-	-	-	-	-
Third or Fourth Degree Laceration	-	-	3.70%	3.63%	3.27%

Northwest Medical Center Oro Valley

1551 E Tangerine Road
Oro Valley, AZ 85737
E-mail: nwmc.orovalley@triadhospitals.com
URL: www.nmcorovalley.com
Ownership: Voluntary non-profit - Private
Emergency Services: Yes

Phone: 520-901-3500
Fax: 520-901-3525
Accredited: Yes
Licensed Beds: 96

Key Personnel:

President/CEO. . . . . Paul Kappelman
Chief Medical Staff. . . . . Robert Cobb, MD
Catheterization Lab . . . . Barbara Hoffman
Emergency Room . . . . Fran Czosnek
ICU . . . . Randy Kesterson
Medical Surgical Nursing . . . . Tim Lorenzen, RN
Respiratory/Cardiopulmonary. . . . . John Worden

Measure	Cases	This Hospital	State Average	U.S. Average	Top Hospital
Heart Attack Care					
ACE Inhibitor or ARB for LVSD[1]	16	94%	83%	82%	100%
Aspirin at Arrival	83	98%	96%	92%	100%
Aspirin at Discharge	70	99%	91%	90%	100%
Beta Blocker at Arrival	60	90%	88%	87%	100%
Beta Blocker at Discharge	70	93%	93%	90%	100%
Fibrinolytic Medication Timing	0	-	10%	31%	100%
PCI Within 90 Minutes of Arrival[1]	4	100%	47%	54%	95%
Smoking Cessation Advice[1]	21	95%	89%	88%	100%
Heart Failure Care					
ACE Inhibitor or ARB for LVSD	41	76%	81%	82%	100%
Discharge Instructions	79	51%	48%	61%	93%

NOTE: Hospital profiles are in alphabetical order by state, then city, then hospital within the city; Rankings are sorted by rate in descending order and exclude hospitals with less than 25 cases; (1) The number of cases is too small (n<25) for purposes of reliably predicting hospital performance; (2) Measure reflects the hospital's indication that its submission was based upon a sample of its relevant discharges; (3) Rate reflects fewer than the maximum possible quarters of data for the measure; (4) Inaccurate information submitted and suppressed for one or more quarters; (5) No data is available from the hospital for this measure; Please refer to the User's Guide for a full explanation of data

Measure	Cases	This Hospital	State Average	U.S. Average	Top Hospital
Evaluation of LVS Function	90	91%	84%	83%	99%
Smoking Cessation Advice[1]	14	79%	76%	82%	100%
Pneumonia Care					
Appropriate Initial Antibiotic	117	91%	84%	83%	94%
Blood Culture Timing	107	94%	87%	90%	100%
Influenza Vaccine	40	58%	61%	70%	100%
Initial Antibiotic Timing	150	79%	73%	80%	93%
Oxygenation Assessment	167	100%	100%	99%	100%
Pneumococcal Vaccine	109	81%	64%	69%	94%
Smoking Cessation Advice	30	90%	69%	80%	100%
Surgical Infection Prevention					
Prophylactic Antibiotic Given	491	91%	74%	77%	95%
Prophylactic Antibiotic Selection	127	96%	88%	90%	100%
Prophylactic Antibiotic Stopped	480	47%	68%	72%	95%
Pregnancy Care					
Inpatient Neonatal Mortality	-	-	-	-	-
Third or Fourth Degree Laceration	-	-	3.70%	3.63%	3.27%

Tucson Heart Hospital

4888 N Stone Ave
Tucson, AZ 85704
Ownership: Proprietary
Emergency Services: Yes
Phone: 520-696-2328
Accredited: Yes

Measure	Cases	This Hospital	State Average	U.S. Average	Top Hospital
Heart Attack Care					
ACE Inhibitor or ARB for LVSD[2]	45	100%	83%	82%	100%
Aspirin at Arrival[2]	140	100%	96%	92%	100%
Aspirin at Discharge[2]	261	98%	91%	90%	100%
Beta Blocker at Arrival[2]	132	100%	88%	87%	100%
Beta Blocker at Discharge[2]	243	100%	93%	90%	100%
Fibrinolytic Medication Timing[2]	0	-	10%	31%	100%
PCI Within 90 Minutes of Arrival[1,2]	2	100%	47%	54%	95%
Smoking Cessation Advice[2]	70	100%	89%	88%	100%
Heart Failure Care					
ACE Inhibitor or ARB for LVSD[2]	98	100%	81%	82%	100%
Discharge Instructions[2]	262	92%	48%	61%	93%
Evaluation of LVS Function[2]	283	95%	84%	83%	99%
Smoking Cessation Advice[1,2]	21	95%	76%	82%	100%
Pneumonia Care					
Appropriate Initial Antibiotic[2]	52	96%	84%	83%	94%
Blood Culture Timing[2]	65	88%	87%	90%	100%
Influenza Vaccine[2]	26	100%	61%	70%	100%
Initial Antibiotic Timing[2]	72	85%	73%	80%	93%
Oxygenation Assessment[2]	84	100%	100%	99%	100%
Pneumococcal Vaccine[2]	64	97%	64%	69%	94%
Smoking Cessation Advice[1,2]	20	100%	69%	80%	100%
Surgical Infection Prevention					
Prophylactic Antibiotic Given[2,3]	107	99%	74%	77%	95%
Prophylactic Antibiotic Selection[2]	37	100%	88%	90%	100%
Prophylactic Antibiotic Stopped[2,3]	107	100%	68%	72%	95%
Pregnancy Care					
Inpatient Neonatal Mortality	-	-	-	-	-
Third or Fourth Degree Laceration	-	-	3.70%	3.63%	3.27%

Tucson Medical Center

5301 E Grant Road
Tucson, AZ 85712
URL: www.tmcaz.com
Ownership: Voluntary non-profit - Other
Emergency Services: Yes
Phone: 520-327-5461
Fax: 520-324-2443
Accredited: Yes
Licensed Beds: 609

Key Personnel:
President/CEO.......................... Frank Alcorez
Chief Medical Staff....................... Richard Rodriquez
Emergency Room .... Keith Kaback, MD
OB/GYN Womens Health.................. David Rhea
Chief Radiology .... Edward Woolsey

Measure	Cases	This Hospital	State Average	U.S. Average	Top Hospital
Heart Attack Care					
ACE Inhibitor or ARB for LVSD	66	85%	83%	82%	100%
Aspirin at Arrival	224	96%	96%	92%	100%
Aspirin at Discharge	270	95%	91%	90%	100%
Beta Blocker at Arrival	202	90%	88%	87%	100%
Beta Blocker at Discharge	271	94%	93%	90%	100%
Fibrinolytic Medication Timing	0	-	10%	31%	100%
PCI Within 90 Minutes of Arrival[1]	4	25%	47%	54%	95%
Smoking Cessation Advice	85	100%	89%	88%	100%
Heart Failure Care					
ACE Inhibitor or ARB for LVSD[2]	95	87%	81%	82%	100%
Discharge Instructions[2]	197	70%	48%	61%	93%
Evaluation of LVS Function[2]	256	96%	84%	83%	99%
Smoking Cessation Advice[2]	42	100%	76%	82%	100%
Pneumonia Care					
Appropriate Initial Antibiotic[2]	72	92%	84%	83%	94%
Blood Culture Timing[2]	74	86%	87%	90%	100%
Influenza Vaccine[4,5]	-	-	61%	70%	100%
Initial Antibiotic Timing[2]	108	62%	73%	80%	93%
Oxygenation Assessment[2]	151	100%	100%	99%	100%
Pneumococcal Vaccine[2]	86	58%	64%	69%	94%
Smoking Cessation Advice[2]	32	100%	69%	80%	100%
Surgical Infection Prevention					
Prophylactic Antibiotic Given[3]	266	79%	74%	77%	95%
Prophylactic Antibiotic Selection	96	96%	88%	90%	100%
Prophylactic Antibiotic Stopped[3]	249	72%	68%	72%	95%
Pregnancy Care					
Inpatient Neonatal Mortality	-	-	-	-	-
Third or Fourth Degree Laceration	-	-	3.70%	3.63%	3.27%

University Medical Center

1501 N Campbell Avenue
Tucson, AZ 85724
URL: www.azumc.com
Ownership: Voluntary non-profit - Private
Emergency Services: Yes
Phone: 520-694-0111
Fax: 520-694-4085
Accredited: Yes
Licensed Beds: 355

Key Personnel:
President/CEO.......................... Gregory Pivirotto
Chief Medical Staff....................... Richard Lemen, MD
Chief Catheterization Laboratory .... Sam Butman
Emergency Room .... Harvey Meislin, MD
Director Infection/Disease Control .... Connie Clasby
Director Medical/Surgical Nursing .... Terry Grzyb-Wysocki
OB/GYN Womens Health.................. Kenneth Hatch, MD
Chief Radiology .... Theron Ovitt, MD
Director Cardio-Pulmonary Services .... Jeff Schaefer

Measure	Cases	This Hospital	State Average	U.S. Average	Top Hospital
Heart Attack Care					
ACE Inhibitor or ARB for LVSD[2]	70	99%	83%	82%	100%
Aspirin at Arrival[2]	192	95%	96%	92%	100%
Aspirin at Discharge[2]	267	100%	91%	90%	100%
Beta Blocker at Arrival[2]	169	92%	88%	87%	100%
Beta Blocker at Discharge[2]	260	99%	93%	90%	100%
Fibrinolytic Medication Timing[2]	0	-	10%	31%	100%
PCI Within 90 Minutes of Arrival[1,2]	6	33%	47%	54%	95%
Smoking Cessation Advice[2]	91	100%	89%	88%	100%
Heart Failure Care					
ACE Inhibitor or ARB for LVSD[2]	183	95%	81%	82%	100%
Discharge Instructions[2]	295	76%	48%	61%	93%
Evaluation of LVS Function[2]	318	99%	84%	83%	99%
Smoking Cessation Advice[2]	59	100%	76%	82%	100%
Pneumonia Care					
Appropriate Initial Antibiotic[2]	73	93%	84%	83%	94%
Blood Culture Timing[2]	45	89%	87%	90%	100%
Influenza Vaccine[1,2]	19	79%	61%	70%	100%
Initial Antibiotic Timing[2]	142	57%	73%	80%	93%
Oxygenation Assessment[2]	188	100%	100%	99%	100%
Pneumococcal Vaccine[2]	74	78%	64%	69%	94%
Smoking Cessation Advice[2]	48	100%	69%	80%	100%
Surgical Infection Prevention					
Prophylactic Antibiotic Given[2,3]	66	76%	74%	77%	95%
Prophylactic Antibiotic Selection[2]	72	60%	88%	90%	100%
Prophylactic Antibiotic Stopped[2,3]	65	58%	68%	72%	95%
Pregnancy Care					
Inpatient Neonatal Mortality	-	-	-	-	-

NOTE: Hospital profiles are in alphabetical order by state, then city, then hospital within the city; Rankings are sorted by rate in descending order and exclude hospitals with less than 25 cases; (1) The number of cases is too small (n<25) for purposes of reliably predicting hospital performance; (2) Measure reflects the hospital's indication that its submission was based upon a sample of its relevant discharges; (3) Rate reflects fewer than the maximum possible quarters of data for the measure; (4) Inaccurate information submitted and suppressed for one or more quarters; (5) No data is available from the hospital for this measure; Please refer to the User's Guide for a full explanation of data

Third or Fourth Degree Laceration	-	-	3.70%	3.63%	3.27%

UPH Hospital at Kino campus

2800 E Ajo Way
Tucson, AZ 85713
URL: ww.uphkino.org
Ownership: Voluntary non-profit - Private
Emergency Services: Yes

Phone: 520-294-4471
Fax: 520-874-4280

Accredited: Yes
Licensed Beds: 190

Key Personnel:
CEO. . . . . Scott Floden
Chief Medical Staff. . . . . Lupe Manriquez
Emergency Room . . . . Candy Simon
Medical/Surgical Nursing . . . . Karen Wilson
OB/GYN Womens Health. . . . . William Meyer, MD
Chief Radiology . . . . Richard Carmody, MD
Director Respiratory Therapy . . . . Anthony Ruiz

Measure	Cases	This Hospital	State Average	U.S. Average	Top Hospital
Heart Attack Care					
ACE Inhibitor or ARB for LVSD[1]	17	71%	83%	82%	100%
Aspirin at Arrival	30	97%	96%	92%	100%
Aspirin at Discharge	26	96%	91%	90%	100%
Beta Blocker at Arrival	32	91%	88%	87%	100%
Beta Blocker at Discharge	26	85%	93%	90%	100%
Fibrinolytic Medication Timing[1]	22	9%	10%	31%	100%
PCI Within 90 Minutes of Arrival	0	-	47%	54%	95%
Smoking Cessation Advice[1]	11	73%	89%	88%	100%
Heart Failure Care					
ACE Inhibitor or ARB for LVSD[1]	16	94%	81%	82%	100%
Discharge Instructions	91	73%	48%	61%	93%
Evaluation of LVS Function	95	92%	84%	83%	99%
Smoking Cessation Advice	47	32%	76%	82%	100%
Pneumonia Care					
Appropriate Initial Antibiotic[2]	107	89%	84%	83%	94%
Blood Culture Timing[2]	62	77%	87%	90%	100%
Influenza Vaccine[1,2]	19	53%	61%	70%	100%
Initial Antibiotic Timing[2]	147	55%	73%	80%	93%
Oxygenation Assessment[2]	161	99%	100%	99%	100%
Pneumococcal Vaccine[2]	58	40%	64%	69%	94%
Smoking Cessation Advice[2]	76	47%	69%	80%	100%
Surgical Infection Prevention					
Prophylactic Antibiotic Given[3]	56	98%	74%	77%	95%
Prophylactic Antibiotic Selection[1]	12	100%	88%	90%	100%
Prophylactic Antibiotic Stopped[3]	56	96%	68%	72%	95%
Pregnancy Care					
Inpatient Neonatal Mortality	-	-	-	-	-
Third or Fourth Degree Laceration	-	-	3.70%	3.63%	3.27%

Whiteriver Indian Hospital

Alternate Name: USPHS Indian Hospital
State Route 73
Box 860
Whiteriver, AZ 85941
URL: www.ihs.gov
Ownership: Government - Federal
Emergency Services: Yes

Phone: 928-338-4911
Fax: 928-338-3522

Accredited: Yes
Licensed Beds: 45

Key Personnel:
Chief Medical Staff. . . . . Dr. David Yost
Emergency Room . . . . Susan Panter
OB/GYN Womens Health. . . . . Martha Jo Billy

Measure	Cases	This Hospital	State Average	U.S. Average	Top Hospital
Heart Attack Care					
ACE Inhibitor or ARB for LVSD[3]	0	-	83%	82%	100%
Aspirin at Arrival[3]	0	-	96%	92%	100%
Aspirin at Discharge[3]	0	-	91%	90%	100%
Beta Blocker at Arrival[3]	0	-	88%	87%	100%
Beta Blocker at Discharge[3]	0	-	93%	90%	100%
Fibrinolytic Medication Timing[3]	0	-	10%	31%	100%
PCI Within 90 Minutes of Arrival	0	-	47%	54%	95%
Smoking Cessation Advice[3]	0	-	89%	88%	100%
Heart Failure Care					
ACE Inhibitor or ARB for LVSD[1,3]	6	67%	81%	82%	100%
Discharge Instructions[1,3]	7	57%	48%	61%	93%
Evaluation of LVS Function[1,3]	7	100%	84%	83%	99%
Smoking Cessation Advice[1,3]	5	0%	76%	82%	100%
Pneumonia Care					
Appropriate Initial Antibiotic	57	79%	84%	83%	94%
Blood Culture Timing	52	79%	87%	90%	100%
Influenza Vaccine[1]	12	100%	61%	70%	100%
Initial Antibiotic Timing	59	83%	73%	80%	93%
Oxygenation Assessment	81	99%	100%	99%	100%
Pneumococcal Vaccine	37	97%	64%	69%	94%
Smoking Cessation Advice[1]	7	57%	69%	80%	100%
Surgical Infection Prevention					
Prophylactic Antibiotic Given[5]	-	-	74%	77%	95%
Prophylactic Antibiotic Selection[5]	-	-	88%	90%	100%
Prophylactic Antibiotic Stopped[5]	-	-	68%	72%	95%
Pregnancy Care					
Inpatient Neonatal Mortality	-	-	-	-	-
Third or Fourth Degree Laceration	-	-	3.70%	3.63%	3.27%

Wickenburg Regional Hospital

520 Rose Lane
Wickenburg, AZ 85390
URL: www.bannerhealth.com
Ownership: Voluntary non-profit - Private
Emergency Services: Yes

Phone: 928-684-5421
Fax: 928-684-5081

Accredited: No
Licensed Beds: 80

Key Personnel:
CEO. . . . . George Larson
Chief Medical Staff. . . . . Diego Cardenaf, MD
Emergency Room . . . . Roger Wilder
Chief Radiology . . . . Tom Rabjohn
Director Respiratory Therapy . . . . James Limon

Measure	Cases	This Hospital	State Average	U.S. Average	Top Hospital
Heart Attack Care					
ACE Inhibitor or ARB for LVSD[5]	-	-	83%	82%	100%
Aspirin at Arrival[5]	-	-	96%	92%	100%
Aspirin at Discharge[5]	-	-	91%	90%	100%
Beta Blocker at Arrival[5]	-	-	88%	87%	100%
Beta Blocker at Discharge[5]	-	-	93%	90%	100%
Fibrinolytic Medication Timing[5]	-	-	10%	31%	100%
PCI Within 90 Minutes of Arrival[5]	-	-	47%	54%	95%
Smoking Cessation Advice[5]	-	-	89%	88%	100%
Heart Failure Care					
ACE Inhibitor or ARB for LVSD[1,3]	3	0%	81%	82%	100%
Discharge Instructions[1,3]	3	0%	48%	61%	93%
Evaluation of LVS Function[1,3]	5	100%	84%	83%	99%
Smoking Cessation Advice[3]	0	-	76%	82%	100%
Pneumonia Care					
Appropriate Initial Antibiotic[3]	33	85%	84%	83%	94%
Blood Culture Timing[1]	16	88%	87%	90%	100%
Influenza Vaccine[1]	13	31%	61%	70%	100%
Initial Antibiotic Timing[3]	33	91%	73%	80%	93%
Oxygenation Assessment[3]	33	88%	100%	99%	100%
Pneumococcal Vaccine[3]	25	24%	64%	69%	94%
Smoking Cessation Advice[1,3]	2	100%	69%	80%	100%
Surgical Infection Prevention					
Prophylactic Antibiotic Given[5]	-	-	74%	77%	95%
Prophylactic Antibiotic Selection[5]	-	-	88%	90%	100%
Prophylactic Antibiotic Stopped[5]	-	-	68%	72%	95%
Pregnancy Care					
Inpatient Neonatal Mortality	-	-	-	-	-
Third or Fourth Degree Laceration	-	-	3.70%	3.63%	3.27%

Northern Cochise Community Hospital

901 W Rex Allen Drive
Willcox, AZ 85643

Toll-Free: 800-696-3541
Phone: 520-384-3541
Fax: 520-384-9212

URL: www.ncch.com
Ownership: Govt - Hospital District or Authority
Emergency Services: No

Accredited: No
Licensed Beds: 24

Key Personnel:
CEO/Administrator. . . . . Chris Cronberg
Chief of Medical Staff . . . . Dawn Walker, DO

NOTE: Hospital profiles are in alphabetical order by state, then city, then hospital within the city; Rankings are sorted by rate in descending order and exclude hospitals with less than 25 cases; (1) The number of cases is too small (n<25) for purposes of reliably predicting hospital performance; (2) Measure reflects the hospital's indication that its submission was based upon a sample of its relevant discharges; (3) Rate reflects fewer than the maximum possible quarters of data for the measure; (4) Inaccurate information submitted and suppressed for one or more quarters; (5) No data is available from the hospital for this measure; Please refer to the User's Guide for a full explanation of data

Emergency Room . . . . Pam Noland, RN
Director Medical/Surgical Nursing . . . . John Hardine, RN
CNO. . . . . Julia Hilton, RN
Director of Pulmonary/Respiratory Care. . . . . . . Shally Newhall

Measure	Cases	This Hospital	State Average	U.S. Average	Top Hospital
Heart Attack Care					
ACE Inhibitor or ARB for LVSD[5]	-	-	83%	82%	100%
Aspirin at Arrival[5]	-	-	96%	92%	100%
Aspirin at Discharge[5]	-	-	91%	90%	100%
Beta Blocker at Arrival[5]	-	-	88%	87%	100%
Beta Blocker at Discharge[5]	-	-	93%	90%	100%
Fibrinolytic Medication Timing[5]	-	-	10%	31%	100%
PCI Within 90 Minutes of Arrival[5]	-	-	47%	54%	95%
Smoking Cessation Advice[5]	-	-	89%	88%	100%
Heart Failure Care					
ACE Inhibitor or ARB for LVSD[1]	7	86%	81%	82%	100%
Discharge Instructions[1]	14	29%	48%	61%	93%
Evaluation of LVS Function[1]	16	69%	84%	83%	99%
Smoking Cessation Advice[1]	3	33%	76%	82%	100%
Pneumonia Care					
Appropriate Initial Antibiotic	42	98%	84%	83%	94%
Blood Culture Timing[1]	9	100%	87%	90%	100%
Influenza Vaccine[1]	15	40%	61%	70%	100%
Initial Antibiotic Timing	53	77%	73%	80%	93%
Oxygenation Assessment	57	100%	100%	99%	100%
Pneumococcal Vaccine	33	70%	64%	69%	94%
Smoking Cessation Advice[1]	16	56%	69%	80%	100%
Surgical Infection Prevention					
Prophylactic Antibiotic Given[5]	-	-	74%	77%	95%
Prophylactic Antibiotic Selection[5]	-	-	88%	90%	100%
Prophylactic Antibiotic Stopped[5]	-	-	68%	72%	95%
Pregnancy Care					
Inpatient Neonatal Mortality	-	-	-	-	-
Third or Fourth Degree Laceration	-	-	3.70%	3.63%	3.27%

Winslow Memorial Hospital

Alternate Name: Little Colorado Medical Center
1501 Williamson Avenue
Winslow, AZ 86047
Phone: 928-289-4691
Fax: 928-289-3855
URL: www.nahealth.com
Ownership: Government - Federal
Accredited: No
Emergency Services: Yes
Licensed Beds: 25

Key Personnel:

CEO. . . . . Jeff Hamblen
Chief Medical Staff. . . . . Perry Mitchell, MD
Infection Control. . . . . Marie Hancock
OB/GYN/Women's Health . . . . Kenneth Ogilvie, MD
Chief Radiology . . . . William Ward
Respiratory/Cardiopulmonary. . . . . Mike Hartnett

Measure	Cases	This Hospital	State Average	U.S. Average	Top Hospital
Heart Attack Care					
ACE Inhibitor or ARB for LVSD[3]	0	-	83%	82%	100%
Aspirin at Arrival[1,3]	1	100%	96%	92%	100%
Aspirin at Discharge[1,3]	1	100%	91%	90%	100%
Beta Blocker at Arrival[1,3]	1	0%	88%	87%	100%
Beta Blocker at Discharge[3]	0	-	93%	90%	100%
Fibrinolytic Medication Timing[1,3]	2	0%	10%	31%	100%
PCI Within 90 Minutes of Arrival	0	-	47%	54%	95%
Smoking Cessation Advice[3]	0	-	89%	88%	100%
Heart Failure Care					
ACE Inhibitor or ARB for LVSD[1,3]	4	75%	81%	82%	100%
Discharge Instructions[1,3]	14	0%	48%	61%	93%
Evaluation of LVS Function[1,3]	17	35%	84%	83%	99%
Smoking Cessation Advice[1,3]	2	0%	76%	82%	100%
Pneumonia Care					
Appropriate Initial Antibiotic[1,3]	21	76%	84%	83%	94%
Blood Culture Timing[1,3]	5	100%	87%	90%	100%
Influenza Vaccine[5]	-	-	61%	70%	100%
Initial Antibiotic Timing[3]	27	81%	73%	80%	93%
Oxygenation Assessment[3]	30	100%	100%	99%	100%
Pneumococcal Vaccine[1,3]	21	5%	64%	69%	94%
Smoking Cessation Advice[1,3]	4	25%	69%	80%	100%
Surgical Infection Prevention					
Prophylactic Antibiotic Given[3]	0	-	74%	77%	95%
Prophylactic Antibiotic Selection	0	-	88%	90%	100%
Prophylactic Antibiotic Stopped[3]	0	-	68%	72%	95%
Pregnancy Care					
Inpatient Neonatal Mortality	-	-	-	-	-
Third or Fourth Degree Laceration	-	-	3.70%	3.63%	3.27%

Yuma Regional Medical Center

2400 S Avenue A
Yuma, AZ 85364
Phone: 928-344-2000
Fax: 928-336-7337
URL: www.yumaregional.org
Ownership: Voluntary non-profit - Other
Accredited: Yes
Emergency Services: Yes
Licensed Beds: 279

Key Personnel:

CEO/President. . . . . Bob Olsen, FACHE
Chief Medical Staff. . . . . Louis K Miller
CEO Heart Center . . . . Scott Bailey
Emergency Room . . . . Phil Richemont
Infection Control Coordinator . . . . Jo Doner
Administrative Director Surgical Service. . . . . . . Phyllis Abbott
Director Cardio-Pulmonary Services . . . . Judith McGinnis

Measure	Cases	This Hospital	State Average	U.S. Average	Top Hospital
Heart Attack Care					
ACE Inhibitor or ARB for LVSD	68	79%	83%	82%	100%
Aspirin at Arrival	277	96%	96%	92%	100%
Aspirin at Discharge	236	94%	91%	90%	100%
Beta Blocker at Arrival	227	89%	88%	87%	100%
Beta Blocker at Discharge	275	85%	93%	90%	100%
Fibrinolytic Medication Timing	30	13%	10%	31%	100%
PCI Within 90 Minutes of Arrival[1]	6	0%	47%	54%	95%
Smoking Cessation Advice	74	92%	89%	88%	100%
Heart Failure Care					
ACE Inhibitor or ARB for LVSD	221	81%	81%	82%	100%
Discharge Instructions	425	55%	48%	61%	93%
Evaluation of LVS Function	488	81%	84%	83%	99%
Smoking Cessation Advice	78	90%	76%	82%	100%
Pneumonia Care					
Appropriate Initial Antibiotic	354	81%	84%	83%	94%
Blood Culture Timing	370	84%	87%	90%	100%
Influenza Vaccine	172	51%	61%	70%	100%
Initial Antibiotic Timing	721	46%	73%	80%	93%
Oxygenation Assessment	848	100%	100%	99%	100%
Pneumococcal Vaccine	545	50%	64%	69%	94%
Smoking Cessation Advice	131	78%	69%	80%	100%
Surgical Infection Prevention					
Prophylactic Antibiotic Given[2]	898	80%	74%	77%	95%
Prophylactic Antibiotic Selection[2]	182	93%	88%	90%	100%
Prophylactic Antibiotic Stopped[2]	886	74%	68%	72%	95%
Pregnancy Care					
Inpatient Neonatal Mortality	3,712	0.24%	-	-	-
Third or Fourth Degree Laceration	2,580	3.02%	3.70%	3.63%	3.27%

NOTE: Hospital profiles are in alphabetical order by state, then city, then hospital within the city; Rankings are sorted by rate in descending order and exclude hospitals with less than 25 cases; (1) The number of cases is too small (n<25) for purposes of reliably predicting hospital performance; (2) Measure reflects the hospital's indication that its submission was based upon a sample of its relevant discharges; (3) Rate reflects fewer than the maximum possible quarters of data for the measure; (4) Inaccurate information submitted and suppressed for one or more quarters; (5) No data is available from the hospital for this measure; Please refer to the User's Guide for a full explanation of data

Heart Attack Care

1. ACE Inhibitor or ARB for LVSD

Hospital Name	City	Rate	Cases
Anaheim Memorial Medical Center	Anaheim	100%	49
Glendale Memorial Hospital and Health Center	Glendale	100%	54
Kaiser Foundation Hospital-South Sacramento	Sacramento	100%	30
Mission Hospital Regional Medical Center	Mission Viejo	100%	29
Oakland Medical Center	Oakland	100%	32
Palomar Medical Center	Escondido	100%	48
Saint Agnes Medical Center	Fresno	100%	71
Cedars-Sinai Medical Center	Los Angeles	98%	54
Grossmont Hospital	La Mesa	98%	66
Mercy Medical Center-Redding	Redding	98%	57
Mercy San Juan Hospital	Carmichael	98%	45
Northridge Hospital Medical Center	Northridge	98%	41
Doctors Medical Center	Modesto	97%	75
Lakewood Regional Medical Center	Lakewood	97%	31
Long Beach Memorial Medical Center	Long Beach	97%	60
Methodist Hospital of Southern California	Arcadia	97%	33
O'Connor Hospital	San Jose	97%	32
Providence Saint Joseph Medical Center	Burbank	97%	37
Saint Mary's Medical Center	San Francisco	97%	32
Seton Medical Center	Daly City	97%	30
Hoag Memorial Hospital Presbyterian	Newport Beach	96%	54
John Muir Medical Center-Concord Campus	Concord	96%	45
Kaiser Permanente San Francisco Med Ctr	San Francisco	96%	69
Kaweah Delta Health Care District	Visalia	96%	57
Saddleback Memorial Medical Center	Laguna Hills	96%	53
Western Medical Center	Santa Ana	96%	26
El Camino Hospital	Mountain View	95%	44
Scripps Mercy Hospital	San Diego	95%	55
Arrowhead Regional Medical Center	Colton	94%	31
Saint Joseph's Medical Center of Stockton	Stockton	94%	48
Shasta Regional Medical Center	Redding	94%	32
Good Samaritan Hospital	San Jose	93%	56
Kaiser Foundation Hospital-San Diego	San Diego	93%	27
Kaiser Permanente Santa Teresa Comm Med Ctr	San Jose	93%	28
Little Company of Mary Hospital	Torrance	93%	43
Saint Francis Medical Center	Lynwood	93%	27
Saint Joseph Hospital	Orange	93%	29
Community Memorial Hospital Ventura	Ventura	92%	37
Kaiser Foundation Hospital	Hayward	92%	25
Providence Holy Cross Medical Center	Mission Hills	92%	39
Salinas Valley Memorial Health Care District	Salinas	92%	40
Alta Bates Summit Medical Center	Oakland	91%	109
California Pacific Medical Center	San Francisco	91%	56
Marin General Hospital	Greenbrae	91%	58
Saint Bernardine Medical Center	San Bernardino	91%	45
Sharp Memorial Hospital	San Diego	91%	56
Sutter General Hospital	Sacramento	91%	87
Sutter Medical Center of Santa Rosa	Santa Rosa	91%	53
Bakersfield Heart Hospital	Bakersfield	90%	80
Glendale Adventist Medical Center	Glendale	90%	81
Huntington Memorial Hospital	Pasadena	90%	51
Mills-Peninsula Health Services	Burlingame	90%	29
Encino-Tarzana Regional Medical Center	Tarzana	89%	47
Fountain Valley Reg Hospital & Med Ctr	Fountain Valley	89%	35
Good Samaritan Hospital	Los Angeles	89%	55
Presbyterian Intercommunity Hospital	Whittier	89%	28
Bakersfield Memorial Hospital	Bakersfield	88%	75
John Muir Medical Center	Walnut Creek	88%	26
Kaiser Foundation Hospital-Fresno	Fresno	88%	34
Lancaster Community Hospital	Lancaster	88%	34
Washington Hospital	Fremont	88%	32
Saint Mary Medical Center	Long Beach	86%	29
Stanford Hospital	Stanford	86%	37
Community Regional Medical Center	Fresno	85%	107
Kaiser Permanente Los Angeles Medical Center	Los Angeles	85%	182
Mercy General Hospital	Sacramento	85%	165
Saint John's Regional Medical Center	Oxnard	85%	40
Sutter Roseville Medical Center	Roseville	85%	33
Dominican Hospital	Santa Cruz	84%	50
Enloe Medical Center	Chico	84%	83
Kaiser Permanente Fontana Medical Center	Fontana	84%	43
Loma Linda University Medical Center	Loma Linda	84%	80
Riverside Community Hospital	Riverside	84%	85
Saint John's Health Center	Santa Monica	84%	25
University of California Irvine Med Ctr	Orange	84%	25
Desert Regional Medical Center	Palm Springs	83%	52
Los Angeles County & USC Medical Center	Los Angeles	83%	66
San Antonio Community Hospital	Upland	83%	54
Beverly Hospital	Montebello	82%	28
Saint Jude Medical Center	Fullerton	81%	47
Tri-City Medical Center	Oceanside	81%	32
Antelope Valley Hospital	Lancaster	80%	56
Eisenhower Medical Center	Rancho Mirage	80%	100
Kaiser Permanente Bellflower Medical Center	Bellflower	80%	30
Pomona Valley Hospital Medical Center	Pomona	80%	98
Redlands Community Hospital	Redlands	80%	30
Scripps Memorial Hospital La Jolla	La Jolla	80%	49
Doctor's Medical Center-San Pablo Campus	San Pablo	78%	63
UCLA Medical Center	Los Angeles	78%	36
Citrus Valley Medical Center	Covina	77%	53
Hemet Valley Medical Center	Hemet	77%	48
Kaiser Permanente South Bay Medical Center	Harbor City	77%	26
Los Robles Regional Medical Center	Thousand Oaks	77%	53
Memorial Medical Center	Modesto	77%	52
Centinela Hospital Medical Center	Inglewood	76%	51
Queen of the Valley Hospital	Napa	76%	55
Torrance Memorial Medical Center	Torrance	76%	58
Valley Presbyterian Hospital	Van Nuys	76%	34
University of California Davis Health System	Sacramento	75%	67
Downey Regional Medical Center	Downey	74%	31
Sharp Chula Vista Medical Center	Chula Vista	73%	66
Kaiser Permanente Santa Clara Medical Center	Santa Clara	72%	29
Saint Mary Medical Center	Apple Valley	72%	50
Santa Barbara Cottage Hospital	Santa Barbara	70%	47
Kaiser Permanente Sacramento Medical Center	Sacramento	69%	45
San Joaquin Community Hospital	Bakersfield	69%	32
Los Angeles County Harbor-UCLA Medical Center	Torrance	67%	39
Rideout Memorial Hospital	Marysville	64%	53
Saint Vincent Medical Center	Los Angeles	64%	25
White Memorial Medical Center	Los Angeles	54%	26

2. Aspirin at Arrival

Hospital Name	City	Rate	Cases
Alameda County Medical Center	Oakland	100%	50
California Hospital Medical Center	Los Angeles	100%	75
Cedars-Sinai Medical Center	Los Angeles	100%	352
Chino Valley Medical Center	Chino	100%	54
Contra Costa Regional Medical Center	Martinez	100%	26
El Camino Hospital	Mountain View	100%	204
El Centro Regional Medical Center	El Centro	100%	85
Enloe Medical Center	Chico	100%	118
Fountain Valley Reg Hospital & Med Ctr	Fountain Valley	100%	174
French Hospital Medical Center	San Luis Obispo	100%	47
John Muir Medical Center	Walnut Creek	100%	157
Kaiser Foundation Hospital	Hayward	100%	340
Kaiser Foundation Hospital-South Sacramento	Sacramento	100%	246
Kaiser Foundation Hospital-Vallejo	Vallejo	100%	217
Kaiser Redwood City Medical Center	Redwood City	100%	104
Lakewood Regional Medical Center	Lakewood	100%	140
Little Company of Mary Hospital	Torrance	100%	246
Memorial Hospital of Gardena	Gardena	100%	59
Mercy Hospital of Folsom	Folsom	100%	25
Mercy Medical Center-Redding	Redding	100%	173
Methodist Hospital of Sacramento	Sacramento	100%	32
Oak Valley Hospital	Oakdale	100%	25
Oakland Medical Center	Oakland	100%	328
Palomar Medical Center	Escondido	100%	278
Pomerado Hospital	Poway	100%	54
Presbyterian Intercommunity Hospital	Whittier	100%	204
Providence Holy Cross Medical Center	Mission Hills	100%	165
Saint Joseph Hospital	Orange	100%	230
Saint Luke's Hospital	San Francisco	100%	43
San Dimas Community Hospital	San Dimas	100%	31
San Francisco General Hospital Medical Center	San Francisco	100%	101
Santa Monica-UCLA Medical Center	Santa Monica	100%	109
Scripps Green Hospital	La Jolla	100%	66
Scripps Mercy Hospital	San Diego	100%	336
Sierra Nevada Memorial Hospital	Grass Valley	100%	45
South Coast Medical Center	Laguna Beach	100%	25
Temple Community Hospital	Los Angeles	100%	33
Tulare District Hospital	Tulare	100%	55
University of California Irvine Med Ctr	Orange	100%	62
University of California San Diego Med Ctr	San Diego	100%	161
Ventura County Medical Center	Ventura	100%	25
Western Medical Center	Santa Ana	100%	86
Alta Bates Summit Medical Center	Oakland	99%	238
Anaheim Memorial Medical Center	Anaheim	99%	204
Bakersfield Heart Hospital	Bakersfield	99%	193
California Pacific Medical Center	San Francisco	99%	147
Desert Valley Hospital	Victorville	99%	106
Dominican Hospital	Santa Cruz	99%	157
Glendale Memorial Hospital and Health Center	Glendale	99%	175
Good Samaritan Hospital	San Jose	99%	166
Hoag Memorial Hospital Presbyterian	Newport Beach	99%	283

NOTE: Hospital profiles are in alphabetical order by state, then city, then hospital within the city; Rankings are sorted by rate in descending order and exclude hospitals with less than 25 cases; (1) The number of cases is too small (n<25) for purposes of reliably predicting hospital performance; (2) Measure reflects the hospital's indication that its submission was based upon a sample of its relevant discharges; (3) Rate reflects fewer than the maximum possible quarters of data for the measure; (4) Inaccurate information submitted and suppressed for one or more quarters; (5) No data is available from the hospital for this measure; Please refer to the User's Guide for a full explanation of data

Irvine Regional Hospital	Irvine	99%	109
John Muir Medical Center-Concord Campus	Concord	99%	183
Kaiser Foundation Hospital	Baldwin Park	99%	104
Kaiser Permanente Bellflower Medical Center	Bellflower	99%	155
Kaiser Permanente Los Angeles Medical Center	Los Angeles	99%	229
Kaiser Permanente San Francisco Med Ctr	San Francisco	99%	75
Kaiser Permanente Santa Clara Medical Center	Santa Clara	99%	149
Kaiser Permanente Santa Teresa Comm Med Ctr	San Jose	99%	204
Kaiser Permanente West Los Angeles Med Ctr	Los Angeles	99%	131
Loma Linda University Medical Center	Loma Linda	99%	123
Long Beach Memorial Medical Center	Long Beach	99%	292
Madera Community Hospital	Madera	99%	74
Marian Medical Center	Santa Maria	99%	141
Mercy General Hospital	Sacramento	99%	233
Mercy San Juan Hospital	Carmichael	99%	295
Mission Hospital Regional Medical Center	Mission Viejo	99%	278
Olive View-UCLA Medical Center	San Fernando	99%	104
Orange Coast Memorial Medical Center	Santa Ana	99%	92
Providence Saint Joseph Medical Center	Burbank	99%	249
Rideout Memorial Hospital	Marysville	99%	204
Saint Agnes Medical Center	Fresno	99%	299
Saint John's Health Center	Santa Monica	99%	153
Saint John's Regional Medical Center	Oxnard	99%	203
Saint Mary's Medical Center	San Francisco	99%	88
San Joaquin Community Hospital	Bakersfield	99%	107
San Joaquin General Hospital	French Camp	99%	70
San Rafael Medical Center	San Rafael	99%	82
Scripps Memorial Hospital-Encinitas	Encinitas	99%	116
Sequoia Hospital	Redwood City	99%	82
Sharp Memorial Hospital	San Diego	99%	275
Shasta Regional Medical Center	Redding	99%	94
Stanford Hospital	Stanford	99%	158
Sutter Roseville Medical Center	Roseville	99%	201
UCLA Medical Center	Los Angeles	99%	103
UCSF Medical Center	San Francisco	99%	138
Alameda Hospital	Alameda	98%	125
Alta Bates Summit Medical Center	Berkeley	98%	100
Arrowhead Regional Medical Center	Colton	98%	87
Dameron Hospital	Stockton	98%	148
Doctors Medical Center	Modesto	98%	192
Downey Regional Medical Center	Downey	98%	174
Garden Grove Hospital and Medical Center	Garden Grove	98%	54
Good Samaritan Hospital	Los Angeles	98%	137
Henry Mayo Newhall Memorial Hospital	Valencia	98%	113
Hollywood Presbyterian Medical Center	Los Angeles	98%	129
Kaiser Foundation Hospital-Riverside	Riverside	98%	140
Kaiser Foundation Hospital-Santa Rosa	Santa Rosa	98%	171
Kaweah Delta Health Care District	Visalia	98%	231
Little Company of Mary-San Pedro Hospital	San Pedro	98%	47
Lodi Memorial Hospital	Lodi	98%	80
Los Alamitos Medical Center	Los Alamitos	98%	129
Mills-Peninsula Health Services	Burlingame	98%	108
Northridge Hospital Medical Center	Northridge	98%	196
Novato Community Hospital	Novato	98%	43
O'Connor Hospital	San Jose	98%	149
Petaluma Valley Hospital	Petaluma	98%	51
Pioneers Memorial Healthcare District	Brawley	98%	42
Saint Bernardine Medical Center	San Bernardino	98%	101
Saint Francis Medical Center	Lynwood	98%	129
Saint Joseph Hospital	Eureka	98%	54
Saint Joseph's Medical Center of Stockton	Stockton	98%	185
Saint Jude Medical Center	Fullerton	98%	265
Saint Louisie Regional Hospital	Gilroy	98%	40
Saint Mary Medical Center	Apple Valley	98%	234
San Antonio Community Hospital	Upland	98%	227
San Gabriel Valley Medical Center	San Gabriel	98%	88
San Gorgonio Memorial Hospital	Banning	98%	81
San Leandro Hospital	San Leandro	98%	49
San Ramon Regional Medical Center	San Ramon	98%	60
Santa Clara Valley Medical Center	San Jose	98%	131
Scripps Memorial Hospital La Jolla	La Jolla	98%	101
S San Francisco Medical Center	S San Francisco	98%	123
Sutter General Hospital	Sacramento	98%	205
Torrance Memorial Medical Center	Torrance	98%	296
University of California Davis Health System	Sacramento	98%	191
Valleycare Medical Center	Livermore	98%	126
Whittier Hospital Medical Center	Whittier	98%	122
Antelope Valley Hospital	Lancaster	97%	301
Arroyo Grande Community Hospital	Arroyo Grande	97%	32
Community Memorial Hospital Ventura	Ventura	97%	181
Desert Regional Medical Center	Palm Springs	97%	180
Doctor's Medical Center-San Pablo Campus	San Pablo	97%	147
Grossmont Hospital	La Mesa	97%	479
Kaiser Foundation Hospital-Fresno	Fresno	97%	183
Kaiser Permanente Anaheim Medical Center	Anaheim	97%	77

Kaiser Permanente South Bay Medical Center	Harbor City	97%	137
Los Angeles County & USC Medical Center	Los Angeles	97%	178
Los Angeles County Harbor-UCLA Medical Center	Torrance	97%	145
Marin General Hospital	Greenbrae	97%	142
Parkview Community Hospital	Riverside	97%	66
Riverside County Regional Medical Center	Moreno Valley	97%	35
Saint Rose Hospital	Hayward	97%	121
Saint Vincent Medical Center	Los Angeles	97%	79
Santa Rosa Memorial Hospital	Santa Rosa	97%	101
Seton Medical Center	Daly City	97%	127
Sharp Chula Vista Medical Center	Chula Vista	97%	279
Sierra Vista Regional Medical Center	San Luis Obispo	97%	60
Sutter Medical Center of Santa Rosa	Santa Rosa	97%	70
Tri-City Medical Center	Oceanside	97%	233
Twin Cities Community Hospital	Templeton	97%	35
Valley Presbyterian Hospital	Van Nuys	97%	119
Washington Hospital	Fremont	97%	207
Watsonville Community Hospital	Watsonville	97%	30
Centinela Freeman Reg Med Ctr-Marina	Marina Del Rey	96%	28
Centinela Hospital Medical Center	Inglewood	96%	207
Community Hospital of San Bernardino	San Bernardino	96%	52
Community Hospital of the Monterey Peninsula	Monterey	96%	138
Community Regional Medical Center	Fresno	96%	342
Encino-Tarzana Regional Medical Center	Encino	96%	47
John F Kennedy Memorial Hospital	Indio	96%	115
Kaiser Foundation Hospital-Manteca	Manteca	96%	49
Kaiser Foundation Hospital-Walnut Creek	Walnut Creek	96%	225
Kaiser Permanente Fontana Medical Center	Fontana	96%	202
Saint Mary Medical Center	Long Beach	96%	137
Barstow Community Hospital	Barstow	95%	43
Community Hospital of Long Beach	Long Beach	95%	39
Corona Regional Medical Center	Corona	95%	110
Glendale Adventist Medical Center	Glendale	95%	236
Kaiser Permanente Sacramento Medical Center	Sacramento	95%	337
Mercy Med Ctr Merced-Community Campus	Merced	95%	101
Methodist Hospital of Southern California	Arcadia	95%	165
Olympia Medical Center	Los Angeles	95%	98
Placentia-Linda Hospital	Placentia	95%	37
Redlands Community Hospital	Redlands	95%	163
Saddleback Memorial Medical Center	Laguna Hills	95%	283
Salinas Valley Memorial Health Care District	Salinas	95%	137
Sierra View District Hospital	Porterville	95%	80
West Hills Hospital and Medical Center	West Hills	95%	92
Beverly Hospital	Montebello	94%	139
Citrus Valley Medical Center	Covina	94%	143
Doctors Hospital of Manteca	Manteca	94%	36
Emanuel Medical Center	Turlock	94%	100
Encino-Tarzana Regional Medical Center	Tarzana	94%	179
Foothill Presbyterian Hospital	Glendora	94%	50
Fresno Heart Hospital	Fresno	94%	33
Huntington Memorial Hospital	Pasadena	94%	249
Kaiser Foundation Hospital	Woodland Hills	94%	100
Kaiser Permanente Panorama City Med Ctr	Panorama City	94%	98
La Palma Intercommunity Hospital	La Palma	94%	69
Marshall Medical Center	Placerville	94%	35
Martin Luther King Jr/Charles R Drew Med Ctr	Los Angeles	94%	108
Memorial Medical Center	Modesto	94%	224
NorthBay Medical Center	Fairfield	94%	50
Queen of the Valley Hospital	Napa	94%	157
Rancho Springs Medical Center	Murrieta	94%	222
Regional Medical Center of San Jose	San Jose	94%	169
Saint John's Pleasant Valley Hospital	Camarillo	94%	34
Santa Barbara Cottage Hospital	Santa Barbara	94%	157
Sonora Regional Medical Center	Sonora	94%	47
Sutter Delta Medical Center	Antioch	94%	154
White Memorial Medical Center	Los Angeles	94%	95
Community Hospital	Huntington Park	93%	28
Greater El Monte Community Hospital	South El Monte	93%	41
Hanford Community Medical Center	Hanford	93%	71
Hemet Valley Medical Center	Hemet	93%	270
Huntington Beach Hospital	Huntington Beach	93%	41
Menifee Valley Medical Center	Sun City	93%	150
Pacifica Hospital of the Valley	Sun Valley	93%	42
Pomona Valley Hospital Medical Center	Pomona	93%	259
Riverside Community Hospital	Riverside	93%	245
VacaValley Hospital	Vacaville	93%	55
West Anaheim Medical Center	Anaheim	93%	98
Bakersfield Memorial Hospital	Bakersfield	92%	210
Eisenhower Medical Center	Rancho Mirage	92%	319
Feather River Hospital	Paradise	92%	62
Kaiser Foundation Hospital-San Diego	San Diego	92%	235
Lancaster Community Hospital	Lancaster	92%	129
Mission Community Hospital	Panorama City	92%	37
Saint Elizabeth Community Hospital	Red Bluff	92%	40
Verdugo Hills Hospital	Glendale	92%	66

NOTE: Hospital profiles are in alphabetical order by state, then city, then hospital within the city; Rankings are sorted by rate in descending order and exclude hospitals with less than 25 cases; (1) The number of cases is too small (n<25) for purposes of reliably predicting hospital performance; (2) Measure reflects the hospital's indication that its submission was based upon a sample of its relevant discharges; (3) Rate reflects fewer than the maximum possible quarters of data for the measure; (4) Inaccurate information submitted and suppressed for one or more quarters; (5) No data is available from the hospital for this measure; Please refer to the User's Guide for a full explanation of data

Paradise Valley Hospital	National City	91%	88
Sutter Solano Medical Center	Vallejo	91%	69
Western Medical Center Hospital Anaheim	Anaheim	91%	34
Citrus Valley Med Ctr Queen Valley Campus	West Covina	90%	62
Eden Medical Center	Castro Valley	90%	63
Garfield Medical Center	Monterey Park	90%	123
Alhambra Hospital Medical Center	Alhambra	89%	36
Community Medical Center-Clovis	Clovis	89%	53
Los Robles Regional Medical Center	Thousand Oaks	89%	202
Hi-Desert Medical Center	Joshua Tree	88%	25
Monterey Park Hospital	Monterey Park	87%	45
Brotman Medical Center	Culver City	86%	122
East Los Angeles Doctors Hospital	Los Angeles	86%	43
Mercy Hospital	Bakersfield	83%	60
Oroville Hospital	Oroville	83%	35
Simi Valley Hospital	Simi Valley	82%	49
Moreno Valley Community Hospital	Moreno Valley	81%	42
Victor Valley Community Hospital	Victorville	81%	63
East Valley Hospital Medical Center	Glendora	74%	43
Pacific Alliance Medical Center	Los Angeles	66%	32

3. Aspirin at Discharge

Hospital Name	City	Rate	Cases
Alta Bates Summit Medical Center	Berkeley	100%	82
Arrowhead Regional Medical Center	Colton	100%	71
California Hospital Medical Center	Los Angeles	100%	40
Cedars-Sinai Medical Center	Los Angeles	100%	347
Community Memorial Hospital Ventura	Ventura	100%	226
Contra Costa Regional Medical Center	Martinez	100%	25
Dominican Hospital	Santa Cruz	100%	160
El Centro Regional Medical Center	El Centro	100%	28
Grossmont Hospital	La Mesa	100%	404
Hoag Memorial Hospital Presbyterian	Newport Beach	100%	287
Hollywood Presbyterian Medical Center	Los Angeles	100%	89
John Muir Medical Center	Walnut Creek	100%	133
Kaiser Permanente Anaheim Medical Center	Anaheim	100%	47
Kaiser Permanente Los Angeles Medical Center	Los Angeles	100%	858
Lodi Memorial Hospital	Lodi	100%	32
Mercy San Juan Hospital	Carmichael	100%	250
Novato Community Hospital	Novato	100%	34
Palomar Medical Center	Escondido	100%	313
Paradise Valley Hospital	National City	100%	40
Saint Helena Hospital	Deer Park	100%	76
Saint Mary's Medical Center	San Francisco	100%	133
Salinas Valley Memorial Health Care District	Salinas	100%	215
San Joaquin General Hospital	French Camp	100%	32
Sharp Memorial Hospital	San Diego	100%	298
Sierra Nevada Memorial Hospital	Grass Valley	100%	26
Temple Community Hospital	Los Angeles	100%	31
USC University Hospital	Los Angeles	100%	31
University of California San Diego Med Ctr	San Diego	100%	208
Alta Bates Summit Medical Center	Oakland	99%	777
Anaheim Memorial Medical Center	Anaheim	99%	396
Beverly Hospital	Montebello	99%	113
California Pacific Medical Center	San Francisco	99%	179
Doctor's Medical Center-San Pablo Campus	San Pablo	99%	171
El Camino Hospital	Mountain View	99%	198
Glendale Memorial Hospital and Health Center	Glendale	99%	201
Good Samaritan Hospital	San Jose	99%	638
Kaiser Foundation Hospital	Hayward	99%	203
Kaiser Foundation Hospital-Vallejo	Vallejo	99%	97
Kaiser Permanente Santa Teresa Comm Med Ctr	San Jose	99%	120
Little Company of Mary Hospital	Torrance	99%	268
Loma Linda University Medical Center	Loma Linda	99%	298
Long Beach Memorial Medical Center	Long Beach	99%	310
Marian Medical Center	Santa Maria	99%	127
Marin General Hospital	Greenbrae	99%	158
Mercy General Hospital	Sacramento	99%	966
Mission Hospital Regional Medical Center	Mission Viejo	99%	254
Northridge Hospital Medical Center	Northridge	99%	169
Saint Agnes Medical Center	Fresno	99%	352
Saint Bernardine Medical Center	San Bernardino	99%	273
Saint Joseph's Medical Center of Stockton	Stockton	99%	270
San Francisco General Hospital Medical Center	San Francisco	99%	67
Santa Monica-UCLA Medical Center	Santa Monica	99%	103
Santa Rosa Memorial Hospital	Santa Rosa	99%	119
Scripps Green Hospital	La Jolla	99%	181
Sequoia Hospital	Redwood City	99%	79
Seton Medical Center	Daly City	99%	130
Stanford Hospital	Stanford	99%	215
Sutter Medical Center of Santa Rosa	Santa Rosa	99%	177
UCLA Medical Center	Los Angeles	99%	77
UCSF Medical Center	San Francisco	99%	149
University of California Davis Health System	Sacramento	99%	220
Western Medical Center	Santa Ana	99%	176
Bakersfield Heart Hospital	Bakersfield	98%	264
Centinela Hospital Medical Center	Inglewood	98%	258
Desert Valley Hospital	Victorville	98%	86
Doctors Medical Center	Modesto	98%	364
Good Samaritan Hospital	Los Angeles	98%	264
Huntington Memorial Hospital	Pasadena	98%	235
John Muir Medical Center-Concord Campus	Concord	98%	281
Kaiser Permanente San Francisco Med Ctr	San Francisco	98%	429
Los Alamitos Medical Center	Los Alamitos	98%	89
Los Angeles County Harbor-UCLA Medical Center	Torrance	98%	161
Memorial Medical Center	Modesto	98%	264
Mills-Peninsula Health Services	Burlingame	98%	131
Presbyterian Intercommunity Hospital	Whittier	98%	196
Providence Holy Cross Medical Center	Mission Hills	98%	200
Providence Saint Joseph Medical Center	Burbank	98%	268
San Antonio Community Hospital	Upland	98%	219
Scripps Memorial Hospital La Jolla	La Jolla	98%	286
Scripps Mercy Hospital	San Diego	98%	307
Sutter General Hospital	Sacramento	98%	501
Alameda County Medical Center	Oakland	97%	30
Alameda Hospital	Alameda	97%	88
Desert Regional Medical Center	Palm Springs	97%	251
Downey Regional Medical Center	Downey	97%	187
Feather River Hospital	Paradise	97%	35
French Hospital Medical Center	San Luis Obispo	97%	117
Kaiser Foundation Hospital-Manteca	Manteca	97%	37
Kaiser Foundation Hospital-South Sacramento	Sacramento	97%	152
Kaiser Foundation Hospital-Walnut Creek	Walnut Creek	97%	86
Kaiser Permanente Fontana Medical Center	Fontana	97%	133
Kaiser Permanente Santa Clara Medical Center	Santa Clara	97%	90
Kaiser Permanente West Los Angeles Med Ctr	Los Angeles	97%	102
Los Angeles County & USC Medical Center	Los Angeles	97%	193
Mercy Medical Center-Redding	Redding	97%	262
O'Connor Hospital	San Jose	97%	151
Oakland Medical Center	Oakland	97%	150
Orange Coast Memorial Medical Center	Santa Ana	97%	70
Saint John's Regional Medical Center	Oxnard	97%	222
Saint Jude Medical Center	Fullerton	97%	245
Saint Mary Medical Center	Long Beach	97%	157
San Leandro Hospital	San Leandro	97%	32
Scripps Memorial Hospital-Encinitas	Encinitas	97%	99
Shasta Regional Medical Center	Redding	97%	114
S San Francisco Medical Center	S San Francisco	97%	38
Enloe Medical Center	Chico	96%	233
Fountain Valley Reg Hospital & Med Ctr	Fountain Valley	96%	218
Glendale Adventist Medical Center	Glendale	96%	249
Irvine Regional Hospital	Irvine	96%	164
Kaiser Permanente Bellflower Medical Center	Bellflower	96%	112
Kaiser Redwood City Medical Center	Redwood City	96%	50
Kaweah Delta Health Care District	Visalia	96%	310
NorthBay Medical Center	Fairfield	96%	25
Olive View-UCLA Medical Center	San Fernando	96%	27
Petaluma Valley Hospital	Petaluma	96%	27
Pomerado Hospital	Poway	96%	25
Pomona Valley Hospital Medical Center	Pomona	96%	265
Saddleback Memorial Medical Center	Laguna Hills	96%	256
Saint Francis Medical Center	Lynwood	96%	115
Saint Joseph Hospital	Orange	96%	234
Santa Barbara Cottage Hospital	Santa Barbara	96%	229
Sierra Vista Regional Medical Center	San Luis Obispo	96%	100
Citrus Valley Medical Center	Covina	95%	276
Community Regional Medical Center	Fresno	95%	347
Kaiser Permanente Panorama City Med Ctr	Panorama City	95%	63
Lakewood Regional Medical Center	Lakewood	95%	171
Madera Community Hospital	Madera	95%	40
Methodist Hospital of Southern California	Arcadia	95%	162
Queen of the Valley Hospital	Napa	95%	206
San Gorgonio Memorial Hospital	Banning	95%	44
San Ramon Regional Medical Center	San Ramon	95%	60
Santa Clara Valley Medical Center	San Jose	95%	134
Sutter Roseville Medical Center	Roseville	95%	129
Tri-City Medical Center	Oceanside	95%	198
Valley Presbyterian Hospital	Van Nuys	95%	138
Valleycare Medical Center	Livermore	95%	94
Community Medical Center-Clovis	Clovis	94%	33
Kaiser Foundation Hospital-Fresno	Fresno	94%	140
Kaiser Permanente South Bay Medical Center	Harbor City	94%	102
Rideout Memorial Hospital	Marysville	94%	191
Saint John's Health Center	Santa Monica	94%	143
University of California Irvine Med Ctr	Orange	94%	63
Washington Hospital	Fremont	94%	216
Antelope Valley Hospital	Lancaster	93%	282
Emanuel Medical Center	Turlock	93%	43
Fresno Heart Hospital	Fresno	93%	101

NOTE: Hospital profiles are in alphabetical order by state, then city, then hospital within the city; Rankings are sorted by rate in descending order and exclude hospitals with less than 25 cases; (1) The number of cases is too small (n<25) for purposes of reliably predicting hospital performance; (2) Measure reflects the hospital's indication that its submission was based upon a sample of its relevant discharges; (3) Rate reflects fewer than the maximum possible quarters of data for the measure; (4) Inaccurate information submitted and suppressed for one or more quarters; (5) No data is available from the hospital for this measure; Please refer to the User's Guide for a full explanation of data

Kaiser Foundation Hospital	Baldwin Park	93%	68
Kaiser Foundation Hospital-San Diego	San Diego	93%	95
Riverside Community Hospital	Riverside	93%	358
Saint Joseph Hospital	Eureka	93%	105
San Rafael Medical Center	San Rafael	93%	45
Sierra View District Hospital	Porterville	93%	44
Torrance Memorial Medical Center	Torrance	93%	287
Bakersfield Memorial Hospital	Bakersfield	92%	277
Little Company of Mary-San Pedro Hospital	San Pedro	92%	25
Redlands Community Hospital	Redlands	92%	88
Regional Medical Center of San Jose	San Jose	92%	138
White Memorial Medical Center	Los Angeles	92%	85
Dameron Hospital	Stockton	91%	145
Eisenhower Medical Center	Rancho Mirage	91%	317
Kaiser Foundation Hospital-Riverside	Riverside	91%	80
Mercy Med Ctr Merced-Community Campus	Merced	91%	46
Parkview Community Hospital	Riverside	91%	35
Saint Mary Medical Center	Apple Valley	91%	254
Saint Rose Hospital	Hayward	91%	87
San Joaquin Community Hospital	Bakersfield	91%	129
Sharp Chula Vista Medical Center	Chula Vista	91%	284
Los Robles Regional Medical Center	Thousand Oaks	90%	212
Martin Luther King Jr/Charles R Drew Med Ctr	Los Angeles	90%	59
West Hills Hospital and Medical Center	West Hills	90%	91
Henry Mayo Newhall Memorial Hospital	Valencia	89%	37
Kaiser Foundation Hospital	Woodland Hills	89%	80
Kaiser Foundation Hospital-Santa Rosa	Santa Rosa	89%	121
Olympia Medical Center	Los Angeles	89%	46
San Gabriel Valley Medical Center	San Gabriel	89%	56
Whittier Hospital Medical Center	Whittier	89%	38
Encino-Tarzana Regional Medical Center	Tarzana	88%	209
La Palma Intercommunity Hospital	La Palma	88%	33
John F Kennedy Memorial Hospital	Indio	87%	84
Kaiser Permanente Sacramento Medical Center	Sacramento	87%	253
Memorial Hospital of Gardena	Gardena	87%	30
Saint Vincent Medical Center	Los Angeles	87%	113
Western Medical Center Hospital Anaheim	Anaheim	87%	132
Eden Medical Center	Castro Valley	86%	36
Corona Regional Medical Center	Corona	85%	74
Community Hospital of the Monterey Peninsula	Monterey	84%	85
Sutter Delta Medical Center	Antioch	84%	73
Verdugo Hills Hospital	Glendale	84%	31
West Anaheim Medical Center	Anaheim	84%	101
Garfield Medical Center	Monterey Park	83%	126
Lancaster Community Hospital	Lancaster	83%	112
Mission Community Hospital	Panorama City	82%	34
Brotman Medical Center	Culver City	81%	116
Foothill Presbyterian Hospital	Glendora	81%	26
Menifee Valley Medical Center	Sun City	81%	52
Rancho Springs Medical Center	Murrieta	80%	84
Hemet Valley Medical Center	Hemet	79%	116
Citrus Valley Med Ctr Queen Valley Campus	West Covina	78%	32
East Los Angeles Doctors Hospital	Los Angeles	73%	26
Encino-Tarzana Regional Medical Center	Encino	70%	30
Hanford Community Medical Center	Hanford	69%	51
Pioneers Memorial Healthcare District	Brawley	67%	33
Mercy Hospital	Bakersfield	64%	39
East Valley Hospital Medical Center	Glendora	61%	31
Victor Valley Community Hospital	Victorville	55%	40
Sutter Solano Medical Center	Vallejo	53%	34
Pacific Alliance Medical Center	Los Angeles	52%	31

4. Beta Blocker at Arrival

Hospital Name	City	Rate	Cases
Anaheim Memorial Medical Center	Anaheim	100%	162
California Hospital Medical Center	Los Angeles	100%	43
Cedars-Sinai Medical Center	Los Angeles	100%	234
Chino Valley Medical Center	Chino	100%	46
El Centro Regional Medical Center	El Centro	100%	76
French Hospital Medical Center	San Luis Obispo	100%	42
Kaiser Foundation Hospital-Vallejo	Vallejo	100%	208
Kaiser Permanente Santa Clara Medical Center	Santa Clara	100%	114
Kaiser Redwood City Medical Center	Redwood City	100%	98
Marian Medical Center	Santa Maria	100%	88
Mercy Med Ctr Merced-Community Campus	Merced	100%	95
Novato Community Hospital	Novato	100%	44
Parkview Community Hospital	Riverside	100%	64
Petaluma Valley Hospital	Petaluma	100%	40
Pomerado Hospital	Poway	100%	50
Saint Mary's Medical Center	San Francisco	100%	73
San Francisco General Hospital Medical Center	San Francisco	100%	87
San Leandro Hospital	San Leandro	100%	28
Santa Monica-UCLA Medical Center	Santa Monica	100%	97
Scripps Green Hospital	La Jolla	100%	60
Sierra Nevada Memorial Hospital	Grass Valley	100%	42
S San Francisco Medical Center	S San Francisco	100%	83
Sutter Medical Center of Santa Rosa	Santa Rosa	100%	65
Temple Community Hospital	Los Angeles	100%	27
UCLA Medical Center	Los Angeles	100%	57
University of California San Diego Med Ctr	San Diego	100%	131
Alameda Hospital	Alameda	99%	125
Desert Valley Hospital	Victorville	99%	102
Dominican Hospital	Santa Cruz	99%	142
Kaiser Foundation Hospital	Baldwin Park	99%	80
Kaiser Foundation Hospital	Hayward	99%	344
Kaiser Foundation Hospital-Walnut Creek	Walnut Creek	99%	197
Little Company of Mary Hospital	Torrance	99%	209
Mercy San Juan Hospital	Carmichael	99%	197
Northridge Hospital Medical Center	Northridge	99%	124
Oakland Medical Center	Oakland	99%	282
Palomar Medical Center	Escondido	99%	253
Presbyterian Intercommunity Hospital	Whittier	99%	194
Saint Agnes Medical Center	Fresno	99%	198
San Rafael Medical Center	San Rafael	99%	76
Scripps Memorial Hospital La Jolla	La Jolla	99%	73
Scripps Mercy Hospital	San Diego	99%	278
Fountain Valley Reg Hospital & Med Ctr	Fountain Valley	98%	152
Good Samaritan Hospital	San Jose	98%	131
Hoag Memorial Hospital Presbyterian	Newport Beach	98%	257
Kaiser Permanente Bellflower Medical Center	Bellflower	98%	149
Kaiser Permanente Los Angeles Medical Center	Los Angeles	98%	219
Kaiser Permanente San Francisco Med Ctr	San Francisco	98%	62
Kaiser Permanente Santa Teresa Comm Med Ctr	San Jose	98%	171
Lodi Memorial Hospital	Lodi	98%	55
Madera Community Hospital	Madera	98%	59
Mercy Medical Center-Redding	Redding	98%	131
Mills-Peninsula Health Services	Burlingame	98%	88
Olive View-UCLA Medical Center	San Fernando	98%	90
Saint John's Regional Medical Center	Oxnard	98%	189
Saint Joseph Hospital	Orange	98%	168
Saint Joseph's Medical Center of Stockton	Stockton	98%	122
San Ramon Regional Medical Center	San Ramon	98%	58
Sharp Memorial Hospital	San Diego	98%	196
Sierra Vista Regional Medical Center	San Luis Obispo	98%	53
University of California Irvine Med Ctr	Orange	98%	46
Good Samaritan Hospital	Los Angeles	97%	106
Hollywood Presbyterian Medical Center	Los Angeles	97%	126
John Muir Medical Center	Walnut Creek	97%	123
John Muir Medical Center-Concord Campus	Concord	97%	155
Kaiser Foundation Hospital-South Sacramento	Sacramento	97%	207
Lakewood Regional Medical Center	Lakewood	97%	120
Little Company of Mary-San Pedro Hospital	San Pedro	97%	36
Los Alamitos Medical Center	Los Alamitos	97%	105
Paradise Valley Hospital	National City	97%	61
Providence Holy Cross Medical Center	Mission Hills	97%	116
Salinas Valley Memorial Health Care District	Salinas	97%	74
Shasta Regional Medical Center	Redding	97%	69
Sutter Roseville Medical Center	Roseville	97%	159
Tri-City Medical Center	Oceanside	97%	157
Alta Bates Summit Medical Center	Oakland	96%	198
Bakersfield Heart Hospital	Bakersfield	96%	141
California Pacific Medical Center	San Francisco	96%	108
Desert Regional Medical Center	Palm Springs	96%	165
Doctors Medical Center	Modesto	96%	163
El Camino Hospital	Mountain View	96%	125
Henry Mayo Newhall Memorial Hospital	Valencia	96%	95
Kaiser Foundation Hospital-Santa Rosa	Santa Rosa	96%	162
Kaiser Permanente West Los Angeles Med Ctr	Los Angeles	96%	128
Long Beach Memorial Medical Center	Long Beach	96%	235
Los Angeles County Harbor-UCLA Medical Center	Torrance	96%	130
Mercy General Hospital	Sacramento	96%	190
Methodist Hospital of Sacramento	Sacramento	96%	28
O'Connor Hospital	San Jose	96%	119
Redlands Community Hospital	Redlands	96%	114
Saint Bernardine Medical Center	San Bernardino	96%	50
Saint John's Pleasant Valley Hospital	Camarillo	96%	26
Saint Jude Medical Center	Fullerton	96%	241
Saint Mary Medical Center	Long Beach	96%	108
San Joaquin General Hospital	French Camp	96%	52
Sequoia Hospital	Redwood City	96%	51
Seton Medical Center	Daly City	96%	107
Stanford Hospital	Stanford	96%	115
UCSF Medical Center	San Francisco	96%	96
Valleycare Medical Center	Livermore	96%	112
Western Medical Center	Santa Ana	96%	79
Alta Bates Summit Medical Center	Berkeley	95%	84
Arrowhead Regional Medical Center	Colton	95%	65
Beverly Hospital	Montebello	95%	111
Citrus Valley Med Ctr Queen Valley Campus	West Covina	95%	41

NOTE: Hospital profiles are in alphabetical order by state, then city, then hospital within the city; Rankings are sorted by rate in descending order and exclude hospitals with less than 25 cases; (1) The number of cases is too small (n<25) for purposes of reliably predicting hospital performance; (2) Measure reflects the hospital's indication that its submission was based upon a sample of its relevant discharges; (3) Rate reflects fewer than the maximum possible quarters of data for the measure; (4) Inaccurate information submitted and suppressed for one or more quarters; (5) No data is available from the hospital for this measure; Please refer to the User's Guide for a full explanation of data

Community Hospital of the Monterey Peninsula	Monterey	95%	93
Doctor's Medical Center-San Pablo Campus	San Pablo	95%	123
Garden Grove Hospital and Medical Center	Garden Grove	95%	39
Grossmont Hospital	La Mesa	95%	433
Irvine Regional Hospital	Irvine	95%	91
Kaiser Foundation Hospital	Woodland Hills	95%	100
Kaiser Foundation Hospital-San Diego	San Diego	95%	215
Kaiser Permanente Anaheim Medical Center	Anaheim	95%	77
Kaiser Permanente Panorama City Med Ctr	Panorama City	95%	100
Loma Linda University Medical Center	Loma Linda	95%	98
Providence Saint Joseph Medical Center	Burbank	95%	199
Saint Francis Medical Center	Lynwood	95%	108
San Antonio Community Hospital	Upland	95%	153
San Gabriel Valley Medical Center	San Gabriel	95%	66
University of California Davis Health System	Sacramento	95%	151
Alameda County Medical Center	Oakland	94%	49
Arroyo Grande Community Hospital	Arroyo Grande	94%	31
Dameron Hospital	Stockton	94%	48
Doctors Hospital of Manteca	Manteca	94%	33
Kaiser Permanente South Bay Medical Center	Harbor City	94%	132
Marshall Medical Center	Placerville	94%	32
Saint Luke's Hospital	San Francisco	94%	34
Santa Rosa Memorial Hospital	Santa Rosa	94%	86
Tulare District Hospital	Tulare	94%	50
Valley Presbyterian Hospital	Van Nuys	94%	79
Barstow Community Hospital	Barstow	93%	29
Huntington Memorial Hospital	Pasadena	93%	170
Kaiser Permanente Fontana Medical Center	Fontana	93%	134
Kaiser Permanente Sacramento Medical Center	Sacramento	93%	287
Kaweah Delta Health Care District	Visalia	93%	196
Orange Coast Memorial Medical Center	Santa Ana	93%	55
Rancho Springs Medical Center	Murrieta	93%	167
Regional Medical Center of San Jose	San Jose	93%	89
Saddleback Memorial Medical Center	Laguna Hills	93%	169
Saint Mary Medical Center	Apple Valley	93%	193
Sharp Chula Vista Medical Center	Chula Vista	93%	243
Sutter General Hospital	Sacramento	93%	183
West Hills Hospital and Medical Center	West Hills	93%	75
Centinela Hospital Medical Center	Inglewood	92%	192
Community Memorial Hospital Ventura	Ventura	92%	165
Eden Medical Center	Castro Valley	92%	39
Glendale Memorial Hospital and Health Center	Glendale	92%	123
Kaiser Foundation Hospital-Riverside	Riverside	92%	125
NorthBay Medical Center	Fairfield	92%	48
Scripps Memorial Hospital-Encinitas	Encinitas	92%	71
Western Medical Center Hospital Anaheim	Anaheim	92%	26
Citrus Valley Medical Center	Covina	91%	99
Community Hospital of San Bernardino	San Bernardino	91%	35
Community Regional Medical Center	Fresno	91%	204
Enloe Medical Center	Chico	91%	75
Kaiser Foundation Hospital-Fresno	Fresno	91%	176
Marin General Hospital	Greenbrae	91%	124
Saint John's Health Center	Santa Monica	91%	145
Santa Clara Valley Medical Center	San Jose	91%	122
Sutter Delta Medical Center	Antioch	91%	148
Whittier Hospital Medical Center	Whittier	91%	101
Antelope Valley Hospital	Lancaster	90%	248
Community Medical Center-Clovis	Clovis	90%	30
Emanuel Medical Center	Turlock	90%	89
Memorial Medical Center	Modesto	90%	170
Methodist Hospital of Southern California	Arcadia	90%	129
Mission Hospital Regional Medical Center	Mission Viejo	90%	188
Rideout Memorial Hospital	Marysville	90%	171
Saint Rose Hospital	Hayward	90%	115
Sonora Regional Medical Center	Sonora	90%	29
Downey Regional Medical Center	Downey	89%	139
Feather River Hospital	Paradise	89%	61
Foothill Presbyterian Hospital	Glendora	89%	45
Mission Community Hospital	Panorama City	89%	36
Saint Joseph Hospital	Eureka	89%	53
Saint Louisie Regional Hospital	Gilroy	89%	27
San Joaquin Community Hospital	Bakersfield	89%	71
Santa Barbara Cottage Hospital	Santa Barbara	89%	116
Contra Costa Regional Medical Center	Martinez	88%	25
Hanford Community Medical Center	Hanford	88%	67
Hemet Valley Medical Center	Hemet	88%	240
John F Kennedy Memorial Hospital	Indio	88%	88
Memorial Hospital of Gardena	Gardena	88%	51
Saint Vincent Medical Center	Los Angeles	88%	74
San Gorgonio Memorial Hospital	Banning	88%	80
Torrance Memorial Medical Center	Torrance	88%	252
Twin Cities Community Hospital	Templeton	88%	33
VacaValley Hospital	Vacaville	88%	42
Corona Regional Medical Center	Corona	87%	103
Glendale Adventist Medical Center	Glendale	87%	174
Kaiser Foundation Hospital-Manteca	Manteca	87%	39
Menifee Valley Medical Center	Sun City	87%	143
Pomona Valley Hospital Medical Center	Pomona	87%	164
Riverside Community Hospital	Riverside	87%	218
Washington Hospital	Fremont	87%	179
East Los Angeles Doctors Hospital	Los Angeles	86%	44
Encino-Tarzana Regional Medical Center	Tarzana	86%	158
La Palma Intercommunity Hospital	La Palma	86%	66
Los Angeles County & USC Medical Center	Los Angeles	86%	142
Pacifica Hospital of the Valley	Sun Valley	86%	36
Simi Valley Hospital	Simi Valley	86%	36
Sutter Solano Medical Center	Vallejo	86%	63
West Anaheim Medical Center	Anaheim	86%	88
Eisenhower Medical Center	Rancho Mirage	85%	182
Encino-Tarzana Regional Medical Center	Encino	85%	46
Olympia Medical Center	Los Angeles	85%	82
Queen of the Valley Hospital	Napa	85%	99
Saint Elizabeth Community Hospital	Red Bluff	85%	39
White Memorial Medical Center	Los Angeles	85%	54
Fresno Heart Hospital	Fresno	84%	32
Bakersfield Memorial Hospital	Bakersfield	83%	145
East Valley Hospital Medical Center	Glendora	83%	41
Huntington Beach Hospital	Huntington Beach	83%	36
Lancaster Community Hospital	Lancaster	81%	122
Oroville Hospital	Oroville	81%	36
Riverside County Regional Medical Center	Moreno Valley	81%	31
Brotman Medical Center	Culver City	80%	111
Garfield Medical Center	Monterey Park	80%	85
Los Robles Regional Medical Center	Thousand Oaks	80%	147
Moreno Valley Community Hospital	Moreno Valley	79%	29
Verdugo Hills Hospital	Glendale	79%	61
San Dimas Community Hospital	San Dimas	78%	32
Hi-Desert Medical Center	Joshua Tree	77%	31
Mercy Hospital	Bakersfield	75%	52
Sierra View District Hospital	Porterville	73%	64
Pioneers Memorial Healthcare District	Brawley	72%	39
Community Hospital	Huntington Park	71%	28
Alhambra Hospital Medical Center	Alhambra	68%	34
Greater El Monte Community Hospital	South El Monte	67%	36
Martin Luther King Jr/Charles R Drew Med Ctr	Los Angeles	66%	102
Monterey Park Hospital	Monterey Park	66%	41
Victor Valley Community Hospital	Victorville	64%	64
Pacific Alliance Medical Center	Los Angeles	43%	30

5. Beta Blocker at Discharge

Hospital Name	City	Rate	Cases
Alameda County Medical Center	Oakland	100%	29
Anaheim Memorial Medical Center	Anaheim	100%	384
California Hospital Medical Center	Los Angeles	100%	44
Cedars-Sinai Medical Center	Los Angeles	100%	312
Feather River Hospital	Paradise	100%	42
John Muir Medical Center	Walnut Creek	100%	126
John Muir Medical Center-Concord Campus	Concord	100%	276
Kaiser Foundation Hospital-Vallejo	Vallejo	100%	103
Kaiser Foundation Hospital-Walnut Creek	Walnut Creek	100%	97
Kaiser Permanente Santa Clara Medical Center	Santa Clara	100%	94
Kaiser Permanente Santa Teresa Comm Med Ctr	San Jose	100%	135
Kaiser Redwood City Medical Center	Redwood City	100%	53
Los Alamitos Medical Center	Los Alamitos	100%	90
Marian Medical Center	Santa Maria	100%	102
Novato Community Hospital	Novato	100%	36
Palomar Medical Center	Escondido	100%	313
Petaluma Valley Hospital	Petaluma	100%	25
Pomerado Hospital	Poway	100%	25
Saint John's Pleasant Valley Hospital	Camarillo	100%	25
Saint Luke's Hospital	San Francisco	100%	25
Saint Mary's Medical Center	San Francisco	100%	141
San Francisco General Hospital Medical Center	San Francisco	100%	63
San Joaquin General Hospital	French Camp	100%	31
San Rafael Medical Center	San Rafael	100%	56
S San Francisco Medical Center	S San Francisco	100%	39
Temple Community Hospital	Los Angeles	100%	34
Alameda Hospital	Alameda	99%	98
Alta Bates Summit Medical Center	Oakland	99%	799
California Pacific Medical Center	San Francisco	99%	181
Dominican Hospital	Santa Cruz	99%	153
Good Samaritan Hospital	San Jose	99%	625
Grossmont Hospital	La Mesa	99%	402
Hoag Memorial Hospital Presbyterian	Newport Beach	99%	284
Kaiser Foundation Hospital	Hayward	99%	216
Kaiser Foundation Hospital	Woodland Hills	99%	87
Kaiser Foundation Hospital-South Sacramento	Sacramento	99%	166
Kaiser Permanente Bellflower Medical Center	Bellflower	99%	118
Kaiser Permanente San Francisco Med Ctr	San Francisco	99%	494

NOTE: Hospital profiles are in alphabetical order by state, then city, then hospital within the city; Rankings are sorted by rate in descending order and exclude hospitals with less than 25 cases; (1) The number of cases is too small (n<25) for purposes of reliably predicting hospital performance; (2) Measure reflects the hospital's indication that its submission was based upon a sample of its relevant discharges; (3) Rate reflects fewer than the maximum possible quarters of data for the measure; (4) Inaccurate information submitted and suppressed for one or more quarters; (5) No data is available from the hospital for this measure; Please refer to the User's Guide for a full explanation of data

Hospital	City	Rate	Cases
Little Company of Mary Hospital	Torrance	99%	260
Loma Linda University Medical Center	Loma Linda	99%	293
Memorial Medical Center	Modesto	99%	287
Mercy San Juan Hospital	Carmichael	99%	284
Oakland Medical Center	Oakland	99%	141
Saint Agnes Medical Center	Fresno	99%	365
Saint Joseph's Medical Center of Stockton	Stockton	99%	261
Salinas Valley Memorial Health Care District	Salinas	99%	226
Sharp Memorial Hospital	San Diego	99%	307
Sutter Roseville Medical Center	Roseville	99%	139
University of California San Diego Med Ctr	San Diego	99%	199
Alta Bates Summit Medical Center	Berkeley	98%	81
Arrowhead Regional Medical Center	Colton	98%	65
Desert Valley Hospital	Victorville	98%	90
El Camino Hospital	Mountain View	98%	169
French Hospital Medical Center	San Luis Obispo	98%	123
Glendale Memorial Hospital and Health Center	Glendale	98%	205
Hollywood Presbyterian Medical Center	Los Angeles	98%	89
Kaiser Foundation Hospital-Santa Rosa	Santa Rosa	98%	123
Los Angeles County Harbor-UCLA Medical Center	Torrance	98%	157
Madera Community Hospital	Madera	98%	42
Mercy General Hospital	Sacramento	98%	997
Mercy Medical Center-Redding	Redding	98%	257
Mission Hospital Regional Medical Center	Mission Viejo	98%	240
Northridge Hospital Medical Center	Northridge	98%	177
Orange Coast Memorial Medical Center	Santa Ana	98%	83
Providence Saint Joseph Medical Center	Burbank	98%	262
Saint Bernardine Medical Center	San Bernardino	98%	248
Saint Joseph Hospital	Orange	98%	233
San Antonio Community Hospital	Upland	98%	209
San Gabriel Valley Medical Center	San Gabriel	98%	49
Santa Monica-UCLA Medical Center	Santa Monica	98%	103
Scripps Green Hospital	La Jolla	98%	167
Seton Medical Center	Daly City	98%	122
Stanford Hospital	Stanford	98%	185
Sutter General Hospital	Sacramento	98%	492
UCSF Medical Center	San Francisco	98%	158
University of California Davis Health System	Sacramento	98%	247
Western Medical Center	Santa Ana	98%	170
Community Medical Center-Clovis	Clovis	97%	34
Doctors Medical Center	Modesto	97%	348
Downey Regional Medical Center	Downey	97%	190
Eden Medical Center	Castro Valley	97%	39
El Centro Regional Medical Center	El Centro	97%	31
Kaiser Foundation Hospital-Manteca	Manteca	97%	35
Kaiser Permanente Los Angeles Medical Center	Los Angeles	97%	874
Kaiser Permanente South Bay Medical Center	Harbor City	97%	109
Kaiser Permanente West Los Angeles Med Ctr	Los Angeles	97%	103
Lakewood Regional Medical Center	Lakewood	97%	165
Long Beach Memorial Medical Center	Long Beach	97%	309
Providence Holy Cross Medical Center	Mission Hills	97%	204
Saddleback Memorial Medical Center	Laguna Hills	97%	258
Saint Helena Hospital	Deer Park	97%	67
Saint John's Regional Medical Center	Oxnard	97%	227
Saint Jude Medical Center	Fullerton	97%	242
Santa Rosa Memorial Hospital	Santa Rosa	97%	120
Scripps Mercy Hospital	San Diego	97%	313
Sequoia Hospital	Redwood City	97%	73
Tri-City Medical Center	Oceanside	97%	184
UCLA Medical Center	Los Angeles	97%	108
University of California Irvine Med Ctr	Orange	97%	61
Valleycare Medical Center	Livermore	97%	97
Community Hospital of the Monterey Peninsula	Monterey	96%	74
Enloe Medical Center	Chico	96%	270
Huntington Memorial Hospital	Pasadena	96%	224
Irvine Regional Hospital	Irvine	96%	174
Kaiser Foundation Hospital	Baldwin Park	96%	72
Kaiser Foundation Hospital-Fresno	Fresno	96%	152
Kaiser Foundation Hospital-San Diego	San Diego	96%	101
Mills-Peninsula Health Services	Burlingame	96%	121
Paradise Valley Hospital	National City	96%	46
Queen of the Valley Hospital	Napa	96%	227
Saint Francis Medical Center	Lynwood	96%	114
Scripps Memorial Hospital La Jolla	La Jolla	96%	280
Shasta Regional Medical Center	Redding	96%	111
Sutter Medical Center of Santa Rosa	Santa Rosa	96%	171
Valley Presbyterian Hospital	Van Nuys	96%	142
Community Regional Medical Center	Fresno	95%	368
Dameron Hospital	Stockton	95%	62
Kaiser Permanente Sacramento Medical Center	Sacramento	95%	263
Marin General Hospital	Greenbrae	95%	150
O'Connor Hospital	San Jose	95%	142
Parkview Community Hospital	Riverside	95%	37
Presbyterian Intercommunity Hospital	Whittier	95%	188
San Leandro Hospital	San Leandro	95%	39
Santa Clara Valley Medical Center	San Jose	95%	137
Sierra View District Hospital	Porterville	95%	40
Sierra Vista Regional Medical Center	San Luis Obispo	95%	94
West Hills Hospital and Medical Center	West Hills	95%	88
Beverly Hospital	Montebello	94%	103
Community Memorial Hospital Ventura	Ventura	94%	220
Desert Regional Medical Center	Palm Springs	94%	249
Doctor's Medical Center-San Pablo Campus	San Pablo	94%	160
Fountain Valley Reg Hospital & Med Ctr	Fountain Valley	94%	226
Kaiser Permanente Fontana Medical Center	Fontana	94%	144
Lodi Memorial Hospital	Lodi	94%	35
Mercy Med Ctr Merced-Community Campus	Merced	94%	53
Methodist Hospital of Southern California	Arcadia	94%	159
Regional Medical Center of San Jose	San Jose	94%	124
Saint John's Health Center	Santa Monica	94%	141
Saint Mary Medical Center	Long Beach	94%	145
Sutter Delta Medical Center	Antioch	94%	81
Centinela Hospital Medical Center	Inglewood	93%	253
Glendale Adventist Medical Center	Glendale	93%	257
Henry Mayo Newhall Memorial Hospital	Valencia	93%	30
Kaiser Permanente Panorama City Med Ctr	Panorama City	93%	71
NorthBay Medical Center	Fairfield	93%	27
Pomona Valley Hospital Medical Center	Pomona	93%	254
Saint Rose Hospital	Hayward	93%	95
Sierra Nevada Memorial Hospital	Grass Valley	93%	28
White Memorial Medical Center	Los Angeles	93%	82
Bakersfield Heart Hospital	Bakersfield	92%	262
Contra Costa Regional Medical Center	Martinez	92%	25
Eisenhower Medical Center	Rancho Mirage	92%	354
Fresno Heart Hospital	Fresno	92%	108
Good Samaritan Hospital	Los Angeles	92%	250
Kaiser Foundation Hospital-Riverside	Riverside	92%	90
Kaiser Permanente Anaheim Medical Center	Anaheim	92%	48
Little Company of Mary-San Pedro Hospital	San Pedro	92%	25
Olive View-UCLA Medical Center	San Fernando	92%	25
Redlands Community Hospital	Redlands	92%	91
Saint Joseph Hospital	Eureka	92%	102
Torrance Memorial Medical Center	Torrance	92%	283
Bakersfield Memorial Hospital	Bakersfield	91%	284
Kaweah Delta Health Care District	Visalia	91%	304
Rancho Springs Medical Center	Murrieta	91%	90
San Ramon Regional Medical Center	San Ramon	91%	55
Citrus Valley Medical Center	Covina	90%	258
Los Angeles County & USC Medical Center	Los Angeles	90%	187
Santa Barbara Cottage Hospital	Santa Barbara	90%	212
Whittier Hospital Medical Center	Whittier	90%	50
John F Kennedy Memorial Hospital	Indio	89%	80
Olympia Medical Center	Los Angeles	89%	46
San Joaquin Community Hospital	Bakersfield	89%	127
Los Robles Regional Medical Center	Thousand Oaks	88%	207
San Gorgonio Memorial Hospital	Banning	88%	50
Sharp Chula Vista Medical Center	Chula Vista	88%	280
Antelope Valley Hospital	Lancaster	87%	280
Rideout Memorial Hospital	Marysville	86%	198
Washington Hospital	Fremont	86%	219
Encino-Tarzana Regional Medical Center	Tarzana	85%	206
Riverside Community Hospital	Riverside	85%	346
USC University Hospital	Los Angeles	85%	27
Scripps Memorial Hospital-Encinitas	Encinitas	84%	93
Western Medical Center Hospital Anaheim	Anaheim	84%	126
La Palma Intercommunity Hospital	La Palma	83%	36
West Anaheim Medical Center	Anaheim	83%	105
Hemet Valley Medical Center	Hemet	81%	149
Corona Regional Medical Center	Corona	80%	74
Lancaster Community Hospital	Lancaster	80%	123
Menifee Valley Medical Center	Sun City	80%	75
Martin Luther King Jr/Charles R Drew Med Ctr	Los Angeles	79%	61
Verdugo Hills Hospital	Glendale	79%	34
Brotman Medical Center	Culver City	78%	120
Garfield Medical Center	Monterey Park	77%	115
Saint Vincent Medical Center	Los Angeles	77%	118
Foothill Presbyterian Hospital	Glendora	76%	25
Saint Elizabeth Community Hospital	Red Bluff	76%	25
Saint Mary Medical Center	Apple Valley	76%	243
Emanuel Medical Center	Turlock	74%	42
Hanford Community Medical Center	Hanford	73%	49
Citrus Valley Med Ctr Queen Valley Campus	West Covina	72%	43
Mission Community Hospital	Panorama City	72%	32
Memorial Hospital of Gardena	Gardena	71%	31
East Los Angeles Doctors Hospital	Los Angeles	70%	27
East Valley Hospital Medical Center	Glendora	69%	32
Pioneers Memorial Healthcare District	Brawley	64%	33
Sutter Solano Medical Center	Vallejo	59%	32
Mercy Hospital	Bakersfield	55%	38
Victor Valley Community Hospital	Victorville	49%	43

NOTE: Hospital profiles are in alphabetical order by state, then city, then hospital within the city; Rankings are sorted by rate in descending order and exclude hospitals with less than 25 cases; (1) The number of cases is too small (n<25) for purposes of reliably predicting hospital performance; (2) Measure reflects the hospital's indication that its submission was based upon a sample of its relevant discharges; (3) Rate reflects fewer than the maximum possible quarters of data for the measure; (4) Inaccurate information submitted and suppressed for one or more quarters; (5) No data is available from the hospital for this measure; Please refer to the User's Guide for a full explanation of data

Hospital Name	City	Rate	Cases
Pacific Alliance Medical Center	Los Angeles	43%	30

6. Fibrinolytic Medication Timing

Hospital Name	City	Rate	Cases
Hemet Valley Medical Center	Hemet	81%	42
Mercy San Juan Hospital	Carmichael	65%	34
Kaiser Permanente Fontana Medical Center	Fontana	64%	44
Oakland Medical Center	Oakland	60%	25
Kaiser Foundation Hospital-Riverside	Riverside	50%	30
Rancho Springs Medical Center	Murrieta	44%	39
Sutter Delta Medical Center	Antioch	34%	32
Kaiser Permanente Sacramento Medical Center	Sacramento	26%	39

7. PCI Within 90 Minutes of Arrival

Hospital Name	City	Rate	Cases
Hoag Memorial Hospital Presbyterian	Newport Beach	93%	27
Palomar Medical Center	Escondido	60%	25
Grossmont Hospital	La Mesa	53%	32

8. Smoking Cessation Advice

Hospital Name	City	Rate	Cases
Alta Bates Summit Medical Center	Oakland	100%	206
Anaheim Memorial Medical Center	Anaheim	100%	108
Cedars-Sinai Medical Center	Los Angeles	100%	72
Desert Valley Hospital	Victorville	100%	29
Doctors Medical Center	Modesto	100%	119
Dominican Hospital	Santa Cruz	100%	39
Downey Regional Medical Center	Downey	100%	37
El Camino Hospital	Mountain View	100%	34
French Hospital Medical Center	San Luis Obispo	100%	35
Glendale Adventist Medical Center	Glendale	100%	83
Glendale Memorial Hospital and Health Center	Glendale	100%	61
John Muir Medical Center	Walnut Creek	100%	25
John Muir Medical Center-Concord Campus	Concord	100%	78
Kaiser Permanente San Francisco Med Ctr	San Francisco	100%	120
Kaiser Permanente Santa Teresa Comm Med Ctr	San Jose	100%	39
Long Beach Memorial Medical Center	Long Beach	100%	87
Marian Medical Center	Santa Maria	100%	35
Mercy Medical Center-Redding	Redding	100%	116
Mercy San Juan Hospital	Carmichael	100%	85
Mills-Peninsula Health Services	Burlingame	100%	40
Mission Hospital Regional Medical Center	Mission Viejo	100%	46
Northridge Hospital Medical Center	Northridge	100%	42
Palomar Medical Center	Escondido	100%	96
Saddleback Memorial Medical Center	Laguna Hills	100%	53
Saint Agnes Medical Center	Fresno	100%	84
Saint Helena Hospital	Deer Park	100%	38
Saint Joseph Hospital	Orange	100%	63
San Antonio Community Hospital	Upland	100%	70
Sharp Memorial Hospital	San Diego	100%	61
Tri-City Medical Center	Oceanside	100%	34
Good Samaritan Hospital	San Jose	99%	133
Grossmont Hospital	La Mesa	99%	144
Mercy General Hospital	Sacramento	99%	329
Pomona Valley Hospital Medical Center	Pomona	99%	78
Saint Bernardine Medical Center	San Bernardino	99%	76
Saint Joseph's Medical Center of Stockton	Stockton	99%	106
Sutter General Hospital	Sacramento	99%	152
Bakersfield Heart Hospital	Bakersfield	98%	103
Bakersfield Memorial Hospital	Bakersfield	98%	88
Fountain Valley Reg Hospital & Med Ctr	Fountain Valley	98%	58
Good Samaritan Hospital	Los Angeles	98%	65
Lakewood Regional Medical Center	Lakewood	98%	47
Little Company of Mary Hospital	Torrance	98%	66
Loma Linda University Medical Center	Loma Linda	98%	108
Memorial Medical Center	Modesto	98%	118
Queen of the Valley Hospital	Napa	98%	64
Saint Mary Medical Center	Apple Valley	98%	85
Santa Barbara Cottage Hospital	Santa Barbara	98%	55
Shasta Regional Medical Center	Redding	98%	47
Sutter Medical Center of Santa Rosa	Santa Rosa	98%	58
University of California San Diego Med Ctr	San Diego	98%	53
Citrus Valley Medical Center	Covina	97%	71
Irvine Regional Hospital	Irvine	97%	37
Kaiser Permanente Fontana Medical Center	Fontana	97%	30
Lancaster Community Hospital	Lancaster	97%	37
Presbyterian Intercommunity Hospital	Whittier	97%	37
Regional Medical Center of San Jose	San Jose	97%	36
Saint Francis Medical Center	Lynwood	97%	34
Saint Jude Medical Center	Fullerton	97%	61
Sierra Vista Regional Medical Center	San Luis Obispo	97%	31
Sutter Roseville Medical Center	Roseville	97%	31
Eisenhower Medical Center	Rancho Mirage	96%	75
Enloe Medical Center	Chico	96%	95
Kaweah Delta Health Care District	Visalia	96%	91
Providence Saint Joseph Medical Center	Burbank	96%	104
University of California Davis Health System	Sacramento	96%	97
University of California Irvine Med Ctr	Orange	96%	27
Washington Hospital	Fremont	96%	55
Antelope Valley Hospital	Lancaster	95%	123
Scripps Mercy Hospital	San Diego	95%	87
Western Medical Center Hospital Anaheim	Anaheim	95%	39
Desert Regional Medical Center	Palm Springs	94%	68
Los Robles Regional Medical Center	Thousand Oaks	94%	48
Providence Holy Cross Medical Center	Mission Hills	94%	64
Saint Mary Medical Center	Long Beach	94%	52
San Joaquin Community Hospital	Bakersfield	94%	48
Scripps Memorial Hospital La Jolla	La Jolla	94%	71
Stanford Hospital	Stanford	94%	33
White Memorial Medical Center	Los Angeles	94%	33
California Pacific Medical Center	San Francisco	93%	46
Encino-Tarzana Regional Medical Center	Tarzana	93%	41
Hoag Memorial Hospital Presbyterian	Newport Beach	93%	58
Huntington Memorial Hospital	Pasadena	93%	60
Methodist Hospital of Southern California	Arcadia	93%	42
Riverside Community Hospital	Riverside	93%	116
Saint John's Health Center	Santa Monica	93%	29
Saint John's Regional Medical Center	Oxnard	93%	46
Kaiser Foundation Hospital-Santa Rosa	Santa Rosa	92%	25
Marin General Hospital	Greenbrae	92%	25
Centinela Hospital Medical Center	Inglewood	91%	81
Community Memorial Hospital Ventura	Ventura	91%	53
Dameron Hospital	Stockton	91%	58
O'Connor Hospital	San Jose	91%	35
Scripps Green Hospital	La Jolla	91%	35
Torrance Memorial Medical Center	Torrance	91%	55
Kaiser Foundation Hospital-South Sacramento	Sacramento	90%	30
Saint Joseph Hospital	Eureka	89%	37
West Anaheim Medical Center	Anaheim	89%	38
Los Angeles County Harbor-UCLA Medical Center	Torrance	87%	68
Saint Mary's Medical Center	San Francisco	86%	29
Kaiser Foundation Hospital-Fresno	Fresno	85%	27
UCSF Medical Center	San Francisco	85%	34
Community Regional Medical Center	Fresno	83%	154
Rideout Memorial Hospital	Marysville	83%	70
Doctor's Medical Center-San Pablo Campus	San Pablo	80%	56
Santa Clara Valley Medical Center	San Jose	80%	50
Kaiser Permanente Los Angeles Medical Center	Los Angeles	79%	207
Western Medical Center	Santa Ana	79%	47
San Francisco General Hospital Medical Center	San Francisco	73%	26
Sharp Chula Vista Medical Center	Chula Vista	72%	57
Los Angeles County & USC Medical Center	Los Angeles	69%	83
Arrowhead Regional Medical Center	Colton	61%	28
Kaiser Permanente Sacramento Medical Center	Sacramento	49%	37

Heart Failure Care

9. ACE Inhibitor or ARB for LVSD

Hospital Name	City	Rate	Cases
California Hospital Medical Center	Los Angeles	100%	218
Desert Valley Hospital	Victorville	100%	64
Doctors Hospital of Manteca	Manteca	100%	30
Hollywood Presbyterian Medical Center	Los Angeles	100%	115
Los Alamitos Medical Center	Los Alamitos	100%	75
Natividad Medical Center	Salinas	100%	28
Pomerado Hospital	Poway	100%	29
San Mateo Medical Center	San Mateo	100%	33
Sutter Tracy Community Hospital	Tracy	100%	26
Ventura County Medical Center	Ventura	100%	39
Cedars-Sinai Medical Center	Los Angeles	99%	336
Community Hospital of San Bernardino	San Bernardino	99%	67
El Centro Regional Medical Center	El Centro	98%	60
John Muir Medical Center	Walnut Creek	98%	88
Kaiser Foundation Hospital-South Sacramento	Sacramento	98%	101
San Joaquin General Hospital	French Camp	98%	109
San Rafael Medical Center	San Rafael	98%	49
Sutter Auburn Faith Hospital	Auburn	98%	45
Chino Valley Medical Center	Chino	97%	31
Community Memorial Hospital Ventura	Ventura	97%	73
Kaiser Permanente San Francisco Med Ctr	San Francisco	97%	134
Kaiser Redwood City Medical Center	Redwood City	97%	37
Lompoc Healthcare District Hospital	Lompoc	97%	29
Olive View-UCLA Medical Center	San Fernando	97%	147
Palomar Medical Center	Escondido	97%	162
Providence Saint Joseph Medical Center	Burbank	97%	99
Tulare District Hospital	Tulare	97%	59
Anaheim Memorial Medical Center	Anaheim	96%	207

NOTE: Hospital profiles are in alphabetical order by state, then city, then hospital within the city; Rankings are sorted by rate in descending order and exclude hospitals with less than 25 cases; (1) The number of cases is too small (n<25) for purposes of reliably predicting hospital performance; (2) Measure reflects the hospital's indication that its submission was based upon a sample of its relevant discharges; (3) Rate reflects fewer than the maximum possible quarters of data for the measure; (4) Inaccurate information submitted and suppressed for one or more quarters; (5) No data is available from the hospital for this measure; Please refer to the User's Guide for a full explanation of data

Contra Costa Regional Medical Center	Martinez	96%	70
Lakewood Regional Medical Center	Lakewood	96%	146
Marian Medical Center	Santa Maria	96%	78
Saint Agnes Medical Center	Fresno	96%	158
Saint Joseph's Medical Center of Stockton	Stockton	96%	119
Saint Mary's Medical Center	San Francisco	96%	78
San Francisco General Hospital Medical Center	San Francisco	96%	200
Ukiah Valley Medical Center	Ukiah	96%	26
Doctors Medical Center	Modesto	95%	165
French Hospital Medical Center	San Luis Obispo	95%	42
Glendale Memorial Hospital and Health Center	Glendale	95%	256
Kern Medical Center	Bakersfield	95%	76
Mercy San Juan Hospital	Carmichael	95%	142
O'Connor Hospital	San Jose	95%	123
Oakland Medical Center	Oakland	95%	169
Saint Bernardine Medical Center	San Bernardino	95%	91
Alameda County Medical Center	Oakland	94%	140
Northridge Hospital Medical Center	Northridge	94%	125
Saddleback Memorial Medical Center	Laguna Hills	94%	219
Sierra View District Hospital	Porterville	94%	47
Sutter General Hospital	Sacramento	94%	124
Woodland Healthcare	Woodland	94%	34
Centinela Freeman Reg Med Ctr-Marina	Marina Del Rey	93%	27
El Camino Hospital	Mountain View	93%	123
John Muir Medical Center-Concord Campus	Concord	93%	106
Kaiser Foundation Hospital-Manteca	Manteca	93%	56
Kaiser Foundation Hospital-Riverside	Riverside	93%	126
Kaiser Foundation Hospital-Walnut Creek	Walnut Creek	93%	41
Mission Hospital Regional Medical Center	Mission Viejo	93%	83
Presbyterian Intercommunity Hospital	Whittier	93%	76
Saint Joseph Hospital	Orange	93%	146
Sierra Nevada Memorial Hospital	Grass Valley	93%	73
Western Medical Center	Santa Ana	93%	101
California Pacific Medical Center	San Francisco	92%	177
Emanuel Medical Center	Turlock	92%	78
Fallbrook Hospital	Fallbrook	92%	25
Loma Linda University Medical Center	Loma Linda	92%	261
Martin Luther King Jr/Charles R Drew Med Ctr	Los Angeles	92%	50
Mills-Peninsula Health Services	Burlingame	92%	76
Olympia Medical Center	Los Angeles	92%	89
Pacific Hospital of Long Beach	Long Beach	92%	26
Regional Medical Center of San Jose	San Jose	92%	113
Saint Luke's Hospital	San Francisco	92%	75
San Joaquin Community Hospital	Bakersfield	92%	169
Scripps Green Hospital	La Jolla	92%	107
Whittier Hospital Medical Center	Whittier	92%	52
Dameron Hospital	Stockton	91%	93
Madera Community Hospital	Madera	91%	47
Memorial Hospital of Gardena	Gardena	91%	82
Methodist Hospital of Sacramento	Sacramento	91%	88
Pioneers Memorial Healthcare District	Brawley	91%	66
Riverside County Regional Medical Center	Moreno Valley	91%	118
Saint Francis Medical Center	Lynwood	91%	258
Saint John's Health Center	Santa Monica	91%	92
Saint John's Regional Medical Center	Oxnard	91%	92
Sequoia Hospital	Redwood City	91%	95
USC University Hospital	Los Angeles	91%	34
Arrowhead Regional Medical Center	Colton	90%	207
Kaiser Permanente Santa Teresa Comm Med Ctr	San Jose	90%	138
Little Company of Mary-San Pedro Hospital	San Pedro	90%	50
Los Angeles County & USC Medical Center	Los Angeles	90%	307
Mercy Med Ctr Merced-Community Campus	Merced	90%	110
Parkview Community Hospital	Riverside	90%	52
Shasta Regional Medical Center	Redding	90%	98
Sierra Vista Regional Medical Center	San Luis Obispo	90%	29
S San Francisco Medical Center	S San Francisco	90%	70
West Hills Hospital and Medical Center	West Hills	90%	49
Grossmont Hospital	La Mesa	89%	254
Mercy General Hospital	Sacramento	89%	269
Mercy Medical Center-Redding	Redding	89%	121
Pomona Valley Hospital Medical Center	Pomona	89%	261
San Gorgonio Memorial Hospital	Banning	89%	37
Santa Rosa Memorial Hospital	Santa Rosa	89%	98
Corona Regional Medical Center	Corona	88%	33
Desert Regional Medical Center	Palm Springs	88%	209
Huntington Beach Hospital	Huntington Beach	88%	26
Little Company of Mary Hospital	Torrance	88%	169
Orange Coast Memorial Medical Center	Santa Ana	88%	103
Saint Joseph Hospital	Eureka	88%	41
Saint Jude Medical Center	Fullerton	88%	171
Salinas Valley Memorial Health Care District	Salinas	88%	142
San Ramon Regional Medical Center	San Ramon	88%	33
Sutter Delta Medical Center	Antioch	88%	78
University of California Irvine Med Ctr	Orange	88%	136
University of California San Diego Med Ctr	San Diego	88%	152

Alta Bates Summit Medical Center	Oakland	87%	85
Fountain Valley Reg Hospital & Med Ctr	Fountain Valley	87%	150
Fresno Heart Hospital	Fresno	87%	52
Good Samaritan Hospital	Los Angeles	87%	197
Hoag Memorial Hospital Presbyterian	Newport Beach	87%	251
Kaiser Permanente Bellflower Medical Center	Bellflower	87%	212
Kaiser Permanente South Bay Medical Center	Harbor City	87%	120
Providence Holy Cross Medical Center	Mission Hills	87%	102
San Gabriel Valley Medical Center	San Gabriel	87%	79
San Leandro Hospital	San Leandro	87%	102
Stanford Hospital	Stanford	87%	150
Sutter Medical Center of Santa Rosa	Santa Rosa	87%	97
Bakersfield Memorial Hospital	Bakersfield	86%	133
Centinela Hospital Medical Center	Inglewood	86%	197
Eisenhower Medical Center	Rancho Mirage	86%	310
Kaiser Foundation Hospital-San Diego	San Diego	86%	242
Mercy Hospital of Folsom	Folsom	86%	43
Rancho Springs Medical Center	Murrieta	86%	146
Scripps Mercy Hospital	San Diego	86%	287
Seton Medical Center	Daly City	86%	151
Valleycare Medical Center	Livermore	86%	66
Garden Grove Hospital and Medical Center	Garden Grove	85%	26
Glendale Adventist Medical Center	Glendale	85%	176
Hi-Desert Medical Center	Joshua Tree	85%	33
Kaiser Foundation Hospital	Woodland Hills	85%	92
Kaiser Foundation Hospital-Santa Rosa	Santa Rosa	85%	48
UCLA Medical Center	Los Angeles	85%	194
Kaiser Foundation Hospital	Baldwin Park	84%	122
Kaiser Foundation Hospital	Hayward	84%	105
Kaiser Permanente Los Angeles Medical Center	Los Angeles	84%	257
Long Beach Memorial Medical Center	Long Beach	84%	330
Oroville Hospital	Oroville	84%	58
Paradise Valley Hospital	National City	84%	161
Rideout Memorial Hospital	Marysville	84%	147
Saint Mary Medical Center	Long Beach	84%	112
Sharp Memorial Hospital	San Diego	84%	161
Alta Bates Summit Medical Center	Berkeley	83%	41
Community Regional Medical Center	Fresno	83%	442
Downey Regional Medical Center	Downey	83%	136
Kaiser Foundation Hospital-Fresno	Fresno	83%	103
Kaiser Permanente Fontana Medical Center	Fontana	83%	301
Los Angeles County Harbor-UCLA Medical Center	Torrance	83%	198
Torrance Memorial Medical Center	Torrance	83%	279
Twin Cities Community Hospital	Templeton	83%	41
Encino-Tarzana Regional Medical Center	Tarzana	82%	130
Kaiser Foundation Hospital-Vallejo	Vallejo	82%	83
Kaiser Permanente Anaheim Medical Center	Anaheim	82%	60
Memorial Medical Center	Modesto	82%	153
Sutter Coast Hospital	Crescent City	82%	34
UCSF Medical Center	San Francisco	82%	136
Marin General Hospital	Greenbrae	81%	104
Riverside Community Hospital	Riverside	81%	193
Saint Rose Hospital	Hayward	81%	113
San Antonio Community Hospital	Upland	81%	207
Santa Monica-UCLA Medical Center	Santa Monica	81%	68
Scripps Memorial Hospital La Jolla	La Jolla	81%	119
Sutter Solano Medical Center	Vallejo	81%	80
Alameda Hospital	Alameda	80%	35
Bakersfield Heart Hospital	Bakersfield	80%	135
Barstow Community Hospital	Barstow	80%	41
Kaiser Permanente West Los Angeles Med Ctr	Los Angeles	80%	134
Ridgecrest Regional Hospital	Ridgecrest	80%	25
Sutter Roseville Medical Center	Roseville	80%	94
La Palma Intercommunity Hospital	La Palma	79%	91
Methodist Hospital of Southern California	Arcadia	79%	189
Redlands Community Hospital	Redlands	79%	110
Tri-City Medical Center	Oceanside	79%	144
VacaValley Hospital	Vacaville	79%	39
Citrus Valley Med Ctr Queen Valley Campus	West Covina	78%	154
Coast Plaza Doctors Hospital	Norwalk	78%	27
Doctor's Medical Center-San Pablo Campus	San Pablo	78%	213
Hanford Community Medical Center	Hanford	77%	30
John F Kennedy Memorial Hospital	Indio	77%	79
Kaweah Delta Health Care District	Visalia	77%	160
Lancaster Community Hospital	Lancaster	77%	105
Santa Barbara Cottage Hospital	Santa Barbara	77%	147
University of California Davis Health System	Sacramento	77%	188
West Anaheim Medical Center	Anaheim	77%	69
Community Hospital of Long Beach	Long Beach	76%	34
Dominican Hospital	Santa Cruz	76%	96
Eden Medical Center	Castro Valley	76%	83
Saint Mary Medical Center	Apple Valley	76%	164
Simi Valley Hospital	Simi Valley	76%	38
White Memorial Medical Center	Los Angeles	76%	175
Henry Mayo Newhall Memorial Hospital	Valencia	75%	69

NOTE: Hospital profiles are in alphabetical order by state, then city, then hospital within the city; Rankings are sorted by rate in descending order and exclude hospitals with less than 25 cases; (1) The number of cases is too small (n<25) for purposes of reliably predicting hospital performance; (2) Measure reflects the hospital's indication that its submission was based upon a sample of its relevant discharges; (3) Rate reflects fewer than the maximum possible quarters of data for the measure; (4) Inaccurate information submitted and suppressed for one or more quarters; (5) No data is available from the hospital for this measure; Please refer to the User's Guide for a full explanation of data

Huntington Memorial Hospital	Pasadena	75%	178
Kaiser Permanente Panorama City Med Ctr	Panorama City	75%	134
Queen of the Valley Hospital	Napa	75%	60
Watsonville Community Hospital	Watsonville	75%	36
Community Hospital	Huntington Park	74%	27
Community Medical Center-Clovis	Clovis	74%	53
Irvine Regional Hospital	Irvine	74%	57
Los Robles Regional Medical Center	Thousand Oaks	74%	89
San Dimas Community Hospital	San Dimas	74%	43
Enloe Medical Center	Chico	73%	112
Kaiser Permanente Sacramento Medical Center	Sacramento	73%	235
Marshall Medical Center	Placerville	73%	55
Washington Hospital	Fremont	73%	81
Brotman Medical Center	Culver City	72%	64
Placentia-Linda Hospital	Placentia	72%	36
Saint Vincent Medical Center	Los Angeles	72%	109
Beverly Hospital	Montebello	71%	127
Lodi Memorial Hospital	Lodi	71%	55
Menifee Valley Medical Center	Sun City	71%	76
Mission Community Hospital	Panorama City	71%	68
NorthBay Medical Center	Fairfield	71%	92
Valley Presbyterian Hospital	Van Nuys	71%	52
Community Hospital of the Monterey Peninsula	Monterey	70%	91
Delano Regional Medical Center	Delano	70%	27
Moreno Valley Community Hospital	Moreno Valley	70%	50
Citrus Valley Medical Center	Covina	69%	151
Santa Clara Valley Medical Center	San Jose	69%	172
Scripps Memorial Hospital-Encinitas	Encinitas	68%	59
Sutter Amador Hospital	Jackson	68%	34
Hemet Valley Medical Center	Hemet	66%	138
Saint Louise Regional Hospital	Gilroy	66%	35
Victor Valley Community Hospital	Victorville	66%	35
Sharp Chula Vista Medical Center	Chula Vista	65%	179
Antelope Valley Hospital	Lancaster	64%	224
Bellflower Medical Center	Bellflower	64%	28
Verdugo Hills Hospital	Glendale	63%	49
Los Angeles Community Hospital	Los Angeles	61%	41
Foothill Presbyterian Hospital	Glendora	60%	55
Good Samaritan Hospital	San Jose	60%	113
Kaiser Permanente Santa Clara Medical Center	Santa Clara	60%	115
Monterey Park Hospital	Monterey Park	59%	76
Mercy Hospital	Bakersfield	57%	63
Garfield Medical Center	Monterey Park	50%	64
City of Angels Medical Center	Los Angeles	48%	27
Pacific Alliance Medical Center	Los Angeles	36%	45

10. Discharge Instructions

Hospital Name	City	Rate	Cases
California Hospital Medical Center	Los Angeles	100%	378
Chino Valley Medical Center	Chino	100%	49
El Centro Regional Medical Center	El Centro	100%	206
San Mateo Medical Center	San Mateo	100%	59
Seton Medical Center	Daly City	100%	71
Sherman Oaks Hospital	Sherman Oaks	100%	32
Coast Plaza Doctors Hospital	Norwalk	99%	90
East Los Angeles Doctors Hospital	Los Angeles	99%	102
Desert Valley Hospital	Victorville	98%	118
Saint Elizabeth Community Hospital	Red Bluff	98%	65
Saint Louise Regional Hospital	Gilroy	98%	84
Sequoia Hospital	Redwood City	98%	262
Marian Medical Center	Santa Maria	97%	223
French Hospital Medical Center	San Luis Obispo	96%	110
Garden Grove Hospital and Medical Center	Garden Grove	96%	71
Saint Jude Medical Center	Fullerton	95%	295
Whittier Hospital Medical Center	Whittier	95%	182
Arroyo Grande Community Hospital	Arroyo Grande	93%	90
Community Hospital of San Bernardino	San Bernardino	93%	227
Doctors Hospital of Manteca	Manteca	93%	90
Twin Cities Community Hospital	Templeton	93%	123
Ventura County Medical Center	Ventura	93%	88
John Muir Medical Center	Walnut Creek	92%	225
Mercy General Hospital	Sacramento	91%	511
Saint Mary Medical Center	Long Beach	91%	236
Sierra Vista Regional Medical Center	San Luis Obispo	91%	64
Doctors Medical Center	Modesto	90%	350
Mercy Medical Center-Mount Shasta	Mount Shasta	90%	40
Palomar Medical Center	Escondido	90%	365
Saint Helena Hospital	Deer Park	90%	67
Anaheim Memorial Medical Center	Anaheim	89%	495
Saint Mary's Medical Center	San Francisco	89%	151
Sutter Auburn Faith Hospital	Auburn	89%	123
Mercy San Juan Hospital	Carmichael	88%	416
Sutter Delta Medical Center	Antioch	88%	253
Alta Bates Summit Medical Center	Oakland	87%	159
Desert Regional Medical Center	Palm Springs	87%	333
Little Company of Mary Hospital	Torrance	87%	349
Mercy Hospital of Folsom	Folsom	87%	100
Presbyterian Intercommunity Hospital	Whittier	86%	218
Salinas Valley Memorial Health Care District	Salinas	86%	78
La Palma Intercommunity Hospital	La Palma	85%	170
Sutter General Hospital	Sacramento	85%	248
Feather River Hospital	Paradise	84%	64
John Muir Medical Center-Concord Campus	Concord	84%	257
Mercy Med Ctr Merced-Community Campus	Merced	84%	247
Placentia-Linda Hospital	Placentia	84%	74
Saint Francis Memorial Hospital	San Francisco	84%	56
Sutter Roseville Medical Center	Roseville	84%	222
Kaiser Foundation Hospital-South Sacramento	Sacramento	83%	255
Mercy Hospital	Bakersfield	83%	149
Mission Hospital Regional Medical Center	Mission Viejo	83%	243
Scripps Green Hospital	La Jolla	83%	247
Stanford Hospital	Stanford	83%	288
Alta Bates Summit Medical Center	Berkeley	82%	94
Dameron Hospital	Stockton	82%	238
Pacific Hospital of Long Beach	Long Beach	82%	34
Saddleback Memorial Medical Center	Laguna Hills	82%	523
San Ramon Regional Medical Center	San Ramon	82%	80
Fresno Heart Hospital	Fresno	81%	123
Long Beach Memorial Medical Center	Long Beach	81%	599
Methodist Hospital of Southern California	Arcadia	81%	480
Pomerado Hospital	Poway	81%	122
Sutter Lakeside Hospital	Lakeport	81%	31
Tri-City Medical Center	Oceanside	81%	339
Tulare District Hospital	Tulare	81%	124
Woodland Healthcare	Woodland	81%	81
Chapman Medical Center	Orange	80%	40
Emanuel Medical Center	Turlock	80%	213
Los Alamitos Medical Center	Los Alamitos	80%	212
Good Samaritan Hospital	Los Angeles	79%	391
Kaiser Permanente San Francisco Med Ctr	San Francisco	79%	336
South Coast Medical Center	Laguna Beach	79%	85
West Anaheim Medical Center	Anaheim	79%	185
San Dimas Community Hospital	San Dimas	78%	83
Watsonville Community Hospital	Watsonville	78%	156
Marin General Hospital	Greenbrae	77%	181
Ridgecrest Regional Hospital	Ridgecrest	77%	74
Sierra Nevada Memorial Hospital	Grass Valley	77%	112
Western Medical Center Hospital Anaheim	Anaheim	77%	35
Kaiser Permanente Santa Teresa Comm Med Ctr	San Jose	76%	346
Lakewood Regional Medical Center	Lakewood	76%	405
Northridge Hospital Medical Center	Northridge	76%	293
Orange Coast Memorial Medical Center	Santa Ana	76%	297
Paradise Valley Hospital	National City	76%	326
Pomona Valley Hospital Medical Center	Pomona	76%	484
Saint Bernardine Medical Center	San Bernardino	76%	275
Torrance Memorial Medical Center	Torrance	76%	467
Novato Community Hospital	Novato	75%	48
San Rafael Medical Center	San Rafael	75%	156
Santa Rosa Memorial Hospital	Santa Rosa	75%	223
Saint Joseph's Medical Center of Stockton	Stockton	74%	216
San Joaquin General Hospital	French Camp	74%	187
Sutter Davis Hospital	Davis	74%	47
Hoag Memorial Hospital Presbyterian	Newport Beach	73%	494
Redlands Community Hospital	Redlands	73%	45
San Gabriel Valley Medical Center	San Gabriel	73%	188
Sierra View District Hospital	Porterville	73%	174
Mercy Medical Center-Redding	Redding	72%	221
Saint Agnes Medical Center	Fresno	72%	357
Sutter Tracy Community Hospital	Tracy	72%	100
Grossmont Hospital	La Mesa	71%	504
San Joaquin Community Hospital	Bakersfield	71%	388
Sutter Solano Medical Center	Vallejo	71%	313
White Memorial Medical Center	Los Angeles	71%	69
Community Hospital of Los Gatos	Los Gatos	70%	63
Community Hospital of the Monterey Peninsula	Monterey	70%	56
Riverside Community Hospital	Riverside	70%	439
Saint Rose Hospital	Hayward	70%	57
Sonora Regional Medical Center	Sonora	70%	80
Sutter Medical Center of Santa Rosa	Santa Rosa	70%	183
Encino-Tarzana Regional Medical Center	Encino	69%	75
Kaiser Permanente Santa Clara Medical Center	Santa Clara	69%	397
Lompoc Healthcare District Hospital	Lompoc	69%	49
Los Angeles County Harbor-UCLA Medical Center	Torrance	69%	323
Methodist Hospital of Sacramento	Sacramento	69%	249
Saint Joseph Hospital	Eureka	69%	101
Scripps Mercy Hospital	San Diego	69%	740
Sharp Chula Vista Medical Center	Chula Vista	69%	478
Ukiah Valley Medical Center	Ukiah	69%	70
Bakersfield Memorial Hospital	Bakersfield	68%	253

NOTE: Hospital profiles are in alphabetical order by state, then city, then hospital within the city; Rankings are sorted by rate in descending order and exclude hospitals with less than 25 cases; (1) The number of cases is too small (n<25) for purposes of reliably predicting hospital performance; (2) Measure reflects the hospital's indication that its submission was based upon a sample of its relevant discharges; (3) Rate reflects fewer than the maximum possible quarters of data for the measure; (4) Inaccurate information submitted and suppressed for one or more quarters; (5) No data is available from the hospital for this measure; Please refer to the User's Guide for a full explanation of data

Hospital Name	City	Rate	Cases
Encino-Tarzana Regional Medical Center	Tarzana	68%	281
Foothill Presbyterian Hospital	Glendora	68%	163
Kaiser Foundation Hospital	Woodland Hills	68%	282
Mills-Peninsula Health Services	Burlingame	68%	217
Sutter Coast Hospital	Crescent City	68%	91
University of California Irvine Med Ctr	Orange	68%	255
Downey Regional Medical Center	Downey	67%	306
Good Samaritan Hospital	San Jose	67%	273
Kaiser Foundation Hospital-Santa Rosa	Santa Rosa	67%	113
Kaiser Permanente Bellflower Medical Center	Bellflower	67%	478
Memorial Hospital Los Banos	Los Banos	67%	43
Pacific Alliance Medical Center	Los Angeles	67%	46
Saint John's Pleasant Valley Hospital	Camarillo	67%	67
Shasta Regional Medical Center	Redding	66%	176
John F Kennedy Memorial Hospital	Indio	65%	162
Pioneers Memorial Healthcare District	Brawley	65%	110
Bakersfield Heart Hospital	Bakersfield	64%	251
Community Hospital of Long Beach	Long Beach	64%	56
Los Robles Regional Medical Center	Thousand Oaks	64%	205
S San Francisco Medical Center	S San Francisco	64%	210
Western Medical Center	Santa Ana	64%	222
Eden Medical Center	Castro Valley	63%	182
Providence Saint Joseph Medical Center	Burbank	63%	241
Saint John's Regional Medical Center	Oxnard	63%	299
Saint Joseph Hospital	Orange	63%	398
Sharp Memorial Hospital	San Diego	63%	365
UCSF Medical Center	San Francisco	63%	292
Chinese Hospital	San Francisco	62%	82
Kaiser Foundation Hospital-Riverside	Riverside	62%	329
Kaiser Permanente Fontana Medical Center	Fontana	62%	607
Little Company of Mary-San Pedro Hospital	San Pedro	62%	166
Saint Francis Medical Center	Lynwood	62%	486
San Leandro Hospital	San Leandro	62%	319
Kaiser Foundation Hospital	Hayward	61%	377
Corona Regional Medical Center	Corona	60%	200
Irvine Regional Hospital	Irvine	60%	173
Kaiser Foundation Hospital-Walnut Creek	Walnut Creek	60%	188
Kaiser Permanente Panorama City Med Ctr	Panorama City	60%	340
Oakland Medical Center	Oakland	60%	534
Saint Mary Medical Center	Apple Valley	60%	401
University of California San Diego Med Ctr	San Diego	60%	270
Fountain Valley Reg Hospital & Med Ctr	Fountain Valley	59%	328
Lodi Memorial Hospital	Lodi	59%	139
Los Angeles Community Hospital	Los Angeles	59%	115
Petaluma Valley Hospital	Petaluma	59%	56
Davies Medical Center	San Francisco	58%	53
Kaiser Foundation Hospital	Baldwin Park	58%	346
Motion Picture & Television Hospital	Woodland Hills	58%	36
Oak Valley Hospital	Oakdale	58%	55
Scripps Memorial Hospital La Jolla	La Jolla	58%	224
Tri-City Regional Medical Center	Hawaiian Gardens	58%	64
Valleycare Medical Center	Livermore	58%	158
Rancho Springs Medical Center	Murrieta	57%	391
Dominican Hospital	Santa Cruz	56%	259
Eisenhower Medical Center	Rancho Mirage	56%	480
Huntington Beach Hospital	Huntington Beach	56%	97
Mark Twain Saint Joseph's Hospital	San Andreas	56%	54
Barstow Community Hospital	Barstow	55%	202
Memorial Medical Center	Modesto	55%	331
Riverside County Regional Medical Center	Moreno Valley	55%	55
Delano Regional Medical Center	Delano	54%	124
Glendale Memorial Hospital and Health Center	Glendale	54%	478
Kaiser Foundation Hospital-Fresno	Fresno	54%	206
Kaiser Permanente Los Angeles Medical Center	Los Angeles	54%	471
Kaiser Permanente South Bay Medical Center	Harbor City	54%	382
Kaiser Permanente West Los Angeles Med Ctr	Los Angeles	54%	335
O'Connor Hospital	San Jose	54%	378
Sharp Coronado Hospital	San Diego	54%	63
Washington Hospital	Fremont	54%	275
Kaiser Foundation Hospital-San Diego	San Diego	53%	575
Menifee Valley Medical Center	Sun City	52%	220
Saint Luke's Hospital	San Francisco	52%	160
UCLA Medical Center	Los Angeles	52%	314
Hazel Hawkins Memorial Hospital	Hollister	51%	59
Enloe Medical Center	Chico	50%	233
Monterey Park Hospital	Monterey Park	50%	193
VacaValley Hospital	Vacaville	50%	107
Hemet Valley Medical Center	Hemet	49%	273
Kaiser Foundation Hospital-Vallejo	Vallejo	49%	267
Parkview Community Hospital	Riverside	49%	159
San Antonio Community Hospital	Upland	49%	380
Community Hospital	Huntington Park	48%	142
Doctor's Medical Center-San Pablo Campus	San Pablo	48%	366
Mission Community Hospital	Panorama City	48%	25
California Pacific Medical Center	San Francisco	47%	384
Santa Barbara Cottage Hospital	Santa Barbara	47%	310
El Camino Hospital	Mountain View	46%	272
Kaweah Delta Health Care District	Visalia	46%	329
Queen of the Valley Hospital	Napa	46%	109
University of California Davis Health System	Sacramento	46%	308
Antelope Valley Hospital	Lancaster	45%	472
Garfield Medical Center	Monterey Park	45%	260
Providence Holy Cross Medical Center	Mission Hills	45%	251
USC University Hospital	Los Angeles	45%	65
Cedars-Sinai Medical Center	Los Angeles	44%	777
Olympia Medical Center	Los Angeles	44%	200
Saint John's Health Center	Santa Monica	44%	197
Olive View-UCLA Medical Center	San Fernando	43%	58
Glendale Adventist Medical Center	Glendale	42%	330
Hollywood Presbyterian Medical Center	Los Angeles	42%	352
Moreno Valley Community Hospital	Moreno Valley	41%	153
San Francisco General Hospital Medical Center	San Francisco	41%	280
Beverly Hospital	Montebello	40%	308
Central Valley General Hospital	Hanford	40%	35
Kaiser Permanente Sacramento Medical Center	Sacramento	40%	654
Kaiser Redwood City Medical Center	Redwood City	40%	112
Santa Clara Valley Medical Center	San Jose	40%	308
Hanford Community Medical Center	Hanford	37%	139
Marshall Medical Center	Placerville	37%	137
Henry Mayo Newhall Memorial Hospital	Valencia	36%	238
Verdugo Hills Hospital	Glendale	34%	107
Community Memorial Hospital Ventura	Ventura	33%	206
Huntington Memorial Hospital	Pasadena	33%	418
Regional Medical Center of San Jose	San Jose	33%	353
Centinela Freeman Reg Med Ctr-Marina	Marina Del Rey	32%	102
Centinela Hospital Medical Center	Inglewood	32%	398
Community Regional Medical Center	Fresno	32%	760
Kaiser Permanente Anaheim Medical Center	Anaheim	32%	137
Loma Linda University Medical Center	Loma Linda	31%	388
Sutter Amador Hospital	Jackson	30%	66
Century City Doctors Hospital	Los Angeles	28%	25
NorthBay Medical Center	Fairfield	28%	163
Fallbrook Hospital	Fallbrook	26%	50
Memorial Hospital of Gardena	Gardena	26%	161
West Hills Hospital and Medical Center	West Hills	26%	138
Sonoma Valley Hospital	Sonoma	25%	32
Coastal Communities Hospital	Santa Ana	24%	54
Redbud Community Hospital	Clearlake	24%	46
Santa Monica-UCLA Medical Center	Santa Monica	24%	176
Scripps Memorial Hospital-Encinitas	Encinitas	24%	120
Saint Vincent Medical Center	Los Angeles	22%	289
Los Angeles County & USC Medical Center	Los Angeles	20%	579
Simi Valley Hospital	Simi Valley	20%	90
Citrus Valley Med Ctr Queen Valley Campus	West Covina	19%	317
Madera Community Hospital	Madera	18%	146
Citrus Valley Medical Center	Covina	16%	306
Community Medical Center-Clovis	Clovis	16%	128
Kaiser Foundation Hospital-Manteca	Manteca	16%	152
Hollywood Community Hospital	Hollywood	15%	27
Natividad Medical Center	Salinas	15%	65
Barton Memorial Hospital	South Lake Tahoe	14%	65
Rideout Memorial Hospital	Marysville	13%	372
Alameda Hospital	Alameda	12%	112
Lancaster Community Hospital	Lancaster	11%	282
Oroville Hospital	Oroville	11%	119
Alhambra Hospital Medical Center	Alhambra	10%	112
Brotman Medical Center	Culver City	10%	210
Greater El Monte Community Hospital	South El Monte	5%	75
Hi-Desert Medical Center	Joshua Tree	5%	65
Arrowhead Regional Medical Center	Colton	4%	322
Los Angeles Metropolitan Med Ctr-LA Campus	Los Angeles	4%	51
Palo Verde Hospital	Blythe	4%	25
Colusa Regional Medical Center	Colusa	3%	36
Alameda County Medical Center	Oakland	2%	266
Martin Luther King Jr/Charles R Drew Med Ctr	Los Angeles	1%	310
Contra Costa Regional Medical Center	Martinez	0%	25
Valley Presbyterian Hospital	Van Nuys	0%	43

11. Evaluation of LVS Function

Hospital Name	City	Rate	Cases
California Hospital Medical Center	Los Angeles	100%	433
Cedars-Sinai Medical Center	Los Angeles	100%	880
Marian Medical Center	Santa Maria	100%	254
Mark Twain Saint Joseph's Hospital	San Andreas	100%	69
Novato Community Hospital	Novato	100%	61
Saint John's Pleasant Valley Hospital	Camarillo	100%	87
San Joaquin General Hospital	French Camp	100%	208
San Mateo Medical Center	San Mateo	100%	68
Scripps Green Hospital	La Jolla	100%	278

NOTE: Hospital profiles are in alphabetical order by state, then city, then hospital within the city; Rankings are sorted by rate in descending order and exclude hospitals with less than 25 cases; (1) The number of cases is too small (n<25) for purposes of reliably predicting hospital performance; (2) Measure reflects the hospital's indication that its submission was based upon a sample of its relevant discharges; (3) Rate reflects fewer than the maximum possible quarters of data for the measure; (4) Inaccurate information submitted and suppressed for one or more quarters; (5) No data is available from the hospital for this measure; Please refer to the User's Guide for a full explanation of data

Hospital	City	Rate	Cases
USC University Hospital	Los Angeles	100%	72
Alameda County Medical Center	Oakland	99%	279
Contra Costa Regional Medical Center	Martinez	99%	151
Kaiser Foundation Hospital-South Sacramento	Sacramento	99%	285
Kaiser Permanente Santa Clara Medical Center	Santa Clara	99%	467
Kaiser Permanente Santa Teresa Comm Med Ctr	San Jose	99%	373
Los Alamitos Medical Center	Los Alamitos	99%	261
Mercy San Juan Hospital	Carmichael	99%	521
Northridge Hospital Medical Center	Northridge	99%	354
Olive View-UCLA Medical Center	San Fernando	99%	297
Palomar Medical Center	Escondido	99%	434
Providence Saint Joseph Medical Center	Burbank	99%	314
Saint John's Regional Medical Center	Oxnard	99%	342
Saint Joseph's Medical Center of Stockton	Stockton	99%	296
Saint Mary's Medical Center	San Francisco	99%	199
San Francisco General Hospital Medical Center	San Francisco	99%	294
Sequoia Hospital	Redwood City	99%	285
Sherman Oaks Hospital	Sherman Oaks	99%	72
S San Francisco Medical Center	S San Francisco	99%	232
Stanford Hospital	Stanford	99%	339
Sutter Auburn Faith Hospital	Auburn	99%	163
Sutter General Hospital	Sacramento	99%	300
Tulare District Hospital	Tulare	99%	144
UCLA Medical Center	Los Angeles	99%	326
UCSF Medical Center	San Francisco	99%	318
University of California Davis Health System	Sacramento	99%	329
Anaheim Memorial Medical Center	Anaheim	98%	576
California Pacific Medical Center	San Francisco	98%	457
Chino Valley Medical Center	Chino	98%	127
Feather River Hospital	Paradise	98%	84
Glendale Memorial Hospital and Health Center	Glendale	98%	578
Kaiser Foundation Hospital-Fresno	Fresno	98%	244
Kaiser Foundation Hospital-Walnut Creek	Walnut Creek	98%	216
Kaiser Permanente Los Angeles Medical Center	Los Angeles	98%	489
Kaiser Redwood City Medical Center	Redwood City	98%	124
Kern Medical Center	Bakersfield	98%	129
Mission Hospital Regional Medical Center	Mission Viejo	98%	283
Pomerado Hospital	Poway	98%	133
Providence Holy Cross Medical Center	Mission Hills	98%	313
Saint Agnes Medical Center	Fresno	98%	430
Saint Helena Hospital	Deer Park	98%	82
Saint Jude Medical Center	Fullerton	98%	369
Scripps Memorial Hospital-Encinitas	Encinitas	98%	170
Temple Community Hospital	Los Angeles	98%	93
University of California Irvine Med Ctr	Orange	98%	265
Ventura County Medical Center	Ventura	98%	102
Davies Medical Center	San Francisco	97%	63
El Centro Regional Medical Center	El Centro	97%	222
Foothill Presbyterian Hospital	Glendora	97%	212
Garden Grove Hospital and Medical Center	Garden Grove	97%	103
Good Samaritan Hospital	Los Angeles	97%	463
Grossmont Hospital	La Mesa	97%	635
Kaiser Foundation Hospital-Vallejo	Vallejo	97%	303
Kaiser Permanente Anaheim Medical Center	Anaheim	97%	155
Kaiser Permanente Sacramento Medical Center	Sacramento	97%	789
Kaiser Permanente San Francisco Med Ctr	San Francisco	97%	353
Loma Linda University Medical Center	Loma Linda	97%	434
Mills-Peninsula Health Services	Burlingame	97%	305
Natividad Medical Center	Salinas	97%	73
Presbyterian Intercommunity Hospital	Whittier	97%	255
Saint Francis Medical Center	Lynwood	97%	539
Saint Francis Memorial Hospital	San Francisco	97%	71
Saint Joseph Hospital	Eureka	97%	106
Saint Joseph Hospital	Orange	97%	470
San Rafael Medical Center	San Rafael	97%	173
San Ramon Regional Medical Center	San Ramon	97%	106
South Coast Medical Center	Laguna Beach	97%	90
Torrance Memorial Medical Center	Torrance	97%	600
Twin Cities Community Hospital	Templeton	97%	142
Woodland Healthcare	Woodland	97%	99
Desert Valley Hospital	Victorville	96%	257
French Hospital Medical Center	San Luis Obispo	96%	131
John Muir Medical Center	Walnut Creek	96%	272
John Muir Medical Center-Concord Campus	Concord	96%	317
Kaiser Foundation Hospital	Baldwin Park	96%	382
Kaiser Foundation Hospital	Woodland Hills	96%	299
Kaiser Foundation Hospital-Santa Rosa	Santa Rosa	96%	123
Mercy General Hospital	Sacramento	96%	562
Motion Picture & Television Hospital	Woodland Hills	96%	49
Oakland Medical Center	Oakland	96%	585
Saddleback Memorial Medical Center	Laguna Hills	96%	642
Santa Clara Valley Medical Center	San Jose	96%	329
Santa Rosa Memorial Hospital	Santa Rosa	96%	255
Seton Medical Center	Daly City	96%	431
University of California San Diego Med Ctr	San Diego	96%	305
Whittier Hospital Medical Center	Whittier	96%	251
Community Memorial Hospital Ventura	Ventura	95%	253
Doctors Medical Center	Modesto	95%	422
Enloe Medical Center	Chico	95%	296
Hoag Memorial Hospital Presbyterian	Newport Beach	95%	598
Hollywood Presbyterian Medical Center	Los Angeles	95%	409
Kaiser Foundation Hospital	Hayward	95%	427
Kaiser Foundation Hospital-Riverside	Riverside	95%	358
Little Company of Mary Hospital	Torrance	95%	501
Los Angeles County Harbor-UCLA Medical Center	Torrance	95%	332
Marin General Hospital	Greenbrae	95%	226
Methodist Hospital of Southern California	Arcadia	95%	634
Saint Bernardine Medical Center	San Bernardino	95%	310
Santa Monica-UCLA Medical Center	Santa Monica	95%	247
Shasta Regional Medical Center	Redding	95%	216
Sutter Lakeside Hospital	Lakeport	95%	39
Sutter Roseville Medical Center	Roseville	95%	279
Western Medical Center Hospital Anaheim	Anaheim	95%	59
Alta Bates Summit Medical Center	Berkeley	94%	109
Arrowhead Regional Medical Center	Colton	94%	337
Bakersfield Heart Hospital	Bakersfield	94%	277
Beverly Hospital	Montebello	94%	385
Chapman Medical Center	Orange	94%	47
Community Hospital of San Bernardino	San Bernardino	94%	247
Kaiser Foundation Hospital-Manteca	Manteca	94%	181
Kaiser Foundation Hospital-San Diego	San Diego	94%	625
Kaiser Permanente Fontana Medical Center	Fontana	94%	644
Mercy Hospital of Folsom	Folsom	94%	125
NorthBay Medical Center	Fairfield	94%	181
Pomona Valley Hospital Medical Center	Pomona	94%	604
San Gabriel Valley Medical Center	San Gabriel	94%	272
Sutter Davis Hospital	Davis	94%	65
White Memorial Medical Center	Los Angeles	94%	416
Alta Bates Summit Medical Center	Oakland	93%	203
Bakersfield Memorial Hospital	Bakersfield	93%	307
Doctor's Medical Center-San Pablo Campus	San Pablo	93%	441
Doctors Hospital of Manteca	Manteca	93%	105
Encino-Tarzana Regional Medical Center	Tarzana	93%	326
Kaiser Permanente South Bay Medical Center	Harbor City	93%	414
Lakewood Regional Medical Center	Lakewood	93%	492
Mercy Medical Center-Mount Shasta	Mount Shasta	93%	44
Orange Coast Memorial Medical Center	Santa Ana	93%	364
Pacifica Hospital of the Valley	Sun Valley	93%	83
Paradise Valley Hospital	National City	93%	370
Queen of the Valley Hospital	Napa	93%	145
Sutter Tracy Community Hospital	Tracy	93%	115
Tri-City Medical Center	Oceanside	93%	432
Centinela Hospital Medical Center	Inglewood	92%	446
Community Hospital of the Monterey Peninsula	Monterey	92%	282
Desert Regional Medical Center	Palm Springs	92%	436
Downey Regional Medical Center	Downey	92%	355
Long Beach Memorial Medical Center	Long Beach	92%	717
Mercy Med Ctr Merced-Community Campus	Merced	92%	285
Mercy Medical Center-Redding	Redding	92%	276
Methodist Hospital of Sacramento	Sacramento	92%	276
Salinas Valley Memorial Health Care District	Salinas	92%	429
San Dimas Community Hospital	San Dimas	92%	120
Scripps Memorial Hospital La Jolla	La Jolla	92%	270
Sonoma Valley Hospital	Sonoma	92%	53
VacaValley Hospital	Vacaville	92%	120
Community Hospital of Long Beach	Long Beach	91%	78
Fountain Valley Reg Hospital & Med Ctr	Fountain Valley	91%	397
Good Samaritan Hospital	San Jose	91%	368
Huntington Beach Hospital	Huntington Beach	91%	128
Los Robles Regional Medical Center	Thousand Oaks	91%	232
Memorial Medical Center	Modesto	91%	388
Monterey Park Hospital	Monterey Park	91%	210
Petaluma Valley Hospital	Petaluma	91%	82
Redlands Community Hospital	Redlands	91%	265
Riverside County Regional Medical Center	Moreno Valley	91%	230
Saint Mary Medical Center	Long Beach	91%	293
Sierra Vista Regional Medical Center	San Luis Obispo	91%	78
Dominican Hospital	Santa Cruz	90%	342
Eisenhower Medical Center	Rancho Mirage	90%	619
Emanuel Medical Center	Turlock	90%	263
Irvine Regional Hospital	Irvine	90%	206
Kaiser Permanente West Los Angeles Med Ctr	Los Angeles	90%	353
Little Company of Mary-San Pedro Hospital	San Pedro	90%	202
Placentia-Linda Hospital	Placentia	90%	110
San Joaquin Community Hospital	Bakersfield	90%	434
Sharp Memorial Hospital	San Diego	90%	454
Sierra Nevada Memorial Hospital	Grass Valley	90%	157
Arroyo Grande Community Hospital	Arroyo Grande	89%	103
Eden Medical Center	Castro Valley	89%	230
Hemet Valley Medical Center	Hemet	89%	375

NOTE: Hospital profiles are in alphabetical order by state, then city, then hospital within the city; Rankings are sorted by rate in descending order and exclude hospitals with less than 25 cases; (1) The number of cases is too small (n<25) for purposes of reliably predicting hospital performance; (2) Measure reflects the hospital's indication that its submission was based upon a sample of its relevant discharges; (3) Rate reflects fewer than the maximum possible quarters of data for the measure; (4) Inaccurate information submitted and suppressed for one or more quarters; (5) No data is available from the hospital for this measure; Please refer to the User's Guide for a full explanation of data

Henry Mayo Newhall Memorial Hospital	Valencia	89%	275
Kaiser Permanente Bellflower Medical Center	Bellflower	89%	525
Marshall Medical Center	Placerville	89%	171
Mercy Hospital	Bakersfield	89%	206
Pacific Hospital of Long Beach	Long Beach	89%	54
Rancho Springs Medical Center	Murrieta	89%	389
Riverside Community Hospital	Riverside	89%	542
San Leandro Hospital	San Leandro	89%	370
Scripps Mercy Hospital	San Diego	89%	860
West Anaheim Medical Center	Anaheim	89%	249
Citrus Valley Med Ctr Queen Valley Campus	West Covina	88%	388
Community Regional Medical Center	Fresno	88%	841
Fallbrook Hospital	Fallbrook	88%	59
Lompoc Healthcare District Hospital	Lompoc	88%	58
O'Connor Hospital	San Jose	88%	471
Olympia Medical Center	Los Angeles	88%	285
Saint Elizabeth Community Hospital	Red Bluff	88%	67
Saint Luke's Hospital	San Francisco	88%	191
San Antonio Community Hospital	Upland	88%	487
Santa Barbara Cottage Hospital	Santa Barbara	88%	382
Valley Presbyterian Hospital	Van Nuys	88%	214
Alameda Hospital	Alameda	87%	173
Antelope Valley Hospital	Lancaster	87%	523
Bellflower Medical Center	Bellflower	87%	94
Chinese Hospital	San Francisco	87%	91
Huntington Memorial Hospital	Pasadena	87%	493
John F Kennedy Memorial Hospital	Indio	87%	195
Kaweah Delta Health Care District	Visalia	87%	399
Menifee Valley Medical Center	Sun City	87%	248
Ridgecrest Regional Hospital	Ridgecrest	87%	82
Sharp Chula Vista Medical Center	Chula Vista	87%	574
Tri-City Regional Medical Center	Hawaiian Gardens	87%	165
Centinela Freeman Reg Med Ctr-Marina	Marina Del Rey	86%	123
Citrus Valley Medical Center	Covina	86%	391
Encino-Tarzana Regional Medical Center	Encino	86%	106
Glendale Adventist Medical Center	Glendale	86%	430
Los Angeles County & USC Medical Center	Los Angeles	86%	617
Memorial Hospital of Gardena	Gardena	86%	200
Saint Rose Hospital	Hayward	86%	276
Sutter Coast Hospital	Crescent City	86%	86
Coastal Communities Hospital	Santa Ana	85%	65
Dameron Hospital	Stockton	85%	297
El Camino Hospital	Mountain View	85%	348
Lodi Memorial Hospital	Lodi	84%	193
Oak Valley Hospital	Oakdale	84%	69
Rideout Memorial Hospital	Marysville	84%	415
Saint Vincent Medical Center	Los Angeles	84%	361
Simi Valley Hospital	Simi Valley	84%	133
Sonora Regional Medical Center	Sonora	84%	93
Sutter Medical Center of Santa Rosa	Santa Rosa	84%	208
Valleycare Medical Center	Livermore	84%	202
Western Medical Center	Santa Ana	84%	283
Century City Doctors Hospital	Los Angeles	83%	35
Kaiser Permanente Panorama City Med Ctr	Panorama City	83%	371
Washington Hospital	Fremont	83%	298
Community Hospital of Los Gatos	Los Gatos	82%	104
La Palma Intercommunity Hospital	La Palma	82%	199
Mission Community Hospital	Panorama City	82%	171
Sutter Solano Medical Center	Vallejo	82%	328
City of Angels Medical Center	Los Angeles	81%	83
Hi-Desert Medical Center	Joshua Tree	81%	106
Saint John's Health Center	Santa Monica	81%	232
Barton Memorial Hospital	South Lake Tahoe	80%	64
Corona Regional Medical Center	Corona	80%	254
Los Angeles Community Hospital	Los Angeles	80%	136
Pioneers Memorial Healthcare District	Brawley	80%	122
Sutter Delta Medical Center	Antioch	80%	300
Fresno Heart Hospital	Fresno	79%	133
Garfield Medical Center	Monterey Park	79%	295
Pacific Alliance Medical Center	Los Angeles	79%	302
East Valley Hospital Medical Center	Glendora	78%	67
Parkview Community Hospital	Riverside	78%	204
West Hills Hospital and Medical Center	West Hills	78%	201
Anaheim General Hospital	Anaheim	77%	35
Oroville Hospital	Oroville	77%	149
Regional Medical Center of San Jose	San Jose	77%	429
Ukiah Valley Medical Center	Ukiah	77%	84
Alhambra Hospital Medical Center	Alhambra	76%	142
Coast Plaza Doctors Hospital	Norwalk	76%	114
Saint Louisie Regional Hospital	Gilroy	76%	110
Verdugo Hills Hospital	Glendale	76%	161
Community Medical Center-Clovis	Clovis	75%	154
Greater El Monte Community Hospital	South El Monte	75%	95
Saint Mary Medical Center	Apple Valley	75%	434
Palm Drive Hospital	Sebastopol	74%	31
Sharp Coronado Hospital	San Diego	74%	74
Brotman Medical Center	Culver City	72%	260
Lancaster Community Hospital	Lancaster	72%	321
Mad River Community Hospital	Arcata	72%	78
Martin Luther King Jr/Charles R Drew Med Ctr	Los Angeles	72%	308
Watsonville Community Hospital	Watsonville	72%	177
Barstow Community Hospital	Barstow	71%	233
Redbud Community Hospital	Clearlake	71%	49
San Gorgonio Memorial Hospital	Banning	71%	164
Moreno Valley Community Hospital	Moreno Valley	70%	158
Madera Community Hospital	Madera	67%	159
Sierra View District Hospital	Porterville	67%	227
Colusa Regional Medical Center	Colusa	66%	41
Hollywood Community Hospital	Hollywood	65%	34
Tahoe Forest Hospital	Truckee	65%	26
Sutter Amador Hospital	Jackson	63%	89
Hazel Hawkins Memorial Hospital	Hollister	59%	79
Delano Regional Medical Center	Delano	58%	146
Victor Valley Community Hospital	Victorville	57%	171
Los Angeles Metropolitan Med Ctr-LA Campus	Los Angeles	56%	72
Tuolumne General Hospital	Sonora	56%	36
Community Hospital	Huntington Park	54%	156
East Los Angeles Doctors Hospital	Los Angeles	53%	116
Memorial Hospital Los Banos	Los Banos	45%	55
Hanford Community Medical Center	Hanford	40%	143
Central Valley General Hospital	Hanford	30%	40
Palo Verde Hospital	Blythe	12%	25
Corcoran District Hospital	Corcoran	10%	40
Healdsburg District Hospital	Healdsburg	8%	25
Good Samaritan Hospital	Bakersfield	7%	69
Sierra Kings District Hospital	Reedley	0%	25

12. Smoking Cessation Advice

Hospital Name	City	Rate	Cases
Alta Bates Summit Medical Center	Oakland	100%	33
Beverly Hospital	Montebello	100%	36
California Hospital Medical Center	Los Angeles	100%	128
Cedars-Sinai Medical Center	Los Angeles	100%	96
Desert Valley Hospital	Victorville	100%	54
Downey Regional Medical Center	Downey	100%	47
John F Kennedy Memorial Hospital	Indio	100%	30
John Muir Medical Center-Concord Campus	Concord	100%	46
Kaiser Permanente Santa Teresa Comm Med Ctr	San Jose	100%	49
La Palma Intercommunity Hospital	La Palma	100%	31
Little Company of Mary Hospital	Torrance	100%	42
Mercy Medical Center-Redding	Redding	100%	65
Methodist Hospital of Sacramento	Sacramento	100%	50
Northridge Hospital Medical Center	Northridge	100%	48
Rancho Springs Medical Center	Murrieta	100%	54
Saint Agnes Medical Center	Fresno	100%	54
Saint Joseph's Medical Center of Stockton	Stockton	100%	43
Saint Jude Medical Center	Fullerton	100%	37
San Antonio Community Hospital	Upland	100%	70
San Leandro Hospital	San Leandro	100%	86
San Mateo Medical Center	San Mateo	100%	28
Shasta Regional Medical Center	Redding	100%	61
Sutter Auburn Faith Hospital	Auburn	100%	32
Sutter General Hospital	Sacramento	100%	53
University of California Irvine Med Ctr	Orange	100%	69
White Memorial Medical Center	Los Angeles	100%	45
Anaheim Memorial Medical Center	Anaheim	99%	82
Community Hospital of San Bernardino	San Bernardino	99%	68
Glendale Memorial Hospital and Health Center	Glendale	99%	80
Mercy General Hospital	Sacramento	99%	127
Mercy Med Ctr Merced-Community Campus	Merced	99%	72
Mercy San Juan Hospital	Carmichael	99%	104
El Camino Hospital	Mountain View	98%	40
Glendale Adventist Medical Center	Glendale	98%	53
Grossmont Hospital	La Mesa	98%	140
Kaiser Permanente San Francisco Med Ctr	San Francisco	98%	41
Orange Coast Memorial Medical Center	Santa Ana	98%	53
Pomona Valley Hospital Medical Center	Pomona	98%	123
Saint Bernardine Medical Center	San Bernardino	98%	55
Saint Francis Medical Center	Lynwood	98%	128
Sutter Delta Medical Center	Antioch	98%	61
Tri-City Medical Center	Oceanside	98%	47
Barstow Community Hospital	Barstow	97%	74
Mission Hospital Regional Medical Center	Mission Viejo	97%	32
Presbyterian Intercommunity Hospital	Whittier	97%	33
Saint Joseph Hospital	Orange	97%	63
San Joaquin Community Hospital	Bakersfield	97%	108
Santa Rosa Memorial Hospital	Santa Rosa	97%	37
Scripps Memorial Hospital La Jolla	La Jolla	97%	31
West Anaheim Medical Center	Anaheim	97%	37

NOTE: Hospital profiles are in alphabetical order by state, then city, then hospital within the city; Rankings are sorted by rate in descending order and exclude hospitals with less than 25 cases; (1) The number of cases is too small (n<25) for purposes of reliably predicting hospital performance; (2) Measure reflects the hospital's indication that its submission was based upon a sample of its relevant discharges; (3) Rate reflects fewer than the maximum possible quarters of data for the measure; (4) Inaccurate information submitted and suppressed for one or more quarters; (5) No data is available from the hospital for this measure; Please refer to the User's Guide for a full explanation of data

Desert Regional Medical Center	Palm Springs	96%	91
Doctors Medical Center	Modesto	96%	105
Fountain Valley Reg Hospital & Med Ctr	Fountain Valley	96%	48
Kaiser Foundation Hospital-South Sacramento	Sacramento	96%	46
Pioneers Memorial Healthcare District	Brawley	96%	26
Providence Saint Joseph Medical Center	Burbank	96%	27
Saddleback Memorial Medical Center	Laguna Hills	96%	55
University of California San Diego Med Ctr	San Diego	96%	77
Bakersfield Heart Hospital	Bakersfield	95%	42
Eisenhower Medical Center	Rancho Mirage	95%	73
Good Samaritan Hospital	Los Angeles	95%	74
Paradise Valley Hospital	National City	95%	96
Saint Mary Medical Center	Apple Valley	95%	112
Sharp Memorial Hospital	San Diego	95%	42
University of California Davis Health System	Sacramento	95%	101
Bakersfield Memorial Hospital	Bakersfield	94%	54
Eden Medical Center	Castro Valley	94%	35
Kaiser Foundation Hospital	Baldwin Park	94%	50
Providence Holy Cross Medical Center	Mission Hills	94%	35
Riverside Community Hospital	Riverside	94%	107
Saint Joseph Hospital	Eureka	94%	33
San Gabriel Valley Medical Center	San Gabriel	94%	36
Sutter Roseville Medical Center	Roseville	94%	32
Enloe Medical Center	Chico	93%	41
Saint Luke's Hospital	San Francisco	93%	44
Scripps Green Hospital	La Jolla	93%	29
Kaiser Foundation Hospital-Fresno	Fresno	92%	38
Lodi Memorial Hospital	Lodi	92%	38
Memorial Medical Center	Modesto	92%	76
Oakland Medical Center	Oakland	92%	92
Saint Mary Medical Center	Long Beach	92%	86
Scripps Mercy Hospital	San Diego	92%	145
Sierra View District Hospital	Porterville	92%	36
Tri-City Regional Medical Center	Hawaiian Gardens	92%	25
UCLA Medical Center	Los Angeles	92%	50
VacaValley Hospital	Vacaville	92%	25
Antelope Valley Hospital	Lancaster	91%	150
Corona Regional Medical Center	Corona	91%	32
Kaiser Foundation Hospital-Riverside	Riverside	91%	47
Lakewood Regional Medical Center	Lakewood	91%	64
Madera Community Hospital	Madera	91%	35
Hanford Community Medical Center	Hanford	90%	29
Parkview Community Hospital	Riverside	90%	29
San Francisco General Hospital Medical Center	San Francisco	90%	122
Doctor's Medical Center-San Pablo Campus	San Pablo	89%	114
Los Angeles County Harbor-UCLA Medical Center	Torrance	89%	111
Torrance Memorial Medical Center	Torrance	89%	63
California Pacific Medical Center	San Francisco	88%	57
Kaiser Permanente South Bay Medical Center	Harbor City	88%	43
Washington Hospital	Fremont	88%	50
Dameron Hospital	Stockton	87%	47
Dominican Hospital	Santa Cruz	87%	47
Kaiser Permanente Fontana Medical Center	Fontana	87%	86
Loma Linda University Medical Center	Loma Linda	87%	62
Palomar Medical Center	Escondido	87%	54
Good Samaritan Hospital	San Jose	86%	29
Huntington Memorial Hospital	Pasadena	86%	72
Kaiser Foundation Hospital-Vallejo	Vallejo	86%	43
Kaweah Delta Health Care District	Visalia	86%	59
Mills-Peninsula Health Services	Burlingame	86%	37
Los Robles Regional Medical Center	Thousand Oaks	85%	27
Saint John's Regional Medical Center	Oxnard	85%	26
Hoag Memorial Hospital Presbyterian	Newport Beach	84%	55
Long Beach Memorial Medical Center	Long Beach	84%	119
NorthBay Medical Center	Fairfield	84%	50
Sharp Chula Vista Medical Center	Chula Vista	84%	56
San Joaquin General Hospital	French Camp	83%	89
Centinela Hospital Medical Center	Inglewood	82%	49
Kaiser Foundation Hospital	Hayward	82%	49
Kaiser Foundation Hospital-San Diego	San Diego	82%	67
Kaiser Permanente Panorama City Med Ctr	Panorama City	82%	45
Kaiser Permanente West Los Angeles Med Ctr	Los Angeles	82%	45
Regional Medical Center of San Jose	San Jose	81%	54
Sutter Medical Center of Santa Rosa	Santa Rosa	81%	43
Hollywood Presbyterian Medical Center	Los Angeles	80%	56
Marin General Hospital	Greenbrae	80%	30
Methodist Hospital of Southern California	Arcadia	79%	63
Sutter Solano Medical Center	Vallejo	79%	106
Kaiser Permanente Santa Clara Medical Center	Santa Clara	78%	27
Menifee Valley Medical Center	Sun City	78%	40
Mercy Hospital	Bakersfield	78%	41
Santa Clara Valley Medical Center	San Jose	77%	112
S San Francisco Medical Center	S San Francisco	77%	48
Lancaster Community Hospital	Lancaster	74%	58
Citrus Valley Medical Center	Covina	73%	48
Santa Barbara Cottage Hospital	Santa Barbara	73%	52
Citrus Valley Med Ctr Queen Valley Campus	West Covina	72%	50
Kaiser Permanente Bellflower Medical Center	Bellflower	72%	82
Stanford Hospital	Stanford	72%	25
Emanuel Medical Center	Turlock	70%	33
Hemet Valley Medical Center	Hemet	69%	58
O'Connor Hospital	San Jose	69%	29
UCSF Medical Center	San Francisco	69%	59
Kaiser Foundation Hospital-Santa Rosa	Santa Rosa	68%	25
Kaiser Permanente Sacramento Medical Center	Sacramento	67%	79
Kaiser Permanente Anaheim Medical Center	Anaheim	65%	26
Western Medical Center	Santa Ana	64%	47
Huntington Beach Hospital	Huntington Beach	63%	27
Kaiser Permanente Los Angeles Medical Center	Los Angeles	63%	59
Watsonville Community Hospital	Watsonville	63%	27
Rideout Memorial Hospital	Marysville	61%	84
Brotman Medical Center	Culver City	60%	42
Community Regional Medical Center	Fresno	58%	178
Olympia Medical Center	Los Angeles	55%	29
Alameda County Medical Center	Oakland	54%	136
Moreno Valley Community Hospital	Moreno Valley	54%	26
Saint Vincent Medical Center	Los Angeles	50%	36
Los Angeles County & USC Medical Center	Los Angeles	47%	211
Memorial Hospital of Gardena	Gardena	42%	36
Arrowhead Regional Medical Center	Colton	34%	124
Oroville Hospital	Oroville	17%	36
Martin Luther King Jr/Charles R Drew Med Ctr	Los Angeles	11%	128
Los Angeles Metropolitan Med Ctr-LA Campus	Los Angeles	7%	29

Pneumonia Care

13. Appropriate Initial Antibiotic

Hospital Name	City	Rate	Cases
Queen of the Valley Hospital	Napa	98%	135
San Rafael Medical Center	San Rafael	97%	135
San Ramon Regional Medical Center	San Ramon	97%	118
NorthBay Medical Center	Fairfield	96%	159
Saint Helena Hospital	Deer Park	96%	27
Oakland Medical Center	Oakland	95%	270
Palomar Medical Center	Escondido	95%	279
Sutter Davis Hospital	Davis	95%	118
Antelope Valley Hospital	Lancaster	94%	340
Cedars-Sinai Medical Center	Los Angeles	94%	334
Chinese Hospital	San Francisco	94%	176
Saint Francis Medical Center	Lynwood	94%	171
Saint Joseph's Medical Center of Stockton	Stockton	94%	126
San Leandro Hospital	San Leandro	94%	114
Scripps Green Hospital	La Jolla	94%	63
Sequoia Hospital	Redwood City	94%	67
Sonoma Valley Hospital	Sonoma	94%	34
Sutter Auburn Faith Hospital	Auburn	94%	104
UCSF Medical Center	San Francisco	94%	94
White Memorial Medical Center	Los Angeles	94%	135
Arrowhead Regional Medical Center	Colton	93%	138
Centinela Freeman Reg Med Ctr-Marina	Marina Del Rey	93%	83
Dameron Hospital	Stockton	93%	121
Desert Regional Medical Center	Palm Springs	93%	244
Fountain Valley Reg Hospital & Med Ctr	Fountain Valley	93%	179
Kaiser Foundation Hospital-Vallejo	Vallejo	93%	118
Kaiser Permanente San Francisco Med Ctr	San Francisco	93%	118
Marian Medical Center	Santa Maria	93%	185
Saint Bernardine Medical Center	San Bernardino	93%	85
VacaValley Hospital	Vacaville	93%	138
Bakersfield Heart Hospital	Bakersfield	92%	89
Doctors Medical Center	Modesto	92%	299
John Muir Medical Center	Walnut Creek	92%	121
Lompoc Healthcare District Hospital	Lompoc	92%	63
Los Alamitos Medical Center	Los Alamitos	92%	201
Methodist Hospital of Sacramento	Sacramento	92%	181
Pioneers Memorial Healthcare District	Brawley	92%	158
Placentia-Linda Hospital	Placentia	92%	146
Saint Agnes Medical Center	Fresno	92%	159
Sierra Nevada Memorial Hospital	Grass Valley	92%	251
Sonora Regional Medical Center	Sonora	92%	113
Alta Bates Summit Medical Center	Berkeley	91%	43
California Hospital Medical Center	Los Angeles	91%	113
Emanuel Medical Center	Turlock	91%	162
Grossmont Hospital	La Mesa	91%	383
Kaiser Foundation Hospital-Fresno	Fresno	91%	105
Lodi Memorial Hospital	Lodi	91%	77
Pomona Valley Hospital Medical Center	Pomona	91%	180
Saint Mary's Medical Center	San Francisco	91%	116
San Joaquin General Hospital	French Camp	91%	164
Scripps Memorial Hospital La Jolla	La Jolla	91%	91

NOTE: Hospital profiles are in alphabetical order by state, then city, then hospital within the city; Rankings are sorted by rate in descending order and exclude hospitals with less than 25 cases; (1) The number of cases is too small (n<25) for purposes of reliably predicting hospital performance; (2) Measure reflects the hospital's indication that its submission was based upon a sample of its relevant discharges; (3) Rate reflects fewer than the maximum possible quarters of data for the measure; (4) Inaccurate information submitted and suppressed for one or more quarters; (5) No data is available from the hospital for this measure; Please refer to the User's Guide for a full explanation of data

Hospital	City	Rate	Cases
Tri-City Medical Center	Oceanside	91%	309
UCLA Medical Center	Los Angeles	91%	77
Alta Bates Summit Medical Center	Oakland	90%	60
Chapman Medical Center	Orange	90%	40
Doctor's Medical Center-San Pablo Campus	San Pablo	90%	205
Kaiser Permanente Santa Teresa Comm Med Ctr	San Jose	90%	105
Lancaster Community Hospital	Lancaster	90%	163
Little Company of Mary-San Pedro Hospital	San Pedro	90%	132
Orange Coast Memorial Medical Center	Santa Ana	90%	200
Pomerado Hospital	Poway	90%	155
Providence Holy Cross Medical Center	Mission Hills	90%	109
Riverside Community Hospital	Riverside	90%	261
Saddleback Memorial Medical Center	Laguna Hills	90%	328
Saint Elizabeth Community Hospital	Red Bluff	90%	152
Saint John's Regional Medical Center	Oxnard	90%	187
Scripps Memorial Hospital-Encinitas	Encinitas	90%	126
Simi Valley Hospital	Simi Valley	90%	105
Sutter General Hospital	Sacramento	90%	111
Twin Cities Community Hospital	Templeton	90%	100
Hoag Memorial Hospital Presbyterian	Newport Beach	89%	320
Irvine Regional Hospital	Irvine	89%	161
John Muir Medical Center-Concord Campus	Concord	89%	116
Kaiser Foundation Hospital-South Sacramento	Sacramento	89%	202
Kaiser Permanente Sacramento Medical Center	Sacramento	89%	298
Kaiser Redwood City Medical Center	Redwood City	89%	96
Mercy Medical Center-Mount Shasta	Mount Shasta	89%	70
Mercy Medical Center-Redding	Redding	89%	274
San Joaquin Community Hospital	Bakersfield	89%	187
Shasta Regional Medical Center	Redding	89%	232
Arroyo Grande Community Hospital	Arroyo Grande	88%	128
Community Medical Center-Clovis	Clovis	88%	119
Dominican Hospital	Santa Cruz	88%	185
Encino-Tarzana Regional Medical Center	Tarzana	88%	200
French Hospital Medical Center	San Luis Obispo	88%	103
Kaiser Foundation Hospital-Walnut Creek	Walnut Creek	88%	108
Mark Twain Saint Joseph's Hospital	San Andreas	88%	82
Memorial Medical Center	Modesto	88%	104
Mercy Hospital of Folsom	Folsom	88%	122
Mercy San Juan Hospital	Carmichael	88%	232
O'Connor Hospital	San Jose	88%	176
Rancho Springs Medical Center	Murrieta	88%	259
Saint Louisie Regional Hospital	Gilroy	88%	86
Tulare District Hospital	Tulare	88%	128
Ukiah Valley Medical Center	Ukiah	88%	102
Whittier Hospital Medical Center	Whittier	88%	191
Banner Lassen Medical Center	Susanville	87%	45
Centinela Hospital Medical Center	Inglewood	87%	149
Citrus Valley Medical Center	Covina	87%	132
Community Regional Medical Center	Fresno	87%	435
Good Samaritan Hospital	San Jose	87%	227
John F Kennedy Memorial Hospital	Indio	87%	216
Kaiser Foundation Hospital-Santa Rosa	Santa Rosa	87%	135
Kaweah Delta Health Care District	Visalia	87%	446
Methodist Hospital of Southern California	Arcadia	87%	341
Mills-Peninsula Health Services	Burlingame	87%	113
Northridge Hospital Medical Center	Northridge	87%	199
Saint Joseph Hospital	Eureka	87%	93
Saint Mary Medical Center	Apple Valley	87%	430
San Dimas Community Hospital	San Dimas	87%	128
Community Hospital of Los Gatos	Los Gatos	86%	80
El Centro Regional Medical Center	El Centro	86%	135
Greater El Monte Community Hospital	South El Monte	86%	98
Kaiser Permanente Fontana Medical Center	Fontana	86%	63
Kaiser Permanente Santa Clara Medical Center	Santa Clara	86%	90
Lakewood Regional Medical Center	Lakewood	86%	168
Little Company of Mary Hospital	Torrance	86%	172
Long Beach Memorial Medical Center	Long Beach	86%	287
Mercy Med Ctr Merced-Community Campus	Merced	86%	92
Monterey Park Hospital	Monterey Park	86%	86
Regional Medical Center of San Jose	San Jose	86%	292
Saint John's Pleasant Valley Hospital	Camarillo	86%	100
San Francisco General Hospital Medical Center	San Francisco	86%	174
Sutter Roseville Medical Center	Roseville	86%	119
Sutter Solano Medical Center	Vallejo	86%	96
Torrance Memorial Medical Center	Torrance	86%	201
Ventura County Medical Center	Ventura	86%	87
Western Medical Center Hospital Anaheim	Anaheim	86%	36
Beverly Hospital	Montebello	85%	200
California Pacific Medical Center	San Francisco	85%	84
Doctors Hospital of Manteca	Manteca	85%	108
Eden Medical Center	Castro Valley	85%	155
Kaiser Foundation Hospital-Riverside	Riverside	85%	86
Natividad Medical Center	Salinas	85%	86
Paradise Valley Hospital	National City	85%	174
Saint Jude Medical Center	Fullerton	85%	236
Salinas Valley Memorial Health Care District	Salinas	85%	26
Sierra Vista Regional Medical Center	San Luis Obispo	85%	85
University of California Davis Health System	Sacramento	85%	105
Washington Hospital	Fremont	85%	123
Central Valley General Hospital	Hanford	84%	67
Citrus Valley Med Ctr Queen Valley Campus	West Covina	84%	207
Downey Regional Medical Center	Downey	84%	128
La Palma Intercommunity Hospital	La Palma	84%	179
Los Robles Regional Medical Center	Thousand Oaks	84%	189
Marin General Hospital	Greenbrae	84%	126
Marshall Medical Center	Placerville	84%	111
Palo Verde Hospital	Blythe	84%	49
Saint Luke's Hospital	San Francisco	84%	116
Saint Mary Medical Center	Long Beach	84%	87
San Antonio Community Hospital	Upland	84%	338
Sharp Chula Vista Medical Center	Chula Vista	84%	270
Sutter Coast Hospital	Crescent City	84%	76
Bakersfield Memorial Hospital	Bakersfield	83%	169
Community Memorial Hospital Ventura	Ventura	83%	181
Feather River Hospital	Paradise	83%	119
Garden Grove Hospital and Medical Center	Garden Grove	83%	162
Glendale Memorial Hospital and Health Center	Glendale	83%	206
Huntington Memorial Hospital	Pasadena	83%	289
Los Angeles County & USC Medical Center	Los Angeles	83%	281
Madera Community Hospital	Madera	83%	112
Mercy General Hospital	Sacramento	83%	166
Mission Hospital Regional Medical Center	Mission Viejo	83%	175
Parkview Community Hospital	Riverside	83%	161
Redbud Community Hospital	Clearlake	83%	93
Davies Medical Center	San Francisco	82%	50
Kaiser Permanente West Los Angeles Med Ctr	Los Angeles	82%	78
Los Angeles County Harbor-UCLA Medical Center	Torrance	82%	132
Moreno Valley Community Hospital	Moreno Valley	82%	127
Oak Valley Hospital	Oakdale	82%	82
Saint Francis Memorial Hospital	San Francisco	82%	38
San Gabriel Valley Medical Center	San Gabriel	82%	200
Santa Barbara Cottage Hospital	Santa Barbara	82%	191
South Coast Medical Center	Laguna Beach	82%	66
Western Medical Center	Santa Ana	82%	101
Enloe Medical Center	Chico	81%	232
Good Samaritan Hospital	Los Angeles	81%	165
Hazel Hawkins Memorial Hospital	Hollister	81%	52
Hi-Desert Medical Center	Joshua Tree	81%	118
Kaiser Foundation Hospital	Baldwin Park	81%	85
Kaiser Foundation Hospital-Manteca	Manteca	81%	113
Mercy Hospital	Bakersfield	81%	427
Ridgecrest Regional Hospital	Ridgecrest	81%	97
Saint Joseph Hospital	Orange	81%	187
Sharp Coronado Hospital	San Diego	81%	70
S San Francisco Medical Center	S San Francisco	81%	108
Sutter Tracy Community Hospital	Tracy	81%	106
Valleycare Medical Center	Livermore	81%	141
Woodland Healthcare	Woodland	81%	62
Community Hospital of San Bernardino	San Bernardino	80%	167
Frank R Howard Memorial Hospital	Willits	80%	40
Kaiser Permanente Los Angeles Medical Center	Los Angeles	80%	66
Oroville Hospital	Oroville	80%	108
Stanford Hospital	Stanford	80%	178
Alameda County Medical Center	Oakland	79%	141
Community Hospital of Long Beach	Long Beach	79%	107
Garfield Medical Center	Monterey Park	79%	103
Sierra View District Hospital	Porterville	79%	160
Anaheim Memorial Medical Center	Anaheim	78%	286
Colusa Regional Medical Center	Colusa	78%	32
Encino-Tarzana Regional Medical Center	Encino	78%	86
Foothill Presbyterian Hospital	Glendora	78%	161
Goleta Valley Cottage Hospital	Santa Barbara	78%	36
Memorial Hospital Los Banos	Los Banos	78%	92
Menifee Valley Medical Center	Sun City	78%	158
Presbyterian Intercommunity Hospital	Whittier	78%	96
Saint John's Health Center	Santa Monica	78%	175
Saint Vincent Medical Center	Los Angeles	78%	159
Sharp Memorial Hospital	San Diego	78%	235
Sutter Medical Center of Santa Rosa	Santa Rosa	78%	126
Eisenhower Medical Center	Rancho Mirage	77%	359
El Camino Hospital	Mountain View	77%	301
Hanford Community Medical Center	Hanford	77%	168
Ojai Valley Community Hospital	Ojai	77%	57
San Mateo Medical Center	San Mateo	77%	43
Santa Monica-UCLA Medical Center	Santa Monica	77%	74
Barstow Community Hospital	Barstow	76%	162
Healdsburg District Hospital	Healdsburg	76%	29
Kaiser Foundation Hospital	Hayward	76%	131
Novato Community Hospital	Novato	76%	71
San Gorgonio Memorial Hospital	Banning	76%	41

NOTE: Hospital profiles are in alphabetical order by state, then city, then hospital within the city; Rankings are sorted by rate in descending order and exclude hospitals with less than 25 cases; (1) The number of cases is too small (n<25) for purposes of reliably predicting hospital performance; (2) Measure reflects the hospital's indication that its submission was based upon a sample of its relevant discharges; (3) Rate reflects fewer than the maximum possible quarters of data for the measure; (4) Inaccurate information submitted and suppressed for one or more quarters; (5) No data is available from the hospital for this measure; Please refer to the User's Guide for a full explanation of data

Sutter Amador Hospital	Jackson	76%	85
Sutter Lakeside Hospital	Lakeport	76%	100
Watsonville Community Hospital	Watsonville	76%	110
Henry Mayo Newhall Memorial Hospital	Valencia	75%	185
Delano Regional Medical Center	Delano	74%	69
Petaluma Valley Hospital	Petaluma	74%	95
Barton Memorial Hospital	South Lake Tahoe	73%	83
Coast Plaza Doctors Hospital	Norwalk	73%	214
Fallbrook Hospital	Fallbrook	73%	62
Rideout Memorial Hospital	Marysville	73%	293
Sutter Delta Medical Center	Antioch	73%	134
Glendale Adventist Medical Center	Glendale	72%	188
Huntington Beach Hospital	Huntington Beach	72%	107
Kaiser Permanente Bellflower Medical Center	Bellflower	72%	95
Loma Linda University Medical Center	Loma Linda	72%	145
Martin Luther King Jr/Charles R Drew Med Ctr	Los Angeles	72%	134
Providence Saint Joseph Medical Center	Burbank	72%	114
Saint Rose Hospital	Hayward	72%	32
Santa Rosa Memorial Hospital	Santa Rosa	72%	213
Alameda Hospital	Alameda	71%	76
University of California Irvine Med Ctr	Orange	71%	76
Alhambra Hospital Medical Center	Alhambra	70%	87
Scripps Mercy Hospital	San Diego	70%	406
Brotman Medical Center	Culver City	69%	86
East Los Angeles Doctors Hospital	Los Angeles	69%	81
Santa Clara Valley Medical Center	San Jose	69%	245
Corona Regional Medical Center	Corona	68%	321
University of California San Diego Med Ctr	San Diego	68%	141
Verdugo Hills Hospital	Glendale	68%	167
Pacific Hospital of Long Beach	Long Beach	67%	39
Tri-City Regional Medical Center	Hawaiian Gardens	66%	44
West Hills Hospital and Medical Center	West Hills	66%	210
Hemet Valley Medical Center	Hemet	65%	220
West Anaheim Medical Center	Anaheim	65%	148
Coastal Communities Hospital	Santa Ana	64%	50
East Valley Hospital Medical Center	Glendora	64%	36
Los Angeles Community Hospital	Los Angeles	64%	72
Community Hospital	Huntington Park	61%	127
Hollywood Presbyterian Medical Center	Los Angeles	61%	354
Kaiser Permanente Anaheim Medical Center	Anaheim	57%	91
Olympia Medical Center	Los Angeles	57%	298
Memorial Hospital of Gardena	Gardena	54%	209
Kaiser Permanente South Bay Medical Center	Harbor City	46%	103
Los Angeles Metropolitan Med Ctr-LA Campus	Los Angeles	40%	40
Kaiser Foundation Hospital	Woodland Hills	37%	76
Kaiser Foundation Hospital-San Diego	San Diego	36%	94
Kaiser Permanente Panorama City Med Ctr	Panorama City	36%	67
Hollywood Community Hospital	Hollywood	29%	35

14. Blood Culture Timing

Hospital Name	City	Rate	Cases
Century City Doctors Hospital	Los Angeles	100%	28
Chapman Medical Center	Orange	100%	52
Garden Grove Hospital and Medical Center	Garden Grove	100%	143
Mark Twain Saint Joseph's Hospital	San Andreas	100%	55
Saint Helena Hospital	Deer Park	100%	27
John Muir Medical Center	Walnut Creek	99%	132
Sutter Auburn Faith Hospital	Auburn	99%	89
Cedars-Sinai Medical Center	Los Angeles	98%	480
Community Hospital of Long Beach	Long Beach	98%	126
San Ramon Regional Medical Center	San Ramon	98%	54
Santa Monica-UCLA Medical Center	Santa Monica	98%	109
California Pacific Medical Center	San Francisco	97%	106
Fountain Valley Reg Hospital & Med Ctr	Fountain Valley	97%	249
French Hospital Medical Center	San Luis Obispo	97%	91
Glendale Adventist Medical Center	Glendale	97%	199
Greater El Monte Community Hospital	South El Monte	97%	134
Los Alamitos Medical Center	Los Alamitos	97%	184
Mercy General Hospital	Sacramento	97%	214
Saint Mary's Medical Center	San Francisco	97%	147
Sonoma Valley Hospital	Sonoma	97%	33
Woodland Healthcare	Woodland	97%	65
Alta Bates Summit Medical Center	Berkeley	96%	72
Barstow Community Hospital	Barstow	96%	112
Doctor's Medical Center-San Pablo Campus	San Pablo	96%	224
Huntington Beach Hospital	Huntington Beach	96%	99
Kaiser Foundation Hospital-Santa Rosa	Santa Rosa	96%	110
Kaiser Foundation Hospital-Vallejo	Vallejo	96%	116
Kaiser Permanente Bellflower Medical Center	Bellflower	96%	75
Marin General Hospital	Greenbrae	96%	160
Mercy Medical Center-Mount Shasta	Mount Shasta	96%	49
Mills-Peninsula Health Services	Burlingame	96%	110
Placentia-Linda Hospital	Placentia	96%	145
Providence Holy Cross Medical Center	Mission Hills	96%	165
Saint Francis Medical Center	Lynwood	96%	203
Saint Joseph Hospital	Orange	96%	169
San Joaquin Community Hospital	Bakersfield	96%	181
Sequoia Hospital	Redwood City	96%	71
Sierra Vista Regional Medical Center	San Luis Obispo	96%	79
Watsonville Community Hospital	Watsonville	96%	92
Anaheim Memorial Medical Center	Anaheim	95%	281
Brotman Medical Center	Culver City	95%	74
Desert Valley Hospital	Victorville	95%	134
Eden Medical Center	Castro Valley	95%	171
Glendale Memorial Hospital and Health Center	Glendale	95%	182
Irvine Regional Hospital	Irvine	95%	133
John F Kennedy Memorial Hospital	Indio	95%	205
John Muir Medical Center-Concord Campus	Concord	95%	122
Kaiser Permanente San Francisco Med Ctr	San Francisco	95%	190
Little Company of Mary Hospital	Torrance	95%	239
Lompoc Healthcare District Hospital	Lompoc	95%	43
Marshall Medical Center	Placerville	95%	120
Mercy Hospital of Folsom	Folsom	95%	104
Mercy Med Ctr Merced-Community Campus	Merced	95%	65
Methodist Hospital of Sacramento	Sacramento	95%	209
Regional Medical Center of San Jose	San Jose	95%	346
Saddleback Memorial Medical Center	Laguna Hills	95%	348
Saint Francis Memorial Hospital	San Francisco	95%	44
Saint Joseph Hospital	Eureka	95%	96
Scripps Memorial Hospital-Encinitas	Encinitas	95%	144
Stanford Hospital	Stanford	95%	199
Tulare District Hospital	Tulare	95%	74
University of California San Diego Med Ctr	San Diego	95%	153
Desert Regional Medical Center	Palm Springs	94%	214
Feather River Hospital	Paradise	94%	128
Hollywood Presbyterian Medical Center	Los Angeles	94%	278
Kaiser Foundation Hospital	Hayward	94%	122
Mission Hospital Regional Medical Center	Mission Viejo	94%	160
Northridge Hospital Medical Center	Northridge	94%	221
S San Francisco Medical Center	S San Francisco	94%	112
Twin Cities Community Hospital	Templeton	94%	100
VacaValley Hospital	Vacaville	94%	160
West Hills Hospital and Medical Center	West Hills	94%	264
Alta Bates Summit Medical Center	Oakland	93%	105
California Hospital Medical Center	Los Angeles	93%	98
Marian Medical Center	Santa Maria	93%	172
Memorial Hospital of Gardena	Gardena	93%	196
Mercy San Juan Hospital	Carmichael	93%	487
Novato Community Hospital	Novato	93%	55
Saint Joseph's Medical Center of Stockton	Stockton	93%	114
Sonora Regional Medical Center	Sonora	93%	74
Sutter Lakeside Hospital	Lakeport	93%	61
Sutter Tracy Community Hospital	Tracy	93%	57
Torrance Memorial Medical Center	Torrance	93%	181
University of California Irvine Med Ctr	Orange	93%	96
West Anaheim Medical Center	Anaheim	93%	115
Whittier Hospital Medical Center	Whittier	93%	219
Bakersfield Heart Hospital	Bakersfield	92%	75
Centinela Hospital Medical Center	Inglewood	92%	135
Community Hospital of Los Gatos	Los Gatos	92%	83
Davies Medical Center	San Francisco	92%	62
Doctors Medical Center	Modesto	92%	360
El Camino Hospital	Mountain View	92%	284
Kaiser Foundation Hospital-South Sacramento	Sacramento	92%	179
Kaiser Permanente Anaheim Medical Center	Anaheim	92%	71
Kaiser Permanente Santa Clara Medical Center	Santa Clara	92%	106
Kaiser Permanente Santa Teresa Comm Med Ctr	San Jose	92%	101
Kaiser Permanente South Bay Medical Center	Harbor City	92%	101
Loma Linda University Medical Center	Loma Linda	92%	166
Long Beach Memorial Medical Center	Long Beach	92%	399
Methodist Hospital of Southern California	Arcadia	92%	260
O'Connor Hospital	San Jose	92%	184
Olympia Medical Center	Los Angeles	92%	279
Presbyterian Intercommunity Hospital	Whittier	92%	101
Queen of the Valley Hospital	Napa	92%	156
Rancho Springs Medical Center	Murrieta	92%	182
Saint Agnes Medical Center	Fresno	92%	213
Saint John's Regional Medical Center	Oxnard	92%	207
Saint Jude Medical Center	Fullerton	92%	238
San Leandro Hospital	San Leandro	92%	111
Santa Barbara Cottage Hospital	Santa Barbara	92%	185
Sharp Coronado Hospital	San Diego	92%	50
Sherman Oaks Hospital	Sherman Oaks	92%	26
White Memorial Medical Center	Los Angeles	92%	185
Chinese Hospital	San Francisco	91%	115
Encino-Tarzana Regional Medical Center	Encino	91%	123
Fallbrook Hospital	Fallbrook	91%	44
Hoag Memorial Hospital Presbyterian	Newport Beach	91%	367
Kaiser Permanente West Los Angeles Med Ctr	Los Angeles	91%	44

NOTE: Hospital profiles are in alphabetical order by state, then city, then hospital within the city; Rankings are sorted by rate in descending order and exclude hospitals with less than 25 cases; (1) The number of cases is too small (n<25) for purposes of reliably predicting hospital performance; (2) Measure reflects the hospital's indication that its submission was based upon a sample of its relevant discharges; (3) Rate reflects fewer than the maximum possible quarters of data for the measure; (4) Inaccurate information submitted and suppressed for one or more quarters; (5) No data is available from the hospital for this measure; Please refer to the User's Guide for a full explanation of data

La Palma Intercommunity Hospital	La Palma	91%	120
Madera Community Hospital	Madera	91%	95
Pacific Hospital of Long Beach	Long Beach	91%	106
Palomar Medical Center	Escondido	91%	264
Parkview Community Hospital	Riverside	91%	197
Providence Saint Joseph Medical Center	Burbank	91%	105
Redbud Community Hospital	Clearlake	91%	64
San Rafael Medical Center	San Rafael	91%	169
Sharp Memorial Hospital	San Diego	91%	216
Valleycare Medical Center	Livermore	91%	124
Arroyo Grande Community Hospital	Arroyo Grande	90%	92
El Centro Regional Medical Center	El Centro	90%	96
Hi-Desert Medical Center	Joshua Tree	90%	142
Huntington Memorial Hospital	Pasadena	90%	391
Kaiser Permanente Sacramento Medical Center	Sacramento	90%	338
Lakewood Regional Medical Center	Lakewood	90%	134
Lodi Memorial Hospital	Lodi	90%	77
Moreno Valley Community Hospital	Moreno Valley	90%	88
Natividad Medical Center	Salinas	90%	69
Paradise Valley Hospital	National City	90%	126
Saint John's Health Center	Santa Monica	90%	162
Saint John's Pleasant Valley Hospital	Camarillo	90%	104
Saint Mary Medical Center	Apple Valley	90%	291
Saint Mary Medical Center	Long Beach	90%	89
Saint Vincent Medical Center	Los Angeles	90%	184
San Dimas Community Hospital	San Dimas	90%	171
San Gabriel Valley Medical Center	San Gabriel	90%	242
Scripps Memorial Hospital La Jolla	La Jolla	90%	107
Shasta Regional Medical Center	Redding	90%	229
Sierra Nevada Memorial Hospital	Grass Valley	90%	191
Sutter Amador Hospital	Jackson	90%	68
Sutter Coast Hospital	Crescent City	90%	78
Sutter Davis Hospital	Davis	90%	96
Sutter General Hospital	Sacramento	90%	135
UCSF Medical Center	San Francisco	90%	141
Ventura County Medical Center	Ventura	90%	71
Beverly Hospital	Montebello	89%	195
Chino Valley Medical Center	Chino	89%	54
Community Hospital of San Bernardino	San Bernardino	89%	151
Doctors Hospital of Manteca	Manteca	89%	96
Foothill Presbyterian Hospital	Glendora	89%	149
Good Samaritan Hospital	San Jose	89%	215
Kaiser Foundation Hospital	Baldwin Park	89%	97
Kaiser Foundation Hospital-Fresno	Fresno	89%	100
Kaiser Redwood City Medical Center	Redwood City	89%	114
Monterey Park Hospital	Monterey Park	89%	63
NorthBay Medical Center	Fairfield	89%	184
Pomerado Hospital	Poway	89%	140
Salinas Valley Memorial Health Care District	Salinas	89%	37
Sutter Medical Center of Santa Rosa	Santa Rosa	89%	89
Western Medical Center	Santa Ana	89%	89
Community Medical Center-Clovis	Clovis	88%	84
Garfield Medical Center	Monterey Park	88%	95
Good Samaritan Hospital	Los Angeles	88%	148
Hemet Valley Medical Center	Hemet	88%	240
Little Company of Mary-San Pedro Hospital	San Pedro	88%	121
Mercy Medical Center-Redding	Redding	88%	180
Oakland Medical Center	Oakland	88%	345
Scripps Mercy Hospital	San Diego	88%	400
Valley Presbyterian Hospital	Van Nuys	88%	32
Western Medical Center Hospital Anaheim	Anaheim	88%	57
Alhambra Hospital Medical Center	Alhambra	87%	130
Centinela Freeman Reg Med Ctr-Marina	Marina Del Rey	87%	39
Coastal Communities Hospital	Santa Ana	87%	113
Community Memorial Hospital Ventura	Ventura	87%	231
Community Regional Medical Center	Fresno	87%	439
Hanford Community Medical Center	Hanford	87%	75
Menifee Valley Medical Center	Sun City	87%	142
Orange Coast Memorial Medical Center	Santa Ana	87%	157
Saint Elizabeth Community Hospital	Red Bluff	87%	89
Saint Luke's Hospital	San Francisco	87%	108
Santa Rosa Memorial Hospital	Santa Rosa	87%	171
Simi Valley Hospital	Simi Valley	87%	107
South Coast Medical Center	Laguna Beach	87%	47
Sutter Roseville Medical Center	Roseville	87%	97
UCLA Medical Center	Los Angeles	87%	85
Washington Hospital	Fremont	87%	105
Alameda Hospital	Alameda	86%	106
Downey Regional Medical Center	Downey	86%	146
Emanuel Medical Center	Turlock	86%	151
Los Robles Regional Medical Center	Thousand Oaks	86%	205
Rideout Memorial Hospital	Marysville	86%	184
Saint Louise Regional Hospital	Gilroy	86%	72
San Antonio Community Hospital	Upland	86%	306
Tri-City Medical Center	Oceanside	86%	325
University of California Davis Health System	Sacramento	86%	112
Dominican Hospital	Santa Cruz	85%	168
Kaiser Foundation Hospital-San Diego	San Diego	85%	71
Oak Valley Hospital	Oakdale	85%	39
Oroville Hospital	Oroville	85%	98
Saint Bernardine Medical Center	San Bernardino	85%	72
San Mateo Medical Center	San Mateo	85%	40
Bakersfield Memorial Hospital	Bakersfield	84%	107
Bellflower Medical Center	Bellflower	84%	32
Enloe Medical Center	Chico	84%	223
Grossmont Hospital	La Mesa	84%	486
Henry Mayo Newhall Memorial Hospital	Valencia	84%	142
Los Angeles County & USC Medical Center	Los Angeles	84%	122
Pomona Valley Hospital Medical Center	Pomona	84%	198
Seton Medical Center	Daly City	84%	32
Sierra View District Hospital	Porterville	84%	160
Tri-City Regional Medical Center	Hawaiian Gardens	84%	77
Ukiah Valley Medical Center	Ukiah	84%	32
Kaiser Foundation Hospital-Manteca	Manteca	83%	100
Kaiser Permanente Los Angeles Medical Center	Los Angeles	83%	92
Riverside Community Hospital	Riverside	83%	308
Verdugo Hills Hospital	Glendale	83%	104
Citrus Valley Medical Center	Covina	82%	148
Kaiser Foundation Hospital-Riverside	Riverside	82%	51
Kaweah Delta Health Care District	Visalia	82%	247
Mercy Hospital	Bakersfield	82%	315
Saint Rose Hospital	Hayward	82%	40
Sharp Chula Vista Medical Center	Chula Vista	82%	283
Encino-Tarzana Regional Medical Center	Tarzana	81%	218
Los Angeles County Harbor-UCLA Medical Center	Torrance	81%	129
Mission Community Hospital	Panorama City	81%	37
Delano Regional Medical Center	Delano	80%	44
Petaluma Valley Hospital	Petaluma	80%	45
San Gorgonio Memorial Hospital	Banning	80%	44
Alameda County Medical Center	Oakland	79%	119
Eisenhower Medical Center	Rancho Mirage	79%	197
San Francisco General Hospital Medical Center	San Francisco	79%	176
Santa Clara Valley Medical Center	San Jose	79%	201
Sutter Delta Medical Center	Antioch	79%	111
Community Hospital	Huntington Park	78%	50
Kern Valley Healthcare District	Lake Isabella	78%	32
Memorial Hospital Los Banos	Los Banos	78%	41
Memorial Medical Center	Modesto	78%	110
Redlands Community Hospital	Redlands	78%	49
Sutter Solano Medical Center	Vallejo	78%	55
Kaiser Foundation Hospital	Woodland Hills	77%	69
San Joaquin General Hospital	French Camp	77%	148
Arrowhead Regional Medical Center	Colton	76%	129
Kaiser Permanente Fontana Medical Center	Fontana	76%	45
Kaiser Permanente Panorama City Med Ctr	Panorama City	75%	51
Lancaster Community Hospital	Lancaster	75%	96
Pioneers Memorial Healthcare District	Brawley	74%	92
Kaiser Foundation Hospital-Walnut Creek	Walnut Creek	73%	113
Dameron Hospital	Stockton	72%	121
Barton Memorial Hospital	South Lake Tahoe	71%	48
Corona Regional Medical Center	Corona	71%	204
East Los Angeles Doctors Hospital	Los Angeles	71%	62
Coast Plaza Doctors Hospital	Norwalk	68%	60
Citrus Valley Med Ctr Queen Valley Campus	West Covina	67%	205
Antelope Valley Hospital	Lancaster	66%	276
Olive View-UCLA Medical Center	San Fernando	63%	30
Hazel Hawkins Memorial Hospital	Hollister	60%	30
Martin Luther King Jr/Charles R Drew Med Ctr	Los Angeles	47%	74

15. Influenza Vaccine

Hospital Name	City	Rate	Cases
Garden Grove Hospital and Medical Center	Garden Grove	100%	32
Saint Joseph Hospital	Eureka	100%	25
San Joaquin Community Hospital	Bakersfield	100%	40
Twin Cities Community Hospital	Templeton	100%	30
Los Alamitos Medical Center	Los Alamitos	98%	54
Centinela Hospital Medical Center	Inglewood	97%	33
John Muir Medical Center	Walnut Creek	96%	28
Saint Jude Medical Center	Fullerton	96%	67
San Dimas Community Hospital	San Dimas	96%	50
Feather River Hospital	Paradise	94%	36
Sutter Davis Hospital	Davis	93%	29
Saddleback Memorial Medical Center	Laguna Hills	92%	113
San Rafael Medical Center	San Rafael	92%	61
Chinese Hospital	San Francisco	91%	44
Mercy Hospital of Folsom	Folsom	91%	34
Stanford Hospital	Stanford	89%	47
Mercy San Juan Hospital	Carmichael	88%	140
Saint Agnes Medical Center	Fresno	88%	56

NOTE: Hospital profiles are in alphabetical order by state, then city, then hospital within the city; Rankings are sorted by rate in descending order and exclude hospitals with less than 25 cases; (1) The number of cases is too small (n<25) for purposes of reliably predicting hospital performance; (2) Measure reflects the hospital's indication that its submission was based upon a sample of its relevant discharges; (3) Rate reflects fewer than the maximum possible quarters of data for the measure; (4) Inaccurate information submitted and suppressed for one or more quarters; (5) No data is available from the hospital for this measure; Please refer to the User's Guide for a full explanation of data

Fountain Valley Reg Hospital & Med Ctr	Fountain Valley	87%	52
Glendale Memorial Hospital and Health Center	Glendale	87%	68
Queen of the Valley Hospital	Napa	87%	47
Saint Elizabeth Community Hospital	Red Bluff	87%	30
Sutter Roseville Medical Center	Roseville	87%	31
Scripps Green Hospital	La Jolla	86%	44
Sequoia Hospital	Redwood City	86%	29
Doctors Hospital of Manteca	Manteca	85%	34
Kaiser Permanente Anaheim Medical Center	Anaheim	85%	27
Little Company of Mary Hospital	Torrance	85%	67
Saint Joseph Hospital	Orange	85%	55
Sierra Vista Regional Medical Center	San Luis Obispo	85%	26
Community Medical Center-Clovis	Clovis	84%	32
Desert Regional Medical Center	Palm Springs	83%	53
Tulare District Hospital	Tulare	83%	36
Doctors Medical Center	Modesto	82%	102
Placentia-Linda Hospital	Placentia	82%	40
Shasta Regional Medical Center	Redding	82%	65
Hoag Memorial Hospital Presbyterian	Newport Beach	81%	84
Kaiser Foundation Hospital-South Sacramento	Sacramento	81%	47
Mercy General Hospital	Sacramento	81%	79
Providence Saint Joseph Medical Center	Burbank	81%	31
Mercy Medical Center-Redding	Redding	80%	66
Sierra Nevada Memorial Hospital	Grass Valley	80%	56
Community Hospital of Los Gatos	Los Gatos	79%	33
El Centro Regional Medical Center	El Centro	79%	39
Northridge Hospital Medical Center	Northridge	79%	70
Petaluma Valley Hospital	Petaluma	79%	28
Valleycare Medical Center	Livermore	79%	43
Whittier Hospital Medical Center	Whittier	79%	66
Bakersfield Heart Hospital	Bakersfield	78%	27
Tri-City Medical Center	Oceanside	78%	85
Kaiser Foundation Hospital	Woodland Hills	77%	30
Orange Coast Memorial Medical Center	Santa Ana	77%	61
San Ramon Regional Medical Center	San Ramon	77%	35
Community Regional Medical Center	Fresno	76%	111
Palomar Medical Center	Escondido	76%	80
Ukiah Valley Medical Center	Ukiah	76%	25
Emanuel Medical Center	Turlock	75%	36
Mission Hospital Regional Medical Center	Mission Viejo	75%	51
Memorial Medical Center	Modesto	74%	35
Sutter Auburn Faith Hospital	Auburn	74%	27
University of California Davis Health System	Sacramento	74%	27
Irvine Regional Hospital	Irvine	72%	58
Marian Medical Center	Santa Maria	72%	69
Washington Hospital	Fremont	72%	29
Beverly Hospital	Montebello	71%	62
Eisenhower Medical Center	Rancho Mirage	71%	96
Los Angeles County Harbor-UCLA Medical Center	Torrance	71%	28
Saint Francis Medical Center	Lynwood	70%	50
Kaiser Foundation Hospital-San Diego	San Diego	69%	29
Kaiser Permanente Santa Clara Medical Center	Santa Clara	69%	26
O'Connor Hospital	San Jose	69%	54
San Leandro Hospital	San Leandro	69%	32
Rancho Springs Medical Center	Murrieta	68%	68
Cedars-Sinai Medical Center	Los Angeles	66%	122
Kaiser Foundation Hospital-Walnut Creek	Walnut Creek	66%	29
Pomona Valley Hospital Medical Center	Pomona	66%	68
Riverside Community Hospital	Riverside	66%	90
Saint John's Pleasant Valley Hospital	Camarillo	66%	32
Saint Vincent Medical Center	Los Angeles	66%	59
Kaiser Redwood City Medical Center	Redwood City	65%	31
Methodist Hospital of Sacramento	Sacramento	65%	51
Sierra View District Hospital	Porterville	65%	60
Simi Valley Hospital	Simi Valley	65%	34
Hi-Desert Medical Center	Joshua Tree	64%	45
Kaiser Permanente Panorama City Med Ctr	Panorama City	64%	25
S San Francisco Medical Center	S San Francisco	64%	25
Anaheim Memorial Medical Center	Anaheim	63%	93
John F Kennedy Memorial Hospital	Indio	63%	62
Kaiser Permanente San Francisco Med Ctr	San Francisco	63%	41
Lakewood Regional Medical Center	Lakewood	63%	46
Santa Rosa Memorial Hospital	Santa Rosa	63%	46
Sutter Tracy Community Hospital	Tracy	63%	38
Dominican Hospital	Santa Cruz	62%	55
Kaiser Foundation Hospital	Hayward	62%	26
Providence Holy Cross Medical Center	Mission Hills	62%	32
Western Medical Center	Santa Ana	62%	29
Marin General Hospital	Greenbrae	61%	41
West Hills Hospital and Medical Center	West Hills	61%	80
Kaiser Foundation Hospital-Fresno	Fresno	60%	30
Encino-Tarzana Regional Medical Center	Encino	59%	44
Good Samaritan Hospital	San Jose	59%	71
Little Company of Mary-San Pedro Hospital	San Pedro	59%	41
Kaiser Foundation Hospital-Santa Rosa	Santa Rosa	58%	38
Kaiser Permanente Sacramento Medical Center	Sacramento	58%	108
Los Angeles County & USC Medical Center	Los Angeles	58%	66
Mills-Peninsula Health Services	Burlingame	58%	31
Oakland Medical Center	Oakland	58%	110
Community Memorial Hospital Ventura	Ventura	57%	60
Kaiser Permanente Santa Teresa Comm Med Ctr	San Jose	57%	28
Paradise Valley Hospital	National City	57%	58
El Camino Hospital	Mountain View	56%	68
Encino-Tarzana Regional Medical Center	Tarzana	55%	75
Loma Linda University Medical Center	Loma Linda	55%	47
Santa Barbara Cottage Hospital	Santa Barbara	54%	72
Downey Regional Medical Center	Downey	53%	32
Hanford Community Medical Center	Hanford	53%	30
Saint John's Regional Medical Center	Oxnard	53%	43
Scripps Memorial Hospital La Jolla	La Jolla	53%	34
Sutter Solano Medical Center	Vallejo	53%	30
Glendale Adventist Medical Center	Glendale	52%	60
John Muir Medical Center-Concord Campus	Concord	52%	29
Menifee Valley Medical Center	Sun City	52%	52
Sharp Memorial Hospital	San Diego	52%	69
UCSF Medical Center	San Francisco	52%	29
Foothill Presbyterian Hospital	Glendora	51%	41
La Palma Intercommunity Hospital	La Palma	50%	58
NorthBay Medical Center	Fairfield	50%	34
Scripps Memorial Hospital-Encinitas	Encinitas	50%	40
Pomerado Hospital	Poway	49%	35
Kaiser Foundation Hospital-Vallejo	Vallejo	47%	32
Regional Medical Center of San Jose	San Jose	45%	100
Kaiser Foundation Hospital-Manteca	Manteca	44%	34
Methodist Hospital of Southern California	Arcadia	44%	108
Saint Mary Medical Center	Apple Valley	44%	75
San Gabriel Valley Medical Center	San Gabriel	44%	85
Doctor's Medical Center-San Pablo Campus	San Pablo	43%	65
Eden Medical Center	Castro Valley	43%	58
Parkview Community Hospital	Riverside	43%	54
Watsonville Community Hospital	Watsonville	43%	30
Saint Mary's Medical Center	San Francisco	42%	36
Coast Plaza Doctors Hospital	Norwalk	40%	25
VacaValley Hospital	Vacaville	39%	31
Citrus Valley Medical Center	Covina	37%	49
University of California Irvine Med Ctr	Orange	36%	28
San Francisco General Hospital Medical Center	San Francisco	35%	26
Dameron Hospital	Stockton	34%	38
Lancaster Community Hospital	Lancaster	34%	41
Santa Monica-UCLA Medical Center	Santa Monica	34%	32
University of California San Diego Med Ctr	San Diego	34%	29
Los Robles Regional Medical Center	Thousand Oaks	33%	82
Sharp Chula Vista Medical Center	Chula Vista	33%	67
Hemet Valley Medical Center	Hemet	32%	78
Long Beach Memorial Medical Center	Long Beach	30%	118
Grossmont Hospital	La Mesa	27%	119
San Antonio Community Hospital	Upland	26%	92
Community Hospital	Huntington Park	24%	29
Olympia Medical Center	Los Angeles	24%	72
Citrus Valley Med Ctr Queen Valley Campus	West Covina	23%	64
Barstow Community Hospital	Barstow	19%	43
Greater El Monte Community Hospital	South El Monte	18%	33
Alameda Hospital	Alameda	16%	38
Huntington Memorial Hospital	Pasadena	14%	132
Delano Regional Medical Center	Delano	12%	26
Saint Luke's Hospital	San Francisco	11%	27
Scripps Mercy Hospital	San Diego	11%	132
Community Hospital of Long Beach	Long Beach	9%	34
Alhambra Hospital Medical Center	Alhambra	8%	59
Verdugo Hills Hospital	Glendale	7%	28
Sutter Medical Center of Santa Rosa	Santa Rosa	6%	32
Torrance Memorial Medical Center	Torrance	5%	86
Bakersfield Memorial Hospital	Bakersfield	4%	50
Saint John's Health Center	Santa Monica	2%	49
Mercy Hospital	Bakersfield	1%	105
Martin Luther King Jr/Charles R Drew Med Ctr	Los Angeles	0%	25
Memorial Hospital of Gardena	Gardena	0%	56
West Anaheim Medical Center	Anaheim	0%	60

16. Initial Antibiotic Timing

Hospital Name	City	Rate	Cases
Sherman Oaks Hospital	Sherman Oaks	98%	43
Sutter Amador Hospital	Jackson	96%	99
Cedars-Sinai Medical Center	Los Angeles	94%	519
French Hospital Medical Center	San Luis Obispo	94%	109
Garden Grove Hospital and Medical Center	Garden Grove	94%	178
Chino Valley Medical Center	Chino	93%	61
Fountain Valley Reg Hospital & Med Ctr	Fountain Valley	93%	281
Saint Helena Hospital	Deer Park	93%	42

NOTE: Hospital profiles are in alphabetical order by state, then city, then hospital within the city; Rankings are sorted by rate in descending order and exclude hospitals with less than 25 cases; (1) The number of cases is too small (n<25) for purposes of reliably predicting hospital performance; (2) Measure reflects the hospital's indication that its submission was based upon a sample of its relevant discharges; (3) Rate reflects fewer than the maximum possible quarters of data for the measure; (4) Inaccurate information submitted and suppressed for one or more quarters; (5) No data is available from the hospital for this measure; Please refer to the User's Guide for a full explanation of data

Hospital	City	Rate	Cases
Saint Joseph Hospital	Eureka	93%	115
Sequoia Hospital	Redwood City	93%	92
Sharp Coronado Hospital	San Diego	93%	84
Chapman Medical Center	Orange	92%	66
Huntington Beach Hospital	Huntington Beach	92%	132
Los Alamitos Medical Center	Los Alamitos	92%	226
Marin General Hospital	Greenbrae	92%	148
Orange Coast Memorial Medical Center	Santa Ana	92%	253
Desert Regional Medical Center	Palm Springs	91%	306
Frank R Howard Memorial Hospital	Willits	91%	47
Healdsburg District Hospital	Healdsburg	91%	32
Pacific Hospital of Long Beach	Long Beach	91%	147
Placentia-Linda Hospital	Placentia	91%	187
Saint Francis Memorial Hospital	San Francisco	91%	56
Woodland Healthcare	Woodland	91%	88
Desert Valley Hospital	Victorville	90%	140
Mad River Community Hospital	Arcata	90%	67
Saddleback Memorial Medical Center	Laguna Hills	90%	429
Saint Bernardine Medical Center	San Bernardino	90%	115
San Dimas Community Hospital	San Dimas	90%	185
Sonora Regional Medical Center	Sonora	90%	149
Sutter Auburn Faith Hospital	Auburn	90%	145
Sutter Davis Hospital	Davis	90%	136
Tuolumne General Hospital	Sonora	90%	72
Twin Cities Community Hospital	Templeton	90%	153
Mercy General Hospital	Sacramento	89%	365
Queen of the Valley Hospital	Napa	89%	194
Saint Elizabeth Community Hospital	Red Bluff	89%	168
San Ramon Regional Medical Center	San Ramon	89%	115
VacaValley Hospital	Vacaville	89%	186
Western Medical Center Hospital Anaheim	Anaheim	89%	85
Arroyo Grande Community Hospital	Arroyo Grande	88%	132
Doctor's Medical Center-San Pablo Campus	San Pablo	88%	295
Novato Community Hospital	Novato	88%	74
Saint Joseph Hospital	Orange	88%	224
Saint Mary's Medical Center	San Francisco	88%	184
South Coast Medical Center	Laguna Beach	88%	81
Anaheim Memorial Medical Center	Anaheim	87%	437
Coastal Communities Hospital	Santa Ana	87%	105
Community Hospital of Long Beach	Long Beach	87%	175
Doctors Hospital of Manteca	Manteca	87%	141
Encino-Tarzana Regional Medical Center	Encino	87%	154
Hoag Memorial Hospital Presbyterian	Newport Beach	87%	376
Little Company of Mary-San Pedro Hospital	San Pedro	87%	174
San Mateo Medical Center	San Mateo	87%	55
Sierra Nevada Memorial Hospital	Grass Valley	87%	276
Chinese Hospital	San Francisco	86%	170
Marian Medical Center	Santa Maria	86%	234
Providence Holy Cross Medical Center	Mission Hills	86%	194
Saint Agnes Medical Center	Fresno	86%	318
Seton Medical Center	Daly City	86%	209
Sierra Vista Regional Medical Center	San Luis Obispo	86%	85
Alameda Hospital	Alameda	85%	158
Community Hospital of Los Gatos	Los Gatos	85%	106
Grossmont Hospital	La Mesa	85%	603
John F Kennedy Memorial Hospital	Indio	85%	229
Kaiser Foundation Hospital-Vallejo	Vallejo	85%	137
Lakewood Regional Medical Center	Lakewood	85%	199
Lompoc Healthcare District Hospital	Lompoc	85%	82
San Gorgonio Memorial Hospital	Banning	85%	259
Ukiah Valley Medical Center	Ukiah	85%	128
Goleta Valley Cottage Hospital	Santa Barbara	84%	38
Irvine Regional Hospital	Irvine	84%	160
Kaiser Redwood City Medical Center	Redwood City	84%	137
Mercy Medical Center-Mount Shasta	Mount Shasta	84%	73
Oak Valley Hospital	Oakdale	84%	91
Saint Louisie Regional Hospital	Gilroy	84%	107
Scripps Green Hospital	La Jolla	84%	88
Scripps Memorial Hospital La Jolla	La Jolla	84%	140
Simi Valley Hospital	Simi Valley	84%	122
S San Francisco Medical Center	S San Francisco	84%	142
Sutter Coast Hospital	Crescent City	84%	105
Western Medical Center	Santa Ana	84%	129
Anaheim General Hospital	Anaheim	83%	53
Bellflower Medical Center	Bellflower	83%	174
East Valley Hospital Medical Center	Glendora	83%	152
Encino-Tarzana Regional Medical Center	Tarzana	83%	246
Hazel Hawkins Memorial Hospital	Hollister	83%	58
Kaiser Permanente San Francisco Med Ctr	San Francisco	83%	222
Methodist Hospital of Southern California	Arcadia	83%	499
Sierra Kings District Hospital	Reedley	83%	109
Torrance Memorial Medical Center	Torrance	83%	299
Tri-City Medical Center	Oceanside	83%	387
Bakersfield Heart Hospital	Bakersfield	82%	112
Community Memorial Hospital Ventura	Ventura	82%	292
Dameron Hospital	Stockton	82%	201
East Los Angeles Doctors Hospital	Los Angeles	82%	96
Feather River Hospital	Paradise	82%	164
Little Company of Mary Hospital	Torrance	82%	290
Monterey Park Hospital	Monterey Park	82%	116
Parkview Community Hospital	Riverside	82%	332
San Rafael Medical Center	San Rafael	82%	210
Santa Rosa Memorial Hospital	Santa Rosa	82%	268
Sonoma Valley Hospital	Sonoma	82%	44
Sutter Lakeside Hospital	Lakeport	82%	107
Sutter Tracy Community Hospital	Tracy	82%	101
Valleycare Medical Center	Livermore	82%	195
John Muir Medical Center-Concord Campus	Concord	81%	152
Marshall Medical Center	Placerville	81%	148
Memorial Hospital Los Banos	Los Banos	81%	98
Olympia Medical Center	Los Angeles	81%	368
Pioneers Memorial Healthcare District	Brawley	81%	157
Saint Jude Medical Center	Fullerton	81%	275
Shasta Regional Medical Center	Redding	81%	313
Sutter General Hospital	Sacramento	81%	180
Ventura County Medical Center	Ventura	81%	73
West Anaheim Medical Center	Anaheim	81%	204
Antelope Valley Hospital	Lancaster	80%	476
Coalinga Regional Medical Center	Coalinga	80%	74
Kaiser Foundation Hospital-South Sacramento	Sacramento	80%	210
Madera Community Hospital	Madera	80%	160
Mercy Medical Center-Redding	Redding	80%	316
Methodist Hospital of Sacramento	Sacramento	80%	255
Pomerado Hospital	Poway	80%	160
Riverside Community Hospital	Riverside	80%	523
Saint Mary Medical Center	Long Beach	80%	141
Saint Vincent Medical Center	Los Angeles	80%	306
Santa Barbara Cottage Hospital	Santa Barbara	80%	256
Santa Ynez Valley Cottage Hospital	Solvang	80%	25
Enloe Medical Center	Chico	79%	416
Garfield Medical Center	Monterey Park	79%	149
Hollywood Community Hospital	Hollywood	79%	48
Mercy Hospital of Folsom	Folsom	79%	138
Palomar Medical Center	Escondido	79%	374
San Joaquin Community Hospital	Bakersfield	79%	251
California Pacific Medical Center	San Francisco	78%	133
Community Hospital of the Monterey Peninsula	Monterey	78%	152
Glendale Memorial Hospital and Health Center	Glendale	78%	285
John Muir Medical Center	Walnut Creek	78%	162
Kaiser Permanente Fontana Medical Center	Fontana	78%	74
Mercy Med Ctr Merced-Community Campus	Merced	78%	129
NorthBay Medical Center	Fairfield	78%	223
O'Connor Hospital	San Jose	78%	238
Oakland Medical Center	Oakland	78%	439
Presbyterian Intercommunity Hospital	Whittier	78%	125
Saint John's Regional Medical Center	Oxnard	78%	268
Saint Mary Medical Center	Apple Valley	78%	454
San Gabriel Valley Medical Center	San Gabriel	78%	398
Coast Plaza Doctors Hospital	Norwalk	77%	219
Davies Medical Center	San Francisco	77%	75
Emanuel Medical Center	Turlock	77%	232
Good Samaritan Hospital	Los Angeles	77%	212
Hollywood Presbyterian Medical Center	Los Angeles	77%	461
Kern Valley Healthcare District	Lake Isabella	77%	30
Mercy San Juan Hospital	Carmichael	77%	598
Palm Drive Hospital	Sebastopol	77%	35
Palo Verde Hospital	Blythe	77%	44
Petaluma Valley Hospital	Petaluma	77%	101
Providence Saint Joseph Medical Center	Burbank	77%	170
Saint Joseph's Medical Center of Stockton	Stockton	77%	154
Scripps Memorial Hospital-Encinitas	Encinitas	77%	145
Whittier Hospital Medical Center	Whittier	77%	292
California Hospital Medical Center	Los Angeles	76%	143
Foothill Presbyterian Hospital	Glendora	76%	208
Mark Twain Saint Joseph's Hospital	San Andreas	76%	89
Mills-Peninsula Health Services	Burlingame	76%	152
Natividad Medical Center	Salinas	76%	89
Regional Medical Center of San Jose	San Jose	76%	417
Saint Luke's Hospital	San Francisco	76%	148
Santa Monica-UCLA Medical Center	Santa Monica	76%	160
Tulare District Hospital	Tulare	76%	158
Washington Hospital	Fremont	76%	152
Dominican Hospital	Santa Cruz	75%	242
Fallbrook Hospital	Fallbrook	75%	89
Henry Mayo Newhall Memorial Hospital	Valencia	75%	234
Long Beach Memorial Medical Center	Long Beach	75%	485
Mercy Hospital	Bakersfield	75%	439
Mission Community Hospital	Panorama City	75%	194
Redlands Community Hospital	Redlands	75%	216
Tri-City Regional Medical Center	Hawaiian Gardens	75%	145

NOTE: Hospital profiles are in alphabetical order by state, then city, then hospital within the city; Rankings are sorted by rate in descending order and exclude hospitals with less than 25 cases; (1) The number of cases is too small (n<25) for purposes of reliably predicting hospital performance; (2) Measure reflects the hospital's indication that its submission was based upon a sample of its relevant discharges; (3) Rate reflects fewer than the maximum possible quarters of data for the measure; (4) Inaccurate information submitted and suppressed for one or more quarters; (5) No data is available from the hospital for this measure; Please refer to the User's Guide for a full explanation of data

Alhambra Hospital Medical Center	Alhambra	74%	231
Barton Memorial Hospital	South Lake Tahoe	74%	61
Colusa Regional Medical Center	Colusa	74%	31
Community Hospital of San Bernardino	San Bernardino	74%	212
Glendale Adventist Medical Center	Glendale	74%	260
Greater El Monte Community Hospital	South El Monte	74%	206
Kaweah Delta Health Care District	Visalia	74%	485
Mission Hospital Regional Medical Center	Mission Viejo	74%	217
Oroville Hospital	Oroville	74%	131
San Leandro Hospital	San Leandro	74%	163
Centinela Freeman Reg Med Ctr-Marina	Marina Del Rey	73%	88
Northridge Hospital Medical Center	Northridge	73%	296
Pacifica Hospital of the Valley	Sun Valley	73%	98
West Hills Hospital and Medical Center	West Hills	73%	339
Central Valley General Hospital	Hanford	72%	65
Good Samaritan Hospital	San Jose	72%	253
Kaiser Foundation Hospital-Manteca	Manteca	72%	119
Kaiser Permanente Los Angeles Medical Center	Los Angeles	72%	95
Kaiser Permanente Santa Teresa Comm Med Ctr	San Jose	72%	130
Moreno Valley Community Hospital	Moreno Valley	72%	164
Saint John's Health Center	Santa Monica	72%	222
Saint John's Pleasant Valley Hospital	Camarillo	72%	120
Brotman Medical Center	Culver City	71%	115
Centinela Hospital Medical Center	Inglewood	71%	181
Corona Regional Medical Center	Corona	71%	315
Downey Regional Medical Center	Downey	71%	192
Huntington Memorial Hospital	Pasadena	71%	462
Kaiser Permanente Santa Clara Medical Center	Santa Clara	71%	132
Menifee Valley Medical Center	Sun City	71%	221
Paradise Valley Hospital	National City	71%	259
Pomona Valley Hospital Medical Center	Pomona	71%	311
Sharp Chula Vista Medical Center	Chula Vista	71%	390
White Memorial Medical Center	Los Angeles	71%	284
Beverly Hospital	Montebello	70%	328
Doctors Medical Center	Modesto	70%	436
Kaiser Foundation Hospital-Santa Rosa	Santa Rosa	70%	156
Sutter Delta Medical Center	Antioch	70%	162
Sutter Roseville Medical Center	Roseville	70%	159
Bakersfield Memorial Hospital	Bakersfield	69%	204
Delano Regional Medical Center	Delano	69%	124
Kaiser Permanente Bellflower Medical Center	Bellflower	69%	108
Lodi Memorial Hospital	Lodi	69%	123
Los Robles Regional Medical Center	Thousand Oaks	69%	270
Redbud Community Hospital	Clearlake	69%	103
Watsonville Community Hospital	Watsonville	69%	151
Alta Bates Summit Medical Center	Berkeley	68%	79
Alta Bates Summit Medical Center	Oakland	68%	125
Kaiser Foundation Hospital	Baldwin Park	68%	98
La Palma Intercommunity Hospital	La Palma	68%	182
Rideout Memorial Hospital	Marysville	68%	353
Ridgecrest Regional Hospital	Ridgecrest	68%	121
Stanford Hospital	Stanford	68%	259
Contra Costa Regional Medical Center	Martinez	67%	99
Eisenhower Medical Center	Rancho Mirage	67%	369
El Camino Hospital	Mountain View	67%	357
Kaiser Foundation Hospital	Hayward	67%	168
Memorial Medical Center	Modesto	67%	163
Rancho Springs Medical Center	Murrieta	67%	321
Salinas Valley Memorial Health Care District	Salinas	67%	280
San Antonio Community Hospital	Upland	67%	427
Sutter Medical Center of Santa Rosa	Santa Rosa	67%	120
Kaiser Foundation Hospital-San Diego	San Diego	66%	112
Kaiser Foundation Hospital-Walnut Creek	Walnut Creek	66%	115
Kaiser Permanente Panorama City Med Ctr	Panorama City	66%	94
Kaiser Permanente Sacramento Medical Center	Sacramento	66%	425
Verdugo Hills Hospital	Glendale	66%	177
UCSF Medical Center	San Francisco	65%	153
University of California San Diego Med Ctr	San Diego	65%	192
Eden Medical Center	Castro Valley	64%	232
Memorial Hospital of Gardena	Gardena	64%	299
Kaiser Foundation Hospital-Fresno	Fresno	63%	121
Kaiser Permanente West Los Angeles Med Ctr	Los Angeles	63%	94
Lancaster Community Hospital	Lancaster	63%	159
Scripps Mercy Hospital	San Diego	63%	552
Sierra View District Hospital	Porterville	63%	240
Sutter Solano Medical Center	Vallejo	63%	131
Citrus Valley Med Ctr Queen Valley Campus	West Covina	62%	300
Community Hospital	Huntington Park	62%	113
Community Medical Center-Clovis	Clovis	62%	129
El Centro Regional Medical Center	El Centro	62%	139
Kaiser Permanente Anaheim Medical Center	Anaheim	62%	101
Martin Luther King Jr/Charles R Drew Med Ctr	Los Angeles	62%	164
Saint Rose Hospital	Hayward	62%	200
Hanford Community Medical Center	Hanford	61%	183
Hi-Desert Medical Center	Joshua Tree	61%	241
Olive View-UCLA Medical Center	San Fernando	61%	158
UCLA Medical Center	Los Angeles	61%	115
Citrus Valley Medical Center	Covina	60%	235
City of Angels Medical Center	Los Angeles	60%	42
Sharp Memorial Hospital	San Diego	60%	308
Arrowhead Regional Medical Center	Colton	59%	184
Barstow Community Hospital	Barstow	59%	165
Saint Francis Medical Center	Lynwood	59%	299
University of California Irvine Med Ctr	Orange	59%	151
Valley Presbyterian Hospital	Van Nuys	59%	199
Hemet Valley Medical Center	Hemet	58%	362
Tustin Hospital and Medical Center	Tustin	58%	26
Los Angeles Community Hospital	Los Angeles	57%	93
Kaiser Foundation Hospital-Riverside	Riverside	56%	94
Santa Clara Valley Medical Center	San Jose	56%	217
Temple Community Hospital	Los Angeles	55%	53
University of California Davis Health System	Sacramento	55%	169
Kaiser Permanente South Bay Medical Center	Harbor City	54%	115
Los Angeles County Harbor-UCLA Medical Center	Torrance	54%	175
Ojai Valley Community Hospital	Ojai	54%	48
Riverside County Regional Medical Center	Moreno Valley	52%	109
San Joaquin General Hospital	French Camp	52%	221
Century City Doctors Hospital	Los Angeles	50%	40
Pacific Alliance Medical Center	Los Angeles	50%	149
San Francisco General Hospital Medical Center	San Francisco	50%	244
Loma Linda University Medical Center	Loma Linda	49%	269
Victor Valley Community Hospital	Victorville	49%	168
Community Regional Medical Center	Fresno	48%	616
Kaiser Foundation Hospital	Woodland Hills	47%	99
Alameda County Medical Center	Oakland	44%	156
Kern Medical Center	Bakersfield	44%	81
Los Angeles County & USC Medical Center	Los Angeles	38%	341
Good Samaritan Hospital	Bakersfield	37%	70
Los Angeles Metropolitan Med Ctr-LA Campus	Los Angeles	26%	53

17. Oxygenation Assessment

Hospital Name	City	Rate	Cases
Alameda County Medical Center	Oakland	100%	220
Alameda Hospital	Alameda	100%	184
Alhambra Hospital Medical Center	Alhambra	100%	397
Alta Bates Summit Medical Center	Berkeley	100%	106
Alta Bates Summit Medical Center	Oakland	100%	146
Anaheim Memorial Medical Center	Anaheim	100%	524
Antelope Valley Hospital	Lancaster	100%	539
Arrowhead Regional Medical Center	Colton	100%	218
Bakersfield Heart Hospital	Bakersfield	100%	161
Bakersfield Memorial Hospital	Bakersfield	100%	281
Banner Lassen Medical Center	Susanville	100%	46
Barstow Community Hospital	Barstow	100%	202
Barton Memorial Hospital	South Lake Tahoe	100%	90
Bellflower Medical Center	Bellflower	100%	205
Brotman Medical Center	Culver City	100%	147
California Hospital Medical Center	Los Angeles	100%	181
California Pacific Medical Center	San Francisco	100%	178
Cedars-Sinai Medical Center	Los Angeles	100%	720
Centinela Hospital Medical Center	Inglewood	100%	230
Central Valley General Hospital	Hanford	100%	71
Chapman Medical Center	Orange	100%	88
Chinese Hospital	San Francisco	100%	203
Chino Valley Medical Center	Chino	100%	81
Coalinga Regional Medical Center	Coalinga	100%	90
Coast Plaza Doctors Hospital	Norwalk	100%	230
Coastal Communities Hospital	Santa Ana	100%	142
Colusa Regional Medical Center	Colusa	100%	35
Community Hospital of Long Beach	Long Beach	100%	226
Community Hospital of Los Gatos	Los Gatos	100%	125
Community Hospital of San Bernardino	San Bernardino	100%	289
Community Hospital of the Monterey Peninsula	Monterey	100%	205
Community Medical Center-Clovis	Clovis	100%	168
Community Memorial Hospital Ventura	Ventura	100%	375
Community Regional Medical Center	Fresno	100%	756
Contra Costa Regional Medical Center	Martinez	100%	117
Dameron Hospital	Stockton	100%	221
Davies Medical Center	San Francisco	100%	101
Desert Regional Medical Center	Palm Springs	100%	354
Desert Valley Hospital	Victorville	100%	185
Doctor's Medical Center-San Pablo Campus	San Pablo	100%	344
Doctors Hospital of Manteca	Manteca	100%	161
Doctors Medical Center	Modesto	100%	560
Dominican Hospital	Santa Cruz	100%	292
Downey Regional Medical Center	Downey	100%	231
East Los Angeles Doctors Hospital	Los Angeles	100%	120
Eden Medical Center	Castro Valley	100%	286
Eisenhower Medical Center	Rancho Mirage	100%	455

NOTE: Hospital profiles are in alphabetical order by state, then city, then hospital within the city; Rankings are sorted by rate in descending order and exclude hospitals with less than 25 cases; (1) The number of cases is too small (n<25) for purposes of reliably predicting hospital performance; (2) Measure reflects the hospital's indication that its submission was based upon a sample of its relevant discharges; (3) Rate reflects fewer than the maximum possible quarters of data for the measure; (4) Inaccurate information submitted and suppressed for one or more quarters; (5) No data is available from the hospital for this measure; Please refer to the User's Guide for a full explanation of data

El Camino Hospital	Mountain View	100%	453
El Centro Regional Medical Center	El Centro	100%	167
Emanuel Medical Center	Turlock	100%	259
Encino-Tarzana Regional Medical Center	Encino	100%	225
Encino-Tarzana Regional Medical Center	Tarzana	100%	344
Enloe Medical Center	Chico	100%	504
Feather River Hospital	Paradise	100%	203
Foothill Presbyterian Hospital	Glendora	100%	259
Fountain Valley Reg Hospital & Med Ctr	Fountain Valley	100%	360
Frank R Howard Memorial Hospital	Willits	100%	60
French Hospital Medical Center	San Luis Obispo	100%	129
Garden Grove Hospital and Medical Center	Garden Grove	100%	225
Garfield Medical Center	Monterey Park	100%	177
Glendale Adventist Medical Center	Glendale	100%	334
Glendale Memorial Hospital and Health Center	Glendale	100%	367
Goleta Valley Cottage Hospital	Santa Barbara	100%	48
Good Samaritan Hospital	San Jose	100%	322
Greater El Monte Community Hospital	South El Monte	100%	247
Grossmont Hospital	La Mesa	100%	686
Healdsburg District Hospital	Healdsburg	100%	38
Hemet Valley Medical Center	Hemet	100%	467
Henry Mayo Newhall Memorial Hospital	Valencia	100%	287
Hi-Desert Medical Center	Joshua Tree	100%	290
Hoag Memorial Hospital Presbyterian	Newport Beach	100%	524
Hollywood Presbyterian Medical Center	Los Angeles	100%	508
Huntington Beach Hospital	Huntington Beach	100%	156
Huntington Memorial Hospital	Pasadena	100%	630
Irvine Regional Hospital	Irvine	100%	244
John F Kennedy Memorial Hospital	Indio	100%	285
John Muir Medical Center	Walnut Creek	100%	207
John Muir Medical Center-Concord Campus	Concord	100%	195
Kaiser Foundation Hospital	Baldwin Park	100%	125
Kaiser Foundation Hospital	Hayward	100%	202
Kaiser Foundation Hospital	Woodland Hills	100%	124
Kaiser Foundation Hospital-Fresno	Fresno	100%	163
Kaiser Foundation Hospital-Manteca	Manteca	100%	164
Kaiser Foundation Hospital-Riverside	Riverside	100%	125
Kaiser Foundation Hospital-San Diego	San Diego	100%	144
Kaiser Foundation Hospital-Santa Rosa	Santa Rosa	100%	190
Kaiser Foundation Hospital-South Sacramento	Sacramento	100%	285
Kaiser Foundation Hospital-Vallejo	Vallejo	100%	171
Kaiser Foundation Hospital-Walnut Creek	Walnut Creek	100%	168
Kaiser Permanente Anaheim Medical Center	Anaheim	100%	121
Kaiser Permanente Bellflower Medical Center	Bellflower	100%	122
Kaiser Permanente Fontana Medical Center	Fontana	100%	102
Kaiser Permanente Los Angeles Medical Center	Los Angeles	100%	127
Kaiser Permanente Sacramento Medical Center	Sacramento	100%	573
Kaiser Permanente San Francisco Med Ctr	San Francisco	100%	263
Kaiser Permanente Santa Clara Medical Center	Santa Clara	100%	173
Kaiser Permanente Santa Teresa Comm Med Ctr	San Jose	100%	160
Kaiser Permanente South Bay Medical Center	Harbor City	100%	138
Kaiser Permanente West Los Angeles Med Ctr	Los Angeles	100%	109
Kaiser Redwood City Medical Center	Redwood City	100%	168
Kaweah Delta Health Care District	Visalia	100%	618
Kern Valley Healthcare District	Lake Isabella	100%	34
Lakewood Regional Medical Center	Lakewood	100%	247
Little Company of Mary Hospital	Torrance	100%	411
Little Company of Mary-San Pedro Hospital	San Pedro	100%	221
Lodi Memorial Hospital	Lodi	100%	158
Loma Linda University Medical Center	Loma Linda	100%	354
Lompoc Healthcare District Hospital	Lompoc	100%	94
Long Beach Memorial Medical Center	Long Beach	100%	619
Los Alamitos Medical Center	Los Alamitos	100%	284
Los Angeles County Harbor-UCLA Medical Center	Torrance	100%	205
Los Robles Regional Medical Center	Thousand Oaks	100%	350
Mad River Community Hospital	Arcata	100%	77
Madera Community Hospital	Madera	100%	193
Marian Medical Center	Santa Maria	100%	307
Marin General Hospital	Greenbrae	100%	218
Mark Twain Saint Joseph's Hospital	San Andreas	100%	122
Marshall Medical Center	Placerville	100%	182
Memorial Hospital Los Banos	Los Banos	100%	112
Memorial Hospital of Gardena	Gardena	100%	323
Menifee Valley Medical Center	Sun City	100%	295
Mercy General Hospital	Sacramento	100%	409
Mercy Hospital	Bakersfield	100%	533
Mercy Hospital of Folsom	Folsom	100%	166
Mercy Med Ctr Merced-Community Campus	Merced	100%	171
Mercy Medical Center-Redding	Redding	100%	410
Mercy San Juan Hospital	Carmichael	100%	704
Methodist Hospital of Sacramento	Sacramento	100%	304
Mills-Peninsula Health Services	Burlingame	100%	186
Mission Hospital Regional Medical Center	Mission Viejo	100%	279
Motion Picture & Television Hospital	Woodland Hills	100%	29
Natividad Medical Center	Salinas	100%	118
NorthBay Medical Center	Fairfield	100%	265
Northridge Hospital Medical Center	Northridge	100%	396
Novato Community Hospital	Novato	100%	92
O'Connor Hospital	San Jose	100%	313
Oak Valley Hospital	Oakdale	100%	107
Oakland Medical Center	Oakland	100%	528
Ojai Valley Community Hospital	Ojai	100%	73
Olive View-UCLA Medical Center	San Fernando	100%	178
Olympia Medical Center	Los Angeles	100%	459
Orange Coast Memorial Medical Center	Santa Ana	100%	310
Oroville Hospital	Oroville	100%	152
Pacifica Hospital of the Valley	Sun Valley	100%	102
Palm Drive Hospital	Sebastopol	100%	42
Palo Verde Hospital	Blythe	100%	64
Palomar Medical Center	Escondido	100%	398
Paradise Valley Hospital	National City	100%	289
Parkview Community Hospital	Riverside	100%	381
Petaluma Valley Hospital	Petaluma	100%	139
Pioneers Memorial Healthcare District	Brawley	100%	183
Placentia-Linda Hospital	Placentia	100%	229
Pomerado Hospital	Poway	100%	206
Pomona Valley Hospital Medical Center	Pomona	100%	406
Presbyterian Intercommunity Hospital	Whittier	100%	156
Providence Holy Cross Medical Center	Mission Hills	100%	236
Providence Saint Joseph Medical Center	Burbank	100%	230
Queen of the Valley Hospital	Napa	100%	245
Rancho Springs Medical Center	Murrieta	100%	384
Redbud Community Hospital	Clearlake	100%	112
Redlands Community Hospital	Redlands	100%	259
Regional Medical Center of San Jose	San Jose	100%	483
Ridgecrest Regional Hospital	Ridgecrest	100%	145
Riverside Community Hospital	Riverside	100%	618
Saddleback Memorial Medical Center	Laguna Hills	100%	539
Saint Agnes Medical Center	Fresno	100%	378
Saint Bernardine Medical Center	San Bernardino	100%	147
Saint Elizabeth Community Hospital	Red Bluff	100%	200
Saint Francis Medical Center	Lynwood	100%	343
Saint Francis Memorial Hospital	San Francisco	100%	67
Saint Helena Hospital	Deer Park	100%	48
Saint John's Health Center	Santa Monica	100%	290
Saint Joseph Hospital	Eureka	100%	147
Saint Joseph Hospital	Orange	100%	300
Saint Joseph's Medical Center of Stockton	Stockton	100%	186
Saint Jude Medical Center	Fullerton	100%	355
Saint Louisie Regional Hospital	Gilroy	100%	129
Saint Luke's Hospital	San Francisco	100%	169
Saint Mary Medical Center	Long Beach	100%	163
Saint Mary's Medical Center	San Francisco	100%	229
Saint Rose Hospital	Hayward	100%	216
Saint Vincent Medical Center	Los Angeles	100%	357
San Dimas Community Hospital	San Dimas	100%	254
San Francisco General Hospital Medical Center	San Francisco	100%	271
San Gabriel Valley Medical Center	San Gabriel	100%	444
San Joaquin Community Hospital	Bakersfield	100%	286
San Joaquin General Hospital	French Camp	100%	241
San Leandro Hospital	San Leandro	100%	193
San Mateo Medical Center	San Mateo	100%	66
San Rafael Medical Center	San Rafael	100%	249
San Ramon Regional Medical Center	San Ramon	100%	143
Santa Barbara Cottage Hospital	Santa Barbara	100%	338
Santa Monica-UCLA Medical Center	Santa Monica	100%	186
Santa Ynez Valley Cottage Hospital	Solvang	100%	32
Scripps Green Hospital	La Jolla	100%	114
Scripps Memorial Hospital La Jolla	La Jolla	100%	176
Scripps Memorial Hospital-Encinitas	Encinitas	100%	205
Scripps Mercy Hospital	San Diego	100%	685
Seneca Hospital	Chester	100%	32
Sequoia Hospital	Redwood City	100%	119
Seton Medical Center	Daly City	100%	243
Sharp Chula Vista Medical Center	Chula Vista	100%	468
Sharp Coronado Hospital	San Diego	100%	104
Sharp Memorial Hospital	San Diego	100%	366
Shasta Regional Medical Center	Redding	100%	381
Sherman Oaks Hospital	Sherman Oaks	100%	56
Sierra Kings District Hospital	Reedley	100%	128
Sierra View District Hospital	Porterville	100%	317
Sierra Vista Regional Medical Center	San Luis Obispo	100%	124
Simi Valley Hospital	Simi Valley	100%	185
Sonoma Valley Hospital	Sonoma	100%	58
Sonora Regional Medical Center	Sonora	100%	172
South Coast Medical Center	Laguna Beach	100%	95
S San Francisco Medical Center	S San Francisco	100%	179
Stanford Hospital	Stanford	100%	351
Sutter Amador Hospital	Jackson	100%	116
Sutter Auburn Faith Hospital	Auburn	100%	170

NOTE: Hospital profiles are in alphabetical order by state, then city, then hospital within the city; Rankings are sorted by rate in descending order and exclude hospitals with less than 25 cases; (1) The number of cases is too small (n<25) for purposes of reliably predicting hospital performance; (2) Measure reflects the hospital's indication that its submission was based upon a sample of its relevant discharges; (3) Rate reflects fewer than the maximum possible quarters of data for the measure; (4) Inaccurate information submitted and suppressed for one or more quarters; (5) No data is available from the hospital for this measure; Please refer to the User's Guide for a full explanation of data

Sutter Coast Hospital	Crescent City	100%	124
Sutter Davis Hospital	Davis	100%	173
Sutter Delta Medical Center	Antioch	100%	195
Sutter General Hospital	Sacramento	100%	207
Sutter Medical Center of Santa Rosa	Santa Rosa	100%	156
Sutter Roseville Medical Center	Roseville	100%	200
Sutter Solano Medical Center	Vallejo	100%	167
Sutter Tracy Community Hospital	Tracy	100%	146
Temple Community Hospital	Los Angeles	100%	75
Torrance Memorial Medical Center	Torrance	100%	394
Tri-City Medical Center	Oceanside	100%	506
Tulare District Hospital	Tulare	100%	197
Tustin Hospital and Medical Center	Tustin	100%	41
UCLA Medical Center	Los Angeles	100%	201
UCSF Medical Center	San Francisco	100%	208
Ukiah Valley Medical Center	Ukiah	100%	150
University of California Davis Health System	Sacramento	100%	200
University of California Irvine Med Ctr	Orange	100%	179
University of California San Diego Med Ctr	San Diego	100%	248
VacaValley Hospital	Vacaville	100%	221
Valley Presbyterian Hospital	Van Nuys	100%	236
Valleycare Medical Center	Livermore	100%	220
Ventura County Medical Center	Ventura	100%	105
Washington Hospital	Fremont	100%	198
Watsonville Community Hospital	Watsonville	100%	163
Western Medical Center Hospital Anaheim	Anaheim	100%	99
White Memorial Medical Center	Los Angeles	100%	325
Whittier Hospital Medical Center	Whittier	100%	353
Woodland Healthcare	Woodland	100%	104
Arroyo Grande Community Hospital	Arroyo Grande	99%	160
Beverly Hospital	Montebello	99%	340
Citrus Valley Medical Center	Covina	99%	300
Citrus Valley Med Ctr Queen Valley Campus	West Covina	99%	378
Corona Regional Medical Center	Corona	99%	375
Delano Regional Medical Center	Delano	99%	157
East Valley Hospital Medical Center	Glendora	99%	165
Fallbrook Hospital	Fallbrook	99%	98
Good Samaritan Hospital	Los Angeles	99%	249
Hanford Community Medical Center	Hanford	99%	207
Kaiser Permanente Panorama City Med Ctr	Panorama City	99%	118
Kern Medical Center	Bakersfield	99%	103
Lancaster Community Hospital	Lancaster	99%	222
Los Angeles County & USC Medical Center	Los Angeles	99%	368
Martin Luther King Jr/Charles R Drew Med Ctr	Los Angeles	99%	202
Memorial Medical Center	Modesto	99%	197
Mercy Medical Center-Mount Shasta	Mount Shasta	99%	85
Methodist Hospital of Southern California	Arcadia	99%	593
Mission Community Hospital	Panorama City	99%	229
Moreno Valley Community Hospital	Moreno Valley	99%	196
Pacific Hospital of Long Beach	Long Beach	99%	158
Riverside County Regional Medical Center	Moreno Valley	99%	138
Saint John's Pleasant Valley Hospital	Camarillo	99%	160
Saint John's Regional Medical Center	Oxnard	99%	326
Saint Mary Medical Center	Apple Valley	99%	536
Salinas Valley Memorial Health Care District	Salinas	99%	296
San Antonio Community Hospital	Upland	99%	551
San Gorgonio Memorial Hospital	Banning	99%	275
Santa Clara Valley Medical Center	San Jose	99%	337
Sierra Nevada Memorial Hospital	Grass Valley	99%	333
Sutter Lakeside Hospital	Lakeport	99%	131
Tri-City Regional Medical Center	Hawaiian Gardens	99%	178
Tuolumne General Hospital	Sonora	99%	80
Twin Cities Community Hospital	Templeton	99%	176
Victor Valley Community Hospital	Victorville	99%	201
West Hills Hospital and Medical Center	West Hills	99%	446
Western Medical Center	Santa Ana	99%	168
Centinela Freeman Reg Med Ctr-Marina	Marina Del Rey	98%	98
Century City Doctors Hospital	Los Angeles	98%	53
Los Angeles Community Hospital	Los Angeles	98%	104
Pacific Alliance Medical Center	Los Angeles	98%	162
Rideout Memorial Hospital	Marysville	98%	400
Santa Rosa Memorial Hospital	Santa Rosa	98%	324
West Anaheim Medical Center	Anaheim	98%	259
City of Angels Medical Center	Los Angeles	97%	86
Community Hospital of Gardena	Gardena	97%	31
Good Samaritan Hospital	Bakersfield	97%	91
Tahoe Forest Hospital	Truckee	97%	29
USC University Hospital	Los Angeles	97%	30
Hazel Hawkins Memorial Hospital	Hollister	96%	77
Anaheim General Hospital	Anaheim	95%	66
La Palma Intercommunity Hospital	La Palma	95%	224
Los Angeles Metropolitan Med Ctr-LA Campus	Los Angeles	95%	62
Monterey Park Hospital	Monterey Park	94%	123
Verdugo Hills Hospital	Glendale	93%	205
Community Hospital	Huntington Park	89%	142
Hollywood Community Hospital	Hollywood	66%	50

18. Pneumococcal Vaccine

Hospital Name	City	Rate	Cases
Temple Community Hospital	Los Angeles	100%	48
Feather River Hospital	Paradise	99%	138
Los Alamitos Medical Center	Los Alamitos	99%	207
Queen of the Valley Hospital	Napa	98%	141
Twin Cities Community Hospital	Templeton	98%	130
California Hospital Medical Center	Los Angeles	96%	83
Kaiser Foundation Hospital-Riverside	Riverside	96%	79
San Rafael Medical Center	San Rafael	96%	189
Sutter Davis Hospital	Davis	96%	104
Saint Elizabeth Community Hospital	Red Bluff	95%	121
Saint Rose Hospital	Hayward	95%	130
San Ramon Regional Medical Center	San Ramon	95%	112
Garden Grove Hospital and Medical Center	Garden Grove	94%	144
Mercy Hospital of Folsom	Folsom	94%	108
Oakland Medical Center	Oakland	94%	367
Colusa Regional Medical Center	Colusa	93%	27
Doctors Hospital of Manteca	Manteca	93%	95
Sutter Auburn Faith Hospital	Auburn	93%	108
El Centro Regional Medical Center	El Centro	92%	108
Kaiser Permanente Anaheim Medical Center	Anaheim	92%	75
Kaiser Permanente South Bay Medical Center	Harbor City	92%	79
San Dimas Community Hospital	San Dimas	92%	158
San Mateo Medical Center	San Mateo	92%	26
Western Medical Center Hospital Anaheim	Anaheim	92%	59
Desert Valley Hospital	Victorville	91%	107
Kaiser Permanente Santa Clara Medical Center	Santa Clara	91%	128
Mercy Medical Center-Mount Shasta	Mount Shasta	91%	58
Saint Agnes Medical Center	Fresno	91%	253
Saint Joseph's Medical Center of Stockton	Stockton	91%	118
Sherman Oaks Hospital	Sherman Oaks	91%	32
Ukiah Valley Medical Center	Ukiah	91%	91
Woodland Healthcare	Woodland	91%	65
Bakersfield Memorial Hospital	Bakersfield	90%	172
Saint Joseph Hospital	Eureka	90%	81
S San Francisco Medical Center	S San Francisco	90%	134
Valleycare Medical Center	Livermore	90%	129
Chino Valley Medical Center	Chino	89%	47
Doctors Medical Center	Modesto	89%	292
French Hospital Medical Center	San Luis Obispo	89%	98
Kaiser Foundation Hospital-South Sacramento	Sacramento	89%	189
Mercy San Juan Hospital	Carmichael	89%	465
Saint Francis Memorial Hospital	San Francisco	89%	36
Cedars-Sinai Medical Center	Los Angeles	88%	455
Chinese Hospital	San Francisco	88%	178
Community Hospital of the Monterey Peninsula	Monterey	88%	147
Glendale Memorial Hospital and Health Center	Glendale	88%	252
Tulare District Hospital	Tulare	88%	113
Chapman Medical Center	Orange	87%	52
Kaiser Foundation Hospital	Baldwin Park	87%	75
Kaiser Permanente Fontana Medical Center	Fontana	87%	70
Desert Regional Medical Center	Palm Springs	86%	234
Fountain Valley Reg Hospital & Med Ctr	Fountain Valley	86%	229
Huntington Beach Hospital	Huntington Beach	86%	96
Kaiser Foundation Hospital-Walnut Creek	Walnut Creek	86%	124
Little Company of Mary Hospital	Torrance	86%	285
Orange Coast Memorial Medical Center	Santa Ana	86%	260
Saint Jude Medical Center	Fullerton	86%	244
Sequoia Hospital	Redwood City	86%	98
Community Hospital of San Bernardino	San Bernardino	85%	134
Lakewood Regional Medical Center	Lakewood	85%	168
Petaluma Valley Hospital	Petaluma	85%	87
Centinela Hospital Medical Center	Inglewood	84%	129
Saddleback Memorial Medical Center	Laguna Hills	84%	447
San Joaquin Community Hospital	Bakersfield	84%	121
Scripps Green Hospital	La Jolla	84%	126
Kaiser Permanente Bellflower Medical Center	Bellflower	83%	76
Mercy General Hospital	Sacramento	83%	286
Kaiser Foundation Hospital-Fresno	Fresno	82%	123
Kaiser Foundation Hospital-Vallejo	Vallejo	82%	106
Kaiser Permanente Sacramento Medical Center	Sacramento	82%	433
Northridge Hospital Medical Center	Northridge	82%	262
Sutter Roseville Medical Center	Roseville	82%	142
Bakersfield Heart Hospital	Bakersfield	81%	112
Community Hospital of Los Gatos	Los Gatos	81%	94
Kaiser Foundation Hospital	Hayward	81%	139
Kaiser Foundation Hospital-San Diego	San Diego	81%	86
Kaiser Foundation Hospital-Santa Rosa	Santa Rosa	81%	140
Kaiser Permanente San Francisco Med Ctr	San Francisco	81%	186
Kaiser Redwood City Medical Center	Redwood City	81%	119
Providence Holy Cross Medical Center	Mission Hills	81%	165

NOTE: Hospital profiles are in alphabetical order by state, then city, then hospital within the city; Rankings are sorted by rate in descending order and exclude hospitals with less than 25 cases; (1) The number of cases is too small (n<25) for purposes of reliably predicting hospital performance; (2) Measure reflects the hospital's indication that its submission was based upon a sample of its relevant discharges; (3) Rate reflects fewer than the maximum possible quarters of data for the measure; (4) Inaccurate information submitted and suppressed for one or more quarters; (5) No data is available from the hospital for this measure; Please refer to the User's Guide for a full explanation of data

Saint Bernardine Medical Center	San Bernardino	81%	77
UCSF Medical Center	San Francisco	81%	106
John Muir Medical Center	Walnut Creek	80%	152
Pacific Hospital of Long Beach	Long Beach	80%	89
Placentia-Linda Hospital	Placentia	80%	164
Shasta Regional Medical Center	Redding	80%	241
Sierra Nevada Memorial Hospital	Grass Valley	80%	254
Sonora Regional Medical Center	Sonora	80%	140
Stanford Hospital	Stanford	80%	223
Sutter Coast Hospital	Crescent City	80%	69
Anaheim Memorial Medical Center	Anaheim	79%	377
Saint Joseph Hospital	Orange	79%	178
Emanuel Medical Center	Turlock	78%	170
Kaiser Permanente Santa Teresa Comm Med Ctr	San Jose	78%	111
Mercy Medical Center-Redding	Redding	78%	260
Riverside Community Hospital	Riverside	78%	321
Salinas Valley Memorial Health Care District	Salinas	78%	206
Sutter General Hospital	Sacramento	78%	130
Whittier Hospital Medical Center	Whittier	78%	229
John Muir Medical Center-Concord Campus	Concord	77%	123
San Leandro Hospital	San Leandro	77%	132
Garfield Medical Center	Monterey Park	76%	124
Irvine Regional Hospital	Irvine	76%	184
Mercy Hospital	Bakersfield	76%	289
Hoag Memorial Hospital Presbyterian	Newport Beach	75%	349
Marian Medical Center	Santa Maria	75%	225
Mercy Med Ctr Merced-Community Campus	Merced	74%	100
California Pacific Medical Center	San Francisco	72%	119
Downey Regional Medical Center	Downey	72%	170
Mark Twain Saint Joseph's Hospital	San Andreas	72%	79
Mills-Peninsula Health Services	Burlingame	72%	155
Mission Hospital Regional Medical Center	Mission Viejo	72%	180
Saint Mary Medical Center	Apple Valley	72%	286
Arroyo Grande Community Hospital	Arroyo Grande	71%	112
Beverly Hospital	Montebello	71%	224
Lodi Memorial Hospital	Lodi	71%	109
Saint Vincent Medical Center	Los Angeles	71%	256
Dominican Hospital	Santa Cruz	70%	194
Kaiser Foundation Hospital	Woodland Hills	70%	96
Kaiser Permanente West Los Angeles Med Ctr	Los Angeles	70%	79
Sierra Vista Regional Medical Center	San Luis Obispo	70%	79
South Coast Medical Center	Laguna Beach	70%	64
Tri-City Medical Center	Oceanside	70%	331
Providence Saint Joseph Medical Center	Burbank	69%	154
University of California Davis Health System	Sacramento	69%	90
Ventura County Medical Center	Ventura	69%	39
Community Medical Center-Clovis	Clovis	68%	103
Frank R Howard Memorial Hospital	Willits	68%	34
Kern Valley Healthcare District	Lake Isabella	68%	25
Palomar Medical Center	Escondido	68%	290
San Francisco General Hospital Medical Center	San Francisco	68%	62
San Gabriel Valley Medical Center	San Gabriel	68%	327
Santa Ynez Valley Cottage Hospital	Solvang	68%	25
Sutter Solano Medical Center	Vallejo	68%	73
Antelope Valley Hospital	Lancaster	67%	263
Barstow Community Hospital	Barstow	67%	118
Centinela Freeman Reg Med Ctr-Marina	Marina Del Rey	67%	60
Davies Medical Center	San Francisco	67%	51
Memorial Medical Center	Modesto	67%	120
Redlands Community Hospital	Redlands	67%	177
Community Regional Medical Center	Fresno	66%	326
Corona Regional Medical Center	Corona	66%	214
San Joaquin General Hospital	French Camp	66%	82
Sierra View District Hospital	Porterville	66%	169
Washington Hospital	Fremont	66%	131
Good Samaritan Hospital	Los Angeles	65%	151
John F Kennedy Memorial Hospital	Indio	65%	178
Kaweah Delta Health Care District	Visalia	65%	370
Little Company of Mary-San Pedro Hospital	San Pedro	65%	142
Santa Rosa Memorial Hospital	Santa Rosa	65%	195
Simi Valley Hospital	Simi Valley	65%	106
Eisenhower Medical Center	Rancho Mirage	64%	342
Hi-Desert Medical Center	Joshua Tree	64%	182
O'Connor Hospital	San Jose	64%	236
Pomerado Hospital	Poway	64%	148
Saint Francis Medical Center	Lynwood	64%	158
Alta Bates Summit Medical Center	Berkeley	63%	51
El Camino Hospital	Mountain View	61%	321
La Palma Intercommunity Hospital	La Palma	61%	142
Los Angeles County Harbor-UCLA Medical Center	Torrance	61%	72
Memorial Hospital Los Banos	Los Banos	61%	71
Saint Mary's Medical Center	San Francisco	61%	162
Sutter Tracy Community Hospital	Tracy	61%	75
VacaValley Hospital	Vacaville	61%	141
Alta Bates Summit Medical Center	Oakland	60%	96
Barton Memorial Hospital	South Lake Tahoe	60%	47
Kaiser Permanente Panorama City Med Ctr	Panorama City	60%	91
Long Beach Memorial Medical Center	Long Beach	60%	373
Methodist Hospital of Sacramento	Sacramento	60%	182
Kaiser Foundation Hospital-Manteca	Manteca	59%	106
Kaiser Permanente Los Angeles Medical Center	Los Angeles	59%	81
Novato Community Hospital	Novato	59%	73
Ridgecrest Regional Hospital	Ridgecrest	59%	80
Santa Barbara Cottage Hospital	Santa Barbara	59%	234
Western Medical Center	Santa Ana	59%	111
Goleta Valley Cottage Hospital	Santa Barbara	58%	36
Pomona Valley Hospital Medical Center	Pomona	58%	226
Pioneers Memorial Healthcare District	Brawley	57%	100
Rancho Springs Medical Center	Murrieta	57%	247
Doctor's Medical Center-San Pablo Campus	San Pablo	56%	213
Los Angeles County & USC Medical Center	Los Angeles	56%	87
Oak Valley Hospital	Oakdale	56%	70
Palo Verde Hospital	Blythe	56%	39
Saint John's Pleasant Valley Hospital	Camarillo	56%	122
University of California San Diego Med Ctr	San Diego	56%	85
Encino-Tarzana Regional Medical Center	Tarzana	55%	246
Hanford Community Medical Center	Hanford	54%	129
Saint John's Regional Medical Center	Oxnard	54%	227
Scripps Memorial Hospital La Jolla	La Jolla	54%	122
Foothill Presbyterian Hospital	Glendora	53%	165
Hazel Hawkins Memorial Hospital	Hollister	53%	59
Saint Louisie Regional Hospital	Gilroy	53%	76
Sierra Kings District Hospital	Reedley	53%	85
Eden Medical Center	Castro Valley	52%	170
Glendale Adventist Medical Center	Glendale	52%	231
Palm Drive Hospital	Sebastopol	52%	29
Scripps Memorial Hospital-Encinitas	Encinitas	52%	130
Sharp Coronado Hospital	San Diego	52%	82
Encino-Tarzana Regional Medical Center	Encino	51%	173
Presbyterian Intercommunity Hospital	Whittier	51%	100
Enloe Medical Center	Chico	50%	345
Paradise Valley Hospital	National City	50%	175
Saint Helena Hospital	Deer Park	50%	46
West Hills Hospital and Medical Center	West Hills	49%	292
Contra Costa Regional Medical Center	Martinez	48%	46
White Memorial Medical Center	Los Angeles	48%	220
Grossmont Hospital	La Mesa	47%	422
Mad River Community Hospital	Arcata	47%	47
Central Valley General Hospital	Hanford	46%	39
Good Samaritan Hospital	San Jose	46%	237
Lancaster Community Hospital	Lancaster	46%	121
NorthBay Medical Center	Fairfield	46%	140
Fallbrook Hospital	Fallbrook	45%	74
Pacific Alliance Medical Center	Los Angeles	45%	114
Madera Community Hospital	Madera	44%	90
Coastal Communities Hospital	Santa Ana	43%	69
Menifee Valley Medical Center	Sun City	42%	211
Seton Medical Center	Daly City	41%	193
Sharp Memorial Hospital	San Diego	41%	237
University of California Irvine Med Ctr	Orange	41%	66
Hollywood Presbyterian Medical Center	Los Angeles	40%	315
Los Robles Regional Medical Center	Thousand Oaks	40%	233
Marin General Hospital	Greenbrae	40%	149
Hemet Valley Medical Center	Hemet	39%	315
Natividad Medical Center	Salinas	39%	36
Sutter Lakeside Hospital	Lakeport	39%	89
Tri-City Regional Medical Center	Hawaiian Gardens	39%	116
Marshall Medical Center	Placerville	38%	125
Sutter Delta Medical Center	Antioch	38%	94
Coast Plaza Doctors Hospital	Norwalk	37%	90
Rideout Memorial Hospital	Marysville	37%	279
San Antonio Community Hospital	Upland	37%	331
Torrance Memorial Medical Center	Torrance	37%	282
Loma Linda University Medical Center	Loma Linda	36%	159
Ojai Valley Community Hospital	Ojai	36%	45
Olympia Medical Center	Los Angeles	36%	295
Saint Mary Medical Center	Long Beach	36%	95
Arrowhead Regional Medical Center	Colton	35%	68
Dameron Hospital	Stockton	33%	138
Olive View-UCLA Medical Center	San Fernando	33%	70
Watsonville Community Hospital	Watsonville	32%	100
Methodist Hospital of Southern California	Arcadia	31%	412
Monterey Park Hospital	Monterey Park	31%	81
Moreno Valley Community Hospital	Moreno Valley	31%	106
Sutter Amador Hospital	Jackson	31%	70
Parkview Community Hospital	Riverside	30%	217
Community Hospital of Long Beach	Long Beach	29%	130
Community Memorial Hospital Ventura	Ventura	29%	266
Saint John's Health Center	Santa Monica	29%	215
Pacifica Hospital of the Valley	Sun Valley	28%	47

NOTE: Hospital profiles are in alphabetical order by state, then city, then hospital within the city; Rankings are sorted by rate in descending order and exclude hospitals with less than 25 cases; (1) The number of cases is too small (n<25) for purposes of reliably predicting hospital performance; (2) Measure reflects the hospital's indication that its submission was based upon a sample of its relevant discharges; (3) Rate reflects fewer than the maximum possible quarters of data for the measure; (4) Inaccurate information submitted and suppressed for one or more quarters; (5) No data is available from the hospital for this measure; Please refer to the User's Guide for a full explanation of data

Regional Medical Center of San Jose	San Jose	28%	349
Kern Medical Center	Bakersfield	27%	30
Brotman Medical Center	Culver City	26%	99
East Valley Hospital Medical Center	Glendora	26%	103
Sonoma Valley Hospital	Sonoma	24%	49
UCLA Medical Center	Los Angeles	24%	105
Alameda Hospital	Alameda	23%	114
Saint Luke's Hospital	San Francisco	23%	102
Sutter Medical Center of Santa Rosa	Santa Rosa	23%	75
Scripps Mercy Hospital	San Diego	22%	402
Sharp Chula Vista Medical Center	Chula Vista	22%	278
Victor Valley Community Hospital	Victorville	21%	107
Century City Doctors Hospital	Los Angeles	20%	44
Citrus Valley Medical Center	Covina	20%	198
Santa Clara Valley Medical Center	San Jose	18%	138
Redbud Community Hospital	Clearlake	17%	53
Riverside County Regional Medical Center	Moreno Valley	17%	36
Alameda County Medical Center	Oakland	16%	58
Valley Presbyterian Hospital	Van Nuys	15%	141
Henry Mayo Newhall Memorial Hospital	Valencia	14%	182
Alhambra Hospital Medical Center	Alhambra	13%	287
Lompoc Healthcare District Hospital	Lompoc	13%	52
Santa Monica-UCLA Medical Center	Santa Monica	13%	134
West Anaheim Medical Center	Anaheim	13%	157
Oroville Hospital	Oroville	12%	73
Citrus Valley Med Ctr Queen Valley Campus	West Covina	11%	207
Delano Regional Medical Center	Delano	11%	104
Bellflower Medical Center	Bellflower	10%	119
Community Hospital	Huntington Park	10%	78
Greater El Monte Community Hospital	South El Monte	9%	150
Huntington Memorial Hospital	Pasadena	9%	443
Los Angeles Metropolitan Med Ctr-LA Campus	Los Angeles	9%	33
Martin Luther King Jr/Charles R Drew Med Ctr	Los Angeles	9%	44
Tuolumne General Hospital	Sonora	9%	47
Verdugo Hills Hospital	Glendale	9%	148
Healdsburg District Hospital	Healdsburg	7%	29
Mission Community Hospital	Panorama City	7%	125
Coalinga Regional Medical Center	Coalinga	6%	32
City of Angels Medical Center	Los Angeles	5%	56
Hollywood Community Hospital	Hollywood	3%	37
San Gorgonio Memorial Hospital	Banning	2%	192
East Los Angeles Doctors Hospital	Los Angeles	1%	73
Memorial Hospital of Gardena	Gardena	1%	170
Anaheim General Hospital	Anaheim	0%	44
Community Hospital of Gardena	Gardena	0%	30
Los Angeles Community Hospital	Los Angeles	0%	53

19. Smoking Cessation Advice

Hospital Name	City	Rate	Cases
Alta Bates Summit Medical Center	Oakland	100%	35
Beverly Hospital	Montebello	100%	26
California Hospital Medical Center	Los Angeles	100%	42
Cedars-Sinai Medical Center	Los Angeles	100%	86
Desert Valley Hospital	Victorville	100%	41
John F Kennedy Memorial Hospital	Indio	100%	37
John Muir Medical Center-Concord Campus	Concord	100%	36
Los Alamitos Medical Center	Los Alamitos	100%	36
Marian Medical Center	Santa Maria	100%	44
Mark Twain Saint Joseph's Hospital	San Andreas	100%	25
Mercy Hospital of Folsom	Folsom	100%	30
Mercy Medical Center-Redding	Redding	100%	111
Queen of the Valley Hospital	Napa	100%	64
Saint Agnes Medical Center	Fresno	100%	55
Saint Elizabeth Community Hospital	Red Bluff	100%	48
Saint Mary's Medical Center	San Francisco	100%	31
San Dimas Community Hospital	San Dimas	100%	26
Sutter Auburn Faith Hospital	Auburn	100%	35
Sutter Coast Hospital	Crescent City	100%	47
University of California Irvine Med Ctr	Orange	100%	36
West Anaheim Medical Center	Anaheim	100%	33
Mercy San Juan Hospital	Carmichael	99%	138
Anaheim Memorial Medical Center	Anaheim	98%	83
Glendale Memorial Hospital and Health Center	Glendale	98%	50
Kaiser Foundation Hospital-South Sacramento	Sacramento	98%	50
Little Company of Mary Hospital	Torrance	98%	51
Mercy General Hospital	Sacramento	98%	64
Sutter General Hospital	Sacramento	98%	50
Sutter Roseville Medical Center	Roseville	98%	43
Centinela Hospital Medical Center	Inglewood	97%	32
Little Company of Mary-San Pedro Hospital	San Pedro	97%	33
Methodist Hospital of Sacramento	Sacramento	97%	38
Northridge Hospital Medical Center	Northridge	97%	62
Palomar Medical Center	Escondido	97%	60
Saddleback Memorial Medical Center	Laguna Hills	97%	58
Saint Joseph's Medical Center of Stockton	Stockton	97%	35
San Joaquin Community Hospital	Bakersfield	97%	78
Simi Valley Hospital	Simi Valley	97%	35
University of California San Diego Med Ctr	San Diego	97%	72
Alameda Hospital	Alameda	96%	27
Saint Mary Medical Center	Long Beach	96%	56
San Antonio Community Hospital	Upland	96%	89
Tri-City Regional Medical Center	Hawaiian Gardens	96%	25
Ventura County Medical Center	Ventura	96%	28
Whittier Hospital Medical Center	Whittier	96%	26
Bakersfield Heart Hospital	Bakersfield	95%	43
Community Hospital of San Bernardino	San Bernardino	95%	65
Doctors Hospital of Manteca	Manteca	95%	38
Long Beach Memorial Medical Center	Long Beach	95%	105
Rancho Springs Medical Center	Murrieta	95%	65
Saint Joseph Hospital	Orange	95%	42
San Gabriel Valley Medical Center	San Gabriel	95%	39
Shasta Regional Medical Center	Redding	95%	153
Tri-City Medical Center	Oceanside	95%	85
Marshall Medical Center	Placerville	94%	33
Mercy Med Ctr Merced-Community Campus	Merced	94%	35
Parkview Community Hospital	Riverside	94%	52
Saint Joseph Hospital	Eureka	94%	49
San Leandro Hospital	San Leandro	94%	36
Tulare District Hospital	Tulare	94%	35
Twin Cities Community Hospital	Templeton	94%	35
El Camino Hospital	Mountain View	93%	45
Feather River Hospital	Paradise	93%	46
Mills-Peninsula Health Services	Burlingame	93%	27
Sierra View District Hospital	Porterville	93%	57
Sutter Delta Medical Center	Antioch	93%	41
White Memorial Medical Center	Los Angeles	93%	57
Doctors Medical Center	Modesto	92%	157
Eisenhower Medical Center	Rancho Mirage	92%	61
Enloe Medical Center	Chico	92%	90
University of California Davis Health System	Sacramento	92%	73
VacaValley Hospital	Vacaville	92%	50
West Hills Hospital and Medical Center	West Hills	92%	36
Providence Saint Joseph Medical Center	Burbank	91%	35
Saint Francis Medical Center	Lynwood	91%	58
Glendale Adventist Medical Center	Glendale	90%	51
Lakewood Regional Medical Center	Lakewood	90%	49
Madera Community Hospital	Madera	90%	52
Desert Regional Medical Center	Palm Springs	89%	89
Menifee Valley Medical Center	Sun City	89%	45
San Rafael Medical Center	San Rafael	89%	38
Sharp Memorial Hospital	San Diego	89%	55
Sutter Solano Medical Center	Vallejo	89%	53
Pomona Valley Hospital Medical Center	Pomona	88%	69
Sutter Davis Hospital	Davis	88%	32
Washington Hospital	Fremont	88%	26
Barstow Community Hospital	Barstow	87%	53
Oakland Medical Center	Oakland	87%	75
Paradise Valley Hospital	National City	87%	53
Grossmont Hospital	La Mesa	85%	104
Hoag Memorial Hospital Presbyterian	Newport Beach	85%	59
Kaiser Foundation Hospital-Vallejo	Vallejo	85%	27
Memorial Hospital Los Banos	Los Banos	85%	26
Providence Holy Cross Medical Center	Mission Hills	85%	46
Sierra Nevada Memorial Hospital	Grass Valley	85%	74
Sonora Regional Medical Center	Sonora	85%	39
Memorial Medical Center	Modesto	84%	51
NorthBay Medical Center	Fairfield	84%	44
Riverside Community Hospital	Riverside	84%	116
Santa Rosa Memorial Hospital	Santa Rosa	84%	64
Sutter Tracy Community Hospital	Tracy	84%	25
Hanford Community Medical Center	Hanford	83%	46
Saint Bernardine Medical Center	San Bernardino	83%	29
Saint Louisie Regional Hospital	Gilroy	83%	29
Stanford Hospital	Stanford	83%	29
Antelope Valley Hospital	Lancaster	82%	149
Lodi Memorial Hospital	Lodi	82%	33
Mercy Hospital	Bakersfield	82%	121
Saint Jude Medical Center	Fullerton	82%	39
Saint Mary Medical Center	Apple Valley	82%	95
UCSF Medical Center	San Francisco	82%	39
Dameron Hospital	Stockton	81%	31
Hi-Desert Medical Center	Joshua Tree	81%	77
Orange Coast Memorial Medical Center	Santa Ana	81%	36
San Francisco General Hospital Medical Center	San Francisco	81%	128
Eden Medical Center	Castro Valley	80%	41
Pacific Hospital of Long Beach	Long Beach	80%	25
Community Medical Center-Clovis	Clovis	79%	38
Davies Medical Center	San Francisco	79%	29
Fountain Valley Reg Hospital & Med Ctr	Fountain Valley	79%	39

NOTE: Hospital profiles are in alphabetical order by state, then city, then hospital within the city; Rankings are sorted by rate in descending order and exclude hospitals with less than 25 cases; (1) The number of cases is too small (n<25) for purposes of reliably predicting hospital performance; (2) Measure reflects the hospital's indication that its submission was based upon a sample of its relevant discharges; (3) Rate reflects fewer than the maximum possible quarters of data for the measure; (4) Inaccurate information submitted and suppressed for one or more quarters; (5) No data is available from the hospital for this measure; Please refer to the User's Guide for a full explanation of data

Good Samaritan Hospital	San Jose	79%	42
Huntington Memorial Hospital	Pasadena	79%	84
Bakersfield Memorial Hospital	Bakersfield	78%	55
Good Samaritan Hospital	Los Angeles	78%	27
Scripps Memorial Hospital La Jolla	La Jolla	78%	27
Sutter Lakeside Hospital	Lakeport	78%	27
Doctor's Medical Center-San Pablo Campus	San Pablo	77%	73
Kaiser Permanente San Francisco Med Ctr	San Francisco	77%	31
Placentia-Linda Hospital	Placentia	77%	30
Pomerado Hospital	Poway	77%	26
Scripps Mercy Hospital	San Diego	77%	146
UCLA Medical Center	Los Angeles	77%	26
Saint Luke's Hospital	San Francisco	76%	46
Kaiser Permanente Sacramento Medical Center	Sacramento	75%	95
Community Hospital of Long Beach	Long Beach	74%	27
Dominican Hospital	Santa Cruz	74%	39
Kaiser Redwood City Medical Center	Redwood City	73%	26
Los Angeles County Harbor-UCLA Medical Center	Torrance	73%	45
Sutter Medical Center of Santa Rosa	Santa Rosa	73%	56
Kaiser Foundation Hospital-Manteca	Manteca	72%	46
La Palma Intercommunity Hospital	La Palma	72%	39
Corona Regional Medical Center	Corona	71%	49
Methodist Hospital of Southern California	Arcadia	70%	57
Sharp Chula Vista Medical Center	Chula Vista	70%	54
Community Memorial Hospital Ventura	Ventura	69%	58
Hollywood Presbyterian Medical Center	Los Angeles	69%	35
Emanuel Medical Center	Turlock	68%	44
Los Robles Regional Medical Center	Thousand Oaks	68%	44
Mission Hospital Regional Medical Center	Mission Viejo	68%	40
Scripps Memorial Hospital-Encinitas	Encinitas	68%	28
Citrus Valley Med Ctr Queen Valley Campus	West Covina	67%	51
Loma Linda University Medical Center	Loma Linda	67%	39
Torrance Memorial Medical Center	Torrance	67%	48
Kaweah Delta Health Care District	Visalia	66%	134
Huntington Beach Hospital	Huntington Beach	64%	25
Kaiser Foundation Hospital-Riverside	Riverside	64%	25
Hemet Valley Medical Center	Hemet	63%	75
Lancaster Community Hospital	Lancaster	63%	60
Ridgecrest Regional Hospital	Ridgecrest	63%	46
Citrus Valley Medical Center	Covina	62%	40
Kaiser Foundation Hospital	Baldwin Park	62%	26
Ukiah Valley Medical Center	Ukiah	62%	37
Moreno Valley Community Hospital	Moreno Valley	61%	33
Verdugo Hills Hospital	Glendale	60%	30
Saint John's Regional Medical Center	Oxnard	58%	43
San Joaquin General Hospital	French Camp	58%	101
Alameda County Medical Center	Oakland	57%	86
Rideout Memorial Hospital	Marysville	56%	126
Regional Medical Center of San Jose	San Jose	55%	53
Redbud Community Hospital	Clearlake	54%	35
Santa Barbara Cottage Hospital	Santa Barbara	54%	57
O'Connor Hospital	San Jose	52%	31
Community Regional Medical Center	Fresno	50%	193
Oak Valley Hospital	Oakdale	50%	30
Memorial Hospital of Gardena	Gardena	48%	29
Arrowhead Regional Medical Center	Colton	47%	76
Santa Clara Valley Medical Center	San Jose	47%	122
Los Angeles Community Hospital	Los Angeles	44%	78
Foothill Presbyterian Hospital	Glendora	42%	36
Oroville Hospital	Oroville	41%	51
Saint Vincent Medical Center	Los Angeles	39%	31
Natividad Medical Center	Salinas	38%	32
Hollywood Community Hospital	Hollywood	32%	34
Los Angeles County & USC Medical Center	Los Angeles	32%	137
Valleycare Medical Center	Livermore	30%	30
Henry Mayo Newhall Memorial Hospital	Valencia	25%	32
Martin Luther King Jr/Charles R Drew Med Ctr	Los Angeles	11%	61
Los Angeles Metropolitan Med Ctr-LA Campus	Los Angeles	0%	25

Surgical Infection Prevention

20. Prophylactic Antibiotic Given

Hospital Name	City	Rate	Cases
Frank R Howard Memorial Hospital	Willits	100%	25
Sierra Nevada Memorial Hospital	Grass Valley	99%	174
Saint Francis Memorial Hospital	San Francisco	97%	118
S San Francisco Medical Center	S San Francisco	97%	282
Cedars-Sinai Medical Center	Los Angeles	96%	2543
Marian Medical Center	Santa Maria	96%	493
Bakersfield Heart Hospital	Bakersfield	95%	185
Saint Helena Hospital	Deer Park	95%	261
Saint Joseph's Medical Center of Stockton	Stockton	95%	189
Oakland Medical Center	Oakland	94%	989
Providence Holy Cross Medical Center	Mission Hills	94%	297
Sharp Coronado Hospital	San Diego	94%	96
University of California Davis Health System	Sacramento	94%	536
Garden Grove Hospital and Medical Center	Garden Grove	93%	163
Saint Jude Medical Center	Fullerton	93%	1253
Santa Monica-UCLA Medical Center	Santa Monica	93%	285
Scripps Green Hospital	La Jolla	93%	259
Scripps Memorial Hospital La Jolla	La Jolla	93%	241
UCLA Medical Center	Los Angeles	93%	387
Alta Bates Summit Medical Center	Berkeley	92%	109
Arrowhead Regional Medical Center	Colton	92%	243
California Pacific Medical Center	San Francisco	92%	244
Kaiser Foundation Hospital-Vallejo	Vallejo	92%	192
Kaiser Permanente San Francisco Med Ctr	San Francisco	92%	631
Providence Saint Joseph Medical Center	Burbank	92%	304
Saint Agnes Medical Center	Fresno	92%	477
Shasta Regional Medical Center	Redding	92%	736
Sutter Roseville Medical Center	Roseville	92%	228
Healdsburg District Hospital	Healdsburg	91%	53
Kaiser Permanente West Los Angeles Med Ctr	Los Angeles	91%	44
Loma Linda University Medical Center	Loma Linda	91%	1147
Pacific Hospital of Long Beach	Long Beach	91%	139
Presbyterian Intercommunity Hospital	Whittier	91%	237
Torrance Memorial Medical Center	Torrance	91%	225
Arroyo Grande Community Hospital	Arroyo Grande	90%	116
Barton Memorial Hospital	South Lake Tahoe	90%	124
Downey Regional Medical Center	Downey	90%	216
El Centro Regional Medical Center	El Centro	90%	244
Hoag Memorial Hospital Presbyterian	Newport Beach	90%	349
Kaiser Foundation Hospital-South Sacramento	Sacramento	90%	735
Kaiser Foundation Hospital-Walnut Creek	Walnut Creek	90%	322
Little Company of Mary Hospital	Torrance	90%	644
Marshall Medical Center	Placerville	90%	197
Patients' Hospital of Redding	Redding	90%	79
Placentia-Linda Hospital	Placentia	90%	145
Rancho Springs Medical Center	Murrieta	90%	798
Saddleback Memorial Medical Center	Laguna Hills	90%	416
San Dimas Community Hospital	San Dimas	90%	318
Century City Doctors Hospital	Los Angeles	89%	206
Mercy Medical Center-Mount Shasta	Mount Shasta	89%	97
Mercy Medical Center-Redding	Redding	89%	274
O'Connor Hospital	San Jose	89%	186
Centinela Freeman Reg Med Ctr-Marina	Marina Del Rey	88%	72
Kaiser Permanente Bellflower Medical Center	Bellflower	88%	42
Los Angeles County Harbor-UCLA Medical Center	Torrance	88%	232
San Ramon Regional Medical Center	San Ramon	88%	325
Sequoia Hospital	Redwood City	88%	248
White Memorial Medical Center	Los Angeles	88%	50
Whittier Hospital Medical Center	Whittier	88%	272
Community Hospital of the Monterey Peninsula	Monterey	87%	191
Eden Medical Center	Castro Valley	87%	418
Enloe Medical Center	Chico	87%	810
Kaiser Foundation Hospital-Fresno	Fresno	87%	161
Orange Coast Memorial Medical Center	Santa Ana	87%	445
Saint Francis Medical Center	Lynwood	87%	122
San Francisco General Hospital Medical Center	San Francisco	87%	121
Sharp Memorial Hospital	San Diego	87%	461
Valleycare Medical Center	Livermore	87%	292
Desert Regional Medical Center	Palm Springs	86%	366
Eisenhower Medical Center	Rancho Mirage	86%	666
French Hospital Medical Center	San Luis Obispo	86%	224
Kaiser Foundation Hospital-Santa Rosa	Santa Rosa	86%	313
Saint Louisie Regional Hospital	Gilroy	86%	97
San Leandro Hospital	San Leandro	86%	196
Scripps Memorial Hospital-Encinitas	Encinitas	86%	94
Sonoma Valley Hospital	Sonoma	86%	91
Tri-City Medical Center	Oceanside	86%	146
California Hospital Medical Center	Los Angeles	85%	152
Huntington Memorial Hospital	Pasadena	85%	319
La Palma Intercommunity Hospital	La Palma	85%	88
Mission Hospital Regional Medical Center	Mission Viejo	85%	186
San Mateo Medical Center	San Mateo	85%	92
San Rafael Medical Center	San Rafael	85%	522
Santa Clara Valley Medical Center	San Jose	85%	422
Sonora Regional Medical Center	Sonora	85%	271
Anaheim Memorial Medical Center	Anaheim	84%	418
Goleta Valley Cottage Hospital	Santa Barbara	84%	108
Good Samaritan Hospital	San Jose	84%	274
Kaiser Foundation Hospital	Woodland Hills	84%	49
Mark Twain Saint Joseph's Hospital	San Andreas	84%	32
Novato Community Hospital	Novato	84%	203
Pomona Valley Hospital Medical Center	Pomona	84%	712
Redlands Community Hospital	Redlands	84%	144
Sutter Davis Hospital	Davis	84%	218
Doctors Hospital of Manteca	Manteca	83%	115
Emanuel Medical Center	Turlock	83%	290

NOTE: Hospital profiles are in alphabetical order by state, then city, then hospital within the city; Rankings are sorted by rate in descending order and exclude hospitals with less than 25 cases; (1) The number of cases is too small (n<25) for purposes of reliably predicting hospital performance; (2) Measure reflects the hospital's indication that its submission was based upon a sample of its relevant discharges; (3) Rate reflects fewer than the maximum possible quarters of data for the measure; (4) Inaccurate information submitted and suppressed for one or more quarters; (5) No data is available from the hospital for this measure; Please refer to the User's Guide for a full explanation of data

Hospital	City	Rate	Cases
Glendale Adventist Medical Center	Glendale	83%	481
Good Samaritan Hospital	Los Angeles	83%	544
Grossmont Hospital	La Mesa	83%	328
John F Kennedy Memorial Hospital	Indio	83%	288
NorthBay Medical Center	Fairfield	83%	179
Saint Mary's Medical Center	San Francisco	83%	173
Sharp Mary Birch Hospital for Women	San Diego	83%	35
Sutter Auburn Faith Hospital	Auburn	83%	202
Sutter General Hospital	Sacramento	83%	370
Twin Cities Community Hospital	Templeton	83%	375
UCSF Medical Center	San Francisco	83%	533
Henry Mayo Newhall Memorial Hospital	Valencia	82%	147
Hollywood Presbyterian Medical Center	Los Angeles	82%	111
Kaiser Foundation Hospital-Riverside	Riverside	82%	50
Kaiser Redwood City Medical Center	Redwood City	82%	367
Kaweah Delta Health Care District	Visalia	82%	68
Los Alamitos Medical Center	Los Alamitos	82%	162
Mercy General Hospital	Sacramento	82%	299
Palomar Medical Center	Escondido	82%	221
Saint Joseph Hospital	Orange	82%	236
Saint Mary Medical Center	Apple Valley	82%	442
Salinas Valley Memorial Health Care District	Salinas	82%	221
San Antonio Community Hospital	Upland	82%	694
Sutter Tracy Community Hospital	Tracy	82%	130
Woodland Healthcare	Woodland	82%	117
Alta Bates Summit Medical Center	Oakland	81%	169
El Camino Hospital	Mountain View	81%	794
John Muir Medical Center	Walnut Creek	81%	181
University of California San Diego Med Ctr	San Diego	81%	336
Washington Hospital	Fremont	81%	70
Lakewood Regional Medical Center	Lakewood	80%	362
Mills-Peninsula Health Services	Burlingame	80%	296
Simi Valley Hospital	Simi Valley	80%	193
VacaValley Hospital	Vacaville	80%	86
West Hills Hospital and Medical Center	West Hills	80%	211
Bakersfield Memorial Hospital	Bakersfield	79%	261
Coastal Communities Hospital	Santa Ana	79%	101
Community Hospital of Los Gatos	Los Gatos	79%	209
Glendale Memorial Hospital and Health Center	Glendale	79%	238
Kaiser Permanente Santa Clara Medical Center	Santa Clara	79%	197
Scripps Mercy Hospital	San Diego	79%	155
South Coast Medical Center	Laguna Beach	79%	71
Stanford Hospital	Stanford	79%	110
West Anaheim Medical Center	Anaheim	79%	84
Centinela Hospital Medical Center	Inglewood	78%	584
Contra Costa Regional Medical Center	Martinez	78%	27
Kaiser Foundation Hospital	Baldwin Park	78%	50
Mercy Hospital of Folsom	Folsom	78%	143
Pioneers Memorial Healthcare District	Brawley	78%	109
Verdugo Hills Hospital	Glendale	78%	117
Fresno Heart Hospital	Fresno	77%	303
John Muir Medical Center-Concord Campus	Concord	77%	231
Queen of the Valley Hospital	Napa	77%	176
Rideout Memorial Hospital	Marysville	77%	269
Saint Rose Hospital	Hayward	77%	39
Seton Medical Center	Daly City	77%	53
Sharp Chula Vista Medical Center	Chula Vista	77%	222
Stanislaus Surgical Hospital	Modesto	77%	35
Tulare District Hospital	Tulare	77%	35
Kaiser Permanente Sacramento Medical Center	Sacramento	76%	622
Kaiser Permanente South Bay Medical Center	Harbor City	76%	51
Lancaster Community Hospital	Lancaster	76%	371
Little Company of Mary-San Pedro Hospital	San Pedro	76%	160
Marin General Hospital	Greenbrae	76%	300
Pomerado Hospital	Poway	76%	146
Regional Medical Center of San Jose	San Jose	76%	127
Saint John's Regional Medical Center	Oxnard	76%	207
Community Hospital of Long Beach	Long Beach	75%	32
Doctors Medical Center	Modesto	75%	607
Encino-Tarzana Regional Medical Center	Encino	75%	121
Fountain Valley Reg Hospital & Med Ctr	Fountain Valley	75%	328
Kern Medical Center	Bakersfield	75%	36
Lompoc Healthcare District Hospital	Lompoc	75%	142
Petaluma Valley Hospital	Petaluma	75%	81
Sierra Vista Regional Medical Center	San Luis Obispo	75%	241
University of California Irvine Med Ctr	Orange	75%	438
Kaiser Foundation Hospital	Hayward	74%	411
Mercy Med Ctr Merced-Community Campus	Merced	74%	140
Natividad Medical Center	Salinas	74%	50
Saint Bernardine Medical Center	San Bernardino	74%	239
Citrus Valley Med Ctr Queen Valley Campus	West Covina	73%	314
Encino-Tarzana Regional Medical Center	Tarzana	73%	152
Irvine Regional Hospital	Irvine	73%	197
Kaiser Permanente Fontana Medical Center	Fontana	73%	48
Lodi Memorial Hospital	Lodi	73%	214
Saint Elizabeth Community Hospital	Red Bluff	73%	168
Citrus Valley Medical Center	Covina	72%	217
Saint John's Pleasant Valley Hospital	Camarillo	72%	120
Watsonville Community Hospital	Watsonville	72%	126
Kaiser Permanente Panorama City Med Ctr	Panorama City	71%	41
Saint John's Health Center	Santa Monica	71%	1293
Sutter Amador Hospital	Jackson	71%	138
Corona Regional Medical Center	Corona	70%	238
Fresno Surgery Center	Fresno	70%	27
Garfield Medical Center	Monterey Park	70%	198
Long Beach Memorial Medical Center	Long Beach	70%	332
Western Medical Center	Santa Ana	70%	33
Brotman Medical Center	Culver City	69%	129
Motion Picture & Television Hospital	Woodland Hills	69%	26
Northridge Hospital Medical Center	Northridge	69%	211
Olympia Medical Center	Los Angeles	69%	114
Beverly Hospital	Montebello	68%	269
Sutter Maternity and Surgery Center	Santa Cruz	68%	222
Fallbrook Hospital	Fallbrook	67%	224
Feather River Hospital	Paradise	67%	119
Saint Mary Medical Center	Long Beach	67%	218
Sutter Medical Center of Santa Rosa	Santa Rosa	67%	507
Los Robles Regional Medical Center	Thousand Oaks	66%	254
Community Hospital of San Bernardino	San Bernardino	65%	68
Ukiah Valley Medical Center	Ukiah	65%	173
Dominican Hospital	Santa Cruz	64%	214
Los Angeles Community Hospital	Los Angeles	64%	25
Methodist Hospital of Southern California	Arcadia	63%	182
Oroville Hospital	Oroville	63%	41
Paradise Valley Hospital	National City	63%	126
Redbud Community Hospital	Clearlake	63%	62
San Joaquin Community Hospital	Bakersfield	63%	139
Foothill Presbyterian Hospital	Glendora	62%	143
Hi-Desert Medical Center	Joshua Tree	62%	61
Kaiser Foundation Hospital-Manteca	Manteca	62%	114
Community Regional Medical Center	Fresno	61%	948
Kaiser Permanente Los Angeles Medical Center	Los Angeles	60%	68
Mercy San Juan Hospital	Carmichael	60%	250
Methodist Hospital of Sacramento	Sacramento	60%	154
Mercy Hospital	Bakersfield	59%	201
Monterey Park Hospital	Monterey Park	59%	71
Parkview Community Hospital	Riverside	59%	126
San Gabriel Valley Medical Center	San Gabriel	59%	127
Kaiser Foundation Hospital-San Diego	San Diego	58%	31
Kaiser Permanente Anaheim Medical Center	Anaheim	58%	43
Memorial Medical Center	Modesto	58%	351
Santa Rosa Memorial Hospital	Santa Rosa	58%	186
Sutter Lakeside Hospital	Lakeport	58%	189
Sutter Solano Medical Center	Vallejo	58%	182
Huntington Beach Hospital	Huntington Beach	56%	68
Thousand Oaks Surgical Hospital	Thousand Oaks	56%	55
Riverside Community Hospital	Riverside	55%	284
Saint Vincent Medical Center	Los Angeles	55%	289
Sutter Coast Hospital	Crescent City	55%	62
Hazel Hawkins Memorial Hospital	Hollister	54%	68
Hemet Valley Medical Center	Hemet	53%	95
Madera Community Hospital	Madera	53%	207
Sierra View District Hospital	Porterville	53%	130
USC University Hospital	Los Angeles	53%	304
Santa Barbara Cottage Hospital	Santa Barbara	52%	254
Saint Luke's Hospital	San Francisco	51%	136
San Joaquin General Hospital	French Camp	49%	136
Sutter Delta Medical Center	Antioch	49%	150
Doctor's Medical Center-San Pablo Campus	San Pablo	48%	225
Ridgecrest Regional Hospital	Ridgecrest	47%	47
Victor Valley Community Hospital	Victorville	47%	38
Antelope Valley Hospital	Lancaster	45%	413
Martin Luther King Jr/Charles R Drew Med Ctr	Los Angeles	45%	77
Community Medical Center-Clovis	Clovis	44%	629
Kaiser Permanente Santa Teresa Comm Med Ctr	San Jose	41%	197
Saint Joseph Hospital	Eureka	41%	256
Dameron Hospital	Stockton	40%	289
Memorial Hospital of Gardena	Gardena	40%	48
Community Hospital	Huntington Park	39%	31
Hanford Community Medical Center	Hanford	39%	84
Central Valley General Hospital	Hanford	35%	34
Valley Presbyterian Hospital	Van Nuys	35%	95
Community Memorial Hospital Ventura	Ventura	34%	127
Oak Valley Hospital	Oakdale	34%	44
Riverside County Regional Medical Center	Moreno Valley	33%	52
Alameda County Medical Center	Oakland	30%	27
Memorial Hospital Los Banos	Los Banos	28%	36
Los Angeles County & USC Medical Center	Los Angeles	15%	995

NOTE: Hospital profiles are in alphabetical order by state, then city, then hospital within the city; Rankings are sorted by rate in descending order and exclude hospitals with less than 25 cases; (1) The number of cases is too small (n<25) for purposes of reliably predicting hospital performance; (2) Measure reflects the hospital's indication that its submission was based upon a sample of its relevant discharges; (3) Rate reflects fewer than the maximum possible quarters of data for the measure; (4) Inaccurate information submitted and suppressed for one or more quarters; (5) No data is available from the hospital for this measure; Please refer to the User's Guide for a full explanation of data

21. Prophylactic Antibiotic Selection

Hospital Name	City	Rate	Cases
Alameda Hospital	Alameda	100%	25
Alta Bates Summit Medical Center	Berkeley	100%	35
Arroyo Grande Community Hospital	Arroyo Grande	100%	37
Barton Memorial Hospital	South Lake Tahoe	100%	34
Feather River Hospital	Paradise	100%	38
Kaiser Foundation Hospital-San Diego	San Diego	100%	30
Mark Twain Saint Joseph's Hospital	San Andreas	100%	32
Mills-Peninsula Health Services	Burlingame	100%	58
Novato Community Hospital	Novato	100%	47
Saint John's Pleasant Valley Hospital	Camarillo	100%	37
Saint Mary's Medical Center	San Francisco	100%	55
San Leandro Hospital	San Leandro	100%	35
San Ramon Regional Medical Center	San Ramon	100%	79
Sutter Amador Hospital	Jackson	100%	37
Sutter Tracy Community Hospital	Tracy	100%	29
Tulare District Hospital	Tulare	100%	35
Scripps Memorial Hospital La Jolla	La Jolla	99%	78
Stanford Hospital	Stanford	99%	68
UCSF Medical Center	San Francisco	99%	81
Beverly Hospital	Montebello	98%	98
California Pacific Medical Center	San Francisco	98%	82
Eden Medical Center	Castro Valley	98%	102
Fresno Heart Hospital	Fresno	98%	163
Glendale Adventist Medical Center	Glendale	98%	156
Kaiser Permanente Bellflower Medical Center	Bellflower	98%	42
Kaiser Permanente Panorama City Med Ctr	Panorama City	98%	41
Kaiser Permanente South Bay Medical Center	Harbor City	98%	50
Loma Linda University Medical Center	Loma Linda	98%	343
Saint Agnes Medical Center	Fresno	98%	151
Scripps Memorial Hospital-Encinitas	Encinitas	98%	50
Sierra View District Hospital	Porterville	98%	63
Sierra Vista Regional Medical Center	San Luis Obispo	98%	57
Sonora Regional Medical Center	Sonora	98%	85
Century City Doctors Hospital	Los Angeles	97%	65
Downey Regional Medical Center	Downey	97%	79
Enloe Medical Center	Chico	97%	198
Fountain Valley Reg Hospital & Med Ctr	Fountain Valley	97%	100
French Hospital Medical Center	San Luis Obispo	97%	75
Kaiser Permanente San Francisco Med Ctr	San Francisco	97%	175
Marin General Hospital	Greenbrae	97%	75
Pacific Hospital of Long Beach	Long Beach	97%	29
Rideout Memorial Hospital	Marysville	97%	68
Saint Helena Hospital	Deer Park	97%	63
Saint Joseph Hospital	Orange	97%	76
Valleycare Medical Center	Livermore	97%	110
Alta Bates Summit Medical Center	Oakland	96%	56
Bakersfield Memorial Hospital	Bakersfield	96%	79
Coastal Communities Hospital	Santa Ana	96%	26
Community Memorial Hospital Ventura	Ventura	96%	114
Eisenhower Medical Center	Rancho Mirage	96%	74
Frank R Howard Memorial Hospital	Willits	96%	26
Hollywood Presbyterian Medical Center	Los Angeles	96%	111
Huntington Memorial Hospital	Pasadena	96%	313
Los Angeles Community Hospital	Los Angeles	96%	25
Providence Holy Cross Medical Center	Mission Hills	96%	76
Saint Joseph Hospital	Eureka	96%	128
San Dimas Community Hospital	San Dimas	96%	74
Santa Barbara Cottage Hospital	Santa Barbara	96%	81
Sutter Roseville Medical Center	Roseville	96%	52
Woodland Healthcare	Woodland	96%	46
Cedars-Sinai Medical Center	Los Angeles	95%	630
Community Medical Center-Clovis	Clovis	95%	141
Kaiser Redwood City Medical Center	Redwood City	95%	82
Little Company of Mary-San Pedro Hospital	San Pedro	95%	40
Los Robles Regional Medical Center	Thousand Oaks	95%	115
O'Connor Hospital	San Jose	95%	65
Palomar Medical Center	Escondido	95%	65
Pomona Valley Hospital Medical Center	Pomona	95%	173
Queen of the Valley Hospital	Napa	95%	73
San Rafael Medical Center	San Rafael	95%	131
Sierra Nevada Memorial Hospital	Grass Valley	95%	57
S San Francisco Medical Center	S San Francisco	95%	58
Centinela Hospital Medical Center	Inglewood	94%	127
Doctors Hospital of Manteca	Manteca	94%	32
Hoag Memorial Hospital Presbyterian	Newport Beach	94%	87
Methodist Hospital of Sacramento	Sacramento	94%	47
Mission Hospital Regional Medical Center	Mission Viejo	94%	62
Parkview Community Hospital	Riverside	94%	81
Presbyterian Intercommunity Hospital	Whittier	94%	64
Saint Jude Medical Center	Fullerton	94%	302
Saint Luke's Hospital	San Francisco	94%	33
San Joaquin Community Hospital	Bakersfield	94%	54
Shasta Regional Medical Center	Redding	94%	189
Sutter Delta Medical Center	Antioch	94%	34
Sutter Lakeside Hospital	Lakeport	94%	53
Tri-City Medical Center	Oceanside	94%	70
Bakersfield Heart Hospital	Bakersfield	93%	69
Community Regional Medical Center	Fresno	93%	234
Desert Regional Medical Center	Palm Springs	93%	88
El Camino Hospital	Mountain View	93%	97
Garden Grove Hospital and Medical Center	Garden Grove	93%	41
Henry Mayo Newhall Memorial Hospital	Valencia	93%	68
Kaiser Foundation Hospital-Fresno	Fresno	93%	42
Kaiser Foundation Hospital-South Sacramento	Sacramento	93%	177
Lakewood Regional Medical Center	Lakewood	93%	74
Mercy Hospital of Folsom	Folsom	93%	42
Mercy Medical Center-Redding	Redding	93%	89
Saddleback Memorial Medical Center	Laguna Hills	93%	104
Torrance Memorial Medical Center	Torrance	93%	81
Twin Cities Community Hospital	Templeton	93%	86
Arrowhead Regional Medical Center	Colton	92%	51
Community Hospital of Los Gatos	Los Gatos	92%	50
Garfield Medical Center	Monterey Park	92%	52
John F Kennedy Memorial Hospital	Indio	92%	78
Kaiser Foundation Hospital	Baldwin Park	92%	51
Little Company of Mary Hospital	Torrance	92%	157
Los Angeles County & USC Medical Center	Los Angeles	92%	211
Marshall Medical Center	Placerville	92%	62
Mercy Medical Center-Mount Shasta	Mount Shasta	92%	38
Oakland Medical Center	Oakland	92%	276
Oroville Hospital	Oroville	92%	36
Riverside Community Hospital	Riverside	92%	136
San Antonio Community Hospital	Upland	92%	241
Ukiah Valley Medical Center	Ukiah	92%	40
Antelope Valley Hospital	Lancaster	91%	134
Doctor's Medical Center-San Pablo Campus	San Pablo	91%	53
Glendale Memorial Hospital and Health Center	Glendale	91%	80
Kaiser Foundation Hospital-Vallejo	Vallejo	91%	46
Kaiser Foundation Hospital-Walnut Creek	Walnut Creek	91%	53
Kaiser Permanente Fontana Medical Center	Fontana	91%	47
Los Angeles County Harbor-UCLA Medical Center	Torrance	91%	53
Marian Medical Center	Santa Maria	91%	172
Mercy San Juan Hospital	Carmichael	91%	80
Saint John's Health Center	Santa Monica	91%	355
Santa Monica-UCLA Medical Center	Santa Monica	91%	46
Scripps Mercy Hospital	San Diego	91%	80
Sharp Memorial Hospital	San Diego	91%	172
Thousand Oaks Surgical Hospital	Thousand Oaks	91%	44
USC University Hospital	Los Angeles	91%	69
University of California Irvine Med Ctr	Orange	91%	126
West Hills Hospital and Medical Center	West Hills	91%	95
Kaiser Foundation Hospital-Riverside	Riverside	90%	49
Kaiser Permanente Los Angeles Medical Center	Los Angeles	90%	72
Memorial Medical Center	Modesto	90%	78
Mercy General Hospital	Sacramento	90%	104
Methodist Hospital of Southern California	Arcadia	90%	181
NorthBay Medical Center	Fairfield	90%	52
Rancho Springs Medical Center	Murrieta	90%	175
Saint Mary Medical Center	Apple Valley	90%	127
Saint Mary Medical Center	Long Beach	90%	41
El Centro Regional Medical Center	El Centro	89%	71
Emanuel Medical Center	Turlock	89%	76
Kaweah Delta Health Care District	Visalia	89%	70
Lompoc Healthcare District Hospital	Lompoc	89%	35
Los Alamitos Medical Center	Los Alamitos	89%	36
Madera Community Hospital	Madera	89%	63
Orange Coast Memorial Medical Center	Santa Ana	89%	105
Sharp Coronado Hospital	San Diego	89%	28
South Coast Medical Center	Laguna Beach	89%	28
Sutter Maternity and Surgery Center	Santa Cruz	89%	37
University of California San Diego Med Ctr	San Diego	89%	65
Watsonville Community Hospital	Watsonville	89%	35
Fallbrook Hospital	Fallbrook	88%	69
Kaiser Permanente West Los Angeles Med Ctr	Los Angeles	88%	43
Lancaster Community Hospital	Lancaster	88%	110
Mercy Med Ctr Merced-Community Campus	Merced	88%	41
Saint Joseph's Medical Center of Stockton	Stockton	88%	64
Scripps Green Hospital	La Jolla	88%	74
Sutter Auburn Faith Hospital	Auburn	88%	52
Citrus Valley Medical Center	Covina	87%	75
Foothill Presbyterian Hospital	Glendora	87%	46
Kaiser Foundation Hospital	Hayward	87%	99
Kaiser Foundation Hospital-Santa Rosa	Santa Rosa	87%	102
Petaluma Valley Hospital	Petaluma	87%	30
Pomerado Hospital	Poway	87%	46
Sutter Davis Hospital	Davis	87%	47
University of California Davis Health System	Sacramento	87%	75

NOTE: Hospital profiles are in alphabetical order by state, then city, then hospital within the city; Rankings are sorted by rate in descending order and exclude hospitals with less than 25 cases; (1) The number of cases is too small (n<25) for purposes of reliably predicting hospital performance; (2) Measure reflects the hospital's indication that its submission was based upon a sample of its relevant discharges; (3) Rate reflects fewer than the maximum possible quarters of data for the measure; (4) Inaccurate information submitted and suppressed for one or more quarters; (5) No data is available from the hospital for this measure; Please refer to the User's Guide for a full explanation of data

Corona Regional Medical Center	Corona	86%	76
Dominican Hospital	Santa Cruz	86%	69
Kaiser Foundation Hospital	Woodland Hills	86%	49
Saint John's Regional Medical Center	Oxnard	86%	65
San Joaquin General Hospital	French Camp	86%	29
Lodi Memorial Hospital	Lodi	85%	52
Placentia-Linda Hospital	Placentia	85%	41
Saint Francis Memorial Hospital	San Francisco	85%	41
Dameron Hospital	Stockton	84%	45
Hi-Desert Medical Center	Joshua Tree	84%	25
Kaiser Permanente Sacramento Medical Center	Sacramento	84%	144
Kaiser Permanente Santa Clara Medical Center	Santa Clara	84%	45
Saint Louise Regional Hospital	Gilroy	84%	43
Saint Vincent Medical Center	Los Angeles	84%	57
Washington Hospital	Fremont	84%	70
California Hospital Medical Center	Los Angeles	83%	54
Mercy Hospital	Bakersfield	83%	65
Whittier Hospital Medical Center	Whittier	83%	69
Paradise Valley Hospital	National City	82%	38
Pioneers Memorial Healthcare District	Brawley	82%	49
Regional Medical Center of San Jose	San Jose	82%	56
San Gabriel Valley Medical Center	San Gabriel	82%	34
Santa Rosa Memorial Hospital	Santa Rosa	82%	57
Providence Saint Joseph Medical Center	Burbank	81%	74
Encino-Tarzana Regional Medical Center	Tarzana	80%	56
Good Samaritan Hospital	Los Angeles	80%	123
Irvine Regional Hospital	Irvine	80%	44
Sutter General Hospital	Sacramento	80%	88
Doctors Medical Center	Modesto	79%	192
Northridge Hospital Medical Center	Northridge	78%	73
Sequoia Hospital	Redwood City	78%	86
Sharp Chula Vista Medical Center	Chula Vista	78%	64
Brotman Medical Center	Culver City	77%	35
Kaiser Permanente Anaheim Medical Center	Anaheim	76%	42
Kaiser Permanente Santa Teresa Comm Med Ctr	San Jose	76%	49
Saint Francis Medical Center	Lynwood	76%	38
Grossmont Hospital	La Mesa	74%	84
Long Beach Memorial Medical Center	Long Beach	74%	92
Santa Clara Valley Medical Center	San Jose	72%	101
Simi Valley Hospital	Simi Valley	71%	38
Sutter Medical Center of Santa Rosa	Santa Rosa	71%	122
Anaheim Memorial Medical Center	Anaheim	69%	64
Saint Bernardine Medical Center	San Bernardino	69%	80
John Muir Medical Center-Concord Campus	Concord	67%	79
Saint Elizabeth Community Hospital	Red Bluff	67%	54
Western Medical Center	Santa Ana	65%	34
San Francisco General Hospital Medical Center	San Francisco	64%	36
Citrus Valley Med Ctr Queen Valley Campus	West Covina	63%	105
Goleta Valley Cottage Hospital	Santa Barbara	62%	40
John Muir Medical Center	Walnut Creek	62%	55
UCLA Medical Center	Los Angeles	62%	55
Good Samaritan Hospital	San Jose	60%	129
Hemet Valley Medical Center	Hemet	52%	94

22. Prophylactic Antibiotic Stopped

Hospital Name	City	Rate	Cases
Mercy Medical Center-Mount Shasta	Mount Shasta	100%	94
Natividad Medical Center	Salinas	100%	54
Oroville Hospital	Oroville	100%	34
Patients' Hospital of Redding	Redding	100%	78
Saint Rose Hospital	Hayward	100%	39
Arroyo Grande Community Hospital	Arroyo Grande	99%	115
Healdsburg District Hospital	Healdsburg	98%	52
Memorial Hospital Los Banos	Los Banos	97%	34
Parkview Community Hospital	Riverside	97%	116
Century City Doctors Hospital	Los Angeles	96%	202
Los Angeles Community Hospital	Los Angeles	96%	25
Mark Twain Saint Joseph's Hospital	San Andreas	94%	31
Oak Valley Hospital	Oakdale	94%	35
Sharp Mary Birch Hospital for Women	San Diego	94%	35
Kaiser Foundation Hospital-Vallejo	Vallejo	91%	180
Tulare District Hospital	Tulare	91%	35
Twin Cities Community Hospital	Templeton	91%	351
Woodland Healthcare	Woodland	91%	113
Martin Luther King Jr/Charles R Drew Med Ctr	Los Angeles	90%	68
Cedars-Sinai Medical Center	Los Angeles	89%	2442
French Hospital Medical Center	San Luis Obispo	89%	217
Sonora Regional Medical Center	Sonora	89%	262
S San Francisco Medical Center	S San Francisco	89%	274
Alta Bates Summit Medical Center	Oakland	87%	157
Sharp Coronado Hospital	San Diego	87%	94
Shasta Regional Medical Center	Redding	87%	714
Thousand Oaks Surgical Hospital	Thousand Oaks	87%	53
West Anaheim Medical Center	Anaheim	87%	82
Kaiser Permanente San Francisco Med Ctr	San Francisco	86%	605
Santa Clara Valley Medical Center	San Jose	86%	410
Sutter Roseville Medical Center	Roseville	86%	224
UCSF Medical Center	San Francisco	86%	466
Kaiser Redwood City Medical Center	Redwood City	85%	367
Palomar Medical Center	Escondido	85%	214
Saint Jude Medical Center	Fullerton	85%	1210
Tri-City Medical Center	Oceanside	85%	133
Frank R Howard Memorial Hospital	Willits	84%	25
Placentia-Linda Hospital	Placentia	84%	139
Riverside County Regional Medical Center	Moreno Valley	84%	50
Saint Agnes Medical Center	Fresno	84%	458
Sutter Davis Hospital	Davis	84%	203
Sutter Maternity and Surgery Center	Santa Cruz	84%	218
Fallbrook Hospital	Fallbrook	83%	216
Hoag Memorial Hospital Presbyterian	Newport Beach	83%	337
Mercy Medical Center-Redding	Redding	82%	271
San Rafael Medical Center	San Rafael	82%	519
Kaiser Foundation Hospital-Walnut Creek	Walnut Creek	81%	313
Pomerado Hospital	Poway	81%	142
Saint Joseph Hospital	Orange	81%	222
Sutter Auburn Faith Hospital	Auburn	81%	194
Bakersfield Heart Hospital	Bakersfield	80%	159
California Pacific Medical Center	San Francisco	80%	242
Feather River Hospital	Paradise	80%	116
Fresno Heart Hospital	Fresno	80%	276
Hazel Hawkins Memorial Hospital	Hollister	80%	64
Kaiser Permanente Los Angeles Medical Center	Los Angeles	80%	65
O'Connor Hospital	San Jose	80%	186
Oakland Medical Center	Oakland	80%	908
Saint Helena Hospital	Deer Park	80%	256
Washington Hospital	Fremont	80%	69
Doctors Hospital of Manteca	Manteca	79%	113
Eden Medical Center	Castro Valley	79%	403
El Camino Hospital	Mountain View	79%	786
Marshall Medical Center	Placerville	79%	188
San Mateo Medical Center	San Mateo	79%	90
Scripps Green Hospital	La Jolla	79%	256
Sequoia Hospital	Redwood City	79%	244
Watsonville Community Hospital	Watsonville	79%	112
Sutter Solano Medical Center	Vallejo	78%	169
White Memorial Medical Center	Los Angeles	78%	41
Arrowhead Regional Medical Center	Colton	77%	226
Saint Elizabeth Community Hospital	Red Bluff	77%	164
Saint Luke's Hospital	San Francisco	77%	128
San Francisco General Hospital Medical Center	San Francisco	77%	113
John Muir Medical Center-Concord Campus	Concord	76%	218
Mercy San Juan Hospital	Carmichael	76%	234
Ridgecrest Regional Hospital	Ridgecrest	76%	46
Sharp Memorial Hospital	San Diego	76%	449
Eisenhower Medical Center	Rancho Mirage	75%	650
Mission Hospital Regional Medical Center	Mission Viejo	75%	186
Saddleback Memorial Medical Center	Laguna Hills	75%	404
San Leandro Hospital	San Leandro	75%	184
Torrance Memorial Medical Center	Torrance	75%	225
Good Samaritan Hospital	Los Angeles	74%	514
Kaiser Foundation Hospital-Fresno	Fresno	74%	159
Kaiser Permanente Santa Clara Medical Center	Santa Clara	74%	193
Kaiser Permanente Santa Teresa Comm Med Ctr	San Jose	74%	183
Madera Community Hospital	Madera	74%	205
Sharp Chula Vista Medical Center	Chula Vista	74%	208
Stanislaus Surgical Hospital	Modesto	74%	35
Community Hospital of the Monterey Peninsula	Monterey	73%	188
Doctors Medical Center	Modesto	73%	578
Kaiser Foundation Hospital	Woodland Hills	73%	48
Los Angeles County & USC Medical Center	Los Angeles	73%	960
Saint John's Health Center	Santa Monica	73%	1265
Scripps Memorial Hospital La Jolla	La Jolla	73%	232
University of California Davis Health System	Sacramento	73%	491
Kaiser Permanente Sacramento Medical Center	Sacramento	72%	614
Saint Francis Memorial Hospital	San Francisco	72%	116
Salinas Valley Memorial Health Care District	Salinas	72%	208
Sutter Delta Medical Center	Antioch	72%	131
Sutter General Hospital	Sacramento	72%	356
Grossmont Hospital	La Mesa	71%	319
Kaiser Foundation Hospital-South Sacramento	Sacramento	71%	730
Sierra Vista Regional Medical Center	San Luis Obispo	71%	232
VacaValley Hospital	Vacaville	71%	85
Alta Bates Summit Medical Center	Berkeley	70%	106
Glendale Adventist Medical Center	Glendale	70%	462
Good Samaritan Hospital	San Jose	70%	259
La Palma Intercommunity Hospital	La Palma	70%	82
Coastal Communities Hospital	Santa Ana	69%	99
Garden Grove Hospital and Medical Center	Garden Grove	69%	162
Mercy General Hospital	Sacramento	69%	285

NOTE: Hospital profiles are in alphabetical order by state, then city, then hospital within the city; Rankings are sorted by rate in descending order and exclude hospitals with less than 25 cases; (1) The number of cases is too small (n<25) for purposes of reliably predicting hospital performance; (2) Measure reflects the hospital's indication that its submission was based upon a sample of its relevant discharges; (3) Rate reflects fewer than the maximum possible quarters of data for the measure; (4) Inaccurate information submitted and suppressed for one or more quarters; (5) No data is available from the hospital for this measure; Please refer to the User's Guide for a full explanation of data

Petaluma Valley Hospital	Petaluma	69%	81
Saint Louisie Regional Hospital	Gilroy	69%	96
San Antonio Community Hospital	Upland	69%	680
Sierra Nevada Memorial Hospital	Grass Valley	69%	170
South Coast Medical Center	Laguna Beach	69%	32
Community Medical Center-Clovis	Clovis	68%	608
Contra Costa Regional Medical Center	Martinez	68%	25
Irvine Regional Hospital	Irvine	68%	199
Lompoc Healthcare District Hospital	Lompoc	68%	142
Paradise Valley Hospital	National City	68%	109
Rideout Memorial Hospital	Marysville	68%	237
University of California Irvine Med Ctr	Orange	68%	430
Antelope Valley Hospital	Lancaster	67%	347
Community Regional Medical Center	Fresno	67%	886
Fresno Surgery Center	Fresno	67%	27
Kaiser Foundation Hospital-Santa Rosa	Santa Rosa	67%	307
Long Beach Memorial Medical Center	Long Beach	67%	316
Los Robles Regional Medical Center	Thousand Oaks	67%	245
Stanford Hospital	Stanford	67%	102
Enloe Medical Center	Chico	66%	775
Kaiser Foundation Hospital-Manteca	Manteca	66%	113
Kern Medical Center	Bakersfield	66%	35
Victor Valley Community Hospital	Victorville	66%	29
Goleta Valley Cottage Hospital	Santa Barbara	65%	102
Hi-Desert Medical Center	Joshua Tree	65%	57
Little Company of Mary Hospital	Torrance	65%	618
Ukiah Valley Medical Center	Ukiah	65%	170
John F Kennedy Memorial Hospital	Indio	64%	280
Presbyterian Intercommunity Hospital	Whittier	64%	225
Sutter Lakeside Hospital	Lakeport	64%	182
Kaiser Permanente South Bay Medical Center	Harbor City	63%	51
Marin General Hospital	Greenbrae	63%	284
Memorial Hospital of Gardena	Gardena	63%	30
NorthBay Medical Center	Fairfield	63%	163
Saint Joseph Hospital	Eureka	63%	252
Kaiser Permanente Bellflower Medical Center	Bellflower	62%	42
Marian Medical Center	Santa Maria	62%	481
Mercy Hospital of Folsom	Folsom	62%	112
Valleycare Medical Center	Livermore	62%	279
Foothill Presbyterian Hospital	Glendora	61%	135
Regional Medical Center of San Jose	San Jose	61%	114
Sutter Medical Center of Santa Rosa	Santa Rosa	61%	473
Lakewood Regional Medical Center	Lakewood	60%	341
Sutter Tracy Community Hospital	Tracy	60%	123
Rancho Springs Medical Center	Murrieta	59%	744
Redbud Community Hospital	Clearlake	59%	61
Saint Joseph's Medical Center of Stockton	Stockton	59%	185
Saint Mary Medical Center	Apple Valley	59%	429
Seton Medical Center	Daly City	59%	51
Sonoma Valley Hospital	Sonoma	58%	88
Dominican Hospital	Santa Cruz	57%	207
Kaiser Foundation Hospital-San Diego	San Diego	57%	28
Queen of the Valley Hospital	Napa	57%	171
Saint Francis Medical Center	Lynwood	57%	122
Saint Mary Medical Center	Long Beach	57%	203
San Joaquin General Hospital	French Camp	57%	120
Scripps Mercy Hospital	San Diego	57%	148
Sutter Amador Hospital	Jackson	57%	137
Encino-Tarzana Regional Medical Center	Tarzana	56%	146
Kaiser Foundation Hospital	Hayward	56%	391
Memorial Medical Center	Modesto	56%	344
Redlands Community Hospital	Redlands	56%	140
Western Medical Center	Santa Ana	56%	32
Community Hospital of Los Gatos	Los Gatos	55%	202
Olympia Medical Center	Los Angeles	55%	113
Saint Bernardine Medical Center	San Bernardino	55%	235
Centinela Freeman Reg Med Ctr-Marina	Marina Del Rey	54%	69
Doctor's Medical Center-San Pablo Campus	San Pablo	54%	216
Providence Holy Cross Medical Center	Mission Hills	54%	273
Santa Rosa Memorial Hospital	Santa Rosa	54%	174
Anaheim Memorial Medical Center	Anaheim	53%	408
Bakersfield Memorial Hospital	Bakersfield	53%	251
John Muir Medical Center	Walnut Creek	53%	171
University of California San Diego Med Ctr	San Diego	53%	318
Downey Regional Medical Center	Downey	52%	213
Kaiser Foundation Hospital	Baldwin Park	52%	46
Kaiser Permanente Panorama City Med Ctr	Panorama City	52%	40
Loma Linda University Medical Center	Loma Linda	52%	1070
Methodist Hospital of Sacramento	Sacramento	52%	154
Pacific Hospital of Long Beach	Long Beach	52%	135
Saint John's Regional Medical Center	Oxnard	52%	203
San Joaquin Community Hospital	Bakersfield	52%	130
San Ramon Regional Medical Center	San Ramon	52%	313
Emanuel Medical Center	Turlock	51%	287
Henry Mayo Newhall Memorial Hospital	Valencia	51%	145
Beverly Hospital	Montebello	50%	263
Centinela Hospital Medical Center	Inglewood	50%	571
Community Memorial Hospital Ventura	Ventura	50%	124
Kaiser Permanente Anaheim Medical Center	Anaheim	50%	38
Kaiser Permanente West Los Angeles Med Ctr	Los Angeles	50%	44
Lancaster Community Hospital	Lancaster	50%	360
UCLA Medical Center	Los Angeles	50%	367
Kaiser Permanente Fontana Medical Center	Fontana	49%	47
Mills-Peninsula Health Services	Burlingame	49%	283
Saint Vincent Medical Center	Los Angeles	49%	269
Dameron Hospital	Stockton	48%	259
Mercy Med Ctr Merced-Community Campus	Merced	48%	133
Riverside Community Hospital	Riverside	48%	255
West Hills Hospital and Medical Center	West Hills	48%	204
Corona Regional Medical Center	Corona	47%	226
Glendale Memorial Hospital and Health Center	Glendale	47%	230
Providence Saint Joseph Medical Center	Burbank	47%	281
Verdugo Hills Hospital	Glendale	47%	108
Sutter Coast Hospital	Crescent City	46%	61
Brotman Medical Center	Culver City	45%	121
Methodist Hospital of Southern California	Arcadia	45%	176
Pomona Valley Hospital Medical Center	Pomona	45%	683
Northridge Hospital Medical Center	Northridge	44%	198
San Dimas Community Hospital	San Dimas	44%	308
Scripps Memorial Hospital-Encinitas	Encinitas	44%	91
Desert Regional Medical Center	Palm Springs	43%	357
California Hospital Medical Center	Los Angeles	42%	147
Huntington Beach Hospital	Huntington Beach	42%	60
Los Alamitos Medical Center	Los Alamitos	42%	154
Orange Coast Memorial Medical Center	Santa Ana	42%	424
Citrus Valley Med Ctr Queen Valley Campus	West Covina	41%	296
Pioneers Memorial Healthcare District	Brawley	41%	109
Simi Valley Hospital	Simi Valley	41%	187
Valley Presbyterian Hospital	Van Nuys	41%	94
Hanford Community Medical Center	Hanford	40%	75
Los Angeles County Harbor-UCLA Medical Center	Torrance	40%	225
San Gabriel Valley Medical Center	San Gabriel	40%	126
Community Hospital of San Bernardino	San Bernardino	39%	64
Sierra View District Hospital	Porterville	39%	113
Kaiser Foundation Hospital-Riverside	Riverside	38%	47
Santa Monica-UCLA Medical Center	Santa Monica	38%	276
Whittier Hospital Medical Center	Whittier	38%	266
Community Hospital of Long Beach	Long Beach	37%	30
El Centro Regional Medical Center	El Centro	37%	71
Little Company of Mary-San Pedro Hospital	San Pedro	37%	149
Novato Community Hospital	Novato	36%	197
Saint John's Pleasant Valley Hospital	Camarillo	36%	118
Fountain Valley Reg Hospital & Med Ctr	Fountain Valley	35%	304
Kaweah Delta Health Care District	Visalia	35%	65
Lodi Memorial Hospital	Lodi	35%	202
Saint Mary's Medical Center	San Francisco	34%	166
Monterey Park Hospital	Monterey Park	33%	69
Huntington Memorial Hospital	Pasadena	30%	315
Mercy Hospital	Bakersfield	29%	201
Santa Barbara Cottage Hospital	Santa Barbara	29%	242
Hollywood Presbyterian Medical Center	Los Angeles	27%	110
USC University Hospital	Los Angeles	26%	300
Citrus Valley Medical Center	Covina	24%	197
Garfield Medical Center	Monterey Park	24%	190
Encino-Tarzana Regional Medical Center	Encino	20%	120
Barton Memorial Hospital	South Lake Tahoe	15%	121
Hemet Valley Medical Center	Hemet	9%	92

Pregnancy Care

23. Inpatient Neonatal Mortality

Hospital Name	City	Rate	Cases
Anaheim General Hospital	Anaheim	0.00%	136
Barton Memorial Hospital	South Lake Tahoe	0.00%	560
East Valley Hospital Medical Center	Glendora	0.00%	398
George L Mee Memorial Hospital	King City	0.00%	590
Goleta Valley Cottage Hospital	Santa Barbara	0.00%	296
Kaiser Foundation Hospital-Fresno	Fresno	0.00%	1345
Kaiser Foundation Hospital-Santa Rosa	Santa Rosa	0.00%	1458
Kaiser Permanente Santa Teresa Comm Med Ctr	San Jose	0.00%	510
Lompoc Healthcare District Hospital	Lompoc	0.00%	473
Mercy Hospital of Folsom	Folsom	0.00%	1084
Orange Coast Memorial Medical Center	Santa Ana	0.00%	1576
Pacific Alliance Medical Center	Los Angeles	0.00%	409
Saint Elizabeth Community Hospital	Red Bluff	0.00%	721
Saint Luke's Hospital	San Francisco	0.00%	255
San Gorgonio Memorial Hospital	Banning	0.00%	415
Scripps Memorial Hospital-Encinitas	Encinitas	0.00%	1530
Sequoia Hospital	Redwood City	0.00%	1088

NOTE: Hospital profiles are in alphabetical order by state, then city, then hospital within the city; Rankings are sorted by rate in descending order and exclude hospitals with less than 25 cases; (1) The number of cases is too small (n<25) for purposes of reliably predicting hospital performance; (2) Measure reflects the hospital's indication that its submission was based upon a sample of its relevant discharges; (3) Rate reflects fewer than the maximum possible quarters of data for the measure; (4) Inaccurate information submitted and suppressed for one or more quarters; (5) No data is available from the hospital for this measure; Please refer to the User's Guide for a full explanation of data

Sierra Kings District Hospital	Reedley	0.00%	1118
South Coast Medical Center	Laguna Beach	0.00%	716
Sutter Maternity and Surgery Center	Santa Cruz	0.00%	874
Kaiser Foundation Hospital-South Sacramento	Sacramento	0.03%	3606
Mercy Medical Center-Redding	Redding	0.04%	2239
Kaiser Foundation Hospital-Riverside	Riverside	0.05%	3785
Scripps Memorial Hospital La Jolla	La Jolla	0.05%	3806
Sutter Roseville Medical Center	Roseville	0.05%	2046
Kaiser Permanente Panorama City Med Ctr	Panorama City	0.06%	1656
Mercy Med Ctr Merced-Community Campus	Merced	0.07%	2764
Methodist Hospital of Sacramento	Sacramento	0.07%	1473
Scripps Mercy Hospital	San Diego	0.07%	4352
Kaiser Foundation Hospital	Baldwin Park	0.10%	3158
Mercy General Hospital	Sacramento	0.12%	2603
Saint Jude Medical Center	Fullerton	0.13%	2255
Sutter Davis Hospital	Davis	0.13%	752
Woodland Healthcare	Woodland	0.13%	771
Hanford Community Medical Center	Hanford	0.14%	733
Kaiser Permanente Santa Clara Medical Center	Santa Clara	0.14%	725
Kaiser Permanente West Los Angeles Med Ctr	Los Angeles	0.14%	1461
Saint Louisie Regional Hospital	Gilroy	0.14%	711
Community Hospital of San Bernardino	San Bernardino	0.16%	2561
John Muir Medical Center	Walnut Creek	0.16%	620
Kaiser Permanente South Bay Medical Center	Harbor City	0.16%	1825
Ventura County Medical Center	Ventura	0.18%	3315
Pomona Valley Hospital Medical Center	Pomona	0.20%	1007
Saddleback Memorial Medical Center	Laguna Hills	0.21%	2890
Saint John's Health Center	Santa Monica	0.22%	915
Kaiser Permanente San Francisco Med Ctr	San Francisco	0.23%	2612
Kaiser Foundation Hospital	Hayward	0.24%	3342
Kaiser Foundation Hospital-Vallejo	Vallejo	0.24%	2510
Kaiser Foundation Hospital-Walnut Creek	Walnut Creek	0.24%	4654
Downey Regional Medical Center	Downey	0.25%	1574
Tri-City Medical Center	Oceanside	0.26%	1948
California Hospital Medical Center	Los Angeles	0.27%	4149
Sutter Coast Hospital	Crescent City	0.27%	376
Kaiser Foundation Hospital	Woodland Hills	0.28%	1761
Central Valley General Hospital	Hanford	0.29%	2062
Tulare District Hospital	Tulare	0.30%	1005
Natividad Medical Center	Salinas	0.31%	2607
Alta Bates Summit Medical Center	Berkeley	0.32%	7706
Bakersfield Memorial Hospital	Bakersfield	0.32%	2854
San Gabriel Valley Medical Center	San Gabriel	0.33%	2142
Parkview Community Hospital	Riverside	0.34%	888
Kaiser Permanente Anaheim Medical Center	Anaheim	0.35%	3398
Mercy Hospital	Bakersfield	0.36%	3587
Sutter Medical Center of Santa Rosa	Santa Rosa	0.37%	818
Anaheim Memorial Medical Center	Anaheim	0.39%	2035
California Pacific Medical Center	San Francisco	0.40%	1003
Kaiser Foundation Hospital-San Diego	San Diego	0.40%	3983
Kaiser Permanente Sacramento Medical Center	Sacramento	0.42%	4283
Kaiser Redwood City Medical Center	Redwood City	0.42%	1430
San Joaquin General Hospital	French Camp	0.42%	3089
Kern Medical Center	Bakersfield	0.43%	932
Santa Clara Valley Medical Center	San Jose	0.43%	6066
Kaiser Permanente Fontana Medical Center	Fontana	0.46%	4777
Sharp Mary Birch Hospital for Women	San Diego	0.46%	8388
Saint Mary Medical Center	Apple Valley	0.49%	2855
White Memorial Medical Center	Los Angeles	0.50%	3828
Queen of the Valley Hospital	Napa	0.56%	1062
Kaiser Permanente Bellflower Medical Center	Bellflower	0.58%	3461
Kaiser Permanente Los Angeles Medical Center	Los Angeles	0.61%	2476
San Antonio Community Hospital	Upland	0.76%	2247
Santa Monica-UCLA Medical Center	Santa Monica	0.81%	369
Redlands Community Hospital	Redlands	1.03%	583
Los Angeles County & USC Medical Center	Los Angeles	1.09%	1566
University of California Davis Health System	Sacramento	1.29%	622
Los Angeles County Harbor-UCLA Medical Center	Torrance	1.40%	285
University of California Irvine Med Ctr	Orange	2.64%	1667

24. Third or Fourth Degree Laceration

Hospital Name	City	Rate	Cases
East Valley Hospital Medical Center	Glendora	0.54%	184
Pacific Alliance Medical Center	Los Angeles	0.71%	282
San Gorgonio Memorial Hospital	Banning	0.75%	266
Central Valley General Hospital	Hanford	1.29%	1319
Woodland Healthcare	Woodland	1.41%	566
San Gabriel Valley Medical Center	San Gabriel	1.45%	1308
Bakersfield Memorial Hospital	Bakersfield	1.71%	2108
Sutter Roseville Medical Center	Roseville	1.74%	1554
Los Angeles County Harbor-UCLA Medical Center	Torrance	1.87%	694
Community Hospital of San Bernardino	San Bernardino	1.91%	1570
Orange Coast Memorial Medical Center	Santa Ana	1.98%	1059
Anaheim General Hospital	Anaheim	2.08%	96
Mercy Medical Center-Redding	Redding	2.09%	1482
Downey Regional Medical Center	Downey	2.18%	1192
Queen of the Valley Hospital	Napa	2.28%	745
Kaiser Permanente Anaheim Medical Center	Anaheim	2.30%	2391
Kaiser Permanente West Los Angeles Med Ctr	Los Angeles	2.34%	1026
Hanford Community Medical Center	Hanford	2.35%	511
Kaiser Foundation Hospital-Riverside	Riverside	2.38%	2733
Sutter Davis Hospital	Davis	2.47%	730
Mercy General Hospital	Sacramento	2.48%	1897
Pomona Valley Hospital Medical Center	Pomona	2.51%	637
California Hospital Medical Center	Los Angeles	2.53%	2841
Goleta Valley Cottage Hospital	Santa Barbara	2.53%	237
Saint Elizabeth Community Hospital	Red Bluff	2.56%	507
Methodist Hospital of Sacramento	Sacramento	2.60%	960
Sierra Kings District Hospital	Reedley	2.61%	690
Los Angeles Metropolitan Med Ctr-LA Campus	Los Angeles	2.63%	571
Kaiser Foundation Hospital	Baldwin Park	2.80%	2211
Ventura County Medical Center	Ventura	2.82%	2412
Kaiser Permanente Sacramento Medical Center	Sacramento	2.85%	2701
Kaiser Permanente Panorama City Med Ctr	Panorama City	2.92%	1026
Kaiser Redwood City Medical Center	Redwood City	3.01%	1131
San Joaquin General Hospital	French Camp	3.04%	2139
Anaheim Memorial Medical Center	Anaheim	3.09%	1457
Alta Bates Summit Medical Center	Berkeley	3.11%	5335
University of California Irvine Med Ctr	Orange	3.15%	1017
Sutter Coast Hospital	Crescent City	3.19%	282
Lompoc Healthcare District Hospital	Lompoc	3.23%	341
Parkview Community Hospital	Riverside	3.25%	584
Tulare District Hospital	Tulare	3.27%	611
Tri-City Medical Center	Oceanside	3.29%	1400
Sequoia Hospital	Redwood City	3.30%	817
South Coast Medical Center	Laguna Beach	3.36%	506
Mercy Med Ctr Merced-Community Campus	Merced	3.38%	2072
Kaiser Permanente Bellflower Medical Center	Bellflower	3.39%	2447
Kaiser Permanente Los Angeles Medical Center	Los Angeles	3.42%	1520
Scripps Memorial Hospital-Encinitas	Encinitas	3.42%	1228
San Antonio Community Hospital	Upland	3.46%	1302
Scripps Mercy Hospital	San Diego	3.49%	2984
Kern Medical Center	Bakersfield	3.50%	742
Barton Memorial Hospital	South Lake Tahoe	3.59%	390
Kaiser Foundation Hospital-Fresno	Fresno	3.63%	910
University of California Davis Health System	Sacramento	3.70%	1893
Kaiser Foundation Hospital-Vallejo	Vallejo	3.71%	1750
Saddleback Memorial Medical Center	Laguna Hills	3.73%	1955
Saint Jude Medical Center	Fullerton	3.74%	1551
Kaiser Foundation Hospital-Walnut Creek	Walnut Creek	3.75%	3228
Kaiser Foundation Hospital	Woodland Hills	3.77%	1219
Kaiser Permanente Fontana Medical Center	Fontana	3.85%	3321
Santa Clara Valley Medical Center	San Jose	3.85%	4627
Saint Louisie Regional Hospital	Gilroy	3.89%	489
California Pacific Medical Center	San Francisco	3.91%	741
Kaiser Foundation Hospital-San Diego	San Diego	3.94%	2640
Kaiser Foundation Hospital-South Sacramento	Sacramento	3.98%	2866
Sutter Medical Center of Santa Rosa	Santa Rosa	4.00%	826
Los Angeles County & USC Medical Center	Los Angeles	4.06%	912
Kaiser Permanente Santa Teresa Comm Med Ctr	San Jose	4.19%	382
Natividad Medical Center	Salinas	4.21%	1853
Redlands Community Hospital	Redlands	4.41%	431
Sharp Mary Birch Hospital for Women	San Diego	4.59%	5165
Santa Monica-UCLA Medical Center	Santa Monica	4.61%	781
Kaiser Permanente South Bay Medical Center	Harbor City	4.82%	1223
Saint Mary Medical Center	Apple Valley	4.96%	2159
Kaiser Foundation Hospital-Santa Rosa	Santa Rosa	5.01%	959
Saint Luke's Hospital	San Francisco	5.05%	376
George L Mee Memorial Hospital	King City	5.15%	408
Mercy Hospital of Folsom	Folsom	5.18%	830
Kaiser Foundation Hospital	Hayward	5.23%	2123
Kaiser Permanente Santa Clara Medical Center	Santa Clara	5.73%	489
Sutter Maternity and Surgery Center	Santa Cruz	5.81%	689
Scripps Memorial Hospital La Jolla	La Jolla	6.04%	2534
Saint John's Health Center	Santa Monica	6.13%	1288
John Muir Medical Center	Walnut Creek	6.19%	679
White Memorial Medical Center	Los Angeles	6.25%	2319
Mercy Hospital	Bakersfield	6.66%	2583
Kaiser Permanente San Francisco Med Ctr	San Francisco	6.87%	1675

NOTE: Hospital profiles are in alphabetical order by state, then city, then hospital within the city; Rankings are sorted by rate in descending order and exclude hospitals with less than 25 cases; (1) The number of cases is too small (n<25) for purposes of reliably predicting hospital performance; (2) Measure reflects the hospital's indication that its submission was based upon a sample of its relevant discharges; (3) Rate reflects fewer than the maximum possible quarters of data for the measure; (4) Inaccurate information submitted and suppressed for one or more quarters; (5) No data is available from the hospital for this measure; Please refer to the User's Guide for a full explanation of data

Alameda Hospital

2070 Clinton Avenue — Phone: 510-522-3700
Alameda, CA 94501 — Fax: 510-814-4005
E-mail: Communityrelations@alamedahospital.org
URL: www.alamedahospital.org
Ownership: Voluntary non-profit - Private — Accredited: Yes
Emergency Services: Yes — Licensed Beds: 135

Key Personnel:
Executive Director . . . . Richard A Warner
CEO. . . . . Stuart Jed
President Medical Staff . . . . Eric Otani, MD
Emergency Room . . . . Cindy Lambdin, RN
Director Respiratory Therapy . . . . Mary Pat Skropeta

Measure	Cases	This Hospital	State Average	U.S. Average	Top Hospital
Heart Attack Care					
ACE Inhibitor or ARB for LVSD[1]	21	71%	82%	82%	100%
Aspirin at Arrival	125	98%	95%	92%	100%
Aspirin at Discharge	88	97%	90%	90%	100%
Beta Blocker at Arrival	125	99%	89%	87%	100%
Beta Blocker at Discharge	98	99%	89%	90%	100%
Fibrinolytic Medication Timing[1]	13	15%	40%	31%	100%
PCI Within 90 Minutes of Arrival	0	-	52%	54%	95%
Smoking Cessation Advice[1]	15	87%	87%	88%	100%
Heart Failure Care					
ACE Inhibitor or ARB for LVSD	35	80%	84%	82%	100%
Discharge Instructions	112	12%	56%	61%	93%
Evaluation of LVS Function	173	87%	84%	83%	99%
Smoking Cessation Advice[1]	21	95%	82%	82%	100%
Pneumonia Care					
Appropriate Initial Antibiotic	76	71%	82%	83%	94%
Blood Culture Timing	106	86%	89%	90%	100%
Influenza Vaccine	38	16%	58%	70%	100%
Initial Antibiotic Timing	158	85%	75%	80%	93%
Oxygenation Assessment	184	100%	99%	99%	100%
Pneumococcal Vaccine	114	23%	58%	69%	94%
Smoking Cessation Advice	27	96%	75%	80%	100%
Surgical Infection Prevention					
Prophylactic Antibiotic Given[1,3]	24	79%	74%	77%	95%
Prophylactic Antibiotic Selection	25	100%	89%	90%	100%
Prophylactic Antibiotic Stopped[1,3]	23	83%	65%	72%	95%
Pregnancy Care					
Inpatient Neonatal Mortality	-	-	-	-	-
Third or Fourth Degree Laceration	-	-	3.58%	3.63%	3.27%

Alhambra Hospital Medical Center

100 South Raymond Avenue — Phone: 626-570-1606
Alhambra, CA 91801 — Fax: 626-570-8825
E-mail: info@alhambrahospital.com
URL: www.alhambrahospital.com
Ownership: Proprietary — Accredited: Yes
Emergency Services: Yes — Licensed Beds: 144

Key Personnel:
CEO. . . . . Lee Fuyenaga
Chief Medical Staff. . . . . Tommy Lu, MD
Director Respiratory Therapy . . . . Jose Ortega

Measure	Cases	This Hospital	State Average	U.S. Average	Top Hospital
Heart Attack Care					
ACE Inhibitor or ARB for LVSD[1]	4	75%	82%	82%	100%
Aspirin at Arrival	36	89%	95%	92%	100%
Aspirin at Discharge[1]	17	59%	90%	90%	100%
Beta Blocker at Arrival	34	68%	89%	87%	100%
Beta Blocker at Discharge[1]	15	60%	89%	90%	100%
Fibrinolytic Medication Timing	0	-	40%	31%	100%
PCI Within 90 Minutes of Arrival	0	-	52%	54%	95%
Smoking Cessation Advice[1]	4	25%	87%	88%	100%
Heart Failure Care					
ACE Inhibitor or ARB for LVSD[1]	23	48%	84%	82%	100%
Discharge Instructions	112	10%	56%	61%	93%
Evaluation of LVS Function	142	76%	84%	83%	99%
Smoking Cessation Advice[1]	6	33%	82%	82%	100%
Pneumonia Care					
Appropriate Initial Antibiotic[2]	87	70%	82%	83%	94%
Blood Culture Timing[2]	130	87%	89%	90%	100%
Influenza Vaccine	59	8%	58%	70%	100%
Initial Antibiotic Timing[2]	231	74%	75%	80%	93%
Oxygenation Assessment[2]	397	100%	99%	99%	100%
Pneumococcal Vaccine[2]	287	13%	58%	69%	94%
Smoking Cessation Advice[1,2]	23	26%	75%	80%	100%
Surgical Infection Prevention					
Prophylactic Antibiotic Given[1,3]	13	69%	74%	77%	95%
Prophylactic Antibiotic Selection[5]	-	-	89%	90%	100%
Prophylactic Antibiotic Stopped[1,3]	13	8%	65%	72%	95%
Pregnancy Care					
Inpatient Neonatal Mortality	-	-	-	-	-
Third or Fourth Degree Laceration	-	-	3.58%	3.63%	3.27%

Modoc Medical Center

228 W McDowell Street — Phone: 530-233-5131
Alturas, CA 96101 — Fax: 530-233-5884
URL: www.modocmedicalcenter.com
Ownership: Voluntary non-profit - Other — Accredited: No
Emergency Services: No — Licensed Beds: 87

Key Personnel:
Chief Executive Officer. Bruce Porter
Chief Medical Staff. . . . . Edward P Richert, MD
Director Infection/Disease Control . . . . Joann Kemble
Director Medical/Surgical Nursing . . . . Delinda Gover
Chief Radiology . . . . William Boland
Director Respiratory Therapy . . . . Michele Marymee

Measure	Cases	This Hospital	State Average	U.S. Average	Top Hospital
Heart Attack Care					
ACE Inhibitor or ARB for LVSD[3]	0	-	82%	82%	100%
Aspirin at Arrival[3]	0	-	95%	92%	100%
Aspirin at Discharge[3]	0	-	90%	90%	100%
Beta Blocker at Arrival[1,3]	1	100%	89%	87%	100%
Beta Blocker at Discharge[3]	0	-	89%	90%	100%
Fibrinolytic Medication Timing[5]	-	-	40%	31%	100%
PCI Within 90 Minutes of Arrival[5]	-	-	52%	54%	95%
Smoking Cessation Advice[5]	-	-	87%	88%	100%
Heart Failure Care					
ACE Inhibitor or ARB for LVSD[3]	0	-	84%	82%	100%
Discharge Instructions[1,3]	1	0%	56%	61%	93%
Evaluation of LVS Function[1,3]	5	20%	84%	83%	99%
Smoking Cessation Advice[1,3]	1	0%	82%	82%	100%
Pneumonia Care					
Appropriate Initial Antibiotic[1,3]	2	100%	82%	83%	94%
Blood Culture Timing[3]	0	-	89%	90%	100%
Influenza Vaccine[5]	-	-	58%	70%	100%
Initial Antibiotic Timing[1,3]	9	44%	75%	80%	93%
Oxygenation Assessment[1,3]	10	100%	99%	99%	100%
Pneumococcal Vaccine[1,3]	5	40%	58%	69%	94%
Smoking Cessation Advice[3]	0	-	75%	80%	100%
Surgical Infection Prevention					
Prophylactic Antibiotic Given[5]	-	-	74%	77%	95%
Prophylactic Antibiotic Selection[5]	-	-	89%	90%	100%
Prophylactic Antibiotic Stopped[5]	-	-	65%	72%	95%
Pregnancy Care					
Inpatient Neonatal Mortality	-	-	-	-	-
Third or Fourth Degree Laceration	-	-	3.58%	3.63%	3.27%

Anaheim General Hospital

3350 W Ball Road — Phone: 714-827-6700
Anaheim, CA 92804 — Fax: 714-821-6537
Ownership: Proprietary — Accredited: Yes
Emergency Services: Yes — Licensed Beds: 143

Key Personnel:
CEO. . . . . Josh Luke
Chief Medical Staff. . . . . C Kim Sang
Emergency Room . . . . Denise Flaws
Emergency Room . . . . Gloria Marston, RN
Director Medical/Surgical Nursing . . . . Ruth Johnson
OB/GYN Womens Health. . . . . Sang C Kim, MD
Chief Radiology . . . . Jason Liu, MD

NOTE: Hospital profiles are in alphabetical order by state, then city, then hospital within the city; Rankings are sorted by rate in descending order and exclude hospitals with less than 25 cases; (1) The number of cases is too small (n<25) for purposes of reliably predicting hospital performance; (2) Measure reflects the hospital's indication that its submission was based upon a sample of its relevant discharges; (3) Rate reflects fewer than the maximum possible quarters of data for the measure; (4) Inaccurate information submitted and suppressed for one or more quarters; (5) No data is available from the hospital for this measure; Please refer to the User's Guide for a full explanation of data

Director Respiratory Therapy . . . . Marcia Bael

Measure	Cases	This Hospital	State Average	U.S. Average	Top Hospital
Heart Attack Care					
ACE Inhibitor or ARB for LVSD[1,3]	1	0%	82%	82%	100%
Aspirin at Arrival[1,3]	6	100%	95%	92%	100%
Aspirin at Discharge[1,3]	7	43%	90%	90%	100%
Beta Blocker at Arrival[1,3]	6	67%	89%	87%	100%
Beta Blocker at Discharge[1,3]	7	0%	89%	90%	100%
Fibrinolytic Medication Timing[3]	0	-	40%	31%	100%
PCI Within 90 Minutes of Arrival	0	-	52%	54%	95%
Smoking Cessation Advice[3]	0	-	87%	88%	100%
Heart Failure Care					
ACE Inhibitor or ARB for LVSD[1]	10	70%	84%	82%	100%
Discharge Instructions[1,3]	5	0%	56%	61%	93%
Evaluation of LVS Function	35	77%	84%	83%	99%
Smoking Cessation Advice[3]	0	-	82%	82%	100%
Pneumonia Care					
Appropriate Initial Antibiotic[1,3]	18	50%	82%	83%	94%
Blood Culture Timing[1,3]	15	73%	89%	90%	100%
Influenza Vaccine[5]	-	-	58%	70%	100%
Initial Antibiotic Timing	53	83%	75%	80%	93%
Oxygenation Assessment	66	95%	99%	99%	100%
Pneumococcal Vaccine	44	0%	58%	69%	94%
Smoking Cessation Advice[1,3]	2	0%	75%	80%	100%
Surgical Infection Prevention					
Prophylactic Antibiotic Given[1,3]	4	25%	74%	77%	95%
Prophylactic Antibiotic Selection[5]	-	-	89%	90%	100%
Prophylactic Antibiotic Stopped[1,3]	2	100%	65%	72%	95%
Pregnancy Care					
Inpatient Neonatal Mortality	136	0.00%	-	-	-
Third or Fourth Degree Laceration	96	2.08%	3.58%	3.63%	3.27%

Anaheim Memorial Medical Center

1111 W LaPalma Avenue
Anaheim, CA 92801
URL: www.memorialcare.org/anaheim
Ownership: Voluntary non-profit - Private
Emergency Services: Yes
Phone: 714-774-1450
Fax: 714-999-6027
Accredited: Yes
Licensed Beds: 217

Key Personnel:

CEO. . . . . Melinda Beswick
Chief Medical Staff. . . . . Mahaveer Kuemka, MD
Director Emergency Services. . . . . Angeli Leggitt
Executive Director Cardiovascular . . . . Donna Nash
Executive Director Cardiovascular Svcs. . . . . . . Donna Nash
Director Women's Services . . . . Pam Moseley
Manager Respiratory Services. . . . . Sherry Blansfield

Measure	Cases	This Hospital	State Average	U.S. Average	Top Hospital
Heart Attack Care					
ACE Inhibitor or ARB for LVSD	49	100%	82%	82%	100%
Aspirin at Arrival	204	99%	95%	92%	100%
Aspirin at Discharge	396	99%	90%	90%	100%
Beta Blocker at Arrival	162	100%	89%	87%	100%
Beta Blocker at Discharge	384	100%	89%	90%	100%
Fibrinolytic Medication Timing[1]	2	50%	40%	31%	100%
PCI Within 90 Minutes of Arrival[1]	15	73%	52%	54%	95%
Smoking Cessation Advice	108	100%	87%	88%	100%
Heart Failure Care					
ACE Inhibitor or ARB for LVSD	207	96%	84%	82%	100%
Discharge Instructions	495	89%	56%	61%	93%
Evaluation of LVS Function	576	98%	84%	83%	99%
Smoking Cessation Advice	82	99%	82%	82%	100%
Pneumonia Care					
Appropriate Initial Antibiotic	286	78%	82%	83%	94%
Blood Culture Timing	281	95%	89%	90%	100%
Influenza Vaccine	93	63%	58%	70%	100%
Initial Antibiotic Timing	437	87%	75%	80%	93%
Oxygenation Assessment	524	100%	99%	99%	100%
Pneumococcal Vaccine	377	79%	58%	69%	94%
Smoking Cessation Advice	83	98%	75%	80%	100%
Surgical Infection Prevention					
Prophylactic Antibiotic Given[2,3]	418	84%	74%	77%	95%
Prophylactic Antibiotic Selection[2]	64	69%	89%	90%	100%
Prophylactic Antibiotic Stopped[2,3]	408	53%	65%	72%	95%
Pregnancy Care					
Inpatient Neonatal Mortality	2,035	0.39%	-	-	-
Third or Fourth Degree Laceration	1,457	3.09%	3.58%	3.63%	3.27%

Kaiser Permanente Anaheim Medical Center

441 N Lakeview Avenue
Anaheim, CA 92807
Ownership: Voluntary non-profit - Other
Emergency Services: Yes
Phone: 714-279-4000
Fax: 714-279-5590
Accredited: Yes
Licensed Beds: 200

Key Personnel:

President/CEO. . . . . Janice Head
Chief Medical Staff. . . . . Edward Ellison, MD
Emergency Room . . . . Mario Cuevas
Emergency Room . . . . Robert Becker, MD
OB/GYN/Women's Health . . . . Maggie Pierce
Director of Pulmonary/Respiratory Care. . . . . . . Eten Bondoc

Measure	Cases	This Hospital	State Average	U.S. Average	Top Hospital
Heart Attack Care					
ACE Inhibitor or ARB for LVSD[1]	16	94%	82%	82%	100%
Aspirin at Arrival	77	97%	95%	92%	100%
Aspirin at Discharge	47	100%	90%	90%	100%
Beta Blocker at Arrival	77	95%	89%	87%	100%
Beta Blocker at Discharge	48	92%	89%	90%	100%
Fibrinolytic Medication Timing[1]	14	64%	40%	31%	100%
PCI Within 90 Minutes of Arrival	0	-	52%	54%	95%
Smoking Cessation Advice[1]	11	64%	87%	88%	100%
Heart Failure Care					
ACE Inhibitor or ARB for LVSD	60	82%	84%	82%	100%
Discharge Instructions	137	32%	56%	61%	93%
Evaluation of LVS Function	155	97%	84%	83%	99%
Smoking Cessation Advice	26	65%	82%	82%	100%
Pneumonia Care					
Appropriate Initial Antibiotic	91	57%	82%	83%	94%
Blood Culture Timing	71	92%	89%	90%	100%
Influenza Vaccine	27	85%	58%	70%	100%
Initial Antibiotic Timing	101	62%	75%	80%	93%
Oxygenation Assessment	121	100%	99%	99%	100%
Pneumococcal Vaccine	75	92%	58%	69%	94%
Smoking Cessation Advice[1]	14	36%	75%	80%	100%
Surgical Infection Prevention					
Prophylactic Antibiotic Given[3]	43	58%	74%	77%	95%
Prophylactic Antibiotic Selection	42	76%	89%	90%	100%
Prophylactic Antibiotic Stopped[3]	38	50%	65%	72%	95%
Pregnancy Care					
Inpatient Neonatal Mortality	3,398	0.35%	-	-	-
Third or Fourth Degree Laceration	2,391	2.30%	3.58%	3.63%	3.27%

West Anaheim Medical Center

3033 W Orange Avenue
Anaheim, CA 92804
E-mail: info@westanaheimmedctr.com
URL: wamc.phcs.us
Ownership: Proprietary
Emergency Services: Yes
Phone: 714-827-3000
Fax: 714-229-4052
Accredited: Yes
Licensed Beds: 219

Key Personnel:

Regional CEO . . . . Virg Narbutas

Measure	Cases	This Hospital	State Average	U.S. Average	Top Hospital
Heart Attack Care					
ACE Inhibitor or ARB for LVSD[1]	24	79%	82%	82%	100%
Aspirin at Arrival	98	93%	95%	92%	100%
Aspirin at Discharge	101	84%	90%	90%	100%
Beta Blocker at Arrival	88	86%	89%	87%	100%
Beta Blocker at Discharge	105	83%	89%	90%	100%
Fibrinolytic Medication Timing[1]	10	30%	40%	31%	100%
PCI Within 90 Minutes of Arrival	0	-	52%	54%	95%
Smoking Cessation Advice	38	89%	87%	88%	100%
Heart Failure Care					

NOTE: Hospital profiles are in alphabetical order by state, then city, then hospital within the city; Rankings are sorted by rate in descending order and exclude hospitals with less than 25 cases; (1) The number of cases is too small (n<25) for purposes of reliably predicting hospital performance; (2) Measure reflects the hospital's indication that its submission was based upon a sample of its relevant discharges; (3) Rate reflects fewer than the maximum possible quarters of data for the measure; (4) Inaccurate information submitted and suppressed for one or more quarters; (5) No data is available from the hospital for this measure; Please refer to the User's Guide for a full explanation of data

ACE Inhibitor or ARB for LVSD[2]	69	77%	84%	82%	100%
Discharge Instructions[2]	185	79%	56%	61%	93%
Evaluation of LVS Function[2]	249	89%	84%	83%	99%
Smoking Cessation Advice[2]	37	97%	82%	82%	100%
Pneumonia Care					
Appropriate Initial Antibiotic[2]	148	65%	82%	83%	94%
Blood Culture Timing[2]	115	93%	89%	90%	100%
Influenza Vaccine[2]	60	0%	58%	70%	100%
Initial Antibiotic Timing[2]	204	81%	75%	80%	93%
Oxygenation Assessment[2]	259	98%	99%	99%	100%
Pneumococcal Vaccine[2]	157	13%	58%	69%	94%
Smoking Cessation Advice[2]	33	100%	75%	80%	100%
Surgical Infection Prevention					
Prophylactic Antibiotic Given[2]	84	79%	74%	77%	95%
Prophylactic Antibiotic Selection[1,2]	16	81%	89%	90%	100%
Prophylactic Antibiotic Stopped[2]	82	87%	65%	72%	95%
Pregnancy Care					
Inpatient Neonatal Mortality	-	-	-	-	-
Third or Fourth Degree Laceration	-	-	3.58%	3.63%	3.27%

Western Medical Center Hospital Anaheim

1025 S Anaheim Boulevard
Anaheim, CA 92805
Phone: 714-533-6220
Fax: 714-563-2839
URL: www.westernmedanaheim.com
Ownership: Proprietary
Accredited: Yes
Emergency Services: Yes
Licensed Beds: 188

Key Personnel:

CEO. . . . . Casey Fatch
Chief Medical Staff. . . . . Jayanti Patel
Emergency Room . . . . Mary Groell, RN
Director Medical/Surgical Nursing . . . . Sue Graves
OB/GYN Womens Health. . . . . Barbara Stebodnick
Director Radiology . . . . Patty Clauson
Manager Respiratory Therapy . . . . Andy Bogy

Measure	Cases	This Hospital	State Average	U.S. Average	Top Hospital
Heart Attack Care					
ACE Inhibitor or ARB for LVSD[1]	14	50%	82%	82%	100%
Aspirin at Arrival	34	91%	95%	92%	100%
Aspirin at Discharge	132	87%	90%	90%	100%
Beta Blocker at Arrival	26	92%	89%	87%	100%
Beta Blocker at Discharge	126	84%	89%	90%	100%
Fibrinolytic Medication Timing[1]	2	50%	40%	31%	100%
PCI Within 90 Minutes of Arrival	0	-	52%	54%	95%
Smoking Cessation Advice	39	95%	87%	88%	100%
Heart Failure Care					
ACE Inhibitor or ARB for LVSD[1]	20	80%	84%	82%	100%
Discharge Instructions	35	77%	56%	61%	93%
Evaluation of LVS Function	59	95%	84%	83%	99%
Smoking Cessation Advice[1]	13	100%	82%	82%	100%
Pneumonia Care					
Appropriate Initial Antibiotic	36	86%	82%	83%	94%
Blood Culture Timing	57	88%	89%	90%	100%
Influenza Vaccine[1]	17	76%	58%	70%	100%
Initial Antibiotic Timing	85	89%	75%	80%	93%
Oxygenation Assessment	99	100%	99%	99%	100%
Pneumococcal Vaccine	59	92%	58%	69%	94%
Smoking Cessation Advice[1]	17	88%	75%	80%	100%
Surgical Infection Prevention					
Prophylactic Antibiotic Given[1,3]	18	61%	74%	77%	95%
Prophylactic Antibiotic Selection[1]	18	94%	89%	90%	100%
Prophylactic Antibiotic Stopped[1,3]	18	44%	65%	72%	95%
Pregnancy Care					
Inpatient Neonatal Mortality	-	-	-	-	-
Third or Fourth Degree Laceration	-	-	3.58%	3.63%	3.27%

Sutter Delta Medical Center

3901 Lone Tree Way
Antioch, CA 94509
Phone: 925-779-7200
Fax: 925-779-7276
E-mail: monfort@sutterdelta.org
URL: www.sutterdelta.org
Ownership: Voluntary non-profit - Private
Accredited: Yes
Emergency Services: Yes
Licensed Beds: 111

Key Personnel:

CEO. . . . . Gary Rapaport
Emergency Room . . . . Allison Mielicke
OB/GYN Womens Health. . . . . Daniel Zimmerman, MD
Chief Radiology . . . . Samuel Choi, MD
Director Respiratory Therapy . . . . Darci Dumford

Measure	Cases	This Hospital	State Average	U.S. Average	Top Hospital
Heart Attack Care					
ACE Inhibitor or ARB for LVSD[1]	19	95%	82%	82%	100%
Aspirin at Arrival	154	94%	95%	92%	100%
Aspirin at Discharge	73	84%	90%	90%	100%
Beta Blocker at Arrival	148	91%	89%	87%	100%
Beta Blocker at Discharge	81	94%	89%	90%	100%
Fibrinolytic Medication Timing	32	34%	40%	31%	100%
PCI Within 90 Minutes of Arrival	0	-	52%	54%	95%
Smoking Cessation Advice[1]	22	100%	87%	88%	100%
Heart Failure Care					
ACE Inhibitor or ARB for LVSD	78	88%	84%	82%	100%
Discharge Instructions	253	88%	56%	61%	93%
Evaluation of LVS Function	300	80%	84%	83%	99%
Smoking Cessation Advice	61	98%	82%	82%	100%
Pneumonia Care					
Appropriate Initial Antibiotic[2]	134	73%	82%	83%	94%
Blood Culture Timing[2]	111	79%	89%	90%	100%
Influenza Vaccine[1,2]	23	13%	58%	70%	100%
Initial Antibiotic Timing[2]	162	70%	75%	80%	93%
Oxygenation Assessment[2]	195	100%	99%	99%	100%
Pneumococcal Vaccine[2]	94	38%	58%	69%	94%
Smoking Cessation Advice[2]	41	93%	75%	80%	100%
Surgical Infection Prevention					
Prophylactic Antibiotic Given[2]	150	49%	74%	77%	95%
Prophylactic Antibiotic Selection[2]	34	94%	89%	90%	100%
Prophylactic Antibiotic Stopped[2]	131	72%	65%	72%	95%
Pregnancy Care					
Inpatient Neonatal Mortality	-	-	-	-	-
Third or Fourth Degree Laceration	-	-	3.58%	3.63%	3.27%

Saint Mary Medical Center

Alternate Name: Saint Mary's Desert Valley Hospital
18300 Highway 18
Apple Valley, CA 92307
Toll-Free: 866-784-5455
Phone: 760-242-2311
Fax: 760-242-9750
URL: www.stmaryapplevalley.com
Ownership: Voluntary non-profit - Church
Accredited: Yes
Emergency Services: Yes
Licensed Beds: 186

Key Personnel:

President/CEO. . . . . Jason Barker
Emergency Room . . . . Rick Smith

Measure	Cases	This Hospital	State Average	U.S. Average	Top Hospital
Heart Attack Care					
ACE Inhibitor or ARB for LVSD	50	72%	82%	82%	100%
Aspirin at Arrival	234	98%	95%	92%	100%
Aspirin at Discharge	254	91%	90%	90%	100%
Beta Blocker at Arrival	193	93%	89%	87%	100%
Beta Blocker at Discharge	243	76%	89%	90%	100%
Fibrinolytic Medication Timing[1]	7	29%	40%	31%	100%
PCI Within 90 Minutes of Arrival[1]	5	60%	52%	54%	95%
Smoking Cessation Advice	85	98%	87%	88%	100%
Heart Failure Care					
ACE Inhibitor or ARB for LVSD	164	76%	84%	82%	100%
Discharge Instructions	401	60%	56%	61%	93%
Evaluation of LVS Function	434	75%	84%	83%	99%
Smoking Cessation Advice	112	95%	82%	82%	100%
Pneumonia Care					

NOTE: Hospital profiles are in alphabetical order by state, then city, then hospital within the city; Rankings are sorted by rate in descending order and exclude hospitals with less than 25 cases; (1) The number of cases is too small (n<25) for purposes of reliably predicting hospital performance; (2) Measure reflects the hospital's indication that its submission was based upon a sample of its relevant discharges; (3) Rate reflects fewer than the maximum possible quarters of data for the measure; (4) Inaccurate information submitted and suppressed for one or more quarters; (5) No data is available from the hospital for this measure; Please refer to the User's Guide for a full explanation of data

Measure	Cases	This Hospital	State Average	U.S. Average	Top Hospital
Appropriate Initial Antibiotic	430	87%	82%	83%	94%
Blood Culture Timing	291	90%	89%	90%	100%
Influenza Vaccine	75	44%	58%	70%	100%
Initial Antibiotic Timing	454	78%	75%	80%	93%
Oxygenation Assessment	536	99%	99%	99%	100%
Pneumococcal Vaccine	286	72%	58%	69%	94%
Smoking Cessation Advice	95	82%	75%	80%	100%
Surgical Infection Prevention					
Prophylactic Antibiotic Given[3]	442	82%	74%	77%	95%
Prophylactic Antibiotic Selection	127	90%	89%	90%	100%
Prophylactic Antibiotic Stopped[3]	429	59%	65%	72%	95%
Pregnancy Care					
Inpatient Neonatal Mortality	2,855	0.49%	-	-	-
Third or Fourth Degree Laceration	2,159	4.96%	3.58%	3.63%	3.27%

Methodist Hospital of Southern California

300 W Huntington Drive
Arcadia, CA 91007
Phone: 626-445-4441
Fax: 626-574-3767
E-mail: info@methodisthospital.org
URL: www.methodisthospital.org
Ownership: Voluntary non-profit - Church
Accredited: Yes
Emergency Services: Yes
Licensed Beds: 460

Key Personnel:
President & CEO . . . . Dennis M Lee
Chief Medical Staff. . . . . Dino Clarizio, MD
Director Infection/Disease Control . . . . Pauline Lopez, RN
CCU Spvg. Nurse . . . . Delia Jervis, RN
Chief OB/GYN . . . . Manjee Kumar, MD
Director Radiology . . . . Joseph Lussier
Director of Respiratory . . . . Denis Ung

Measure	Cases	This Hospital	State Average	U.S. Average	Top Hospital
Heart Attack Care					
ACE Inhibitor or ARB for LVSD	33	97%	82%	82%	100%
Aspirin at Arrival	165	95%	95%	92%	100%
Aspirin at Discharge	162	95%	90%	90%	100%
Beta Blocker at Arrival	129	90%	89%	87%	100%
Beta Blocker at Discharge	159	94%	89%	90%	100%
Fibrinolytic Medication Timing	0	-	40%	31%	100%
PCI Within 90 Minutes of Arrival[1]	17	59%	52%	54%	95%
Smoking Cessation Advice	42	93%	87%	88%	100%
Heart Failure Care					
ACE Inhibitor or ARB for LVSD	189	79%	84%	82%	100%
Discharge Instructions	480	81%	56%	61%	93%
Evaluation of LVS Function	634	95%	84%	83%	99%
Smoking Cessation Advice	63	79%	82%	82%	100%
Pneumonia Care					
Appropriate Initial Antibiotic	341	87%	82%	83%	94%
Blood Culture Timing	260	92%	89%	90%	100%
Influenza Vaccine	108	44%	58%	70%	100%
Initial Antibiotic Timing	499	83%	75%	80%	93%
Oxygenation Assessment	593	99%	99%	99%	100%
Pneumococcal Vaccine	412	31%	58%	69%	94%
Smoking Cessation Advice	57	70%	75%	80%	100%
Surgical Infection Prevention					
Prophylactic Antibiotic Given[3]	182	63%	74%	77%	95%
Prophylactic Antibiotic Selection	181	90%	89%	90%	100%
Prophylactic Antibiotic Stopped[3]	176	45%	65%	72%	95%
Pregnancy Care					
Inpatient Neonatal Mortality	-	-	-	-	-
Third or Fourth Degree Laceration	-	-	3.58%	3.63%	3.27%

Mad River Community Hospital

3800 Janes Road
Arcata, CA 95521
Phone: 707-822-3621
Fax: 707-822-6311
E-mail: mrch@madriverhospital.com
URL: www.madriverhospital.com
Ownership: Proprietary
Accredited: No
Emergency Services: Yes
Licensed Beds: 78

Key Personnel:
President/CEO. . . . . Douglas Shaw
Chief Medical Staff. . . . . Timothy Nicely
Emergency Room . . . . Tina Wood
Infection Control. . . . . Jennifer Cox
ICU . . . . Margery Young
Intensive/Coronary Care . . . . Margery Young
Medical/Surgical Nursing . . . . Margery Young
OB/GYN Womens Health. . . . . Patricia Ehlert-Abler
Surgical Servicves . . . . Margery Young
Respiratory/Cardiopulmonary. . . . . Jennie Potter

Measure	Cases	This Hospital	State Average	U.S. Average	Top Hospital
Heart Attack Care					
ACE Inhibitor or ARB for LVSD[1]	2	50%	82%	82%	100%
Aspirin at Arrival[1]	19	95%	95%	92%	100%
Aspirin at Discharge[1]	13	85%	90%	90%	100%
Beta Blocker at Arrival[1]	15	100%	89%	87%	100%
Beta Blocker at Discharge[1]	17	94%	89%	90%	100%
Fibrinolytic Medication Timing[3]	0	-	40%	31%	100%
PCI Within 90 Minutes of Arrival	0	-	52%	54%	95%
Smoking Cessation Advice[1,3]	2	100%	87%	88%	100%
Heart Failure Care					
ACE Inhibitor or ARB for LVSD[1]	24	88%	84%	82%	100%
Discharge Instructions[1,3]	10	60%	56%	61%	93%
Evaluation of LVS Function	78	72%	84%	83%	99%
Smoking Cessation Advice[1,3]	3	100%	82%	82%	100%
Pneumonia Care					
Appropriate Initial Antibiotic[1,3]	3	67%	82%	83%	94%
Blood Culture Timing[1,3]	6	100%	89%	90%	100%
Influenza Vaccine[5]	-	-	58%	70%	100%
Initial Antibiotic Timing	67	90%	75%	80%	93%
Oxygenation Assessment	77	100%	99%	99%	100%
Pneumococcal Vaccine	47	47%	58%	69%	94%
Smoking Cessation Advice[1,3]	1	100%	75%	80%	100%
Surgical Infection Prevention					
Prophylactic Antibiotic Given[1,3]	22	55%	74%	77%	95%
Prophylactic Antibiotic Selection[5]	-	-	89%	90%	100%
Prophylactic Antibiotic Stopped[1,3]	21	57%	65%	72%	95%
Pregnancy Care					
Inpatient Neonatal Mortality	-	-	-	-	-
Third or Fourth Degree Laceration	-	-	3.58%	3.63%	3.27%

Arroyo Grande Community Hospital

345 S Halcyon Road
Arroyo Grande, CA 93420
Phone: 805-489-4261
Fax: 805-473-7603
URL: www.arroyograndehospital.org
Ownership: Voluntary non-profit - Private
Accredited: Yes
Emergency Services: Yes
Licensed Beds: 65

Key Personnel:
President/CEO. . . . . Lloyd H Dean
Emergency Room . . . . Dan Culhane
Emergency Room . . . . Eugene Keller
Director Respiratory Therapy . . . . Steve Goss

Measure	Cases	This Hospital	State Average	U.S. Average	Top Hospital
Heart Attack Care					
ACE Inhibitor or ARB for LVSD[1]	6	100%	82%	82%	100%
Aspirin at Arrival	32	97%	95%	92%	100%
Aspirin at Discharge[1]	21	90%	90%	90%	100%
Beta Blocker at Arrival	31	94%	89%	87%	100%
Beta Blocker at Discharge[1]	21	90%	89%	90%	100%
Fibrinolytic Medication Timing	0	-	40%	31%	100%
PCI Within 90 Minutes of Arrival	0	-	52%	54%	95%
Smoking Cessation Advice[1]	2	100%	87%	88%	100%
Heart Failure Care					
ACE Inhibitor or ARB for LVSD[1]	24	92%	84%	82%	100%
Discharge Instructions	90	93%	56%	61%	93%
Evaluation of LVS Function	103	89%	84%	83%	99%
Smoking Cessation Advice[1]	12	100%	82%	82%	100%
Pneumonia Care					
Appropriate Initial Antibiotic	128	88%	82%	83%	94%
Blood Culture Timing	92	90%	89%	90%	100%
Influenza Vaccine[1]	24	88%	58%	70%	100%
Initial Antibiotic Timing	132	88%	75%	80%	93%
Oxygenation Assessment	160	99%	99%	99%	100%

NOTE: Hospital profiles are in alphabetical order by state, then city, then hospital within the city; Rankings are sorted by rate in descending order and exclude hospitals with less than 25 cases; (1) The number of cases is too small (n<25) for purposes of reliably predicting hospital performance; (2) Measure reflects the hospital's indication that its submission was based upon a sample of its relevant discharges; (3) Rate reflects fewer than the maximum possible quarters of data for the measure; (4) Inaccurate information submitted and suppressed for one or more quarters; (5) No data is available from the hospital for this measure; Please refer to the User's Guide for a full explanation of data

Measure	Cases	This Hospital	State Average	U.S. Average	Top Hospital
Pneumococcal Vaccine	112	71%	58%	69%	94%
Smoking Cessation Advice[1]	24	88%	75%	80%	100%
Surgical Infection Prevention					
Prophylactic Antibiotic Given[2,3]	116	90%	74%	77%	95%
Prophylactic Antibiotic Selection[2]	37	100%	89%	90%	100%
Prophylactic Antibiotic Stopped[2,3]	115	99%	65%	72%	95%
Pregnancy Care					
Inpatient Neonatal Mortality	-	-	-	-	-
Third or Fourth Degree Laceration	-	-	3.58%	3.63%	3.27%

Sutter Auburn Faith Hospital

11815 Education Street
Auburn, CA 95602
URL: www.sutterauburnfaith.org
Ownership: Voluntary non-profit - Other
Emergency Services: Yes
Phone: 530-888-4500
Fax: 530-889-6054
Accredited: Yes
Licensed Beds: 98

Key Personnel:
President/CEO . . . . Patrick Fry
Emergency Room . . . . Lisa Ralston
Director Medical/Surgical Nursing . . . . Reberta Mori
Chief Radiology . . . . Bob Brearley
Director Respiratory Therapy . . . . Ronna Davis

Measure	Cases	This Hospital	State Average	U.S. Average	Top Hospital
Heart Attack Care					
ACE Inhibitor or ARB for LVSD[1]	2	100%	82%	82%	100%
Aspirin at Arrival[1]	22	100%	95%	92%	100%
Aspirin at Discharge[1]	10	90%	90%	90%	100%
Beta Blocker at Arrival[1]	15	100%	89%	87%	100%
Beta Blocker at Discharge[1]	9	100%	89%	90%	100%
Fibrinolytic Medication Timing[1]	4	75%	40%	31%	100%
PCI Within 90 Minutes of Arrival	0	-	52%	54%	95%
Smoking Cessation Advice	0	-	87%	88%	100%
Heart Failure Care					
ACE Inhibitor or ARB for LVSD	45	98%	84%	82%	100%
Discharge Instructions	123	89%	56%	61%	93%
Evaluation of LVS Function	163	99%	84%	83%	99%
Smoking Cessation Advice	32	100%	82%	82%	100%
Pneumonia Care					
Appropriate Initial Antibiotic[2]	104	94%	82%	83%	94%
Blood Culture Timing[2]	89	99%	89%	90%	100%
Influenza Vaccine[2]	27	74%	58%	70%	100%
Initial Antibiotic Timing[2]	145	90%	75%	80%	93%
Oxygenation Assessment[2]	170	100%	99%	99%	100%
Pneumococcal Vaccine[2]	108	93%	58%	69%	94%
Smoking Cessation Advice[2]	35	100%	75%	80%	100%
Surgical Infection Prevention					
Prophylactic Antibiotic Given[2]	202	83%	74%	77%	95%
Prophylactic Antibiotic Selection[2]	52	88%	89%	90%	100%
Prophylactic Antibiotic Stopped[2]	194	81%	65%	72%	95%
Pregnancy Care					
Inpatient Neonatal Mortality	-	-	-	-	-
Third or Fourth Degree Laceration	-	-	3.58%	3.63%	3.27%

Catalina Island Medical Center

100 Falls Canyon Road
PO Box 1563
Avalon, CA 90704
Ownership: Voluntary non-profit - Private
Emergency Services: Yes
Phone: 310-510-0700
Fax: 310-510-2938
Accredited: No
Licensed Beds: 12

Key Personnel:
President/CEO . . . . William M Greene, FACHE
Chief Medical Staff . . . . Peter Trottier, MD
Medical/Surgical Nursing . . . . Doreen Macktal, RN

Measure	Cases	This Hospital	State Average	U.S. Average	Top Hospital
Heart Attack Care					
ACE Inhibitor or ARB for LVSD[5]	-	-	82%	82%	100%
Aspirin at Arrival[5]	-	-	95%	92%	100%
Aspirin at Discharge[5]	-	-	90%	90%	100%
Beta Blocker at Arrival[5]	-	-	89%	87%	100%
Beta Blocker at Discharge[5]	-	-	89%	90%	100%
Fibrinolytic Medication Timing[5]	-	-	40%	31%	100%
PCI Within 90 Minutes of Arrival[5]	-	-	52%	54%	95%
Smoking Cessation Advice[5]	-	-	87%	88%	100%
Heart Failure Care					
ACE Inhibitor or ARB for LVSD[5]	-	-	84%	82%	100%
Discharge Instructions[5]	-	-	56%	61%	93%
Evaluation of LVS Function[5]	-	-	84%	83%	99%
Smoking Cessation Advice[5]	-	-	82%	82%	100%
Pneumonia Care					
Appropriate Initial Antibiotic[5]	-	-	82%	83%	94%
Blood Culture Timing[5]	-	-	89%	90%	100%
Influenza Vaccine[5]	-	-	58%	70%	100%
Initial Antibiotic Timing[5]	-	-	75%	80%	93%
Oxygenation Assessment[5]	-	-	99%	99%	100%
Pneumococcal Vaccine[5]	-	-	58%	69%	94%
Smoking Cessation Advice[5]	-	-	75%	80%	100%
Surgical Infection Prevention					
Prophylactic Antibiotic Given[5]	-	-	74%	77%	95%
Prophylactic Antibiotic Selection[5]	-	-	89%	90%	100%
Prophylactic Antibiotic Stopped[5]	-	-	65%	72%	95%
Pregnancy Care					
Inpatient Neonatal Mortality	-	-	-	-	-
Third or Fourth Degree Laceration	-	-	3.58%	3.63%	3.27%

Bakersfield Heart Hospital

3001 Sillect Avenue
Bakersfield, CA 93308
URL: www.bakersfieldhearthospital.com
Ownership: Proprietary
Emergency Services: Yes
Phone: 661-316-6000
Accredited: Yes
Licensed Beds: 47

Key Personnel:
President . . . . Randall H Rolfe

Measure	Cases	This Hospital	State Average	U.S. Average	Top Hospital
Heart Attack Care					
ACE Inhibitor or ARB for LVSD[2]	80	90%	82%	82%	100%
Aspirin at Arrival[2]	193	99%	95%	92%	100%
Aspirin at Discharge[2]	264	98%	90%	90%	100%
Beta Blocker at Arrival[2]	141	96%	89%	87%	100%
Beta Blocker at Discharge[2]	262	92%	89%	90%	100%
Fibrinolytic Medication Timing[2]	0	-	40%	31%	100%
PCI Within 90 Minutes of Arrival[1,2]	11	27%	52%	54%	95%
Smoking Cessation Advice[2]	103	98%	87%	88%	100%
Heart Failure Care					
ACE Inhibitor or ARB for LVSD[2]	135	80%	84%	82%	100%
Discharge Instructions[2]	251	64%	56%	61%	93%
Evaluation of LVS Function[2]	277	94%	84%	83%	99%
Smoking Cessation Advice[2]	42	95%	82%	82%	100%
Pneumonia Care					
Appropriate Initial Antibiotic[2]	89	92%	82%	83%	94%
Blood Culture Timing[2]	75	92%	89%	90%	100%
Influenza Vaccine[2]	27	78%	58%	70%	100%
Initial Antibiotic Timing[2]	112	82%	75%	80%	93%
Oxygenation Assessment[2]	161	100%	99%	99%	100%
Pneumococcal Vaccine[2]	112	81%	58%	69%	94%
Smoking Cessation Advice[2]	43	95%	75%	80%	100%
Surgical Infection Prevention					
Prophylactic Antibiotic Given[3]	185	95%	74%	77%	95%
Prophylactic Antibiotic Selection	69	93%	89%	90%	100%
Prophylactic Antibiotic Stopped[3]	159	80%	65%	72%	95%
Pregnancy Care					
Inpatient Neonatal Mortality	-	-	-	-	-
Third or Fourth Degree Laceration	-	-	3.58%	3.63%	3.27%

Bakersfield Memorial Hospital

420 34th Street
Bakersfield, CA 93301
URL: www.bakersfieldmemorial.org
Ownership: Voluntary non-profit - Private
Emergency Services: Yes
Phone: 661-327-4647
Fax: 661-327-8061
Accredited: Yes
Licensed Beds: 355

Key Personnel:
President . . . . Jon Van Boening

NOTE: Hospital profiles are in alphabetical order by state, then city, then hospital within the city; Rankings are sorted by rate in descending order and exclude hospitals with less than 25 cases; (1) The number of cases is too small (n<25) for purposes of reliably predicting hospital performance; (2) Measure reflects the hospital's indication that its submission was based upon a sample of its relevant discharges; (3) Rate reflects fewer than the maximum possible quarters of data for the measure; (4) Inaccurate information submitted and suppressed for one or more quarters; (5) No data is available from the hospital for this measure; Please refer to the User's Guide for a full explanation of data

Chief Medical Staff . . . . Robert Marshall, MD
CCU Spvg. Nurse . . . . Terri Totzke, RN
OB/GYN Womens Health. . . . . Kurt Finberg, MD
Respiratory Care . . . . Kathie Genter

Measure	Cases	This Hospital	State Average	U.S. Average	Top Hospital
Heart Attack Care					
ACE Inhibitor or ARB for LVSD	75	88%	82%	82%	100%
Aspirin at Arrival	210	92%	95%	92%	100%
Aspirin at Discharge	277	92%	90%	90%	100%
Beta Blocker at Arrival	145	83%	89%	87%	100%
Beta Blocker at Discharge	284	91%	89%	90%	100%
Fibrinolytic Medication Timing	0	-	40%	31%	100%
PCI Within 90 Minutes of Arrival[1]	8	75%	52%	54%	95%
Smoking Cessation Advice	88	98%	87%	88%	100%
Heart Failure Care					
ACE Inhibitor or ARB for LVSD	133	86%	84%	82%	100%
Discharge Instructions	253	68%	56%	61%	93%
Evaluation of LVS Function	307	93%	84%	83%	99%
Smoking Cessation Advice	54	94%	82%	82%	100%
Pneumonia Care					
Appropriate Initial Antibiotic	169	83%	82%	83%	94%
Blood Culture Timing	107	84%	89%	90%	100%
Influenza Vaccine	50	4%	58%	70%	100%
Initial Antibiotic Timing	204	69%	75%	80%	93%
Oxygenation Assessment	281	100%	99%	99%	100%
Pneumococcal Vaccine	172	90%	58%	69%	94%
Smoking Cessation Advice	55	78%	75%	80%	100%
Surgical Infection Prevention					
Prophylactic Antibiotic Given[2,3]	261	79%	74%	77%	95%
Prophylactic Antibiotic Selection[2]	79	96%	89%	90%	100%
Prophylactic Antibiotic Stopped[2,3]	251	53%	65%	72%	95%
Pregnancy Care					
Inpatient Neonatal Mortality	2,854	0.32%	-	-	-
Third or Fourth Degree Laceration	2,108	1.71%	3.58%	3.63%	3.27%

Good Samaritan Hospital

901 Olive Drive
Bakersfield, CA 93308
Phone: 661-399-4461
Fax: 661-399-4224
Ownership: Proprietary
Accredited: Yes
Emergency Services: No
Licensed Beds: 64

Key Personnel:

President . . . . Tim Kollars
Chief Medical Staff. . . . . Ronnie Claiborne
Infection Control. . . . . Linda Head, RN
Medical/Surgery Nurse Manager . . . . Grace Biden, RN
Surgery . . . . Edgare Sangueza
Respiratory Therapy Manager . . . . Henry Delacruz
Medical Surgery Discharge . . . . Emmanuel Okpala

Measure	Cases	This Hospital	State Average	U.S. Average	Top Hospital
Heart Attack Care					
ACE Inhibitor or ARB for LVSD[5]	-	-	82%	82%	100%
Aspirin at Arrival[5]	-	-	95%	92%	100%
Aspirin at Discharge[5]	-	-	90%	90%	100%
Beta Blocker at Arrival[5]	-	-	89%	87%	100%
Beta Blocker at Discharge[5]	-	-	89%	90%	100%
Fibrinolytic Medication Timing[5]	-	-	40%	31%	100%
PCI Within 90 Minutes of Arrival[5]	-	-	52%	54%	95%
Smoking Cessation Advice[5]	-	-	87%	88%	100%
Heart Failure Care					
ACE Inhibitor or ARB for LVSD	0	-	84%	82%	100%
Discharge Instructions[1,3]	15	0%	56%	61%	93%
Evaluation of LVS Function	69	7%	84%	83%	99%
Smoking Cessation Advice[1,3]	5	40%	82%	82%	100%
Pneumonia Care					
Appropriate Initial Antibiotic[1,3]	7	86%	82%	83%	94%
Blood Culture Timing[1,3]	2	100%	89%	90%	100%
Influenza Vaccine[5]	-	-	58%	70%	100%
Initial Antibiotic Timing	70	37%	75%	80%	93%
Oxygenation Assessment	91	97%	99%	99%	100%
Pneumococcal Vaccine[1]	18	44%	58%	69%	94%
Smoking Cessation Advice[1,3]	2	50%	75%	80%	100%
Surgical Infection Prevention					
Prophylactic Antibiotic Given[5]	-	-	74%	77%	95%
Prophylactic Antibiotic Selection[5]	-	-	89%	90%	100%
Prophylactic Antibiotic Stopped[5]	-	-	65%	72%	95%
Pregnancy Care					
Inpatient Neonatal Mortality	-	-	-	-	-
Third or Fourth Degree Laceration	-	-	3.58%	3.63%	3.27%

Kern Medical Center

1830 Flower Street
Bakersfield, CA 93305
Phone: 661-326-2640
Fax: 661-862-7630
E-mail: ewaldm@kernmedctr.com
URL: www.kernmedicalcenter.com
Ownership: Government - Local
Accredited: Yes
Emergency Services: Yes
Licensed Beds: 243

Key Personnel:

CEO. . . . . Peter K Bryan
Chief of Medical Staff . . . . Erwin Harris
Emergency Room . . . . Ugene Kercher
Director of Pulmonary . . . . Lon Lancaster

Measure	Cases	This Hospital	State Average	U.S. Average	Top Hospital
Heart Attack Care					
ACE Inhibitor or ARB for LVSD[1]	3	67%	82%	82%	100%
Aspirin at Arrival[1]	15	100%	95%	92%	100%
Aspirin at Discharge[1]	8	100%	90%	90%	100%
Beta Blocker at Arrival[1]	13	85%	89%	87%	100%
Beta Blocker at Discharge[1]	8	100%	89%	90%	100%
Fibrinolytic Medication Timing[3]	0	-	40%	31%	100%
PCI Within 90 Minutes of Arrival	0	-	52%	54%	95%
Smoking Cessation Advice[3]	0	-	87%	88%	100%
Heart Failure Care					
ACE Inhibitor or ARB for LVSD	76	95%	84%	82%	100%
Discharge Instructions[1,3]	23	0%	56%	61%	93%
Evaluation of LVS Function	129	98%	84%	83%	99%
Smoking Cessation Advice[1,3]	8	25%	82%	82%	100%
Pneumonia Care					
Appropriate Initial Antibiotic[1,3]	12	100%	82%	83%	94%
Blood Culture Timing[1,3]	16	81%	89%	90%	100%
Influenza Vaccine[5]	-	-	58%	70%	100%
Initial Antibiotic Timing	81	44%	75%	80%	93%
Oxygenation Assessment	103	99%	99%	99%	100%
Pneumococcal Vaccine	30	27%	58%	69%	94%
Smoking Cessation Advice[1,3]	8	12%	75%	80%	100%
Surgical Infection Prevention					
Prophylactic Antibiotic Given[2,3]	36	75%	74%	77%	95%
Prophylactic Antibiotic Selection[5]	-	-	89%	90%	100%
Prophylactic Antibiotic Stopped[2,3]	35	66%	65%	72%	95%
Pregnancy Care					
Inpatient Neonatal Mortality[2]	932	0.43%	-	-	-
Third or Fourth Degree Laceration[2]	742	3.50%	3.58%	3.63%	3.27%

Mercy Hospital

2215 Truxtun Avenue
Bakersfield, CA 93301
Phone: 661-632-5000
Fax: 661-322-8543
URL: www.mercybakersfield.org
Ownership: Voluntary non-profit - Church
Accredited: Yes
Emergency Services: Yes
Licensed Beds: 260

Key Personnel:

President . . . . Russell Judd
Chief Medical Officer . . . . Dr Mitesh Patel

Measure	Cases	This Hospital	State Average	U.S. Average	Top Hospital
Heart Attack Care					
ACE Inhibitor or ARB for LVSD[1]	7	71%	82%	82%	100%
Aspirin at Arrival	60	83%	95%	92%	100%
Aspirin at Discharge	39	64%	90%	90%	100%
Beta Blocker at Arrival	52	75%	89%	87%	100%
Beta Blocker at Discharge	38	55%	89%	90%	100%
Fibrinolytic Medication Timing	0	-	40%	31%	100%
PCI Within 90 Minutes of Arrival	0	-	52%	54%	95%

NOTE: Hospital profiles are in alphabetical order by state, then city, then hospital within the city; Rankings are sorted by rate in descending order and exclude hospitals with less than 25 cases; (1) The number of cases is too small (n<25) for purposes of reliably predicting hospital performance; (2) Measure reflects the hospital's indication that its submission was based upon a sample of its relevant discharges; (3) Rate reflects fewer than the maximum possible quarters of data for the measure; (4) Inaccurate information submitted and suppressed for one or more quarters; (5) No data is available from the hospital for this measure; Please refer to the User's Guide for a full explanation of data

Measure	Cases	This Hospital	State Average	U.S. Average	Top Hospital
Smoking Cessation Advice[1]	9	89%	87%	88%	100%
Heart Failure Care					
ACE Inhibitor or ARB for LVSD	63	57%	84%	82%	100%
Discharge Instructions	149	83%	56%	61%	93%
Evaluation of LVS Function	206	89%	84%	83%	99%
Smoking Cessation Advice	41	78%	82%	82%	100%
Pneumonia Care					
Appropriate Initial Antibiotic	427	81%	82%	83%	94%
Blood Culture Timing	315	82%	89%	90%	100%
Influenza Vaccine	105	1%	58%	70%	100%
Initial Antibiotic Timing	439	75%	75%	80%	93%
Oxygenation Assessment	533	100%	99%	99%	100%
Pneumococcal Vaccine	289	76%	58%	69%	94%
Smoking Cessation Advice	121	82%	75%	80%	100%
Surgical Infection Prevention					
Prophylactic Antibiotic Given[2,3]	201	59%	74%	77%	95%
Prophylactic Antibiotic Selection[2]	65	83%	89%	90%	100%
Prophylactic Antibiotic Stopped[2,3]	201	29%	65%	72%	95%
Pregnancy Care					
Inpatient Neonatal Mortality	3,587	0.36%	-	-	-
Third or Fourth Degree Laceration	2,583	6.66%	3.58%	3.63%	3.27%

San Joaquin Community Hospital

2615 Eye Street
Bakersfield, CA 93301
URL: www.sanjoaquinhospital.org
Ownership: Voluntary non-profit - Church
Emergency Services: Yes

Phone: 661-395-3000
Fax: 661-324-5162
Accredited: Yes
Licensed Beds: 252

Key Personnel:

CEO. . . . . Doug Lafferty
Chief Medical Staff. . . . . Shawn Shambaugh
Emergency Room . . . . Jackie Laws
Director Medical/Surgical Nursing . . . . Bob Lawson
OB/GYN Womens Health. . . . . John Owens

Measure	Cases	This Hospital	State Average	U.S. Average	Top Hospital
Heart Attack Care					
ACE Inhibitor or ARB for LVSD	32	69%	82%	82%	100%
Aspirin at Arrival	107	99%	95%	92%	100%
Aspirin at Discharge	129	91%	90%	90%	100%
Beta Blocker at Arrival	71	89%	89%	87%	100%
Beta Blocker at Discharge	127	89%	89%	90%	100%
Fibrinolytic Medication Timing[1]	2	100%	40%	31%	100%
PCI Within 90 Minutes of Arrival[1]	4	75%	52%	54%	95%
Smoking Cessation Advice	48	94%	87%	88%	100%
Heart Failure Care					
ACE Inhibitor or ARB for LVSD	169	92%	84%	82%	100%
Discharge Instructions	388	71%	56%	61%	93%
Evaluation of LVS Function	434	90%	84%	83%	99%
Smoking Cessation Advice	108	97%	82%	82%	100%
Pneumonia Care					
Appropriate Initial Antibiotic	187	89%	82%	83%	94%
Blood Culture Timing	181	96%	89%	90%	100%
Influenza Vaccine	40	100%	58%	70%	100%
Initial Antibiotic Timing	251	79%	75%	80%	93%
Oxygenation Assessment	286	100%	99%	99%	100%
Pneumococcal Vaccine	121	84%	58%	69%	94%
Smoking Cessation Advice	78	97%	75%	80%	100%
Surgical Infection Prevention					
Prophylactic Antibiotic Given[2,3]	139	63%	74%	77%	95%
Prophylactic Antibiotic Selection[2]	54	94%	89%	90%	100%
Prophylactic Antibiotic Stopped[2,3]	130	52%	65%	72%	95%
Pregnancy Care					
Inpatient Neonatal Mortality	-	-	-	-	-
Third or Fourth Degree Laceration	-	-	3.58%	3.63%	3.27%

Kaiser Foundation Hospital

1011 Baldwin Park Blvd
Baldwin Park, CA 91706
Ownership: Voluntary non-profit - Other
Emergency Services: Yes

Phone: 626-851-1011
Accredited: Yes

Measure	Cases	This Hospital	State Average	U.S. Average	Top Hospital
Heart Attack Care					
ACE Inhibitor or ARB for LVSD[1]	12	83%	82%	82%	100%
Aspirin at Arrival	104	99%	95%	92%	100%
Aspirin at Discharge	68	93%	90%	90%	100%
Beta Blocker at Arrival	80	99%	89%	87%	100%
Beta Blocker at Discharge	72	96%	89%	90%	100%
Fibrinolytic Medication Timing[1]	17	71%	40%	31%	100%
PCI Within 90 Minutes of Arrival	0	-	52%	54%	95%
Smoking Cessation Advice[1]	11	91%	87%	88%	100%
Heart Failure Care					
ACE Inhibitor or ARB for LVSD	122	84%	84%	82%	100%
Discharge Instructions	346	58%	56%	61%	93%
Evaluation of LVS Function	382	96%	84%	83%	99%
Smoking Cessation Advice	50	94%	82%	82%	100%
Pneumonia Care					
Appropriate Initial Antibiotic	85	81%	82%	83%	94%
Blood Culture Timing	97	89%	89%	90%	100%
Influenza Vaccine[4,5]	-	-	58%	70%	100%
Initial Antibiotic Timing	98	68%	75%	80%	93%
Oxygenation Assessment	125	100%	99%	99%	100%
Pneumococcal Vaccine	75	87%	58%	69%	94%
Smoking Cessation Advice	26	62%	75%	80%	100%
Surgical Infection Prevention					
Prophylactic Antibiotic Given[3]	50	78%	74%	77%	95%
Prophylactic Antibiotic Selection	51	92%	89%	90%	100%
Prophylactic Antibiotic Stopped[3]	46	52%	65%	72%	95%
Pregnancy Care					
Inpatient Neonatal Mortality	3,158	0.10%	-	-	-
Third or Fourth Degree Laceration	2,211	2.80%	3.58%	3.63%	3.27%

San Gorgonio Memorial Hospital

600 N Highland Springs Avenue
Banning, CA 92220
E-mail: info@sgmh.org
URL: www.sgmh.org
Ownership: Govt - Hospital District or Authority
Emergency Services: Yes

Phone: 951-845-1121
Fax: 951-845-2836
Accredited: Yes
Licensed Beds: 70

Key Personnel:

CEO. . . . . Don N Larkin
Chief Medical Staff. . . . . Sherif Khalil, MD
Director Emergency Room. . . . . Ludwig Cibelli, MD
Coordinator Emergency Room. . . . . Pat Brown, RN
Coordinator Obstetrics . . . . Carrie Echols, RN
Coordinator Surgery. . . . . Hilary Falconer, RN
Coordinator Respiratory Therapy . . . . David Anderson

Measure	Cases	This Hospital	State Average	U.S. Average	Top Hospital
Heart Attack Care					
ACE Inhibitor or ARB for LVSD[1]	15	73%	82%	82%	100%
Aspirin at Arrival	81	98%	95%	92%	100%
Aspirin at Discharge	44	95%	90%	90%	100%
Beta Blocker at Arrival	80	88%	89%	87%	100%
Beta Blocker at Discharge	50	88%	89%	90%	100%
Fibrinolytic Medication Timing[3]	0	-	40%	31%	100%
PCI Within 90 Minutes of Arrival	0	-	52%	54%	95%
Smoking Cessation Advice[1,3]	1	0%	87%	88%	100%
Heart Failure Care					
ACE Inhibitor or ARB for LVSD	37	89%	84%	82%	100%
Discharge Instructions[1,3]	23	0%	56%	61%	93%
Evaluation of LVS Function	164	71%	84%	83%	99%
Smoking Cessation Advice[1,3]	7	29%	82%	82%	100%
Pneumonia Care					
Appropriate Initial Antibiotic[3]	41	76%	82%	83%	94%
Blood Culture Timing[3]	44	80%	89%	90%	100%
Influenza Vaccine[5]	-	-	58%	70%	100%
Initial Antibiotic Timing	259	85%	75%	80%	93%

NOTE: Hospital profiles are in alphabetical order by state, then city, then hospital within the city; Rankings are sorted by rate in descending order and exclude hospitals with less than 25 cases; (1) The number of cases is too small (n<25) for purposes of reliably predicting hospital performance; (2) Measure reflects the hospital's indication that its submission was based upon a sample of its relevant discharges; (3) Rate reflects fewer than the maximum possible quarters of data for the measure; (4) Inaccurate information submitted and suppressed for one or more quarters; (5) No data is available from the hospital for this measure; Please refer to the User's Guide for a full explanation of data

Oxygenation Assessment	275	99%	99%	99%	100%
Pneumococcal Vaccine	192	2%	58%	69%	94%
Smoking Cessation Advice[1,3]	8	62%	75%	80%	100%
Surgical Infection Prevention					
Prophylactic Antibiotic Given[1,3]	9	11%	74%	77%	95%
Prophylactic Antibiotic Selection[5]	-	-	89%	90%	100%
Prophylactic Antibiotic Stopped[1,3]	7	0%	65%	72%	95%
Pregnancy Care					
Inpatient Neonatal Mortality	415	0.00%	-	-	-
Third or Fourth Degree Laceration	266	0.75%	3.58%	3.63%	3.27%

Barstow Community Hospital

555 South Seventh Avenue
Barstow, CA 92311
URL: www.barstowhospital.com
Ownership: Government - Local
Emergency Services: Yes

Phone: 760-256-1761
Fax: 760-957-3359
Accredited: Yes
Licensed Beds: 56

Key Personnel:

CEO. . . . . Randall Hempling
President Medical Staff . . . . Charles Taylor, MD
Director Medical/Surgical Nursing . . . . Chris Thorn, RN
OB/GYN Womens Health. . . . . Alejandro Vicente, MD
Chief Radiology . . . . Larry Givens, MD
Chief Cardio-Pulmonary Services . . . . Rabani Zaheer, MD

Measure	Cases	This Hospital	State Average	U.S. Average	Top Hospital
Heart Attack Care					
ACE Inhibitor or ARB for LVSD[1]	3	67%	82%	82%	100%
Aspirin at Arrival	43	95%	95%	92%	100%
Aspirin at Discharge[1]	11	82%	90%	90%	100%
Beta Blocker at Arrival	29	93%	89%	87%	100%
Beta Blocker at Discharge[1]	12	83%	89%	90%	100%
Fibrinolytic Medication Timing[1]	16	19%	40%	31%	100%
PCI Within 90 Minutes of Arrival	0	-	52%	54%	95%
Smoking Cessation Advice[1]	6	100%	87%	88%	100%
Heart Failure Care					
ACE Inhibitor or ARB for LVSD	41	80%	84%	82%	100%
Discharge Instructions	202	55%	56%	61%	93%
Evaluation of LVS Function	233	71%	84%	83%	99%
Smoking Cessation Advice	74	97%	82%	82%	100%
Pneumonia Care					
Appropriate Initial Antibiotic	162	76%	82%	83%	94%
Blood Culture Timing	112	96%	89%	90%	100%
Influenza Vaccine	43	19%	58%	70%	100%
Initial Antibiotic Timing	165	59%	75%	80%	93%
Oxygenation Assessment	202	100%	99%	99%	100%
Pneumococcal Vaccine	118	67%	58%	69%	94%
Smoking Cessation Advice	53	87%	75%	80%	100%
Surgical Infection Prevention					
Prophylactic Antibiotic Given[1,2,3]	23	26%	74%	77%	95%
Prophylactic Antibiotic Selection[1,2]	9	67%	89%	90%	100%
Prophylactic Antibiotic Stopped[1,2,3]	20	65%	65%	72%	95%
Pregnancy Care					
Inpatient Neonatal Mortality	-	-	-	-	-
Third or Fourth Degree Laceration	-	-	3.58%	3.63%	3.27%

Bellflower Medical Center

Alternate Name: Bellflower Doctors Hospital
9542 E Artesia Boulevard
Bellflower, CA 90706
URL: www.bellflowermedicalctr.com
Ownership: Proprietary
Emergency Services: Yes

Phone: 562-925-8355
Fax: 562-925-4413
Accredited: Yes
Licensed Beds: 144

Key Personnel:

CEO. . . . . James Linhare
Chief of Medical Staff. . . . . D Pangamiban, MD
Head Emergency Room. . . . . Pam Gavanus
Director Medical/Surgical Nursing . . . . John North, RN
Supervisor Respiratory Therapy. . . . . Joyce Eggleston

Measure	Cases	This Hospital	State Average	U.S. Average	Top Hospital
Heart Attack Care					
ACE Inhibitor or ARB for LVSD[1]	3	33%	82%	82%	100%
Aspirin at Arrival[1]	11	82%	95%	92%	100%
Aspirin at Discharge[1]	5	40%	90%	90%	100%
Beta Blocker at Arrival[1]	8	75%	89%	87%	100%
Beta Blocker at Discharge[1]	6	33%	89%	90%	100%
Fibrinolytic Medication Timing[1,3]	1	0%	40%	31%	100%
PCI Within 90 Minutes of Arrival	0	-	52%	54%	95%
Smoking Cessation Advice[3]	0	-	87%	88%	100%
Heart Failure Care					
ACE Inhibitor or ARB for LVSD	28	64%	84%	82%	100%
Discharge Instructions[1,3]	14	50%	56%	61%	93%
Evaluation of LVS Function	94	87%	84%	83%	99%
Smoking Cessation Advice[1,3]	4	100%	82%	82%	100%
Pneumonia Care					
Appropriate Initial Antibiotic[1,3]	11	73%	82%	83%	94%
Blood Culture Timing[3]	32	84%	89%	90%	100%
Influenza Vaccine[4,5]	-	-	58%	70%	100%
Initial Antibiotic Timing	174	83%	75%	80%	93%
Oxygenation Assessment	205	100%	99%	99%	100%
Pneumococcal Vaccine	119	10%	58%	69%	94%
Smoking Cessation Advice[1,3]	6	67%	75%	80%	100%
Surgical Infection Prevention					
Prophylactic Antibiotic Given[1,3]	18	72%	74%	77%	95%
Prophylactic Antibiotic Selection[5]	-	-	89%	90%	100%
Prophylactic Antibiotic Stopped[1,3]	18	56%	65%	72%	95%
Pregnancy Care					
Inpatient Neonatal Mortality	-	-	-	-	-
Third or Fourth Degree Laceration	-	-	3.58%	3.63%	3.27%

Kaiser Permanente Bellflower Medical Center

9400 E Rosencrans Ave
Bellflower, CA 90706
URL: www.kaiserpermanente.org
Ownership: Voluntary non-profit - Other
Emergency Services: Yes

Phone: 562-461-3000
Fax: 510-625-6398
Accredited: Yes
Licensed Beds: 453

Key Personnel:

CEO/President. . . . . Jude North
Chief Medical Staff. . . . . HS Kim
Emergency Room . . . . Jeff Miller
OB/GYN Womens Health. . . . . Gerald Karten

Measure	Cases	This Hospital	State Average	U.S. Average	Top Hospital
Heart Attack Care					
ACE Inhibitor or ARB for LVSD	30	80%	82%	82%	100%
Aspirin at Arrival	155	99%	95%	92%	100%
Aspirin at Discharge	112	96%	90%	90%	100%
Beta Blocker at Arrival	149	98%	89%	87%	100%
Beta Blocker at Discharge	118	99%	89%	90%	100%
Fibrinolytic Medication Timing[1]	24	46%	40%	31%	100%
PCI Within 90 Minutes of Arrival	0	-	52%	54%	95%
Smoking Cessation Advice[1]	17	82%	87%	88%	100%
Heart Failure Care					
ACE Inhibitor or ARB for LVSD	212	87%	84%	82%	100%
Discharge Instructions	478	67%	56%	61%	93%
Evaluation of LVS Function	525	89%	84%	83%	99%
Smoking Cessation Advice	82	72%	82%	82%	100%
Pneumonia Care					
Appropriate Initial Antibiotic	95	72%	82%	83%	94%
Blood Culture Timing	75	96%	89%	90%	100%
Influenza Vaccine[1]	24	54%	58%	70%	100%
Initial Antibiotic Timing	108	69%	75%	80%	93%
Oxygenation Assessment	122	100%	99%	99%	100%
Pneumococcal Vaccine	76	83%	58%	69%	94%
Smoking Cessation Advice[1]	13	69%	75%	80%	100%
Surgical Infection Prevention					
Prophylactic Antibiotic Given[3]	42	88%	74%	77%	95%
Prophylactic Antibiotic Selection	42	98%	89%	90%	100%
Prophylactic Antibiotic Stopped[3]	42	62%	65%	72%	95%
Pregnancy Care					
Inpatient Neonatal Mortality	3,461	0.58%	-	-	-
Third or Fourth Degree Laceration	2,447	3.39%	3.58%	3.63%	3.27%

NOTE: Hospital profiles are in alphabetical order by state, then city, then hospital within the city; Rankings are sorted by rate in descending order and exclude hospitals with less than 25 cases; (1) The number of cases is too small (n<25) for purposes of reliably predicting hospital performance; (2) Measure reflects the hospital's indication that its submission was based upon a sample of its relevant discharges; (3) Rate reflects fewer than the maximum possible quarters of data for the measure; (4) Inaccurate information submitted and suppressed for one or more quarters; (5) No data is available from the hospital for this measure; Please refer to the User's Guide for a full explanation of data

Alta Bates Summit Medical Center

2450 Ashby Avenue
Berkeley, CA 94705
Phone: 510-204-4444
Fax: 510-204-5203
URL: www.altabates.com
Ownership: Voluntary non-profit - Other
Accredited: Yes
Emergency Services: Yes
Licensed Beds: 551

Key Personnel:

President/CEO . . . . Warren J Kirk

Measure	Cases	This Hospital	State Average	U.S. Average	Top Hospital
Heart Attack Care					
ACE Inhibitor or ARB for LVSD[1]	13	85%	82%	82%	100%
Aspirin at Arrival	100	98%	95%	92%	100%
Aspirin at Discharge	82	100%	90%	90%	100%
Beta Blocker at Arrival	84	95%	89%	87%	100%
Beta Blocker at Discharge	81	98%	89%	90%	100%
Fibrinolytic Medication Timing	0	-	40%	31%	100%
PCI Within 90 Minutes of Arrival[1]	1	100%	52%	54%	95%
Smoking Cessation Advice[1]	20	100%	87%	88%	100%
Heart Failure Care					
ACE Inhibitor or ARB for LVSD[2]	41	83%	84%	82%	100%
Discharge Instructions[2]	94	82%	56%	61%	93%
Evaluation of LVS Function[2]	109	94%	84%	83%	99%
Smoking Cessation Advice[1,2]	23	100%	82%	82%	100%
Pneumonia Care					
Appropriate Initial Antibiotic[2]	43	91%	82%	83%	94%
Blood Culture Timing[2]	72	96%	89%	90%	100%
Influenza Vaccine[1]	12	67%	58%	70%	100%
Initial Antibiotic Timing[2]	79	68%	75%	80%	93%
Oxygenation Assessment[2]	106	100%	99%	99%	100%
Pneumococcal Vaccine[2]	51	63%	58%	69%	94%
Smoking Cessation Advice[1,2]	23	100%	75%	80%	100%
Surgical Infection Prevention					
Prophylactic Antibiotic Given[2,3]	109	92%	74%	77%	95%
Prophylactic Antibiotic Selection[2]	35	100%	89%	90%	100%
Prophylactic Antibiotic Stopped[2,3]	106	70%	65%	72%	95%
Pregnancy Care					
Inpatient Neonatal Mortality	7,706	0.32%	-	-	-
Third or Fourth Degree Laceration	5,335	3.11%	3.58%	3.63%	3.27%

Bear Valley Community Hospital

Alternate Name: Bear Valley Community Healthcare District
41870 Garstin Drive
PO Box 1649
Big Bear Lake, CA 92315
Phone: 909-866-6501
Fax: 909-878-8282
E-mail: garstin@excite.com
URL: www.bvchd.com
Ownership: Voluntary non-profit - Church
Accredited: Yes
Emergency Services: Yes
Licensed Beds: 30

Key Personnel:

CEO. . . . . Mary Norman
Chief Medical Staff. . . . . Michael Norman, DO
Director Emergency . . . . Ines Tedford, RN
Infection Control. . . . . Ann Haggard, RN
Chief Radiology . . . . S Dand, MD
Director Respiratory Therapy . . . . Sue Cliffords

Measure	Cases	This Hospital	State Average	U.S. Average	Top Hospital
Heart Attack Care					
ACE Inhibitor or ARB for LVSD[3]	0	-	82%	82%	100%
Aspirin at Arrival[1,3]	1	100%	95%	92%	100%
Aspirin at Discharge[1,3]	1	0%	90%	90%	100%
Beta Blocker at Arrival[3]	0	-	89%	87%	100%
Beta Blocker at Discharge[1,3]	1	100%	89%	90%	100%
Fibrinolytic Medication Timing[5]	-	-	40%	31%	100%
PCI Within 90 Minutes of Arrival[5]	-	-	52%	54%	95%
Smoking Cessation Advice[5]	-	-	87%	88%	100%
Heart Failure Care					
ACE Inhibitor or ARB for LVSD[3]	0	-	84%	82%	100%
Discharge Instructions[1,3]	5	100%	56%	61%	93%
Evaluation of LVS Function[1,3]	10	10%	84%	83%	99%
Smoking Cessation Advice[3]	0	-	82%	82%	100%
Pneumonia Care					
Appropriate Initial Antibiotic[1,3]	4	100%	82%	83%	94%
Blood Culture Timing[1,3]	2	100%	89%	90%	100%
Influenza Vaccine[5]	-	-	58%	70%	100%
Initial Antibiotic Timing[1,3]	8	100%	75%	80%	93%
Oxygenation Assessment[1,3]	10	100%	99%	99%	100%
Pneumococcal Vaccine[1,3]	6	17%	58%	69%	94%
Smoking Cessation Advice[3]	0	-	75%	80%	100%
Surgical Infection Prevention					
Prophylactic Antibiotic Given[5]	-	-	74%	77%	95%
Prophylactic Antibiotic Selection[5]	-	-	89%	90%	100%
Prophylactic Antibiotic Stopped[5]	-	-	65%	72%	95%
Pregnancy Care					
Inpatient Neonatal Mortality	-	-	-	-	-
Third or Fourth Degree Laceration	-	-	3.58%	3.63%	3.27%

Palo Verde Hospital

250 North First Street
Blythe, CA 92225
Phone: 760-922-4115
Fax: 760-921-5201
URL: paloverdehospital.org
Ownership: Proprietary
Accredited: Yes
Emergency Services: Yes
Licensed Beds: 51

Key Personnel:

President . . . . Derek Copple
CEO. . . . . Jeff Flood
Emergency Room . . . . Chuck Noden
Infection Control. . . . . Leida Meek
ICU . . . . Andrea Barrera
Medical/Surgical Nursing . . . . Barbara Lancastor

Measure	Cases	This Hospital	State Average	U.S. Average	Top Hospital
Heart Attack Care					
ACE Inhibitor or ARB for LVSD[3]	0	-	82%	82%	100%
Aspirin at Arrival[1,3]	3	0%	95%	92%	100%
Aspirin at Discharge[1,3]	2	100%	90%	90%	100%
Beta Blocker at Arrival[1,3]	5	40%	89%	87%	100%
Beta Blocker at Discharge[1,3]	2	100%	89%	90%	100%
Fibrinolytic Medication Timing[1,3]	1	100%	40%	31%	100%
PCI Within 90 Minutes of Arrival[5]	-	-	52%	54%	95%
Smoking Cessation Advice[1,3]	1	0%	87%	88%	100%
Heart Failure Care					
ACE Inhibitor or ARB for LVSD	0	-	84%	82%	100%
Discharge Instructions	25	4%	56%	61%	93%
Evaluation of LVS Function	25	12%	84%	83%	99%
Smoking Cessation Advice[1]	7	29%	82%	82%	100%
Pneumonia Care					
Appropriate Initial Antibiotic	49	84%	82%	83%	94%
Blood Culture Timing[1]	20	90%	89%	90%	100%
Influenza Vaccine[1]	11	55%	58%	70%	100%
Initial Antibiotic Timing	44	77%	75%	80%	93%
Oxygenation Assessment	64	100%	99%	99%	100%
Pneumococcal Vaccine	39	56%	58%	69%	94%
Smoking Cessation Advice[1]	17	24%	75%	80%	100%
Surgical Infection Prevention					
Prophylactic Antibiotic Given[1,3]	10	50%	74%	77%	95%
Prophylactic Antibiotic Selection[1]	2	100%	89%	90%	100%
Prophylactic Antibiotic Stopped[1,3]	5	60%	65%	72%	95%
Pregnancy Care					
Inpatient Neonatal Mortality	-	-	-	-	-
Third or Fourth Degree Laceration	-	-	3.58%	3.63%	3.27%

Pioneers Memorial Healthcare District

Alternate Name: Pioneers Memorial Hospital District
207 W Legion Road
Brawley, CA 92227
Phone: 760-351-3333
Fax: 760-344-4401
URL: www.pmhd.org
Ownership: Govt - Hospital District or Authority
Accredited: Yes
Emergency Services: Yes
Licensed Beds: 99

Key Personnel:

CEO. . . . . Richard Mendoza
Chief of Medical Staff. Horacio Rogiles
Emergency Room . . . . Robin Atadero
Director Infection/Disease Control . . . . Kathleen Messerschmidt, BSN

NOTE: Hospital profiles are in alphabetical order by state, then city, then hospital within the city; Rankings are sorted by rate in descending order and exclude hospitals with less than 25 cases; (1) The number of cases is too small (n<25) for purposes of reliably predicting hospital performance; (2) Measure reflects the hospital's indication that its submission was based upon a sample of its relevant discharges; (3) Rate reflects fewer than the maximum possible quarters of data for the measure; (4) Inaccurate information submitted and suppressed for one or more quarters; (5) No data is available from the hospital for this measure; Please refer to the User's Guide for a full explanation of data

Director Medical/Surgical Nursing . . . . Tina Pendley, RN
Chief Radiology . . . . Ceasar Trillanes, MD
Director Respiratory Therapy . . . . Mike Gilbert

Measure	Cases	This Hospital	State Average	U.S. Average	Top Hospital
Heart Attack Care					
ACE Inhibitor or ARB for LVSD[1]	18	44%	82%	82%	100%
Aspirin at Arrival	42	98%	95%	92%	100%
Aspirin at Discharge	33	67%	90%	90%	100%
Beta Blocker at Arrival	39	72%	89%	87%	100%
Beta Blocker at Discharge	33	64%	89%	90%	100%
Fibrinolytic Medication Timing[1]	6	50%	40%	31%	100%
PCI Within 90 Minutes of Arrival	0	-	52%	54%	95%
Smoking Cessation Advice[1]	15	87%	87%	88%	100%
Heart Failure Care					
ACE Inhibitor or ARB for LVSD	66	91%	84%	82%	100%
Discharge Instructions	110	65%	56%	61%	93%
Evaluation of LVS Function	122	80%	84%	83%	99%
Smoking Cessation Advice	26	96%	82%	82%	100%
Pneumonia Care					
Appropriate Initial Antibiotic	158	92%	82%	83%	94%
Blood Culture Timing	92	74%	89%	90%	100%
Influenza Vaccine[4,5]	-	-	58%	70%	100%
Initial Antibiotic Timing	157	81%	75%	80%	93%
Oxygenation Assessment	183	100%	99%	99%	100%
Pneumococcal Vaccine	100	57%	58%	69%	94%
Smoking Cessation Advice[1]	20	80%	75%	80%	100%
Surgical Infection Prevention					
Prophylactic Antibiotic Given[3]	109	78%	74%	77%	95%
Prophylactic Antibiotic Selection	49	82%	89%	90%	100%
Prophylactic Antibiotic Stopped[3]	109	41%	65%	72%	95%
Pregnancy Care					
Inpatient Neonatal Mortality	-	-	-	-	-
Third or Fourth Degree Laceration	-	-	3.58%	3.63%	3.27%

Providence Saint Joseph Medical Center

501 South Buena Vista — Phone: 818-843-5111
Burbank, CA 91505
Ownership: Voluntary non-profit - Church — Accredited: Yes
Emergency Services: Yes

Measure	Cases	This Hospital	State Average	U.S. Average	Top Hospital
Heart Attack Care					
ACE Inhibitor or ARB for LVSD[2]	37	97%	82%	82%	100%
Aspirin at Arrival[2]	249	99%	95%	92%	100%
Aspirin at Discharge[2]	268	98%	90%	90%	100%
Beta Blocker at Arrival[2]	199	95%	89%	87%	100%
Beta Blocker at Discharge[2]	262	98%	89%	90%	100%
Fibrinolytic Medication Timing[2]	0	-	40%	31%	100%
PCI Within 90 Minutes of Arrival[1,2]	20	75%	52%	54%	95%
Smoking Cessation Advice[2]	104	96%	87%	88%	100%
Heart Failure Care					
ACE Inhibitor or ARB for LVSD[2]	99	97%	84%	82%	100%
Discharge Instructions[2]	241	63%	56%	61%	93%
Evaluation of LVS Function[2]	314	99%	84%	83%	99%
Smoking Cessation Advice[2]	27	96%	82%	82%	100%
Pneumonia Care					
Appropriate Initial Antibiotic[2]	114	72%	82%	83%	94%
Blood Culture Timing[2]	105	91%	89%	90%	100%
Influenza Vaccine	31	81%	58%	70%	100%
Initial Antibiotic Timing[2]	170	77%	75%	80%	93%
Oxygenation Assessment[2]	230	100%	99%	99%	100%
Pneumococcal Vaccine[2]	154	69%	58%	69%	94%
Smoking Cessation Advice[2]	35	91%	75%	80%	100%
Surgical Infection Prevention					
Prophylactic Antibiotic Given[2]	304	92%	74%	77%	95%
Prophylactic Antibiotic Selection[2]	74	81%	89%	90%	100%
Prophylactic Antibiotic Stopped[2]	281	47%	65%	72%	95%
Pregnancy Care					
Inpatient Neonatal Mortality	-	-	-	-	-
Third or Fourth Degree Laceration	-	-	3.58%	3.63%	3.27%

Mills-Peninsula Health Services

Alternate Name: Peninsula Medical Center
1783 El Camino Real — Phone: 650-696-5400
Burlingame, CA 94010 — Fax: 650-696-5487
URL: www.mills-peninsula.org
Ownership: Voluntary non-profit - Other — Accredited: Yes
Emergency Services: Yes — Licensed Beds: 403
Key Personnel:
CEO. . . . . Robert W Merwin
Chief Medical Staff . . . . Donald Ho, MD
Emergency Room . . . . Dan Ovenin, MD
Intensive/Coronary Care . . . . Isabel Rink, RN
Director Respiratory Therapy . . . . Chris Comstock

Measure	Cases	This Hospital	State Average	U.S. Average	Top Hospital
Heart Attack Care					
ACE Inhibitor or ARB for LVSD	29	90%	82%	82%	100%
Aspirin at Arrival	108	98%	95%	92%	100%
Aspirin at Discharge	131	98%	90%	90%	100%
Beta Blocker at Arrival	88	98%	89%	87%	100%
Beta Blocker at Discharge	121	96%	89%	90%	100%
Fibrinolytic Medication Timing	0	-	40%	31%	100%
PCI Within 90 Minutes of Arrival[1]	9	11%	52%	54%	95%
Smoking Cessation Advice	40	100%	87%	88%	100%
Heart Failure Care					
ACE Inhibitor or ARB for LVSD	76	92%	84%	82%	100%
Discharge Instructions	217	68%	56%	61%	93%
Evaluation of LVS Function	305	97%	84%	83%	99%
Smoking Cessation Advice	37	86%	82%	82%	100%
Pneumonia Care					
Appropriate Initial Antibiotic[2]	113	87%	82%	83%	94%
Blood Culture Timing[2]	110	96%	89%	90%	100%
Influenza Vaccine[2]	31	58%	58%	70%	100%
Initial Antibiotic Timing[2]	152	76%	75%	80%	93%
Oxygenation Assessment[2]	186	100%	99%	99%	100%
Pneumococcal Vaccine[2]	155	72%	58%	69%	94%
Smoking Cessation Advice[2]	27	93%	75%	80%	100%
Surgical Infection Prevention					
Prophylactic Antibiotic Given[2]	296	80%	74%	77%	95%
Prophylactic Antibiotic Selection[2]	58	100%	89%	90%	100%
Prophylactic Antibiotic Stopped[2]	283	49%	65%	72%	95%
Pregnancy Care					
Inpatient Neonatal Mortality	-	-	-	-	-
Third or Fourth Degree Laceration	-	-	3.58%	3.63%	3.27%

Saint John's Pleasant Valley Hospital

Alternate Name: Pleasant Valley Hospital
2309 Antonio Avenue — Phone: 805-389-5800
Camarillo, CA 93010 — Fax: 805-383-7450
URL: www.stjohnshealth.org
Ownership: Voluntary non-profit - Church — Accredited: Yes
Emergency Services: Yes — Licensed Beds: 187
Key Personnel:
President/CEO. . . . . Lloyd H Dean
Emergency Room . . . . Becky Hansen
OB/GYN Womens Health. . . . . M Belzar, MD

Measure	Cases	This Hospital	State Average	U.S. Average	Top Hospital
Heart Attack Care					
ACE Inhibitor or ARB for LVSD[1]	8	62%	82%	82%	100%
Aspirin at Arrival	34	94%	95%	92%	100%
Aspirin at Discharge[1]	22	86%	90%	90%	100%
Beta Blocker at Arrival	26	96%	89%	87%	100%
Beta Blocker at Discharge	25	100%	89%	90%	100%
Fibrinolytic Medication Timing	0	-	40%	31%	100%
PCI Within 90 Minutes of Arrival	0	-	52%	54%	95%
Smoking Cessation Advice[1]	4	75%	87%	88%	100%
Heart Failure Care					
ACE Inhibitor or ARB for LVSD[1]	18	94%	84%	82%	100%
Discharge Instructions	67	67%	56%	61%	93%
Evaluation of LVS Function	87	100%	84%	83%	99%
Smoking Cessation Advice[1]	4	100%	82%	82%	100%
Pneumonia Care					

NOTE: Hospital profiles are in alphabetical order by state, then city, then hospital within the city; Rankings are sorted by rate in descending order and exclude hospitals with less than 25 cases; (1) The number of cases is too small (n<25) for purposes of reliably predicting hospital performance; (2) Measure reflects the hospital's indication that its submission was based upon a sample of its relevant discharges; (3) Rate reflects fewer than the maximum possible quarters of data for the measure; (4) Inaccurate information submitted and suppressed for one or more quarters; (5) No data is available from the hospital for this measure; Please refer to the User's Guide for a full explanation of data

Measure	Cases	This Hospital	State Average	U.S. Average	Top Hospital
Appropriate Initial Antibiotic	100	86%	82%	83%	94%
Blood Culture Timing	104	90%	89%	90%	100%
Influenza Vaccine	32	66%	58%	70%	100%
Initial Antibiotic Timing	120	72%	75%	80%	93%
Oxygenation Assessment	160	99%	99%	99%	100%
Pneumococcal Vaccine	122	56%	58%	69%	94%
Smoking Cessation Advice[1]	15	53%	75%	80%	100%
Surgical Infection Prevention					
Prophylactic Antibiotic Given[2,3]	120	72%	74%	77%	95%
Prophylactic Antibiotic Selection[2]	37	100%	89%	90%	100%
Prophylactic Antibiotic Stopped[2,3]	118	36%	65%	72%	95%
Pregnancy Care					
Inpatient Neonatal Mortality	-	-	-	-	-
Third or Fourth Degree Laceration	-	-	3.58%	3.63%	3.27%

Mercy San Juan Hospital

Alternate Name: Mercy American River
6501 Coyle Avenue — Phone: 916-537-5000
Carmichael, CA 95608 — Fax: 916-537-5111
E-mail: bgaron@chw.edu
URL: www.mercysanjuan.org
Ownership: Voluntary non-profit - Other — Accredited: Yes
Emergency Services: Yes — Licensed Beds: 260

Key Personnel:
President . . . . Michael J Uboldi
Chief Medical Staff . . . . Kuldip Sandhu, MD
Catheterization Lab . . . . Bill Colditz
Manager Emergency Room . . . . Rogeren Lloydugh, RN
Infection Control . . . . Jane Nelson
Manager OB/GYN Womens Health . . . . Cecelia Kilpatrick
Manager Radiology . . . . Ed Oliyarrs
Cardiopulmonary . . . . Quincy Mitchell

Measure	Cases	This Hospital	State Average	U.S. Average	Top Hospital
Heart Attack Care					
ACE Inhibitor or ARB for LVSD	45	98%	82%	82%	100%
Aspirin at Arrival	295	99%	95%	92%	100%
Aspirin at Discharge	250	100%	90%	90%	100%
Beta Blocker at Arrival	197	99%	89%	87%	100%
Beta Blocker at Discharge	284	99%	89%	90%	100%
Fibrinolytic Medication Timing	34	65%	40%	31%	100%
PCI Within 90 Minutes of Arrival[1]	11	27%	52%	54%	95%
Smoking Cessation Advice	85	100%	87%	88%	100%
Heart Failure Care					
ACE Inhibitor or ARB for LVSD	142	95%	84%	82%	100%
Discharge Instructions	416	88%	56%	61%	93%
Evaluation of LVS Function	521	99%	84%	83%	99%
Smoking Cessation Advice	104	99%	82%	82%	100%
Pneumonia Care					
Appropriate Initial Antibiotic	232	88%	82%	83%	94%
Blood Culture Timing	487	93%	89%	90%	100%
Influenza Vaccine	140	88%	58%	70%	100%
Initial Antibiotic Timing	598	77%	75%	80%	93%
Oxygenation Assessment	704	100%	99%	99%	100%
Pneumococcal Vaccine	465	89%	58%	69%	94%
Smoking Cessation Advice	138	99%	75%	80%	100%
Surgical Infection Prevention					
Prophylactic Antibiotic Given[2,3]	250	60%	74%	77%	95%
Prophylactic Antibiotic Selection[2]	80	91%	89%	90%	100%
Prophylactic Antibiotic Stopped[2,3]	234	76%	65%	72%	95%
Pregnancy Care					
Inpatient Neonatal Mortality	-	-	-	-	-
Third or Fourth Degree Laceration	-	-	3.58%	3.63%	3.27%

Eden Medical Center

20103 Lake Chabot Road — Phone: 510-537-1234
Castro Valley, CA 94546
Ownership: Govt - Hospital District or Authority — Accredited: Yes
Emergency Services: Yes

Measure	Cases	This Hospital	State Average	U.S. Average	Top Hospital
Heart Attack Care					
ACE Inhibitor or ARB for LVSD[1]	9	78%	82%	82%	100%
Aspirin at Arrival	63	90%	95%	92%	100%
Aspirin at Discharge	36	86%	90%	90%	100%
Beta Blocker at Arrival	39	92%	89%	87%	100%
Beta Blocker at Discharge	39	97%	89%	90%	100%
Fibrinolytic Medication Timing[1]	1	0%	40%	31%	100%
PCI Within 90 Minutes of Arrival	0	-	52%	54%	95%
Smoking Cessation Advice[1]	8	75%	87%	88%	100%
Heart Failure Care					
ACE Inhibitor or ARB for LVSD	83	76%	84%	82%	100%
Discharge Instructions	182	63%	56%	61%	93%
Evaluation of LVS Function	230	89%	84%	83%	99%
Smoking Cessation Advice	35	94%	82%	82%	100%
Pneumonia Care					
Appropriate Initial Antibiotic	155	85%	82%	83%	94%
Blood Culture Timing	171	95%	89%	90%	100%
Influenza Vaccine	58	43%	58%	70%	100%
Initial Antibiotic Timing	232	64%	75%	80%	93%
Oxygenation Assessment	286	100%	99%	99%	100%
Pneumococcal Vaccine	170	52%	58%	69%	94%
Smoking Cessation Advice	41	80%	75%	80%	100%
Surgical Infection Prevention					
Prophylactic Antibiotic Given[2]	418	87%	74%	77%	95%
Prophylactic Antibiotic Selection[2]	102	98%	89%	90%	100%
Prophylactic Antibiotic Stopped[2]	403	79%	65%	72%	95%
Pregnancy Care					
Inpatient Neonatal Mortality	-	-	-	-	-
Third or Fourth Degree Laceration	-	-	3.58%	3.63%	3.27%

Laurel Grove Hosp Acute Rehab Facility

19933 Lake Chabot Road — Phone: 510-537-1234
Hayward, CA 94546 — Fax: 510-537-3530
URL: www.edenmedcenter.org
Ownership: Proprietary — Accredited: Yes
Emergency Services: No — Licensed Beds: 31

Key Personnel:
President/CEO . . . . Patrick Fry

Measure	Cases	This Hospital	State Average	U.S. Average	Top Hospital
Heart Attack Care					
ACE Inhibitor or ARB for LVSD[5]	-	-	82%	82%	100%
Aspirin at Arrival[5]	-	-	95%	92%	100%
Aspirin at Discharge[5]	-	-	90%	90%	100%
Beta Blocker at Arrival[5]	-	-	89%	87%	100%
Beta Blocker at Discharge[5]	-	-	89%	90%	100%
Fibrinolytic Medication Timing[5]	-	-	40%	31%	100%
PCI Within 90 Minutes of Arrival[5]	-	-	52%	54%	95%
Smoking Cessation Advice[5]	-	-	87%	88%	100%
Heart Failure Care					
ACE Inhibitor or ARB for LVSD[5]	-	-	84%	82%	100%
Discharge Instructions[5]	-	-	56%	61%	93%
Evaluation of LVS Function[5]	-	-	84%	83%	99%
Smoking Cessation Advice[5]	-	-	82%	82%	100%
Pneumonia Care					
Appropriate Initial Antibiotic[5]	-	-	82%	83%	94%
Blood Culture Timing[5]	-	-	89%	90%	100%
Influenza Vaccine[5]	-	-	58%	70%	100%
Initial Antibiotic Timing[5]	-	-	75%	80%	93%
Oxygenation Assessment[5]	-	-	99%	99%	100%
Pneumococcal Vaccine[5]	-	-	58%	69%	94%
Smoking Cessation Advice[5]	-	-	75%	80%	100%
Surgical Infection Prevention					
Prophylactic Antibiotic Given[5]	-	-	74%	77%	95%
Prophylactic Antibiotic Selection[5]	-	-	89%	90%	100%
Prophylactic Antibiotic Stopped[5]	-	-	65%	72%	95%
Pregnancy Care					
Inpatient Neonatal Mortality	-	-	-	-	-
Third or Fourth Degree Laceration	-	-	3.58%	3.63%	3.27%

NOTE: Hospital profiles are in alphabetical order by state, then city, then hospital within the city; Rankings are sorted by rate in descending order and exclude hospitals with less than 25 cases; (1) The number of cases is too small (n<25) for purposes of reliably predicting hospital performance; (2) Measure reflects the hospital's indication that its submission was based upon a sample of its relevant discharges; (3) Rate reflects fewer than the maximum possible quarters of data for the measure; (4) Inaccurate information submitted and suppressed for one or more quarters; (5) No data is available from the hospital for this measure; Please refer to the User's Guide for a full explanation of data

Surprise Valley Healthcare District

Main & Washington
Cedarville, CA 96104
Ownership: Govt - Hospital District or Authority
Emergency Services: Yes

Phone: 530-279-6111
Fax: 530-279-2680
Accredited: No
Licensed Beds: 26

Key Personnel:

CEO . . . . Joyce I Gysin
Chief Radiology . . . . DT Matthews, MD
Director Respiratory Therapy . . . . Cheryl Azevedo

Measure	Cases	This Hospital	State Average	U.S. Average	Top Hospital
Heart Attack Care					
ACE Inhibitor or ARB for LVSD[5]	-	-	82%	82%	100%
Aspirin at Arrival[5]	-	-	95%	92%	100%
Aspirin at Discharge[5]	-	-	90%	90%	100%
Beta Blocker at Arrival[5]	-	-	89%	87%	100%
Beta Blocker at Discharge[5]	-	-	89%	90%	100%
Fibrinolytic Medication Timing[5]	-	-	40%	31%	100%
PCI Within 90 Minutes of Arrival[5]	-	-	52%	54%	95%
Smoking Cessation Advice[5]	-	-	87%	88%	100%
Heart Failure Care					
ACE Inhibitor or ARB for LVSD[5]	-	-	84%	82%	100%
Discharge Instructions[5]	-	-	56%	61%	93%
Evaluation of LVS Function[5]	-	-	84%	83%	99%
Smoking Cessation Advice[5]	-	-	82%	82%	100%
Pneumonia Care					
Appropriate Initial Antibiotic[3]	0	-	82%	83%	94%
Blood Culture Timing[1,3]	1	100%	89%	90%	100%
Influenza Vaccine[5]	-	-	58%	70%	100%
Initial Antibiotic Timing[1,3]	1	100%	75%	80%	93%
Oxygenation Assessment[1,3]	1	100%	99%	99%	100%
Pneumococcal Vaccine[1,3]	1	100%	58%	69%	94%
Smoking Cessation Advice[3]	0	-	75%	80%	100%
Surgical Infection Prevention					
Prophylactic Antibiotic Given[5]	-	-	74%	77%	95%
Prophylactic Antibiotic Selection[5]	-	-	89%	90%	100%
Prophylactic Antibiotic Stopped[5]	-	-	65%	72%	95%
Pregnancy Care					
Inpatient Neonatal Mortality	-	-	-	-	-
Third or Fourth Degree Laceration	-	-	3.58%	3.63%	3.27%

Seneca Hospital

130 Brentwood Drive
PO Box 737
Chester, CA 96020
URL: www.senecahospital.org
Ownership: Govt - Hospital District or Authority
Emergency Services: Yes

Phone: 530-258-2151
Fax: 530-258-3836
Accredited: No
Licensed Beds: 26

Key Personnel:

CEO . . . . Warren Benincosa
Chief of Medical Staff . . . . Chris Ward, MD
Manager Respiratory Care . . . . Lee Cargile

Measure	Cases	This Hospital	State Average	U.S. Average	Top Hospital
Heart Attack Care					
ACE Inhibitor or ARB for LVSD[5]	-	-	82%	82%	100%
Aspirin at Arrival[5]	-	-	95%	92%	100%
Aspirin at Discharge[5]	-	-	90%	90%	100%
Beta Blocker at Arrival[5]	-	-	89%	87%	100%
Beta Blocker at Discharge[5]	-	-	89%	90%	100%
Fibrinolytic Medication Timing[5]	-	-	40%	31%	100%
PCI Within 90 Minutes of Arrival[5]	-	-	52%	54%	95%
Smoking Cessation Advice[5]	-	-	87%	88%	100%
Heart Failure Care					
ACE Inhibitor or ARB for LVSD[1]	1	100%	84%	82%	100%
Discharge Instructions[1,3]	4	0%	56%	61%	93%
Evaluation of LVS Function[1]	17	0%	84%	83%	99%
Smoking Cessation Advice[1,3]	1	0%	82%	82%	100%
Pneumonia Care					
Appropriate Initial Antibiotic[1,3]	3	67%	82%	83%	94%
Blood Culture Timing[1,3]	2	50%	89%	90%	100%
Influenza Vaccine[5]	-	-	58%	70%	100%
Initial Antibiotic Timing[1]	20	85%	75%	80%	93%
Oxygenation Assessment	32	100%	99%	99%	100%
Pneumococcal Vaccine[1]	21	14%	58%	69%	94%
Smoking Cessation Advice[1,3]	2	50%	75%	80%	100%
Surgical Infection Prevention					
Prophylactic Antibiotic Given[5]	-	-	74%	77%	95%
Prophylactic Antibiotic Selection[5]	-	-	89%	90%	100%
Prophylactic Antibiotic Stopped[5]	-	-	65%	72%	95%
Pregnancy Care					
Inpatient Neonatal Mortality	-	-	-	-	-
Third or Fourth Degree Laceration	-	-	3.58%	3.63%	3.27%

Enloe Medical Center

1531 Esplanade
Chico, CA 95926

Toll-Free: 800-822-8102
Phone: 530-332-7300
Fax: 530-899-2026

URL: www.enloe.org
Ownership: Voluntary non-profit - Private
Emergency Services: Yes

Accredited: Yes
Licensed Beds: 369

Key Personnel:

CEO . . . . Deborah A Yancer
Chief Medical Staff . . . . Bonnie Perry
Chief Catheterization Laboratory . . . . Darrell Fuller
Emergency Room . . . . Cory Boyles, RN
Director Infection/Disease Control . . . . Alivia Strawn, RN
CCU Spvg. Nurse . . . . Lee Zweifel, RN
Director Medical/Surgical Nursing . . . . Lee Zweifel, RN
Director Respiratory Therapy . . . . Bob Morejohn

Measure	Cases	This Hospital	State Average	U.S. Average	Top Hospital
Heart Attack Care					
ACE Inhibitor or ARB for LVSD	83	84%	82%	82%	100%
Aspirin at Arrival	118	100%	95%	92%	100%
Aspirin at Discharge	233	96%	90%	90%	100%
Beta Blocker at Arrival	75	91%	89%	87%	100%
Beta Blocker at Discharge	270	96%	89%	90%	100%
Fibrinolytic Medication Timing[1]	1	100%	40%	31%	100%
PCI Within 90 Minutes of Arrival[1]	7	57%	52%	54%	95%
Smoking Cessation Advice	95	96%	87%	88%	100%
Heart Failure Care					
ACE Inhibitor or ARB for LVSD	112	73%	84%	82%	100%
Discharge Instructions	233	50%	56%	61%	93%
Evaluation of LVS Function	296	95%	84%	83%	99%
Smoking Cessation Advice	41	93%	82%	82%	100%
Pneumonia Care					
Appropriate Initial Antibiotic	232	81%	82%	83%	94%
Blood Culture Timing	223	84%	89%	90%	100%
Influenza Vaccine[4,5]	-	-	58%	70%	100%
Initial Antibiotic Timing	416	79%	75%	80%	93%
Oxygenation Assessment	504	100%	99%	99%	100%
Pneumococcal Vaccine	345	50%	58%	69%	94%
Smoking Cessation Advice	90	92%	75%	80%	100%
Surgical Infection Prevention					
Prophylactic Antibiotic Given[2]	810	87%	74%	77%	95%
Prophylactic Antibiotic Selection[2]	198	97%	89%	90%	100%
Prophylactic Antibiotic Stopped[2]	775	66%	65%	72%	95%
Pregnancy Care					
Inpatient Neonatal Mortality	-	-	-	-	-
Third or Fourth Degree Laceration	-	-	3.58%	3.63%	3.27%

Chino Valley Medical Center

5451 Walnut Avenue
Chino, CA 91710
URL: www.cvmc.com
Ownership: Proprietary
Emergency Services: Yes

Phone: 909-464-8600
Fax: 909-464-8882
Accredited: Yes
Licensed Beds: 126

Key Personnel:

Emergency Room . . . . Linda Ruggil
Infection Control . . . . Jeanine Martin
ICU . . . . Kim Jones
Medical/Surgical Nursing . . . . Anne Marie Robertson
OB/GYN Womens Health . . . . Janel Hinman
Manager of Respiratory . . . . Joseph Carrillo

NOTE: Hospital profiles are in alphabetical order by state, then city, then hospital within the city; Rankings are sorted by rate in descending order and exclude hospitals with less than 25 cases; (1) The number of cases is too small (n<25) for purposes of reliably predicting hospital performance; (2) Measure reflects the hospital's indication that its submission was based upon a sample of its relevant discharges; (3) Rate reflects fewer than the maximum possible quarters of data for the measure; (4) Inaccurate information submitted and suppressed for one or more quarters; (5) No data is available from the hospital for this measure; Please refer to the User's Guide for a full explanation of data

Measure	Cases	This Hospital	State Average	U.S. Average	Top Hospital
Heart Attack Care					
ACE Inhibitor or ARB for LVSD[1]	9	100%	82%	82%	100%
Aspirin at Arrival	54	100%	95%	92%	100%
Aspirin at Discharge[1]	19	100%	90%	90%	100%
Beta Blocker at Arrival	46	100%	89%	87%	100%
Beta Blocker at Discharge[1]	21	100%	89%	90%	100%
Fibrinolytic Medication Timing[1,3]	3	100%	40%	31%	100%
PCI Within 90 Minutes of Arrival	0	-	52%	54%	95%
Smoking Cessation Advice[1]	3	100%	87%	88%	100%
Heart Failure Care					
ACE Inhibitor or ARB for LVSD	31	97%	84%	82%	100%
Discharge Instructions[3]	49	100%	56%	61%	93%
Evaluation of LVS Function	127	98%	84%	83%	99%
Smoking Cessation Advice[1]	21	100%	82%	82%	100%
Pneumonia Care					
Appropriate Initial Antibiotic[1,3]	8	100%	82%	83%	94%
Blood Culture Timing	54	89%	89%	90%	100%
Influenza Vaccine[5]	-	-	58%	70%	100%
Initial Antibiotic Timing	61	93%	75%	80%	93%
Oxygenation Assessment	81	100%	99%	99%	100%
Pneumococcal Vaccine	47	89%	58%	69%	94%
Smoking Cessation Advice[1]	20	100%	75%	80%	100%
Surgical Infection Prevention					
Prophylactic Antibiotic Given[1,3]	2	100%	74%	77%	95%
Prophylactic Antibiotic Selection	0	-	89%	90%	100%
Prophylactic Antibiotic Stopped[3]	0	-	65%	72%	95%
Pregnancy Care					
Inpatient Neonatal Mortality	-	-	-	-	-
Third or Fourth Degree Laceration	-	-	3.58%	3.63%	3.27%

Chowchilla Memorial Hospital District

1104 Ventura Avenue
Chowchilla, CA 93610
Phone: 559-665-3781
Fax: 559-665-0391
E-mail: npencecdmh@yahoo.com
Ownership: Govt - Hospital District or Authority
Accredited: No
Emergency Services: No
Licensed Beds: 24

Key Personnel:

Administrator/CEO. . . . . Cathy J Flores
Chief of Medical Staff. . . . . Satwant Samaro, MD
Infection Control. . . . . Dianne Collier, LVN

Measure	Cases	This Hospital	State Average	U.S. Average	Top Hospital
Heart Attack Care					
ACE Inhibitor or ARB for LVSD[5]	-	-	82%	82%	100%
Aspirin at Arrival[5]	-	-	95%	92%	100%
Aspirin at Discharge[5]	-	-	90%	90%	100%
Beta Blocker at Arrival[5]	-	-	89%	87%	100%
Beta Blocker at Discharge[5]	-	-	89%	90%	100%
Fibrinolytic Medication Timing[5]	-	-	40%	31%	100%
PCI Within 90 Minutes of Arrival[5]	-	-	52%	54%	95%
Smoking Cessation Advice[5]	-	-	87%	88%	100%
Heart Failure Care					
ACE Inhibitor or ARB for LVSD[5]	-	-	84%	82%	100%
Discharge Instructions[5]	-	-	56%	61%	93%
Evaluation of LVS Function[5]	-	-	84%	83%	99%
Smoking Cessation Advice[5]	-	-	82%	82%	100%
Pneumonia Care					
Appropriate Initial Antibiotic[5]	-	-	82%	83%	94%
Blood Culture Timing[5]	-	-	89%	90%	100%
Influenza Vaccine[5]	-	-	58%	70%	100%
Initial Antibiotic Timing[5]	-	-	75%	80%	93%
Oxygenation Assessment[5]	-	-	99%	99%	100%
Pneumococcal Vaccine[5]	-	-	58%	69%	94%
Smoking Cessation Advice[5]	-	-	75%	80%	100%
Surgical Infection Prevention					
Prophylactic Antibiotic Given[5]	-	-	74%	77%	95%
Prophylactic Antibiotic Selection[5]	-	-	89%	90%	100%
Prophylactic Antibiotic Stopped[5]	-	-	65%	72%	95%
Pregnancy Care					
Inpatient Neonatal Mortality	-	-	-	-	-
Third or Fourth Degree Laceration	-	-	3.58%	3.63%	3.27%

Sharp Chula Vista Medical Center

Alternate Name: Community Hospital of Chula Vista
751 Medical Center Court
Chula Vista, CA 91911
Toll-Free: 800-827-4277
Phone: 619-482-5800
Fax: 619-482-3535
E-mail: info@sharp.com
URL: www.sharp.com
Ownership: Voluntary non-profit - Other
Accredited: Yes
Emergency Services: Yes
Licensed Beds: 330

Key Personnel:

CEO. . . . . Christopher L Boyd
Chief Medical Staff. . . . . Seung-Yi T Song, MD
Medical Director of Cardiology Services. . . . . . . Daniel Copin, MD
Medical Dir, Cardiac Catheterization Lab . . . . . . H Mehrdad Sadeghi, MD
Chief of Emergency Services. . . . . Andres Smith, MD
Director Infection/Disease Control . . . . Linda Riley
Manager, Medical/Surgical. . . . . Deanna White
Director OB/GYN . . . . Christine Basillere
Manager Radiology . . . . Jeffrey Liebesman
Manager, Respiratory/Cardiology. . . . . Carmen Kasmauski

Measure	Cases	This Hospital	State Average	U.S. Average	Top Hospital
Heart Attack Care					
ACE Inhibitor or ARB for LVSD	66	73%	82%	82%	100%
Aspirin at Arrival	279	97%	95%	92%	100%
Aspirin at Discharge	284	91%	90%	90%	100%
Beta Blocker at Arrival	243	93%	89%	87%	100%
Beta Blocker at Discharge	280	88%	89%	90%	100%
Fibrinolytic Medication Timing[1]	2	0%	40%	31%	100%
PCI Within 90 Minutes of Arrival[1]	10	50%	52%	54%	95%
Smoking Cessation Advice	57	72%	87%	88%	100%
Heart Failure Care					
ACE Inhibitor or ARB for LVSD	179	65%	84%	82%	100%
Discharge Instructions	478	69%	56%	61%	93%
Evaluation of LVS Function	574	87%	84%	83%	99%
Smoking Cessation Advice	56	84%	82%	82%	100%
Pneumonia Care					
Appropriate Initial Antibiotic[2]	270	84%	82%	83%	94%
Blood Culture Timing[2]	283	82%	89%	90%	100%
Influenza Vaccine[2]	67	33%	58%	70%	100%
Initial Antibiotic Timing[2]	390	71%	75%	80%	93%
Oxygenation Assessment[2]	468	100%	99%	99%	100%
Pneumococcal Vaccine[2]	278	22%	58%	69%	94%
Smoking Cessation Advice[2]	54	70%	75%	80%	100%
Surgical Infection Prevention					
Prophylactic Antibiotic Given[2,3]	222	77%	74%	77%	95%
Prophylactic Antibiotic Selection[2]	64	78%	89%	90%	100%
Prophylactic Antibiotic Stopped[2,3]	208	74%	65%	72%	95%
Pregnancy Care					
Inpatient Neonatal Mortality	-	-	-	-	-
Third or Fourth Degree Laceration	-	-	3.58%	3.63%	3.27%

Redbud Community Hospital

15630 18th Avenue
Clearlake, CA 95422
Phone: 707-994-6486
Fax: 707-995-3516
URL: www.redbudhospital.org
Ownership: Voluntary non-profit - Private
Accredited: Yes
Emergency Services: No
Licensed Beds: 32

Key Personnel:

CEO. . . . . Kendall R Fults
Chief Medical Staff. . . . . Steve Schpper
Emergency Room . . . . Vicky Lentz
Infection Control Nurse. . . . . Maureen Milligan
ICU Director. . . . . Vicky Lentz
Director Cardiopulmonary Services . . . . Ilona Horton
Respiratory Care . . . . Penny Nichols

Measure	Cases	This Hospital	State Average	U.S. Average	Top Hospital
Heart Attack Care					
ACE Inhibitor or ARB for LVSD[3]	0	-	82%	82%	100%
Aspirin at Arrival[1,3]	4	50%	95%	92%	100%

NOTE: Hospital profiles are in alphabetical order by state, then city, then hospital within the city; Rankings are sorted by rate in descending order and exclude hospitals with less than 25 cases; (1) The number of cases is too small (n<25) for purposes of reliably predicting hospital performance; (2) Measure reflects the hospital's indication that its submission was based upon a sample of its relevant discharges; (3) Rate reflects fewer than the maximum possible quarters of data for the measure; (4) Inaccurate information submitted and suppressed for one or more quarters; (5) No data is available from the hospital for this measure; Please refer to the User's Guide for a full explanation of data

Aspirin at Discharge[1,3]	2	50%	90%	90%	100%
Beta Blocker at Arrival[1,3]	3	33%	89%	87%	100%
Beta Blocker at Discharge[1,3]	2	50%	89%	90%	100%
Fibrinolytic Medication Timing[3]	0	-	40%	31%	100%
PCI Within 90 Minutes of Arrival[5]	-	-	52%	54%	95%
Smoking Cessation Advice[3]	0	-	87%	88%	100%
Heart Failure Care					
ACE Inhibitor or ARB for LVSD[1]	13	69%	84%	82%	100%
Discharge Instructions	46	24%	56%	61%	93%
Evaluation of LVS Function	49	71%	84%	83%	99%
Smoking Cessation Advice[1]	16	56%	82%	82%	100%
Pneumonia Care					
Appropriate Initial Antibiotic	93	83%	82%	83%	94%
Blood Culture Timing	64	91%	89%	90%	100%
Influenza Vaccine[1]	15	27%	58%	70%	100%
Initial Antibiotic Timing	103	69%	75%	80%	93%
Oxygenation Assessment	112	100%	99%	99%	100%
Pneumococcal Vaccine	53	17%	58%	69%	94%
Smoking Cessation Advice	35	54%	75%	80%	100%
Surgical Infection Prevention					
Prophylactic Antibiotic Given[3]	62	63%	74%	77%	95%
Prophylactic Antibiotic Selection[1]	20	100%	89%	90%	100%
Prophylactic Antibiotic Stopped[3]	61	59%	65%	72%	95%
Pregnancy Care					
Inpatient Neonatal Mortality	-	-	-	-	-
Third or Fourth Degree Laceration	-	-	3.58%	3.63%	3.27%

Community Medical Center-Clovis

2755 Herndon Avenue Phone: 559-324-4000
Clovis, CA 93611 Fax: 559-459-3851
URL: www.communitymedical.org
Ownership: Voluntary non-profit - Other Accredited: Yes
Emergency Services: Yes Licensed Beds: 109

Key Personnel:

CEO. . . . . Tim A Joslin
Emergency Room Director. . . . . Kan Coon
Director Medical/Surgical Nursing . . . . Vic Gaitan

Measure	Cases	This Hospital	State Average	U.S. Average	Top Hospital
Heart Attack Care					
ACE Inhibitor or ARB for LVSD[1]	5	100%	82%	82%	100%
Aspirin at Arrival	53	89%	95%	92%	100%
Aspirin at Discharge	33	94%	90%	90%	100%
Beta Blocker at Arrival	30	90%	89%	87%	100%
Beta Blocker at Discharge	34	97%	89%	90%	100%
Fibrinolytic Medication Timing	0	-	40%	31%	100%
PCI Within 90 Minutes of Arrival[1]	1	0%	52%	54%	95%
Smoking Cessation Advice[1]	14	79%	87%	88%	100%
Heart Failure Care					
ACE Inhibitor or ARB for LVSD	53	74%	84%	82%	100%
Discharge Instructions	128	16%	56%	61%	93%
Evaluation of LVS Function	154	75%	84%	83%	99%
Smoking Cessation Advice[1]	14	36%	82%	82%	100%
Pneumonia Care					
Appropriate Initial Antibiotic	119	88%	82%	83%	94%
Blood Culture Timing	84	88%	89%	90%	100%
Influenza Vaccine	32	84%	58%	70%	100%
Initial Antibiotic Timing	129	62%	75%	80%	93%
Oxygenation Assessment	168	100%	99%	99%	100%
Pneumococcal Vaccine	103	68%	58%	69%	94%
Smoking Cessation Advice	38	79%	75%	80%	100%
Surgical Infection Prevention					
Prophylactic Antibiotic Given	629	44%	74%	77%	95%
Prophylactic Antibiotic Selection	141	95%	89%	90%	100%
Prophylactic Antibiotic Stopped	608	68%	65%	72%	95%
Pregnancy Care					
Inpatient Neonatal Mortality	-	-	-	-	-
Third or Fourth Degree Laceration	-	-	3.58%	3.63%	3.27%

Coalinga Regional Medical Center

Alternate Name: Coalinga District Hospital
1191 Phelps Avenue Phone: 559-935-6400
Coalinga, CA 93210 Fax: 559-935-6596
E-mail: admincrmc@onemain.com
URL: www.coalingamedicalcenter.com
Ownership: Govt - Hospital District or Authority Accredited: No
Emergency Services: Yes Licensed Beds: 78

Key Personnel:

Interim CEO. . . . . Sharon Spurgeon
Chief Medical Staff. . . . . H J Zwang, MD
Director Infection/Disease Control . . . . Lori Bryan, RN, DON
Surgical Services . . . . Nina Williams
Chief Radiology . . . . Richard B Peterson, MD
Manager Respiratory Therapy . . . . Thomas Lowrey

Measure	Cases	This Hospital	State Average	U.S. Average	Top Hospital
Heart Attack Care					
ACE Inhibitor or ARB for LVSD[5]	-	-	82%	82%	100%
Aspirin at Arrival[5]	-	-	95%	92%	100%
Aspirin at Discharge[5]	-	-	90%	90%	100%
Beta Blocker at Arrival[5]	-	-	89%	87%	100%
Beta Blocker at Discharge[5]	-	-	89%	90%	100%
Fibrinolytic Medication Timing[5]	-	-	40%	31%	100%
PCI Within 90 Minutes of Arrival[5]	-	-	52%	54%	95%
Smoking Cessation Advice[5]	-	-	87%	88%	100%
Heart Failure Care					
ACE Inhibitor or ARB for LVSD[3]	0	-	84%	82%	100%
Discharge Instructions[1,3]	2	0%	56%	61%	93%
Evaluation of LVS Function[1,3]	1	0%	84%	83%	99%
Smoking Cessation Advice[3]	0	-	82%	82%	100%
Pneumonia Care					
Appropriate Initial Antibiotic[1,3]	19	79%	82%	83%	94%
Blood Culture Timing[1,3]	7	14%	89%	90%	100%
Influenza Vaccine[5]	-	-	58%	70%	100%
Initial Antibiotic Timing	74	80%	75%	80%	93%
Oxygenation Assessment	90	100%	99%	99%	100%
Pneumococcal Vaccine	32	6%	58%	69%	94%
Smoking Cessation Advice[1,3]	2	0%	75%	80%	100%
Surgical Infection Prevention					
Prophylactic Antibiotic Given[5]	-	-	74%	77%	95%
Prophylactic Antibiotic Selection[5]	-	-	89%	90%	100%
Prophylactic Antibiotic Stopped[5]	-	-	65%	72%	95%
Pregnancy Care					
Inpatient Neonatal Mortality	-	-	-	-	-
Third or Fourth Degree Laceration	-	-	3.58%	3.63%	3.27%

Arrowhead Regional Medical Center

Alternate Name: San Bernardino County Medical Center
400 N Pepper Avenue Phone: 909-580-1000
Colton, CA 92324 Fax: 909-580-1388
URL: www.arrowheadmedcenter.org
Ownership: Government - Local Accredited: Yes
Emergency Services: Yes Licensed Beds: 283

Key Personnel:

CEO. . . . . June Griffith-Collso
Cardiac Lab . . . . Aslam Mohammed, MD
Chairman Emergency Room . . . . Rodney Borger
OB/GYN Womens Health. . . . . Guillermo Valenzuela, MD
Director Respiratory Therapy . . . . Paula Meares-Conrad

Measure	Cases	This Hospital	State Average	U.S. Average	Top Hospital
Heart Attack Care					
ACE Inhibitor or ARB for LVSD[2]	31	94%	82%	82%	100%
Aspirin at Arrival[2]	87	98%	95%	92%	100%
Aspirin at Discharge[2]	71	100%	90%	90%	100%
Beta Blocker at Arrival[2]	65	95%	89%	87%	100%
Beta Blocker at Discharge[2]	65	98%	89%	90%	100%
Fibrinolytic Medication Timing[1,2]	17	12%	40%	31%	100%
PCI Within 90 Minutes of Arrival[1,2]	3	0%	52%	54%	95%
Smoking Cessation Advice[2]	28	61%	87%	88%	100%
Heart Failure Care					
ACE Inhibitor or ARB for LVSD[2]	207	90%	84%	82%	100%
Discharge Instructions[2]	322	4%	56%	61%	93%
Evaluation of LVS Function[2]	337	94%	84%	83%	99%

NOTE: Hospital profiles are in alphabetical order by state, then city, then hospital within the city; Rankings are sorted by rate in descending order and exclude hospitals with less than 25 cases; (1) The number of cases is too small (n<25) for purposes of reliably predicting hospital performance; (2) Measure reflects the hospital's indication that its submission was based upon a sample of its relevant discharges; (3) Rate reflects fewer than the maximum possible quarters of data for the measure; (4) Inaccurate information submitted and suppressed for one or more quarters; (5) No data is available from the hospital for this measure; Please refer to the User's Guide for a full explanation of data

Measure	Cases	This Hospital	State Average	U.S. Average	Top Hospital
Smoking Cessation Advice[2]	124	34%	82%	82%	100%
Pneumonia Care					
Appropriate Initial Antibiotic[2]	138	93%	82%	83%	94%
Blood Culture Timing[2]	129	76%	89%	90%	100%
Influenza Vaccine[4,5]	-	-	58%	70%	100%
Initial Antibiotic Timing[2]	184	59%	75%	80%	93%
Oxygenation Assessment[2]	218	100%	99%	99%	100%
Pneumococcal Vaccine[2]	68	35%	58%	69%	94%
Smoking Cessation Advice[2]	76	47%	75%	80%	100%
Surgical Infection Prevention					
Prophylactic Antibiotic Given	243	92%	74%	77%	95%
Prophylactic Antibiotic Selection	51	92%	89%	90%	100%
Prophylactic Antibiotic Stopped	226	77%	65%	72%	95%
Pregnancy Care					
Inpatient Neonatal Mortality	-	-	-	-	-
Third or Fourth Degree Laceration	-	-	3.58%	3.63%	3.27%

Colusa Regional Medical Center

199 East Webster Street — Phone: 530-458-5821
Colusa, CA 95932 — Fax: 530-458-3210
URL: www.colusamedicalcenter.org
Ownership: Voluntary non-profit - Other — Accredited: Yes
Emergency Services: Yes — Licensed Beds: 48

Key Personnel:

CEO . . . . Dale Kirby
Chief Medical Staff . . . . Julian Delgado, MD
Emergency Room . . . . Samuel Medrano, MD
Infection Control . . . . Katherine Hughes, RN
ICU . . . . Christine Gregory, RN
Respiratory/Cardiopulmonary . . . . Cory Jamison

Measure	Cases	This Hospital	State Average	U.S. Average	Top Hospital
Heart Attack Care					
ACE Inhibitor or ARB for LVSD	0	-	82%	82%	100%
Aspirin at Arrival[1]	3	100%	95%	92%	100%
Aspirin at Discharge[1]	2	50%	90%	90%	100%
Beta Blocker at Arrival[1]	2	50%	89%	87%	100%
Beta Blocker at Discharge[1]	1	100%	89%	90%	100%
Fibrinolytic Medication Timing	0	-	40%	31%	100%
PCI Within 90 Minutes of Arrival	0	-	52%	54%	95%
Smoking Cessation Advice	0	-	87%	88%	100%
Heart Failure Care					
ACE Inhibitor or ARB for LVSD[1]	6	50%	84%	82%	100%
Discharge Instructions	36	3%	56%	61%	93%
Evaluation of LVS Function	41	66%	84%	83%	99%
Smoking Cessation Advice[1]	4	50%	82%	82%	100%
Pneumonia Care					
Appropriate Initial Antibiotic	32	78%	82%	83%	94%
Blood Culture Timing[1]	10	70%	89%	90%	100%
Influenza Vaccine[1]	3	33%	58%	70%	100%
Initial Antibiotic Timing	31	74%	75%	80%	93%
Oxygenation Assessment	35	100%	99%	99%	100%
Pneumococcal Vaccine	27	93%	58%	69%	94%
Smoking Cessation Advice[1]	4	25%	75%	80%	100%
Surgical Infection Prevention					
Prophylactic Antibiotic Given[5]	-	-	74%	77%	95%
Prophylactic Antibiotic Selection[5]	-	-	89%	90%	100%
Prophylactic Antibiotic Stopped[5]	-	-	65%	72%	95%
Pregnancy Care					
Inpatient Neonatal Mortality	-	-	-	-	-
Third or Fourth Degree Laceration	-	-	3.58%	3.63%	3.27%

John Muir Medical Center-Concord Campus

2540 E Street — Phone: 925-682-8200
PO Box 4110 — Fax: 925-674-2009
Concord, CA 94520
URL: www.johnmuirhealth.com
Ownership: Govt - Hospital District or Authority — Accredited: Yes
Emergency Services: Yes

Key Personnel:

CEO . . . . J Kendall Anderson
Chief Medical Staff . . . . Roy Kaplan, MD
Emergency Room . . . . Kathy Hester, RN
Director Medical/Surgical Nursing . . . . Elaine Shingleton
OB/GYN Womens Health . . . . Anita Rama, MD
Chief Radiology . . . . Robert Schick, MD
Director Respiratory Therapy . . . . Kathy Hester

Measure	Cases	This Hospital	State Average	U.S. Average	Top Hospital
Heart Attack Care					
ACE Inhibitor or ARB for LVSD	45	96%	82%	82%	100%
Aspirin at Arrival	183	99%	95%	92%	100%
Aspirin at Discharge	281	98%	90%	90%	100%
Beta Blocker at Arrival	155	97%	89%	87%	100%
Beta Blocker at Discharge	276	100%	89%	90%	100%
Fibrinolytic Medication Timing[1]	1	100%	40%	31%	100%
PCI Within 90 Minutes of Arrival[1]	5	40%	52%	54%	95%
Smoking Cessation Advice	78	100%	87%	88%	100%
Heart Failure Care					
ACE Inhibitor or ARB for LVSD[2]	106	93%	84%	82%	100%
Discharge Instructions[2]	257	84%	56%	61%	93%
Evaluation of LVS Function[2]	317	96%	84%	83%	99%
Smoking Cessation Advice[2]	46	100%	82%	82%	100%
Pneumonia Care					
Appropriate Initial Antibiotic[2]	116	89%	82%	83%	94%
Blood Culture Timing[2]	122	95%	89%	90%	100%
Influenza Vaccine[2]	29	52%	58%	70%	100%
Initial Antibiotic Timing[2]	152	81%	75%	80%	93%
Oxygenation Assessment[2]	195	100%	99%	99%	100%
Pneumococcal Vaccine[2]	123	77%	58%	69%	94%
Smoking Cessation Advice[2]	36	100%	75%	80%	100%
Surgical Infection Prevention					
Prophylactic Antibiotic Given[2,3]	231	77%	74%	77%	95%
Prophylactic Antibiotic Selection[2]	79	67%	89%	90%	100%
Prophylactic Antibiotic Stopped[2,3]	218	76%	65%	72%	95%
Pregnancy Care					
Inpatient Neonatal Mortality	-	-	-	-	-
Third or Fourth Degree Laceration	-	-	3.58%	3.63%	3.27%

Corcoran District Hospital

1310 Hanna Avenue — Phone: 559-992-5051
Corcoran, CA 93212 — Fax: 559-992-3972
Ownership: Govt - Hospital District or Authority — Accredited: No
Emergency Services: Yes — Licensed Beds: 32

Key Personnel:

CEO . . . . Evan J Rayner
Chief Medical Staff . . . . Thomas Lambert, MD
Emergency Room . . . . Terry Cardona
Emergency Room . . . . Thomas Lambert, MD
Infection Control . . . . Judy Wofford
Director Medical/Surgical Nursing . . . . Susan Fairchild
Chief Radiology . . . . Armando Tajum
Director Respiratory Therapy . . . . Mitchell Denham

Measure	Cases	This Hospital	State Average	U.S. Average	Top Hospital
Heart Attack Care					
ACE Inhibitor or ARB for LVSD[5]	-	-	82%	82%	100%
Aspirin at Arrival[5]	-	-	95%	92%	100%
Aspirin at Discharge[5]	-	-	90%	90%	100%
Beta Blocker at Arrival[5]	-	-	89%	87%	100%
Beta Blocker at Discharge[5]	-	-	89%	90%	100%
Fibrinolytic Medication Timing[5]	-	-	40%	31%	100%
PCI Within 90 Minutes of Arrival[5]	-	-	52%	54%	95%
Smoking Cessation Advice[5]	-	-	87%	88%	100%
Heart Failure Care					
ACE Inhibitor or ARB for LVSD[1]	3	33%	84%	82%	100%
Discharge Instructions[1,3]	8	12%	56%	61%	93%
Evaluation of LVS Function	40	10%	84%	83%	99%
Smoking Cessation Advice[3]	0	-	82%	82%	100%
Pneumonia Care					
Appropriate Initial Antibiotic[1,3]	1	100%	82%	83%	94%
Blood Culture Timing[3]	0	-	89%	90%	100%
Influenza Vaccine[5]	-	-	58%	70%	100%
Initial Antibiotic Timing[1]	18	44%	75%	80%	93%
Oxygenation Assessment[1]	23	83%	99%	99%	100%

NOTE: Hospital profiles are in alphabetical order by state, then city, then hospital within the city; Rankings are sorted by rate in descending order and exclude hospitals with less than 25 cases; (1) The number of cases is too small (n<25) for purposes of reliably predicting hospital performance; (2) Measure reflects the hospital's indication that its submission was based upon a sample of its relevant discharges; (3) Rate reflects fewer than the maximum possible quarters of data for the measure; (4) Inaccurate information submitted and suppressed for one or more quarters; (5) No data is available from the hospital for this measure; Please refer to the User's Guide for a full explanation of data

Measure	Cases	This Hospital	State Average	U.S. Average	Top Hospital
Pneumococcal Vaccine[1]	9	0%	58%	69%	94%
Smoking Cessation Advice[3]	0	-	75%	80%	100%
Surgical Infection Prevention					
Prophylactic Antibiotic Given[5]	-	-	74%	77%	95%
Prophylactic Antibiotic Selection[5]	-	-	89%	90%	100%
Prophylactic Antibiotic Stopped[5]	-	-	65%	72%	95%
Pregnancy Care					
Inpatient Neonatal Mortality	-	-	-	-	-
Third or Fourth Degree Laceration	-	-	3.58%	3.63%	3.27%

Corona Regional Medical Center

Alternate Name: Corona Community Hospital
800 South Main Street
Corona, CA 92882
URL: www.coronaregional.com
Ownership: Proprietary
Emergency Services: Yes
Phone: 951-737-4343
Fax: 951-736-6334
Accredited: Yes
Licensed Beds: 228

Key Personnel:
CEO. . . . . Ken Rivers
Chief Medical Staff. . . . . Anoop Maheshwari, MD
Emergency Room . . . . Nancy Bakewell
Director Medical/Surgical Nursing . . . . Marlene Cole, RN
OB/GYN Womens Health. . . . . Allyn Pierce, DO
Chief Radiology . . . . Michael Brand
Director Respiratory Therapy . . . . Lisa Pierce

Measure	Cases	This Hospital	State Average	U.S. Average	Top Hospital
Heart Attack Care					
ACE Inhibitor or ARB for LVSD[1]	5	60%	82%	82%	100%
Aspirin at Arrival	110	95%	95%	92%	100%
Aspirin at Discharge	74	85%	90%	90%	100%
Beta Blocker at Arrival	103	87%	89%	87%	100%
Beta Blocker at Discharge	74	80%	89%	90%	100%
Fibrinolytic Medication Timing[1]	14	29%	40%	31%	100%
PCI Within 90 Minutes of Arrival	0	-	52%	54%	95%
Smoking Cessation Advice[1]	17	76%	87%	88%	100%
Heart Failure Care					
ACE Inhibitor or ARB for LVSD	33	88%	84%	82%	100%
Discharge Instructions	200	60%	56%	61%	93%
Evaluation of LVS Function	254	80%	84%	83%	99%
Smoking Cessation Advice	32	91%	82%	82%	100%
Pneumonia Care					
Appropriate Initial Antibiotic	321	68%	82%	83%	94%
Blood Culture Timing	204	71%	89%	90%	100%
Influenza Vaccine[4,5]	-	-	58%	70%	100%
Initial Antibiotic Timing	315	71%	75%	80%	93%
Oxygenation Assessment	375	99%	99%	99%	100%
Pneumococcal Vaccine	214	66%	58%	69%	94%
Smoking Cessation Advice	49	71%	75%	80%	100%
Surgical Infection Prevention					
Prophylactic Antibiotic Given[3]	238	70%	74%	77%	95%
Prophylactic Antibiotic Selection	76	86%	89%	90%	100%
Prophylactic Antibiotic Stopped[3]	226	47%	65%	72%	95%
Pregnancy Care					
Inpatient Neonatal Mortality	-	-	-	-	-
Third or Fourth Degree Laceration	-	-	3.58%	3.63%	3.27%

Sharp Coronado Hospital

Alternate Name: Coronado Hospital
250 Prospect Place
San Diego, CA 92118
URL: www.sharp.com/coronado
Ownership: Voluntary non-profit - Other
Emergency Services: Yes
Phone: 619-522-3600
Fax: 619-522-3777
Accredited: Yes
Licensed Beds: 204

Key Personnel:
CEO. . . . . Marcia K Hall
Chief Medical Staff. . . . . Matthew Horn, MD

Measure	Cases	This Hospital	State Average	U.S. Average	Top Hospital
Heart Attack Care					
ACE Inhibitor or ARB for LVSD[1]	2	100%	82%	82%	100%
Aspirin at Arrival[1]	16	100%	95%	92%	100%
Aspirin at Discharge[1]	5	100%	90%	90%	100%
Beta Blocker at Arrival[1]	14	100%	89%	87%	100%
Beta Blocker at Discharge[1]	7	100%	89%	90%	100%
Fibrinolytic Medication Timing[1]	3	33%	40%	31%	100%
PCI Within 90 Minutes of Arrival	0	-	52%	54%	95%
Smoking Cessation Advice[1]	1	100%	87%	88%	100%
Heart Failure Care					
ACE Inhibitor or ARB for LVSD[1]	7	100%	84%	82%	100%
Discharge Instructions	63	54%	56%	61%	93%
Evaluation of LVS Function	74	74%	84%	83%	99%
Smoking Cessation Advice[1]	4	75%	82%	82%	100%
Pneumonia Care					
Appropriate Initial Antibiotic	70	81%	82%	83%	94%
Blood Culture Timing	50	92%	89%	90%	100%
Influenza Vaccine[1]	22	55%	58%	70%	100%
Initial Antibiotic Timing	84	93%	75%	80%	93%
Oxygenation Assessment	104	100%	99%	99%	100%
Pneumococcal Vaccine	82	52%	58%	69%	94%
Smoking Cessation Advice[1]	19	95%	75%	80%	100%
Surgical Infection Prevention					
Prophylactic Antibiotic Given[2,3]	96	94%	74%	77%	95%
Prophylactic Antibiotic Selection[2]	28	89%	89%	90%	100%
Prophylactic Antibiotic Stopped[2,3]	94	87%	65%	72%	95%
Pregnancy Care					
Inpatient Neonatal Mortality	-	-	-	-	-
Third or Fourth Degree Laceration	-	-	3.58%	3.63%	3.27%

College Hospital Costa Mesa

Alternate Name: Costa Mesa Medical Center
301 Victoria Street
Costa Mesa, CA 92627
URL: www.collegehospitals.com
Ownership: Proprietary
Emergency Services: No
Phone: 949-642-2734
Fax: 949-574-3695
Accredited: Yes
Licensed Beds: 122

Key Personnel:
CEO. . . . . Wayne Lingenfelter
Chief Medical Staff. . . . . Craig Ross
Director Medical/Surgical Nursing . . . . Jasmine Rodriguez, RN
Chief Radiology . . . . Alexander Lin, MD
Director Respiratory Therapy . . . . Maud Johansson

Measure	Cases	This Hospital	State Average	U.S. Average	Top Hospital
Heart Attack Care					
ACE Inhibitor or ARB for LVSD[5]	-	-	82%	82%	100%
Aspirin at Arrival[5]	-	-	95%	92%	100%
Aspirin at Discharge[5]	-	-	90%	90%	100%
Beta Blocker at Arrival[5]	-	-	89%	87%	100%
Beta Blocker at Discharge[5]	-	-	89%	90%	100%
Fibrinolytic Medication Timing[5]	-	-	40%	31%	100%
PCI Within 90 Minutes of Arrival[5]	-	-	52%	54%	95%
Smoking Cessation Advice[5]	-	-	87%	88%	100%
Heart Failure Care					
ACE Inhibitor or ARB for LVSD[3]	0	-	84%	82%	100%
Discharge Instructions[3]	0	-	56%	61%	93%
Evaluation of LVS Function[1,3]	1	100%	84%	83%	99%
Smoking Cessation Advice[3]	0	-	82%	82%	100%
Pneumonia Care					
Appropriate Initial Antibiotic[5]	-	-	82%	83%	94%
Blood Culture Timing[5]	-	-	89%	90%	100%
Influenza Vaccine[5]	-	-	58%	70%	100%
Initial Antibiotic Timing[1,3]	4	75%	75%	80%	93%
Oxygenation Assessment[1,3]	4	100%	99%	99%	100%
Pneumococcal Vaccine[3]	0	-	58%	69%	94%
Smoking Cessation Advice[5]	-	-	75%	80%	100%
Surgical Infection Prevention					
Prophylactic Antibiotic Given[5]	-	-	74%	77%	95%
Prophylactic Antibiotic Selection[5]	-	-	89%	90%	100%
Prophylactic Antibiotic Stopped[5]	-	-	65%	72%	95%
Pregnancy Care					
Inpatient Neonatal Mortality	-	-	-	-	-
Third or Fourth Degree Laceration	-	-	3.58%	3.63%	3.27%

NOTE: Hospital profiles are in alphabetical order by state, then city, then hospital within the city; Rankings are sorted by rate in descending order and exclude hospitals with less than 25 cases; (1) The number of cases is too small (n<25) for purposes of reliably predicting hospital performance; (2) Measure reflects the hospital's indication that its submission was based upon a sample of its relevant discharges; (3) Rate reflects fewer than the maximum possible quarters of data for the measure; (4) Inaccurate information submitted and suppressed for one or more quarters; (5) No data is available from the hospital for this measure; Please refer to the User's Guide for a full explanation of data

Citrus Valley Medical Center

Alternate Name: Inter-Community Campus
210 W San Bernardino Road — Phone: 626-331-7331
Covina, CA 91723 — Fax: 626-814-2428
URL: www.cvhp.org
Ownership: Voluntary non-profit - Other — Accredited: Yes
Emergency Services: Yes — Licensed Beds: 208

Key Personnel:

President/CEO. . . . . James T Yoshioka
Chief of Medical Staff . . . . Robinson Barron
OB/GYN Womens Health. . . . . Elie Shuhaibar, MD
Chief Radiology . . . . David Underwood, MD
Director Cardio-Respiratory Services . . . . Fred Lopez

Measure	Cases	This Hospital	State Average	U.S. Average	Top Hospital
Heart Attack Care					
ACE Inhibitor or ARB for LVSD	53	77%	82%	82%	100%
Aspirin at Arrival	143	94%	95%	92%	100%
Aspirin at Discharge	276	95%	90%	90%	100%
Beta Blocker at Arrival	99	91%	89%	87%	100%
Beta Blocker at Discharge	258	90%	89%	90%	100%
Fibrinolytic Medication Timing	0	-	40%	31%	100%
PCI Within 90 Minutes of Arrival[1]	7	14%	52%	54%	95%
Smoking Cessation Advice	71	97%	87%	88%	100%
Heart Failure Care					
ACE Inhibitor or ARB for LVSD	151	69%	84%	82%	100%
Discharge Instructions	306	16%	56%	61%	93%
Evaluation of LVS Function	391	86%	84%	83%	99%
Smoking Cessation Advice	48	73%	82%	82%	100%
Pneumonia Care					
Appropriate Initial Antibiotic	132	87%	82%	83%	94%
Blood Culture Timing	148	82%	89%	90%	100%
Influenza Vaccine	49	37%	58%	70%	100%
Initial Antibiotic Timing	235	60%	75%	80%	93%
Oxygenation Assessment	300	99%	99%	99%	100%
Pneumococcal Vaccine	198	20%	58%	69%	94%
Smoking Cessation Advice	40	62%	75%	80%	100%
Surgical Infection Prevention					
Prophylactic Antibiotic Given[2,3]	217	72%	74%	77%	95%
Prophylactic Antibiotic Selection[2]	75	87%	89%	90%	100%
Prophylactic Antibiotic Stopped[2,3]	197	24%	65%	72%	95%
Pregnancy Care					
Inpatient Neonatal Mortality	-	-	-	-	-
Third or Fourth Degree Laceration	-	-	3.58%	3.63%	3.27%

Sutter Coast Hospital

800 E Washington Boulevard — Phone: 707-464-8511
Crescent City, CA 95531 — Fax: 707-464-8941
E-mail: SutterCoast@Sutterhealth.org
URL: www.suttercoast.org
Ownership: Govt - Hospital District or Authority — Accredited: Yes
Emergency Services: Yes — Licensed Beds: 59

Key Personnel:

CEO. . . . . John E Menaugh
Chief Medical Staff. . . . . Gregory Higgins, MD
Director Medical/Surgical Nursing . . . . Phyllis Speir
OB/GYN Womens Health. . . . . W Christopher Slater, MD

Measure	Cases	This Hospital	State Average	U.S. Average	Top Hospital
Heart Attack Care					
ACE Inhibitor or ARB for LVSD	0	-	82%	82%	100%
Aspirin at Arrival[1]	14	93%	95%	92%	100%
Aspirin at Discharge[1]	6	100%	90%	90%	100%
Beta Blocker at Arrival[1]	7	100%	89%	87%	100%
Beta Blocker at Discharge[1]	6	100%	89%	90%	100%
Fibrinolytic Medication Timing[1]	1	0%	40%	31%	100%
PCI Within 90 Minutes of Arrival	0	-	52%	54%	95%
Smoking Cessation Advice[1]	2	100%	87%	88%	100%
Heart Failure Care					
ACE Inhibitor or ARB for LVSD	34	82%	84%	82%	100%
Discharge Instructions	91	68%	56%	61%	93%
Evaluation of LVS Function	86	86%	84%	83%	99%
Smoking Cessation Advice[1]	21	100%	82%	82%	100%
Pneumonia Care					
Appropriate Initial Antibiotic	76	84%	82%	83%	94%
Blood Culture Timing	78	90%	89%	90%	100%
Influenza Vaccine[1]	21	52%	58%	70%	100%
Initial Antibiotic Timing	105	84%	75%	80%	93%
Oxygenation Assessment	124	100%	99%	99%	100%
Pneumococcal Vaccine	69	80%	58%	69%	94%
Smoking Cessation Advice	47	100%	75%	80%	100%
Surgical Infection Prevention					
Prophylactic Antibiotic Given	62	55%	74%	77%	95%
Prophylactic Antibiotic Selection[1]	11	55%	89%	90%	100%
Prophylactic Antibiotic Stopped	61	46%	65%	72%	95%
Pregnancy Care					
Inpatient Neonatal Mortality	376	0.27%	-	-	-
Third or Fourth Degree Laceration	282	3.19%	3.58%	3.63%	3.27%

Brotman Medical Center

3828 Delmas Terrace — Phone: 310-836-7000
Culver City, CA 90232 — Fax: 310-202-4141
URL: www.brotmanmedicalcenter.com
Ownership: Proprietary — Accredited: Yes
Emergency Services: Yes — Licensed Beds: 420

Key Personnel:

CEO. . . . . Maurine Cate
Chief Medical Staff. . . . . Jordan Goodstien, MD
Cardiac Lab . . . . Mark Raffaele, RN
Catheterization Lab . . . . Mark Raffaele
Emergency Room . . . . Cindy Calvillo, RN
Emergency Room . . . . Pat McCusker
Infection Control. . . . . Alfonso Torress-Cook
ICU . . . . Kate Begley
Medical/Surgical Nursing . . . . Cindy Calvillo
Respiratory/Cardiopulmonary. . . . . John Woodard

Measure	Cases	This Hospital	State Average	U.S. Average	Top Hospital
Heart Attack Care					
ACE Inhibitor or ARB for LVSD[1]	22	82%	82%	82%	100%
Aspirin at Arrival	122	86%	95%	92%	100%
Aspirin at Discharge	116	81%	90%	90%	100%
Beta Blocker at Arrival	111	80%	89%	87%	100%
Beta Blocker at Discharge	120	78%	89%	90%	100%
Fibrinolytic Medication Timing[1]	3	0%	40%	31%	100%
PCI Within 90 Minutes of Arrival[1]	4	25%	52%	54%	95%
Smoking Cessation Advice[1]	21	71%	87%	88%	100%
Heart Failure Care					
ACE Inhibitor or ARB for LVSD	64	72%	84%	82%	100%
Discharge Instructions	210	10%	56%	61%	93%
Evaluation of LVS Function	260	72%	84%	83%	99%
Smoking Cessation Advice	42	60%	82%	82%	100%
Pneumonia Care					
Appropriate Initial Antibiotic	86	69%	82%	83%	94%
Blood Culture Timing	74	95%	89%	90%	100%
Influenza Vaccine[1]	18	22%	58%	70%	100%
Initial Antibiotic Timing	115	71%	75%	80%	93%
Oxygenation Assessment	147	100%	99%	99%	100%
Pneumococcal Vaccine	99	26%	58%	69%	94%
Smoking Cessation Advice[1]	19	47%	75%	80%	100%
Surgical Infection Prevention					
Prophylactic Antibiotic Given	129	69%	74%	77%	95%
Prophylactic Antibiotic Selection	35	77%	89%	90%	100%
Prophylactic Antibiotic Stopped	121	45%	65%	72%	95%
Pregnancy Care					
Inpatient Neonatal Mortality	-	-	-	-	-
Third or Fourth Degree Laceration	-	-	3.58%	3.63%	3.27%

Seton Medical Center

1900 Sullivan Avenue — Phone: 650-992-4000
Daly City, CA 94015 — Fax: 650-991-6025
URL: www.setonmedicalcenter.org
Ownership: Voluntary non-profit - Church — Accredited: Yes
Emergency Services: Yes — Licensed Beds: 357

Key Personnel:

CEO. . . . . John Williams

NOTE: Hospital profiles are in alphabetical order by state, then city, then hospital within the city; Rankings are sorted by rate in descending order and exclude hospitals with less than 25 cases; (1) The number of cases is too small (n<25) for purposes of reliably predicting hospital performance; (2) Measure reflects the hospital's indication that its submission was based upon a sample of its relevant discharges; (3) Rate reflects fewer than the maximum possible quarters of data for the measure; (4) Inaccurate information submitted and suppressed for one or more quarters; (5) No data is available from the hospital for this measure; Please refer to the User's Guide for a full explanation of data

Chief Medical Staff. . . . . Robert Dunlap, MD
Emergency Room . . . . Jeff Clingan
Manager Infection Control . . . . Robert Grisnak
CCU Spvg. Nurse . . . . Jeanne Lee
Director Medical/Surgical Nursing . . . . Judy Cook
Director Respiratory Therapy . . . . Gene Ann La Moria

Measure	Cases	This Hospital	State Average	U.S. Average	Top Hospital
Heart Attack Care					
ACE Inhibitor or ARB for LVSD	30	97%	82%	82%	100%
Aspirin at Arrival	127	97%	95%	92%	100%
Aspirin at Discharge	130	99%	90%	90%	100%
Beta Blocker at Arrival	107	96%	89%	87%	100%
Beta Blocker at Discharge	122	98%	89%	90%	100%
Fibrinolytic Medication Timing[3]	0	-	40%	31%	100%
PCI Within 90 Minutes of Arrival[1]	9	89%	52%	54%	95%
Smoking Cessation Advice[1,3]	8	100%	87%	88%	100%
Heart Failure Care					
ACE Inhibitor or ARB for LVSD	151	86%	84%	82%	100%
Discharge Instructions[3]	71	100%	56%	61%	93%
Evaluation of LVS Function	431	96%	84%	83%	99%
Smoking Cessation Advice[1,3]	6	100%	82%	82%	100%
Pneumonia Care					
Appropriate Initial Antibiotic[1,3]	23	87%	82%	83%	94%
Blood Culture Timing[3]	32	84%	89%	90%	100%
Influenza Vaccine[5]	-	-	58%	70%	100%
Initial Antibiotic Timing	209	86%	75%	80%	93%
Oxygenation Assessment	243	100%	99%	99%	100%
Pneumococcal Vaccine	193	41%	58%	69%	94%
Smoking Cessation Advice[1,3]	3	100%	75%	80%	100%
Surgical Infection Prevention					
Prophylactic Antibiotic Given[2,3]	53	77%	74%	77%	95%
Prophylactic Antibiotic Selection[5]	-	-	89%	90%	100%
Prophylactic Antibiotic Stopped[2,3]	51	59%	65%	72%	95%
Pregnancy Care					
Inpatient Neonatal Mortality	-	-	-	-	-
Third or Fourth Degree Laceration	-	-	3.58%	3.63%	3.27%

Sutter Davis Hospital

2000 Sutter Place
Davis, CA 95616
URL: www.sutterdavis.org
Ownership: Proprietary
Emergency Services: Yes
Phone: 530-756-6440
Fax: 530-757-5779
Accredited: Yes
Licensed Beds: 48

Key Personnel:
President/CEO. . . . . Sarah Krevans

Measure	Cases	This Hospital	State Average	U.S. Average	Top Hospital
Heart Attack Care					
ACE Inhibitor or ARB for LVSD	0	-	82%	82%	100%
Aspirin at Arrival[1]	7	100%	95%	92%	100%
Aspirin at Discharge[1]	5	100%	90%	90%	100%
Beta Blocker at Arrival[1]	6	100%	89%	87%	100%
Beta Blocker at Discharge[1]	4	100%	89%	90%	100%
Fibrinolytic Medication Timing[1]	1	100%	40%	31%	100%
PCI Within 90 Minutes of Arrival	0	-	52%	54%	95%
Smoking Cessation Advice	0	-	87%	88%	100%
Heart Failure Care					
ACE Inhibitor or ARB for LVSD[1]	15	87%	84%	82%	100%
Discharge Instructions	47	74%	56%	61%	93%
Evaluation of LVS Function	65	94%	84%	83%	99%
Smoking Cessation Advice[1]	9	89%	82%	82%	100%
Pneumonia Care					
Appropriate Initial Antibiotic	118	95%	82%	83%	94%
Blood Culture Timing	96	90%	89%	90%	100%
Influenza Vaccine	29	93%	58%	70%	100%
Initial Antibiotic Timing	136	90%	75%	80%	93%
Oxygenation Assessment	173	100%	99%	99%	100%
Pneumococcal Vaccine	104	96%	58%	69%	94%
Smoking Cessation Advice	32	88%	75%	80%	100%
Surgical Infection Prevention					
Prophylactic Antibiotic Given[2]	218	84%	74%	77%	95%
Prophylactic Antibiotic Selection[2]	47	87%	89%	90%	100%
Prophylactic Antibiotic Stopped[2]	203	84%	65%	72%	95%
Pregnancy Care					
Inpatient Neonatal Mortality[2]	752	0.13%	-	-	-
Third or Fourth Degree Laceration[2]	730	2.47%	3.58%	3.63%	3.27%

Delano Regional Medical Center

1401 Garces Highway
Delano, CA 93215
URL: www.drmc.com
Ownership: Proprietary
Emergency Services: Yes
Phone: 661-725-4800
Fax: 661-721-5355
Accredited: Yes
Licensed Beds: 156

Key Personnel:
Executive Director . . . . Allan G Komarek, MD
Chief of Medical Staff. Radhey Bansel
Emergency Room . . . . Shanthi Margoschis
Emergency Room . . . . Barbara Faller
Director of Pulmonary/Respiratory Care. . . . . . . Sukhmander Dhillon

Measure	Cases	This Hospital	State Average	U.S. Average	Top Hospital
Heart Attack Care					
ACE Inhibitor or ARB for LVSD[3]	0	-	82%	82%	100%
Aspirin at Arrival[1,3]	14	86%	95%	92%	100%
Aspirin at Discharge[1,3]	5	100%	90%	90%	100%
Beta Blocker at Arrival[1,3]	10	70%	89%	87%	100%
Beta Blocker at Discharge[1,3]	5	60%	89%	90%	100%
Fibrinolytic Medication Timing[3]	0	-	40%	31%	100%
PCI Within 90 Minutes of Arrival[5]	-	-	52%	54%	95%
Smoking Cessation Advice[3]	0	-	87%	88%	100%
Heart Failure Care					
ACE Inhibitor or ARB for LVSD	27	70%	84%	82%	100%
Discharge Instructions	124	54%	56%	61%	93%
Evaluation of LVS Function	146	58%	84%	83%	99%
Smoking Cessation Advice[1]	22	45%	82%	82%	100%
Pneumonia Care					
Appropriate Initial Antibiotic	69	74%	82%	83%	94%
Blood Culture Timing	44	80%	89%	90%	100%
Influenza Vaccine	26	12%	58%	70%	100%
Initial Antibiotic Timing	124	69%	75%	80%	93%
Oxygenation Assessment	157	99%	99%	99%	100%
Pneumococcal Vaccine	104	11%	58%	69%	94%
Smoking Cessation Advice[1]	17	29%	75%	80%	100%
Surgical Infection Prevention					
Prophylactic Antibiotic Given[1,3]	13	69%	74%	77%	95%
Prophylactic Antibiotic Selection[1]	13	77%	89%	90%	100%
Prophylactic Antibiotic Stopped[1,3]	13	46%	65%	72%	95%
Pregnancy Care					
Inpatient Neonatal Mortality	-	-	-	-	-
Third or Fourth Degree Laceration	-	-	3.58%	3.63%	3.27%

Downey Regional Medical Center

Alternate Name: Downey Community Hospital
11500 Brookshire Avenue
Downey, CA 90241
URL: www.drmci.org
Ownership: Voluntary non-profit - Private
Emergency Services: Yes
Phone: 562-904-5000
Fax: 562-904-5309
Accredited: Yes
Licensed Beds: 199

Key Personnel:
President/CEO. . . . . Allen Korneff
Emergency Room . . . . Richard Guess, MD
Director Infection/Disease Control . . . . Mary Stevens
Medical/Surgical Nursing . . . . Millie Cervantes
Director Respiratory Therapy . . . . Cathy Blackwood

Measure	Cases	This Hospital	State Average	U.S. Average	Top Hospital
Heart Attack Care					
ACE Inhibitor or ARB for LVSD	31	74%	82%	82%	100%
Aspirin at Arrival	174	98%	95%	92%	100%
Aspirin at Discharge	187	97%	90%	90%	100%
Beta Blocker at Arrival	139	89%	89%	87%	100%
Beta Blocker at Discharge	190	97%	89%	90%	100%
Fibrinolytic Medication Timing[1]	8	38%	40%	31%	100%

NOTE: Hospital profiles are in alphabetical order by state, then city, then hospital within the city; Rankings are sorted by rate in descending order and exclude hospitals with less than 25 cases; (1) The number of cases is too small (n<25) for purposes of reliably predicting hospital performance; (2) Measure reflects the hospital's indication that its submission was based upon a sample of its relevant discharges; (3) Rate reflects fewer than the maximum possible quarters of data for the measure; (4) Inaccurate information submitted and suppressed for one or more quarters; (5) No data is available from the hospital for this measure; Please refer to the User's Guide for a full explanation of data

PCI Within 90 Minutes of Arrival[1]	6	0%	52%	54%	95%
Smoking Cessation Advice	37	100%	87%	88%	100%
Heart Failure Care					
ACE Inhibitor or ARB for LVSD[2]	136	83%	84%	82%	100%
Discharge Instructions[2]	306	67%	56%	61%	93%
Evaluation of LVS Function[2]	355	92%	84%	83%	99%
Smoking Cessation Advice[2]	47	100%	82%	82%	100%
Pneumonia Care					
Appropriate Initial Antibiotic[2]	128	84%	82%	83%	94%
Blood Culture Timing[2]	146	86%	89%	90%	100%
Influenza Vaccine[2]	32	53%	58%	70%	100%
Initial Antibiotic Timing[2]	192	71%	75%	80%	93%
Oxygenation Assessment[2]	231	100%	99%	99%	100%
Pneumococcal Vaccine[2]	170	72%	58%	69%	94%
Smoking Cessation Advice[1,2]	23	70%	75%	80%	100%
Surgical Infection Prevention					
Prophylactic Antibiotic Given[2,3]	216	90%	74%	77%	95%
Prophylactic Antibiotic Selection[2]	79	97%	89%	90%	100%
Prophylactic Antibiotic Stopped[2,3]	213	52%	65%	72%	95%
Pregnancy Care					
Inpatient Neonatal Mortality	1,574	0.25%	-	-	-
Third or Fourth Degree Laceration	1,192	2.18%	3.58%	3.63%	3.27%

Ranchos Los Amigos Nat'l Rehab Ctr

Alternate Name: Ranchos Los Amigos Medical Center
7601 E Imperial Highway — Phone: 562-401-7111
Downey, CA 90242 — Fax: 562-803-3486
URL: www.rancho.org
Ownership: Government - Local — Accredited: Yes
Emergency Services: No — Licensed Beds: 395

Key Personnel:
CEO/President . . . . Valerie Orange
Chief Medical Staff . . . . Henry Gong, MD
Director Infection/Disease Control . . . . Francisco Sapico, MD
Director Medical/Surgical Nursing . . . . Karen Wunch, RN
Chief Radiology . . . . Charles A Stewart, MD
Director Respiratory Therapy . . . . Glynis Frederick

Measure	Cases	This Hospital	State Average	U.S. Average	Top Hospital
Heart Attack Care					
ACE Inhibitor or ARB for LVSD[5]	-	-	82%	82%	100%
Aspirin at Arrival[5]	-	-	95%	92%	100%
Aspirin at Discharge[5]	-	-	90%	90%	100%
Beta Blocker at Arrival[5]	-	-	89%	87%	100%
Beta Blocker at Discharge[5]	-	-	89%	90%	100%
Fibrinolytic Medication Timing[5]	-	-	40%	31%	100%
PCI Within 90 Minutes of Arrival[5]	-	-	52%	54%	95%
Smoking Cessation Advice[5]	-	-	87%	88%	100%
Heart Failure Care					
ACE Inhibitor or ARB for LVSD[1]	6	100%	84%	82%	100%
Discharge Instructions[1,3]	3	0%	56%	61%	93%
Evaluation of LVS Function[1]	22	64%	84%	83%	99%
Smoking Cessation Advice[3]	0	-	82%	82%	100%
Pneumonia Care					
Appropriate Initial Antibiotic[3]	0	-	82%	83%	94%
Blood Culture Timing[3]	0	-	89%	90%	100%
Influenza Vaccine[5]	-	-	58%	70%	100%
Initial Antibiotic Timing[1]	2	100%	75%	80%	93%
Oxygenation Assessment[1]	8	100%	99%	99%	100%
Pneumococcal Vaccine[1]	4	0%	58%	69%	94%
Smoking Cessation Advice[1,3]	1	0%	75%	80%	100%
Surgical Infection Prevention					
Prophylactic Antibiotic Given[1,3]	4	50%	74%	77%	95%
Prophylactic Antibiotic Selection[5]	-	-	89%	90%	100%
Prophylactic Antibiotic Stopped[1,3]	4	100%	65%	72%	95%
Pregnancy Care					
Inpatient Neonatal Mortality	-	-	-	-	-
Third or Fourth Degree Laceration	-	-	3.58%	3.63%	3.27%

El Centro Regional Medical Center

Alternate Name: El Centro Community Hospital
1415 Ross Avenue — Phone: 760-339-7100
El Centro, CA 92243 — Fax: 760-339-7363
E-mail: wecare@ecrmc.org
URL: www.ecrmc.org
Ownership: Government - Local — Accredited: Yes
Emergency Services: Yes — Licensed Beds: 165

Key Personnel:
President . . . . Jennifer McGrew-Thomason
CEO . . . . David R Green
Cardiology Medical Director . . . . Randy Steffen
Emergency Room . . . . George Rodriguez, MD
Emergency Room . . . . Tomas Virgen, RN
Director of Medical Surgical . . . . Suzanne Martinez, RN
Obstetrics/Gynecology Chair . . . . Elias Moukarzel, MD
Director of Surgical Services . . . . Karen Timmerman, RN
Cardiopulmonary . . . . Randy Steffen

Measure	Cases	This Hospital	State Average	U.S. Average	Top Hospital
Heart Attack Care					
ACE Inhibitor or ARB for LVSD[1]	10	90%	82%	82%	100%
Aspirin at Arrival	85	100%	95%	92%	100%
Aspirin at Discharge	28	100%	90%	90%	100%
Beta Blocker at Arrival	76	100%	89%	87%	100%
Beta Blocker at Discharge	31	97%	89%	90%	100%
Fibrinolytic Medication Timing[1]	7	43%	40%	31%	100%
PCI Within 90 Minutes of Arrival	0	-	52%	54%	95%
Smoking Cessation Advice[1]	5	100%	87%	88%	100%
Heart Failure Care					
ACE Inhibitor or ARB for LVSD	60	98%	84%	82%	100%
Discharge Instructions	206	100%	56%	61%	93%
Evaluation of LVS Function	222	97%	84%	83%	99%
Smoking Cessation Advice[1]	8	100%	82%	82%	100%
Pneumonia Care					
Appropriate Initial Antibiotic	135	86%	82%	83%	94%
Blood Culture Timing	96	90%	89%	90%	100%
Influenza Vaccine	39	79%	58%	70%	100%
Initial Antibiotic Timing	139	62%	75%	80%	93%
Oxygenation Assessment	167	100%	99%	99%	100%
Pneumococcal Vaccine	108	92%	58%	69%	94%
Smoking Cessation Advice[1]	16	100%	75%	80%	100%
Surgical Infection Prevention					
Prophylactic Antibiotic Given[3]	244	90%	74%	77%	95%
Prophylactic Antibiotic Selection	71	89%	89%	90%	100%
Prophylactic Antibiotic Stopped[3]	71	37%	65%	72%	95%
Pregnancy Care					
Inpatient Neonatal Mortality	-	-	-	-	-
Third or Fourth Degree Laceration	-	-	3.58%	3.63%	3.27%

Sonoma Developmental Center

15000 Arnold Drive — Phone: 707-938-6000
Eldridge, CA 95431 — Fax: 707-938-6574
URL: www.dds.ca.gov/sonoma/sonoma.cfm
Ownership: Government - State — Accredited: No
Emergency Services: No — Licensed Beds: 1,421

Key Personnel:
Executive Director . . . . Jim Rogers
Chief Medical Staff . . . . Judith Bjorndal
Emergency Room . . . . David Grey
Chief Radiology . . . . Ted Hansen

Measure	Cases	This Hospital	State Average	U.S. Average	Top Hospital
Heart Attack Care					
ACE Inhibitor or ARB for LVSD[5]	-	-	82%	82%	100%
Aspirin at Arrival[5]	-	-	95%	92%	100%
Aspirin at Discharge[5]	-	-	90%	90%	100%
Beta Blocker at Arrival[5]	-	-	89%	87%	100%
Beta Blocker at Discharge[5]	-	-	89%	90%	100%
Fibrinolytic Medication Timing[5]	-	-	40%	31%	100%
PCI Within 90 Minutes of Arrival[5]	-	-	52%	54%	95%
Smoking Cessation Advice[5]	-	-	87%	88%	100%
Heart Failure Care					
ACE Inhibitor or ARB for LVSD[1,3]	3	0%	84%	82%	100%
Discharge Instructions[3]	0	-	56%	61%	93%

NOTE: Hospital profiles are in alphabetical order by state, then city, then hospital within the city; Rankings are sorted by rate in descending order and exclude hospitals with less than 25 cases; (1) The number of cases is too small (n<25) for purposes of reliably predicting hospital performance; (2) Measure reflects the hospital's indication that its submission was based upon a sample of its relevant discharges; (3) Rate reflects fewer than the maximum possible quarters of data for the measure; (4) Inaccurate information submitted and suppressed for one or more quarters; (5) No data is available from the hospital for this measure; Please refer to the User's Guide for a full explanation of data

Measure	Cases	This Hospital	State Average	U.S. Average	Top Hospital
Evaluation of LVS Function[1,3]	4	100%	84%	83%	99%
Smoking Cessation Advice[3]	0	-	82%	82%	100%
Pneumonia Care					
Appropriate Initial Antibiotic[3]	0	-	82%	83%	94%
Blood Culture Timing[3]	0	-	89%	90%	100%
Influenza Vaccine[5]	-	-	58%	70%	100%
Initial Antibiotic Timing[1]	4	100%	75%	80%	93%
Oxygenation Assessment[1]	9	100%	99%	99%	100%
Pneumococcal Vaccine[1]	2	100%	58%	69%	94%
Smoking Cessation Advice[3]	0	-	75%	80%	100%
Surgical Infection Prevention					
Prophylactic Antibiotic Given[5]	-	-	74%	77%	95%
Prophylactic Antibiotic Selection[5]	-	-	89%	90%	100%
Prophylactic Antibiotic Stopped[5]	-	-	65%	72%	95%
Pregnancy Care					
Inpatient Neonatal Mortality	-	-	-	-	-
Third or Fourth Degree Laceration	-	-	3.58%	3.63%	3.27%

Scripps Memorial Hospital-Encinitas

354 Santa Fe Drive
Encinitas, CA 92024
Phone: 760-633-6501
Fax: 760-633-7356
Ownership: Voluntary non-profit - Private
Accredited: Yes
Emergency Services: Yes
Licensed Beds: 140

Key Personnel:

CEO/Administrator . . . . John Schleif
Chief Medical Staff . . . . James LaBelle
Emergency Room . . . . Jan Zachary

Measure	Cases	This Hospital	State Average	U.S. Average	Top Hospital
Heart Attack Care					
ACE Inhibitor or ARB for LVSD[1]	16	100%	82%	82%	100%
Aspirin at Arrival	116	99%	95%	92%	100%
Aspirin at Discharge	99	97%	90%	90%	100%
Beta Blocker at Arrival	71	92%	89%	87%	100%
Beta Blocker at Discharge	93	84%	89%	90%	100%
Fibrinolytic Medication Timing[1]	2	0%	40%	31%	100%
PCI Within 90 Minutes of Arrival[1]	7	29%	52%	54%	95%
Smoking Cessation Advice[1]	21	95%	87%	88%	100%
Heart Failure Care					
ACE Inhibitor or ARB for LVSD	59	68%	84%	82%	100%
Discharge Instructions	120	24%	56%	61%	93%
Evaluation of LVS Function	170	98%	84%	83%	99%
Smoking Cessation Advice[1]	11	73%	82%	82%	100%
Pneumonia Care					
Appropriate Initial Antibiotic	126	90%	82%	83%	94%
Blood Culture Timing	144	95%	89%	90%	100%
Influenza Vaccine	40	50%	58%	70%	100%
Initial Antibiotic Timing	145	77%	75%	80%	93%
Oxygenation Assessment	205	100%	99%	99%	100%
Pneumococcal Vaccine	130	52%	58%	69%	94%
Smoking Cessation Advice	28	68%	75%	80%	100%
Surgical Infection Prevention					
Prophylactic Antibiotic Given[2,3]	94	86%	74%	77%	95%
Prophylactic Antibiotic Selection[2]	50	98%	89%	90%	100%
Prophylactic Antibiotic Stopped[2,3]	91	44%	65%	72%	95%
Pregnancy Care					
Inpatient Neonatal Mortality	1,530	0.00%	-	-	-
Third or Fourth Degree Laceration	1,228	3.42%	3.58%	3.63%	3.27%

Encino-Tarzana Regional Medical Center

Alternate Name: Encino Hospital/Campus
16237 Ventura Boulevard
Encino, CA 91436
Toll-Free: 800-227-3669
Phone: 818-995-5000
Fax: 818-907-8630
E-mail: etrmcpublicrelations@tenethealth.com
URL: www.encino-tarzana.com
Ownership: Proprietary
Accredited: Yes
Emergency Services: Yes
Licensed Beds: 151

Key Personnel:

CEO . . . . Dale Surowitz
Chief Staff . . . . Glenn Irani, MD
Infection Control . . . . Hala Mashed
ICU . . . . Brenda Scott Manzur
Director Womens Services . . . . Diane Galati
Director Respiratory Therapy . . . . George Torres

Measure	Cases	This Hospital	State Average	U.S. Average	Top Hospital
Heart Attack Care					
ACE Inhibitor or ARB for LVSD[1]	7	57%	82%	82%	100%
Aspirin at Arrival	47	96%	95%	92%	100%
Aspirin at Discharge	30	70%	90%	90%	100%
Beta Blocker at Arrival	46	85%	89%	87%	100%
Beta Blocker at Discharge[1]	23	52%	89%	90%	100%
Fibrinolytic Medication Timing	0	-	40%	31%	100%
PCI Within 90 Minutes of Arrival	0	-	52%	54%	95%
Smoking Cessation Advice	0	-	87%	88%	100%
Heart Failure Care					
ACE Inhibitor or ARB for LVSD[1]	15	67%	84%	82%	100%
Discharge Instructions	75	69%	56%	61%	93%
Evaluation of LVS Function	106	86%	84%	83%	99%
Smoking Cessation Advice[1]	4	75%	82%	82%	100%
Pneumonia Care					
Appropriate Initial Antibiotic	86	78%	82%	83%	94%
Blood Culture Timing	123	91%	89%	90%	100%
Influenza Vaccine	44	59%	58%	70%	100%
Initial Antibiotic Timing	154	87%	75%	80%	93%
Oxygenation Assessment	225	100%	99%	99%	100%
Pneumococcal Vaccine	173	51%	58%	69%	94%
Smoking Cessation Advice[1]	10	70%	75%	80%	100%
Surgical Infection Prevention					
Prophylactic Antibiotic Given[2]	121	75%	74%	77%	95%
Prophylactic Antibiotic Selection[1,2]	24	83%	89%	90%	100%
Prophylactic Antibiotic Stopped[2]	120	20%	65%	72%	95%
Pregnancy Care					
Inpatient Neonatal Mortality	-	-	-	-	-
Third or Fourth Degree Laceration	-	-	3.58%	3.63%	3.27%

Palomar Medical Center

555 E Valley Parkway
Escondido, CA 92025
Phone: 760-739-3000
Fax: 760-739-3108
E-mail: tlc@pph.org
URL: www.pph.org
Ownership: Govt - Hospital District or Authority
Accredited: Yes
Emergency Services: Yes
Licensed Beds: 332

Key Personnel:

President & CEO . . . . Michael H Covert, FACHE
Chief Medical Staff . . . . Charles Smith, MD
Chief Catheterization Laboratory . . . . Robert Stein, MD
Director Infection/Disease Control . . . . Lina Mendenhall
CCU Spvg. Nurse . . . . Lorrie Shoemaker, RN
Director Medical/Surgical Nursing . . . . Ruth Baer
Chief OB/GYN . . . . Robert Trifunovic, MD
Chief Radiology . . . . Earl Shultz, MD
Director Respiratory Therapy . . . . Diana Faugno

Measure	Cases	This Hospital	State Average	U.S. Average	Top Hospital
Heart Attack Care					
ACE Inhibitor or ARB for LVSD	48	100%	82%	82%	100%
Aspirin at Arrival	278	100%	95%	92%	100%
Aspirin at Discharge	313	100%	90%	90%	100%
Beta Blocker at Arrival	253	99%	89%	87%	100%
Beta Blocker at Discharge	313	100%	89%	90%	100%
Fibrinolytic Medication Timing	0	-	40%	31%	100%
PCI Within 90 Minutes of Arrival	25	60%	52%	54%	95%
Smoking Cessation Advice	96	100%	87%	88%	100%
Heart Failure Care					
ACE Inhibitor or ARB for LVSD	162	97%	84%	82%	100%
Discharge Instructions	365	90%	56%	61%	93%
Evaluation of LVS Function	434	99%	84%	83%	99%
Smoking Cessation Advice	54	87%	82%	82%	100%
Pneumonia Care					
Appropriate Initial Antibiotic	279	95%	82%	83%	94%
Blood Culture Timing	264	91%	89%	90%	100%
Influenza Vaccine	80	76%	58%	70%	100%
Initial Antibiotic Timing	374	79%	75%	80%	93%

NOTE: Hospital profiles are in alphabetical order by state, then city, then hospital within the city; Rankings are sorted by rate in descending order and exclude hospitals with less than 25 cases; (1) The number of cases is too small (n<25) for purposes of reliably predicting hospital performance; (2) Measure reflects the hospital's indication that its submission was based upon a sample of its relevant discharges; (3) Rate reflects fewer than the maximum possible quarters of data for the measure; (4) Inaccurate information submitted and suppressed for one or more quarters; (5) No data is available from the hospital for this measure; Please refer to the User's Guide for a full explanation of data

Oxygenation Assessment	398	100%	99%	99%	100%
Pneumococcal Vaccine	290	68%	58%	69%	94%
Smoking Cessation Advice	60	97%	75%	80%	100%
Surgical Infection Prevention					
Prophylactic Antibiotic Given[2,3]	221	82%	74%	77%	95%
Prophylactic Antibiotic Selection[2]	65	95%	89%	90%	100%
Prophylactic Antibiotic Stopped[2,3]	214	85%	65%	72%	95%
Pregnancy Care					
Inpatient Neonatal Mortality	-	-	-	-	-
Third or Fourth Degree Laceration	-	-	3.58%	3.63%	3.27%

Saint Joseph Hospital

2700 Dolbeer Street
Eureka, CA 95501
URL: www.stjosepheureka.org
Ownership: Voluntary non-profit - Church
Emergency Services: Yes

Phone: 707-269-4223
Fax: 707-269-3897
Accredited: Yes
Licensed Beds: 189

Key Personnel:

CEO. . . . . Joseph Mark
Cardiac Lab . . . . Debi Clark
Emergency Room . . . . Linda Fitzpatrick
Manager Infection Control . . . . Torg Starr
ICU . . . . Debi Clark
OB/GYN/Women's Health . . . . Ruth Howell
Director Respiratory Therapy . . . . Jack Scott

Measure	Cases	This Hospital	State Average	U.S. Average	Top Hospital
Heart Attack Care					
ACE Inhibitor or ARB for LVSD[1]	24	79%	82%	82%	100%
Aspirin at Arrival	54	98%	95%	92%	100%
Aspirin at Discharge	105	93%	90%	90%	100%
Beta Blocker at Arrival	53	89%	89%	87%	100%
Beta Blocker at Discharge	102	92%	89%	90%	100%
Fibrinolytic Medication Timing	0	-	40%	31%	100%
PCI Within 90 Minutes of Arrival[1]	2	0%	52%	54%	95%
Smoking Cessation Advice	37	89%	87%	88%	100%
Heart Failure Care					
ACE Inhibitor or ARB for LVSD	41	88%	84%	82%	100%
Discharge Instructions	101	69%	56%	61%	93%
Evaluation of LVS Function	106	97%	84%	83%	99%
Smoking Cessation Advice	33	94%	82%	82%	100%
Pneumonia Care					
Appropriate Initial Antibiotic	93	87%	82%	83%	94%
Blood Culture Timing	96	95%	89%	90%	100%
Influenza Vaccine	25	100%	58%	70%	100%
Initial Antibiotic Timing	115	93%	75%	80%	93%
Oxygenation Assessment	147	100%	99%	99%	100%
Pneumococcal Vaccine	81	90%	58%	69%	94%
Smoking Cessation Advice	49	94%	75%	80%	100%
Surgical Infection Prevention					
Prophylactic Antibiotic Given[2,3]	256	41%	74%	77%	95%
Prophylactic Antibiotic Selection[2]	128	96%	89%	90%	100%
Prophylactic Antibiotic Stopped[2,3]	252	63%	65%	72%	95%
Pregnancy Care					
Inpatient Neonatal Mortality	-	-	-	-	-
Third or Fourth Degree Laceration	-	-	3.58%	3.63%	3.27%

NorthBay Medical Center

1200 B Gale Wilson Blvd
Fairfield, CA 94533
URL: www.northbay.org
Ownership: Voluntary non-profit - Other
Emergency Services: Yes

Phone: 707-429-3600
Fax: 707-426-5287
Accredited: Yes
Licensed Beds: 132

Key Personnel:

CEO. . . . . Gary Passama
Emergency Room . . . . Ed Ballerine

Measure	Cases	This Hospital	State Average	U.S. Average	Top Hospital
Heart Attack Care					
ACE Inhibitor or ARB for LVSD[1]	6	83%	82%	82%	100%
Aspirin at Arrival	50	94%	95%	92%	100%
Aspirin at Discharge	25	96%	90%	90%	100%
Beta Blocker at Arrival	48	92%	89%	87%	100%
Beta Blocker at Discharge	27	93%	89%	90%	100%
Fibrinolytic Medication Timing[1]	16	44%	40%	31%	100%
PCI Within 90 Minutes of Arrival	0	-	52%	54%	95%
Smoking Cessation Advice[1]	5	40%	87%	88%	100%
Heart Failure Care					
ACE Inhibitor or ARB for LVSD	92	71%	84%	82%	100%
Discharge Instructions	163	28%	56%	61%	93%
Evaluation of LVS Function	181	94%	84%	83%	99%
Smoking Cessation Advice	50	84%	82%	82%	100%
Pneumonia Care					
Appropriate Initial Antibiotic	159	96%	82%	83%	94%
Blood Culture Timing	184	89%	89%	90%	100%
Influenza Vaccine	34	50%	58%	70%	100%
Initial Antibiotic Timing	223	78%	75%	80%	93%
Oxygenation Assessment	265	100%	99%	99%	100%
Pneumococcal Vaccine	140	46%	58%	69%	94%
Smoking Cessation Advice	44	84%	75%	80%	100%
Surgical Infection Prevention					
Prophylactic Antibiotic Given	179	83%	74%	77%	95%
Prophylactic Antibiotic Selection	52	90%	89%	90%	100%
Prophylactic Antibiotic Stopped	163	63%	65%	72%	95%
Pregnancy Care					
Inpatient Neonatal Mortality	-	-	-	-	-
Third or Fourth Degree Laceration	-	-	3.58%	3.63%	3.27%

Mayers Memorial Hospital District

43563 State Highway 299e
PO Box 459
Fall River Mills, CA 96028
E-mail: mmhl@shasta.com
URL: www.mayersmemorial.com
Ownership: Govt - Hospital District or Authority
Emergency Services: Yes

Phone: 530-336-5511
Fax: 530-336-5755
Accredited: No
Licensed Beds: 121

Key Personnel:

CEO. . . . . Jerry Fikes
Chief Medical Staff. . . . . Dr. Steven Scharps
Infection Control. . . . . Terry Sampson
Director Medical/Surgical Nursing . . . . Anna Engman, RN
OB/GYN Womens Health. . . . . Tom Watson, MD

Measure	Cases	This Hospital	State Average	U.S. Average	Top Hospital
Heart Attack Care					
ACE Inhibitor or ARB for LVSD[5]	-	-	82%	82%	100%
Aspirin at Arrival[5]	-	-	95%	92%	100%
Aspirin at Discharge[5]	-	-	90%	90%	100%
Beta Blocker at Arrival[5]	-	-	89%	87%	100%
Beta Blocker at Discharge[5]	-	-	89%	90%	100%
Fibrinolytic Medication Timing[5]	-	-	40%	31%	100%
PCI Within 90 Minutes of Arrival[5]	-	-	52%	54%	95%
Smoking Cessation Advice[5]	-	-	87%	88%	100%
Heart Failure Care					
ACE Inhibitor or ARB for LVSD[5]	-	-	84%	82%	100%
Discharge Instructions[5]	-	-	56%	61%	93%
Evaluation of LVS Function[5]	-	-	84%	83%	99%
Smoking Cessation Advice[5]	-	-	82%	82%	100%
Pneumonia Care					
Appropriate Initial Antibiotic[1,3]	4	100%	82%	83%	94%
Blood Culture Timing[1,3]	2	50%	89%	90%	100%
Influenza Vaccine[5]	-	-	58%	70%	100%
Initial Antibiotic Timing[1,3]	3	100%	75%	80%	93%
Oxygenation Assessment[1,3]	5	100%	99%	99%	100%
Pneumococcal Vaccine[1,3]	4	50%	58%	69%	94%
Smoking Cessation Advice[1,3]	2	100%	75%	80%	100%
Surgical Infection Prevention					
Prophylactic Antibiotic Given[5]	-	-	74%	77%	95%
Prophylactic Antibiotic Selection[5]	-	-	89%	90%	100%
Prophylactic Antibiotic Stopped[5]	-	-	65%	72%	95%
Pregnancy Care					
Inpatient Neonatal Mortality	-	-	-	-	-
Third or Fourth Degree Laceration	-	-	3.58%	3.63%	3.27%

NOTE: Hospital profiles are in alphabetical order by state, then city, then hospital within the city; Rankings are sorted by rate in descending order and exclude hospitals with less than 25 cases; (1) The number of cases is too small (n<25) for purposes of reliably predicting hospital performance; (2) Measure reflects the hospital's indication that its submission was based upon a sample of its relevant discharges; (3) Rate reflects fewer than the maximum possible quarters of data for the measure; (4) Inaccurate information submitted and suppressed for one or more quarters; (5) No data is available from the hospital for this measure; Please refer to the User's Guide for a full explanation of data

Fallbrook Hospital

624 E Elder Street Phone: 760-728-1191
Fallbrook, CA 92028 Fax: 760-723-6214
URL: www.fallbrook.com
Ownership: Govt - Hospital District or Authority Accredited: Yes
Emergency Services: Yes Licensed Beds: 140

Key Personnel:

CEO . . . . Larry W Payton
Chief Medical Staff . . . . Anthony Bianchi
Director Medical/Surgical Nursing . . . . Marvina Kramer
Director of Pulmonary . . . . Munis Salek

Measure	Cases	This Hospital	State Average	U.S. Average	Top Hospital
Heart Attack Care					
ACE Inhibitor or ARB for LVSD[1]	2	100%	82%	82%	100%
Aspirin at Arrival[1]	16	94%	95%	92%	100%
Aspirin at Discharge[1]	4	75%	90%	90%	100%
Beta Blocker at Arrival[1]	11	91%	89%	87%	100%
Beta Blocker at Discharge[1]	5	80%	89%	90%	100%
Fibrinolytic Medication Timing[1]	2	0%	40%	31%	100%
PCI Within 90 Minutes of Arrival	0	-	52%	54%	95%
Smoking Cessation Advice[1]	2	100%	87%	88%	100%
Heart Failure Care					
ACE Inhibitor or ARB for LVSD	25	92%	84%	82%	100%
Discharge Instructions	50	26%	56%	61%	93%
Evaluation of LVS Function	59	88%	84%	83%	99%
Smoking Cessation Advice[1]	5	100%	82%	82%	100%
Pneumonia Care					
Appropriate Initial Antibiotic	62	73%	82%	83%	94%
Blood Culture Timing	44	91%	89%	90%	100%
Influenza Vaccine[1]	19	37%	58%	70%	100%
Initial Antibiotic Timing	89	75%	75%	80%	93%
Oxygenation Assessment	98	99%	99%	99%	100%
Pneumococcal Vaccine	74	45%	58%	69%	94%
Smoking Cessation Advice[1]	10	100%	75%	80%	100%
Surgical Infection Prevention					
Prophylactic Antibiotic Given[2,3]	224	67%	74%	77%	95%
Prophylactic Antibiotic Selection[2]	69	88%	89%	90%	100%
Prophylactic Antibiotic Stopped[2,3]	216	83%	65%	72%	95%
Pregnancy Care					
Inpatient Neonatal Mortality	-	-	-	-	-
Third or Fourth Degree Laceration	-	-	3.58%	3.63%	3.27%

Mercy Hospital of Folsom

1650 Creekside Drive Phone: 916-983-7400
Folsom, CA 95630 Fax: 916-983-7406
URL: www.mercyfolsom.org
Ownership: Proprietary Accredited: Yes
Emergency Services: Yes Licensed Beds: 85

Key Personnel:

President . . . . Donald C Hudson

Measure	Cases	This Hospital	State Average	U.S. Average	Top Hospital
Heart Attack Care					
ACE Inhibitor or ARB for LVSD	0	-	82%	82%	100%
Aspirin at Arrival	25	100%	95%	92%	100%
Aspirin at Discharge[1]	12	100%	90%	90%	100%
Beta Blocker at Arrival[1]	24	88%	89%	87%	100%
Beta Blocker at Discharge[1]	12	100%	89%	90%	100%
Fibrinolytic Medication Timing[1]	2	0%	40%	31%	100%
PCI Within 90 Minutes of Arrival	0	-	52%	54%	95%
Smoking Cessation Advice[1]	1	100%	87%	88%	100%
Heart Failure Care					
ACE Inhibitor or ARB for LVSD	43	86%	84%	82%	100%
Discharge Instructions	100	87%	56%	61%	93%
Evaluation of LVS Function	125	94%	84%	83%	99%
Smoking Cessation Advice[1]	19	89%	82%	82%	100%
Pneumonia Care					
Appropriate Initial Antibiotic	122	88%	82%	83%	94%
Blood Culture Timing	104	95%	89%	90%	100%
Influenza Vaccine	34	91%	58%	70%	100%
Initial Antibiotic Timing	138	79%	75%	80%	93%
Oxygenation Assessment	166	100%	99%	99%	100%
Pneumococcal Vaccine	108	94%	58%	69%	94%
Smoking Cessation Advice	30	100%	75%	80%	100%
Surgical Infection Prevention					
Prophylactic Antibiotic Given[2,3]	143	78%	74%	77%	95%
Prophylactic Antibiotic Selection[2]	42	93%	89%	90%	100%
Prophylactic Antibiotic Stopped[2,3]	112	62%	65%	72%	95%
Pregnancy Care					
Inpatient Neonatal Mortality	1,084	0.00%	-	-	-
Third or Fourth Degree Laceration	830	5.18%	3.58%	3.63%	3.27%

Kaiser Permanente Fontana Medical Center

9961 Sierra Avenue Phone: 909-427-5000
Fontana, CA 92335 Fax: 909-427-7359
URL: www.kaiserpermanente.com
Ownership: Voluntary non-profit - Other Accredited: Yes
Emergency Services: Yes Licensed Beds: 444

Key Personnel:

Administrator . . . . Greg Chirstian
Administrator . . . . Gerald McCall
Chief Catheterization Laboratory . . . . Tyan Lee, MD
Emergency Room . . . . Gary McLarty, MD
Infection Control . . . . Mike Lynd
Intensive/Coronary Care . . . . Diane Kehler - Bird
Director Medical/Surgical Nursing . . . . Debra Bourgette, RN
OB/GYN Womens Health . . . . Berneda Adams, MD
Chief Radiology . . . . Johan D'Abreo, MD
Director Respiratory Therapy . . . . Pamela Hansen

Measure	Cases	This Hospital	State Average	U.S. Average	Top Hospital
Heart Attack Care					
ACE Inhibitor or ARB for LVSD	43	84%	82%	82%	100%
Aspirin at Arrival	202	96%	95%	92%	100%
Aspirin at Discharge	133	97%	90%	90%	100%
Beta Blocker at Arrival	134	93%	89%	87%	100%
Beta Blocker at Discharge	144	94%	89%	90%	100%
Fibrinolytic Medication Timing	44	64%	40%	31%	100%
PCI Within 90 Minutes of Arrival	0	-	52%	54%	95%
Smoking Cessation Advice	30	97%	87%	88%	100%
Heart Failure Care					
ACE Inhibitor or ARB for LVSD	301	83%	84%	82%	100%
Discharge Instructions	607	62%	56%	61%	93%
Evaluation of LVS Function	644	94%	84%	83%	99%
Smoking Cessation Advice	86	87%	82%	82%	100%
Pneumonia Care					
Appropriate Initial Antibiotic	63	86%	82%	83%	94%
Blood Culture Timing	45	76%	89%	90%	100%
Influenza Vaccine[4,5]	-	-	58%	70%	100%
Initial Antibiotic Timing	74	78%	75%	80%	93%
Oxygenation Assessment	102	100%	99%	99%	100%
Pneumococcal Vaccine	70	87%	58%	69%	94%
Smoking Cessation Advice[1]	22	77%	75%	80%	100%
Surgical Infection Prevention					
Prophylactic Antibiotic Given[3]	48	73%	74%	77%	95%
Prophylactic Antibiotic Selection	47	91%	89%	90%	100%
Prophylactic Antibiotic Stopped[3]	47	49%	65%	72%	95%
Pregnancy Care					
Inpatient Neonatal Mortality	4,777	0.46%	-	-	-
Third or Fourth Degree Laceration	3,321	3.85%	3.58%	3.63%	3.27%

Fountain Valley Reg Hospital & Med Ctr

17100 Euclid Street Phone: 714-966-7200
Fountain Valley, CA 92708 Fax: 714-966-8039
URL: www.fountainvalleyhospital.com
Ownership: Proprietary Accredited: Yes
Emergency Services: Yes Licensed Beds: 413

Key Personnel:

CEO . . . . Debbie Keel
Emergency Room . . . . Cess Canson
Infection Control . . . . Barbara Goss
Surgical Services . . . . Mary Meola
Chief Radiology . . . . Bob McKewen
Director Respiratory Therapy . . . . Joe Giordano

NOTE: Hospital profiles are in alphabetical order by state, then city, then hospital within the city; Rankings are sorted by rate in descending order and exclude hospitals with less than 25 cases; (1) The number of cases is too small (n<25) for purposes of reliably predicting hospital performance; (2) Measure reflects the hospital's indication that its submission was based upon a sample of its relevant discharges; (3) Rate reflects fewer than the maximum possible quarters of data for the measure; (4) Inaccurate information submitted and suppressed for one or more quarters; (5) No data is available from the hospital for this measure; Please refer to the User's Guide for a full explanation of data

Measure	Cases	This Hospital	State Average	U.S. Average	Top Hospital
Heart Attack Care					
ACE Inhibitor or ARB for LVSD	35	89%	82%	82%	100%
Aspirin at Arrival	174	100%	95%	92%	100%
Aspirin at Discharge	218	96%	90%	90%	100%
Beta Blocker at Arrival	152	98%	89%	87%	100%
Beta Blocker at Discharge	226	94%	89%	90%	100%
Fibrinolytic Medication Timing	0	-	40%	31%	100%
PCI Within 90 Minutes of Arrival[1]	10	80%	52%	54%	95%
Smoking Cessation Advice	58	98%	87%	88%	100%
Heart Failure Care					
ACE Inhibitor or ARB for LVSD	150	87%	84%	82%	100%
Discharge Instructions	328	59%	56%	61%	93%
Evaluation of LVS Function	397	91%	84%	83%	99%
Smoking Cessation Advice	48	96%	82%	82%	100%
Pneumonia Care					
Appropriate Initial Antibiotic	179	93%	82%	83%	94%
Blood Culture Timing	249	97%	89%	90%	100%
Influenza Vaccine	52	87%	58%	70%	100%
Initial Antibiotic Timing	281	93%	75%	80%	93%
Oxygenation Assessment	360	100%	99%	99%	100%
Pneumococcal Vaccine	229	86%	58%	69%	94%
Smoking Cessation Advice	39	79%	75%	80%	100%
Surgical Infection Prevention					
Prophylactic Antibiotic Given[2]	328	75%	74%	77%	95%
Prophylactic Antibiotic Selection[2]	100	97%	89%	90%	100%
Prophylactic Antibiotic Stopped[2]	304	35%	65%	72%	95%
Pregnancy Care					
Inpatient Neonatal Mortality	-	-	-	-	-
Third or Fourth Degree Laceration	-	-	3.58%	3.63%	3.27%

Orange Coast Memorial Medical Center

9920 Talbert Avenue | Phone: 714-378-7410
Santa Ana, CA 92708 | Fax: 714-378-7474
Ownership: Voluntary non-profit - Private | Accredited: Yes
Emergency Services: Yes | Licensed Beds: 230

Key Personnel:

CEO.................................. Marcia Mauker
Emergency Room .... Dale Vital
Director Medical/Surgical Nursing .... Brenda Miller
Chief Radiology .... T Walden
Director Respiratory Therapy .... Jim Nicol

Measure	Cases	This Hospital	State Average	U.S. Average	Top Hospital
Heart Attack Care					
ACE Inhibitor or ARB for LVSD[1]	15	100%	82%	82%	100%
Aspirin at Arrival	92	99%	95%	92%	100%
Aspirin at Discharge	70	97%	90%	90%	100%
Beta Blocker at Arrival	55	93%	89%	87%	100%
Beta Blocker at Discharge	83	98%	89%	90%	100%
Fibrinolytic Medication Timing	0	-	40%	31%	100%
PCI Within 90 Minutes of Arrival[1]	5	80%	52%	54%	95%
Smoking Cessation Advice[1]	9	100%	87%	88%	100%
Heart Failure Care					
ACE Inhibitor or ARB for LVSD	103	88%	84%	82%	100%
Discharge Instructions	297	76%	56%	61%	93%
Evaluation of LVS Function	364	93%	84%	83%	99%
Smoking Cessation Advice	53	98%	82%	82%	100%
Pneumonia Care					
Appropriate Initial Antibiotic	200	90%	82%	83%	94%
Blood Culture Timing	157	87%	89%	90%	100%
Influenza Vaccine	61	77%	58%	70%	100%
Initial Antibiotic Timing	253	92%	75%	80%	93%
Oxygenation Assessment	310	100%	99%	99%	100%
Pneumococcal Vaccine	260	86%	58%	69%	94%
Smoking Cessation Advice	36	81%	75%	80%	100%
Surgical Infection Prevention					
Prophylactic Antibiotic Given[2,3]	445	87%	74%	77%	95%
Prophylactic Antibiotic Selection[2]	105	89%	89%	90%	100%
Prophylactic Antibiotic Stopped[2,3]	424	42%	65%	72%	95%
Pregnancy Care					
Inpatient Neonatal Mortality	1,576	0.00%	-	-	-
Third or Fourth Degree Laceration	1,059	1.98%	3.58%	3.63%	3.27%

Washington Hospital

2000 Mowry Avenue | Phone: 510-797-1111
Fremont, CA 94538 | Fax: 510-791-3496
URL: www.whhs.com
Ownership: Govt - Hospital District or Authority | Accredited: Yes
Emergency Services: Yes | Licensed Beds: 337

Key Personnel:

CEO.................................. Nancy Farber
Chief of Medical Staff..................... Ahmed Sadiq
Emergency Room .... Brenda Brennan, RN
Chief Radiology .... Bruce Nixon
Director Respiratory Therapy .... Tom Wagner

Measure	Cases	This Hospital	State Average	U.S. Average	Top Hospital
Heart Attack Care					
ACE Inhibitor or ARB for LVSD	32	88%	82%	82%	100%
Aspirin at Arrival	207	97%	95%	92%	100%
Aspirin at Discharge	216	94%	90%	90%	100%
Beta Blocker at Arrival	179	87%	89%	87%	100%
Beta Blocker at Discharge	219	86%	89%	90%	100%
Fibrinolytic Medication Timing	0	-	40%	31%	100%
PCI Within 90 Minutes of Arrival[1]	14	93%	52%	54%	95%
Smoking Cessation Advice	55	96%	87%	88%	100%
Heart Failure Care					
ACE Inhibitor or ARB for LVSD[2]	81	73%	84%	82%	100%
Discharge Instructions[2]	275	54%	56%	61%	93%
Evaluation of LVS Function[2]	298	83%	84%	83%	99%
Smoking Cessation Advice[2]	50	88%	82%	82%	100%
Pneumonia Care					
Appropriate Initial Antibiotic[2]	123	85%	82%	83%	94%
Blood Culture Timing[2]	105	87%	89%	90%	100%
Influenza Vaccine[2]	29	72%	58%	70%	100%
Initial Antibiotic Timing[2]	152	76%	75%	80%	93%
Oxygenation Assessment[2]	198	100%	99%	99%	100%
Pneumococcal Vaccine[2]	131	66%	58%	69%	94%
Smoking Cessation Advice[2]	26	88%	75%	80%	100%
Surgical Infection Prevention					
Prophylactic Antibiotic Given[2,3]	70	81%	74%	77%	95%
Prophylactic Antibiotic Selection[2]	70	84%	89%	90%	100%
Prophylactic Antibiotic Stopped[2,3]	69	80%	65%	72%	95%
Pregnancy Care					
Inpatient Neonatal Mortality	-	-	-	-	-
Third or Fourth Degree Laceration	-	-	3.58%	3.63%	3.27%

San Joaquin General Hospital

500 W Hospital Road | Phone: 209-468-6000
French Camp, CA 95231
URL: www.sjgeneralhospital.com
Ownership: Government - Local | Accredited: Yes
Emergency Services: Yes | Licensed Beds: 234

Key Personnel:

President/CEO........................... Kenneth B. Cohen
Chief Medical Staff........................ Lawrence Frank, MD
Director Medical/Surgical Nursing .... Linda Bacigalupi
Chief Radiology .... Dennis Jacobson, MD
Director Respiratory Therapy .... Pat Melton

Measure	Cases	This Hospital	State Average	U.S. Average	Top Hospital
Heart Attack Care					
ACE Inhibitor or ARB for LVSD[1]	7	100%	82%	82%	100%
Aspirin at Arrival	70	99%	95%	92%	100%
Aspirin at Discharge	32	100%	90%	90%	100%
Beta Blocker at Arrival	52	96%	89%	87%	100%
Beta Blocker at Discharge	31	100%	89%	90%	100%
Fibrinolytic Medication Timing[1]	12	67%	40%	31%	100%
PCI Within 90 Minutes of Arrival	0	-	52%	54%	95%
Smoking Cessation Advice[1]	13	77%	87%	88%	100%
Heart Failure Care					
ACE Inhibitor or ARB for LVSD	109	98%	84%	82%	100%

NOTE: Hospital profiles are in alphabetical order by state, then city, then hospital within the city; Rankings are sorted by rate in descending order and exclude hospitals with less than 25 cases; (1) The number of cases is too small (n<25) for purposes of reliably predicting hospital performance; (2) Measure reflects the hospital's indication that its submission was based upon a sample of its relevant discharges; (3) Rate reflects fewer than the maximum possible quarters of data for the measure; (4) Inaccurate information submitted and suppressed for one or more quarters; (5) No data is available from the hospital for this measure; Please refer to the User's Guide for a full explanation of data

Measure	Cases	This Hospital	State Average	U.S. Average	Top Hospital
Discharge Instructions	187	74%	56%	61%	93%
Evaluation of LVS Function	208	100%	84%	83%	99%
Smoking Cessation Advice	89	83%	82%	82%	100%
Pneumonia Care					
Appropriate Initial Antibiotic	164	91%	82%	83%	94%
Blood Culture Timing	148	77%	89%	90%	100%
Influenza Vaccine[4,5]	-	-	58%	70%	100%
Initial Antibiotic Timing	221	52%	75%	80%	93%
Oxygenation Assessment	241	100%	99%	99%	100%
Pneumococcal Vaccine	82	66%	58%	69%	94%
Smoking Cessation Advice	101	58%	75%	80%	100%
Surgical Infection Prevention					
Prophylactic Antibiotic Given	136	49%	74%	77%	95%
Prophylactic Antibiotic Selection	29	86%	89%	90%	100%
Prophylactic Antibiotic Stopped	120	57%	65%	72%	95%
Pregnancy Care					
Inpatient Neonatal Mortality	3,089	0.42%	-	-	-
Third or Fourth Degree Laceration	2,139	3.04%	3.58%	3.63%	3.27%

Community Regional Medical Center

2823 Fresno Street
Fresno, CA 93721
Phone: 559-459-2425
Fax: 559-459-2450
URL: www.communitymedical.org
Ownership: Voluntary non-profit - Other
Accredited: Yes
Emergency Services: Yes
Licensed Beds: 408
Key Personnel:
CEO. . . . . Tim A Josling
Chief Medical Staff. . . . . William Feaster

Measure	Cases	This Hospital	State Average	U.S. Average	Top Hospital
Heart Attack Care					
ACE Inhibitor or ARB for LVSD	107	85%	82%	82%	100%
Aspirin at Arrival	342	96%	95%	92%	100%
Aspirin at Discharge	347	95%	90%	90%	100%
Beta Blocker at Arrival	204	91%	89%	87%	100%
Beta Blocker at Discharge	368	95%	89%	90%	100%
Fibrinolytic Medication Timing	0	-	40%	31%	100%
PCI Within 90 Minutes of Arrival[1]	11	18%	52%	54%	95%
Smoking Cessation Advice	154	83%	87%	88%	100%
Heart Failure Care					
ACE Inhibitor or ARB for LVSD	442	83%	84%	82%	100%
Discharge Instructions	760	32%	56%	61%	93%
Evaluation of LVS Function	841	88%	84%	83%	99%
Smoking Cessation Advice	178	58%	82%	82%	100%
Pneumonia Care					
Appropriate Initial Antibiotic	435	87%	82%	83%	94%
Blood Culture Timing	439	87%	89%	90%	100%
Influenza Vaccine	111	76%	58%	70%	100%
Initial Antibiotic Timing	616	48%	75%	80%	93%
Oxygenation Assessment	756	100%	99%	99%	100%
Pneumococcal Vaccine	326	66%	58%	69%	94%
Smoking Cessation Advice	193	50%	75%	80%	100%
Surgical Infection Prevention					
Prophylactic Antibiotic Given	948	61%	74%	77%	95%
Prophylactic Antibiotic Selection	234	93%	89%	90%	100%
Prophylactic Antibiotic Stopped	886	67%	65%	72%	95%
Pregnancy Care					
Inpatient Neonatal Mortality	-	-	-	-	-
Third or Fourth Degree Laceration	-	-	3.58%	3.63%	3.27%

Fresno Heart Hospital

15 East Audobon Drive
Fresno, CA 93720
Phone: 559-433-8000
Fax: 559-433-8125
URL: www.fresnoheart.com
Ownership: Proprietary
Accredited: No
Emergency Services: No
Licensed Beds: 48
Key Personnel:
CEO. . . . . Carolyn Webster
Director Invasive Cardiovascular Service . . . . . . Marleen Meister Anderson, RN/MSN
Director Surgery. . . . . Debi Stephen-Lesser, RN
Manager Respiratory Care Services . . . . LeAnn Murray

Measure	Cases	This Hospital	State Average	U.S. Average	Top Hospital
Heart Attack Care					
ACE Inhibitor or ARB for LVSD[1]	22	86%	82%	82%	100%
Aspirin at Arrival	33	94%	95%	92%	100%
Aspirin at Discharge	101	93%	90%	90%	100%
Beta Blocker at Arrival	32	84%	89%	87%	100%
Beta Blocker at Discharge	108	92%	89%	90%	100%
Fibrinolytic Medication Timing	0	-	40%	31%	100%
PCI Within 90 Minutes of Arrival	0	-	52%	54%	95%
Smoking Cessation Advice[1]	23	100%	87%	88%	100%
Heart Failure Care					
ACE Inhibitor or ARB for LVSD	52	87%	84%	82%	100%
Discharge Instructions	123	81%	56%	61%	93%
Evaluation of LVS Function	133	79%	84%	83%	99%
Smoking Cessation Advice[1]	9	100%	82%	82%	100%
Pneumonia Care					
Appropriate Initial Antibiotic[1,3]	1	100%	82%	83%	94%
Blood Culture Timing[1,3]	1	100%	89%	90%	100%
Influenza Vaccine	0	-	58%	70%	100%
Initial Antibiotic Timing[1,3]	1	0%	75%	80%	93%
Oxygenation Assessment[1,3]	2	100%	99%	99%	100%
Pneumococcal Vaccine[1,3]	1	0%	58%	69%	94%
Smoking Cessation Advice[1,3]	1	100%	75%	80%	100%
Surgical Infection Prevention					
Prophylactic Antibiotic Given[2]	303	77%	74%	77%	95%
Prophylactic Antibiotic Selection[2]	163	98%	89%	90%	100%
Prophylactic Antibiotic Stopped[2]	276	80%	65%	72%	95%
Pregnancy Care					
Inpatient Neonatal Mortality	-	-	-	-	-
Third or Fourth Degree Laceration	-	-	3.58%	3.63%	3.27%

Fresno Surgery Center

6125 N Fresno Street
Fresno, CA 93710
Toll-Free: 800-431-8455
Phone: 559-431-8000
Fax: 559-431-8242
URL: www.fresnosurgerycenter.com
Ownership: Voluntary non-profit - Private
Accredited: No
Emergency Services: No
Key Personnel:
Administrator . . . . Barbara Anderson

Measure	Cases	This Hospital	State Average	U.S. Average	Top Hospital
Heart Attack Care					
ACE Inhibitor or ARB for LVSD[5]	-	-	82%	82%	100%
Aspirin at Arrival[5]	-	-	95%	92%	100%
Aspirin at Discharge[5]	-	-	90%	90%	100%
Beta Blocker at Arrival[5]	-	-	89%	87%	100%
Beta Blocker at Discharge[5]	-	-	89%	90%	100%
Fibrinolytic Medication Timing[5]	-	-	40%	31%	100%
PCI Within 90 Minutes of Arrival[5]	-	-	52%	54%	95%
Smoking Cessation Advice[5]	-	-	87%	88%	100%
Heart Failure Care					
ACE Inhibitor or ARB for LVSD[5]	-	-	84%	82%	100%
Discharge Instructions[5]	-	-	56%	61%	93%
Evaluation of LVS Function[5]	-	-	84%	83%	99%
Smoking Cessation Advice[5]	-	-	82%	82%	100%
Pneumonia Care					
Appropriate Initial Antibiotic[5]	-	-	82%	83%	94%
Blood Culture Timing[5]	-	-	89%	90%	100%
Influenza Vaccine[5]	-	-	58%	70%	100%
Initial Antibiotic Timing[5]	-	-	75%	80%	93%
Oxygenation Assessment[5]	-	-	99%	99%	100%
Pneumococcal Vaccine[5]	-	-	58%	69%	94%
Smoking Cessation Advice[5]	-	-	75%	80%	100%
Surgical Infection Prevention					
Prophylactic Antibiotic Given[3]	27	70%	74%	77%	95%
Prophylactic Antibiotic Selection[5]	-	-	89%	90%	100%
Prophylactic Antibiotic Stopped[3]	27	67%	65%	72%	95%
Pregnancy Care					
Inpatient Neonatal Mortality	-	-	-	-	-
Third or Fourth Degree Laceration	-	-	3.58%	3.63%	3.27%

NOTE: Hospital profiles are in alphabetical order by state, then city, then hospital within the city; Rankings are sorted by rate in descending order and exclude hospitals with less than 25 cases; (1) The number of cases is too small (n<25) for purposes of reliably predicting hospital performance; (2) Measure reflects the hospital's indication that its submission was based upon a sample of its relevant discharges; (3) Rate reflects fewer than the maximum possible quarters of data for the measure; (4) Inaccurate information submitted and suppressed for one or more quarters; (5) No data is available from the hospital for this measure; Please refer to the User's Guide for a full explanation of data

Kaiser Foundation Hospital-Fresno

7300 North Fresno St
Fresno, CA 93720
Phone: 559-448-4500
Ownership: Voluntary non-profit - Private
Accredited: Yes
Emergency Services: Yes

Measure	Cases	This Hospital	State Average	U.S. Average	Top Hospital
Heart Attack Care					
ACE Inhibitor or ARB for LVSD	34	88%	82%	82%	100%
Aspirin at Arrival	183	97%	95%	92%	100%
Aspirin at Discharge	140	94%	90%	90%	100%
Beta Blocker at Arrival	176	91%	89%	87%	100%
Beta Blocker at Discharge	152	96%	89%	90%	100%
Fibrinolytic Medication Timing[1]	14	43%	40%	31%	100%
PCI Within 90 Minutes of Arrival	0	-	52%	54%	95%
Smoking Cessation Advice	27	85%	87%	88%	100%
Heart Failure Care					
ACE Inhibitor or ARB for LVSD	103	83%	84%	82%	100%
Discharge Instructions	206	54%	56%	61%	93%
Evaluation of LVS Function	244	98%	84%	83%	99%
Smoking Cessation Advice	38	92%	82%	82%	100%
Pneumonia Care					
Appropriate Initial Antibiotic	105	91%	82%	83%	94%
Blood Culture Timing	100	89%	89%	90%	100%
Influenza Vaccine	30	60%	58%	70%	100%
Initial Antibiotic Timing	121	63%	75%	80%	93%
Oxygenation Assessment	163	100%	99%	99%	100%
Pneumococcal Vaccine	123	82%	58%	69%	94%
Smoking Cessation Advice[1]	21	100%	75%	80%	100%
Surgical Infection Prevention					
Prophylactic Antibiotic Given	161	87%	74%	77%	95%
Prophylactic Antibiotic Selection	42	93%	89%	90%	100%
Prophylactic Antibiotic Stopped	159	74%	65%	72%	95%
Pregnancy Care					
Inpatient Neonatal Mortality	1,345	0.00%	-	-	-
Third or Fourth Degree Laceration	910	3.63%	3.58%	3.63%	3.27%

Saint Agnes Medical Center

1303 E Herndon Ave
Fresno, CA 93710
Phone: 559-449-3000
Ownership: Voluntary non-profit - Church
Accredited: Yes
Emergency Services: Yes

Measure	Cases	This Hospital	State Average	U.S. Average	Top Hospital
Heart Attack Care					
ACE Inhibitor or ARB for LVSD[2]	71	100%	82%	82%	100%
Aspirin at Arrival[2]	299	99%	95%	92%	100%
Aspirin at Discharge[2]	352	99%	90%	90%	100%
Beta Blocker at Arrival[2]	198	99%	89%	87%	100%
Beta Blocker at Discharge[2]	365	99%	89%	90%	100%
Fibrinolytic Medication Timing[2]	0	-	40%	31%	100%
PCI Within 90 Minutes of Arrival[1,2]	12	75%	52%	54%	95%
Smoking Cessation Advice[2]	84	100%	87%	88%	100%
Heart Failure Care					
ACE Inhibitor or ARB for LVSD[2]	158	96%	84%	82%	100%
Discharge Instructions[2]	357	72%	56%	61%	93%
Evaluation of LVS Function[2]	430	98%	84%	83%	99%
Smoking Cessation Advice[2]	54	100%	82%	82%	100%
Pneumonia Care					
Appropriate Initial Antibiotic[2]	159	92%	82%	83%	94%
Blood Culture Timing[2]	213	92%	89%	90%	100%
Influenza Vaccine[2]	56	88%	58%	70%	100%
Initial Antibiotic Timing[2]	318	86%	75%	80%	93%
Oxygenation Assessment[2]	378	100%	99%	99%	100%
Pneumococcal Vaccine[2]	253	91%	58%	69%	94%
Smoking Cessation Advice[2]	55	100%	75%	80%	100%
Surgical Infection Prevention					
Prophylactic Antibiotic Given[2,3]	477	92%	74%	77%	95%
Prophylactic Antibiotic Selection[2]	151	98%	89%	90%	100%
Prophylactic Antibiotic Stopped[2,3]	458	84%	65%	72%	95%
Pregnancy Care					
Inpatient Neonatal Mortality	-	-	-	-	-
Third or Fourth Degree Laceration	-	-	3.58%	3.63%	3.27%

Saint Jude Medical Center

101 E Valencia Mesa Drive
Fullerton, CA 92835
Phone: 714-871-3280
Fax: 714-992-3029
URL: www.stjudemedicalcenter.org
Ownership: Voluntary non-profit - Church
Accredited: Yes
Emergency Services: Yes
Licensed Beds: 347

Key Personnel:

CEO. . . . . Robert J Fraschetti
Chief Medical Staff. . . . . Mark Song
Emergency Room . . . . Janet Magnani, RN
Director Medical/Surgical Nursing . . . . Barbar Miller
OB/GYN Womens Health. . . . . Donald Henderson, MD
Chief Radiology . . . . Robert Morten, MD
Director Respiratory Therapy . . . . Martha Lomeli

Measure	Cases	This Hospital	State Average	U.S. Average	Top Hospital
Heart Attack Care					
ACE Inhibitor or ARB for LVSD	47	81%	82%	82%	100%
Aspirin at Arrival	265	98%	95%	92%	100%
Aspirin at Discharge	245	97%	90%	90%	100%
Beta Blocker at Arrival	241	96%	89%	87%	100%
Beta Blocker at Discharge	242	97%	89%	90%	100%
Fibrinolytic Medication Timing	0	-	40%	31%	100%
PCI Within 90 Minutes of Arrival[1]	14	71%	52%	54%	95%
Smoking Cessation Advice	61	97%	87%	88%	100%
Heart Failure Care					
ACE Inhibitor or ARB for LVSD	171	88%	84%	82%	100%
Discharge Instructions	295	95%	56%	61%	93%
Evaluation of LVS Function	369	98%	84%	83%	99%
Smoking Cessation Advice	37	100%	82%	82%	100%
Pneumonia Care					
Appropriate Initial Antibiotic	236	85%	82%	83%	94%
Blood Culture Timing	238	92%	89%	90%	100%
Influenza Vaccine	67	96%	58%	70%	100%
Initial Antibiotic Timing	275	81%	75%	80%	93%
Oxygenation Assessment	355	100%	99%	99%	100%
Pneumococcal Vaccine	244	86%	58%	69%	94%
Smoking Cessation Advice	39	82%	75%	80%	100%
Surgical Infection Prevention					
Prophylactic Antibiotic Given	1,253	93%	74%	77%	95%
Prophylactic Antibiotic Selection	302	94%	89%	90%	100%
Prophylactic Antibiotic Stopped	1,210	85%	65%	72%	95%
Pregnancy Care					
Inpatient Neonatal Mortality	2,255	0.13%	-	-	-
Third or Fourth Degree Laceration	1,551	3.74%	3.58%	3.63%	3.27%

Jerold Phelps Community Hospital

Alternate Name: Southern Humboldt Community Hospital
733 Cedar Street
Garberville, CA 95542
Phone: 707-923-3921
Fax: 707-923-9352
E-mail: shchadmin@asis.com
URL: www.shchd.org
Ownership: Govt - Hospital District or Authority
Accredited: No
Emergency Services: Yes
Licensed Beds: 9

Key Personnel:

CEO. . . . . Steven G Cherry, RN
Director Medical/Surgical Nursing . . . . Dana Heald, RN
OB/GYN Womens Health. . . . . Mark H Phelps, MD
Chief Radiology . . . . David Huang, MD

Measure	Cases	This Hospital	State Average	U.S. Average	Top Hospital
Heart Attack Care					
ACE Inhibitor or ARB for LVSD[5]	-	-	82%	82%	100%
Aspirin at Arrival[5]	-	-	95%	92%	100%
Aspirin at Discharge[5]	-	-	90%	90%	100%
Beta Blocker at Arrival[5]	-	-	89%	87%	100%
Beta Blocker at Discharge[5]	-	-	89%	90%	100%
Fibrinolytic Medication Timing[5]	-	-	40%	31%	100%
PCI Within 90 Minutes of Arrival[5]	-	-	52%	54%	95%
Smoking Cessation Advice[5]	-	-	87%	88%	100%
Heart Failure Care					

NOTE: Hospital profiles are in alphabetical order by state, then city, then hospital within the city; Rankings are sorted by rate in descending order and exclude hospitals with less than 25 cases; (1) The number of cases is too small (n<25) for purposes of reliably predicting hospital performance; (2) Measure reflects the hospital's indication that its submission was based upon a sample of its relevant discharges; (3) Rate reflects fewer than the maximum possible quarters of data for the measure; (4) Inaccurate information submitted and suppressed for one or more quarters; (5) No data is available from the hospital for this measure; Please refer to the User's Guide for a full explanation of data

ACE Inhibitor or ARB for LVSD[5]	-	-	84%	82%	100%
Discharge Instructions[5]	-	-	56%	61%	93%
Evaluation of LVS Function[5]	-	-	84%	83%	99%
Smoking Cessation Advice[5]	-	-	82%	82%	100%
Pneumonia Care					
Appropriate Initial Antibiotic[1,3]	1	100%	82%	83%	94%
Blood Culture Timing[1,3]	1	100%	89%	90%	100%
Influenza Vaccine[5]	-	-	58%	70%	100%
Initial Antibiotic Timing[1,3]	2	100%	75%	80%	93%
Oxygenation Assessment[1,3]	2	100%	99%	99%	100%
Pneumococcal Vaccine[3]	0	-	58%	69%	94%
Smoking Cessation Advice[3]	0	-	75%	80%	100%
Surgical Infection Prevention					
Prophylactic Antibiotic Given[5]	-	-	74%	77%	95%
Prophylactic Antibiotic Selection[5]	-	-	89%	90%	100%
Prophylactic Antibiotic Stopped[5]	-	-	65%	72%	95%
Pregnancy Care					
Inpatient Neonatal Mortality	-	-	-	-	-
Third or Fourth Degree Laceration	-	-	3.58%	3.63%	3.27%

Garden Grove Hospital and Medical Center

Alternate Name: Medical Center of Garden Grove
12601 Garden Grove Boulevard
Garden Grove, CA 92843
Phone: 714-537-5160
Fax: 714-741-3332
URL: www.gardengrovehospital.com
Ownership: Proprietary
Emergency Services: Yes
Accredited: Yes
Licensed Beds: 167

Key Personnel:

CEO/President.......................... Maxine Cooper
Chief Medical Staff....................... Peter Wang
Cardiac Lab............................ Ed Barrus
Emergency Room .... Leslie Koch
Infection Control......................... Jose Cartagener
Director Medical/Surgical Nursing .... Leslie Koch
Director Medical/Surgical Nursing .... Jackie Pham
OB/GYN Womens Health.................. Joseph Perkins, MD
Chief Radiology .... Bernard Louvet
Director Respiratory Therapy .... Ed Barrus

Measure	Cases	This Hospital	State Average	U.S. Average	Top Hospital
Heart Attack Care					
ACE Inhibitor or ARB for LVSD[1]	7	100%	82%	82%	100%
Aspirin at Arrival	54	98%	95%	92%	100%
Aspirin at Discharge[1]	24	92%	90%	90%	100%
Beta Blocker at Arrival	39	95%	89%	87%	100%
Beta Blocker at Discharge[1]	23	96%	89%	90%	100%
Fibrinolytic Medication Timing[1]	2	0%	40%	31%	100%
PCI Within 90 Minutes of Arrival	0	-	52%	54%	95%
Smoking Cessation Advice[1]	3	100%	87%	88%	100%
Heart Failure Care					
ACE Inhibitor or ARB for LVSD	26	85%	84%	82%	100%
Discharge Instructions	71	96%	56%	61%	93%
Evaluation of LVS Function	103	97%	84%	83%	99%
Smoking Cessation Advice[1]	17	100%	82%	82%	100%
Pneumonia Care					
Appropriate Initial Antibiotic	162	83%	82%	83%	94%
Blood Culture Timing	143	100%	89%	90%	100%
Influenza Vaccine	32	100%	58%	70%	100%
Initial Antibiotic Timing	178	94%	75%	80%	93%
Oxygenation Assessment	225	100%	99%	99%	100%
Pneumococcal Vaccine	144	94%	58%	69%	94%
Smoking Cessation Advice[1]	17	100%	75%	80%	100%
Surgical Infection Prevention					
Prophylactic Antibiotic Given[2]	163	93%	74%	77%	95%
Prophylactic Antibiotic Selection[2]	41	93%	89%	90%	100%
Prophylactic Antibiotic Stopped[2]	162	69%	65%	72%	95%
Pregnancy Care					
Inpatient Neonatal Mortality	-	-	-	-	-
Third or Fourth Degree Laceration	-	-	3.58%	3.63%	3.27%

Community Hospital of Gardena

1246 W 155th Street
Gardena, CA 90247
Phone: 310-323-5330
Fax: 310-327-0952
URL: www.gardenahospital.com
Ownership: Proprietary
Emergency Services: No
Accredited: Yes
Licensed Beds: 58

Key Personnel:

CEO................................. Raymond N Smith
Chief Medical Staff...................... Toshiyuki Tanaka, MD
Director Medical/Surgical Nursing .... Richard Yap
Chief Radiology .... Fred Grossman, MD
Director Respiratory Therapy .... Coreen Saito

Measure	Cases	This Hospital	State Average	U.S. Average	Top Hospital
Heart Attack Care					
ACE Inhibitor or ARB for LVSD[5]	-	-	82%	82%	100%
Aspirin at Arrival[5]	-	-	95%	92%	100%
Aspirin at Discharge[5]	-	-	90%	90%	100%
Beta Blocker at Arrival[5]	-	-	89%	87%	100%
Beta Blocker at Discharge[5]	-	-	89%	90%	100%
Fibrinolytic Medication Timing[5]	-	-	40%	31%	100%
PCI Within 90 Minutes of Arrival[5]	-	-	52%	54%	95%
Smoking Cessation Advice[5]	-	-	87%	88%	100%
Heart Failure Care					
ACE Inhibitor or ARB for LVSD[1,3]	2	100%	84%	82%	100%
Discharge Instructions[5]	-	-	56%	61%	93%
Evaluation of LVS Function[1,3]	6	17%	84%	83%	99%
Smoking Cessation Advice[5]	-	-	82%	82%	100%
Pneumonia Care					
Appropriate Initial Antibiotic[5]	-	-	82%	83%	94%
Blood Culture Timing[5]	-	-	89%	90%	100%
Influenza Vaccine[5]	-	-	58%	70%	100%
Initial Antibiotic Timing[1,3]	14	71%	75%	80%	93%
Oxygenation Assessment[3]	31	97%	99%	99%	100%
Pneumococcal Vaccine[3]	30	0%	58%	69%	94%
Smoking Cessation Advice[5]	-	-	75%	80%	100%
Surgical Infection Prevention					
Prophylactic Antibiotic Given[5]	-	-	74%	77%	95%
Prophylactic Antibiotic Selection[5]	-	-	89%	90%	100%
Prophylactic Antibiotic Stopped[5]	-	-	65%	72%	95%
Pregnancy Care					
Inpatient Neonatal Mortality	-	-	-	-	-
Third or Fourth Degree Laceration	-	-	3.58%	3.63%	3.27%

Memorial Hospital of Gardena

1145 W Redondo Beach Boulevard
Gardena, CA 90247
Phone: 310-532-4200
Fax: 310-538-6680
Ownership: Proprietary
Emergency Services: Yes
Accredited: Yes
Licensed Beds: 173

Key Personnel:

CEO................................. Steve Popkin
Chief of Medical Staff..................... Alfonso Bayz
Emergency Room .... Mickey Kolodny
Director Medical/Surgical Nursing .... Kelly Miyake, RN
OB/GYN Womens Health.................. Everett Campbell, MD
Chief Radiology .... Laura Thompson, MD
Director Respiratory Therapy .... Denise Anderson

Measure	Cases	This Hospital	State Average	U.S. Average	Top Hospital
Heart Attack Care					
ACE Inhibitor or ARB for LVSD[1]	7	86%	82%	82%	100%
Aspirin at Arrival	59	100%	95%	92%	100%
Aspirin at Discharge	30	87%	90%	90%	100%
Beta Blocker at Arrival	51	88%	89%	87%	100%
Beta Blocker at Discharge	31	71%	89%	90%	100%
Fibrinolytic Medication Timing[1]	15	0%	40%	31%	100%
PCI Within 90 Minutes of Arrival	0	-	52%	54%	95%
Smoking Cessation Advice[1]	12	67%	87%	88%	100%
Heart Failure Care					
ACE Inhibitor or ARB for LVSD	82	91%	84%	82%	100%
Discharge Instructions	161	26%	56%	61%	93%
Evaluation of LVS Function	200	86%	84%	83%	99%
Smoking Cessation Advice	36	42%	82%	82%	100%

NOTE: Hospital profiles are in alphabetical order by state, then city, then hospital within the city; Rankings are sorted by rate in descending order and exclude hospitals with less than 25 cases; (1) The number of cases is too small (n<25) for purposes of reliably predicting hospital performance; (2) Measure reflects the hospital's indication that its submission was based upon a sample of its relevant discharges; (3) Rate reflects fewer than the maximum possible quarters of data for the measure; (4) Inaccurate information submitted and suppressed for one or more quarters; (5) No data is available from the hospital for this measure; Please refer to the User's Guide for a full explanation of data

Measure	Cases	This Hospital	State Average	U.S. Average	Top Hospital
Pneumonia Care					
Appropriate Initial Antibiotic	209	54%	82%	83%	94%
Blood Culture Timing	196	93%	89%	90%	100%
Influenza Vaccine	56	0%	58%	70%	100%
Initial Antibiotic Timing	299	64%	75%	80%	93%
Oxygenation Assessment	323	100%	99%	99%	100%
Pneumococcal Vaccine	170	1%	58%	69%	94%
Smoking Cessation Advice	29	48%	75%	80%	100%
Surgical Infection Prevention					
Prophylactic Antibiotic Given[3]	48	40%	74%	77%	95%
Prophylactic Antibiotic Selection[1]	14	57%	89%	90%	100%
Prophylactic Antibiotic Stopped[3]	30	63%	65%	72%	95%
Pregnancy Care					
Inpatient Neonatal Mortality	-	-	-	-	-
Third or Fourth Degree Laceration	-	-	3.58%	3.63%	3.27%

Saint Louisie Regional Hospital

Alternate Name: South Valley Hospital
9400 No Name Uno
Gilroy, CA 95020
Toll-Free: 800-423-2032
Phone: 408-848-2000
Fax: 408-842-2155
Ownership: Voluntary non-profit - Church
Emergency Services: Yes
Accredited: Yes
Licensed Beds: 93

Key Personnel:

CEO . . . . Ted Fox
Chief Medical Staff . . . . Bakri Musa
Emergency Room . . . . Kelly Jackson

Measure	Cases	This Hospital	State Average	U.S. Average	Top Hospital
Heart Attack Care					
ACE Inhibitor or ARB for LVSD[1]	4	75%	82%	82%	100%
Aspirin at Arrival	40	98%	95%	92%	100%
Aspirin at Discharge[1]	13	69%	90%	90%	100%
Beta Blocker at Arrival	27	89%	89%	87%	100%
Beta Blocker at Discharge[1]	13	92%	89%	90%	100%
Fibrinolytic Medication Timing[1]	2	50%	40%	31%	100%
PCI Within 90 Minutes of Arrival	0	-	52%	54%	95%
Smoking Cessation Advice[1]	1	100%	87%	88%	100%
Heart Failure Care					
ACE Inhibitor or ARB for LVSD	35	66%	84%	82%	100%
Discharge Instructions	84	98%	56%	61%	93%
Evaluation of LVS Function	110	76%	84%	83%	99%
Smoking Cessation Advice[1]	13	92%	82%	82%	100%
Pneumonia Care					
Appropriate Initial Antibiotic	86	88%	82%	83%	94%
Blood Culture Timing	72	86%	89%	90%	100%
Influenza Vaccine[1]	15	80%	58%	70%	100%
Initial Antibiotic Timing	107	84%	75%	80%	93%
Oxygenation Assessment	129	100%	99%	99%	100%
Pneumococcal Vaccine	76	53%	58%	69%	94%
Smoking Cessation Advice	29	83%	75%	80%	100%
Surgical Infection Prevention					
Prophylactic Antibiotic Given[2,3]	97	86%	74%	77%	95%
Prophylactic Antibiotic Selection[2]	43	84%	89%	90%	100%
Prophylactic Antibiotic Stopped[2,3]	96	69%	65%	72%	95%
Pregnancy Care					
Inpatient Neonatal Mortality	711	0.14%	-	-	-
Third or Fourth Degree Laceration	489	3.89%	3.58%	3.63%	3.27%

Glendale Adventist Medical Center

1509 Wilson Terrace
Glendale, CA 91206
Phone: 818-409-8000
Fax: 818-546-5600
URL: www.glendaleadventist.com
Ownership: Voluntary non-profit - Church
Emergency Services: Yes
Accredited: Yes
Licensed Beds: 448

Key Personnel:

President/CEO . . . . Scott Reiner
Chief Medical Staff . . . . Carl B Ermshar, MD
Cardiac Lab . . . . Robert Marchuck
Catheterization Lab . . . . Robert Marchuk
Emergency Room . . . . Bonita Hulin
Emergency Room . . . . Edmund Noll, MD
Director Infection/Disease Control . . . . Michelle Garcia
ICU . . . . Punnoose Varghese
Intensive/Coronary Care . . . . Punnoose Varghese
Director Medical/Surgical Nursing . . . . Lynn Cameron
OB/GYN Womens Health . . . . Barry Schifrin, MD
Director Radiology . . . . Robert McKay, MD

Measure	Cases	This Hospital	State Average	U.S. Average	Top Hospital
Heart Attack Care					
ACE Inhibitor or ARB for LVSD	81	90%	82%	82%	100%
Aspirin at Arrival	236	95%	95%	92%	100%
Aspirin at Discharge	249	96%	90%	90%	100%
Beta Blocker at Arrival	174	87%	89%	87%	100%
Beta Blocker at Discharge	257	93%	89%	90%	100%
Fibrinolytic Medication Timing	0	-	40%	31%	100%
PCI Within 90 Minutes of Arrival[1]	13	54%	52%	54%	95%
Smoking Cessation Advice	83	100%	87%	88%	100%
Heart Failure Care					
ACE Inhibitor or ARB for LVSD	176	85%	84%	82%	100%
Discharge Instructions	330	42%	56%	61%	93%
Evaluation of LVS Function	430	86%	84%	83%	99%
Smoking Cessation Advice	53	98%	82%	82%	100%
Pneumonia Care					
Appropriate Initial Antibiotic	188	72%	82%	83%	94%
Blood Culture Timing	199	97%	89%	90%	100%
Influenza Vaccine	60	52%	58%	70%	100%
Initial Antibiotic Timing	260	74%	75%	80%	93%
Oxygenation Assessment	334	100%	99%	99%	100%
Pneumococcal Vaccine	231	52%	58%	69%	94%
Smoking Cessation Advice	51	90%	75%	80%	100%
Surgical Infection Prevention					
Prophylactic Antibiotic Given[3]	481	83%	74%	77%	95%
Prophylactic Antibiotic Selection	156	98%	89%	90%	100%
Prophylactic Antibiotic Stopped[3]	462	70%	65%	72%	95%
Pregnancy Care					
Inpatient Neonatal Mortality	-	-	-	-	-
Third or Fourth Degree Laceration	-	-	3.58%	3.63%	3.27%

Glendale Memorial Hospital and Health Center

1420 South Central Avenue
Glendale, CA 91204
Phone: 818-502-1900
Fax: 818-409-7688
URL: www.glendalememorial.com
Ownership: Voluntary non-profit - Private
Emergency Services: Yes
Accredited: Yes
Licensed Beds: 334

Key Personnel:

President . . . . Catherine M Pelley
Catheterization Lab . . . . Nassib Abdul Karim
Emergency Room . . . . Michael Agron, MD
Infection Control . . . . Kaye Baymiller, RN
Respiratory/Cardiopulmonary . . . . Jill Mathison

Measure	Cases	This Hospital	State Average	U.S. Average	Top Hospital
Heart Attack Care					
ACE Inhibitor or ARB for LVSD	54	100%	82%	82%	100%
Aspirin at Arrival	175	99%	95%	92%	100%
Aspirin at Discharge	201	99%	90%	90%	100%
Beta Blocker at Arrival	123	92%	89%	87%	100%
Beta Blocker at Discharge	205	98%	89%	90%	100%
Fibrinolytic Medication Timing	0	-	40%	31%	100%
PCI Within 90 Minutes of Arrival[1]	9	56%	52%	54%	95%
Smoking Cessation Advice	61	100%	87%	88%	100%
Heart Failure Care					
ACE Inhibitor or ARB for LVSD	256	95%	84%	82%	100%
Discharge Instructions	478	54%	56%	61%	93%
Evaluation of LVS Function	578	98%	84%	83%	99%
Smoking Cessation Advice	80	99%	82%	82%	100%
Pneumonia Care					
Appropriate Initial Antibiotic	206	83%	82%	83%	94%
Blood Culture Timing	182	95%	89%	90%	100%
Influenza Vaccine	68	87%	58%	70%	100%
Initial Antibiotic Timing	285	78%	75%	80%	93%
Oxygenation Assessment	367	100%	99%	99%	100%
Pneumococcal Vaccine	252	88%	58%	69%	94%

NOTE: Hospital profiles are in alphabetical order by state, then city, then hospital within the city; Rankings are sorted by rate in descending order and exclude hospitals with less than 25 cases; (1) The number of cases is too small (n<25) for purposes of reliably predicting hospital performance; (2) Measure reflects the hospital's indication that its submission was based upon a sample of its relevant discharges; (3) Rate reflects fewer than the maximum possible quarters of data for the measure; (4) Inaccurate information submitted and suppressed for one or more quarters; (5) No data is available from the hospital for this measure; Please refer to the User's Guide for a full explanation of data

Measure	Cases	This Hospital	State Average	U.S. Average	Top Hospital
Smoking Cessation Advice	50	98%	75%	80%	100%
Surgical Infection Prevention					
Prophylactic Antibiotic Given[2,3]	238	79%	74%	77%	95%
Prophylactic Antibiotic Selection[2]	80	91%	89%	90%	100%
Prophylactic Antibiotic Stopped[2,3]	230	47%	65%	72%	95%
Pregnancy Care					
Inpatient Neonatal Mortality	-	-	-	-	-
Third or Fourth Degree Laceration	-	-	3.58%	3.63%	3.27%

Verdugo Hills Hospital

1812 Verdugo Boulevard
Glendale, CA 91208
Phone: 818-790-7100
Fax: 818-952-3597
URL: www.verdugohillshospital.org
Ownership: Voluntary non-profit - Other
Accredited: Yes
Emergency Services: Yes
Licensed Beds: 158

Key Personnel:

President/CEO . . . . Leonard Labbella
Chief of Medical Staff . . . . Steven L Hartford, MD
Emergency Room . . . . Leo E Berkenbile, MD
Emergency Room . . . . Kevin Traber, RN
Director Radiology . . . . Michael Gomhar
Director Respiratory Therapy . . . . Monte Schachner

Measure	Cases	This Hospital	State Average	U.S. Average	Top Hospital
Heart Attack Care					
ACE Inhibitor or ARB for LVSD[1]	12	50%	82%	82%	100%
Aspirin at Arrival	66	92%	95%	92%	100%
Aspirin at Discharge	31	84%	90%	90%	100%
Beta Blocker at Arrival	61	79%	89%	87%	100%
Beta Blocker at Discharge	34	79%	89%	90%	100%
Fibrinolytic Medication Timing[1]	1	0%	40%	31%	100%
PCI Within 90 Minutes of Arrival	0	-	52%	54%	95%
Smoking Cessation Advice[1]	4	75%	87%	88%	100%
Heart Failure Care					
ACE Inhibitor or ARB for LVSD	49	63%	84%	82%	100%
Discharge Instructions	107	34%	56%	61%	93%
Evaluation of LVS Function	161	76%	84%	83%	99%
Smoking Cessation Advice[1]	21	29%	82%	82%	100%
Pneumonia Care					
Appropriate Initial Antibiotic	167	68%	82%	83%	94%
Blood Culture Timing	104	83%	89%	90%	100%
Influenza Vaccine	28	7%	58%	70%	100%
Initial Antibiotic Timing	177	66%	75%	80%	93%
Oxygenation Assessment	205	93%	99%	99%	100%
Pneumococcal Vaccine	148	9%	58%	69%	94%
Smoking Cessation Advice	30	60%	75%	80%	100%
Surgical Infection Prevention					
Prophylactic Antibiotic Given[3]	117	78%	74%	77%	95%
Prophylactic Antibiotic Selection[1]	10	60%	89%	90%	100%
Prophylactic Antibiotic Stopped[3]	108	47%	65%	72%	95%
Pregnancy Care					
Inpatient Neonatal Mortality	-	-	-	-	-
Third or Fourth Degree Laceration	-	-	3.58%	3.63%	3.27%

East Valley Hospital Medical Center

Alternate Name: Glendora Community Hospital/Huntington East Valley
150 West Route 66
Glendora, CA 91740
Phone: 626-852-5000
Fax: 626-852-5022
URL: www.eastvalleyhospital.org
Ownership: Voluntary non-profit - Private
Accredited: Yes
Emergency Services: Yes
Licensed Beds: 128

Key Personnel:

President/CEO . . . . C Joseph Chang
Chief Medical Staff . . . . Marc Domaguing, MD
Emergency Room . . . . Richard MacDonald, RN
Infection Control . . . . Milad Shokair
ICU . . . . Richard MacDonald, RN
CNO . . . . Liz Dreisbach, RN
OB/GYN Womens Health . . . . Dennice Morris, RN
Respiratory Therapy . . . . Rick Rezkalla

Measure	Cases	This Hospital	State Average	U.S. Average	Top Hospital
Heart Attack Care					
ACE Inhibitor or ARB for LVSD[1]	6	50%	82%	82%	100%
Aspirin at Arrival	43	74%	95%	92%	100%
Aspirin at Discharge	31	61%	90%	90%	100%
Beta Blocker at Arrival	41	83%	89%	87%	100%
Beta Blocker at Discharge	32	69%	89%	90%	100%
Fibrinolytic Medication Timing[3]	0	-	40%	31%	100%
PCI Within 90 Minutes of Arrival	0	-	52%	54%	95%
Smoking Cessation Advice[1,3]	1	0%	87%	88%	100%
Heart Failure Care					
ACE Inhibitor or ARB for LVSD[1]	20	65%	84%	82%	100%
Discharge Instructions[1,3]	8	38%	56%	61%	93%
Evaluation of LVS Function	67	78%	84%	83%	99%
Smoking Cessation Advice[3]	0	-	82%	82%	100%
Pneumonia Care					
Appropriate Initial Antibiotic[3]	36	64%	82%	83%	94%
Blood Culture Timing[1,3]	18	67%	89%	90%	100%
Influenza Vaccine[4,5]	-	-	58%	70%	100%
Initial Antibiotic Timing	152	83%	75%	80%	93%
Oxygenation Assessment	165	99%	99%	99%	100%
Pneumococcal Vaccine	103	26%	58%	69%	94%
Smoking Cessation Advice[1,3]	1	100%	75%	80%	100%
Surgical Infection Prevention					
Prophylactic Antibiotic Given[3]	0	-	74%	77%	95%
Prophylactic Antibiotic Selection[5]	-	-	89%	90%	100%
Prophylactic Antibiotic Stopped[3]	0	-	65%	72%	95%
Pregnancy Care					
Inpatient Neonatal Mortality	398	0.00%	-	-	-
Third or Fourth Degree Laceration	184	0.54%	3.58%	3.63%	3.27%

Foothill Presbyterian Hospital

Alternate Name: Morris L Johnston Memorial
250 S Grand Avenue
Glendora, CA 91741
Phone: 626-963-8411
Fax: 626-814-2428
URL: www.cvhp.org
Ownership: Voluntary non-profit - Private
Accredited: Yes
Emergency Services: Yes
Licensed Beds: 106

Key Personnel:

Administrator . . . . Larry S Fetters
Chief Medical Staff . . . . Ihsan Hikimah', MD
Director Medical/Surgical Nursing . . . . Susan Benson
OB/GYN Womens Health . . . . Richard Williams, MD
Director Respiratory Therapy . . . . Cindy Ghandour

Measure	Cases	This Hospital	State Average	U.S. Average	Top Hospital
Heart Attack Care					
ACE Inhibitor or ARB for LVSD[1]	7	71%	82%	82%	100%
Aspirin at Arrival	50	94%	95%	92%	100%
Aspirin at Discharge	26	81%	90%	90%	100%
Beta Blocker at Arrival	45	89%	89%	87%	100%
Beta Blocker at Discharge	25	76%	89%	90%	100%
Fibrinolytic Medication Timing	0	-	40%	31%	100%
PCI Within 90 Minutes of Arrival	0	-	52%	54%	95%
Smoking Cessation Advice[1]	1	100%	87%	88%	100%
Heart Failure Care					
ACE Inhibitor or ARB for LVSD	55	60%	84%	82%	100%
Discharge Instructions	163	68%	56%	61%	93%
Evaluation of LVS Function	212	97%	84%	83%	99%
Smoking Cessation Advice[1]	23	96%	82%	82%	100%
Pneumonia Care					
Appropriate Initial Antibiotic	161	78%	82%	83%	94%
Blood Culture Timing	149	89%	89%	90%	100%
Influenza Vaccine	41	51%	58%	70%	100%
Initial Antibiotic Timing	208	76%	75%	80%	93%
Oxygenation Assessment	259	100%	99%	99%	100%
Pneumococcal Vaccine	165	53%	58%	69%	94%
Smoking Cessation Advice	36	42%	75%	80%	100%
Surgical Infection Prevention					
Prophylactic Antibiotic Given[3]	143	62%	74%	77%	95%
Prophylactic Antibiotic Selection	46	87%	89%	90%	100%
Prophylactic Antibiotic Stopped[3]	135	61%	65%	72%	95%
Pregnancy Care					
Inpatient Neonatal Mortality	-	-	-	-	-

NOTE: Hospital profiles are in alphabetical order by state, then city, then hospital within the city; Rankings are sorted by rate in descending order and exclude hospitals with less than 25 cases; (1) The number of cases is too small (n<25) for purposes of reliably predicting hospital performance; (2) Measure reflects the hospital's indication that its submission was based upon a sample of its relevant discharges; (3) Rate reflects fewer than the maximum possible quarters of data for the measure; (4) Inaccurate information submitted and suppressed for one or more quarters; (5) No data is available from the hospital for this measure; Please refer to the User's Guide for a full explanation of data

Third or Fourth Degree Laceration	-	-	3.58%	3.63%	3.27%

Sierra Nevada Memorial Hospital

155 Glasson Way — Phone: 530-274-6000
Grass Valley, CA 95945 — Fax: 530-274-6614
E-mail: info@snmh.org
URL: www.snmh.org
Ownership: Voluntary non-profit - Other — Accredited: Yes
Emergency Services: Yes — Licensed Beds: 75

Key Personnel:

Interim President/CEO.................... Mary L Gish
Chief of Medical Staff..................... Robert Lowe
Emergency Room........................ Roger Loid
OB/GYN Womens Health.................. Michael Dahle
Director of Pulmonary/Cardiology............ John Mallery

Measure	Cases	This Hospital	State Average	U.S. Average	Top Hospital
Heart Attack Care					
ACE Inhibitor or ARB for LVSD[1]	2	100%	82%	82%	100%
Aspirin at Arrival	45	100%	95%	92%	100%
Aspirin at Discharge	26	100%	90%	90%	100%
Beta Blocker at Arrival	42	100%	89%	87%	100%
Beta Blocker at Discharge	28	93%	89%	90%	100%
Fibrinolytic Medication Timing[1]	2	50%	40%	31%	100%
PCI Within 90 Minutes of Arrival	0	-	52%	54%	95%
Smoking Cessation Advice[1]	3	100%	87%	88%	100%
Heart Failure Care					
ACE Inhibitor or ARB for LVSD	73	93%	84%	82%	100%
Discharge Instructions	112	77%	56%	61%	93%
Evaluation of LVS Function	157	90%	84%	83%	99%
Smoking Cessation Advice[1]	21	76%	82%	82%	100%
Pneumonia Care					
Appropriate Initial Antibiotic[2]	251	92%	82%	83%	94%
Blood Culture Timing[2]	191	90%	89%	90%	100%
Influenza Vaccine	56	80%	58%	70%	100%
Initial Antibiotic Timing[2]	276	87%	75%	80%	93%
Oxygenation Assessment[2]	333	99%	99%	99%	100%
Pneumococcal Vaccine[2]	254	80%	58%	69%	94%
Smoking Cessation Advice[2]	74	85%	75%	80%	100%
Surgical Infection Prevention					
Prophylactic Antibiotic Given[2,3]	174	99%	74%	77%	95%
Prophylactic Antibiotic Selection[2]	57	95%	89%	90%	100%
Prophylactic Antibiotic Stopped[2,3]	170	69%	65%	72%	95%
Pregnancy Care					
Inpatient Neonatal Mortality	-	-	-	-	-
Third or Fourth Degree Laceration	-	-	3.58%	3.63%	3.27%

Marin General Hospital

250 Bon Air Road — Phone: 415-925-7000
Greenbrae, CA 94904 — Fax: 415-925-7518
URL: www.maringeneral.sutterhealth.org
Ownership: Govt - Hospital District or Authority — Accredited: Yes
Emergency Services: Yes — Licensed Beds: 235

Key Personnel:

CEO................................. David Bradley
Chief Medical Staff........................ Gerald Wilner, MD
Director Intensive Coronary................ Mark Kobe

Measure	Cases	This Hospital	State Average	U.S. Average	Top Hospital
Heart Attack Care					
ACE Inhibitor or ARB for LVSD	58	91%	82%	82%	100%
Aspirin at Arrival	142	97%	95%	92%	100%
Aspirin at Discharge	158	99%	90%	90%	100%
Beta Blocker at Arrival	124	91%	89%	87%	100%
Beta Blocker at Discharge	150	95%	89%	90%	100%
Fibrinolytic Medication Timing	0	-	40%	31%	100%
PCI Within 90 Minutes of Arrival[1]	5	100%	52%	54%	95%
Smoking Cessation Advice	25	92%	87%	88%	100%
Heart Failure Care					
ACE Inhibitor or ARB for LVSD	104	81%	84%	82%	100%
Discharge Instructions	181	77%	56%	61%	93%
Evaluation of LVS Function	226	95%	84%	83%	99%
Smoking Cessation Advice	30	80%	82%	82%	100%
Pneumonia Care					
Appropriate Initial Antibiotic	126	84%	82%	83%	94%
Blood Culture Timing	160	96%	89%	90%	100%
Influenza Vaccine	41	61%	58%	70%	100%
Initial Antibiotic Timing	148	92%	75%	80%	93%
Oxygenation Assessment	218	100%	99%	99%	100%
Pneumococcal Vaccine	149	40%	58%	69%	94%
Smoking Cessation Advice[1]	20	95%	75%	80%	100%
Surgical Infection Prevention					
Prophylactic Antibiotic Given[2]	300	76%	74%	77%	95%
Prophylactic Antibiotic Selection[2]	75	97%	89%	90%	100%
Prophylactic Antibiotic Stopped[2]	284	63%	65%	72%	95%
Pregnancy Care					
Inpatient Neonatal Mortality	-	-	-	-	-
Third or Fourth Degree Laceration	-	-	3.58%	3.63%	3.27%

Indian Valley Hospital

184 Hot Springs Road — Phone: 530-284-7191
Greenville, CA 95947
Ownership: Govt - Hospital District or Authority — Accredited: No
Emergency Services: Yes

Measure	Cases	This Hospital	State Average	U.S. Average	Top Hospital
Heart Attack Care					
ACE Inhibitor or ARB for LVSD[5]	-	-	82%	82%	100%
Aspirin at Arrival[5]	-	-	95%	92%	100%
Aspirin at Discharge[5]	-	-	90%	90%	100%
Beta Blocker at Arrival[5]	-	-	89%	87%	100%
Beta Blocker at Discharge[5]	-	-	89%	90%	100%
Fibrinolytic Medication Timing[5]	-	-	40%	31%	100%
PCI Within 90 Minutes of Arrival[5]	-	-	52%	54%	95%
Smoking Cessation Advice[5]	-	-	87%	88%	100%
Heart Failure Care					
ACE Inhibitor or ARB for LVSD[5]	-	-	84%	82%	100%
Discharge Instructions[5]	-	-	56%	61%	93%
Evaluation of LVS Function[5]	-	-	84%	83%	99%
Smoking Cessation Advice[5]	-	-	82%	82%	100%
Pneumonia Care					
Appropriate Initial Antibiotic[5]	-	-	82%	83%	94%
Blood Culture Timing[5]	-	-	89%	90%	100%
Influenza Vaccine[5]	-	-	58%	70%	100%
Initial Antibiotic Timing[5]	-	-	75%	80%	93%
Oxygenation Assessment[5]	-	-	99%	99%	100%
Pneumococcal Vaccine[5]	-	-	58%	69%	94%
Smoking Cessation Advice[5]	-	-	75%	80%	100%
Surgical Infection Prevention					
Prophylactic Antibiotic Given[5]	-	-	74%	77%	95%
Prophylactic Antibiotic Selection[5]	-	-	89%	90%	100%
Prophylactic Antibiotic Stopped[5]	-	-	65%	72%	95%
Pregnancy Care					
Inpatient Neonatal Mortality	-	-	-	-	-
Third or Fourth Degree Laceration	-	-	3.58%	3.63%	3.27%

Central Valley General Hospital

1025 N Douty Street — Phone: 559-583-2100
Hanford, CA 93230 — Fax: 559-583-2225
URL: www.hanfordhealth.com
Ownership: Voluntary non-profit - Church — Accredited: Yes
Emergency Services: Yes — Licensed Beds: 49

Key Personnel:

President/CEO.......................... Rick Rawson
Chief Medical Staff....................... Charles Craft
Director of Cardiology/Cardiac Lab........... Anita Anivigate
Emergency Room........................ Gladys Barnes
Director Infection/Disease Control........... Kathy Palusko
Director Medical/Surgical Nursing........... Gladys Barnes
OB/GYN Womens Health.................. Kris Johnson

Measure	Cases	This Hospital	State Average	U.S. Average	Top Hospital
Heart Attack Care					
ACE Inhibitor or ARB for LVSD[3]	0	-	82%	82%	100%

NOTE: Hospital profiles are in alphabetical order by state, then city, then hospital within the city; Rankings are sorted by rate in descending order and exclude hospitals with less than 25 cases; (1) The number of cases is too small (n<25) for purposes of reliably predicting hospital performance; (2) Measure reflects the hospital's indication that its submission was based upon a sample of its relevant discharges; (3) Rate reflects fewer than the maximum possible quarters of data for the measure; (4) Inaccurate information submitted and suppressed for one or more quarters; (5) No data is available from the hospital for this measure; Please refer to the User's Guide for a full explanation of data

Aspirin at Arrival[1,3]	2	100%	95%	92%	100%
Aspirin at Discharge[1,3]	1	0%	90%	90%	100%
Beta Blocker at Arrival[1,3]	2	100%	89%	87%	100%
Beta Blocker at Discharge[1,3]	1	100%	89%	90%	100%
Fibrinolytic Medication Timing[3]	0	-	40%	31%	100%
PCI Within 90 Minutes of Arrival	0	-	52%	54%	95%
Smoking Cessation Advice[3]	0	-	87%	88%	100%
Heart Failure Care					
ACE Inhibitor or ARB for LVSD[1]	8	75%	84%	82%	100%
Discharge Instructions	35	40%	56%	61%	93%
Evaluation of LVS Function	40	30%	84%	83%	99%
Smoking Cessation Advice[1]	12	92%	82%	82%	100%
Pneumonia Care					
Appropriate Initial Antibiotic	67	84%	82%	83%	94%
Blood Culture Timing[1]	20	90%	89%	90%	100%
Influenza Vaccine[1]	9	78%	58%	70%	100%
Initial Antibiotic Timing	65	72%	75%	80%	93%
Oxygenation Assessment	71	100%	99%	99%	100%
Pneumococcal Vaccine	39	46%	58%	69%	94%
Smoking Cessation Advice[1]	14	86%	75%	80%	100%
Surgical Infection Prevention					
Prophylactic Antibiotic Given[2,3]	34	35%	74%	77%	95%
Prophylactic Antibiotic Selection[1,2]	3	67%	89%	90%	100%
Prophylactic Antibiotic Stopped[1,2,3]	23	91%	65%	72%	95%
Pregnancy Care					
Inpatient Neonatal Mortality	2,062	0.29%	-	-	-
Third or Fourth Degree Laceration	1,319	1.29%	3.58%	3.63%	3.27%

Hanford Community Medical Center

450 Greenfield Avenue — Phone: 559-582-9000
Hanford, CA 93230 — Fax: 559-584-7401
URL: www.hanfordhealth.com
Ownership: Voluntary non-profit - Church — Accredited: Yes
Emergency Services: Yes — Licensed Beds: 60

Key Personnel:

President/CEO . . . . Rick Rawson
Chief Medical Staff . . . . MR Goodman, MD
Emergency Room Director . . . . Scott Lethi
Emergency Room . . . . Trini Juarez
Director Medical/Surgical Nursing . . . . Marilyn Harris
OB/GYN Womens Health . . . . David Nelson, MD
Chief Radiology . . . . David Baca

Measure	Cases	This Hospital	State Average	U.S. Average	Top Hospital
Heart Attack Care					
ACE Inhibitor or ARB for LVSD[1]	5	20%	82%	82%	100%
Aspirin at Arrival	71	93%	95%	92%	100%
Aspirin at Discharge	51	69%	90%	90%	100%
Beta Blocker at Arrival	67	88%	89%	87%	100%
Beta Blocker at Discharge	49	73%	89%	90%	100%
Fibrinolytic Medication Timing[1]	12	17%	40%	31%	100%
PCI Within 90 Minutes of Arrival	0	-	52%	54%	95%
Smoking Cessation Advice[1]	17	82%	87%	88%	100%
Heart Failure Care					
ACE Inhibitor or ARB for LVSD	30	77%	84%	82%	100%
Discharge Instructions	139	37%	56%	61%	93%
Evaluation of LVS Function	143	40%	84%	83%	99%
Smoking Cessation Advice	29	90%	82%	82%	100%
Pneumonia Care					
Appropriate Initial Antibiotic	168	77%	82%	83%	94%
Blood Culture Timing	75	87%	89%	90%	100%
Influenza Vaccine	30	53%	58%	70%	100%
Initial Antibiotic Timing	183	61%	75%	80%	93%
Oxygenation Assessment	207	99%	99%	99%	100%
Pneumococcal Vaccine	129	54%	58%	69%	94%
Smoking Cessation Advice	46	83%	75%	80%	100%
Surgical Infection Prevention					
Prophylactic Antibiotic Given[2,3]	84	39%	74%	77%	95%
Prophylactic Antibiotic Selection[1,2]	24	88%	89%	90%	100%
Prophylactic Antibiotic Stopped[2,3]	75	40%	65%	72%	95%
Pregnancy Care					
Inpatient Neonatal Mortality	733	0.14%	-	-	-
Third or Fourth Degree Laceration	511	2.35%	3.58%	3.63%	3.27%

Kaiser Permanente South Bay Medical Center

25825 S Vermont Avenue — Phone: 310-325-5111
Harbor City, CA 90710 — Fax: 310-517-2234
URL: www.kaiserpermanente.org
Ownership: Voluntary non-profit - Other — Accredited: Yes
Emergency Services: Yes — Licensed Beds: 251

Key Personnel:

CEO . . . . George Halvorson
Chief Medical Staff . . . . Randel King, MD
OB/GYN Womens Health . . . . Jamshid Moossazadeh, MD
Chief Radiology . . . . Augusto Salceda, MD
Director Respiratory Therapy . . . . Kirk Rinella

Measure	Cases	This Hospital	State Average	U.S. Average	Top Hospital
Heart Attack Care					
ACE Inhibitor or ARB for LVSD	26	77%	82%	82%	100%
Aspirin at Arrival	137	97%	95%	92%	100%
Aspirin at Discharge	102	94%	90%	90%	100%
Beta Blocker at Arrival	132	94%	89%	87%	100%
Beta Blocker at Discharge	109	97%	89%	90%	100%
Fibrinolytic Medication Timing[1]	14	29%	40%	31%	100%
PCI Within 90 Minutes of Arrival	0	-	52%	54%	95%
Smoking Cessation Advice[1]	13	100%	87%	88%	100%
Heart Failure Care					
ACE Inhibitor or ARB for LVSD	120	87%	84%	82%	100%
Discharge Instructions	382	54%	56%	61%	93%
Evaluation of LVS Function	414	93%	84%	83%	99%
Smoking Cessation Advice	43	88%	82%	82%	100%
Pneumonia Care					
Appropriate Initial Antibiotic	103	46%	82%	83%	94%
Blood Culture Timing	101	92%	89%	90%	100%
Influenza Vaccine[1]	21	52%	58%	70%	100%
Initial Antibiotic Timing	115	54%	75%	80%	93%
Oxygenation Assessment	138	100%	99%	99%	100%
Pneumococcal Vaccine	79	92%	58%	69%	94%
Smoking Cessation Advice[1]	22	64%	75%	80%	100%
Surgical Infection Prevention					
Prophylactic Antibiotic Given[3]	51	76%	74%	77%	95%
Prophylactic Antibiotic Selection	50	98%	89%	90%	100%
Prophylactic Antibiotic Stopped[3]	51	63%	65%	72%	95%
Pregnancy Care					
Inpatient Neonatal Mortality	1,825	0.16%	-	-	-
Third or Fourth Degree Laceration	1,223	4.82%	3.58%	3.63%	3.27%

Tri-City Regional Medical Center

21530 S Pioneer Boulevard — Phone: 562-860-0401
Hawaiian Gardens, CA 90716 — Fax: 562-924-5871
URL: www.tri-cityrmc.org
Ownership: Govt - Hospital District or Authority — Accredited: Yes
Emergency Services: Yes — Licensed Beds: 137

Key Personnel:

CEO . . . . Arthur J Gerrick
Chief Medical Staff . . . . Hyun J Lee, MD
Emergency Room . . . . Amable Aguiluz, MD
OB/GYN . . . . William Caldwell, MD
Surgical Services . . . . Sioney Querubin, RN
Director Respiratory Therapy . . . . Wali Muhammad

Measure	Cases	This Hospital	State Average	U.S. Average	Top Hospital
Heart Attack Care					
ACE Inhibitor or ARB for LVSD[1]	4	75%	82%	82%	100%
Aspirin at Arrival[1]	10	80%	95%	92%	100%
Aspirin at Discharge[1]	7	86%	90%	90%	100%
Beta Blocker at Arrival[1]	7	57%	89%	87%	100%
Beta Blocker at Discharge[1]	6	67%	89%	90%	100%
Fibrinolytic Medication Timing[1]	1	100%	40%	31%	100%
PCI Within 90 Minutes of Arrival	0	-	52%	54%	95%
Smoking Cessation Advice[1]	2	50%	87%	88%	100%
Heart Failure Care					
ACE Inhibitor or ARB for LVSD[1]	21	62%	84%	82%	100%
Discharge Instructions	64	58%	56%	61%	93%
Evaluation of LVS Function	165	87%	84%	83%	99%
Smoking Cessation Advice	25	92%	82%	82%	100%

NOTE: Hospital profiles are in alphabetical order by state, then city, then hospital within the city; Rankings are sorted by rate in descending order and exclude hospitals with less than 25 cases; (1) The number of cases is too small (n<25) for purposes of reliably predicting hospital performance; (2) Measure reflects the hospital's indication that its submission was based upon a sample of its relevant discharges; (3) Rate reflects fewer than the maximum possible quarters of data for the measure; (4) Inaccurate information submitted and suppressed for one or more quarters; (5) No data is available from the hospital for this measure; Please refer to the User's Guide for a full explanation of data

Pneumonia Care					
Appropriate Initial Antibiotic	44	66%	82%	83%	94%
Blood Culture Timing	77	84%	89%	90%	100%
Influenza Vaccine[4,5]	-	-	58%	70%	100%
Initial Antibiotic Timing	145	75%	75%	80%	93%
Oxygenation Assessment	178	99%	99%	99%	100%
Pneumococcal Vaccine	116	39%	58%	69%	94%
Smoking Cessation Advice	25	96%	75%	80%	100%
Surgical Infection Prevention					
Prophylactic Antibiotic Given[1,3]	16	25%	74%	77%	95%
Prophylactic Antibiotic Selection[1]	7	86%	89%	90%	100%
Prophylactic Antibiotic Stopped[1,3]	8	38%	65%	72%	95%
Pregnancy Care					
Inpatient Neonatal Mortality	-	-	-	-	-
Third or Fourth Degree Laceration	-	-	3.58%	3.63%	3.27%

Kaiser Foundation Hospital

27400 Hesperian Boulevard — Phone: 510-784-4000
Hayward, CA 94545 — Fax: 510-784-2791
URL: www.kaiserpermanente.org
Ownership: Voluntary non-profit - Other — Accredited: Yes
Emergency Services: Yes — Licensed Beds: 224

Key Personnel:

Chief Medical Staff . . . . Anabel Andarson Imberg
Asst Director of Emergency . . . . Doug Lumkin
Emergency Room . . . . Terri Pillow-Noriega
OB/GYN Womens Health. . . . . Steven Young, MD
Chief Radiology . . . . Laurre Mazzara, MD
Manager of Respiratory . . . . Thomas Wagner

Measure	Cases	This Hospital	State Average	U.S. Average	Top Hospital
Heart Attack Care					
ACE Inhibitor or ARB for LVSD	25	92%	82%	82%	100%
Aspirin at Arrival	340	100%	95%	92%	100%
Aspirin at Discharge	203	99%	90%	90%	100%
Beta Blocker at Arrival	344	99%	89%	87%	100%
Beta Blocker at Discharge	216	99%	89%	90%	100%
Fibrinolytic Medication Timing[1]	10	60%	40%	31%	100%
PCI Within 90 Minutes of Arrival	0	-	52%	54%	95%
Smoking Cessation Advice[1]	20	95%	87%	88%	100%
Heart Failure Care					
ACE Inhibitor or ARB for LVSD	105	84%	84%	82%	100%
Discharge Instructions	377	61%	56%	61%	93%
Evaluation of LVS Function	427	95%	84%	83%	99%
Smoking Cessation Advice	49	82%	82%	82%	100%
Pneumonia Care					
Appropriate Initial Antibiotic	131	76%	82%	83%	94%
Blood Culture Timing	122	94%	89%	90%	100%
Influenza Vaccine	26	62%	58%	70%	100%
Initial Antibiotic Timing	168	67%	75%	80%	93%
Oxygenation Assessment	202	100%	99%	99%	100%
Pneumococcal Vaccine	139	81%	58%	69%	94%
Smoking Cessation Advice[1]	24	67%	75%	80%	100%
Surgical Infection Prevention					
Prophylactic Antibiotic Given	411	74%	74%	77%	95%
Prophylactic Antibiotic Selection	99	87%	89%	90%	100%
Prophylactic Antibiotic Stopped	391	56%	65%	72%	95%
Pregnancy Care					
Inpatient Neonatal Mortality	3,342	0.24%	-	-	-
Third or Fourth Degree Laceration	2,123	5.23%	3.58%	3.63%	3.27%

Saint Rose Hospital

27200 Calaroga Avenue — Phone: 510-264-4000
Hayward, CA 94545 — Fax: 510-264-4076
URL: www.strosehospital.org
Ownership: Voluntary non-profit - Church — Accredited: Yes
Emergency Services: Yes — Licensed Beds: 175

Key Personnel:

CEO. . . . . Michael P Mahoney
Chief Medical Staff. . . . . Vasiliki Economou, MD
Emergency Room . . . . Patrick Evangelista

Measure	Cases	This Hospital	State Average	U.S. Average	Top Hospital
Heart Attack Care					
ACE Inhibitor or ARB for LVSD[1]	20	90%	82%	82%	100%
Aspirin at Arrival	121	97%	95%	92%	100%
Aspirin at Discharge	87	91%	90%	90%	100%
Beta Blocker at Arrival	115	90%	89%	87%	100%
Beta Blocker at Discharge	95	93%	89%	90%	100%
Fibrinolytic Medication Timing[3]	0	-	40%	31%	100%
PCI Within 90 Minutes of Arrival[1]	15	47%	52%	54%	95%
Smoking Cessation Advice[1,3]	12	92%	87%	88%	100%
Heart Failure Care					
ACE Inhibitor or ARB for LVSD	113	81%	84%	82%	100%
Discharge Instructions[3]	57	70%	56%	61%	93%
Evaluation of LVS Function	276	86%	84%	83%	99%
Smoking Cessation Advice[1,3]	12	100%	82%	82%	100%
Pneumonia Care					
Appropriate Initial Antibiotic[3]	32	72%	82%	83%	94%
Blood Culture Timing[3]	40	82%	89%	90%	100%
Influenza Vaccine[5]	-	-	58%	70%	100%
Initial Antibiotic Timing	200	62%	75%	80%	93%
Oxygenation Assessment	216	100%	99%	99%	100%
Pneumococcal Vaccine	130	95%	58%	69%	94%
Smoking Cessation Advice[1,3]	5	100%	75%	80%	100%
Surgical Infection Prevention					
Prophylactic Antibiotic Given[3]	39	77%	74%	77%	95%
Prophylactic Antibiotic Selection[5]	-	-	89%	90%	100%
Prophylactic Antibiotic Stopped[3]	39	100%	65%	72%	95%
Pregnancy Care					
Inpatient Neonatal Mortality	-	-	-	-	-
Third or Fourth Degree Laceration	-	-	3.58%	3.63%	3.27%

Healdsburg District Hospital

1375 University Avenue — Phone: 707-431-6500
Healdsburg, CA 95448 — Fax: 707-431-6588
URL: www.h-g-h.org
Ownership: Govt - Hospital District or Authority — Accredited: No
Emergency Services: Yes — Licensed Beds: 43

Key Personnel:

CEO. . . . . Dale E Iverson
Emergency Room . . . . Walter Maack, MD
Infection Control. . . . . Mary Daniels

Measure	Cases	This Hospital	State Average	U.S. Average	Top Hospital
Heart Attack Care					
ACE Inhibitor or ARB for LVSD[3]	0	-	82%	82%	100%
Aspirin at Arrival[1,3]	2	50%	95%	92%	100%
Aspirin at Discharge[3]	0	-	90%	90%	100%
Beta Blocker at Arrival[1,3]	2	0%	89%	87%	100%
Beta Blocker at Discharge[3]	0	-	89%	90%	100%
Fibrinolytic Medication Timing[3]	0	-	40%	31%	100%
PCI Within 90 Minutes of Arrival[5]	-	-	52%	54%	95%
Smoking Cessation Advice[3]	0	-	87%	88%	100%
Heart Failure Care					
ACE Inhibitor or ARB for LVSD[1]	1	100%	84%	82%	100%
Discharge Instructions[1]	17	0%	56%	61%	93%
Evaluation of LVS Function	25	8%	84%	83%	99%
Smoking Cessation Advice[1]	1	0%	82%	82%	100%
Pneumonia Care					
Appropriate Initial Antibiotic[3]	29	76%	82%	83%	94%
Blood Culture Timing[1]	11	73%	89%	90%	100%
Influenza Vaccine[1]	10	0%	58%	70%	100%
Initial Antibiotic Timing	32	91%	75%	80%	93%
Oxygenation Assessment	38	100%	99%	99%	100%
Pneumococcal Vaccine	29	7%	58%	69%	94%
Smoking Cessation Advice[1]	7	0%	75%	80%	100%
Surgical Infection Prevention					
Prophylactic Antibiotic Given[2]	53	91%	74%	77%	95%
Prophylactic Antibiotic Selection[1,2]	4	100%	89%	90%	100%
Prophylactic Antibiotic Stopped[2]	52	98%	65%	72%	95%
Pregnancy Care					
Inpatient Neonatal Mortality	-	-	-	-	-

NOTE: Hospital profiles are in alphabetical order by state, then city, then hospital within the city; Rankings are sorted by rate in descending order and exclude hospitals with less than 25 cases; (1) The number of cases is too small (n<25) for purposes of reliably predicting hospital performance; (2) Measure reflects the hospital's indication that its submission was based upon a sample of its relevant discharges; (3) Rate reflects fewer than the maximum possible quarters of data for the measure; (4) Inaccurate information submitted and suppressed for one or more quarters; (5) No data is available from the hospital for this measure; Please refer to the User's Guide for a full explanation of data

Third or Fourth Degree Laceration	-	-	3.58%	3.63%	3.27%

Hemet Valley Medical Center

1117 E Devonshire Ave
Hemet, CA 92543
Phone: 951-652-2811
Fax: 951-766-6415
URL: www.valleyhealthsystem.com
Ownership: Govt - Hospital District or Authority
Accredited: Yes
Emergency Services: Yes
Licensed Beds: 240
Key Personnel:
CEO. . . . . James W Maki

Measure	Cases	This Hospital	State Average	U.S. Average	Top Hospital
Heart Attack Care					
ACE Inhibitor or ARB for LVSD	48	77%	82%	82%	100%
Aspirin at Arrival	270	93%	95%	92%	100%
Aspirin at Discharge	116	79%	90%	90%	100%
Beta Blocker at Arrival	240	88%	89%	87%	100%
Beta Blocker at Discharge	149	81%	89%	90%	100%
Fibrinolytic Medication Timing	42	81%	40%	31%	100%
PCI Within 90 Minutes of Arrival	0	-	52%	54%	95%
Smoking Cessation Advice[1]	21	43%	87%	88%	100%
Heart Failure Care					
ACE Inhibitor or ARB for LVSD	138	66%	84%	82%	100%
Discharge Instructions	273	49%	56%	61%	93%
Evaluation of LVS Function	375	89%	84%	83%	99%
Smoking Cessation Advice	58	69%	82%	82%	100%
Pneumonia Care					
Appropriate Initial Antibiotic	220	65%	82%	83%	94%
Blood Culture Timing	240	88%	89%	90%	100%
Influenza Vaccine	78	32%	58%	70%	100%
Initial Antibiotic Timing	362	58%	75%	80%	93%
Oxygenation Assessment	467	100%	99%	99%	100%
Pneumococcal Vaccine	315	39%	58%	69%	94%
Smoking Cessation Advice	75	63%	75%	80%	100%
Surgical Infection Prevention					
Prophylactic Antibiotic Given[3]	95	53%	74%	77%	95%
Prophylactic Antibiotic Selection	94	52%	89%	90%	100%
Prophylactic Antibiotic Stopped[3]	92	9%	65%	72%	95%
Pregnancy Care					
Inpatient Neonatal Mortality	-	-	-	-	-
Third or Fourth Degree Laceration	-	-	3.58%	3.63%	3.27%

Hazel Hawkins Memorial Hospital

911 Sunset Drive
Hollister, CA 95023
Phone: 831-637-5711
Fax: 831-636-2668
E-mail: fvalent@hazelhawkins.com
URL: www.hazelhawkins.com
Ownership: Govt - Hospital District or Authority
Accredited: Yes
Emergency Services: Yes
Licensed Beds: 101
Key Personnel:
CEO. . . . . Ken S Underwood
Chief Medical Staff . . . . Leonard Catuto, MD
Emergency Room . . . . Marian Anderson, RN
Director Medical/Surgical Nursing . . . . . B Gatcomb, RN
OB/GYN Womens Health. . . . . A Barra, MD
Chief Radiology . . . . RL Darby, MD

Measure	Cases	This Hospital	State Average	U.S. Average	Top Hospital
Heart Attack Care					
ACE Inhibitor or ARB for LVSD[1]	1	0%	82%	82%	100%
Aspirin at Arrival[1]	8	88%	95%	92%	100%
Aspirin at Discharge[1]	3	100%	90%	90%	100%
Beta Blocker at Arrival[1]	8	75%	89%	87%	100%
Beta Blocker at Discharge[1]	6	83%	89%	90%	100%
Fibrinolytic Medication Timing	0	-	40%	31%	100%
PCI Within 90 Minutes of Arrival	0	-	52%	54%	95%
Smoking Cessation Advice[1]	1	100%	87%	88%	100%
Heart Failure Care					
ACE Inhibitor or ARB for LVSD[1]	7	100%	84%	82%	100%
Discharge Instructions	59	51%	56%	61%	93%
Evaluation of LVS Function	79	59%	84%	83%	99%
Smoking Cessation Advice[1]	8	50%	82%	82%	100%
Pneumonia Care					
Appropriate Initial Antibiotic	52	81%	82%	83%	94%
Blood Culture Timing	30	60%	89%	90%	100%
Influenza Vaccine[1]	23	70%	58%	70%	100%
Initial Antibiotic Timing	58	83%	75%	80%	93%
Oxygenation Assessment	77	96%	99%	99%	100%
Pneumococcal Vaccine	59	53%	58%	69%	94%
Smoking Cessation Advice[1]	9	33%	75%	80%	100%
Surgical Infection Prevention					
Prophylactic Antibiotic Given	68	54%	74%	77%	95%
Prophylactic Antibiotic Selection[1]	12	92%	89%	90%	100%
Prophylactic Antibiotic Stopped	64	80%	65%	72%	95%
Pregnancy Care					
Inpatient Neonatal Mortality	-	-	-	-	-
Third or Fourth Degree Laceration	-	-	3.58%	3.63%	3.27%

Hollywood Community Hospital

6245 De Longpre Avenue
Hollywood, CA 90028
Phone: 323-462-2271
Fax: 323-461-9278
URL: www.hollywoodcommunityhospital.com
Ownership: Voluntary non-profit - Other
Accredited: Yes
Emergency Services: Yes
Licensed Beds: 100
Key Personnel:
CEO. . . . . Casey Fatch

Measure	Cases	This Hospital	State Average	U.S. Average	Top Hospital
Heart Attack Care					
ACE Inhibitor or ARB for LVSD[1]	4	75%	82%	82%	100%
Aspirin at Arrival[1]	3	100%	95%	92%	100%
Aspirin at Discharge[1]	5	100%	90%	90%	100%
Beta Blocker at Arrival[1]	3	67%	89%	87%	100%
Beta Blocker at Discharge[1]	5	80%	89%	90%	100%
Fibrinolytic Medication Timing	0	-	40%	31%	100%
PCI Within 90 Minutes of Arrival	0	-	52%	54%	95%
Smoking Cessation Advice[1]	4	75%	87%	88%	100%
Heart Failure Care					
ACE Inhibitor or ARB for LVSD[1]	11	82%	84%	82%	100%
Discharge Instructions	27	15%	56%	61%	93%
Evaluation of LVS Function	34	65%	84%	83%	99%
Smoking Cessation Advice[1]	16	75%	82%	82%	100%
Pneumonia Care					
Appropriate Initial Antibiotic	35	29%	82%	83%	94%
Blood Culture Timing[1]	3	67%	89%	90%	100%
Influenza Vaccine[1]	12	0%	58%	70%	100%
Initial Antibiotic Timing	48	79%	75%	80%	93%
Oxygenation Assessment	50	66%	99%	99%	100%
Pneumococcal Vaccine	37	3%	58%	69%	94%
Smoking Cessation Advice	34	32%	75%	80%	100%
Surgical Infection Prevention					
Prophylactic Antibiotic Given[1,3]	6	100%	74%	77%	95%
Prophylactic Antibiotic Selection[1]	6	100%	89%	90%	100%
Prophylactic Antibiotic Stopped[1,3]	6	100%	65%	72%	95%
Pregnancy Care					
Inpatient Neonatal Mortality	-	-	-	-	-
Third or Fourth Degree Laceration	-	-	3.58%	3.63%	3.27%

Huntington Beach Hospital

Alternate Name: Huntington Beach Medical Center
17772 Beach Boulevard
Huntington Beach, CA 92647
Phone: 714-842-1473
Fax: 714-843-5038
URL: www.hbhospital.com
Ownership: Proprietary
Accredited: Yes
Emergency Services: Yes
Licensed Beds: 134
Key Personnel:
CEO. . . . . Mary Botticelia

Measure	Cases	This Hospital	State Average	U.S. Average	Top Hospital
Heart Attack Care					
ACE Inhibitor or ARB for LVSD[1]	7	43%	82%	82%	100%
Aspirin at Arrival	41	93%	95%	92%	100%
Aspirin at Discharge[1]	16	94%	90%	90%	100%
Beta Blocker at Arrival	36	83%	89%	87%	100%

NOTE: Hospital profiles are in alphabetical order by state, then city, then hospital within the city; Rankings are sorted by rate in descending order and exclude hospitals with less than 25 cases; (1) The number of cases is too small (n<25) for purposes of reliably predicting hospital performance; (2) Measure reflects the hospital's indication that its submission was based upon a sample of its relevant discharges; (3) Rate reflects fewer than the maximum possible quarters of data for the measure; (4) Inaccurate information submitted and suppressed for one or more quarters; (5) No data is available from the hospital for this measure; Please refer to the User's Guide for a full explanation of data

Measure	Cases	This Hospital	State Average	U.S. Average	Top Hospital
Beta Blocker at Discharge[1]	23	78%	89%	90%	100%
Fibrinolytic Medication Timing[1]	3	33%	40%	31%	100%
PCI Within 90 Minutes of Arrival	0	-	52%	54%	95%
Smoking Cessation Advice[1]	5	20%	87%	88%	100%
Heart Failure Care					
ACE Inhibitor or ARB for LVSD	26	88%	84%	82%	100%
Discharge Instructions	97	56%	56%	61%	93%
Evaluation of LVS Function	128	91%	84%	83%	99%
Smoking Cessation Advice	27	63%	82%	82%	100%
Pneumonia Care					
Appropriate Initial Antibiotic	107	72%	82%	83%	94%
Blood Culture Timing	99	96%	89%	90%	100%
Influenza Vaccine[1]	20	70%	58%	70%	100%
Initial Antibiotic Timing	132	92%	75%	80%	93%
Oxygenation Assessment	156	100%	99%	99%	100%
Pneumococcal Vaccine	96	86%	58%	69%	94%
Smoking Cessation Advice	25	64%	75%	80%	100%
Surgical Infection Prevention					
Prophylactic Antibiotic Given	68	56%	74%	77%	95%
Prophylactic Antibiotic Selection[1]	16	94%	89%	90%	100%
Prophylactic Antibiotic Stopped	60	42%	65%	72%	95%
Pregnancy Care					
Inpatient Neonatal Mortality	-	-	-	-	-
Third or Fourth Degree Laceration	-	-	3.58%	3.63%	3.27%

Community Hospital

2623 E Slauson Avenue
Huntington Park, CA 90255
Phone: 323-583-1931
Fax: 323-582-8179
Ownership: Voluntary non-profit - Private
Accredited: Yes
Emergency Services: Yes
Licensed Beds: 81

Key Personnel:

CEO. . . . . Charles Martinez
Chief Medical Staff. . . . . Jesus Ramirez
Chief Radiology . . . . Mark Brown
Director Respiratory Therapy . . . . Sean Boulouki

Measure	Cases	This Hospital	State Average	U.S. Average	Top Hospital
Heart Attack Care					
ACE Inhibitor or ARB for LVSD[1]	4	100%	82%	82%	100%
Aspirin at Arrival	28	93%	95%	92%	100%
Aspirin at Discharge[1]	13	69%	90%	90%	100%
Beta Blocker at Arrival	28	71%	89%	87%	100%
Beta Blocker at Discharge[1]	13	46%	89%	90%	100%
Fibrinolytic Medication Timing	0	-	40%	31%	100%
PCI Within 90 Minutes of Arrival	0	-	52%	54%	95%
Smoking Cessation Advice	0	-	87%	88%	100%
Heart Failure Care					
ACE Inhibitor or ARB for LVSD	27	74%	84%	82%	100%
Discharge Instructions	142	48%	56%	61%	93%
Evaluation of LVS Function	156	54%	84%	83%	99%
Smoking Cessation Advice[1]	7	43%	82%	82%	100%
Pneumonia Care					
Appropriate Initial Antibiotic	127	61%	82%	83%	94%
Blood Culture Timing	50	78%	89%	90%	100%
Influenza Vaccine	29	24%	58%	70%	100%
Initial Antibiotic Timing	113	62%	75%	80%	93%
Oxygenation Assessment	142	89%	99%	99%	100%
Pneumococcal Vaccine	78	10%	58%	69%	94%
Smoking Cessation Advice[1]	13	23%	75%	80%	100%
Surgical Infection Prevention					
Prophylactic Antibiotic Given[2]	31	39%	74%	77%	95%
Prophylactic Antibiotic Selection[1,2]	4	75%	89%	90%	100%
Prophylactic Antibiotic Stopped[1,2]	22	95%	65%	72%	95%
Pregnancy Care					
Inpatient Neonatal Mortality	-	-	-	-	-
Third or Fourth Degree Laceration	-	-	3.58%	3.63%	3.27%

John F Kennedy Memorial Hospital

47111 Monroe Street
Indio, CA 92201
Phone: 760-347-6191
Fax: 760-775-8014
URL: www.jfkmemorialhosp.com
Ownership: Proprietary
Accredited: Yes
Emergency Services: Yes
Licensed Beds: 145

Key Personnel:

CEO. . . . . John Ferrelli
Chief Medical Officer . . . . Dr Jennifer Daley
Emergency Room . . . . Reiner Jakel
Director Medical/Surgical Nursing . . . . Marge Doyle
Director of Respiratory . . . . Dave Mohlenhoff

Measure	Cases	This Hospital	State Average	U.S. Average	Top Hospital
Heart Attack Care					
ACE Inhibitor or ARB for LVSD[1]	19	68%	82%	82%	100%
Aspirin at Arrival	115	96%	95%	92%	100%
Aspirin at Discharge	84	87%	90%	90%	100%
Beta Blocker at Arrival	88	88%	89%	87%	100%
Beta Blocker at Discharge	80	89%	89%	90%	100%
Fibrinolytic Medication Timing[1]	14	64%	40%	31%	100%
PCI Within 90 Minutes of Arrival[1]	3	67%	52%	54%	95%
Smoking Cessation Advice[1]	20	100%	87%	88%	100%
Heart Failure Care					
ACE Inhibitor or ARB for LVSD	79	77%	84%	82%	100%
Discharge Instructions	162	65%	56%	61%	93%
Evaluation of LVS Function	195	87%	84%	83%	99%
Smoking Cessation Advice	30	100%	82%	82%	100%
Pneumonia Care					
Appropriate Initial Antibiotic	216	87%	82%	83%	94%
Blood Culture Timing	205	95%	89%	90%	100%
Influenza Vaccine	62	63%	58%	70%	100%
Initial Antibiotic Timing	229	85%	75%	80%	93%
Oxygenation Assessment	285	100%	99%	99%	100%
Pneumococcal Vaccine	178	65%	58%	69%	94%
Smoking Cessation Advice	37	100%	75%	80%	100%
Surgical Infection Prevention					
Prophylactic Antibiotic Given[2]	288	83%	74%	77%	95%
Prophylactic Antibiotic Selection[2]	78	92%	89%	90%	100%
Prophylactic Antibiotic Stopped[2]	280	64%	65%	72%	95%
Pregnancy Care					
Inpatient Neonatal Mortality	-	-	-	-	-
Third or Fourth Degree Laceration	-	-	3.58%	3.63%	3.27%

Centinela Hospital Medical Center

555 E Hardy Street
Inglewood, CA 90301
Phone: 310-673-4660
Fax: 310-674-9604
URL: www.centinelafreeman.com
Ownership: Proprietary
Accredited: Yes
Emergency Services: Yes
Licensed Beds: 400

Key Personnel:

CEO. . . . . Michael Rembis
Chief Medical Staff. . . . . Rama Chandran, MD
Director Infection/Disease Control . . . . Geri Braddock, RN

Measure	Cases	This Hospital	State Average	U.S. Average	Top Hospital
Heart Attack Care					
ACE Inhibitor or ARB for LVSD	51	76%	82%	82%	100%
Aspirin at Arrival	207	96%	95%	92%	100%
Aspirin at Discharge	258	98%	90%	90%	100%
Beta Blocker at Arrival	192	92%	89%	87%	100%
Beta Blocker at Discharge	253	93%	89%	90%	100%
Fibrinolytic Medication Timing[1]	10	50%	40%	31%	100%
PCI Within 90 Minutes of Arrival[1]	8	0%	52%	54%	95%
Smoking Cessation Advice	81	91%	87%	88%	100%
Heart Failure Care					
ACE Inhibitor or ARB for LVSD	197	86%	84%	82%	100%
Discharge Instructions	398	32%	56%	61%	93%
Evaluation of LVS Function	446	92%	84%	83%	99%
Smoking Cessation Advice	49	82%	82%	82%	100%
Pneumonia Care					
Appropriate Initial Antibiotic	149	87%	82%	83%	94%
Blood Culture Timing	135	92%	89%	90%	100%

NOTE: Hospital profiles are in alphabetical order by state, then city, then hospital within the city; Rankings are sorted by rate in descending order and exclude hospitals with less than 25 cases; (1) The number of cases is too small (n<25) for purposes of reliably predicting hospital performance; (2) Measure reflects the hospital's indication that its submission was based upon a sample of its relevant discharges; (3) Rate reflects fewer than the maximum possible quarters of data for the measure; (4) Inaccurate information submitted and suppressed for one or more quarters; (5) No data is available from the hospital for this measure; Please refer to the User's Guide for a full explanation of data

Influenza Vaccine	33	97%	58%	70%	100%
Initial Antibiotic Timing	181	71%	75%	80%	93%
Oxygenation Assessment	230	100%	99%	99%	100%
Pneumococcal Vaccine	129	84%	58%	69%	94%
Smoking Cessation Advice	32	97%	75%	80%	100%
Surgical Infection Prevention					
Prophylactic Antibiotic Given	584	78%	74%	77%	95%
Prophylactic Antibiotic Selection	127	94%	89%	90%	100%
Prophylactic Antibiotic Stopped	571	50%	65%	72%	95%
Pregnancy Care					
Inpatient Neonatal Mortality	-	-	-	-	-
Third or Fourth Degree Laceration	-	-	3.58%	3.63%	3.27%

Irvine Regional Hospital

16200 Sand Canyon Avenue
Irvine, CA 92618
Phone: 949-753-2000
Fax: 949-753-2077
URL: www.irvineregionalhospital.com
Ownership: Proprietary
Accredited: Yes
Emergency Services: Yes
Licensed Beds: 176
Key Personnel:
CEO. . . . . Donald A Lorack Jr

Measure	Cases	This Hospital	State Average	U.S. Average	Top Hospital
Heart Attack Care					
ACE Inhibitor or ARB for LVSD[1]	24	79%	82%	82%	100%
Aspirin at Arrival	109	99%	95%	92%	100%
Aspirin at Discharge	164	96%	90%	90%	100%
Beta Blocker at Arrival	91	95%	89%	87%	100%
Beta Blocker at Discharge	174	96%	89%	90%	100%
Fibrinolytic Medication Timing[1]	3	67%	40%	31%	100%
PCI Within 90 Minutes of Arrival[1]	6	83%	52%	54%	95%
Smoking Cessation Advice	37	97%	87%	88%	100%
Heart Failure Care					
ACE Inhibitor or ARB for LVSD	57	74%	84%	82%	100%
Discharge Instructions	173	60%	56%	61%	93%
Evaluation of LVS Function	206	90%	84%	83%	99%
Smoking Cessation Advice[1]	13	85%	82%	82%	100%
Pneumonia Care					
Appropriate Initial Antibiotic	161	89%	82%	83%	94%
Blood Culture Timing	133	95%	89%	90%	100%
Influenza Vaccine	58	72%	58%	70%	100%
Initial Antibiotic Timing	160	84%	75%	80%	93%
Oxygenation Assessment	244	100%	99%	99%	100%
Pneumococcal Vaccine	184	76%	58%	69%	94%
Smoking Cessation Advice[1]	22	73%	75%	80%	100%
Surgical Infection Prevention					
Prophylactic Antibiotic Given[2]	197	73%	74%	77%	95%
Prophylactic Antibiotic Selection[2]	44	80%	89%	90%	100%
Prophylactic Antibiotic Stopped[2]	199	68%	65%	72%	95%
Pregnancy Care					
Inpatient Neonatal Mortality	-	-	-	-	-
Third or Fourth Degree Laceration	-	-	3.58%	3.63%	3.27%

Sutter Amador Hospital

Alternate Name: Amador Hospital
200 Mission Boulevard
Jackson, CA 95642
Phone: 209-223-7500
Fax: 209-223-7509
E-mail: boetzej@sutterhealth.org
URL: www.sutteramador.org
Ownership: Government - Local
Accredited: Yes
Emergency Services: Yes
Licensed Beds: 66
Key Personnel:
CEO. . . . . Anne Platt
Director Medical/Surgical Nursing . . . . Denise Sammons
Director Pulmonary Services . . . . Tim Sammons

Measure	Cases	This Hospital	State Average	U.S. Average	Top Hospital
Heart Attack Care					
ACE Inhibitor or ARB for LVSD[1]	5	40%	82%	82%	100%
Aspirin at Arrival[1]	15	80%	95%	92%	100%
Aspirin at Discharge[1]	7	86%	90%	90%	100%
Beta Blocker at Arrival[1]	11	100%	89%	87%	100%
Beta Blocker at Discharge[1]	8	100%	89%	90%	100%
Fibrinolytic Medication Timing	0	-	40%	31%	100%
PCI Within 90 Minutes of Arrival	0	-	52%	54%	95%
Smoking Cessation Advice[1]	1	100%	87%	88%	100%
Heart Failure Care					
ACE Inhibitor or ARB for LVSD	34	68%	84%	82%	100%
Discharge Instructions	66	30%	56%	61%	93%
Evaluation of LVS Function	89	63%	84%	83%	99%
Smoking Cessation Advice[1]	20	80%	82%	82%	100%
Pneumonia Care					
Appropriate Initial Antibiotic	85	76%	82%	83%	94%
Blood Culture Timing	68	90%	89%	90%	100%
Influenza Vaccine[1]	21	0%	58%	70%	100%
Initial Antibiotic Timing	99	96%	75%	80%	93%
Oxygenation Assessment	116	100%	99%	99%	100%
Pneumococcal Vaccine	70	31%	58%	69%	94%
Smoking Cessation Advice[1]	24	75%	75%	80%	100%
Surgical Infection Prevention					
Prophylactic Antibiotic Given[2]	138	71%	74%	77%	95%
Prophylactic Antibiotic Selection[2]	37	100%	89%	90%	100%
Prophylactic Antibiotic Stopped[2]	137	57%	65%	72%	95%
Pregnancy Care					
Inpatient Neonatal Mortality	-	-	-	-	-
Third or Fourth Degree Laceration	-	-	3.58%	3.63%	3.27%

Hi-Desert Medical Center

6601 White Feather Road
Joshua Tree, CA 92252
Phone: 760-366-3711
Fax: 760-366-6136
URL: www.hdmc.org
Ownership: Govt - Hospital District or Authority
Accredited: Yes
Emergency Services: Yes
Licensed Beds: 59
Key Personnel:
CEO. . . . . Keith Mesmer
Cardiopulmonary . . . . Jackie Combs
Emergency Room . . . . Donna Johnson
Infection Control. . . . . Peggy Ventura
Surgery . . . . Sandy Teets

Measure	Cases	This Hospital	State Average	U.S. Average	Top Hospital
Heart Attack Care					
ACE Inhibitor or ARB for LVSD[1]	1	100%	82%	82%	100%
Aspirin at Arrival	25	88%	95%	92%	100%
Aspirin at Discharge[1]	13	92%	90%	90%	100%
Beta Blocker at Arrival	31	77%	89%	87%	100%
Beta Blocker at Discharge[1]	15	87%	89%	90%	100%
Fibrinolytic Medication Timing	0	-	40%	31%	100%
PCI Within 90 Minutes of Arrival	0	-	52%	54%	95%
Smoking Cessation Advice[1]	7	100%	87%	88%	100%
Heart Failure Care					
ACE Inhibitor or ARB for LVSD	33	85%	84%	82%	100%
Discharge Instructions	65	5%	56%	61%	93%
Evaluation of LVS Function	106	81%	84%	83%	99%
Smoking Cessation Advice[1]	23	83%	82%	82%	100%
Pneumonia Care					
Appropriate Initial Antibiotic	118	81%	82%	83%	94%
Blood Culture Timing	142	90%	89%	90%	100%
Influenza Vaccine	45	64%	58%	70%	100%
Initial Antibiotic Timing	241	61%	75%	80%	93%
Oxygenation Assessment	290	100%	99%	99%	100%
Pneumococcal Vaccine	182	64%	58%	69%	94%
Smoking Cessation Advice	77	81%	75%	80%	100%
Surgical Infection Prevention					
Prophylactic Antibiotic Given[3]	61	62%	74%	77%	95%
Prophylactic Antibiotic Selection	25	84%	89%	90%	100%
Prophylactic Antibiotic Stopped[3]	57	65%	65%	72%	95%
Pregnancy Care					
Inpatient Neonatal Mortality	-	-	-	-	-
Third or Fourth Degree Laceration	-	-	3.58%	3.63%	3.27%

NOTE: Hospital profiles are in alphabetical order by state, then city, then hospital within the city; Rankings are sorted by rate in descending order and exclude hospitals with less than 25 cases; (1) The number of cases is too small (n<25) for purposes of reliably predicting hospital performance; (2) Measure reflects the hospital's indication that its submission was based upon a sample of its relevant discharges; (3) Rate reflects fewer than the maximum possible quarters of data for the measure; (4) Inaccurate information submitted and suppressed for one or more quarters; (5) No data is available from the hospital for this measure; Please refer to the User's Guide for a full explanation of data

George L Mee Memorial Hospital

300 Canal Street
King City, CA 93930
Phone: 831-385-6000
Fax: 831-385-7171
E-mail: info@meememorial.com
URL: www.meememorial.com
Ownership: Voluntary non-profit - Other
Accredited: Yes
Emergency Services: Yes
Licensed Beds: 123

Key Personnel:

President/CEO. . . . . Walt Beck
Director Medical/Surgical Nursing . . . . Virginia Rojas, RN
Chief Radiology . . . . Kevin Jenkins
Director Respiratory Therapy . . . . Brian Fischer

Measure	Cases	This Hospital	State Average	U.S. Average	Top Hospital
Heart Attack Care					
ACE Inhibitor or ARB for LVSD[3]	0	-	82%	82%	100%
Aspirin at Arrival[1,3]	4	100%	95%	92%	100%
Aspirin at Discharge[1,3]	3	100%	90%	90%	100%
Beta Blocker at Arrival[1,3]	3	100%	89%	87%	100%
Beta Blocker at Discharge[1,3]	2	50%	89%	90%	100%
Fibrinolytic Medication Timing[3]	0	-	40%	31%	100%
PCI Within 90 Minutes of Arrival	0	-	52%	54%	95%
Smoking Cessation Advice[3]	0	-	87%	88%	100%
Heart Failure Care					
ACE Inhibitor or ARB for LVSD[1]	4	100%	84%	82%	100%
Discharge Instructions[1,3]	6	33%	56%	61%	93%
Evaluation of LVS Function[1]	20	65%	84%	83%	99%
Smoking Cessation Advice[3]	0	-	82%	82%	100%
Pneumonia Care					
Appropriate Initial Antibiotic[1,3]	6	50%	82%	83%	94%
Blood Culture Timing[3]	0	-	89%	90%	100%
Influenza Vaccine[5]	-	-	58%	70%	100%
Initial Antibiotic Timing[1]	19	63%	75%	80%	93%
Oxygenation Assessment[1]	23	100%	99%	99%	100%
Pneumococcal Vaccine[1]	16	31%	58%	69%	94%
Smoking Cessation Advice[1,3]	1	100%	75%	80%	100%
Surgical Infection Prevention					
Prophylactic Antibiotic Given[3]	0	-	74%	77%	95%
Prophylactic Antibiotic Selection[5]	-	-	89%	90%	100%
Prophylactic Antibiotic Stopped[3]	0	-	65%	72%	95%
Pregnancy Care					
Inpatient Neonatal Mortality	590	0.00%	-	-	-
Third or Fourth Degree Laceration	408	5.15%	3.58%	3.63%	3.27%

Kingsburg District Hospital

Alternate Name: Kingsburg General Hospital
1200 Smith Street
Kingsburg, CA 93631
Phone: 559-897-5841
Fax: 559-897-8645
Ownership: Voluntary non-profit - Private
Accredited: No
Emergency Services: Yes
Licensed Beds: 35

Key Personnel:

Administrator/CEO. . . . . Doug Skubitz
Chief Medical Staff. . . . . David Hadden
Infection Control. . . . . Mary Lynn Baker
Medical/Surgical Nursing . . . . Garth Wade
Surgical Services . . . . Tom Stoeckel
Respiratory/Cardiopulmonary. . . . . Mary Lynn Baker

Measure	Cases	This Hospital	State Average	U.S. Average	Top Hospital
Heart Attack Care					
ACE Inhibitor or ARB for LVSD[5]	-	-	82%	82%	100%
Aspirin at Arrival[5]	-	-	95%	92%	100%
Aspirin at Discharge[5]	-	-	90%	90%	100%
Beta Blocker at Arrival[5]	-	-	89%	87%	100%
Beta Blocker at Discharge[5]	-	-	89%	90%	100%
Fibrinolytic Medication Timing[5]	-	-	40%	31%	100%
PCI Within 90 Minutes of Arrival[5]	-	-	52%	54%	95%
Smoking Cessation Advice[5]	-	-	87%	88%	100%
Heart Failure Care					
ACE Inhibitor or ARB for LVSD[3]	0	-	84%	82%	100%
Discharge Instructions[1,3]	3	0%	56%	61%	93%
Evaluation of LVS Function[1,3]	5	0%	84%	83%	99%
Smoking Cessation Advice[1,3]	1	100%	82%	82%	100%
Pneumonia Care					
Appropriate Initial Antibiotic[1,3]	1	0%	82%	83%	94%
Blood Culture Timing[1,3]	1	100%	89%	90%	100%
Influenza Vaccine[5]	-	-	58%	70%	100%
Initial Antibiotic Timing[1,3]	14	36%	75%	80%	93%
Oxygenation Assessment[1,3]	17	82%	99%	99%	100%
Pneumococcal Vaccine[1,3]	8	0%	58%	69%	94%
Smoking Cessation Advice[3]	0	-	75%	80%	100%
Surgical Infection Prevention					
Prophylactic Antibiotic Given[5]	-	-	74%	77%	95%
Prophylactic Antibiotic Selection[5]	-	-	89%	90%	100%
Prophylactic Antibiotic Stopped[5]	-	-	65%	72%	95%
Pregnancy Care					
Inpatient Neonatal Mortality	-	-	-	-	-
Third or Fourth Degree Laceration	-	-	3.58%	3.63%	3.27%

Scripps Green Hospital

10666 N Torrey Pines Road
La Jolla, CA 92037
Phone: 858-554-9100
Fax: 858-554-3170
URL: www.scrippshealth.org
Ownership: Voluntary non-profit - Other
Accredited: Yes
Emergency Services: No
Licensed Beds: 173

Key Personnel:

Director Radiology . . . . Linda Comfort
Supervisor Respiratory Therapy. . . . . William Holliday

Measure	Cases	This Hospital	State Average	U.S. Average	Top Hospital
Heart Attack Care					
ACE Inhibitor or ARB for LVSD[1]	22	100%	82%	82%	100%
Aspirin at Arrival	66	100%	95%	92%	100%
Aspirin at Discharge	181	99%	90%	90%	100%
Beta Blocker at Arrival	60	100%	89%	87%	100%
Beta Blocker at Discharge	167	98%	89%	90%	100%
Fibrinolytic Medication Timing	0	-	40%	31%	100%
PCI Within 90 Minutes of Arrival[1]	3	33%	52%	54%	95%
Smoking Cessation Advice	35	91%	87%	88%	100%
Heart Failure Care					
ACE Inhibitor or ARB for LVSD	107	92%	84%	82%	100%
Discharge Instructions	247	83%	56%	61%	93%
Evaluation of LVS Function	278	100%	84%	83%	99%
Smoking Cessation Advice	29	93%	82%	82%	100%
Pneumonia Care					
Appropriate Initial Antibiotic	63	94%	82%	83%	94%
Blood Culture Timing[1]	23	100%	89%	90%	100%
Influenza Vaccine	44	86%	58%	70%	100%
Initial Antibiotic Timing	88	84%	75%	80%	93%
Oxygenation Assessment	114	100%	99%	99%	100%
Pneumococcal Vaccine	126	84%	58%	69%	94%
Smoking Cessation Advice[1]	18	94%	75%	80%	100%
Surgical Infection Prevention					
Prophylactic Antibiotic Given[2,3]	259	93%	74%	77%	95%
Prophylactic Antibiotic Selection[2]	74	88%	89%	90%	100%
Prophylactic Antibiotic Stopped[2,3]	256	79%	65%	72%	95%
Pregnancy Care					
Inpatient Neonatal Mortality	-	-	-	-	-
Third or Fourth Degree Laceration	-	-	3.58%	3.63%	3.27%

Scripps Memorial Hospital La Jolla

9888 Genesee Avenue
La Jolla, CA 92037
Phone: 858-626-4123
Fax: 858-678-6900
URL: www.scrippshealth.org
Ownership: Voluntary non-profit - Private
Accredited: Yes
Emergency Services: Yes
Licensed Beds: 293

Key Personnel:

Director Infection/Disease Control . . . . Stephanie Meyers, RN
Admin. Dir. CCU . . . . Linda Hodges, RN
Director Medical/Surgical Nursing . . . . Richard Peterson, RN
Director Medical/Surgical Nursing . . . . A Brent Eastman, MD
OB/GYN Womens Health. . . . . S Demarzo

Measure	Cases	This Hospital	State Average	U.S. Average	Top Hospital
Heart Attack Care					

NOTE: Hospital profiles are in alphabetical order by state, then city, then hospital within the city; Rankings are sorted by rate in descending order and exclude hospitals with less than 25 cases; (1) The number of cases is too small (n<25) for purposes of reliably predicting hospital performance; (2) Measure reflects the hospital's indication that its submission was based upon a sample of its relevant discharges; (3) Rate reflects fewer than the maximum possible quarters of data for the measure; (4) Inaccurate information submitted and suppressed for one or more quarters; (5) No data is available from the hospital for this measure; Please refer to the User's Guide for a full explanation of data

ACE Inhibitor or ARB for LVSD[2]	49	80%	82%	82%	100%
Aspirin at Arrival[2]	101	98%	95%	92%	100%
Aspirin at Discharge[2]	286	98%	90%	90%	100%
Beta Blocker at Arrival[2]	73	99%	89%	87%	100%
Beta Blocker at Discharge[2]	280	96%	89%	90%	100%
Fibrinolytic Medication Timing[1,2]	3	67%	40%	31%	100%
PCI Within 90 Minutes of Arrival[1,2]	7	71%	52%	54%	95%
Smoking Cessation Advice[2]	71	94%	87%	88%	100%
Heart Failure Care					
ACE Inhibitor or ARB for LVSD	119	81%	84%	82%	100%
Discharge Instructions	224	58%	56%	61%	93%
Evaluation of LVS Function	270	92%	84%	83%	99%
Smoking Cessation Advice	31	97%	82%	82%	100%
Pneumonia Care					
Appropriate Initial Antibiotic[2]	91	91%	82%	83%	94%
Blood Culture Timing[2]	107	90%	89%	90%	100%
Influenza Vaccine[2]	34	53%	58%	70%	100%
Initial Antibiotic Timing[2]	140	84%	75%	80%	93%
Oxygenation Assessment[2]	176	100%	99%	99%	100%
Pneumococcal Vaccine[2]	122	54%	58%	69%	94%
Smoking Cessation Advice[2]	27	78%	75%	80%	100%
Surgical Infection Prevention					
Prophylactic Antibiotic Given[2,3]	241	93%	74%	77%	95%
Prophylactic Antibiotic Selection[2]	78	99%	89%	90%	100%
Prophylactic Antibiotic Stopped[2,3]	232	73%	65%	72%	95%
Pregnancy Care					
Inpatient Neonatal Mortality	3,806	0.05%	-	-	-
Third or Fourth Degree Laceration	2,534	6.04%	3.58%	3.63%	3.27%

Grossmont Hospital

5555 Grossmont Center Drive
La Mesa, CA 91942
Phone: 619-740-6000
Fax: 619-740-4255
URL: www.sharp.com
Ownership: Govt - Hospital District or Authority
Accredited: Yes
Emergency Services: Yes
Licensed Beds: 450

Key Personnel:

CEO. . . . . Michele T Tarbet
Chief Medical Staff. . . . . Margret Elizando
Emergency Room . . . . Kenny Davis
Emergency Room . . . . Dale Fox
OB/GYN Womens Health. . . . . Frank Goicoechea
Director Respiratory Therapy . . . . Ron Owens

Measure	Cases	This Hospital	State Average	U.S. Average	Top Hospital
Heart Attack Care					
ACE Inhibitor or ARB for LVSD	66	98%	82%	82%	100%
Aspirin at Arrival	479	97%	95%	92%	100%
Aspirin at Discharge	404	100%	90%	90%	100%
Beta Blocker at Arrival	433	95%	89%	87%	100%
Beta Blocker at Discharge	402	99%	89%	90%	100%
Fibrinolytic Medication Timing[1]	3	0%	40%	31%	100%
PCI Within 90 Minutes of Arrival	32	53%	52%	54%	95%
Smoking Cessation Advice	144	99%	87%	88%	100%
Heart Failure Care					
ACE Inhibitor or ARB for LVSD	254	89%	84%	82%	100%
Discharge Instructions	504	71%	56%	61%	93%
Evaluation of LVS Function	635	97%	84%	83%	99%
Smoking Cessation Advice	140	98%	82%	82%	100%
Pneumonia Care					
Appropriate Initial Antibiotic[2]	383	91%	82%	83%	94%
Blood Culture Timing[2]	486	84%	89%	90%	100%
Influenza Vaccine	119	27%	58%	70%	100%
Initial Antibiotic Timing[2]	603	85%	75%	80%	93%
Oxygenation Assessment[2]	686	100%	99%	99%	100%
Pneumococcal Vaccine[2]	422	47%	58%	69%	94%
Smoking Cessation Advice[2]	104	85%	75%	80%	100%
Surgical Infection Prevention					
Prophylactic Antibiotic Given[2,3]	328	83%	74%	77%	95%
Prophylactic Antibiotic Selection[2]	84	74%	89%	90%	100%
Prophylactic Antibiotic Stopped[2,3]	319	71%	65%	72%	95%
Pregnancy Care					
Inpatient Neonatal Mortality	-	-	-	-	-
Third or Fourth Degree Laceration	-	-	3.58%	3.63%	3.27%

La Palma Intercommunity Hospital

7901 Walker Street
La Palma, CA 90623
Phone: 714-670-7400
Fax: 714-670-6004
URL: www.lapalmaintercommunityhospital.com
Ownership: Proprietary
Accredited: Yes
Emergency Services: Yes
Licensed Beds: 139

Key Personnel:

President . . . . Steve Dixon
Administrator/CEO . . . . Pat Wolfram
Chief Medical Staff. . . . . S Shouikair, MD
Emergency Room . . . . H Schumaker, MD
Director Medical/Surgical Nursing . . . . Sylvia Ventura, R
Chief Radiology . . . . J Liu, MD
Director Respiratory Therapy . . . . Joe Hamai

Measure	Cases	This Hospital	State Average	U.S. Average	Top Hospital
Heart Attack Care					
ACE Inhibitor or ARB for LVSD[1]	19	63%	82%	82%	100%
Aspirin at Arrival	69	94%	95%	92%	100%
Aspirin at Discharge	33	88%	90%	90%	100%
Beta Blocker at Arrival	66	86%	89%	87%	100%
Beta Blocker at Discharge	36	83%	89%	90%	100%
Fibrinolytic Medication Timing[1]	11	73%	40%	31%	100%
PCI Within 90 Minutes of Arrival	0	-	52%	54%	95%
Smoking Cessation Advice[1]	9	100%	87%	88%	100%
Heart Failure Care					
ACE Inhibitor or ARB for LVSD	91	79%	84%	82%	100%
Discharge Instructions	170	85%	56%	61%	93%
Evaluation of LVS Function	199	82%	84%	83%	99%
Smoking Cessation Advice	31	100%	82%	82%	100%
Pneumonia Care					
Appropriate Initial Antibiotic	179	84%	82%	83%	94%
Blood Culture Timing	120	91%	89%	90%	100%
Influenza Vaccine	58	50%	58%	70%	100%
Initial Antibiotic Timing	182	68%	75%	80%	93%
Oxygenation Assessment	224	95%	99%	99%	100%
Pneumococcal Vaccine	142	61%	58%	69%	94%
Smoking Cessation Advice	39	72%	75%	80%	100%
Surgical Infection Prevention					
Prophylactic Antibiotic Given	88	85%	74%	77%	95%
Prophylactic Antibiotic Selection[1]	18	94%	89%	90%	100%
Prophylactic Antibiotic Stopped	82	70%	65%	72%	95%
Pregnancy Care					
Inpatient Neonatal Mortality	-	-	-	-	-
Third or Fourth Degree Laceration	-	-	3.58%	3.63%	3.27%

South Coast Medical Center

31872 Coast Highway
Laguna Beach, CA 92651
Phone: 949-499-1311
Fax: 949-499-8644
E-mail: info@southcoastmedcenter.com
URL: www.southcoastmedcenter.com
Ownership: Voluntary non-profit - Other
Accredited: Yes
Emergency Services: Yes

Key Personnel:

Administrator . . . . Bob Carmen
CEO. . . . . Gary Irish
Chief Medical Staff. . . . . William Anderson, MD
Emergency Room . . . . Joni Taylor, RN
Emergency Room . . . . Marc Taub, MD
Infection Control. . . . . Debbie Mulligan, RN
ICU . . . . Danyce Mills, RN
Intensive Coronary. . . . . Sonya Williams, RN
Medical Surgical Nursing . . . . Danyce Mills, RN
OB/GYN/Women's Health . . . . Donna Carney, RN
Supervisor Respiratory Therapy. . . . . Jeff Miller

Measure	Cases	This Hospital	State Average	U.S. Average	Top Hospital
Heart Attack Care					
ACE Inhibitor or ARB for LVSD[1]	4	75%	82%	82%	100%
Aspirin at Arrival	25	100%	95%	92%	100%
Aspirin at Discharge[1]	10	100%	90%	90%	100%

NOTE: Hospital profiles are in alphabetical order by state, then city, then hospital within the city; Rankings are sorted by rate in descending order and exclude hospitals with less than 25 cases; (1) The number of cases is too small (n<25) for purposes of reliably predicting hospital performance; (2) Measure reflects the hospital's indication that its submission was based upon a sample of its relevant discharges; (3) Rate reflects fewer than the maximum possible quarters of data for the measure; (4) Inaccurate information submitted and suppressed for one or more quarters; (5) No data is available from the hospital for this measure; Please refer to the User's Guide for a full explanation of data

Beta Blocker at Arrival[1]	14	93%	89%	87%	100%
Beta Blocker at Discharge[1]	11	100%	89%	90%	100%
Fibrinolytic Medication Timing[1]	1	0%	40%	31%	100%
PCI Within 90 Minutes of Arrival	0	-	52%	54%	95%
Smoking Cessation Advice[1]	1	100%	87%	88%	100%
Heart Failure Care					
ACE Inhibitor or ARB for LVSD[1]	23	87%	84%	82%	100%
Discharge Instructions	85	79%	56%	61%	93%
Evaluation of LVS Function	90	97%	84%	83%	99%
Smoking Cessation Advice[1]	10	80%	82%	82%	100%
Pneumonia Care					
Appropriate Initial Antibiotic	66	82%	82%	83%	94%
Blood Culture Timing	47	87%	89%	90%	100%
Influenza Vaccine[1]	11	64%	58%	70%	100%
Initial Antibiotic Timing	81	88%	75%	80%	93%
Oxygenation Assessment	95	100%	99%	99%	100%
Pneumococcal Vaccine	64	70%	58%	69%	94%
Smoking Cessation Advice[1]	17	65%	75%	80%	100%
Surgical Infection Prevention					
Prophylactic Antibiotic Given[2,3]	71	79%	74%	77%	95%
Prophylactic Antibiotic Selection[2]	28	89%	89%	90%	100%
Prophylactic Antibiotic Stopped[2,3]	32	69%	65%	72%	95%
Pregnancy Care					
Inpatient Neonatal Mortality	716	0.00%	-	-	-
Third or Fourth Degree Laceration	506	3.36%	3.58%	3.63%	3.27%

Saddleback Memorial Medical Center

24451 Health Center Drive
Laguna Hills, CA 92653
URL: www.memorialcare.org
Phone: 949-837-4500
Fax: 949-452-3549
Ownership: Voluntary non-profit - Private
Emergency Services: Yes
Accredited: Yes
Licensed Beds: 252

Key Personnel:

CEO. . . . . Steve Geidt
Chief Medical Staff. . . . . David Lagrew

Measure	Cases	This Hospital	State Average	U.S. Average	Top Hospital
Heart Attack Care					
ACE Inhibitor or ARB for LVSD	53	96%	82%	82%	100%
Aspirin at Arrival	283	95%	95%	92%	100%
Aspirin at Discharge	256	96%	90%	90%	100%
Beta Blocker at Arrival	169	93%	89%	87%	100%
Beta Blocker at Discharge	258	97%	89%	90%	100%
Fibrinolytic Medication Timing[1]	5	40%	40%	31%	100%
PCI Within 90 Minutes of Arrival[1]	13	46%	52%	54%	95%
Smoking Cessation Advice	53	100%	87%	88%	100%
Heart Failure Care					
ACE Inhibitor or ARB for LVSD	219	94%	84%	82%	100%
Discharge Instructions	523	82%	56%	61%	93%
Evaluation of LVS Function	642	96%	84%	83%	99%
Smoking Cessation Advice	55	96%	82%	82%	100%
Pneumonia Care					
Appropriate Initial Antibiotic	328	90%	82%	83%	94%
Blood Culture Timing	348	95%	89%	90%	100%
Influenza Vaccine	113	92%	58%	70%	100%
Initial Antibiotic Timing	429	90%	75%	80%	93%
Oxygenation Assessment	539	100%	99%	99%	100%
Pneumococcal Vaccine	447	84%	58%	69%	94%
Smoking Cessation Advice	58	97%	75%	80%	100%
Surgical Infection Prevention					
Prophylactic Antibiotic Given[2,3]	416	90%	74%	77%	95%
Prophylactic Antibiotic Selection[2]	104	93%	89%	90%	100%
Prophylactic Antibiotic Stopped[2,3]	404	75%	65%	72%	95%
Pregnancy Care					
Inpatient Neonatal Mortality	2,890	0.21%	-	-	-
Third or Fourth Degree Laceration	1,955	3.73%	3.58%	3.63%	3.27%

Mountains Community Hospital

29101 Hospital Road
PO Box 70
Lake Arrowhead, CA 92352
URL: www.mchcares.com
Phone: 909-336-3651
Fax: 909-336-1179
Ownership: Govt - Hospital District or Authority
Emergency Services: Yes
Accredited: Yes
Licensed Beds: 35

Key Personnel:

Executive Director . . . . Jim Hoss
Emergency Department Manager . . . . Terri Montgomery
Infection Control Manager . . . . Terri Montgomery
Med/Surg Manager . . . . Sarah D'Antonio
Surgery Department Manager . . . . Terri Montgomery, RN
Respiratory Department Manager . . . . Charlie Anderson

Measure	Cases	This Hospital	State Average	U.S. Average	Top Hospital
Heart Attack Care					
ACE Inhibitor or ARB for LVSD[5]	-	-	82%	82%	100%
Aspirin at Arrival[5]	-	-	95%	92%	100%
Aspirin at Discharge[5]	-	-	90%	90%	100%
Beta Blocker at Arrival[5]	-	-	89%	87%	100%
Beta Blocker at Discharge[5]	-	-	89%	90%	100%
Fibrinolytic Medication Timing[5]	-	-	40%	31%	100%
PCI Within 90 Minutes of Arrival[5]	-	-	52%	54%	95%
Smoking Cessation Advice[5]	-	-	87%	88%	100%
Heart Failure Care					
ACE Inhibitor or ARB for LVSD[5]	-	-	84%	82%	100%
Discharge Instructions[5]	-	-	56%	61%	93%
Evaluation of LVS Function[5]	-	-	84%	83%	99%
Smoking Cessation Advice[5]	-	-	82%	82%	100%
Pneumonia Care					
Appropriate Initial Antibiotic[5]	-	-	82%	83%	94%
Blood Culture Timing[5]	-	-	89%	90%	100%
Influenza Vaccine[5]	-	-	58%	70%	100%
Initial Antibiotic Timing[5]	-	-	75%	80%	93%
Oxygenation Assessment[5]	-	-	99%	99%	100%
Pneumococcal Vaccine[5]	-	-	58%	69%	94%
Smoking Cessation Advice[5]	-	-	75%	80%	100%
Surgical Infection Prevention					
Prophylactic Antibiotic Given[5]	-	-	74%	77%	95%
Prophylactic Antibiotic Selection[5]	-	-	89%	90%	100%
Prophylactic Antibiotic Stopped[5]	-	-	65%	72%	95%
Pregnancy Care					
Inpatient Neonatal Mortality	-	-	-	-	-
Third or Fourth Degree Laceration	-	-	3.58%	3.63%	3.27%

Kern Valley Healthcare District

Alternate Name: Kern Valley Hospital District
6412 Laurel Avenue
PO Box 1628
Lake Isabella, CA 93240
E-mail: MicheleRosato@kvhd.org
URL: www.kvhd.org
Phone: 760-379-2681
Fax: 760-379-0066
Ownership: Govt - Hospital District or Authority
Emergency Services: Yes
Accredited: No
Licensed Beds: 101

Key Personnel:

CEO. . . . . Pamela Ott
Chief Medical Staff. . . . . Gary Finstad, MD
Director Infection/Disease Control . . . . Carol Bradshaw
Chief Radiology . . . . Eleanor Fraser, MD
Director Respiratory Therapy . . . . Tom Wright

Measure	Cases	This Hospital	State Average	U.S. Average	Top Hospital
Heart Attack Care					
ACE Inhibitor or ARB for LVSD[5]	-	-	82%	82%	100%
Aspirin at Arrival[5]	-	-	95%	92%	100%
Aspirin at Discharge[5]	-	-	90%	90%	100%
Beta Blocker at Arrival[5]	-	-	89%	87%	100%
Beta Blocker at Discharge[5]	-	-	89%	90%	100%
Fibrinolytic Medication Timing[5]	-	-	40%	31%	100%
PCI Within 90 Minutes of Arrival[5]	-	-	52%	54%	95%
Smoking Cessation Advice[5]	-	-	87%	88%	100%
Heart Failure Care					

NOTE: Hospital profiles are in alphabetical order by state, then city, then hospital within the city; Rankings are sorted by rate in descending order and exclude hospitals with less than 25 cases; (1) The number of cases is too small (n<25) for purposes of reliably predicting hospital performance; (2) Measure reflects the hospital's indication that its submission was based upon a sample of its relevant discharges; (3) Rate reflects fewer than the maximum possible quarters of data for the measure; (4) Inaccurate information submitted and suppressed for one or more quarters; (5) No data is available from the hospital for this measure; Please refer to the User's Guide for a full explanation of data

Measure	Cases	This Hospital	State Average	U.S. Average	Top Hospital
ACE Inhibitor or ARB for LVSD[5]	-	-	84%	82%	100%
Discharge Instructions[5]	-	-	56%	61%	93%
Evaluation of LVS Function[5]	-	-	84%	83%	99%
Smoking Cessation Advice[5]	-	-	82%	82%	100%
Pneumonia Care					
Appropriate Initial Antibiotic[1,2,3]	20	100%	82%	83%	94%
Blood Culture Timing[2,3]	32	78%	89%	90%	100%
Influenza Vaccine[5]	-	-	58%	70%	100%
Initial Antibiotic Timing[2,3]	30	77%	75%	80%	93%
Oxygenation Assessment[2,3]	34	100%	99%	99%	100%
Pneumococcal Vaccine[2,3]	25	68%	58%	69%	94%
Smoking Cessation Advice[1,2,3]	6	33%	75%	80%	100%
Surgical Infection Prevention					
Prophylactic Antibiotic Given[5]	-	-	74%	77%	95%
Prophylactic Antibiotic Selection[5]	-	-	89%	90%	100%
Prophylactic Antibiotic Stopped[5]	-	-	65%	72%	95%
Pregnancy Care					
Inpatient Neonatal Mortality	-	-	-	-	-
Third or Fourth Degree Laceration	-	-	3.58%	3.63%	3.27%

Sutter Lakeside Hospital

5176 Hill Road E
Lakeport, CA 95453
URL: www.sutterlake.org
Ownership: Voluntary non-profit - Other
Emergency Services: Yes

Phone: 707-262-5000
Fax: 707-262-5003
Accredited: Yes
Licensed Beds: 53

Key Personnel:

CEO . . . . Kelly Mather
CNO . . . . Cherie Hensley
Emergency Room . . . . John Gorbenko, RN
Infection Control . . . . Susan Meyers, RN
Director of Cardiopulmonary Rehab . . . . Dennis Stanley

Measure	Cases	This Hospital	State Average	U.S. Average	Top Hospital
Heart Attack Care					
ACE Inhibitor or ARB for LVSD[1]	2	100%	82%	82%	100%
Aspirin at Arrival[1]	19	95%	95%	92%	100%
Aspirin at Discharge[1]	9	89%	90%	90%	100%
Beta Blocker at Arrival[1]	18	89%	89%	87%	100%
Beta Blocker at Discharge[1]	8	88%	89%	90%	100%
Fibrinolytic Medication Timing[1]	2	0%	40%	31%	100%
PCI Within 90 Minutes of Arrival	0	-	52%	54%	95%
Smoking Cessation Advice[1]	3	67%	87%	88%	100%
Heart Failure Care					
ACE Inhibitor or ARB for LVSD[1]	15	80%	84%	82%	100%
Discharge Instructions	31	81%	56%	61%	93%
Evaluation of LVS Function	39	95%	84%	83%	99%
Smoking Cessation Advice[1]	11	73%	82%	82%	100%
Pneumonia Care					
Appropriate Initial Antibiotic	100	76%	82%	83%	94%
Blood Culture Timing	61	93%	89%	90%	100%
Influenza Vaccine[4,5]	-	-	58%	70%	100%
Initial Antibiotic Timing	107	82%	75%	80%	93%
Oxygenation Assessment	131	99%	99%	99%	100%
Pneumococcal Vaccine	89	39%	58%	69%	94%
Smoking Cessation Advice	27	78%	75%	80%	100%
Surgical Infection Prevention					
Prophylactic Antibiotic Given[2]	189	58%	74%	77%	95%
Prophylactic Antibiotic Selection[2]	53	94%	89%	90%	100%
Prophylactic Antibiotic Stopped[2]	182	64%	65%	72%	95%
Pregnancy Care					
Inpatient Neonatal Mortality	-	-	-	-	-
Third or Fourth Degree Laceration	-	-	3.58%	3.63%	3.27%

Lakewood Regional Medical Center

3700 East South Street
Lakewood, CA 90712
URL: www.lakewoodregional.com
Ownership: Proprietary
Emergency Services: Yes

Phone: 562-531-2550
Fax: 562-602-0083
Accredited: Yes
Licensed Beds: 161

Key Personnel:

CEO . . . . Michael Hunn
Chief of Medical Staff . . . . Carl Hartman, MD
Cardiac Lab Chair . . . . Miguel Sanmarco, MD
Infection Control Chair . . . . Stuart Finklestein, MD
Chair Coronary Care Committee . . . . Joel Epstien, MD

Measure	Cases	This Hospital	State Average	U.S. Average	Top Hospital
Heart Attack Care					
ACE Inhibitor or ARB for LVSD	31	97%	82%	82%	100%
Aspirin at Arrival	140	100%	95%	92%	100%
Aspirin at Discharge	171	95%	90%	90%	100%
Beta Blocker at Arrival	120	97%	89%	87%	100%
Beta Blocker at Discharge	165	97%	89%	90%	100%
Fibrinolytic Medication Timing[1]	9	22%	40%	31%	100%
PCI Within 90 Minutes of Arrival[1]	7	29%	52%	54%	95%
Smoking Cessation Advice	47	98%	87%	88%	100%
Heart Failure Care					
ACE Inhibitor or ARB for LVSD	146	96%	84%	82%	100%
Discharge Instructions	405	76%	56%	61%	93%
Evaluation of LVS Function	492	93%	84%	83%	99%
Smoking Cessation Advice	64	91%	82%	82%	100%
Pneumonia Care					
Appropriate Initial Antibiotic	168	86%	82%	83%	94%
Blood Culture Timing	134	90%	89%	90%	100%
Influenza Vaccine	46	63%	58%	70%	100%
Initial Antibiotic Timing	199	85%	75%	80%	93%
Oxygenation Assessment	247	100%	99%	99%	100%
Pneumococcal Vaccine	168	85%	58%	69%	94%
Smoking Cessation Advice	49	90%	75%	80%	100%
Surgical Infection Prevention					
Prophylactic Antibiotic Given[2]	362	80%	74%	77%	95%
Prophylactic Antibiotic Selection[2]	74	93%	89%	90%	100%
Prophylactic Antibiotic Stopped[2]	341	60%	65%	72%	95%
Pregnancy Care					
Inpatient Neonatal Mortality	-	-	-	-	-
Third or Fourth Degree Laceration	-	-	3.58%	3.63%	3.27%

Antelope Valley Hospital

1600 West Avenue J
Lancaster, CA 93534
URL: www.avhospital.org
Ownership: Govt - Hospital District or Authority
Emergency Services: Yes

Phone: 661-949-5000
Accredited: Yes
Licensed Beds: 378

Key Personnel:

CEO . . . . Les Wong
Emergency Room . . . . Linda Lawson
Emergency Room . . . . John Lynn, MD
ICU . . . . Brenda Burns
Intensive/Coronary Care . . . . Brenda Burns
OB/GYN Womens Health . . . . Bonnie Daniel

Measure	Cases	This Hospital	State Average	U.S. Average	Top Hospital
Heart Attack Care					
ACE Inhibitor or ARB for LVSD	56	80%	82%	82%	100%
Aspirin at Arrival	301	97%	95%	92%	100%
Aspirin at Discharge	282	93%	90%	90%	100%
Beta Blocker at Arrival	248	90%	89%	87%	100%
Beta Blocker at Discharge	280	87%	89%	90%	100%
Fibrinolytic Medication Timing[1]	4	75%	40%	31%	100%
PCI Within 90 Minutes of Arrival[1]	21	90%	52%	54%	95%
Smoking Cessation Advice	123	95%	87%	88%	100%
Heart Failure Care					
ACE Inhibitor or ARB for LVSD	224	64%	84%	82%	100%
Discharge Instructions	472	45%	56%	61%	93%
Evaluation of LVS Function	523	87%	84%	83%	99%
Smoking Cessation Advice	150	91%	82%	82%	100%
Pneumonia Care					
Appropriate Initial Antibiotic	340	94%	82%	83%	94%
Blood Culture Timing	276	66%	89%	90%	100%
Influenza Vaccine[4,5]	-	-	58%	70%	100%
Initial Antibiotic Timing	476	80%	75%	80%	93%
Oxygenation Assessment	539	100%	99%	99%	100%
Pneumococcal Vaccine	263	67%	58%	69%	94%
Smoking Cessation Advice	149	82%	75%	80%	100%

NOTE: Hospital profiles are in alphabetical order by state, then city, then hospital within the city; Rankings are sorted by rate in descending order and exclude hospitals with less than 25 cases; (1) The number of cases is too small (n<25) for purposes of reliably predicting hospital performance; (2) Measure reflects the hospital's indication that its submission was based upon a sample of its relevant discharges; (3) Rate reflects fewer than the maximum possible quarters of data for the measure; (4) Inaccurate information submitted and suppressed for one or more quarters; (5) No data is available from the hospital for this measure; Please refer to the User's Guide for a full explanation of data

Surgical Infection Prevention					
Prophylactic Antibiotic Given[3]	413	45%	74%	77%	95%
Prophylactic Antibiotic Selection	134	91%	89%	90%	100%
Prophylactic Antibiotic Stopped[3]	347	67%	65%	72%	95%
Pregnancy Care					
Inpatient Neonatal Mortality	-	-	-	-	-
Third or Fourth Degree Laceration	-	-	3.58%	3.63%	3.27%

Lancaster Community Hospital

43830 N Tenth Street W — Phone: 661-948-4781
Lancaster, CA 93534 — Fax: 661-949-9783
URL: www.lancastercommunityhospital.net
Ownership: Proprietary — Accredited: Yes
Emergency Services: Yes — Licensed Beds: 117

Key Personnel:

CEO . . . . . Robert J Trautman
Chief Medical Staff . . . . . P Damle, MD
Director of Cardiology/Cardiac Lab . . . . . Jim Guton
Emergency Room . . . . . Shona Smart
Director Medical/Surgical Nursing . . . . . Lyn DiBernardo
CNO . . . . . Jusya White
Chief Radiology . . . . . Sam Moses, MD
Director of Pulmonary/Respiratory Care . . . . . Glenn Dabatos

Measure	Cases	This Hospital	State Average	U.S. Average	Top Hospital
Heart Attack Care					
ACE Inhibitor or ARB for LVSD	34	88%	82%	82%	100%
Aspirin at Arrival	129	92%	95%	92%	100%
Aspirin at Discharge	112	83%	90%	90%	100%
Beta Blocker at Arrival	122	81%	89%	87%	100%
Beta Blocker at Discharge	123	80%	89%	90%	100%
Fibrinolytic Medication Timing	0	-	40%	31%	100%
PCI Within 90 Minutes of Arrival[1]	4	75%	52%	54%	95%
Smoking Cessation Advice	37	97%	87%	88%	100%
Heart Failure Care					
ACE Inhibitor or ARB for LVSD	105	77%	84%	82%	100%
Discharge Instructions	282	11%	56%	61%	93%
Evaluation of LVS Function	321	72%	84%	83%	99%
Smoking Cessation Advice	58	74%	82%	82%	100%
Pneumonia Care					
Appropriate Initial Antibiotic	163	90%	82%	83%	94%
Blood Culture Timing	96	75%	89%	90%	100%
Influenza Vaccine	41	34%	58%	70%	100%
Initial Antibiotic Timing	159	63%	75%	80%	93%
Oxygenation Assessment	222	99%	99%	99%	100%
Pneumococcal Vaccine	121	46%	58%	69%	94%
Smoking Cessation Advice	60	63%	75%	80%	100%
Surgical Infection Prevention					
Prophylactic Antibiotic Given	371	76%	74%	77%	95%
Prophylactic Antibiotic Selection	110	88%	89%	90%	100%
Prophylactic Antibiotic Stopped	360	50%	65%	72%	95%
Pregnancy Care					
Inpatient Neonatal Mortality	-	-	-	-	-
Third or Fourth Degree Laceration	-	-	3.58%	3.63%	3.27%

Valleycare Medical Center

1111 East Stanley Blvd — Phone: 925-447-7000
Livermore, CA 94550
Ownership: Voluntary non-profit - Private — Accredited: Yes
Emergency Services: Yes

Key Personnel:

Chief of Medical Staff . . . . . Michael Alper, MD

Measure	Cases	This Hospital	State Average	U.S. Average	Top Hospital
Heart Attack Care					
ACE Inhibitor or ARB for LVSD[1]	6	83%	82%	82%	100%
Aspirin at Arrival	126	98%	95%	92%	100%
Aspirin at Discharge	94	95%	90%	90%	100%
Beta Blocker at Arrival	112	96%	89%	87%	100%
Beta Blocker at Discharge	97	97%	89%	90%	100%
Fibrinolytic Medication Timing	0	-	40%	31%	100%
PCI Within 90 Minutes of Arrival[1]	6	83%	52%	54%	95%
Smoking Cessation Advice[1]	18	94%	87%	88%	100%
Heart Failure Care					
ACE Inhibitor or ARB for LVSD	66	86%	84%	82%	100%
Discharge Instructions	158	58%	56%	61%	93%
Evaluation of LVS Function	202	84%	84%	83%	99%
Smoking Cessation Advice[1]	23	83%	82%	82%	100%
Pneumonia Care					
Appropriate Initial Antibiotic	141	81%	82%	83%	94%
Blood Culture Timing	124	91%	89%	90%	100%
Influenza Vaccine	43	79%	58%	70%	100%
Initial Antibiotic Timing	195	82%	75%	80%	93%
Oxygenation Assessment	220	100%	99%	99%	100%
Pneumococcal Vaccine	129	90%	58%	69%	94%
Smoking Cessation Advice	30	30%	75%	80%	100%
Surgical Infection Prevention					
Prophylactic Antibiotic Given[3]	292	87%	74%	77%	95%
Prophylactic Antibiotic Selection	110	97%	89%	90%	100%
Prophylactic Antibiotic Stopped[3]	279	62%	65%	72%	95%
Pregnancy Care					
Inpatient Neonatal Mortality	-	-	-	-	-
Third or Fourth Degree Laceration	-	-	3.58%	3.63%	3.27%

Lodi Memorial Hospital

Alternate Name: Community Hospital of Lodi
975 S Fairmont Avenue — Toll-Free: 800-323-3360
Lodi, CA 95240 — Phone: 209-334-3411
Fax: 209-368-3745
URL: www.lodihealth.org
Ownership: Voluntary non-profit - Other — Accredited: Yes
Emergency Services: Yes — Licensed Beds: 181

Key Personnel:

President/CEO . . . . . Joseph Harrington
Chief Medical Staff . . . . . Mary Brown, MD
Director Cardiology . . . . . Willis Marvolf
Emergency Room . . . . . Kelly Stunt
Director Medical/Surgical Nursing . . . . . Lynn McCarty
OB/GYN Womens Health . . . . . Leslie Sackschewsky, MD
Director Respiratory Therapy . . . . . Michael Mericle

Measure	Cases	This Hospital	State Average	U.S. Average	Top Hospital
Heart Attack Care					
ACE Inhibitor or ARB for LVSD[1]	13	77%	82%	82%	100%
Aspirin at Arrival	80	98%	95%	92%	100%
Aspirin at Discharge	32	100%	90%	90%	100%
Beta Blocker at Arrival	55	98%	89%	87%	100%
Beta Blocker at Discharge	35	94%	89%	90%	100%
Fibrinolytic Medication Timing[1]	20	70%	40%	31%	100%
PCI Within 90 Minutes of Arrival	0	-	52%	54%	95%
Smoking Cessation Advice[1]	9	78%	87%	88%	100%
Heart Failure Care					
ACE Inhibitor or ARB for LVSD[2]	55	71%	84%	82%	100%
Discharge Instructions[2]	139	59%	56%	61%	93%
Evaluation of LVS Function[2]	193	84%	84%	83%	99%
Smoking Cessation Advice[2]	38	92%	82%	82%	100%
Pneumonia Care					
Appropriate Initial Antibiotic[2]	77	91%	82%	83%	94%
Blood Culture Timing[2]	77	90%	89%	90%	100%
Influenza Vaccine[1,2]	24	75%	58%	70%	100%
Initial Antibiotic Timing[2]	123	69%	75%	80%	93%
Oxygenation Assessment[2]	158	100%	99%	99%	100%
Pneumococcal Vaccine[2]	109	71%	58%	69%	94%
Smoking Cessation Advice[2]	33	82%	75%	80%	100%
Surgical Infection Prevention					
Prophylactic Antibiotic Given[2]	214	73%	74%	77%	95%
Prophylactic Antibiotic Selection[2]	52	85%	89%	90%	100%
Prophylactic Antibiotic Stopped[2]	202	35%	65%	72%	95%
Pregnancy Care					
Inpatient Neonatal Mortality	-	-	-	-	-
Third or Fourth Degree Laceration	-	-	3.58%	3.63%	3.27%

NOTE: Hospital profiles are in alphabetical order by state, then city, then hospital within the city; Rankings are sorted by rate in descending order and exclude hospitals with less than 25 cases; (1) The number of cases is too small (n<25) for purposes of reliably predicting hospital performance; (2) Measure reflects the hospital's indication that its submission was based upon a sample of its relevant discharges; (3) Rate reflects fewer than the maximum possible quarters of data for the measure; (4) Inaccurate information submitted and suppressed for one or more quarters; (5) No data is available from the hospital for this measure; Please refer to the User's Guide for a full explanation of data

Loma Linda University Medical Center

11234 Anderson Street
Loma Linda, CA 92354
Toll-Free: 800-558-6297
Phone: 909-558-4000
Fax: 909-558-4058

URL: www.llumc.edu
Ownership: Voluntary non-profit - Church
Accredited: Yes
Emergency Services: Yes
Licensed Beds: 724

Key Personnel:

CEO/Administrator . . . . . Ruthita J Fike, MA
Administration Director/Emergency Room . . . . . Connie Cunningham
ICU . . . . . Helen Jenks
Medical Surgical Nursing . . . . . Jan Kroetz
Administrative Director/Radiology . . . . . Brenda Holden
Director Respiratory Care . . . . . Randy Scott

Measure	Cases	This Hospital	State Average	U.S. Average	Top Hospital
Heart Attack Care					
ACE Inhibitor or ARB for LVSD	80	84%	82%	82%	100%
Aspirin at Arrival	123	99%	95%	92%	100%
Aspirin at Discharge	298	99%	90%	90%	100%
Beta Blocker at Arrival	98	95%	89%	87%	100%
Beta Blocker at Discharge	293	99%	89%	90%	100%
Fibrinolytic Medication Timing[1]	1	100%	40%	31%	100%
PCI Within 90 Minutes of Arrival[1]	5	20%	52%	54%	95%
Smoking Cessation Advice	108	98%	87%	88%	100%
Heart Failure Care					
ACE Inhibitor or ARB for LVSD	261	92%	84%	82%	100%
Discharge Instructions	388	31%	56%	61%	93%
Evaluation of LVS Function	434	97%	84%	83%	99%
Smoking Cessation Advice	62	87%	82%	82%	100%
Pneumonia Care					
Appropriate Initial Antibiotic	145	72%	82%	83%	94%
Blood Culture Timing	166	92%	89%	90%	100%
Influenza Vaccine	47	55%	58%	70%	100%
Initial Antibiotic Timing	269	49%	75%	80%	93%
Oxygenation Assessment	354	100%	99%	99%	100%
Pneumococcal Vaccine	159	36%	58%	69%	94%
Smoking Cessation Advice	39	67%	75%	80%	100%
Surgical Infection Prevention					
Prophylactic Antibiotic Given	1,147	91%	74%	77%	95%
Prophylactic Antibiotic Selection	343	98%	89%	90%	100%
Prophylactic Antibiotic Stopped	1,070	52%	65%	72%	95%
Pregnancy Care					
Inpatient Neonatal Mortality	-	-	-	-	-
Third or Fourth Degree Laceration	-	-	3.58%	3.63%	3.27%

Lompoc Healthcare District Hospital

508 East Hickory
Lompoc, CA 93436
Phone: 805-737-3300
Fax: 805-735-8591
E-mail: webmaster@lompochospital.org
URL: lompochospital.org
Ownership: Govt - Hospital District or Authority
Accredited: Yes
Emergency Services: Yes
Licensed Beds: 170

Key Personnel:

CEO . . . . . Jim Raggio
Chief Medical Staff . . . . . Rollin Bailey, MD
Director of Cardiology/Cardiac Lab . . . . . Larry Coughlin
Emergency Room . . . . . David Tusenkin
Emergency Room . . . . . Glenn Wollman, MD
Director Medical/Surgical Nursing . . . . . Erika Hirsch
OB/GYN Womens Health . . . . . Rodney Huss, MD
Director Respiratory Therapy . . . . . Mark Hadley

Measure	Cases	This Hospital	State Average	U.S. Average	Top Hospital
Heart Attack Care					
ACE Inhibitor or ARB for LVSD[1]	3	100%	82%	82%	100%
Aspirin at Arrival[1]	4	100%	95%	92%	100%
Aspirin at Discharge[1]	2	100%	90%	90%	100%
Beta Blocker at Arrival[1]	1	0%	89%	87%	100%
Beta Blocker at Discharge[1]	3	67%	89%	90%	100%
Fibrinolytic Medication Timing	0	-	40%	31%	100%
PCI Within 90 Minutes of Arrival	0	-	52%	54%	95%
Smoking Cessation Advice[1]	1	100%	87%	88%	100%
Heart Failure Care					
ACE Inhibitor or ARB for LVSD[2]	29	97%	84%	82%	100%
Discharge Instructions[2]	49	69%	56%	61%	93%
Evaluation of LVS Function[2]	58	88%	84%	83%	99%
Smoking Cessation Advice[1,2]	13	77%	82%	82%	100%
Pneumonia Care					
Appropriate Initial Antibiotic	63	92%	82%	83%	94%
Blood Culture Timing	43	95%	89%	90%	100%
Influenza Vaccine[1]	14	7%	58%	70%	100%
Initial Antibiotic Timing	82	85%	75%	80%	93%
Oxygenation Assessment	94	100%	99%	99%	100%
Pneumococcal Vaccine	52	13%	58%	69%	94%
Smoking Cessation Advice[1]	22	50%	75%	80%	100%
Surgical Infection Prevention					
Prophylactic Antibiotic Given[2]	142	75%	74%	77%	95%
Prophylactic Antibiotic Selection[2]	35	89%	89%	90%	100%
Prophylactic Antibiotic Stopped[2]	142	68%	65%	72%	95%
Pregnancy Care					
Inpatient Neonatal Mortality	473	0.00%	-	-	-
Third or Fourth Degree Laceration	341	3.23%	3.58%	3.63%	3.27%

Southern Inyo Healthcare District

Alternate Name: Southern Inyo Hospital
501 E Locust Street
PO Box 1009
Lone Pine, CA 93545
Phone: 760-876-5501
Fax: 760-876-4388
URL: www.sihd.org
Ownership: Govt - Hospital District or Authority
Accredited: No
Emergency Services: Yes
Licensed Beds: 37

Key Personnel:

Administrator/CEO . . . . . Lee Barron
Chief Medical Staff . . . . . Michael Dillon, MD
Emergency Room . . . . . Sandy Manning
Head of Radiology . . . . . Sharon Cumming

Measure	Cases	This Hospital	State Average	U.S. Average	Top Hospital
Heart Attack Care					
ACE Inhibitor or ARB for LVSD[5]	-	-	82%	82%	100%
Aspirin at Arrival[5]	-	-	95%	92%	100%
Aspirin at Discharge[5]	-	-	90%	90%	100%
Beta Blocker at Arrival[5]	-	-	89%	87%	100%
Beta Blocker at Discharge[5]	-	-	89%	90%	100%
Fibrinolytic Medication Timing[5]	-	-	40%	31%	100%
PCI Within 90 Minutes of Arrival[5]	-	-	52%	54%	95%
Smoking Cessation Advice[5]	-	-	87%	88%	100%
Heart Failure Care					
ACE Inhibitor or ARB for LVSD[5]	-	-	84%	82%	100%
Discharge Instructions[5]	-	-	56%	61%	93%
Evaluation of LVS Function[5]	-	-	84%	83%	99%
Smoking Cessation Advice[5]	-	-	82%	82%	100%
Pneumonia Care					
Appropriate Initial Antibiotic[5]	-	-	82%	83%	94%
Blood Culture Timing[5]	-	-	89%	90%	100%
Influenza Vaccine[5]	-	-	58%	70%	100%
Initial Antibiotic Timing[5]	-	-	75%	80%	93%
Oxygenation Assessment[5]	-	-	99%	99%	100%
Pneumococcal Vaccine[5]	-	-	58%	69%	94%
Smoking Cessation Advice[5]	-	-	75%	80%	100%
Surgical Infection Prevention					
Prophylactic Antibiotic Given[5]	-	-	74%	77%	95%
Prophylactic Antibiotic Selection[5]	-	-	89%	90%	100%
Prophylactic Antibiotic Stopped[5]	-	-	65%	72%	95%
Pregnancy Care					
Inpatient Neonatal Mortality	-	-	-	-	-
Third or Fourth Degree Laceration	-	-	3.58%	3.63%	3.27%

NOTE: Hospital profiles are in alphabetical order by state, then city, then hospital within the city; Rankings are sorted by rate in descending order and exclude hospitals with less than 25 cases; (1) The number of cases is too small (n<25) for purposes of reliably predicting hospital performance; (2) Measure reflects the hospital's indication that its submission was based upon a sample of its relevant discharges; (3) Rate reflects fewer than the maximum possible quarters of data for the measure; (4) Inaccurate information submitted and suppressed for one or more quarters; (5) No data is available from the hospital for this measure; Please refer to the User's Guide for a full explanation of data

Community Hospital of Long Beach

1720 Termino Avenue
Long Beach, CA 90804
URL: www.chlb.org
Ownership: Voluntary non-profit - Private
Emergency Services: Yes

Phone: 562-498-1000
Fax: 562-498-4434
Accredited: Yes
Licensed Beds: 256

Key Personnel:

President/CEO . . . . Raymond M Jankowski, MD
Chief Medical Staff . . . . Andrew Manos, DO
Catheterization Lab . . . . Vicki Kral
Emergency Room . . . . Barbara Neel, RN
Infection Control . . . . Bill Reeder
ICU . . . . Barbara Neel, RN
Medical/Surgical Nursing . . . . Linda Basile, RN
Respiratory/Cardiopulmonary . . . . Josie Obligacion

Measure	Cases	This Hospital	State Average	U.S. Average	Top Hospital
Heart Attack Care					
ACE Inhibitor or ARB for LVSD[1]	2	50%	82%	82%	100%
Aspirin at Arrival	39	95%	95%	92%	100%
Aspirin at Discharge[1]	17	76%	90%	90%	100%
Beta Blocker at Arrival[1]	24	83%	89%	87%	100%
Beta Blocker at Discharge[1]	16	81%	89%	90%	100%
Fibrinolytic Medication Timing[1]	14	36%	40%	31%	100%
PCI Within 90 Minutes of Arrival	0	-	52%	54%	95%
Smoking Cessation Advice[1]	4	75%	87%	88%	100%
Heart Failure Care					
ACE Inhibitor or ARB for LVSD	34	76%	84%	82%	100%
Discharge Instructions	56	64%	56%	61%	93%
Evaluation of LVS Function	78	91%	84%	83%	99%
Smoking Cessation Advice[1]	18	78%	82%	82%	100%
Pneumonia Care					
Appropriate Initial Antibiotic	107	79%	82%	83%	94%
Blood Culture Timing	126	98%	89%	90%	100%
Influenza Vaccine	34	9%	58%	70%	100%
Initial Antibiotic Timing	175	87%	75%	80%	93%
Oxygenation Assessment	226	100%	99%	99%	100%
Pneumococcal Vaccine	130	29%	58%	69%	94%
Smoking Cessation Advice	27	74%	75%	80%	100%
Surgical Infection Prevention					
Prophylactic Antibiotic Given	32	75%	74%	77%	95%
Prophylactic Antibiotic Selection[1]	4	100%	89%	90%	100%
Prophylactic Antibiotic Stopped	30	37%	65%	72%	95%
Pregnancy Care					
Inpatient Neonatal Mortality	-	-	-	-	-
Third or Fourth Degree Laceration	-	-	3.58%	3.63%	3.27%

Long Beach Memorial Medical Center

2801 Atlantic Avenue
Long Beach, CA 90806
URL: www.memorialcare.com/long_beach
Ownership: Voluntary non-profit - Other
Emergency Services: Yes

Phone: 562-933-2000
Fax: 562-933-1299
Accredited: Yes
Licensed Beds: 816

Key Personnel:

CEO . . . . Byron F Schweigert
Chief Medical Staff . . . . Barry Zamost, MD
Chief Catheterization Laboratory . . . . Clyde Smith, MD
Emergency Room . . . . Daniel Whitcraft, MD
Director Infection/Disease Control . . . . Harriett Pitt
Director Medical/Surgical Nursing . . . . Jane Rutherfer, RN
OB/GYN Womens Health . . . . Barbara Schwartz, MD
Chief Radiology . . . . Paul Berger, MD
Director Respiratory Therapy . . . . David Calder

Measure	Cases	This Hospital	State Average	U.S. Average	Top Hospital
Heart Attack Care					
ACE Inhibitor or ARB for LVSD	60	97%	82%	82%	100%
Aspirin at Arrival	292	99%	95%	92%	100%
Aspirin at Discharge	310	99%	90%	90%	100%
Beta Blocker at Arrival	235	96%	89%	87%	100%
Beta Blocker at Discharge	309	97%	89%	90%	100%
Fibrinolytic Medication Timing	0	-	40%	31%	100%
PCI Within 90 Minutes of Arrival[1]	5	40%	52%	54%	95%
Smoking Cessation Advice	87	100%	87%	88%	100%
Heart Failure Care					
ACE Inhibitor or ARB for LVSD	330	84%	84%	82%	100%
Discharge Instructions	599	81%	56%	61%	93%
Evaluation of LVS Function	717	92%	84%	83%	99%
Smoking Cessation Advice	119	84%	82%	82%	100%
Pneumonia Care					
Appropriate Initial Antibiotic	287	86%	82%	83%	94%
Blood Culture Timing	399	92%	89%	90%	100%
Influenza Vaccine	118	30%	58%	70%	100%
Initial Antibiotic Timing	485	75%	75%	80%	93%
Oxygenation Assessment	619	100%	99%	99%	100%
Pneumococcal Vaccine	373	60%	58%	69%	94%
Smoking Cessation Advice	105	95%	75%	80%	100%
Surgical Infection Prevention					
Prophylactic Antibiotic Given[2,3]	332	70%	74%	77%	95%
Prophylactic Antibiotic Selection[2]	92	74%	89%	90%	100%
Prophylactic Antibiotic Stopped[2,3]	316	67%	65%	72%	95%
Pregnancy Care					
Inpatient Neonatal Mortality	-	-	-	-	-
Third or Fourth Degree Laceration	-	-	3.58%	3.63%	3.27%

Pacific Hospital of Long Beach

2776 Pacific Avenue
Long Beach, CA 90806
URL: www.phlb.org
Ownership: Voluntary non-profit - Private
Emergency Services: Yes

Phone: 562-997-2000
Fax: 562-492-1363
Accredited: Yes
Licensed Beds: 184

Key Personnel:

Administrator/President . . . . Michael D Drobot
Chief Medical Staff . . . . Luke Watson, MD
Emergency Room . . . . Stanley Williams, MD
Emergency Room . . . . Theresa Cesiro, RN
Director Infection/Disease Control . . . . Alfonso Torres-Cook
OB/GYN Womens Health . . . . Irene Thibault
Director Radiology . . . . Jasonn Lui, MD
Director Respiratory Therapy . . . . Scott Llewellyn

Measure	Cases	This Hospital	State Average	U.S. Average	Top Hospital
Heart Attack Care					
ACE Inhibitor or ARB for LVSD[1,3]	2	50%	82%	82%	100%
Aspirin at Arrival[1,3]	10	100%	95%	92%	100%
Aspirin at Discharge[1,3]	4	100%	90%	90%	100%
Beta Blocker at Arrival[1,3]	10	90%	89%	87%	100%
Beta Blocker at Discharge[1,3]	6	83%	89%	90%	100%
Fibrinolytic Medication Timing[1,3]	2	50%	40%	31%	100%
PCI Within 90 Minutes of Arrival	0	-	52%	54%	95%
Smoking Cessation Advice[1,3]	1	100%	87%	88%	100%
Heart Failure Care					
ACE Inhibitor or ARB for LVSD	26	92%	84%	82%	100%
Discharge Instructions	34	82%	56%	61%	93%
Evaluation of LVS Function	54	89%	84%	83%	99%
Smoking Cessation Advice[1]	12	67%	82%	82%	100%
Pneumonia Care					
Appropriate Initial Antibiotic	39	67%	82%	83%	94%
Blood Culture Timing	106	91%	89%	90%	100%
Influenza Vaccine[1]	20	50%	58%	70%	100%
Initial Antibiotic Timing	147	91%	75%	80%	93%
Oxygenation Assessment	158	99%	99%	99%	100%
Pneumococcal Vaccine	89	80%	58%	69%	94%
Smoking Cessation Advice	25	80%	75%	80%	100%
Surgical Infection Prevention					
Prophylactic Antibiotic Given	139	91%	74%	77%	95%
Prophylactic Antibiotic Selection	29	97%	89%	90%	100%
Prophylactic Antibiotic Stopped	135	52%	65%	72%	95%
Pregnancy Care					
Inpatient Neonatal Mortality	-	-	-	-	-
Third or Fourth Degree Laceration	-	-	3.58%	3.63%	3.27%

NOTE: Hospital profiles are in alphabetical order by state, then city, then hospital within the city; Rankings are sorted by rate in descending order and exclude hospitals with less than 25 cases; (1) The number of cases is too small (n<25) for purposes of reliably predicting hospital performance; (2) Measure reflects the hospital's indication that its submission was based upon a sample of its relevant discharges; (3) Rate reflects fewer than the maximum possible quarters of data for the measure; (4) Inaccurate information submitted and suppressed for one or more quarters; (5) No data is available from the hospital for this measure; Please refer to the User's Guide for a full explanation of data

Saint Mary Medical Center

1050 Linden Avenue Phone: 562-491-9000
Long Beach, CA 90813 Fax: 562-436-6378
URL: www.sc.chw.edu
Ownership: Voluntary non-profit - Church Accredited: Yes
Emergency Services: Yes Licensed Beds: 551

Key Personnel:
President/CEO. . . . . Christopher DiCicco, MD
Chief Medical Staff. . . . . Merrill Knopf, MD
Cardiology . . . . Pam Fair, RN
Emergency Room . . . . Stephen Shea, MD
Director Infection/Disease Control . . . . Jerry Pennington, RN
Manager Respiratory Therapy . . . . Sharon Sauser

Measure	Cases	This Hospital	State Average	U.S. Average	Top Hospital
Heart Attack Care					
ACE Inhibitor or ARB for LVSD	29	86%	82%	82%	100%
Aspirin at Arrival	137	96%	95%	92%	100%
Aspirin at Discharge	157	97%	90%	90%	100%
Beta Blocker at Arrival	108	96%	89%	87%	100%
Beta Blocker at Discharge	145	94%	89%	90%	100%
Fibrinolytic Medication Timing[1]	5	0%	40%	31%	100%
PCI Within 90 Minutes of Arrival[1]	2	50%	52%	54%	95%
Smoking Cessation Advice	52	94%	87%	88%	100%
Heart Failure Care					
ACE Inhibitor or ARB for LVSD[2]	112	84%	84%	82%	100%
Discharge Instructions[2]	236	91%	56%	61%	93%
Evaluation of LVS Function[2]	293	91%	84%	83%	99%
Smoking Cessation Advice[2]	86	92%	82%	82%	100%
Pneumonia Care					
Appropriate Initial Antibiotic[2]	87	84%	82%	83%	94%
Blood Culture Timing[2]	89	90%	89%	90%	100%
Influenza Vaccine[1,2]	24	33%	58%	70%	100%
Initial Antibiotic Timing[2]	141	80%	75%	80%	93%
Oxygenation Assessment[2]	163	100%	99%	99%	100%
Pneumococcal Vaccine[2]	95	36%	58%	69%	94%
Smoking Cessation Advice[2]	56	96%	75%	80%	100%
Surgical Infection Prevention					
Prophylactic Antibiotic Given[2]	218	67%	74%	77%	95%
Prophylactic Antibiotic Selection[2]	41	90%	89%	90%	100%
Prophylactic Antibiotic Stopped[2]	203	57%	65%	72%	95%
Pregnancy Care					
Inpatient Neonatal Mortality	-	-	-	-	-
Third or Fourth Degree Laceration	-	-	3.58%	3.63%	3.27%

Los Alamitos Medical Center

3751 Katella Avenue Phone: 562-598-1311
Los Alamitos, CA 90720 Fax: 562-493-2812
URL: www.losalamitosmedctr.com
Ownership: Proprietary Accredited: Yes
Emergency Services: Yes Licensed Beds: 167

Key Personnel:
CEO. . . . . Michele Finney
Chief Medical Officer . . . . Dr Jennifer Daley
Chief Catheterization Laboratory . . . . Alan Gold, MD
Director Infection/Disease Control . . . . Joan Blake
CCU Spvg. Nurse . . . . Janet Bracha
Director Medical/Surgical Nursing . . . . Vicki Stec
Chief OB/GYN . . . . Kenneth Farhang
Chief Radiology . . . . Paul Kamin, MD
Director Respiratory Therapy . . . . Mary Ann Walker

Measure	Cases	This Hospital	State Average	U.S. Average	Top Hospital
Heart Attack Care					
ACE Inhibitor or ARB for LVSD[1]	14	100%	82%	82%	100%
Aspirin at Arrival	129	98%	95%	92%	100%
Aspirin at Discharge	89	98%	90%	90%	100%
Beta Blocker at Arrival	105	97%	89%	87%	100%
Beta Blocker at Discharge	90	100%	89%	90%	100%
Fibrinolytic Medication Timing	0	-	40%	31%	100%
PCI Within 90 Minutes of Arrival[1]	8	100%	52%	54%	95%
Smoking Cessation Advice[1]	16	100%	87%	88%	100%
Heart Failure Care					
ACE Inhibitor or ARB for LVSD	75	100%	84%	82%	100%
Discharge Instructions	212	80%	56%	61%	93%
Evaluation of LVS Function	261	99%	84%	83%	99%
Smoking Cessation Advice[1]	20	100%	82%	82%	100%
Pneumonia Care					
Appropriate Initial Antibiotic	201	92%	82%	83%	94%
Blood Culture Timing	184	97%	89%	90%	100%
Influenza Vaccine	54	98%	58%	70%	100%
Initial Antibiotic Timing	226	92%	75%	80%	93%
Oxygenation Assessment	284	100%	99%	99%	100%
Pneumococcal Vaccine	207	99%	58%	69%	94%
Smoking Cessation Advice	36	100%	75%	80%	100%
Surgical Infection Prevention					
Prophylactic Antibiotic Given[2]	162	82%	74%	77%	95%
Prophylactic Antibiotic Selection[2]	36	89%	89%	90%	100%
Prophylactic Antibiotic Stopped[2]	154	42%	65%	72%	95%
Pregnancy Care					
Inpatient Neonatal Mortality	-	-	-	-	-
Third or Fourth Degree Laceration	-	-	3.58%	3.63%	3.27%

California Hospital Medical Center

Alternate Name: California Medical Center-Los Angeles
1401 S Grand Avenue Phone: 213-748-2411
Los Angeles, CA 90015 Fax: 213-742-5913
URL: www.chmcla.org
Ownership: Voluntary non-profit - Other Accredited: Yes
Emergency Services: Yes Licensed Beds: 313

Key Personnel:
President . . . . Mark A Meyers
Director of Cardiology/Cardiac Lab. . . . . Phil Fairchild
Emergency Room Director. . . . . Robert Swan
Chief Respiratory Care. Bill Melon

Measure	Cases	This Hospital	State Average	U.S. Average	Top Hospital
Heart Attack Care					
ACE Inhibitor or ARB for LVSD[1]	12	100%	82%	82%	100%
Aspirin at Arrival	75	100%	95%	92%	100%
Aspirin at Discharge	40	100%	90%	90%	100%
Beta Blocker at Arrival	43	100%	89%	87%	100%
Beta Blocker at Discharge	44	100%	89%	90%	100%
Fibrinolytic Medication Timing[1]	3	33%	40%	31%	100%
PCI Within 90 Minutes of Arrival	0	-	52%	54%	95%
Smoking Cessation Advice[1]	9	100%	87%	88%	100%
Heart Failure Care					
ACE Inhibitor or ARB for LVSD	218	100%	84%	82%	100%
Discharge Instructions	378	100%	56%	61%	93%
Evaluation of LVS Function	433	100%	84%	83%	99%
Smoking Cessation Advice	128	100%	82%	82%	100%
Pneumonia Care					
Appropriate Initial Antibiotic	113	91%	82%	83%	94%
Blood Culture Timing	98	93%	89%	90%	100%
Influenza Vaccine[1]	19	100%	58%	70%	100%
Initial Antibiotic Timing	143	76%	75%	80%	93%
Oxygenation Assessment	181	100%	99%	99%	100%
Pneumococcal Vaccine	83	96%	58%	69%	94%
Smoking Cessation Advice	42	100%	75%	80%	100%
Surgical Infection Prevention					
Prophylactic Antibiotic Given[2,3]	152	85%	74%	77%	95%
Prophylactic Antibiotic Selection[2]	54	83%	89%	90%	100%
Prophylactic Antibiotic Stopped[2,3]	147	42%	65%	72%	95%
Pregnancy Care					
Inpatient Neonatal Mortality	4,149	0.27%	-	-	-
Third or Fourth Degree Laceration	2,841	2.53%	3.58%	3.63%	3.27%

Cedars-Sinai Medical Center

8700 Beverly Boulevard Phone: 310-423-3277
Los Angeles, CA 90048 Fax: 310-423-0470
URL: www.cedars-sinai.edu
Ownership: Voluntary non-profit - Other Accredited: Yes
Emergency Services: Yes Licensed Beds: 1,012

Key Personnel:
President/CEO. . . . . Thomas M Priselac
Chief Medical Staff. . . . . Glenn Braunstein, MD

NOTE: Hospital profiles are in alphabetical order by state, then city, then hospital within the city; Rankings are sorted by rate in descending order and exclude hospitals with less than 25 cases; (1) The number of cases is too small (n<25) for purposes of reliably predicting hospital performance; (2) Measure reflects the hospital's indication that its submission was based upon a sample of its relevant discharges; (3) Rate reflects fewer than the maximum possible quarters of data for the measure; (4) Inaccurate information submitted and suppressed for one or more quarters; (5) No data is available from the hospital for this measure; Please refer to the User's Guide for a full explanation of data

Chief Catheterization Laboratory . . . . Neil Eigler, MD
Emergency Room . . . . James Loftus, MD
Director Infection/Disease Control . . . . Eric Daar, MD
VP Medical/Surgical Nursing . . . . Linda Procci
OB/GYN Womens Health. . . . . Lawrence Platt, MD
Chief Radiology . . . . Barry Pressman, MD
Director Respiratory Therapy . . . . Zab Mohsenifar, MD

Measure	Cases	This Hospital	State Average	U.S. Average	Top Hospital
Heart Attack Care					
ACE Inhibitor or ARB for LVSD	54	98%	82%	82%	100%
Aspirin at Arrival	352	100%	95%	92%	100%
Aspirin at Discharge	347	100%	90%	90%	100%
Beta Blocker at Arrival	234	100%	89%	87%	100%
Beta Blocker at Discharge	312	100%	89%	90%	100%
Fibrinolytic Medication Timing[1]	1	0%	40%	31%	100%
PCI Within 90 Minutes of Arrival[1]	13	85%	52%	54%	95%
Smoking Cessation Advice	72	100%	87%	88%	100%
Heart Failure Care					
ACE Inhibitor or ARB for LVSD	336	99%	84%	82%	100%
Discharge Instructions	777	44%	56%	61%	93%
Evaluation of LVS Function	880	100%	84%	83%	99%
Smoking Cessation Advice	96	100%	82%	82%	100%
Pneumonia Care					
Appropriate Initial Antibiotic	334	94%	82%	83%	94%
Blood Culture Timing	480	98%	89%	90%	100%
Influenza Vaccine	122	66%	58%	70%	100%
Initial Antibiotic Timing	519	94%	75%	80%	93%
Oxygenation Assessment	720	100%	99%	99%	100%
Pneumococcal Vaccine	455	88%	58%	69%	94%
Smoking Cessation Advice	86	100%	75%	80%	100%
Surgical Infection Prevention					
Prophylactic Antibiotic Given[2]	2,543	96%	74%	77%	95%
Prophylactic Antibiotic Selection[2]	630	95%	89%	90%	100%
Prophylactic Antibiotic Stopped[2]	2,442	89%	65%	72%	95%
Pregnancy Care					
Inpatient Neonatal Mortality	-	-	-	-	-
Third or Fourth Degree Laceration	-	-	3.58%	3.63%	3.27%

Century City Doctors Hospital

2070 Century Park East
Los Angeles, CA 90067
Ownership: Proprietary
Emergency Services: Yes
Phone: 310-772-4915
Accredited: Yes

Measure	Cases	This Hospital	State Average	U.S. Average	Top Hospital
Heart Attack Care					
ACE Inhibitor or ARB for LVSD[1,3]	2	100%	82%	82%	100%
Aspirin at Arrival[1,3]	6	100%	95%	92%	100%
Aspirin at Discharge[1,3]	4	100%	90%	90%	100%
Beta Blocker at Arrival[1,3]	9	100%	89%	87%	100%
Beta Blocker at Discharge[1,3]	5	80%	89%	90%	100%
Fibrinolytic Medication Timing[1,3]	1	100%	40%	31%	100%
PCI Within 90 Minutes of Arrival	0	-	52%	54%	95%
Smoking Cessation Advice[3]	0	-	87%	88%	100%
Heart Failure Care					
ACE Inhibitor or ARB for LVSD[1,3]	5	80%	84%	82%	100%
Discharge Instructions[3]	25	28%	56%	61%	93%
Evaluation of LVS Function[3]	35	83%	84%	83%	99%
Smoking Cessation Advice[1,3]	3	33%	82%	82%	100%
Pneumonia Care					
Appropriate Initial Antibiotic[1,3]	22	64%	82%	83%	94%
Blood Culture Timing	28	100%	89%	90%	100%
Influenza Vaccine[1]	8	38%	58%	70%	100%
Initial Antibiotic Timing[3]	40	50%	75%	80%	93%
Oxygenation Assessment[3]	53	98%	99%	99%	100%
Pneumococcal Vaccine[3]	44	20%	58%	69%	94%
Smoking Cessation Advice[1,3]	3	33%	75%	80%	100%
Surgical Infection Prevention					
Prophylactic Antibiotic Given[3]	206	89%	74%	77%	95%
Prophylactic Antibiotic Selection	65	97%	89%	90%	100%
Prophylactic Antibiotic Stopped[3]	202	96%	65%	72%	95%
Pregnancy Care					
Inpatient Neonatal Mortality	-	-	-	-	-
Third or Fourth Degree Laceration	-	-	3.58%	3.63%	3.27%

City of Angels Medical Center

1711 West Temple Street
Los Angeles, CA 90026
Ownership: Proprietary
Emergency Services: No
Phone: 213-989-6100
Fax: 626-795-6999
Accredited: Yes
Licensed Beds: 187

Key Personnel:
President/CEO. . . . . Rudra Sabaratnam
Chief Medical Staff. . . . . Louis Acosta

Measure	Cases	This Hospital	State Average	U.S. Average	Top Hospital
Heart Attack Care					
ACE Inhibitor or ARB for LVSD[1]	2	50%	82%	82%	100%
Aspirin at Arrival[1]	12	83%	95%	92%	100%
Aspirin at Discharge[1]	9	44%	90%	90%	100%
Beta Blocker at Arrival[1]	12	42%	89%	87%	100%
Beta Blocker at Discharge[1]	9	33%	89%	90%	100%
Fibrinolytic Medication Timing[3]	0	-	40%	31%	100%
PCI Within 90 Minutes of Arrival	0	-	52%	54%	95%
Smoking Cessation Advice[3]	0	-	87%	88%	100%
Heart Failure Care					
ACE Inhibitor or ARB for LVSD	27	48%	84%	82%	100%
Discharge Instructions[1,3]	21	0%	56%	61%	93%
Evaluation of LVS Function	83	81%	84%	83%	99%
Smoking Cessation Advice[1,3]	6	33%	82%	82%	100%
Pneumonia Care					
Appropriate Initial Antibiotic[1,2,3]	2	50%	82%	83%	94%
Blood Culture Timing[2,3]	0	-	89%	90%	100%
Influenza Vaccine[5]	-	-	58%	70%	100%
Initial Antibiotic Timing[2]	42	60%	75%	80%	93%
Oxygenation Assessment[2]	86	97%	99%	99%	100%
Pneumococcal Vaccine[2]	56	5%	58%	69%	94%
Smoking Cessation Advice[1,2,3]	1	100%	75%	80%	100%
Surgical Infection Prevention					
Prophylactic Antibiotic Given[3]	0	-	74%	77%	95%
Prophylactic Antibiotic Selection[5]	-	-	89%	90%	100%
Prophylactic Antibiotic Stopped[3]	0	-	65%	72%	95%
Pregnancy Care					
Inpatient Neonatal Mortality	-	-	-	-	-
Third or Fourth Degree Laceration	-	-	3.58%	3.63%	3.27%

East Los Angeles Doctors Hospital

4060 Whittier Boulevard
Los Angeles, CA 90023
Ownership: Proprietary
Emergency Services: Yes
Phone: 323-268-5514
Fax: 323-266-1256
Accredited: Yes
Licensed Beds: 127

Key Personnel:
CEO. . . . . Araceli Longeran
Chief Medical Staff. . . . . Masad Arbid, MD
Cardiac Lab . . . . Carlos Nunez
Emergency Room . . . . Margarel Villagran
Emergency Room . . . . Susan Salazar
Infection Control. . . . . Barbara Edmonds
OB/GYN Womens Health. . . . . Knuaya Tabora
Surgical Services . . . . Anita Esteban, RN
Director Respiratory Therapy . . . . Carlos Nunez

Measure	Cases	This Hospital	State Average	U.S. Average	Top Hospital
Heart Attack Care					
ACE Inhibitor or ARB for LVSD[1]	4	75%	82%	82%	100%
Aspirin at Arrival	43	86%	95%	92%	100%
Aspirin at Discharge	26	73%	90%	90%	100%
Beta Blocker at Arrival	44	86%	89%	87%	100%
Beta Blocker at Discharge	27	70%	89%	90%	100%
Fibrinolytic Medication Timing[1]	3	33%	40%	31%	100%
PCI Within 90 Minutes of Arrival	0	-	52%	54%	95%
Smoking Cessation Advice[1]	8	88%	87%	88%	100%
Heart Failure Care					
ACE Inhibitor or ARB for LVSD[1]	20	85%	84%	82%	100%

NOTE: Hospital profiles are in alphabetical order by state, then city, then hospital within the city; Rankings are sorted by rate in descending order and exclude hospitals with less than 25 cases; (1) The number of cases is too small (n<25) for purposes of reliably predicting hospital performance; (2) Measure reflects the hospital's indication that its submission was based upon a sample of its relevant discharges; (3) Rate reflects fewer than the maximum possible quarters of data for the measure; (4) Inaccurate information submitted and suppressed for one or more quarters; (5) No data is available from the hospital for this measure; Please refer to the User's Guide for a full explanation of data

Discharge Instructions	102	99%	56%	61%	93%
Evaluation of LVS Function	116	53%	84%	83%	99%
Smoking Cessation Advice[1]	13	100%	82%	82%	100%
Pneumonia Care					
Appropriate Initial Antibiotic	81	69%	82%	83%	94%
Blood Culture Timing	62	71%	89%	90%	100%
Influenza Vaccine[4,5]	-	-	58%	70%	100%
Initial Antibiotic Timing	96	82%	75%	80%	93%
Oxygenation Assessment	120	100%	99%	99%	100%
Pneumococcal Vaccine	73	1%	58%	69%	94%
Smoking Cessation Advice[1]	4	75%	75%	80%	100%
Surgical Infection Prevention					
Prophylactic Antibiotic Given[1,3]	10	10%	74%	77%	95%
Prophylactic Antibiotic Selection[1]	1	100%	89%	90%	100%
Prophylactic Antibiotic Stopped[1,3]	9	78%	65%	72%	95%
Pregnancy Care					
Inpatient Neonatal Mortality	-	-	-	-	-
Third or Fourth Degree Laceration	-	-	3.58%	3.63%	3.27%

Good Samaritan Hospital

1225 Wilshire Boulevard
Los Angeles, CA 90017
E-mail: info@goodsam.org
URL: www.goodsam.org
Ownership: Proprietary
Emergency Services: Yes

Phone: 213-977-2121
Fax: 213-482-2770
Accredited: Yes
Licensed Beds: 408

Key Personnel:

President/CEO . . . . Andrew B Leeka
Chief Medical Staff . . . . Thomas Shook, MD
Medical Director Cardiology . . . . David Cannon, MD
Emergency Room . . . . Kevin Traber, RN
Emergency Room . . . . Philip Fagan, MD
Medical Surgical Nursing . . . . Richard Brock
OB/GYN/Women's Health . . . . Connie Von Kohler, RN
Respiratory/Cardiopulmonary . . . . Bill Millon

Measure	Cases	This Hospital	State Average	U.S. Average	Top Hospital
Heart Attack Care					
ACE Inhibitor or ARB for LVSD	55	89%	82%	82%	100%
Aspirin at Arrival	137	98%	95%	92%	100%
Aspirin at Discharge	264	98%	90%	90%	100%
Beta Blocker at Arrival	106	97%	89%	87%	100%
Beta Blocker at Discharge	250	92%	89%	90%	100%
Fibrinolytic Medication Timing[1]	13	0%	40%	31%	100%
PCI Within 90 Minutes of Arrival[1]	6	67%	52%	54%	95%
Smoking Cessation Advice	65	98%	87%	88%	100%
Heart Failure Care					
ACE Inhibitor or ARB for LVSD	197	87%	84%	82%	100%
Discharge Instructions	391	79%	56%	61%	93%
Evaluation of LVS Function	463	97%	84%	83%	99%
Smoking Cessation Advice	74	95%	82%	82%	100%
Pneumonia Care					
Appropriate Initial Antibiotic	165	81%	82%	83%	94%
Blood Culture Timing	148	88%	89%	90%	100%
Influenza Vaccine[4,5]	-	-	58%	70%	100%
Initial Antibiotic Timing	212	77%	75%	80%	93%
Oxygenation Assessment	249	99%	99%	99%	100%
Pneumococcal Vaccine	151	65%	58%	69%	94%
Smoking Cessation Advice	27	78%	75%	80%	100%
Surgical Infection Prevention					
Prophylactic Antibiotic Given	544	83%	74%	77%	95%
Prophylactic Antibiotic Selection	123	80%	89%	90%	100%
Prophylactic Antibiotic Stopped	514	74%	65%	72%	95%
Pregnancy Care					
Inpatient Neonatal Mortality	-	-	-	-	-
Third or Fourth Degree Laceration	-	-	3.58%	3.63%	3.27%

Hollywood Presbyterian Medical Center

1300 N Vermont Ave
Los Angeles, CA 90027
URL: www.hollywoodpresbyterian.com
Ownership: Voluntary non-profit - Church
Emergency Services: Yes

Phone: 323-413-3000
Fax: 323-644-4411
Accredited: Yes
Licensed Beds: 434

Key Personnel:

Interim CEO . . . . Shawn Bolouki
Director Cardiology . . . . Rose Gumadi
Director Emergency Room . . . . Julie Tatico
Manager Medical/Surgical Nursing . . . . Saundra Timmons
CNO . . . . Beverly Quaye
Surgical Services . . . . Lee Craig
Respiratory . . . . Rose Gumadi

Measure	Cases	This Hospital	State Average	U.S. Average	Top Hospital
Heart Attack Care					
ACE Inhibitor or ARB for LVSD[1]	19	100%	82%	82%	100%
Aspirin at Arrival	129	98%	95%	92%	100%
Aspirin at Discharge	89	100%	90%	90%	100%
Beta Blocker at Arrival	126	97%	89%	87%	100%
Beta Blocker at Discharge	89	98%	89%	90%	100%
Fibrinolytic Medication Timing[1]	9	22%	40%	31%	100%
PCI Within 90 Minutes of Arrival	0	-	52%	54%	95%
Smoking Cessation Advice[1]	19	89%	87%	88%	100%
Heart Failure Care					
ACE Inhibitor or ARB for LVSD	115	100%	84%	82%	100%
Discharge Instructions	352	42%	56%	61%	93%
Evaluation of LVS Function	409	95%	84%	83%	99%
Smoking Cessation Advice	56	80%	82%	82%	100%
Pneumonia Care					
Appropriate Initial Antibiotic	354	61%	82%	83%	94%
Blood Culture Timing	278	94%	89%	90%	100%
Influenza Vaccine[4,5]	-	-	58%	70%	100%
Initial Antibiotic Timing	461	77%	75%	80%	93%
Oxygenation Assessment	508	100%	99%	99%	100%
Pneumococcal Vaccine	315	40%	58%	69%	94%
Smoking Cessation Advice	35	69%	75%	80%	100%
Surgical Infection Prevention					
Prophylactic Antibiotic Given[3]	111	82%	74%	77%	95%
Prophylactic Antibiotic Selection	111	96%	89%	90%	100%
Prophylactic Antibiotic Stopped[3]	110	27%	65%	72%	95%
Pregnancy Care					
Inpatient Neonatal Mortality	-	-	-	-	-
Third or Fourth Degree Laceration	-	-	3.58%	3.63%	3.27%

Kaiser Permanente Los Angeles Medical Center

4867 Sunset Boulevard
Los Angeles, CA 90027
URL: www.kaiserpermanente.org
Ownership: Voluntary non-profit - Other
Emergency Services: Yes

Phone: 323-783-4011
Fax: 323-783-7946
Accredited: Yes
Licensed Beds: 737

Key Personnel:

CEO . . . . Anthony Armada
Chief Medical Staff . . . . Maureen Spell, MD
Chief Catheterization Laboratory . . . . V Aharonian, MD
Emergency Room . . . . Robert Ungar, MD
Director Infection/Disease Control . . . . Joel Ruskin, MD
OB/GYN Womens Health . . . . Tina Nevarrez, MD
Chief Radiology . . . . Morley Slote, MD
Director Respiratory Therapy . . . . Rob West

Measure	Cases	This Hospital	State Average	U.S. Average	Top Hospital
Heart Attack Care					
ACE Inhibitor or ARB for LVSD	182	85%	82%	82%	100%
Aspirin at Arrival	229	99%	95%	92%	100%
Aspirin at Discharge	858	100%	90%	90%	100%
Beta Blocker at Arrival	219	98%	89%	87%	100%
Beta Blocker at Discharge	874	97%	89%	90%	100%
Fibrinolytic Medication Timing[1]	14	71%	40%	31%	100%
PCI Within 90 Minutes of Arrival[1]	4	100%	52%	54%	95%
Smoking Cessation Advice	207	79%	87%	88%	100%
Heart Failure Care					

NOTE: Hospital profiles are in alphabetical order by state, then city, then hospital within the city; Rankings are sorted by rate in descending order and exclude hospitals with less than 25 cases; (1) The number of cases is too small (n<25) for purposes of reliably predicting hospital performance; (2) Measure reflects the hospital's indication that its submission was based upon a sample of its relevant discharges; (3) Rate reflects fewer than the maximum possible quarters of data for the measure; (4) Inaccurate information submitted and suppressed for one or more quarters; (5) No data is available from the hospital for this measure; Please refer to the User's Guide for a full explanation of data

ACE Inhibitor or ARB for LVSD	257	84%	84%	82%	100%
Discharge Instructions	471	54%	56%	61%	93%
Evaluation of LVS Function	489	98%	84%	83%	99%
Smoking Cessation Advice	59	63%	82%	82%	100%
Pneumonia Care					
Appropriate Initial Antibiotic	66	80%	82%	83%	94%
Blood Culture Timing	92	83%	89%	90%	100%
Influenza Vaccine[4,5]	-	-	58%	70%	100%
Initial Antibiotic Timing	95	72%	75%	80%	93%
Oxygenation Assessment	127	100%	99%	99%	100%
Pneumococcal Vaccine	81	59%	58%	69%	94%
Smoking Cessation Advice[1]	15	53%	75%	80%	100%
Surgical Infection Prevention					
Prophylactic Antibiotic Given[3]	68	60%	74%	77%	95%
Prophylactic Antibiotic Selection	72	90%	89%	90%	100%
Prophylactic Antibiotic Stopped[3]	65	80%	65%	72%	95%
Pregnancy Care					
Inpatient Neonatal Mortality	2,476	0.61%	-	-	-
Third or Fourth Degree Laceration	1,520	3.42%	3.58%	3.63%	3.27%

Kaiser Permanente West Los Angeles Med Ctr

6041 Cadillac Avenue — Phone: 323-857-2201
Los Angeles, CA 90034 — Fax: 323-857-4051
URL: www.kaiserpermanente.org
Ownership: Voluntary non-profit - Private — Accredited: Yes
Emergency Services: Yes — Licensed Beds: 306

Key Personnel:

President/CEO . . . . Janice Head
Chief Medical Staff. . . . . Edward Ellison, MD
Department Administrator ER Services . . . . Teresa Siaca
Emergency Room . . . . Robert Becker, MD
OB/GYN. . . . . Maggie Pierce
Director Respiratory Therapy . . . . Jesus Alamillo

Measure	Cases	This Hospital	State Average	U.S. Average	Top Hospital
Heart Attack Care					
ACE Inhibitor or ARB for LVSD[1]	20	90%	82%	82%	100%
Aspirin at Arrival	131	99%	95%	92%	100%
Aspirin at Discharge	102	97%	90%	90%	100%
Beta Blocker at Arrival	128	96%	89%	87%	100%
Beta Blocker at Discharge	103	97%	89%	90%	100%
Fibrinolytic Medication Timing[1]	18	56%	40%	31%	100%
PCI Within 90 Minutes of Arrival	0	-	52%	54%	95%
Smoking Cessation Advice[1]	13	85%	87%	88%	100%
Heart Failure Care					
ACE Inhibitor or ARB for LVSD	134	80%	84%	82%	100%
Discharge Instructions	335	54%	56%	61%	93%
Evaluation of LVS Function	353	90%	84%	83%	99%
Smoking Cessation Advice	45	82%	82%	82%	100%
Pneumonia Care					
Appropriate Initial Antibiotic	78	82%	82%	83%	94%
Blood Culture Timing	44	91%	89%	90%	100%
Influenza Vaccine[1]	20	70%	58%	70%	100%
Initial Antibiotic Timing	94	63%	75%	80%	93%
Oxygenation Assessment	109	100%	99%	99%	100%
Pneumococcal Vaccine	79	70%	58%	69%	94%
Smoking Cessation Advice[1]	12	67%	75%	80%	100%
Surgical Infection Prevention					
Prophylactic Antibiotic Given[3]	44	91%	74%	77%	95%
Prophylactic Antibiotic Selection	43	88%	89%	90%	100%
Prophylactic Antibiotic Stopped[3]	44	50%	65%	72%	95%
Pregnancy Care					
Inpatient Neonatal Mortality	1,461	0.14%	-	-	-
Third or Fourth Degree Laceration	1,026	2.34%	3.58%	3.63%	3.27%

Los Angeles Community Hospital

4081 E Olympic Blvd — Phone: 323-367-0477
Los Angeles, CA 90023
Ownership: Proprietary — Accredited: Yes
Emergency Services: Yes

Measure	Cases	This Hospital	State Average	U.S. Average	Top Hospital
Heart Attack Care					
ACE Inhibitor or ARB for LVSD[1]	3	67%	82%	82%	100%
Aspirin at Arrival[1]	8	100%	95%	92%	100%
Aspirin at Discharge[1]	7	100%	90%	90%	100%
Beta Blocker at Arrival[1]	9	78%	89%	87%	100%
Beta Blocker at Discharge[1]	8	75%	89%	90%	100%
Fibrinolytic Medication Timing[1]	5	20%	40%	31%	100%
PCI Within 90 Minutes of Arrival	0	-	52%	54%	95%
Smoking Cessation Advice[1]	1	0%	87%	88%	100%
Heart Failure Care					
ACE Inhibitor or ARB for LVSD	41	61%	84%	82%	100%
Discharge Instructions	115	59%	56%	61%	93%
Evaluation of LVS Function	136	80%	84%	83%	99%
Smoking Cessation Advice[1]	23	96%	82%	82%	100%
Pneumonia Care					
Appropriate Initial Antibiotic	72	64%	82%	83%	94%
Blood Culture Timing[1]	16	75%	89%	90%	100%
Influenza Vaccine[1]	16	0%	58%	70%	100%
Initial Antibiotic Timing	93	57%	75%	80%	93%
Oxygenation Assessment	104	98%	99%	99%	100%
Pneumococcal Vaccine	53	0%	58%	69%	94%
Smoking Cessation Advice	78	44%	75%	80%	100%
Surgical Infection Prevention					
Prophylactic Antibiotic Given[3]	25	64%	74%	77%	95%
Prophylactic Antibiotic Selection	25	96%	89%	90%	100%
Prophylactic Antibiotic Stopped[3]	25	96%	65%	72%	95%
Pregnancy Care					
Inpatient Neonatal Mortality	-	-	-	-	-
Third or Fourth Degree Laceration	-	-	3.58%	3.63%	3.27%

Los Angeles County & USC Medical Center

1200 N State Street — Phone: 323-226-2622
Los Angeles, CA 90033 — Fax: 323-226-6518
E-mail: webinformatics@ladhs.org
URL: www.ladhs.org
Ownership: Government - Local — Accredited: Yes
Emergency Services: Yes — Licensed Beds: 1,395

Key Personnel:

CEO. . . . . Pete Delgado
Chief of Medical Staff. . . . . Peter Gruen
Emergency Room . . . . Gail Anderson, MD
ICU . . . . Steve Giannotta, MD
OB/GYN Womens Health. . . . . Daniel Mishell, MD
Chief Radiology . . . . James Halls, MD

Measure	Cases	This Hospital	State Average	U.S. Average	Top Hospital
Heart Attack Care					
ACE Inhibitor or ARB for LVSD	66	83%	82%	82%	100%
Aspirin at Arrival	178	97%	95%	92%	100%
Aspirin at Discharge	193	97%	90%	90%	100%
Beta Blocker at Arrival	142	86%	89%	87%	100%
Beta Blocker at Discharge	187	90%	89%	90%	100%
Fibrinolytic Medication Timing	0	-	40%	31%	100%
PCI Within 90 Minutes of Arrival[1]	13	0%	52%	54%	95%
Smoking Cessation Advice	83	69%	87%	88%	100%
Heart Failure Care					
ACE Inhibitor or ARB for LVSD	307	90%	84%	82%	100%
Discharge Instructions	579	20%	56%	61%	93%
Evaluation of LVS Function	617	86%	84%	83%	99%
Smoking Cessation Advice	211	47%	82%	82%	100%
Pneumonia Care					
Appropriate Initial Antibiotic	281	83%	82%	83%	94%
Blood Culture Timing	122	84%	89%	90%	100%
Influenza Vaccine	66	58%	58%	70%	100%
Initial Antibiotic Timing	341	38%	75%	80%	93%
Oxygenation Assessment	368	99%	99%	99%	100%
Pneumococcal Vaccine	87	56%	58%	69%	94%
Smoking Cessation Advice	137	32%	75%	80%	100%
Surgical Infection Prevention					
Prophylactic Antibiotic Given[2]	995	15%	74%	77%	95%
Prophylactic Antibiotic Selection[2]	211	92%	89%	90%	100%
Prophylactic Antibiotic Stopped[2]	960	73%	65%	72%	95%
Pregnancy Care					

NOTE: Hospital profiles are in alphabetical order by state, then city, then hospital within the city; Rankings are sorted by rate in descending order and exclude hospitals with less than 25 cases; (1) The number of cases is too small (n<25) for purposes of reliably predicting hospital performance; (2) Measure reflects the hospital's indication that its submission was based upon a sample of its relevant discharges; (3) Rate reflects fewer than the maximum possible quarters of data for the measure; (4) Inaccurate information submitted and suppressed for one or more quarters; (5) No data is available from the hospital for this measure; Please refer to the User's Guide for a full explanation of data

Inpatient Neonatal Mortality	1,566	1.09%	-	-	-
Third or Fourth Degree Laceration	912	4.06%	3.58%	3.63%	3.27%

Los Angeles Metropolitan Med Ctr-LA Campus

2231 S Western Avenue
Los Angeles, CA 90018
URL: www.lammc.com
Ownership: Proprietary
Emergency Services: No
Phone: 323-730-7300
Fax: 323-734-0963
Accredited: No
Licensed Beds: 191

Key Personnel:

President/CEO . . . . John V Fenton
Chief Medical Staff . . . . Lowell Theard, MD
Director Infection/Disease Control . . . . Pat Rutherford, RN
Director Medical/Surgical Nursing . . . . Kelly Miyake, RN
OB/GYN Womens Health . . . . Lucien Cox, MD

Measure	Cases	This Hospital	State Average	U.S. Average	Top Hospital
Heart Attack Care					
ACE Inhibitor or ARB for LVSD[3]	0	-	82%	82%	100%
Aspirin at Arrival[1,3]	1	0%	95%	92%	100%
Aspirin at Discharge[1,3]	1	0%	90%	90%	100%
Beta Blocker at Arrival[1,3]	1	0%	89%	87%	100%
Beta Blocker at Discharge[1,3]	1	0%	89%	90%	100%
Fibrinolytic Medication Timing[3]	0	-	40%	31%	100%
PCI Within 90 Minutes of Arrival	0	-	52%	54%	95%
Smoking Cessation Advice[3]	0	-	87%	88%	100%
Heart Failure Care					
ACE Inhibitor or ARB for LVSD[1,3]	8	25%	84%	82%	100%
Discharge Instructions[3]	51	4%	56%	61%	93%
Evaluation of LVS Function[3]	72	56%	84%	83%	99%
Smoking Cessation Advice[3]	29	7%	82%	82%	100%
Pneumonia Care					
Appropriate Initial Antibiotic[3]	40	40%	82%	83%	94%
Blood Culture Timing[1]	4	100%	89%	90%	100%
Influenza Vaccine[1]	20	0%	58%	70%	100%
Initial Antibiotic Timing[3]	53	26%	75%	80%	93%
Oxygenation Assessment[3]	62	95%	99%	99%	100%
Pneumococcal Vaccine[3]	33	9%	58%	69%	94%
Smoking Cessation Advice[3]	25	0%	75%	80%	100%
Surgical Infection Prevention					
Prophylactic Antibiotic Given[5]	-	-	74%	77%	95%
Prophylactic Antibiotic Selection[5]	-	-	89%	90%	100%
Prophylactic Antibiotic Stopped[5]	-	-	65%	72%	95%
Pregnancy Care					
Inpatient Neonatal Mortality[5]	0	0.00%	-	-	-
Third or Fourth Degree Laceration	571	2.63%	3.58%	3.63%	3.27%

Martin Luther King Jr/Charles R Drew Med Ctr

12021 S Wilmington Avenue
Los Angeles, CA 90059
URL: www.ladhs.org/mlk
Ownership: Government - Federal
Emergency Services: Yes
Phone: 310-668-4321
Fax: 310-635-1449
Accredited: Yes
Licensed Beds: 537

Key Personnel:

Administrator . . . . Randy Foster
CEO/President . . . . Linda McCouley
Chief of Medical Staff . . . . Roger Keith
Emergency Room . . . . Samuel Harden, MD
Director Infection/Disease Control . . . . Jessie Sherrod, MD
Director Medical/Surgical Nursing . . . . Rosemary Haggins, RN
OB/GYN Womens Health . . . . Techiro Fukushima, MD
Chief Radiology . . . . Jack I Eisenman

Measure	Cases	This Hospital	State Average	U.S. Average	Top Hospital
Heart Attack Care					
ACE Inhibitor or ARB for LVSD[1,2]	6	83%	82%	82%	100%
Aspirin at Arrival[2]	108	94%	95%	92%	100%
Aspirin at Discharge[2]	59	90%	90%	90%	100%
Beta Blocker at Arrival[2]	102	66%	89%	87%	100%
Beta Blocker at Discharge[2]	61	79%	89%	90%	100%
Fibrinolytic Medication Timing[1,2]	10	0%	40%	31%	100%
PCI Within 90 Minutes of Arrival[2]	0	-	52%	54%	95%
Smoking Cessation Advice[1,2]	10	10%	87%	88%	100%
Heart Failure Care					
ACE Inhibitor or ARB for LVSD[2]	50	92%	84%	82%	100%
Discharge Instructions[2]	310	1%	56%	61%	93%
Evaluation of LVS Function[2]	308	72%	84%	83%	99%
Smoking Cessation Advice[2]	128	11%	82%	82%	100%
Pneumonia Care					
Appropriate Initial Antibiotic[2]	134	72%	82%	83%	94%
Blood Culture Timing[2]	74	47%	89%	90%	100%
Influenza Vaccine[2]	25	0%	58%	70%	100%
Initial Antibiotic Timing[2]	164	62%	75%	80%	93%
Oxygenation Assessment[2]	202	99%	99%	99%	100%
Pneumococcal Vaccine[2]	44	9%	58%	69%	94%
Smoking Cessation Advice[2]	61	11%	75%	80%	100%
Surgical Infection Prevention					
Prophylactic Antibiotic Given[2,3]	77	45%	74%	77%	95%
Prophylactic Antibiotic Selection[1,2]	16	62%	89%	90%	100%
Prophylactic Antibiotic Stopped[2,3]	68	90%	65%	72%	95%
Pregnancy Care					
Inpatient Neonatal Mortality	-	-	-	-	-
Third or Fourth Degree Laceration	-	-	3.58%	3.63%	3.27%

Miracle Mile Medical Center

6000 San Vicente Blvd
Los Angeles, CA 90036
Ownership: Proprietary
Emergency Services: No
Phone: 323-930-1040
Accredited: Yes

Measure	Cases	This Hospital	State Average	U.S. Average	Top Hospital
Heart Attack Care					
ACE Inhibitor or ARB for LVSD[5]	-	-	82%	82%	100%
Aspirin at Arrival[5]	-	-	95%	92%	100%
Aspirin at Discharge[5]	-	-	90%	90%	100%
Beta Blocker at Arrival[5]	-	-	89%	87%	100%
Beta Blocker at Discharge[5]	-	-	89%	90%	100%
Fibrinolytic Medication Timing[5]	-	-	40%	31%	100%
PCI Within 90 Minutes of Arrival[5]	-	-	52%	54%	95%
Smoking Cessation Advice[5]	-	-	87%	88%	100%
Heart Failure Care					
ACE Inhibitor or ARB for LVSD[5]	-	-	84%	82%	100%
Discharge Instructions[5]	-	-	56%	61%	93%
Evaluation of LVS Function[5]	-	-	84%	83%	99%
Smoking Cessation Advice[5]	-	-	82%	82%	100%
Pneumonia Care					
Appropriate Initial Antibiotic[5]	-	-	82%	83%	94%
Blood Culture Timing[5]	-	-	89%	90%	100%
Influenza Vaccine[5]	-	-	58%	70%	100%
Initial Antibiotic Timing[5]	-	-	75%	80%	93%
Oxygenation Assessment[5]	-	-	99%	99%	100%
Pneumococcal Vaccine[5]	-	-	58%	69%	94%
Smoking Cessation Advice[5]	-	-	75%	80%	100%
Surgical Infection Prevention					
Prophylactic Antibiotic Given[5]	-	-	74%	77%	95%
Prophylactic Antibiotic Selection[5]	-	-	89%	90%	100%
Prophylactic Antibiotic Stopped[5]	-	-	65%	72%	95%
Pregnancy Care					
Inpatient Neonatal Mortality	-	-	-	-	-
Third or Fourth Degree Laceration	-	-	3.58%	3.63%	3.27%

Olympia Medical Center

5900 West Olympic Boulevard
Los Angeles, CA 90036
Ownership: Proprietary
Emergency Services: Yes
Phone: 310-657-5900
Accredited: Yes

Measure	Cases	This Hospital	State Average	U.S. Average	Top Hospital
Heart Attack Care					
ACE Inhibitor or ARB for LVSD[1]	10	70%	82%	82%	100%
Aspirin at Arrival	98	95%	95%	92%	100%
Aspirin at Discharge	46	89%	90%	90%	100%
Beta Blocker at Arrival	82	85%	89%	87%	100%
Beta Blocker at Discharge	46	89%	89%	90%	100%
Fibrinolytic Medication Timing[1]	4	50%	40%	31%	100%

NOTE: Hospital profiles are in alphabetical order by state, then city, then hospital within the city; Rankings are sorted by rate in descending order and exclude hospitals with less than 25 cases; (1) The number of cases is too small (n<25) for purposes of reliably predicting hospital performance; (2) Measure reflects the hospital's indication that its submission was based upon a sample of its relevant discharges; (3) Rate reflects fewer than the maximum possible quarters of data for the measure; (4) Inaccurate information submitted and suppressed for one or more quarters; (5) No data is available from the hospital for this measure; Please refer to the User's Guide for a full explanation of data

PCI Within 90 Minutes of Arrival	0	-	52%	54%	95%
Smoking Cessation Advice[1]	5	80%	87%	88%	100%
Heart Failure Care					
ACE Inhibitor or ARB for LVSD	89	92%	84%	82%	100%
Discharge Instructions	200	44%	56%	61%	93%
Evaluation of LVS Function	285	88%	84%	83%	99%
Smoking Cessation Advice	29	55%	82%	82%	100%
Pneumonia Care					
Appropriate Initial Antibiotic	298	57%	82%	83%	94%
Blood Culture Timing	279	92%	89%	90%	100%
Influenza Vaccine	72	24%	58%	70%	100%
Initial Antibiotic Timing	368	81%	75%	80%	93%
Oxygenation Assessment	459	100%	99%	99%	100%
Pneumococcal Vaccine	295	36%	58%	69%	94%
Smoking Cessation Advice[1]	21	67%	75%	80%	100%
Surgical Infection Prevention					
Prophylactic Antibiotic Given	114	69%	74%	77%	95%
Prophylactic Antibiotic Selection[1]	24	88%	89%	90%	100%
Prophylactic Antibiotic Stopped	113	55%	65%	72%	95%
Pregnancy Care					
Inpatient Neonatal Mortality	-	-	-	-	-
Third or Fourth Degree Laceration	-	-	3.58%	3.63%	3.27%

Pacific Alliance Medical Center

531 W College Street
Los Angeles, CA 90012
URL: www.pamc.net
Ownership: Proprietary
Emergency Services: No
Phone: 213-624-8411
Fax: 213-626-3107
Accredited: Yes
Licensed Beds: 122

Key Personnel:
Administrator/CEO . . . . John R Edwards
Chief Medical Staff . . . . Martha Maleon
Emergency Room . . . . Ruby Blak

Measure	Cases	This Hospital	State Average	U.S. Average	Top Hospital
Heart Attack Care					
ACE Inhibitor or ARB for LVSD[1]	3	67%	82%	82%	100%
Aspirin at Arrival	32	66%	95%	92%	100%
Aspirin at Discharge	31	52%	90%	90%	100%
Beta Blocker at Arrival	30	43%	89%	87%	100%
Beta Blocker at Discharge	30	43%	89%	90%	100%
Fibrinolytic Medication Timing[3]	0	-	40%	31%	100%
PCI Within 90 Minutes of Arrival	0	-	52%	54%	95%
Smoking Cessation Advice[1,3]	1	100%	87%	88%	100%
Heart Failure Care					
ACE Inhibitor or ARB for LVSD	45	36%	84%	82%	100%
Discharge Instructions[3]	46	67%	56%	61%	93%
Evaluation of LVS Function	302	79%	84%	83%	99%
Smoking Cessation Advice[1,3]	2	50%	82%	82%	100%
Pneumonia Care					
Appropriate Initial Antibiotic[1,3]	3	0%	82%	83%	94%
Blood Culture Timing[1,3]	11	100%	89%	90%	100%
Influenza Vaccine[5]	-	-	58%	70%	100%
Initial Antibiotic Timing	149	50%	75%	80%	93%
Oxygenation Assessment	162	98%	99%	99%	100%
Pneumococcal Vaccine	114	45%	58%	69%	94%
Smoking Cessation Advice[1,3]	2	50%	75%	80%	100%
Surgical Infection Prevention					
Prophylactic Antibiotic Given[1,3]	12	67%	74%	77%	95%
Prophylactic Antibiotic Selection[5]	-	-	89%	90%	100%
Prophylactic Antibiotic Stopped[1,3]	12	67%	65%	72%	95%
Pregnancy Care					
Inpatient Neonatal Mortality[2]	409	0.00%	-	-	-
Third or Fourth Degree Laceration[2]	282	0.71%	3.58%	3.63%	3.27%

Saint Vincent Medical Center

2131 W 3rd Street
Los Angeles, CA 90057
Ownership: Voluntary non-profit - Church
Emergency Services: No
Phone: 213-484-7111
Fax: 213-484-7036
Accredited: Yes
Licensed Beds: 386

Key Personnel:
President/CEO . . . . Gustavo Valdestano
Chief Medical Staff . . . . D Hart, MD
Director Infection/Disease Control . . . . Katherine Keil
CCU Spvg. Nurse . . . . Toni Shewell
Chief Radiology . . . . E Michael McMonigle, MD

Measure	Cases	This Hospital	State Average	U.S. Average	Top Hospital
Heart Attack Care					
ACE Inhibitor or ARB for LVSD	25	64%	82%	82%	100%
Aspirin at Arrival	79	97%	95%	92%	100%
Aspirin at Discharge	113	87%	90%	90%	100%
Beta Blocker at Arrival	74	88%	89%	87%	100%
Beta Blocker at Discharge	118	77%	89%	90%	100%
Fibrinolytic Medication Timing	0	-	40%	31%	100%
PCI Within 90 Minutes of Arrival	0	-	52%	54%	95%
Smoking Cessation Advice[1]	20	50%	87%	88%	100%
Heart Failure Care					
ACE Inhibitor or ARB for LVSD	109	72%	84%	82%	100%
Discharge Instructions	289	22%	56%	61%	93%
Evaluation of LVS Function	361	84%	84%	83%	99%
Smoking Cessation Advice	36	50%	82%	82%	100%
Pneumonia Care					
Appropriate Initial Antibiotic	159	78%	82%	83%	94%
Blood Culture Timing	184	90%	89%	90%	100%
Influenza Vaccine	59	66%	58%	70%	100%
Initial Antibiotic Timing	306	80%	75%	80%	93%
Oxygenation Assessment	357	100%	99%	99%	100%
Pneumococcal Vaccine	256	71%	58%	69%	94%
Smoking Cessation Advice	31	39%	75%	80%	100%
Surgical Infection Prevention					
Prophylactic Antibiotic Given[2]	289	55%	74%	77%	95%
Prophylactic Antibiotic Selection[2]	57	84%	89%	90%	100%
Prophylactic Antibiotic Stopped[2]	269	49%	65%	72%	95%
Pregnancy Care					
Inpatient Neonatal Mortality	-	-	-	-	-
Third or Fourth Degree Laceration	-	-	3.58%	3.63%	3.27%

Temple Community Hospital

235 N Hoover Street
Los Angeles, CA 90004
URL: www.templecommunityhospital.com
Ownership: Proprietary
Emergency Services: No
Phone: 213-382-7252
Fax: 213-389-4559
Accredited: Yes
Licensed Beds: 170

Key Personnel:
CEO . . . . Herbert Needman
Chief Medical Staff . . . . I Y Kim
Director Infection/Disease Control . . . . Terry McCabe
Chief Radiology . . . . Viktor Naiman
Director Respiratory Therapy . . . . Alan Guzman

Measure	Cases	This Hospital	State Average	U.S. Average	Top Hospital
Heart Attack Care					
ACE Inhibitor or ARB for LVSD[1]	2	100%	82%	82%	100%
Aspirin at Arrival	33	100%	95%	92%	100%
Aspirin at Discharge	31	100%	90%	90%	100%
Beta Blocker at Arrival	27	100%	89%	87%	100%
Beta Blocker at Discharge	34	100%	89%	90%	100%
Fibrinolytic Medication Timing[3]	0	-	40%	31%	100%
PCI Within 90 Minutes of Arrival	0	-	52%	54%	95%
Smoking Cessation Advice[3]	0	-	87%	88%	100%
Heart Failure Care					
ACE Inhibitor or ARB for LVSD[1]	13	100%	84%	82%	100%
Discharge Instructions[1,3]	24	100%	56%	61%	93%
Evaluation of LVS Function	93	98%	84%	83%	99%
Smoking Cessation Advice[1,3]	4	100%	82%	82%	100%
Pneumonia Care					
Appropriate Initial Antibiotic[1,3]	3	100%	82%	83%	94%
Blood Culture Timing[3]	0	-	89%	90%	100%
Influenza Vaccine[5]	-	-	58%	70%	100%
Initial Antibiotic Timing	53	55%	75%	80%	93%
Oxygenation Assessment	75	100%	99%	99%	100%
Pneumococcal Vaccine	48	100%	58%	69%	94%
Smoking Cessation Advice[1,3]	4	100%	75%	80%	100%

NOTE: Hospital profiles are in alphabetical order by state, then city, then hospital within the city; Rankings are sorted by rate in descending order and exclude hospitals with less than 25 cases; (1) The number of cases is too small (n<25) for purposes of reliably predicting hospital performance; (2) Measure reflects the hospital's indication that its submission was based upon a sample of its relevant discharges; (3) Rate reflects fewer than the maximum possible quarters of data for the measure; (4) Inaccurate information submitted and suppressed for one or more quarters; (5) No data is available from the hospital for this measure; Please refer to the User's Guide for a full explanation of data

Measure	Cases	This Hospital	State Average	U.S. Average	Top Hospital
Surgical Infection Prevention					
Prophylactic Antibiotic Given[1,3]	4	100%	74%	77%	95%
Prophylactic Antibiotic Selection[5]	-	-	89%	90%	100%
Prophylactic Antibiotic Stopped[1,3]	4	25%	65%	72%	95%
Pregnancy Care					
Inpatient Neonatal Mortality	-	-	-	-	-
Third or Fourth Degree Laceration	-	-	3.58%	3.63%	3.27%

UCLA Medical Center

10833 Le Conte Avenue
Los Angeles, CA 90095
URL: www.healthcare.ucla.edu
Ownership: Government - State
Emergency Services: Yes

Phone: 310-825-6301
Fax: 310-794-0530

Accredited: Yes
Licensed Beds: 592

Key Personnel:

CEO. . . . . David L Callender, MD
Chief Medical Staff. . . . . Robert Ettenger
Director Cardiology . . . . James Weiss
Head Emergency Room. . . . . Marshall Morgan
Chief Respiratory Care. Paul Bellamy

Measure	Cases	This Hospital	State Average	U.S. Average	Top Hospital
Heart Attack Care					
ACE Inhibitor or ARB for LVSD	36	78%	82%	82%	100%
Aspirin at Arrival	103	99%	95%	92%	100%
Aspirin at Discharge	77	99%	90%	90%	100%
Beta Blocker at Arrival	57	100%	89%	87%	100%
Beta Blocker at Discharge	108	97%	89%	90%	100%
Fibrinolytic Medication Timing	0	-	40%	31%	100%
PCI Within 90 Minutes of Arrival[1]	2	0%	52%	54%	95%
Smoking Cessation Advice[1]	20	90%	87%	88%	100%
Heart Failure Care					
ACE Inhibitor or ARB for LVSD[2]	194	85%	84%	82%	100%
Discharge Instructions[2]	314	52%	56%	61%	93%
Evaluation of LVS Function[2]	326	99%	84%	83%	99%
Smoking Cessation Advice[2]	50	92%	82%	82%	100%
Pneumonia Care					
Appropriate Initial Antibiotic[2]	77	91%	82%	83%	94%
Blood Culture Timing[2]	85	87%	89%	90%	100%
Influenza Vaccine[1,2]	23	26%	58%	70%	100%
Initial Antibiotic Timing[2]	115	61%	75%	80%	93%
Oxygenation Assessment[2]	201	100%	99%	99%	100%
Pneumococcal Vaccine[2]	105	24%	58%	69%	94%
Smoking Cessation Advice[2]	26	77%	75%	80%	100%
Surgical Infection Prevention					
Prophylactic Antibiotic Given[2]	387	93%	74%	77%	95%
Prophylactic Antibiotic Selection[2]	55	62%	89%	90%	100%
Prophylactic Antibiotic Stopped[2]	367	50%	65%	72%	95%
Pregnancy Care					
Inpatient Neonatal Mortality	-	-	-	-	-
Third or Fourth Degree Laceration	-	-	3.58%	3.63%	3.27%

USC University Hospital

1500 San Pablo St
Los Angeles, CA 90033
Ownership: Proprietary
Emergency Services: No

Phone: 323-442-8656

Accredited: Yes

Measure	Cases	This Hospital	State Average	U.S. Average	Top Hospital
Heart Attack Care					
ACE Inhibitor or ARB for LVSD[1]	10	80%	82%	82%	100%
Aspirin at Arrival[1]	5	100%	95%	92%	100%
Aspirin at Discharge	31	100%	90%	90%	100%
Beta Blocker at Arrival[1]	4	100%	89%	87%	100%
Beta Blocker at Discharge	27	85%	89%	90%	100%
Fibrinolytic Medication Timing	0	-	40%	31%	100%
PCI Within 90 Minutes of Arrival	0	-	52%	54%	95%
Smoking Cessation Advice[1]	5	80%	87%	88%	100%
Heart Failure Care					
ACE Inhibitor or ARB for LVSD	34	91%	84%	82%	100%
Discharge Instructions	65	45%	56%	61%	93%
Evaluation of LVS Function	72	100%	84%	83%	99%
Smoking Cessation Advice[1]	3	67%	82%	82%	100%
Pneumonia Care					
Appropriate Initial Antibiotic[1]	20	75%	82%	83%	94%
Blood Culture Timing[1]	2	100%	89%	90%	100%
Influenza Vaccine[1]	4	75%	58%	70%	100%
Initial Antibiotic Timing[1]	18	67%	75%	80%	93%
Oxygenation Assessment	30	97%	99%	99%	100%
Pneumococcal Vaccine[1]	24	79%	58%	69%	94%
Smoking Cessation Advice[1]	3	33%	75%	80%	100%
Surgical Infection Prevention					
Prophylactic Antibiotic Given[2]	304	53%	74%	77%	95%
Prophylactic Antibiotic Selection[2]	69	91%	89%	90%	100%
Prophylactic Antibiotic Stopped[2]	300	26%	65%	72%	95%
Pregnancy Care					
Inpatient Neonatal Mortality	-	-	-	-	-
Third or Fourth Degree Laceration	-	-	3.58%	3.63%	3.27%

White Memorial Medical Center

1720 Cesar E Chavez Avenue
Los Angeles, CA 90033
URL: www.whitememorial.com
Ownership: Voluntary non-profit - Church
Emergency Services: Yes

Phone: 323-268-5000
Fax: 323-881-8605

Accredited: Yes
Licensed Beds: 369

Key Personnel:

President/CEO. . . . . Beth D Zachary
Chief Medical Staff. . . . . Brian D Johnston, MD
Cardiac Lab . . . . Crystal Davis
Catheterization Lab . . . . Marcellin Simard, MD
Emergency Room . . . . Brian Johnson, MD
Emergency Room . . . . Rebecca Sales
Infection Control. . . . . Rebecca Berberian
ICU . . . . Diane Freeman
Intensive/Coronary Care . . . . Diane Freeman
Medical Surgical Nursing . . . . Diane Freeman
OB/GYN/Women's Health . . . . Anne Marie Floyd
Respiratory/Cardiopulmonary. . . . . Steve Engle, MD

Measure	Cases	This Hospital	State Average	U.S. Average	Top Hospital
Heart Attack Care					
ACE Inhibitor or ARB for LVSD	26	54%	82%	82%	100%
Aspirin at Arrival	95	94%	95%	92%	100%
Aspirin at Discharge	85	92%	90%	90%	100%
Beta Blocker at Arrival	54	85%	89%	87%	100%
Beta Blocker at Discharge	82	93%	89%	90%	100%
Fibrinolytic Medication Timing	0	-	40%	31%	100%
PCI Within 90 Minutes of Arrival[1]	2	100%	52%	54%	95%
Smoking Cessation Advice	33	94%	87%	88%	100%
Heart Failure Care					
ACE Inhibitor or ARB for LVSD	175	76%	84%	82%	100%
Discharge Instructions[3]	69	71%	56%	61%	93%
Evaluation of LVS Function	416	94%	84%	83%	99%
Smoking Cessation Advice	45	100%	82%	82%	100%
Pneumonia Care					
Appropriate Initial Antibiotic	135	94%	82%	83%	94%
Blood Culture Timing	185	92%	89%	90%	100%
Influenza Vaccine[5]	-	-	58%	70%	100%
Initial Antibiotic Timing	284	71%	75%	80%	93%
Oxygenation Assessment	325	100%	99%	99%	100%
Pneumococcal Vaccine	220	48%	58%	69%	94%
Smoking Cessation Advice	57	93%	75%	80%	100%
Surgical Infection Prevention					
Prophylactic Antibiotic Given[2,3]	50	88%	74%	77%	95%
Prophylactic Antibiotic Selection[5]	-	-	89%	90%	100%
Prophylactic Antibiotic Stopped[2,3]	41	78%	65%	72%	95%
Pregnancy Care					
Inpatient Neonatal Mortality	3,828	0.50%	-	-	-
Third or Fourth Degree Laceration	2,319	6.25%	3.58%	3.63%	3.27%

Memorial Hospital Los Banos

Alternate Name: A Sutter Health Affiliate

NOTE: Hospital profiles are in alphabetical order by state, then city, then hospital within the city; Rankings are sorted by rate in descending order and exclude hospitals with less than 25 cases; (1) The number of cases is too small (n<25) for purposes of reliably predicting hospital performance; (2) Measure reflects the hospital's indication that its submission was based upon a sample of its relevant discharges; (3) Rate reflects fewer than the maximum possible quarters of data for the measure; (4) Inaccurate information submitted and suppressed for one or more quarters; (5) No data is available from the hospital for this measure; Please refer to the User's Guide for a full explanation of data

520 West I Street
Los Banos, CA 93635
E-mail: MHALosBanos@sutterhealth.org
URL: www.memoriallosbanos.org
Ownership: Voluntary non-profit - Other
Emergency Services: Yes
Phone: 209-826-0591
Fax: 209-826-1943
Accredited: Yes
Licensed Beds: 48

Key Personnel:
Administrator . . . . Richard S Liszewski
Chief Medical Staff. . . . . Daniel Hardy, MD
Emergency Room . . . . Alan Gottlieb, MD
Infection Control. . . . . Carolyn Nazabal, RN
ICU . . . . Susan Benson, RN
Intensive/Coronary Care . . . . Susan Benson, RN
Medical/Surgical Nursing . . . . Misty Worthy, RN
Director Medical/Surgical Nursing . . . . Karen Norris
OB/GYN Womens Health. . . . . Helen Sadar, RN
Director Respiratory Therapy . . . . Sharon Stevens

Measure	Cases	This Hospital	State Average	U.S. Average	Top Hospital
Heart Attack Care					
ACE Inhibitor or ARB for LVSD	0	-	82%	82%	100%
Aspirin at Arrival[1]	8	75%	95%	92%	100%
Aspirin at Discharge[1]	5	80%	90%	90%	100%
Beta Blocker at Arrival[1]	8	50%	89%	87%	100%
Beta Blocker at Discharge[1]	5	40%	89%	90%	100%
Fibrinolytic Medication Timing	0	-	40%	31%	100%
PCI Within 90 Minutes of Arrival	0	-	52%	54%	95%
Smoking Cessation Advice[1]	1	100%	87%	88%	100%
Heart Failure Care					
ACE Inhibitor or ARB for LVSD[1]	8	62%	84%	82%	100%
Discharge Instructions	43	67%	56%	61%	93%
Evaluation of LVS Function	55	45%	84%	83%	99%
Smoking Cessation Advice[1]	10	90%	82%	82%	100%
Pneumonia Care					
Appropriate Initial Antibiotic	92	78%	82%	83%	94%
Blood Culture Timing	41	78%	89%	90%	100%
Influenza Vaccine[1]	17	18%	58%	70%	100%
Initial Antibiotic Timing	98	81%	75%	80%	93%
Oxygenation Assessment	112	100%	99%	99%	100%
Pneumococcal Vaccine	71	61%	58%	69%	94%
Smoking Cessation Advice	26	85%	75%	80%	100%
Surgical Infection Prevention					
Prophylactic Antibiotic Given[2]	36	28%	74%	77%	95%
Prophylactic Antibiotic Selection[1,2]	10	90%	89%	90%	100%
Prophylactic Antibiotic Stopped[2]	34	97%	65%	72%	95%
Pregnancy Care					
Inpatient Neonatal Mortality	-	-	-	-	-
Third or Fourth Degree Laceration	-	-	3.58%	3.63%	3.27%

Community Hospital of Los Gatos

815 Pollard Road
Los Gatos, CA 95030
URL: www.communityhospitallg.com
Ownership: Proprietary
Emergency Services: Yes
Phone: 408-378-6131
Fax: 408-866-4003
Accredited: Yes
Licensed Beds: 143

Key Personnel:
Administrator/CEO. . . . . Daniel P Doore
Chief Medical Staff. . . . . Donald Silcox, MD
Emergency Room . . . . Judy Dethiefs, MD
Director Emergency Room. . . . . Pat Erbst
Infection Control. . . . . Suzanne Cistulli, RN
ICU . . . . Kris Hoover
Director Medical/Surgical Nursing . . . . Dierdre Hegarty
OB/GYN Womens Health. . . . . Linda Teagle, MD
Director Respiratory Therapy . . . . Barbara Van Amburg

Measure	Cases	This Hospital	State Average	U.S. Average	Top Hospital
Heart Attack Care					
ACE Inhibitor or ARB for LVSD[1]	5	60%	82%	82%	100%
Aspirin at Arrival[1]	21	86%	95%	92%	100%
Aspirin at Discharge[1]	14	93%	90%	90%	100%
Beta Blocker at Arrival[1]	22	86%	89%	87%	100%
Beta Blocker at Discharge[1]	15	87%	89%	90%	100%
Fibrinolytic Medication Timing[1]	1	0%	40%	31%	100%
PCI Within 90 Minutes of Arrival	0	-	52%	54%	95%
Smoking Cessation Advice[1]	2	100%	87%	88%	100%
Heart Failure Care					
ACE Inhibitor or ARB for LVSD[1]	17	76%	84%	82%	100%
Discharge Instructions	63	70%	56%	61%	93%
Evaluation of LVS Function	104	82%	84%	83%	99%
Smoking Cessation Advice[1]	6	50%	82%	82%	100%
Pneumonia Care					
Appropriate Initial Antibiotic	80	86%	82%	83%	94%
Blood Culture Timing	83	92%	89%	90%	100%
Influenza Vaccine	33	79%	58%	70%	100%
Initial Antibiotic Timing	106	85%	75%	80%	93%
Oxygenation Assessment	125	100%	99%	99%	100%
Pneumococcal Vaccine	94	81%	58%	69%	94%
Smoking Cessation Advice[1]	5	60%	75%	80%	100%
Surgical Infection Prevention					
Prophylactic Antibiotic Given[2]	209	79%	74%	77%	95%
Prophylactic Antibiotic Selection[2]	50	92%	89%	90%	100%
Prophylactic Antibiotic Stopped[2]	202	55%	65%	72%	95%
Pregnancy Care					
Inpatient Neonatal Mortality	-	-	-	-	-
Third or Fourth Degree Laceration	-	-	3.58%	3.63%	3.27%

Saint Francis Medical Center

3630 E Imperial Highway
Lynwood, CA 90262
Ownership: Voluntary non-profit - Church
Emergency Services: Yes
Phone: 310-900-8900
Fax: 310-604-0864
Accredited: Yes
Licensed Beds: 328

Key Personnel:
CEO/President. . . . . Gerald Kozai
Chief Medical Staff. . . . . Jose Stiwak
Emergency Room . . . . Mark Louden, MD
Manager Infection/Disease Control . . . . Ana Torres
Chief OB/GYN . . . . Silas Thomas, MD
Chief Radiology . . . . Dan Schimmel
Director of Respiratory . . . . Steve Vinbrough

Measure	Cases	This Hospital	State Average	U.S. Average	Top Hospital
Heart Attack Care					
ACE Inhibitor or ARB for LVSD	27	93%	82%	82%	100%
Aspirin at Arrival	129	98%	95%	92%	100%
Aspirin at Discharge	115	96%	90%	90%	100%
Beta Blocker at Arrival	108	95%	89%	87%	100%
Beta Blocker at Discharge	114	96%	89%	90%	100%
Fibrinolytic Medication Timing[1]	18	39%	40%	31%	100%
PCI Within 90 Minutes of Arrival[1]	1	0%	52%	54%	95%
Smoking Cessation Advice	34	97%	87%	88%	100%
Heart Failure Care					
ACE Inhibitor or ARB for LVSD	258	91%	84%	82%	100%
Discharge Instructions	486	62%	56%	61%	93%
Evaluation of LVS Function	539	97%	84%	83%	99%
Smoking Cessation Advice	128	98%	82%	82%	100%
Pneumonia Care					
Appropriate Initial Antibiotic	171	94%	82%	83%	94%
Blood Culture Timing	203	96%	89%	90%	100%
Influenza Vaccine	50	70%	58%	70%	100%
Initial Antibiotic Timing	299	59%	75%	80%	93%
Oxygenation Assessment	343	100%	99%	99%	100%
Pneumococcal Vaccine	158	64%	58%	69%	94%
Smoking Cessation Advice	58	91%	75%	80%	100%
Surgical Infection Prevention					
Prophylactic Antibiotic Given[2,3]	122	87%	74%	77%	95%
Prophylactic Antibiotic Selection[2]	38	76%	89%	90%	100%
Prophylactic Antibiotic Stopped[2,3]	122	57%	65%	72%	95%
Pregnancy Care					
Inpatient Neonatal Mortality	-	-	-	-	-
Third or Fourth Degree Laceration	-	-	3.58%	3.63%	3.27%

NOTE: Hospital profiles are in alphabetical order by state, then city, then hospital within the city; Rankings are sorted by rate in descending order and exclude hospitals with less than 25 cases; (1) The number of cases is too small (n<25) for purposes of reliably predicting hospital performance; (2) Measure reflects the hospital's indication that its submission was based upon a sample of its relevant discharges; (3) Rate reflects fewer than the maximum possible quarters of data for the measure; (4) Inaccurate information submitted and suppressed for one or more quarters; (5) No data is available from the hospital for this measure; Please refer to the User's Guide for a full explanation of data

Madera Community Hospital

1250 E Almond Avenue
Madera, CA 93637
E-mail: rkelley@maderahospital.org
URL: www.maderahospital.org
Ownership: Voluntary non-profit - Other
Emergency Services: Yes

Phone: 559-675-5501
Fax: 559-675-5509
Accredited: Yes
Licensed Beds: 106

Key Personnel:

CEO. . . . . John W Frye, JR
Chief of Medical Staff . . . . . Todd Spencer
Emergency Room . . . . . Robert Toman
Director Respiratory Therapy . . . . . Pat Young

Measure	Cases	This Hospital	State Average	U.S. Average	Top Hospital
Heart Attack Care					
ACE Inhibitor or ARB for LVSD[1]	20	100%	82%	82%	100%
Aspirin at Arrival	74	99%	95%	92%	100%
Aspirin at Discharge	40	95%	90%	90%	100%
Beta Blocker at Arrival	59	98%	89%	87%	100%
Beta Blocker at Discharge	42	98%	89%	90%	100%
Fibrinolytic Medication Timing[1]	10	40%	40%	31%	100%
PCI Within 90 Minutes of Arrival	0	-	52%	54%	95%
Smoking Cessation Advice[1]	19	100%	87%	88%	100%
Heart Failure Care					
ACE Inhibitor or ARB for LVSD	47	91%	84%	82%	100%
Discharge Instructions	146	18%	56%	61%	93%
Evaluation of LVS Function	159	67%	84%	83%	99%
Smoking Cessation Advice	35	91%	82%	82%	100%
Pneumonia Care					
Appropriate Initial Antibiotic	112	83%	82%	83%	94%
Blood Culture Timing	95	91%	89%	90%	100%
Influenza Vaccine[4,5]	-	-	58%	70%	100%
Initial Antibiotic Timing	160	80%	75%	80%	93%
Oxygenation Assessment	193	100%	99%	99%	100%
Pneumococcal Vaccine	90	44%	58%	69%	94%
Smoking Cessation Advice	52	90%	75%	80%	100%
Surgical Infection Prevention					
Prophylactic Antibiotic Given	207	53%	74%	77%	95%
Prophylactic Antibiotic Selection	63	89%	89%	90%	100%
Prophylactic Antibiotic Stopped	205	74%	65%	72%	95%
Pregnancy Care					
Inpatient Neonatal Mortality	-	-	-	-	-
Third or Fourth Degree Laceration	-	-	3.58%	3.63%	3.27%

Mammoth Hospital

Alternate Name: Centinela Mammoth Hospital
85 Sierra Park Road
PO Box 660
Mammoth Lakes, CA 93546
E-mail: hillmo@mammothhospital.com
URL: www.mammothhospital.com
Ownership: Govt - Hospital District or Authority
Emergency Services: Yes

Phone: 760-934-3311
Fax: 760-924-4006
Accredited: No
Licensed Beds: 15

Key Personnel:

CEO. . . . . Gary Myers
Chief Medical Staff . . . . . Kyle Howell, MD
Emergency Room . . . . . Chris Hummel, MD
Infection Control . . . . . Antonette Ciccarelli, MD
Director Medical/Surgical Nursing . . . . . Lori Pernerilli, RN
Chief Radiology . . . . . Ronald Frug, MD
Director Respiratory Therapy . . . . . Christie McMillan, RT

Measure	Cases	This Hospital	State Average	U.S. Average	Top Hospital
Heart Attack Care					
ACE Inhibitor or ARB for LVSD[5]	-	-	82%	82%	100%
Aspirin at Arrival[5]	-	-	95%	92%	100%
Aspirin at Discharge[5]	-	-	90%	90%	100%
Beta Blocker at Arrival[5]	-	-	89%	87%	100%
Beta Blocker at Discharge[5]	-	-	89%	90%	100%
Fibrinolytic Medication Timing[5]	-	-	40%	31%	100%
PCI Within 90 Minutes of Arrival[5]	-	-	52%	54%	95%
Smoking Cessation Advice[5]	-	-	87%	88%	100%
Heart Failure Care					
ACE Inhibitor or ARB for LVSD[3]	0	-	84%	82%	100%
Discharge Instructions[1,3]	1	0%	56%	61%	93%
Evaluation of LVS Function[1,3]	1	0%	84%	83%	99%
Smoking Cessation Advice[3]	0	-	82%	82%	100%
Pneumonia Care					
Appropriate Initial Antibiotic[5]	-	-	82%	83%	94%
Blood Culture Timing[5]	-	-	89%	90%	100%
Influenza Vaccine[5]	-	-	58%	70%	100%
Initial Antibiotic Timing[5]	-	-	75%	80%	93%
Oxygenation Assessment[5]	-	-	99%	99%	100%
Pneumococcal Vaccine[5]	-	-	58%	69%	94%
Smoking Cessation Advice[5]	-	-	75%	80%	100%
Surgical Infection Prevention					
Prophylactic Antibiotic Given[5]	-	-	74%	77%	95%
Prophylactic Antibiotic Selection[5]	-	-	89%	90%	100%
Prophylactic Antibiotic Stopped[5]	-	-	65%	72%	95%
Pregnancy Care					
Inpatient Neonatal Mortality	-	-	-	-	-
Third or Fourth Degree Laceration	-	-	3.58%	3.63%	3.27%

Doctors Hospital of Manteca

1205 E N Street
Manteca, CA 95336
E-mail: gregg.bixel@tenethelp.com
URL: www.doctorsmanteca.com
Ownership: Proprietary
Emergency Services: Yes

Phone: 209-823-3111
Fax: 209-824-4907
Accredited: Yes
Licensed Beds: 73

Key Personnel:

CEO. . . . . Katherine Medeiros
Chief Medical Staff . . . . . Michael Davis, MD
Emergency Room . . . . . Amy Alillaroya
Emergency Room . . . . . Susan Pepe, RN
Director Medical/Surgical Nursing . . . . . Jan Gambs
Director of Pulmonary Therapy. . . . . D Lammey

Measure	Cases	This Hospital	State Average	U.S. Average	Top Hospital
Heart Attack Care					
ACE Inhibitor or ARB for LVSD[1]	1	100%	82%	82%	100%
Aspirin at Arrival	36	94%	95%	92%	100%
Aspirin at Discharge[1]	16	94%	90%	90%	100%
Beta Blocker at Arrival	33	94%	89%	87%	100%
Beta Blocker at Discharge[1]	17	94%	89%	90%	100%
Fibrinolytic Medication Timing[1]	4	25%	40%	31%	100%
PCI Within 90 Minutes of Arrival	0	-	52%	54%	95%
Smoking Cessation Advice[1]	3	100%	87%	88%	100%
Heart Failure Care					
ACE Inhibitor or ARB for LVSD	30	100%	84%	82%	100%
Discharge Instructions	90	93%	56%	61%	93%
Evaluation of LVS Function	105	93%	84%	83%	99%
Smoking Cessation Advice[1]	23	100%	82%	82%	100%
Pneumonia Care					
Appropriate Initial Antibiotic	108	85%	82%	83%	94%
Blood Culture Timing	96	89%	89%	90%	100%
Influenza Vaccine	34	85%	58%	70%	100%
Initial Antibiotic Timing	141	87%	75%	80%	93%
Oxygenation Assessment	161	100%	99%	99%	100%
Pneumococcal Vaccine	95	93%	58%	69%	94%
Smoking Cessation Advice	38	95%	75%	80%	100%
Surgical Infection Prevention					
Prophylactic Antibiotic Given[2]	115	83%	74%	77%	95%
Prophylactic Antibiotic Selection[2]	32	94%	89%	90%	100%
Prophylactic Antibiotic Stopped[2]	113	79%	65%	72%	95%
Pregnancy Care					
Inpatient Neonatal Mortality	-	-	-	-	-
Third or Fourth Degree Laceration	-	-	3.58%	3.63%	3.27%

NOTE: Hospital profiles are in alphabetical order by state, then city, then hospital within the city; Rankings are sorted by rate in descending order and exclude hospitals with less than 25 cases; (1) The number of cases is too small (n<25) for purposes of reliably predicting hospital performance; (2) Measure reflects the hospital's indication that its submission was based upon a sample of its relevant discharges; (3) Rate reflects fewer than the maximum possible quarters of data for the measure; (4) Inaccurate information submitted and suppressed for one or more quarters; (5) No data is available from the hospital for this measure; Please refer to the User's Guide for a full explanation of data

Kaiser Foundation Hospital-Manteca

1777 West Yosemite Ave Phone: 209-825-3700
Manteca, CA 95337
Ownership: Voluntary non-profit - Private Accredited: Yes
Emergency Services: Yes

Measure	Cases	This Hospital	State Average	U.S. Average	Top Hospital
Heart Attack Care					
ACE Inhibitor or ARB for LVSD[1]	9	89%	82%	82%	100%
Aspirin at Arrival	49	96%	95%	92%	100%
Aspirin at Discharge	37	97%	90%	90%	100%
Beta Blocker at Arrival	39	87%	89%	87%	100%
Beta Blocker at Discharge	35	97%	89%	90%	100%
Fibrinolytic Medication Timing[1]	3	67%	40%	31%	100%
PCI Within 90 Minutes of Arrival	0	-	52%	54%	95%
Smoking Cessation Advice[1]	9	78%	87%	88%	100%
Heart Failure Care					
ACE Inhibitor or ARB for LVSD	56	93%	84%	82%	100%
Discharge Instructions	152	16%	56%	61%	93%
Evaluation of LVS Function	181	94%	84%	83%	99%
Smoking Cessation Advice[1]	22	86%	82%	82%	100%
Pneumonia Care					
Appropriate Initial Antibiotic	113	81%	82%	83%	94%
Blood Culture Timing	100	83%	89%	90%	100%
Influenza Vaccine	34	44%	58%	70%	100%
Initial Antibiotic Timing	119	72%	75%	80%	93%
Oxygenation Assessment	164	100%	99%	99%	100%
Pneumococcal Vaccine	106	59%	58%	69%	94%
Smoking Cessation Advice	46	72%	75%	80%	100%
Surgical Infection Prevention					
Prophylactic Antibiotic Given	114	62%	74%	77%	95%
Prophylactic Antibiotic Selection[1]	14	100%	89%	90%	100%
Prophylactic Antibiotic Stopped	113	66%	65%	72%	95%
Pregnancy Care					
Inpatient Neonatal Mortality	-	-	-	-	-
Third or Fourth Degree Laceration	-	-	3.58%	3.63%	3.27%

Centinela Freeman Reg Med Ctr-Marina

4650 Lincoln Blvd Phone: 310-823-8911
Marina Del Rey, CA 90291
Ownership: Proprietary Accredited: Yes
Emergency Services: Yes

Measure	Cases	This Hospital	State Average	U.S. Average	Top Hospital
Heart Attack Care					
ACE Inhibitor or ARB for LVSD	0	-	82%	82%	100%
Aspirin at Arrival	28	96%	95%	92%	100%
Aspirin at Discharge[1]	11	100%	90%	90%	100%
Beta Blocker at Arrival[1]	22	86%	89%	87%	100%
Beta Blocker at Discharge[1]	9	89%	89%	90%	100%
Fibrinolytic Medication Timing[1]	2	0%	40%	31%	100%
PCI Within 90 Minutes of Arrival	0	-	52%	54%	95%
Smoking Cessation Advice[1]	1	100%	87%	88%	100%
Heart Failure Care					
ACE Inhibitor or ARB for LVSD	27	93%	84%	82%	100%
Discharge Instructions	102	32%	56%	61%	93%
Evaluation of LVS Function	123	86%	84%	83%	99%
Smoking Cessation Advice[1]	11	91%	82%	82%	100%
Pneumonia Care					
Appropriate Initial Antibiotic	83	93%	82%	83%	94%
Blood Culture Timing	39	87%	89%	90%	100%
Influenza Vaccine[1]	16	56%	58%	70%	100%
Initial Antibiotic Timing	88	73%	75%	80%	93%
Oxygenation Assessment	98	98%	99%	99%	100%
Pneumococcal Vaccine	60	67%	58%	69%	94%
Smoking Cessation Advice[1]	11	100%	75%	80%	100%
Surgical Infection Prevention					
Prophylactic Antibiotic Given	72	88%	74%	77%	95%
Prophylactic Antibiotic Selection[1]	19	95%	89%	90%	100%
Prophylactic Antibiotic Stopped	69	54%	65%	72%	95%
Pregnancy Care					
Inpatient Neonatal Mortality	-	-	-	-	-
Third or Fourth Degree Laceration	-	-	3.58%	3.63%	3.27%

John C Fremont Healthcare District

Alternate Name: John C Fremont Hospital
5189 Hospital Road Phone: 209-966-3631
PO Box 216 Fax: 209-966-3776
Mariposa, CA 95338
E-mail: jcfadm@jcfhospital.com
URL: www.jcfhospital.com
Ownership: Govt - Hospital District or Authority Accredited: No
Emergency Services: Yes Licensed Beds: 34
Key Personnel:
Administrator/CEO/CFO. . . . . Elnora George
Chief Medical Staff. . . . . Joseph Rogers
Emergency Room . . . . G McCallum, MD
Director Infection/Disease Control . . . . Theresa Loya
Respiratory/Cardiopulmonary. . . . . Chris Miller

Measure	Cases	This Hospital	State Average	U.S. Average	Top Hospital
Heart Attack Care					
ACE Inhibitor or ARB for LVSD[5]	-	-	82%	82%	100%
Aspirin at Arrival[5]	-	-	95%	92%	100%
Aspirin at Discharge[5]	-	-	90%	90%	100%
Beta Blocker at Arrival[5]	-	-	89%	87%	100%
Beta Blocker at Discharge[5]	-	-	89%	90%	100%
Fibrinolytic Medication Timing[5]	-	-	40%	31%	100%
PCI Within 90 Minutes of Arrival[5]	-	-	52%	54%	95%
Smoking Cessation Advice[5]	-	-	87%	88%	100%
Heart Failure Care					
ACE Inhibitor or ARB for LVSD[5]	-	-	84%	82%	100%
Discharge Instructions[5]	-	-	56%	61%	93%
Evaluation of LVS Function[5]	-	-	84%	83%	99%
Smoking Cessation Advice[5]	-	-	82%	82%	100%
Pneumonia Care					
Appropriate Initial Antibiotic[5]	-	-	82%	83%	94%
Blood Culture Timing[5]	-	-	89%	90%	100%
Influenza Vaccine[5]	-	-	58%	70%	100%
Initial Antibiotic Timing[5]	-	-	75%	80%	93%
Oxygenation Assessment[5]	-	-	99%	99%	100%
Pneumococcal Vaccine[5]	-	-	58%	69%	94%
Smoking Cessation Advice[5]	-	-	75%	80%	100%
Surgical Infection Prevention					
Prophylactic Antibiotic Given[5]	-	-	74%	77%	95%
Prophylactic Antibiotic Selection[5]	-	-	89%	90%	100%
Prophylactic Antibiotic Stopped[5]	-	-	65%	72%	95%
Pregnancy Care					
Inpatient Neonatal Mortality	-	-	-	-	-
Third or Fourth Degree Laceration	-	-	3.58%	3.63%	3.27%

Contra Costa Regional Medical Center

2500 Alhambra Avenue Phone: 925-370-5000
Martinez, CA 94553 Fax: 925-370-5138
URL: www.cchealth.org/medical-center
Ownership: Government - Local Accredited: Yes
Emergency Services: Yes Licensed Beds: 166

Measure	Cases	This Hospital	State Average	U.S. Average	Top Hospital
Heart Attack Care					
ACE Inhibitor or ARB for LVSD	0	-	82%	82%	100%
Aspirin at Arrival	26	100%	95%	92%	100%
Aspirin at Discharge	25	100%	90%	90%	100%
Beta Blocker at Arrival	25	88%	89%	87%	100%
Beta Blocker at Discharge	25	92%	89%	90%	100%
Fibrinolytic Medication Timing[1,3]	2	50%	40%	31%	100%
PCI Within 90 Minutes of Arrival	0	-	52%	54%	95%
Smoking Cessation Advice[1,3]	5	80%	87%	88%	100%
Heart Failure Care					
ACE Inhibitor or ARB for LVSD	70	96%	84%	82%	100%
Discharge Instructions[3]	25	0%	56%	61%	93%
Evaluation of LVS Function	151	99%	84%	83%	99%
Smoking Cessation Advice[1,3]	11	18%	82%	82%	100%
Pneumonia Care					

NOTE: Hospital profiles are in alphabetical order by state, then city, then hospital within the city; Rankings are sorted by rate in descending order and exclude hospitals with less than 25 cases; (1) The number of cases is too small (n<25) for purposes of reliably predicting hospital performance; (2) Measure reflects the hospital's indication that its submission was based upon a sample of its relevant discharges; (3) Rate reflects fewer than the maximum possible quarters of data for the measure; (4) Inaccurate information submitted and suppressed for one or more quarters; (5) No data is available from the hospital for this measure; Please refer to the User's Guide for a full explanation of data

Appropriate Initial Antibiotic[1,3]	19	84%	82%	83%	94%
Blood Culture Timing[1,3]	23	78%	89%	90%	100%
Influenza Vaccine[5]	-	-	58%	70%	100%
Initial Antibiotic Timing	99	67%	75%	80%	93%
Oxygenation Assessment	117	100%	99%	99%	100%
Pneumococcal Vaccine	46	48%	58%	69%	94%
Smoking Cessation Advice[1,3]	8	50%	75%	80%	100%
Surgical Infection Prevention					
Prophylactic Antibiotic Given[3]	27	78%	74%	77%	95%
Prophylactic Antibiotic Selection[5]	-	-	89%	90%	100%
Prophylactic Antibiotic Stopped[3]	25	68%	65%	72%	95%
Pregnancy Care					
Inpatient Neonatal Mortality	-	-	-	-	-
Third or Fourth Degree Laceration	-	-	3.58%	3.63%	3.27%

Rideout Memorial Hospital

726 4th Street
Marysville, CA 95901
URL: www.frhg.org
Ownership: Voluntary non-profit - Other
Emergency Services: Yes

Phone: 530-749-4300
Fax: 530-751-4226
Accredited: Yes
Licensed Beds: 164

Key Personnel:

CEO . . . . Thomas P Hayes
Chief Medical Staff . . . . Michael Fahey, MD
Chief Radiology . . . . Robert White
Director Respiratory Therapy . . . . Linda Alexander

Measure	Cases	This Hospital	State Average	U.S. Average	Top Hospital
Heart Attack Care					
ACE Inhibitor or ARB for LVSD	53	64%	82%	82%	100%
Aspirin at Arrival	204	99%	95%	92%	100%
Aspirin at Discharge	191	94%	90%	90%	100%
Beta Blocker at Arrival	171	90%	89%	87%	100%
Beta Blocker at Discharge	198	86%	89%	90%	100%
Fibrinolytic Medication Timing[1]	18	33%	40%	31%	100%
PCI Within 90 Minutes of Arrival[1]	3	0%	52%	54%	95%
Smoking Cessation Advice	70	83%	87%	88%	100%
Heart Failure Care					
ACE Inhibitor or ARB for LVSD	147	84%	84%	82%	100%
Discharge Instructions	372	13%	56%	61%	93%
Evaluation of LVS Function	415	84%	84%	83%	99%
Smoking Cessation Advice	84	61%	82%	82%	100%
Pneumonia Care					
Appropriate Initial Antibiotic	293	73%	82%	83%	94%
Blood Culture Timing	184	86%	89%	90%	100%
Influenza Vaccine[4,5]	-	-	58%	70%	100%
Initial Antibiotic Timing	353	68%	75%	80%	93%
Oxygenation Assessment	400	98%	99%	99%	100%
Pneumococcal Vaccine	279	37%	58%	69%	94%
Smoking Cessation Advice	126	56%	75%	80%	100%
Surgical Infection Prevention					
Prophylactic Antibiotic Given[2]	269	77%	74%	77%	95%
Prophylactic Antibiotic Selection[2]	68	97%	89%	90%	100%
Prophylactic Antibiotic Stopped[2]	237	68%	65%	72%	95%
Pregnancy Care					
Inpatient Neonatal Mortality	-	-	-	-	-
Third or Fourth Degree Laceration	-	-	3.58%	3.63%	3.27%

Mercy Med Ctr Merced-Community Campus

Alternate Name: Merced Community Medical Center
301 E 13th Street
Merced, CA 95340
URL: www.mercymercedcares.org
Ownership: Government - Local
Emergency Services: Yes

Phone: 209-385-7100
Fax: 209-385-7062
Accredited: Yes
Licensed Beds: 174

Key Personnel:

President . . . . David S Dunham
Chief of Medical Staff . . . . Lynn Cooman
Chief Radiology . . . . Duane Richey, MD
Director Respiratory Therapy . . . . Adam William

Measure	Cases	This Hospital	State Average	U.S. Average	Top Hospital
Heart Attack Care					
ACE Inhibitor or ARB for LVSD[1]	8	88%	82%	82%	100%
Aspirin at Arrival	101	95%	95%	92%	100%
Aspirin at Discharge	46	91%	90%	90%	100%
Beta Blocker at Arrival	95	100%	89%	87%	100%
Beta Blocker at Discharge	53	94%	89%	90%	100%
Fibrinolytic Medication Timing[1]	10	20%	40%	31%	100%
PCI Within 90 Minutes of Arrival	0	-	52%	54%	95%
Smoking Cessation Advice[1]	11	82%	87%	88%	100%
Heart Failure Care					
ACE Inhibitor or ARB for LVSD[2]	110	90%	84%	82%	100%
Discharge Instructions[2]	247	84%	56%	61%	93%
Evaluation of LVS Function[2]	285	92%	84%	83%	99%
Smoking Cessation Advice[2]	72	99%	82%	82%	100%
Pneumonia Care					
Appropriate Initial Antibiotic[2]	92	86%	82%	83%	94%
Blood Culture Timing[2]	65	95%	89%	90%	100%
Influenza Vaccine[1,2]	21	29%	58%	70%	100%
Initial Antibiotic Timing[2]	129	78%	75%	80%	93%
Oxygenation Assessment[2]	171	100%	99%	99%	100%
Pneumococcal Vaccine[2]	100	74%	58%	69%	94%
Smoking Cessation Advice[2]	35	94%	75%	80%	100%
Surgical Infection Prevention					
Prophylactic Antibiotic Given[2,3]	140	74%	74%	77%	95%
Prophylactic Antibiotic Selection[2]	41	88%	89%	90%	100%
Prophylactic Antibiotic Stopped[2,3]	133	48%	65%	72%	95%
Pregnancy Care					
Inpatient Neonatal Mortality	2,764	0.07%	-	-	-
Third or Fourth Degree Laceration	2,072	3.38%	3.58%	3.63%	3.27%

Providence Holy Cross Medical Center

Alternate Name: Holy Cross Medical Center
15031 Rinaldi Street
Mission Hills, CA 91346
URL: www.providence.org
Ownership: Voluntary non-profit - Church
Emergency Services: Yes

Phone: 818-365-8051
Fax: 818-898-4569
Accredited: Yes
Licensed Beds: 254

Key Personnel:

Administrator . . . . Kerry Carmody
Chief Medical Staff . . . . Robert Titcher, MD
Emergency Room . . . . Linda Coale, RN

Measure	Cases	This Hospital	State Average	U.S. Average	Top Hospital
Heart Attack Care					
ACE Inhibitor or ARB for LVSD[2]	39	92%	82%	82%	100%
Aspirin at Arrival[2]	165	100%	95%	92%	100%
Aspirin at Discharge[2]	200	98%	90%	90%	100%
Beta Blocker at Arrival[2]	116	97%	89%	87%	100%
Beta Blocker at Discharge[2]	204	97%	89%	90%	100%
Fibrinolytic Medication Timing[2]	0	-	40%	31%	100%
PCI Within 90 Minutes of Arrival[1,2]	13	69%	52%	54%	95%
Smoking Cessation Advice[2]	64	94%	87%	88%	100%
Heart Failure Care					
ACE Inhibitor or ARB for LVSD[2]	102	87%	84%	82%	100%
Discharge Instructions[2]	251	45%	56%	61%	93%
Evaluation of LVS Function[2]	313	98%	84%	83%	99%
Smoking Cessation Advice[2]	35	94%	82%	82%	100%
Pneumonia Care					
Appropriate Initial Antibiotic[2]	109	90%	82%	83%	94%
Blood Culture Timing[2]	165	96%	89%	90%	100%
Influenza Vaccine	32	62%	58%	70%	100%
Initial Antibiotic Timing[2]	194	86%	75%	80%	93%
Oxygenation Assessment[2]	236	100%	99%	99%	100%
Pneumococcal Vaccine[2]	165	81%	58%	69%	94%
Smoking Cessation Advice[2]	46	85%	75%	80%	100%
Surgical Infection Prevention					
Prophylactic Antibiotic Given[2]	297	94%	74%	77%	95%
Prophylactic Antibiotic Selection[2]	76	96%	89%	90%	100%
Prophylactic Antibiotic Stopped[2]	273	54%	65%	72%	95%
Pregnancy Care					
Inpatient Neonatal Mortality	-	-	-	-	-
Third or Fourth Degree Laceration	-	-	3.58%	3.63%	3.27%

NOTE: Hospital profiles are in alphabetical order by state, then city, then hospital within the city; Rankings are sorted by rate in descending order and exclude hospitals with less than 25 cases; (1) The number of cases is too small (n<25) for purposes of reliably predicting hospital performance; (2) Measure reflects the hospital's indication that its submission was based upon a sample of its relevant discharges; (3) Rate reflects fewer than the maximum possible quarters of data for the measure; (4) Inaccurate information submitted and suppressed for one or more quarters; (5) No data is available from the hospital for this measure; Please refer to the User's Guide for a full explanation of data

Mission Hospital Regional Medical Center

27700 Medical Center Road
Mission Viejo, CA 92691
URL: www.mission4health.com
Ownership: Proprietary
Emergency Services: Yes
Phone: 818-787-2222
Fax: 818-904-3529
Accredited: Yes
Licensed Beds: 331

Key Personnel:
CEO. . . . . Peter Bastone
Director Medical/Surgical Nursing . . . . Jeanne Caldwell

Measure	Cases	This Hospital	State Average	U.S. Average	Top Hospital
Heart Attack Care					
ACE Inhibitor or ARB for LVSD	29	100%	82%	82%	100%
Aspirin at Arrival	278	99%	95%	92%	100%
Aspirin at Discharge	254	99%	90%	90%	100%
Beta Blocker at Arrival	188	90%	89%	87%	100%
Beta Blocker at Discharge	240	98%	89%	90%	100%
Fibrinolytic Medication Timing	0	-	40%	31%	100%
PCI Within 90 Minutes of Arrival[1]	16	62%	52%	54%	95%
Smoking Cessation Advice	46	100%	87%	88%	100%
Heart Failure Care					
ACE Inhibitor or ARB for LVSD	83	93%	84%	82%	100%
Discharge Instructions	243	83%	56%	61%	93%
Evaluation of LVS Function	283	98%	84%	83%	99%
Smoking Cessation Advice	32	97%	82%	82%	100%
Pneumonia Care					
Appropriate Initial Antibiotic	175	83%	82%	83%	94%
Blood Culture Timing	160	94%	89%	90%	100%
Influenza Vaccine	51	75%	58%	70%	100%
Initial Antibiotic Timing	217	74%	75%	80%	93%
Oxygenation Assessment	279	100%	99%	99%	100%
Pneumococcal Vaccine	180	72%	58%	69%	94%
Smoking Cessation Advice	40	68%	75%	80%	100%
Surgical Infection Prevention					
Prophylactic Antibiotic Given[2,3]	186	85%	74%	77%	95%
Prophylactic Antibiotic Selection[2]	62	94%	89%	90%	100%
Prophylactic Antibiotic Stopped[2,3]	186	75%	65%	72%	95%
Pregnancy Care					
Inpatient Neonatal Mortality	-	-	-	-	-
Third or Fourth Degree Laceration	-	-	3.58%	3.63%	3.27%

Doctors Medical Center

Alternate Name: Modesto City Hospital
1441 Florida Avenue
Modesto, CA 95350
E-mail: catherine.larson@tenethealth.com
URL: www.dmc-modesto.com
Ownership: Proprietary
Emergency Services: Yes
Phone: 209-578-1211
Fax: 209-342-3123
Accredited: Yes
Licensed Beds: 397

Key Personnel:
CEO. . . . . Tim Joslin
Director Emergency Services. . . . . Laura List
Director Surgical Services . . . . Syd Fuentes
Director Radiology . . . . Roberta Edge

Measure	Cases	This Hospital	State Average	U.S. Average	Top Hospital
Heart Attack Care					
ACE Inhibitor or ARB for LVSD	75	97%	82%	82%	100%
Aspirin at Arrival	192	98%	95%	92%	100%
Aspirin at Discharge	364	98%	90%	90%	100%
Beta Blocker at Arrival	163	96%	89%	87%	100%
Beta Blocker at Discharge	348	97%	89%	90%	100%
Fibrinolytic Medication Timing[1]	9	22%	40%	31%	100%
PCI Within 90 Minutes of Arrival[1]	11	27%	52%	54%	95%
Smoking Cessation Advice	119	100%	87%	88%	100%
Heart Failure Care					
ACE Inhibitor or ARB for LVSD	165	95%	84%	82%	100%
Discharge Instructions	350	90%	56%	61%	93%
Evaluation of LVS Function	422	95%	84%	83%	99%
Smoking Cessation Advice	105	96%	82%	82%	100%
Pneumonia Care					
Appropriate Initial Antibiotic	299	92%	82%	83%	94%
Blood Culture Timing	360	92%	89%	90%	100%
Influenza Vaccine	102	82%	58%	70%	100%
Initial Antibiotic Timing	436	70%	75%	80%	93%
Oxygenation Assessment	560	100%	99%	99%	100%
Pneumococcal Vaccine	292	89%	58%	69%	94%
Smoking Cessation Advice	157	92%	75%	80%	100%
Surgical Infection Prevention					
Prophylactic Antibiotic Given[2]	607	75%	74%	77%	95%
Prophylactic Antibiotic Selection[2]	192	79%	89%	90%	100%
Prophylactic Antibiotic Stopped[2]	578	73%	65%	72%	95%
Pregnancy Care					
Inpatient Neonatal Mortality	-	-	-	-	-
Third or Fourth Degree Laceration	-	-	3.58%	3.63%	3.27%

Memorial Medical Center

1700 Coffee Road
Modesto, CA 95355
URL: www.memorialmedicalcenter.org
Ownership: Voluntary non-profit - Other
Emergency Services: Yes
Phone: 209-526-4500
Fax: 209-576-7385
Accredited: Yes
Licensed Beds: 112

Key Personnel:
CEO. . . . . David P Benn

Measure	Cases	This Hospital	State Average	U.S. Average	Top Hospital
Heart Attack Care					
ACE Inhibitor or ARB for LVSD	52	77%	82%	82%	100%
Aspirin at Arrival	224	94%	95%	92%	100%
Aspirin at Discharge	264	98%	90%	90%	100%
Beta Blocker at Arrival	170	90%	89%	87%	100%
Beta Blocker at Discharge	287	99%	89%	90%	100%
Fibrinolytic Medication Timing[1]	6	50%	40%	31%	100%
PCI Within 90 Minutes of Arrival[1]	7	71%	52%	54%	95%
Smoking Cessation Advice	118	98%	87%	88%	100%
Heart Failure Care					
ACE Inhibitor or ARB for LVSD[2]	153	82%	84%	82%	100%
Discharge Instructions[2]	331	55%	56%	61%	93%
Evaluation of LVS Function[2]	388	91%	84%	83%	99%
Smoking Cessation Advice[2]	76	92%	82%	82%	100%
Pneumonia Care					
Appropriate Initial Antibiotic[2]	104	88%	82%	83%	94%
Blood Culture Timing[2]	110	78%	89%	90%	100%
Influenza Vaccine[2]	35	74%	58%	70%	100%
Initial Antibiotic Timing[2]	163	67%	75%	80%	93%
Oxygenation Assessment[2]	197	99%	99%	99%	100%
Pneumococcal Vaccine[2]	120	67%	58%	69%	94%
Smoking Cessation Advice[2]	51	84%	75%	80%	100%
Surgical Infection Prevention					
Prophylactic Antibiotic Given[2]	351	58%	74%	77%	95%
Prophylactic Antibiotic Selection[2]	78	90%	89%	90%	100%
Prophylactic Antibiotic Stopped[2]	344	56%	65%	72%	95%
Pregnancy Care					
Inpatient Neonatal Mortality	-	-	-	-	-
Third or Fourth Degree Laceration	-	-	3.58%	3.63%	3.27%

Stanislaus Surgical Hospital

1421 Oakdale Road
Modesto, CA 95355
Ownership: Proprietary
Emergency Services: No
Phone: 209-572-2700
Accredited: No

Key Personnel:
CEO. . . . . Michael J Lipomi

Measure	Cases	This Hospital	State Average	U.S. Average	Top Hospital
Heart Attack Care					
ACE Inhibitor or ARB for LVSD[5]	-	-	82%	82%	100%
Aspirin at Arrival[5]	-	-	95%	92%	100%
Aspirin at Discharge[5]	-	-	90%	90%	100%
Beta Blocker at Arrival[5]	-	-	89%	87%	100%
Beta Blocker at Discharge[5]	-	-	89%	90%	100%
Fibrinolytic Medication Timing[5]	-	-	40%	31%	100%
PCI Within 90 Minutes of Arrival[5]	-	-	52%	54%	95%
Smoking Cessation Advice[5]	-	-	87%	88%	100%
Heart Failure Care					

NOTE: Hospital profiles are in alphabetical order by state, then city, then hospital within the city; Rankings are sorted by rate in descending order and exclude hospitals with less than 25 cases; (1) The number of cases is too small (n<25) for purposes of reliably predicting hospital performance; (2) Measure reflects the hospital's indication that its submission was based upon a sample of its relevant discharges; (3) Rate reflects fewer than the maximum possible quarters of data for the measure; (4) Inaccurate information submitted and suppressed for one or more quarters; (5) No data is available from the hospital for this measure; Please refer to the User's Guide for a full explanation of data

ACE Inhibitor or ARB for LVSD[5]	-	-	84%	82%	100%
Discharge Instructions[5]	-	-	56%	61%	93%
Evaluation of LVS Function[5]	-	-	84%	83%	99%
Smoking Cessation Advice[5]	-	-	82%	82%	100%
Pneumonia Care					
Appropriate Initial Antibiotic[5]	-	-	82%	83%	94%
Blood Culture Timing[5]	-	-	89%	90%	100%
Influenza Vaccine[5]	-	-	58%	70%	100%
Initial Antibiotic Timing[5]	-	-	75%	80%	93%
Oxygenation Assessment[5]	-	-	99%	99%	100%
Pneumococcal Vaccine[5]	-	-	58%	69%	94%
Smoking Cessation Advice[5]	-	-	75%	80%	100%
Surgical Infection Prevention					
Prophylactic Antibiotic Given[2,3]	35	77%	74%	77%	95%
Prophylactic Antibiotic Selection[5]	-	-	89%	90%	100%
Prophylactic Antibiotic Stopped[2,3]	35	74%	65%	72%	95%
Pregnancy Care					
Inpatient Neonatal Mortality	-	-	-	-	-
Third or Fourth Degree Laceration	-	-	3.58%	3.63%	3.27%

Beverly Hospital

309 West Beverly Boulevard
Montebello, CA 90640
URL: www.beverly.org
Phone: 323-726-1222
Fax: 323-837-3481
Ownership: Voluntary non-profit - Private
Emergency Services: Yes
Accredited: Yes
Licensed Beds: 223

Key Personnel:

President/CEO. . . . . Gary V Kiff
Director Catheterization Lab. . . . . Ruth Johnson, RN
Director Emergency Room. . . . . Karen Rodgers, RN
Emergency Room . . . . John Uphold, MD
Director Intensive Coronary Care. . . . . Ruth Johnson, RN
Director Medical/Surgical Nursing . . . . Lynda Mansfield, RN
Manager OB/GYN Womens Health . . . . Kristie Beach, RN
Director Radiology . . . . Rick McLaughlin
Director Respiratory Therapy. . . . . Carlos Garza

Measure	Cases	This Hospital	State Average	U.S. Average	Top Hospital
Heart Attack Care					
ACE Inhibitor or ARB for LVSD	28	82%	82%	82%	100%
Aspirin at Arrival	139	94%	95%	92%	100%
Aspirin at Discharge	113	99%	90%	90%	100%
Beta Blocker at Arrival	111	95%	89%	87%	100%
Beta Blocker at Discharge	103	94%	89%	90%	100%
Fibrinolytic Medication Timing[1]	2	50%	40%	31%	100%
PCI Within 90 Minutes of Arrival[1]	3	67%	52%	54%	95%
Smoking Cessation Advice[1]	22	100%	87%	88%	100%
Heart Failure Care					
ACE Inhibitor or ARB for LVSD	127	71%	84%	82%	100%
Discharge Instructions	308	40%	56%	61%	93%
Evaluation of LVS Function	385	94%	84%	83%	99%
Smoking Cessation Advice	36	100%	82%	82%	100%
Pneumonia Care					
Appropriate Initial Antibiotic	200	85%	82%	83%	94%
Blood Culture Timing	195	89%	89%	90%	100%
Influenza Vaccine	62	71%	58%	70%	100%
Initial Antibiotic Timing	328	70%	75%	80%	93%
Oxygenation Assessment	340	99%	99%	99%	100%
Pneumococcal Vaccine	224	71%	58%	69%	94%
Smoking Cessation Advice	26	100%	75%	80%	100%
Surgical Infection Prevention					
Prophylactic Antibiotic Given[3]	269	68%	74%	77%	95%
Prophylactic Antibiotic Selection	98	98%	89%	90%	100%
Prophylactic Antibiotic Stopped[3]	263	50%	65%	72%	95%
Pregnancy Care					
Inpatient Neonatal Mortality	-	-	-	-	-
Third or Fourth Degree Laceration	-	-	3.58%	3.63%	3.27%

Community Hospital of the Monterey Peninsula

23625 Holman Highway
PO Box HH
Monterey, CA 93942
E-mail: information@chomp.org
URL: www.chomp.org
Phone: 831-624-5311
Fax: 831-624-0497
Ownership: Voluntary non-profit - Private
Emergency Services: Yes
Accredited: Yes
Licensed Beds: 205

Key Personnel:

CEO. . . . . Steven J Packer, MD
Chief of Medical Staff. . . . . Dr Anthony Chavis
Emergency Room . . . . Jodi Schafer

Measure	Cases	This Hospital	State Average	U.S. Average	Top Hospital
Heart Attack Care					
ACE Inhibitor or ARB for LVSD[1]	24	83%	82%	82%	100%
Aspirin at Arrival	138	96%	95%	92%	100%
Aspirin at Discharge	85	84%	90%	90%	100%
Beta Blocker at Arrival	93	95%	89%	87%	100%
Beta Blocker at Discharge	74	96%	89%	90%	100%
Fibrinolytic Medication Timing[3]	0	-	40%	31%	100%
PCI Within 90 Minutes of Arrival[1]	5	60%	52%	54%	95%
Smoking Cessation Advice[1,3]	3	100%	87%	88%	100%
Heart Failure Care					
ACE Inhibitor or ARB for LVSD	91	70%	84%	82%	100%
Discharge Instructions[3]	56	70%	56%	61%	93%
Evaluation of LVS Function	282	92%	84%	83%	99%
Smoking Cessation Advice[1,3]	11	100%	82%	82%	100%
Pneumonia Care					
Appropriate Initial Antibiotic[1,3]	21	76%	82%	83%	94%
Blood Culture Timing[1,3]	24	100%	89%	90%	100%
Influenza Vaccine[5]	-	-	58%	70%	100%
Initial Antibiotic Timing	152	78%	75%	80%	93%
Oxygenation Assessment	205	100%	99%	99%	100%
Pneumococcal Vaccine	147	88%	58%	69%	94%
Smoking Cessation Advice[1,3]	2	100%	75%	80%	100%
Surgical Infection Prevention					
Prophylactic Antibiotic Given[3]	191	87%	74%	77%	95%
Prophylactic Antibiotic Selection[5]	-	-	89%	90%	100%
Prophylactic Antibiotic Stopped[3]	188	73%	65%	72%	95%
Pregnancy Care					
Inpatient Neonatal Mortality	-	-	-	-	-
Third or Fourth Degree Laceration	-	-	3.58%	3.63%	3.27%

Garfield Medical Center

525 N Garfield Avenue
Monterey Park, CA 91754
URL: www.garfieldmedicalcenter.com
Phone: 626-573-2222
Fax: 626-571-8972
Ownership: Proprietary
Emergency Services: Yes
Accredited: Yes
Licensed Beds: 210

Key Personnel:

CEO. . . . . Philip A Cohen
Chief Medical Staff. . . . . Tim Ker
Director Emergency Room. . . . . Saskia Dekoomen
Director Infection Control . . . . Alicia Pettles
Director Medical/Surgical Nursing . . . . Chanju Yoo
Director Surgery. . . . . Un Hee Song
Chief Radiology . . . . Gordon Boroditsky

Measure	Cases	This Hospital	State Average	U.S. Average	Top Hospital
Heart Attack Care					
ACE Inhibitor or ARB for LVSD[1,2]	23	74%	82%	82%	100%
Aspirin at Arrival[2]	123	90%	95%	92%	100%
Aspirin at Discharge[2]	126	83%	90%	90%	100%
Beta Blocker at Arrival[2]	85	80%	89%	87%	100%
Beta Blocker at Discharge[2]	115	77%	89%	90%	100%
Fibrinolytic Medication Timing[1,2]	1	0%	40%	31%	100%
PCI Within 90 Minutes of Arrival[1,2]	3	33%	52%	54%	95%
Smoking Cessation Advice[1,2]	21	86%	87%	88%	100%
Heart Failure Care					
ACE Inhibitor or ARB for LVSD[2]	64	50%	84%	82%	100%
Discharge Instructions[2]	260	45%	56%	61%	93%
Evaluation of LVS Function[2]	295	79%	84%	83%	99%

NOTE: Hospital profiles are in alphabetical order by state, then city, then hospital within the city; Rankings are sorted by rate in descending order and exclude hospitals with less than 25 cases; (1) The number of cases is too small (n<25) for purposes of reliably predicting hospital performance; (2) Measure reflects the hospital's indication that its submission was based upon a sample of its relevant discharges; (3) Rate reflects fewer than the maximum possible quarters of data for the measure; (4) Inaccurate information submitted and suppressed for one or more quarters; (5) No data is available from the hospital for this measure; Please refer to the User's Guide for a full explanation of data

Measure	Cases	This Hospital	State Average	U.S. Average	Top Hospital
Smoking Cessation Advice[1,2]	9	100%	82%	82%	100%
Pneumonia Care					
Appropriate Initial Antibiotic[2]	103	79%	82%	83%	94%
Blood Culture Timing[2]	95	88%	89%	90%	100%
Influenza Vaccine[1]	18	94%	58%	70%	100%
Initial Antibiotic Timing[2]	149	79%	75%	80%	93%
Oxygenation Assessment[2]	177	100%	99%	99%	100%
Pneumococcal Vaccine[2]	124	76%	58%	69%	94%
Smoking Cessation Advice[1,2]	11	91%	75%	80%	100%
Surgical Infection Prevention					
Prophylactic Antibiotic Given[2]	198	70%	74%	77%	95%
Prophylactic Antibiotic Selection[2]	52	92%	89%	90%	100%
Prophylactic Antibiotic Stopped[2]	190	24%	65%	72%	95%
Pregnancy Care					
Inpatient Neonatal Mortality	-	-	-	-	-
Third or Fourth Degree Laceration	-	-	3.58%	3.63%	3.27%

Monterey Park Hospital

900 South Atlantic Boulevard Phone: 626-570-9000
Monterey Park, CA 91754 Fax: 626-281-4719
URL: www.montereyparkhosp.com
Ownership: Proprietary Accredited: Yes
Emergency Services: Yes Licensed Beds: 101

Key Personnel:

CEO . . . . . Philip A Cohen
Cardiac Lab . . . . . Remedio Raguiza, MD
Catheterization Lab . . . . . Richard Garrovillo
Emergency Room . . . . . Ewa Hunter
Chief Emergency . . . . . Joe Englanoff
Infection Control . . . . . Sheila Segura
ICU . . . . . Jeanie Cervantes, RN
Intensive Coronary . . . . . Jeanie Cervantes, RN
Medical Surgical Nursing . . . . . Bert Basconcillo, RN
Chief OB/GYN . . . . . Margaret Warez, MD
Respiratory/Cardiopulmonary . . . . . Richard Garrorillo

Measure	Cases	This Hospital	State Average	U.S. Average	Top Hospital
Heart Attack Care					
ACE Inhibitor or ARB for LVSD[1,2]	8	75%	82%	82%	100%
Aspirin at Arrival[2]	45	87%	95%	92%	100%
Aspirin at Discharge[1,2]	19	68%	90%	90%	100%
Beta Blocker at Arrival[2]	41	66%	89%	87%	100%
Beta Blocker at Discharge[1,2]	20	60%	89%	90%	100%
Fibrinolytic Medication Timing[1,2]	3	33%	40%	31%	100%
PCI Within 90 Minutes of Arrival[2]	0	-	52%	54%	95%
Smoking Cessation Advice[1,2]	3	100%	87%	88%	100%
Heart Failure Care					
ACE Inhibitor or ARB for LVSD[2]	76	59%	84%	82%	100%
Discharge Instructions[2]	193	50%	56%	61%	93%
Evaluation of LVS Function[2]	210	91%	84%	83%	99%
Smoking Cessation Advice[1,2]	11	100%	82%	82%	100%
Pneumonia Care					
Appropriate Initial Antibiotic[2]	86	86%	82%	83%	94%
Blood Culture Timing[2]	63	89%	89%	90%	100%
Influenza Vaccine[1]	18	33%	58%	70%	100%
Initial Antibiotic Timing[2]	116	82%	75%	80%	93%
Oxygenation Assessment[2]	123	94%	99%	99%	100%
Pneumococcal Vaccine[2]	81	31%	58%	69%	94%
Smoking Cessation Advice[1,2]	8	88%	75%	80%	100%
Surgical Infection Prevention					
Prophylactic Antibiotic Given[2]	71	59%	74%	77%	95%
Prophylactic Antibiotic Selection[1,2]	18	100%	89%	90%	100%
Prophylactic Antibiotic Stopped[2]	69	33%	65%	72%	95%
Pregnancy Care					
Inpatient Neonatal Mortality	-	-	-	-	-
Third or Fourth Degree Laceration	-	-	3.58%	3.63%	3.27%

Moreno Valley Community Hospital

27300 Iris Avenue Phone: 951-243-0811
Moreno Valley, CA 92555
Ownership: Govt - Hospital District or Authority Accredited: Yes
Emergency Services: Yes

Measure	Cases	This Hospital	State Average	U.S. Average	Top Hospital
Heart Attack Care					
ACE Inhibitor or ARB for LVSD[1]	3	33%	82%	82%	100%
Aspirin at Arrival	42	81%	95%	92%	100%
Aspirin at Discharge[1]	13	46%	90%	90%	100%
Beta Blocker at Arrival	29	79%	89%	87%	100%
Beta Blocker at Discharge[1]	13	54%	89%	90%	100%
Fibrinolytic Medication Timing[1]	4	25%	40%	31%	100%
PCI Within 90 Minutes of Arrival	0	-	52%	54%	95%
Smoking Cessation Advice[1]	1	0%	87%	88%	100%
Heart Failure Care					
ACE Inhibitor or ARB for LVSD	50	70%	84%	82%	100%
Discharge Instructions	153	41%	56%	61%	93%
Evaluation of LVS Function	158	70%	84%	83%	99%
Smoking Cessation Advice	26	54%	82%	82%	100%
Pneumonia Care					
Appropriate Initial Antibiotic	127	82%	82%	83%	94%
Blood Culture Timing	88	90%	89%	90%	100%
Influenza Vaccine[4,5]	-	-	58%	70%	100%
Initial Antibiotic Timing	164	72%	75%	80%	93%
Oxygenation Assessment	196	99%	99%	99%	100%
Pneumococcal Vaccine	106	31%	58%	69%	94%
Smoking Cessation Advice	33	61%	75%	80%	100%
Surgical Infection Prevention					
Prophylactic Antibiotic Given[1,3]	20	45%	74%	77%	95%
Prophylactic Antibiotic Selection[1]	15	47%	89%	90%	100%
Prophylactic Antibiotic Stopped[1,3]	16	19%	65%	72%	95%
Pregnancy Care					
Inpatient Neonatal Mortality	-	-	-	-	-
Third or Fourth Degree Laceration	-	-	3.58%	3.63%	3.27%

Riverside County Regional Medical Center

26520 Cactus Avenue Phone: 951-486-4000
Moreno Valley, CA 92555
Ownership: Proprietary Accredited: Yes
Emergency Services: Yes

Measure	Cases	This Hospital	State Average	U.S. Average	Top Hospital
Heart Attack Care					
ACE Inhibitor or ARB for LVSD[1]	5	80%	82%	82%	100%
Aspirin at Arrival	35	97%	95%	92%	100%
Aspirin at Discharge[1]	18	67%	90%	90%	100%
Beta Blocker at Arrival	31	81%	89%	87%	100%
Beta Blocker at Discharge[1]	17	82%	89%	90%	100%
Fibrinolytic Medication Timing[3]	0	-	40%	31%	100%
PCI Within 90 Minutes of Arrival	0	-	52%	54%	95%
Smoking Cessation Advice[1,3]	3	100%	87%	88%	100%
Heart Failure Care					
ACE Inhibitor or ARB for LVSD	118	91%	84%	82%	100%
Discharge Instructions[3]	55	55%	56%	61%	93%
Evaluation of LVS Function	230	91%	84%	83%	99%
Smoking Cessation Advice[1,3]	19	63%	82%	82%	100%
Pneumonia Care					
Appropriate Initial Antibiotic[1,3]	20	90%	82%	83%	94%
Blood Culture Timing[1,3]	18	78%	89%	90%	100%
Influenza Vaccine[4,5]	-	-	58%	70%	100%
Initial Antibiotic Timing	109	52%	75%	80%	93%
Oxygenation Assessment	138	99%	99%	99%	100%
Pneumococcal Vaccine	36	17%	58%	69%	94%
Smoking Cessation Advice[1,3]	5	80%	75%	80%	100%
Surgical Infection Prevention					
Prophylactic Antibiotic Given[3]	52	33%	74%	77%	95%
Prophylactic Antibiotic Selection[5]	-	-	89%	90%	100%
Prophylactic Antibiotic Stopped[3]	50	84%	65%	72%	95%
Pregnancy Care					
Inpatient Neonatal Mortality	-	-	-	-	-

NOTE: Hospital profiles are in alphabetical order by state, then city, then hospital within the city; Rankings are sorted by rate in descending order and exclude hospitals with less than 25 cases; (1) The number of cases is too small (n<25) for purposes of reliably predicting hospital performance; (2) Measure reflects the hospital's indication that its submission was based upon a sample of its relevant discharges; (3) Rate reflects fewer than the maximum possible quarters of data for the measure; (4) Inaccurate information submitted and suppressed for one or more quarters; (5) No data is available from the hospital for this measure; Please refer to the User's Guide for a full explanation of data

Third or Fourth Degree Laceration	-	-	3.58%	3.63%	3.27%

Mercy Medical Center-Mount Shasta

914 Pine Street Phone: 530-926-6111
Mount Shasta, CA 96067 Fax: 530-926-0517
URL: www.mercymtshasta.org
Ownership: Voluntary non-profit - Other Accredited: Yes
Emergency Services: Yes Licensed Beds: 80
Key Personnel:
Director Infection/Disease Control . . . . Sharon Piva, RN
Director Respiratory Therapy . . . . Craig Hanna

Measure	Cases	This Hospital	State Average	U.S. Average	Top Hospital
Heart Attack Care					
ACE Inhibitor or ARB for LVSD[1]	3	67%	82%	82%	100%
Aspirin at Arrival[1]	8	100%	95%	92%	100%
Aspirin at Discharge[1]	7	86%	90%	90%	100%
Beta Blocker at Arrival[1]	9	100%	89%	87%	100%
Beta Blocker at Discharge[1]	6	83%	89%	90%	100%
Fibrinolytic Medication Timing[1]	1	0%	40%	31%	100%
PCI Within 90 Minutes of Arrival	0	-	52%	54%	95%
Smoking Cessation Advice	0	-	87%	88%	100%
Heart Failure Care					
ACE Inhibitor or ARB for LVSD[1]	24	92%	84%	82%	100%
Discharge Instructions	40	90%	56%	61%	93%
Evaluation of LVS Function	44	93%	84%	83%	99%
Smoking Cessation Advice[1]	8	100%	82%	82%	100%
Pneumonia Care					
Appropriate Initial Antibiotic	70	89%	82%	83%	94%
Blood Culture Timing	49	96%	89%	90%	100%
Influenza Vaccine[1]	10	70%	58%	70%	100%
Initial Antibiotic Timing	73	84%	75%	80%	93%
Oxygenation Assessment	85	99%	99%	99%	100%
Pneumococcal Vaccine	58	91%	58%	69%	94%
Smoking Cessation Advice[1]	15	100%	75%	80%	100%
Surgical Infection Prevention					
Prophylactic Antibiotic Given[2,3]	97	89%	74%	77%	95%
Prophylactic Antibiotic Selection[2]	38	92%	89%	90%	100%
Prophylactic Antibiotic Stopped[2,3]	94	100%	65%	72%	95%
Pregnancy Care					
Inpatient Neonatal Mortality	-	-	-	-	-
Third or Fourth Degree Laceration	-	-	3.58%	3.63%	3.27%

El Camino Hospital

2500 Grant Road Toll-Free: 800-216-5556
Mountain View, CA 94040 Phone: 650-940-7000
Fax: 650-988-8100
URL: www.elcaminohospital.org
Ownership: Voluntary non-profit - Other Accredited: Yes
Emergency Services: Yes Licensed Beds: 395
Key Personnel:
Head of Emergency . . . . Mary Anderson
Director of Respiratory . . . . Judy Pantages

Measure	Cases	This Hospital	State Average	U.S. Average	Top Hospital
Heart Attack Care					
ACE Inhibitor or ARB for LVSD	44	95%	82%	82%	100%
Aspirin at Arrival	204	100%	95%	92%	100%
Aspirin at Discharge	198	99%	90%	90%	100%
Beta Blocker at Arrival	125	96%	89%	87%	100%
Beta Blocker at Discharge	169	98%	89%	90%	100%
Fibrinolytic Medication Timing[1]	1	0%	40%	31%	100%
PCI Within 90 Minutes of Arrival[1]	14	29%	52%	54%	95%
Smoking Cessation Advice	34	100%	87%	88%	100%
Heart Failure Care					
ACE Inhibitor or ARB for LVSD[2]	123	93%	84%	82%	100%
Discharge Instructions[2]	272	46%	56%	61%	93%
Evaluation of LVS Function[2]	348	85%	84%	83%	99%
Smoking Cessation Advice[2]	40	98%	82%	82%	100%
Pneumonia Care					
Appropriate Initial Antibiotic	301	77%	82%	83%	94%
Blood Culture Timing	284	92%	89%	90%	100%

Influenza Vaccine	68	56%	58%	70%	100%
Initial Antibiotic Timing	357	67%	75%	80%	93%
Oxygenation Assessment	453	100%	99%	99%	100%
Pneumococcal Vaccine	321	61%	58%	69%	94%
Smoking Cessation Advice	45	93%	75%	80%	100%
Surgical Infection Prevention					
Prophylactic Antibiotic Given[2]	794	81%	74%	77%	95%
Prophylactic Antibiotic Selection[2]	97	93%	89%	90%	100%
Prophylactic Antibiotic Stopped[2]	786	79%	65%	72%	95%
Pregnancy Care					
Inpatient Neonatal Mortality	-	-	-	-	-
Third or Fourth Degree Laceration	-	-	3.58%	3.63%	3.27%

Rancho Springs Medical Center

25500 Medical Center Drive Phone: 951-696-6000
Murrieta, CA 92562 Fax: 951-698-7721
URL: www.ivrmc-rsmc.com
Ownership: Voluntary non-profit - Private Accredited: Yes
Emergency Services: Yes Licensed Beds: 96
Key Personnel:
CEO. . . . . Linda Bradley

Measure	Cases	This Hospital	State Average	U.S. Average	Top Hospital
Heart Attack Care					
ACE Inhibitor or ARB for LVSD[1]	23	74%	82%	82%	100%
Aspirin at Arrival	222	94%	95%	92%	100%
Aspirin at Discharge	84	80%	90%	90%	100%
Beta Blocker at Arrival	167	93%	89%	87%	100%
Beta Blocker at Discharge	90	91%	89%	90%	100%
Fibrinolytic Medication Timing	39	44%	40%	31%	100%
PCI Within 90 Minutes of Arrival	0	-	52%	54%	95%
Smoking Cessation Advice[1]	18	100%	87%	88%	100%
Heart Failure Care					
ACE Inhibitor or ARB for LVSD	146	86%	84%	82%	100%
Discharge Instructions	391	57%	56%	61%	93%
Evaluation of LVS Function	389	89%	84%	83%	99%
Smoking Cessation Advice	54	100%	82%	82%	100%
Pneumonia Care					
Appropriate Initial Antibiotic	259	88%	82%	83%	94%
Blood Culture Timing	182	92%	89%	90%	100%
Influenza Vaccine	68	68%	58%	70%	100%
Initial Antibiotic Timing	321	67%	75%	80%	93%
Oxygenation Assessment	384	100%	99%	99%	100%
Pneumococcal Vaccine	247	57%	58%	69%	94%
Smoking Cessation Advice	65	95%	75%	80%	100%
Surgical Infection Prevention					
Prophylactic Antibiotic Given[2]	798	90%	74%	77%	95%
Prophylactic Antibiotic Selection[2]	175	90%	89%	90%	100%
Prophylactic Antibiotic Stopped[2]	744	59%	65%	72%	95%
Pregnancy Care					
Inpatient Neonatal Mortality	-	-	-	-	-
Third or Fourth Degree Laceration	-	-	3.58%	3.63%	3.27%

Queen of the Valley Hospital

1000 Trancas Street Phone: 707-252-4411
Napa, CA 94558 Fax: 707-257-7221
URL: www.thequeen.org
Ownership: Voluntary non-profit - Church Accredited: Yes
Emergency Services: Yes Licensed Beds: 166
Key Personnel:
President/CEO. . . . . Dennis Sisto
Chief of Medical Staff . . . . Daniel Maslope
Director Respiratory Therapy . . . . Steve Hepenstreit

Measure	Cases	This Hospital	State Average	U.S. Average	Top Hospital
Heart Attack Care					
ACE Inhibitor or ARB for LVSD	55	76%	82%	82%	100%
Aspirin at Arrival	157	94%	95%	92%	100%
Aspirin at Discharge	206	95%	90%	90%	100%
Beta Blocker at Arrival	99	85%	89%	87%	100%
Beta Blocker at Discharge	227	96%	89%	90%	100%
Fibrinolytic Medication Timing[1]	1	100%	40%	31%	100%

NOTE: Hospital profiles are in alphabetical order by state, then city, then hospital within the city; Rankings are sorted by rate in descending order and exclude hospitals with less than 25 cases; (1) The number of cases is too small (n<25) for purposes of reliably predicting hospital performance; (2) Measure reflects the hospital's indication that its submission was based upon a sample of its relevant discharges; (3) Rate reflects fewer than the maximum possible quarters of data for the measure; (4) Inaccurate information submitted and suppressed for one or more quarters; (5) No data is available from the hospital for this measure; Please refer to the User's Guide for a full explanation of data

PCI Within 90 Minutes of Arrival[1]	9	100%	52%	54%	95%
Smoking Cessation Advice	64	98%	87%	88%	100%
Heart Failure Care					
ACE Inhibitor or ARB for LVSD	60	75%	84%	82%	100%
Discharge Instructions	109	46%	56%	61%	93%
Evaluation of LVS Function	145	93%	84%	83%	99%
Smoking Cessation Advice[1]	18	100%	82%	82%	100%
Pneumonia Care					
Appropriate Initial Antibiotic	135	98%	82%	83%	94%
Blood Culture Timing	156	92%	89%	90%	100%
Influenza Vaccine	47	87%	58%	70%	100%
Initial Antibiotic Timing	194	89%	75%	80%	93%
Oxygenation Assessment	245	100%	99%	99%	100%
Pneumococcal Vaccine	141	98%	58%	69%	94%
Smoking Cessation Advice	64	100%	75%	80%	100%
Surgical Infection Prevention					
Prophylactic Antibiotic Given[2,3]	176	77%	74%	77%	95%
Prophylactic Antibiotic Selection[2]	73	95%	89%	90%	100%
Prophylactic Antibiotic Stopped[2,3]	171	57%	65%	72%	95%
Pregnancy Care					
Inpatient Neonatal Mortality	1,062	0.56%	-	-	-
Third or Fourth Degree Laceration	745	2.28%	3.58%	3.63%	3.27%

Paradise Valley Hospital

2400 E Fourth Street — Phone: 619-470-4321
National City, CA 91950 — Fax: 619-470-4249
URL: www.paradisevalleyhospital.org
Ownership: Voluntary non-profit - Church — Accredited: Yes
Emergency Services: Yes — Licensed Beds: 301

Key Personnel:
CEO . . . . Terrence A Hansen
Administrator . . . . Suzanne Perdy, MD
Chief Medical Staff . . . . Morton Jorgensen, MD
Manager Catheterization Laboratory . . . . Mario Guerro
Director Emergency Services . . . . Stephanie Baker, RN
Manager Infection Control . . . . Sue Parini
Director Medical/Surgical Nursing . . . . Linda Krusen
Medical/Surgical Nursing . . . . Walter Fahsing, MD
Director OB/GYN Womens Health . . . . Ann O'Neil
Director Radiology . . . . Charles Fraley
Manager Respiratory . . . . Mike Collins

Measure	Cases	This Hospital	State Average	U.S. Average	Top Hospital
Heart Attack Care					
ACE Inhibitor or ARB for LVSD[1]	17	88%	82%	82%	100%
Aspirin at Arrival	88	91%	95%	92%	100%
Aspirin at Discharge	40	100%	90%	90%	100%
Beta Blocker at Arrival	61	97%	89%	87%	100%
Beta Blocker at Discharge	46	96%	89%	90%	100%
Fibrinolytic Medication Timing[1]	4	50%	40%	31%	100%
PCI Within 90 Minutes of Arrival	0	-	52%	54%	95%
Smoking Cessation Advice[1]	14	86%	87%	88%	100%
Heart Failure Care					
ACE Inhibitor or ARB for LVSD	161	84%	84%	82%	100%
Discharge Instructions	326	76%	56%	61%	93%
Evaluation of LVS Function	370	93%	84%	83%	99%
Smoking Cessation Advice	96	95%	82%	82%	100%
Pneumonia Care					
Appropriate Initial Antibiotic	174	85%	82%	83%	94%
Blood Culture Timing	126	90%	89%	90%	100%
Influenza Vaccine	58	57%	58%	70%	100%
Initial Antibiotic Timing	259	71%	75%	80%	93%
Oxygenation Assessment	289	100%	99%	99%	100%
Pneumococcal Vaccine	175	50%	58%	69%	94%
Smoking Cessation Advice	53	87%	75%	80%	100%
Surgical Infection Prevention					
Prophylactic Antibiotic Given[3]	126	63%	74%	77%	95%
Prophylactic Antibiotic Selection	38	82%	89%	90%	100%
Prophylactic Antibiotic Stopped[3]	109	68%	65%	72%	95%
Pregnancy Care					
Inpatient Neonatal Mortality	-	-	-	-	-
Third or Fourth Degree Laceration	-	-	3.58%	3.63%	3.27%

Hoag Memorial Hospital Presbyterian

One Hoag Drive — Phone: 949-764-4624
PO Box 6100 — Fax: 949-760-2138
Newport Beach, CA 92658
URL: www.hoaghospital.org
Ownership: Voluntary non-profit - Other — Accredited: Yes
Emergency Services: Yes

Key Personnel:
President/CEO . . . . Richard Afable, MD
Chief of Medical Staff . . . . J. Paul Curry, MD
Executive Director . . . . Bret Kelsey
Chief Catheterization Laboratory . . . . Joel Manchester, MD
Emergency Room . . . . Gregory Super, MD
Director Infection/Disease Control . . . . Rosalie DeSantis, RN
Chief Radiology . . . . Michael Brandt-Zawadski, MD
Director Respiratory Therapy . . . . Michael Gonzalez

Measure	Cases	This Hospital	State Average	U.S. Average	Top Hospital
Heart Attack Care					
ACE Inhibitor or ARB for LVSD	54	96%	82%	82%	100%
Aspirin at Arrival	283	99%	95%	92%	100%
Aspirin at Discharge	287	100%	90%	90%	100%
Beta Blocker at Arrival	257	98%	89%	87%	100%
Beta Blocker at Discharge	284	99%	89%	90%	100%
Fibrinolytic Medication Timing	0	-	40%	31%	100%
PCI Within 90 Minutes of Arrival	27	93%	52%	54%	95%
Smoking Cessation Advice	58	93%	87%	88%	100%
Heart Failure Care					
ACE Inhibitor or ARB for LVSD	251	87%	84%	82%	100%
Discharge Instructions	494	73%	56%	61%	93%
Evaluation of LVS Function	598	95%	84%	83%	99%
Smoking Cessation Advice	55	84%	82%	82%	100%
Pneumonia Care					
Appropriate Initial Antibiotic	320	89%	82%	83%	94%
Blood Culture Timing	367	91%	89%	90%	100%
Influenza Vaccine	84	81%	58%	70%	100%
Initial Antibiotic Timing	376	87%	75%	80%	93%
Oxygenation Assessment	524	100%	99%	99%	100%
Pneumococcal Vaccine	349	75%	58%	69%	94%
Smoking Cessation Advice	59	85%	75%	80%	100%
Surgical Infection Prevention					
Prophylactic Antibiotic Given[2]	349	90%	74%	77%	95%
Prophylactic Antibiotic Selection[2]	87	94%	89%	90%	100%
Prophylactic Antibiotic Stopped[2]	337	83%	65%	72%	95%
Pregnancy Care					
Inpatient Neonatal Mortality	-	-	-	-	-
Third or Fourth Degree Laceration	-	-	3.58%	3.63%	3.27%

Northridge Hospital Medical Center

18300 Roscoe Boulevard — Phone: 818-885-8500
Northridge, CA 91328 — Fax: 818-885-5439
URL: www.northridgehospital.org
Ownership: Voluntary non-profit - Other — Accredited: Yes
Emergency Services: Yes — Licensed Beds: 411

Key Personnel:
President . . . . Michael Wall
Chief Medical Staff . . . . Lamya Jarjour, MD
Medical Director Emergency Department . . . . Stephen Jones, MD
Manager Infection Control . . . . Vicki Kelley, RN
Clinical Director ICU/CCU . . . . Elsie Crowninshield, RN
Director Womens Center . . . . Nana Deeb
Clinical Director Women/Children Svcs . . . . Kathy Alfe
Director Radiology . . . . Nana Deeb
Manager Respiratory Services . . . . Ed Lopez

Measure	Cases	This Hospital	State Average	U.S. Average	Top Hospital
Heart Attack Care					
ACE Inhibitor or ARB for LVSD	41	98%	82%	82%	100%
Aspirin at Arrival	196	98%	95%	92%	100%
Aspirin at Discharge	169	99%	90%	90%	100%
Beta Blocker at Arrival	124	99%	89%	87%	100%
Beta Blocker at Discharge	177	98%	89%	90%	100%

NOTE: Hospital profiles are in alphabetical order by state, then city, then hospital within the city; Rankings are sorted by rate in descending order and exclude hospitals with less than 25 cases; (1) The number of cases is too small (n<25) for purposes of reliably predicting hospital performance; (2) Measure reflects the hospital's indication that its submission was based upon a sample of its relevant discharges; (3) Rate reflects fewer than the maximum possible quarters of data for the measure; (4) Inaccurate information submitted and suppressed for one or more quarters; (5) No data is available from the hospital for this measure; Please refer to the User's Guide for a full explanation of data

Fibrinolytic Medication Timing[1]	4	25%	40%	31%	100%
PCI Within 90 Minutes of Arrival[1]	3	33%	52%	54%	95%
Smoking Cessation Advice	42	100%	87%	88%	100%
Heart Failure Care					
ACE Inhibitor or ARB for LVSD	125	94%	84%	82%	100%
Discharge Instructions	293	76%	56%	61%	93%
Evaluation of LVS Function	354	99%	84%	83%	99%
Smoking Cessation Advice	48	100%	82%	82%	100%
Pneumonia Care					
Appropriate Initial Antibiotic	199	87%	82%	83%	94%
Blood Culture Timing	221	94%	89%	90%	100%
Influenza Vaccine	70	79%	58%	70%	100%
Initial Antibiotic Timing	296	73%	75%	80%	93%
Oxygenation Assessment	396	100%	99%	99%	100%
Pneumococcal Vaccine	262	82%	58%	69%	94%
Smoking Cessation Advice	62	97%	75%	80%	100%
Surgical Infection Prevention					
Prophylactic Antibiotic Given[2,3]	211	69%	74%	77%	95%
Prophylactic Antibiotic Selection[2]	73	78%	89%	90%	100%
Prophylactic Antibiotic Stopped[2,3]	198	44%	65%	72%	95%
Pregnancy Care					
Inpatient Neonatal Mortality	-	-	-	-	-
Third or Fourth Degree Laceration	-	-	3.58%	3.63%	3.27%

Coast Plaza Doctors Hospital

Alternate Name: Coast Plaza Medical Center
13100 Studebaker Road
Norwalk, CA 90650
Phone: 562-868-3751
Fax: 562-868-3198
URL: www.coastplazahospital.com
Ownership: Voluntary non-profit - Private
Accredited: Yes
Emergency Services: Yes
Licensed Beds: 123

Key Personnel:
CEO. . . . . Craig Boyd Garner
Chief Medical Staff. . . . . Galal S Gough, MD
Administrator . . . . Linda Roman
Emergency Room . . . . Thomas A Gionis, MD
Respiratory/Cardiopulmonary. . . . . Abraham George

Measure	Cases	This Hospital	State Average	U.S. Average	Top Hospital
Heart Attack Care					
ACE Inhibitor or ARB for LVSD	0	-	82%	82%	100%
Aspirin at Arrival[1]	17	94%	95%	92%	100%
Aspirin at Discharge[1]	4	50%	90%	90%	100%
Beta Blocker at Arrival[1]	17	88%	89%	87%	100%
Beta Blocker at Discharge[1]	4	50%	89%	90%	100%
Fibrinolytic Medication Timing[1]	1	100%	40%	31%	100%
PCI Within 90 Minutes of Arrival	0	-	52%	54%	95%
Smoking Cessation Advice[1]	2	100%	87%	88%	100%
Heart Failure Care					
ACE Inhibitor or ARB for LVSD	27	78%	84%	82%	100%
Discharge Instructions	90	99%	56%	61%	93%
Evaluation of LVS Function	114	76%	84%	83%	99%
Smoking Cessation Advice[1]	18	100%	82%	82%	100%
Pneumonia Care					
Appropriate Initial Antibiotic	214	73%	82%	83%	94%
Blood Culture Timing	60	68%	89%	90%	100%
Influenza Vaccine	25	40%	58%	70%	100%
Initial Antibiotic Timing	219	77%	75%	80%	93%
Oxygenation Assessment	230	100%	99%	99%	100%
Pneumococcal Vaccine	90	37%	58%	69%	94%
Smoking Cessation Advice[1]	15	100%	75%	80%	100%
Surgical Infection Prevention					
Prophylactic Antibiotic Given[1,3]	5	0%	74%	77%	95%
Prophylactic Antibiotic Selection[1]	5	80%	89%	90%	100%
Prophylactic Antibiotic Stopped[1,3]	5	80%	65%	72%	95%
Pregnancy Care					
Inpatient Neonatal Mortality	-	-	-	-	-
Third or Fourth Degree Laceration	-	-	3.58%	3.63%	3.27%

Novato Community Hospital

180 Rowland Way
Novato, CA 94945
Phone: 415-209-1300
Fax: 415-492-4751
URL: www.novatocommunity.sutterhealth.org
Ownership: Voluntary non-profit - Other
Accredited: Yes
Emergency Services: Yes

Key Personnel:
CEO. . . . . David Bradley
Chief of Medical Staff . . . . Timothy Murphy, MD
Emergency Room . . . . Peggy Parenti, RN
OB/GYN Womens Health. . . . . Michael Maioriello, MD

Measure	Cases	This Hospital	State Average	U.S. Average	Top Hospital
Heart Attack Care					
ACE Inhibitor or ARB for LVSD[1]	5	100%	82%	82%	100%
Aspirin at Arrival	43	98%	95%	92%	100%
Aspirin at Discharge	34	100%	90%	90%	100%
Beta Blocker at Arrival	44	100%	89%	87%	100%
Beta Blocker at Discharge	36	100%	89%	90%	100%
Fibrinolytic Medication Timing	0	-	40%	31%	100%
PCI Within 90 Minutes of Arrival	0	-	52%	54%	95%
Smoking Cessation Advice[1]	4	100%	87%	88%	100%
Heart Failure Care					
ACE Inhibitor or ARB for LVSD[1]	16	94%	84%	82%	100%
Discharge Instructions	48	75%	56%	61%	93%
Evaluation of LVS Function	61	100%	84%	83%	99%
Smoking Cessation Advice[1]	6	100%	82%	82%	100%
Pneumonia Care					
Appropriate Initial Antibiotic	71	76%	82%	83%	94%
Blood Culture Timing	55	93%	89%	90%	100%
Influenza Vaccine[1]	23	52%	58%	70%	100%
Initial Antibiotic Timing	74	88%	75%	80%	93%
Oxygenation Assessment	92	100%	99%	99%	100%
Pneumococcal Vaccine	73	59%	58%	69%	94%
Smoking Cessation Advice[1]	11	82%	75%	80%	100%
Surgical Infection Prevention					
Prophylactic Antibiotic Given	203	84%	74%	77%	95%
Prophylactic Antibiotic Selection	47	100%	89%	90%	100%
Prophylactic Antibiotic Stopped	197	36%	65%	72%	95%
Pregnancy Care					
Inpatient Neonatal Mortality	-	-	-	-	-
Third or Fourth Degree Laceration	-	-	3.58%	3.63%	3.27%

Oak Valley Hospital

350 S Oak Street
Oakdale, CA 95361
Phone: 209-847-3011
Fax: 209-848-4110
URL: www.oakvalleycares.org
Ownership: Govt - Hospital District or Authority
Accredited: Yes
Emergency Services: Yes
Licensed Beds: 141

Key Personnel:
President . . . . Bob Wickoff
Emergency Room . . . . Vivian Thompson, RN
Director Medical/Surgical Nursing . . . . Jan Nickerson, RN
OB/GYN Womens Health. . . . . Lawrence Podolsky, MD
Chief Radiology . . . . Chuck Canterbury
Director Respiratory Therapy . . . . Charles Groves

Measure	Cases	This Hospital	State Average	U.S. Average	Top Hospital
Heart Attack Care					
ACE Inhibitor or ARB for LVSD[1]	2	0%	82%	82%	100%
Aspirin at Arrival	25	100%	95%	92%	100%
Aspirin at Discharge[1]	8	75%	90%	90%	100%
Beta Blocker at Arrival[1]	23	100%	89%	87%	100%
Beta Blocker at Discharge[1]	8	88%	89%	90%	100%
Fibrinolytic Medication Timing[1]	2	50%	40%	31%	100%
PCI Within 90 Minutes of Arrival	0	-	52%	54%	95%
Smoking Cessation Advice[1]	1	100%	87%	88%	100%
Heart Failure Care					
ACE Inhibitor or ARB for LVSD[1]	23	91%	84%	82%	100%
Discharge Instructions	55	58%	56%	61%	93%
Evaluation of LVS Function	69	84%	84%	83%	99%
Smoking Cessation Advice[1]	11	55%	82%	82%	100%
Pneumonia Care					

NOTE: Hospital profiles are in alphabetical order by state, then city, then hospital within the city; Rankings are sorted by rate in descending order and exclude hospitals with less than 25 cases; (1) The number of cases is too small (n<25) for purposes of reliably predicting hospital performance; (2) Measure reflects the hospital's indication that its submission was based upon a sample of its relevant discharges; (3) Rate reflects fewer than the maximum possible quarters of data for the measure; (4) Inaccurate information submitted and suppressed for one or more quarters; (5) No data is available from the hospital for this measure; Please refer to the User's Guide for a full explanation of data

Measure	Cases	This Hospital	State Average	U.S. Average	Top Hospital
Appropriate Initial Antibiotic	82	82%	82%	83%	94%
Blood Culture Timing	39	85%	89%	90%	100%
Influenza Vaccine[1]	14	71%	58%	70%	100%
Initial Antibiotic Timing	91	84%	75%	80%	93%
Oxygenation Assessment	107	100%	99%	99%	100%
Pneumococcal Vaccine	70	56%	58%	69%	94%
Smoking Cessation Advice	30	50%	75%	80%	100%
Surgical Infection Prevention					
Prophylactic Antibiotic Given[2,3]	44	34%	74%	77%	95%
Prophylactic Antibiotic Selection[1,2]	13	100%	89%	90%	100%
Prophylactic Antibiotic Stopped[2,3]	35	94%	65%	72%	95%
Pregnancy Care					
Inpatient Neonatal Mortality	-	-	-	-	-
Third or Fourth Degree Laceration	-	-	3.58%	3.63%	3.27%

Alameda County Medical Center

Alternate Name: Highland General Hospital
1411 E 31st Street — Phone: 510-437-4800
Oakland, CA 94602 — Fax: 510-535-7759
E-mail: btate@acmedctr.org
URL: www.acmedctr.org
Ownership: Government - Local — Accredited: Yes
Emergency Services: Yes — Licensed Beds: 308

Key Personnel:

CEO. . . . . Kenneth Cohen
Chief Medical Staff. . . . . Parry Zorthian, MD
OB/GYN Womens Health. . . . . James Jackson, MD
Chief Radiology . . . . Ronald Eisenberg, MD
Director Respiratory Therapy . . . . Paulette Walls

Measure	Cases	This Hospital	State Average	U.S. Average	Top Hospital
Heart Attack Care					
ACE Inhibitor or ARB for LVSD[1]	10	100%	82%	82%	100%
Aspirin at Arrival	50	100%	95%	92%	100%
Aspirin at Discharge	30	97%	90%	90%	100%
Beta Blocker at Arrival	49	94%	89%	87%	100%
Beta Blocker at Discharge	29	100%	89%	90%	100%
Fibrinolytic Medication Timing[1]	1	0%	40%	31%	100%
PCI Within 90 Minutes of Arrival	0	-	52%	54%	95%
Smoking Cessation Advice[1]	9	44%	87%	88%	100%
Heart Failure Care					
ACE Inhibitor or ARB for LVSD	140	94%	84%	82%	100%
Discharge Instructions	266	2%	56%	61%	93%
Evaluation of LVS Function	279	99%	84%	83%	99%
Smoking Cessation Advice	136	54%	82%	82%	100%
Pneumonia Care					
Appropriate Initial Antibiotic	141	79%	82%	83%	94%
Blood Culture Timing	119	79%	89%	90%	100%
Influenza Vaccine[4,5]	-	-	58%	70%	100%
Initial Antibiotic Timing	156	44%	75%	80%	93%
Oxygenation Assessment	220	100%	99%	99%	100%
Pneumococcal Vaccine	58	16%	58%	69%	94%
Smoking Cessation Advice	86	57%	75%	80%	100%
Surgical Infection Prevention					
Prophylactic Antibiotic Given[3]	27	30%	74%	77%	95%
Prophylactic Antibiotic Selection[1]	23	61%	89%	90%	100%
Prophylactic Antibiotic Stopped[1,3]	23	91%	65%	72%	95%
Pregnancy Care					
Inpatient Neonatal Mortality	-	-	-	-	-
Third or Fourth Degree Laceration	-	-	3.58%	3.63%	3.27%

Alta Bates Summit Medical Center

Merritt Pavilion — Phone: 510-655-4000
350 Hawthorne Avenue — Fax: 510-869-8980
Oakland, CA 94609
URL: www.altabates.com
Ownership: Voluntary non-profit - Other — Accredited: Yes
Emergency Services: Yes — Licensed Beds: 517

Key Personnel:

Administrator/President . . . . Warren Kirk
Chief Medical Staff. . . . . Samuel Dong, MD
Emergency Room . . . . Patrick Evendalista
Emergency Room . . . . Ellie Pecora

Measure	Cases	This Hospital	State Average	U.S. Average	Top Hospital
Heart Attack Care					
ACE Inhibitor or ARB for LVSD	109	91%	82%	82%	100%
Aspirin at Arrival	238	99%	95%	92%	100%
Aspirin at Discharge	777	99%	90%	90%	100%
Beta Blocker at Arrival	198	96%	89%	87%	100%
Beta Blocker at Discharge	799	99%	89%	90%	100%
Fibrinolytic Medication Timing	0	-	40%	31%	100%
PCI Within 90 Minutes of Arrival[1]	19	63%	52%	54%	95%
Smoking Cessation Advice	206	100%	87%	88%	100%
Heart Failure Care					
ACE Inhibitor or ARB for LVSD[2]	85	87%	84%	82%	100%
Discharge Instructions[2]	159	87%	56%	61%	93%
Evaluation of LVS Function[2]	203	93%	84%	83%	99%
Smoking Cessation Advice[2]	33	100%	82%	82%	100%
Pneumonia Care					
Appropriate Initial Antibiotic[2]	60	90%	82%	83%	94%
Blood Culture Timing[2]	105	93%	89%	90%	100%
Influenza Vaccine[1]	20	70%	58%	70%	100%
Initial Antibiotic Timing[2]	125	68%	75%	80%	93%
Oxygenation Assessment[2]	146	100%	99%	99%	100%
Pneumococcal Vaccine[2]	96	60%	58%	69%	94%
Smoking Cessation Advice[2]	35	100%	75%	80%	100%
Surgical Infection Prevention					
Prophylactic Antibiotic Given[2,3]	169	81%	74%	77%	95%
Prophylactic Antibiotic Selection[2]	56	96%	89%	90%	100%
Prophylactic Antibiotic Stopped[2,3]	157	87%	65%	72%	95%
Pregnancy Care					
Inpatient Neonatal Mortality	-	-	-	-	-
Third or Fourth Degree Laceration	-	-	3.58%	3.63%	3.27%

Oakland Medical Center

280 West MacArthur Boulevard — Toll-Free: 888-499-1500
Oakland, CA 94611 — Phone: 510-752-1000
Fax: 408-366-4182
E-mail: Oakland-Webmaster@kp.org
URL: www.oakland.kaiser.org
Ownership: Voluntary non-profit - Other — Accredited: Yes
Emergency Services: Yes — Licensed Beds: 348

Key Personnel:

CEO. . . . . Mary Holland

Measure	Cases	This Hospital	State Average	U.S. Average	Top Hospital
Heart Attack Care					
ACE Inhibitor or ARB for LVSD	32	100%	82%	82%	100%
Aspirin at Arrival	328	100%	95%	92%	100%
Aspirin at Discharge	150	97%	90%	90%	100%
Beta Blocker at Arrival	282	99%	89%	87%	100%
Beta Blocker at Discharge	141	99%	89%	90%	100%
Fibrinolytic Medication Timing	25	60%	40%	31%	100%
PCI Within 90 Minutes of Arrival	0	-	52%	54%	95%
Smoking Cessation Advice[1]	20	95%	87%	88%	100%
Heart Failure Care					
ACE Inhibitor or ARB for LVSD	169	95%	84%	82%	100%
Discharge Instructions	534	60%	56%	61%	93%
Evaluation of LVS Function	585	96%	84%	83%	99%
Smoking Cessation Advice	92	92%	82%	82%	100%
Pneumonia Care					
Appropriate Initial Antibiotic	270	95%	82%	83%	94%
Blood Culture Timing	345	88%	89%	90%	100%
Influenza Vaccine	110	58%	58%	70%	100%
Initial Antibiotic Timing	439	78%	75%	80%	93%
Oxygenation Assessment	528	100%	99%	99%	100%
Pneumococcal Vaccine	367	94%	58%	69%	94%
Smoking Cessation Advice	75	87%	75%	80%	100%
Surgical Infection Prevention					
Prophylactic Antibiotic Given	989	94%	74%	77%	95%
Prophylactic Antibiotic Selection	276	92%	89%	90%	100%
Prophylactic Antibiotic Stopped	908	80%	65%	72%	95%
Pregnancy Care					
Inpatient Neonatal Mortality	-	-	-	-	-
Third or Fourth Degree Laceration	-	-	3.58%	3.63%	3.27%

NOTE: Hospital profiles are in alphabetical order by state, then city, then hospital within the city; Rankings are sorted by rate in descending order and exclude hospitals with less than 25 cases; (1) The number of cases is too small (n<25) for purposes of reliably predicting hospital performance; (2) Measure reflects the hospital's indication that its submission was based upon a sample of its relevant discharges; (3) Rate reflects fewer than the maximum possible quarters of data for the measure; (4) Inaccurate information submitted and suppressed for one or more quarters; (5) No data is available from the hospital for this measure; Please refer to the User's Guide for a full explanation of data

Tri-City Medical Center

4002 Vista Way
Oceanside, CA 92056
URL: www.tricitymed.org
Phone: 760-724-8411
Ownership: Govt - Hospital District or Authority
Emergency Services: Yes
Accredited: Yes
Licensed Beds: 397

Key Personnel:

President/CEO. . . . . Dr Arthur Gonzalez, FACHE PH
Chief Medical Staff. . . . . Ken Iwaoka, MD
Director Cardio-Pulmonary. . . . . Linda Acklin
Emergency Room . . . . Stephe Karas
OB/GYN Womens Health. . . . . Nancy Graver
Chief Radiology . . . . Stephen Dorros
Director Cardio-Pulmonary. . . . . Linda Acklin

Measure	Cases	This Hospital	State Average	U.S. Average	Top Hospital
Heart Attack Care					
ACE Inhibitor or ARB for LVSD	32	81%	82%	82%	100%
Aspirin at Arrival	233	97%	95%	92%	100%
Aspirin at Discharge	198	95%	90%	90%	100%
Beta Blocker at Arrival	157	97%	89%	87%	100%
Beta Blocker at Discharge	184	97%	89%	90%	100%
Fibrinolytic Medication Timing[1]	8	25%	40%	31%	100%
PCI Within 90 Minutes of Arrival[1]	12	50%	52%	54%	95%
Smoking Cessation Advice	34	100%	87%	88%	100%
Heart Failure Care					
ACE Inhibitor or ARB for LVSD	144	79%	84%	82%	100%
Discharge Instructions	339	81%	56%	61%	93%
Evaluation of LVS Function	432	93%	84%	83%	99%
Smoking Cessation Advice	47	98%	82%	82%	100%
Pneumonia Care					
Appropriate Initial Antibiotic	309	91%	82%	83%	94%
Blood Culture Timing	325	86%	89%	90%	100%
Influenza Vaccine	85	78%	58%	70%	100%
Initial Antibiotic Timing	387	83%	75%	80%	93%
Oxygenation Assessment	506	100%	99%	99%	100%
Pneumococcal Vaccine	331	70%	58%	69%	94%
Smoking Cessation Advice	85	95%	75%	80%	100%
Surgical Infection Prevention					
Prophylactic Antibiotic Given[2,3]	146	86%	74%	77%	95%
Prophylactic Antibiotic Selection[2]	70	94%	89%	90%	100%
Prophylactic Antibiotic Stopped[2,3]	133	85%	65%	72%	95%
Pregnancy Care					
Inpatient Neonatal Mortality	1,948	0.26%	-	-	-
Third or Fourth Degree Laceration	1,400	3.29%	3.58%	3.63%	3.27%

Ojai Valley Community Hospital

1306 Maricopa Highway
Ojai, CA 93023
E-mail: Foundation@ojaihospital.org
URL: www.ojaihospital.org
Phone: 805-646-1401
Fax: 805-640-2204
Ownership: Proprietary
Emergency Services: Yes
Accredited: Yes
Licensed Beds: 110

Key Personnel:

CEO. . . . . Victoria A Alexander
Chief of Medical Staff. . . . . Gordon Clawson, MD
Emergency Room Manager . . . . Kristi Cain, RN
Infection Control. . . . . Anne Borchard, RN ICP
Cardio-Pulmonary Manager. . . . . Aaron McColpin, RT RN

Measure	Cases	This Hospital	State Average	U.S. Average	Top Hospital
Heart Attack Care					
ACE Inhibitor or ARB for LVSD[1]	6	67%	82%	82%	100%
Aspirin at Arrival[1]	21	81%	95%	92%	100%
Aspirin at Discharge[1]	18	67%	90%	90%	100%
Beta Blocker at Arrival[1]	20	40%	89%	87%	100%
Beta Blocker at Discharge[1]	20	65%	89%	90%	100%
Fibrinolytic Medication Timing	0	-	40%	31%	100%
PCI Within 90 Minutes of Arrival	0	-	52%	54%	95%
Smoking Cessation Advice[1]	5	40%	87%	88%	100%
Heart Failure Care					
ACE Inhibitor or ARB for LVSD[1]	1	100%	84%	82%	100%
Discharge Instructions[1]	12	0%	56%	61%	93%
Evaluation of LVS Function[1]	17	53%	84%	83%	99%
Smoking Cessation Advice[1]	1	0%	82%	82%	100%
Pneumonia Care					
Appropriate Initial Antibiotic	57	77%	82%	83%	94%
Blood Culture Timing[1]	17	88%	89%	90%	100%
Influenza Vaccine[1]	12	58%	58%	70%	100%
Initial Antibiotic Timing	48	54%	75%	80%	93%
Oxygenation Assessment	73	100%	99%	99%	100%
Pneumococcal Vaccine	45	36%	58%	69%	94%
Smoking Cessation Advice[1]	15	27%	75%	80%	100%
Surgical Infection Prevention					
Prophylactic Antibiotic Given[1,3]	8	50%	74%	77%	95%
Prophylactic Antibiotic Selection[1]	10	90%	89%	90%	100%
Prophylactic Antibiotic Stopped[1,3]	8	100%	65%	72%	95%
Pregnancy Care					
Inpatient Neonatal Mortality	-	-	-	-	-
Third or Fourth Degree Laceration	-	-	3.58%	3.63%	3.27%

Chapman Medical Center

2601 E Chapman Avenue
Orange, CA 92869
URL: www.chapmanmedicalcenter.com
Phone: 714-633-0011
Fax: 714-532-4345
Ownership: Proprietary
Emergency Services: Yes
Accredited: Yes
Licensed Beds: 114

Key Personnel:

CEO. . . . . Doug Norris
Chief of Medical Staff . . . . John Luster, MD
Director Medical/Surgical Nursing . . . . Nancy McKinney, RN
Director Radiology . . . . Joe Sonntag
Director Respiratory . . . . Joe Sonntag

Measure	Cases	This Hospital	State Average	U.S. Average	Top Hospital
Heart Attack Care					
ACE Inhibitor or ARB for LVSD[1]	3	100%	82%	82%	100%
Aspirin at Arrival[1]	8	100%	95%	92%	100%
Aspirin at Discharge[1]	3	100%	90%	90%	100%
Beta Blocker at Arrival[1]	3	100%	89%	87%	100%
Beta Blocker at Discharge[1]	5	100%	89%	90%	100%
Fibrinolytic Medication Timing[1]	2	100%	40%	31%	100%
PCI Within 90 Minutes of Arrival	0	-	52%	54%	95%
Smoking Cessation Advice	0	-	87%	88%	100%
Heart Failure Care					
ACE Inhibitor or ARB for LVSD[1]	15	80%	84%	82%	100%
Discharge Instructions	40	80%	56%	61%	93%
Evaluation of LVS Function	47	94%	84%	83%	99%
Smoking Cessation Advice[1]	8	100%	82%	82%	100%
Pneumonia Care					
Appropriate Initial Antibiotic	40	90%	82%	83%	94%
Blood Culture Timing	52	100%	89%	90%	100%
Influenza Vaccine[1]	10	100%	58%	70%	100%
Initial Antibiotic Timing	66	92%	75%	80%	93%
Oxygenation Assessment	88	100%	99%	99%	100%
Pneumococcal Vaccine	52	87%	58%	69%	94%
Smoking Cessation Advice[1]	6	100%	75%	80%	100%
Surgical Infection Prevention					
Prophylactic Antibiotic Given[1,3]	7	100%	74%	77%	95%
Prophylactic Antibiotic Selection[1]	7	86%	89%	90%	100%
Prophylactic Antibiotic Stopped[1,3]	6	83%	65%	72%	95%
Pregnancy Care					
Inpatient Neonatal Mortality	-	-	-	-	-
Third or Fourth Degree Laceration	-	-	3.58%	3.63%	3.27%

Saint Joseph Hospital

1100 West Steware Drive
Orange, CA 92868
URL: www.sjo.org
Phone: 714-633-9111
Fax: 714-744-8551
Ownership: Voluntary non-profit - Church
Emergency Services: Yes
Accredited: Yes
Licensed Beds: 412

Key Personnel:

CEO/President. . . . . Larry K Ainsworth
Chief Medical Staff. . . . . Robert Armen, MD
Executive Director . . . . Sonoma Van Brunt

NOTE: Hospital profiles are in alphabetical order by state, then city, then hospital within the city; Rankings are sorted by rate in descending order and exclude hospitals with less than 25 cases; (1) The number of cases is too small (n<25) for purposes of reliably predicting hospital performance; (2) Measure reflects the hospital's indication that its submission was based upon a sample of its relevant discharges; (3) Rate reflects fewer than the maximum possible quarters of data for the measure; (4) Inaccurate information submitted and suppressed for one or more quarters; (5) No data is available from the hospital for this measure; Please refer to the User's Guide for a full explanation of data

Executive Director . . . . Jan Grankowski
Executive Director . . . . Pat Brydges
Executive Director . . . . Dennis Kmetz
Emergency Room . . . . James Pierog, MD
Executive Director . . . . Kathy Penzes
OB/GYN Womens Health. . . . . E Peter Anzaldo, MD
Executive Director . . . . Beth Padilla
Chief Radiology . . . . Wallace Peck, MD

Measure	Cases	This Hospital	State Average	U.S. Average	Top Hospital
Heart Attack Care					
ACE Inhibitor or ARB for LVSD	29	93%	82%	82%	100%
Aspirin at Arrival	230	100%	95%	92%	100%
Aspirin at Discharge	234	96%	90%	90%	100%
Beta Blocker at Arrival	168	98%	89%	87%	100%
Beta Blocker at Discharge	233	98%	89%	90%	100%
Fibrinolytic Medication Timing[1]	2	100%	40%	31%	100%
PCI Within 90 Minutes of Arrival[1]	6	83%	52%	54%	95%
Smoking Cessation Advice	63	100%	87%	88%	100%
Heart Failure Care					
ACE Inhibitor or ARB for LVSD	146	93%	84%	82%	100%
Discharge Instructions	398	63%	56%	61%	93%
Evaluation of LVS Function	470	97%	84%	83%	99%
Smoking Cessation Advice	63	97%	82%	82%	100%
Pneumonia Care					
Appropriate Initial Antibiotic	187	81%	82%	83%	94%
Blood Culture Timing	169	96%	89%	90%	100%
Influenza Vaccine	55	85%	58%	70%	100%
Initial Antibiotic Timing	224	88%	75%	80%	93%
Oxygenation Assessment	300	100%	99%	99%	100%
Pneumococcal Vaccine	178	79%	58%	69%	94%
Smoking Cessation Advice	42	95%	75%	80%	100%
Surgical Infection Prevention					
Prophylactic Antibiotic Given[2,3]	236	82%	74%	77%	95%
Prophylactic Antibiotic Selection[2]	76	97%	89%	90%	100%
Prophylactic Antibiotic Stopped[2,3]	222	81%	65%	72%	95%
Pregnancy Care					
Inpatient Neonatal Mortality	-	-	-	-	-
Third or Fourth Degree Laceration	-	-	3.58%	3.63%	3.27%

University of California Irvine Med Ctr

Alternate Name: UCI Medical Center
101 The City Drive S
Orange, CA 92868
Toll-Free: 877-824-3627
Phone: 714-456-7890
Fax: 714-456-7927
E-mail: ucihealth@uci.edu
URL: www.ucihealth.com
Ownership: Government - State
Accredited: Yes
Emergency Services: Yes
Licensed Beds: 453

Key Personnel:

CEO. . . . . Ralph Cygan, MD
Chief Medical Officer . . . . Eugene Spiritus, MD
Emergency Room . . . . Mark Langdorf, MD
Emergency Room . . . . Darlene Bradley, RN
Director Infection/Disease Control . . . . Linda Dickey, RN
ICU . . . . Sonia Ramos Lane, RN
OB/GYN Womens Health. . . . . Manuel Porto, MD
Respiratory . . . . Carol Buffington

Measure	Cases	This Hospital	State Average	U.S. Average	Top Hospital
Heart Attack Care					
ACE Inhibitor or ARB for LVSD	25	84%	82%	82%	100%
Aspirin at Arrival	62	100%	95%	92%	100%
Aspirin at Discharge	63	94%	90%	90%	100%
Beta Blocker at Arrival	46	98%	89%	87%	100%
Beta Blocker at Discharge	61	97%	89%	90%	100%
Fibrinolytic Medication Timing	0	-	40%	31%	100%
PCI Within 90 Minutes of Arrival[1]	4	50%	52%	54%	95%
Smoking Cessation Advice	27	96%	87%	88%	100%
Heart Failure Care					
ACE Inhibitor or ARB for LVSD	136	88%	84%	82%	100%
Discharge Instructions	255	68%	56%	61%	93%
Evaluation of LVS Function	265	98%	84%	83%	99%
Smoking Cessation Advice	69	100%	82%	82%	100%
Pneumonia Care					
Appropriate Initial Antibiotic[2]	76	71%	82%	83%	94%
Blood Culture Timing[2]	96	93%	89%	90%	100%
Influenza Vaccine	28	36%	58%	70%	100%
Initial Antibiotic Timing[2]	151	59%	75%	80%	93%
Oxygenation Assessment[2]	179	100%	99%	99%	100%
Pneumococcal Vaccine[2]	66	41%	58%	69%	94%
Smoking Cessation Advice[2]	36	100%	75%	80%	100%
Surgical Infection Prevention					
Prophylactic Antibiotic Given[2]	438	75%	74%	77%	95%
Prophylactic Antibiotic Selection[2]	126	91%	89%	90%	100%
Prophylactic Antibiotic Stopped[2]	430	68%	65%	72%	95%
Pregnancy Care					
Inpatient Neonatal Mortality	1,667	2.64%	-	-	-
Third or Fourth Degree Laceration	1,017	3.15%	3.58%	3.63%	3.27%

Oroville Hospital

2767 Olive Highway
Oroville, CA 95966
Phone: 530-533-8500
Fax: 530-532-8433
E-mail: info@orovillehospital.com
URL: www.orovillehospital.com
Ownership: Voluntary non-profit - Private
Accredited: No
Emergency Services: Yes
Licensed Beds: 153

Key Personnel:

CEO/President. . . . . Robert J Wentz
Chief Medical Staff. . . . . Mark Heinrich, DO
Emergency Room . . . . Leslie Mann
Infection Control. . . . . Kimberly Nixon, RN
Intensive Coronary Care . . . . Darla Epperson, RN
Director Medical/Surgical Nursing . . . . Carol Speer-Smith, RN
Surgery Clinical Advisor. . . . . Robyn North, RN
Director Radiology . . . . William Moe, MD
Director Respiratory Therapy . . . . Steve Whiteman

Measure	Cases	This Hospital	State Average	U.S. Average	Top Hospital
Heart Attack Care					
ACE Inhibitor or ARB for LVSD[1]	4	75%	82%	82%	100%
Aspirin at Arrival	35	83%	95%	92%	100%
Aspirin at Discharge[1]	11	91%	90%	90%	100%
Beta Blocker at Arrival	36	81%	89%	87%	100%
Beta Blocker at Discharge[1]	11	73%	89%	90%	100%
Fibrinolytic Medication Timing[1]	3	0%	40%	31%	100%
PCI Within 90 Minutes of Arrival	0	-	52%	54%	95%
Smoking Cessation Advice[1]	3	0%	87%	88%	100%
Heart Failure Care					
ACE Inhibitor or ARB for LVSD	58	84%	84%	82%	100%
Discharge Instructions	119	11%	56%	61%	93%
Evaluation of LVS Function	149	77%	84%	83%	99%
Smoking Cessation Advice	36	17%	82%	82%	100%
Pneumonia Care					
Appropriate Initial Antibiotic	108	80%	82%	83%	94%
Blood Culture Timing	98	85%	89%	90%	100%
Influenza Vaccine[1]	21	24%	58%	70%	100%
Initial Antibiotic Timing	131	74%	75%	80%	93%
Oxygenation Assessment	152	100%	99%	99%	100%
Pneumococcal Vaccine	73	12%	58%	69%	94%
Smoking Cessation Advice	51	41%	75%	80%	100%
Surgical Infection Prevention					
Prophylactic Antibiotic Given[3]	41	63%	74%	77%	95%
Prophylactic Antibiotic Selection	36	92%	89%	90%	100%
Prophylactic Antibiotic Stopped[3]	34	100%	65%	72%	95%
Pregnancy Care					
Inpatient Neonatal Mortality	-	-	-	-	-
Third or Fourth Degree Laceration	-	-	3.58%	3.63%	3.27%

NOTE: Hospital profiles are in alphabetical order by state, then city, then hospital within the city; Rankings are sorted by rate in descending order and exclude hospitals with less than 25 cases; (1) The number of cases is too small (n<25) for purposes of reliably predicting hospital performance; (2) Measure reflects the hospital's indication that its submission was based upon a sample of its relevant discharges; (3) Rate reflects fewer than the maximum possible quarters of data for the measure; (4) Inaccurate information submitted and suppressed for one or more quarters; (5) No data is available from the hospital for this measure; Please refer to the User's Guide for a full explanation of data

Saint John's Regional Medical Center

1600 N Rose Avenue
Oxnard, CA 93030
URL: www.stjohnshealth.org
Ownership: Voluntary non-profit - Church
Emergency Services: Yes
Phone: 805-988-2500
Fax: 805-981-4440
Accredited: Yes
Licensed Beds: 230

Key Personnel:
CEO.................................. Michael Merray
Chief Medical Staff......................... Zack Rotenderg
Emergency Room .... Elleen Hooper
OB/GYN Womens Health.................. Maynard Belzer, MD

Measure	Cases	This Hospital	State Average	U.S. Average	Top Hospital
Heart Attack Care					
ACE Inhibitor or ARB for LVSD	40	85%	82%	82%	100%
Aspirin at Arrival	203	99%	95%	92%	100%
Aspirin at Discharge	222	97%	90%	90%	100%
Beta Blocker at Arrival	189	98%	89%	87%	100%
Beta Blocker at Discharge	227	97%	89%	90%	100%
Fibrinolytic Medication Timing	0	-	40%	31%	100%
PCI Within 90 Minutes of Arrival[1]	5	40%	52%	54%	95%
Smoking Cessation Advice	46	93%	87%	88%	100%
Heart Failure Care					
ACE Inhibitor or ARB for LVSD	92	91%	84%	82%	100%
Discharge Instructions	299	63%	56%	61%	93%
Evaluation of LVS Function	342	99%	84%	83%	99%
Smoking Cessation Advice	26	85%	82%	82%	100%
Pneumonia Care					
Appropriate Initial Antibiotic	187	90%	82%	83%	94%
Blood Culture Timing	207	92%	89%	90%	100%
Influenza Vaccine	43	53%	58%	70%	100%
Initial Antibiotic Timing	268	78%	75%	80%	93%
Oxygenation Assessment	326	99%	99%	99%	100%
Pneumococcal Vaccine	227	54%	58%	69%	94%
Smoking Cessation Advice	43	58%	75%	80%	100%
Surgical Infection Prevention					
Prophylactic Antibiotic Given[2,3]	207	76%	74%	77%	95%
Prophylactic Antibiotic Selection[2]	65	86%	89%	90%	100%
Prophylactic Antibiotic Stopped[2,3]	203	52%	65%	72%	95%
Pregnancy Care					
Inpatient Neonatal Mortality	-	-	-	-	-
Third or Fourth Degree Laceration	-	-	3.58%	3.63%	3.27%

Desert Regional Medical Center

Alternate Name: Desert Hospital
1150 N Indian Canon Drive
Palm Springs, CA 92262
Toll-Free: 800-443-3076
Phone: 760-323-6511
Fax: 760-323-6330
URL: www.tenethealth.com
Ownership: Govt - Hospital District or Authority
Emergency Services: Yes
Accredited: Yes
Licensed Beds: 398

Key Personnel:
Administrator .... Steve Schmidt
CEO.................................. Truman Gates

Measure	Cases	This Hospital	State Average	U.S. Average	Top Hospital
Heart Attack Care					
ACE Inhibitor or ARB for LVSD	52	83%	82%	82%	100%
Aspirin at Arrival	180	97%	95%	92%	100%
Aspirin at Discharge	251	97%	90%	90%	100%
Beta Blocker at Arrival	165	96%	89%	87%	100%
Beta Blocker at Discharge	249	94%	89%	90%	100%
Fibrinolytic Medication Timing	0	-	40%	31%	100%
PCI Within 90 Minutes of Arrival[1]	5	80%	52%	54%	95%
Smoking Cessation Advice	68	94%	87%	88%	100%
Heart Failure Care					
ACE Inhibitor or ARB for LVSD	209	88%	84%	82%	100%
Discharge Instructions	333	87%	56%	61%	93%
Evaluation of LVS Function	436	92%	84%	83%	99%
Smoking Cessation Advice	91	96%	82%	82%	100%
Pneumonia Care					
Appropriate Initial Antibiotic	244	93%	82%	83%	94%
Blood Culture Timing	214	94%	89%	90%	100%
Influenza Vaccine	53	83%	58%	70%	100%
Initial Antibiotic Timing	306	91%	75%	80%	93%
Oxygenation Assessment	354	100%	99%	99%	100%
Pneumococcal Vaccine	234	86%	58%	69%	94%
Smoking Cessation Advice	89	89%	75%	80%	100%
Surgical Infection Prevention					
Prophylactic Antibiotic Given[2]	366	86%	74%	77%	95%
Prophylactic Antibiotic Selection[2]	88	93%	89%	90%	100%
Prophylactic Antibiotic Stopped[2]	357	43%	65%	72%	95%
Pregnancy Care					
Inpatient Neonatal Mortality	-	-	-	-	-
Third or Fourth Degree Laceration	-	-	3.58%	3.63%	3.27%

Kaiser Permanente Panorama City Med Ctr

13652 Cantara Street
Panorama City, CA 91402
URL: www.kaiserpermanente.org
Ownership: Voluntary non-profit - Private
Emergency Services: Yes
Phone: 818-375-2000
Fax: 818-375-2728
Accredited: Yes
Licensed Beds: 325

Key Personnel:
CEO.................................. Dev Mahadevan
OB/GYN Womens Health.................. Nabeel Atalla, MD
Director Respiratory Therapy .... John LaCombe

Measure	Cases	This Hospital	State Average	U.S. Average	Top Hospital
Heart Attack Care					
ACE Inhibitor or ARB for LVSD[1]	17	82%	82%	82%	100%
Aspirin at Arrival	98	94%	95%	92%	100%
Aspirin at Discharge	63	95%	90%	90%	100%
Beta Blocker at Arrival	100	95%	89%	87%	100%
Beta Blocker at Discharge	71	93%	89%	90%	100%
Fibrinolytic Medication Timing[1]	17	71%	40%	31%	100%
PCI Within 90 Minutes of Arrival	0	-	52%	54%	95%
Smoking Cessation Advice[1]	10	90%	87%	88%	100%
Heart Failure Care					
ACE Inhibitor or ARB for LVSD	134	75%	84%	82%	100%
Discharge Instructions	340	60%	56%	61%	93%
Evaluation of LVS Function	371	83%	84%	83%	99%
Smoking Cessation Advice	45	82%	82%	82%	100%
Pneumonia Care					
Appropriate Initial Antibiotic	67	36%	82%	83%	94%
Blood Culture Timing	51	75%	89%	90%	100%
Influenza Vaccine	25	64%	58%	70%	100%
Initial Antibiotic Timing	94	66%	75%	80%	93%
Oxygenation Assessment	118	99%	99%	99%	100%
Pneumococcal Vaccine	91	60%	58%	69%	94%
Smoking Cessation Advice[1]	15	67%	75%	80%	100%
Surgical Infection Prevention					
Prophylactic Antibiotic Given[3]	41	71%	74%	77%	95%
Prophylactic Antibiotic Selection	41	98%	89%	90%	100%
Prophylactic Antibiotic Stopped[3]	40	52%	65%	72%	95%
Pregnancy Care					
Inpatient Neonatal Mortality	1,656	0.06%	-	-	-
Third or Fourth Degree Laceration	1,026	2.92%	3.58%	3.63%	3.27%

Mission Community Hospital

Alternate Name: Panorama Community Hospital
14850 Roscoe Boulevard
Panorama City, CA 91402
Toll-Free: 800-608-4624
Phone: 818-787-2222
Fax: 818-904-3529
E-mail: info@mchonline.org
URL: www.mcchonline.org
Ownership: Voluntary non-profit - Private
Emergency Services: Yes
Accredited: Yes
Licensed Beds: 120

Key Personnel:
CEO.................................. Heidi Lennartz
Chief of Medical Staff....................... Ravi Gupta
Emergency Room .... James Webb
CNO.................................. Camila Muirey
ICU .... Camila Mulrey
Intensive Coronary......................... Camila Mulrey
Director Medical/Surgical Nursing .... Carmela Tellez
Director of Pulmonary/Respiratory Care....... Steve Pritchett

NOTE: Hospital profiles are in alphabetical order by state, then city, then hospital within the city; Rankings are sorted by rate in descending order and exclude hospitals with less than 25 cases; (1) The number of cases is too small (n<25) for purposes of reliably predicting hospital performance; (2) Measure reflects the hospital's indication that its submission was based upon a sample of its relevant discharges; (3) Rate reflects fewer than the maximum possible quarters of data for the measure; (4) Inaccurate information submitted and suppressed for one or more quarters; (5) No data is available from the hospital for this measure; Please refer to the User's Guide for a full explanation of data

Measure	Cases	This Hospital	State Average	U.S. Average	Top Hospital
Heart Attack Care					
ACE Inhibitor or ARB for LVSD[1]	15	53%	82%	82%	100%
Aspirin at Arrival	37	92%	95%	92%	100%
Aspirin at Discharge	34	82%	90%	90%	100%
Beta Blocker at Arrival	36	89%	89%	87%	100%
Beta Blocker at Discharge	32	72%	89%	90%	100%
Fibrinolytic Medication Timing[1,3]	2	0%	40%	31%	100%
PCI Within 90 Minutes of Arrival	0	-	52%	54%	95%
Smoking Cessation Advice[1,3]	3	0%	87%	88%	100%
Heart Failure Care					
ACE Inhibitor or ARB for LVSD	68	71%	84%	82%	100%
Discharge Instructions[3]	25	48%	56%	61%	93%
Evaluation of LVS Function	171	82%	84%	83%	99%
Smoking Cessation Advice[1,3]	7	57%	82%	82%	100%
Pneumonia Care					
Appropriate Initial Antibiotic[1,3]	21	57%	82%	83%	94%
Blood Culture Timing[3]	37	81%	89%	90%	100%
Influenza Vaccine[5]	-	-	58%	70%	100%
Initial Antibiotic Timing	194	75%	75%	80%	93%
Oxygenation Assessment	229	99%	99%	99%	100%
Pneumococcal Vaccine	125	7%	58%	69%	94%
Smoking Cessation Advice[1,3]	4	75%	75%	80%	100%
Surgical Infection Prevention					
Prophylactic Antibiotic Given[1,3]	5	20%	74%	77%	95%
Prophylactic Antibiotic Selection[5]	-	-	89%	90%	100%
Prophylactic Antibiotic Stopped[1,3]	4	25%	65%	72%	95%
Pregnancy Care					
Inpatient Neonatal Mortality	-	-	-	-	-
Third or Fourth Degree Laceration	-	-	3.58%	3.63%	3.27%

Feather River Hospital

5974 Pentz Road
Paradise, CA 95969
Phone: 530-877-9361
Fax: 530-876-2157
E-mail: wisenemm@ah.org
URL: www.frhosp.org
Ownership: Voluntary non-profit - Church
Accredited: Yes
Emergency Services: Yes
Licensed Beds: 122

Key Personnel:

President/CEO.......................... Wayne Ferch
Director Catheterization .... Sue Hancock
Director Emergency Room................. Bruce Broyer, RN
Infection Control......................... Carole Farmer
Director OB/GYN Womens Health .... Linda Edwards, RN
Director Radiology .... Sue Hancock
Director Respiratory/Cardiopulmonary .... Laurie Taggert

Measure	Cases	This Hospital	State Average	U.S. Average	Top Hospital
Heart Attack Care					
ACE Inhibitor or ARB for LVSD[1]	11	91%	82%	82%	100%
Aspirin at Arrival	62	92%	95%	92%	100%
Aspirin at Discharge	35	97%	90%	90%	100%
Beta Blocker at Arrival	61	89%	89%	87%	100%
Beta Blocker at Discharge	42	100%	89%	90%	100%
Fibrinolytic Medication Timing[1]	1	100%	40%	31%	100%
PCI Within 90 Minutes of Arrival	0	-	52%	54%	95%
Smoking Cessation Advice[1]	5	80%	87%	88%	100%
Heart Failure Care					
ACE Inhibitor or ARB for LVSD[1]	22	91%	84%	82%	100%
Discharge Instructions	64	84%	56%	61%	93%
Evaluation of LVS Function	84	98%	84%	83%	99%
Smoking Cessation Advice[1]	10	90%	82%	82%	100%
Pneumonia Care					
Appropriate Initial Antibiotic	119	83%	82%	83%	94%
Blood Culture Timing	128	94%	89%	90%	100%
Influenza Vaccine	36	94%	58%	70%	100%
Initial Antibiotic Timing	164	82%	75%	80%	93%
Oxygenation Assessment	203	100%	99%	99%	100%
Pneumococcal Vaccine	138	99%	58%	69%	94%
Smoking Cessation Advice	46	93%	75%	80%	100%
Surgical Infection Prevention					
Prophylactic Antibiotic Given[2,3]	119	67%	74%	77%	95%
Prophylactic Antibiotic Selection[2]	38	100%	89%	90%	100%
Prophylactic Antibiotic Stopped[2,3]	116	80%	65%	72%	95%
Pregnancy Care					
Inpatient Neonatal Mortality	-	-	-	-	-
Third or Fourth Degree Laceration	-	-	3.58%	3.63%	3.27%

Huntington Memorial Hospital

100 W California Boulevard
Pasadena, CA 91105
Phone: 626-397-5000
Fax: 626-397-2903
URL: www.huntingtonhospital.com
Ownership: Voluntary non-profit - Private
Accredited: Yes
Emergency Services: Yes
Licensed Beds: 525

Key Personnel:

President/CEO.......................... Steven A Ralph
Chief Medical Staff....................... Vande Polich
Emergency Room .... Stanley Kalter, MD
OB/GYN Womens Health................... James Cailloutte, MD
Director Radiology .... John Kassabian

Measure	Cases	This Hospital	State Average	U.S. Average	Top Hospital
Heart Attack Care					
ACE Inhibitor or ARB for LVSD	51	90%	82%	82%	100%
Aspirin at Arrival	249	94%	95%	92%	100%
Aspirin at Discharge	235	98%	90%	90%	100%
Beta Blocker at Arrival	170	93%	89%	87%	100%
Beta Blocker at Discharge	224	96%	89%	90%	100%
Fibrinolytic Medication Timing	0	-	40%	31%	100%
PCI Within 90 Minutes of Arrival[1]	11	64%	52%	54%	95%
Smoking Cessation Advice	60	93%	87%	88%	100%
Heart Failure Care					
ACE Inhibitor or ARB for LVSD	178	75%	84%	82%	100%
Discharge Instructions	418	33%	56%	61%	93%
Evaluation of LVS Function	493	87%	84%	83%	99%
Smoking Cessation Advice	72	86%	82%	82%	100%
Pneumonia Care					
Appropriate Initial Antibiotic	289	83%	82%	83%	94%
Blood Culture Timing	391	90%	89%	90%	100%
Influenza Vaccine	132	14%	58%	70%	100%
Initial Antibiotic Timing	462	71%	75%	80%	93%
Oxygenation Assessment	630	100%	99%	99%	100%
Pneumococcal Vaccine	443	9%	58%	69%	94%
Smoking Cessation Advice	84	79%	75%	80%	100%
Surgical Infection Prevention					
Prophylactic Antibiotic Given[2,3]	319	85%	74%	77%	95%
Prophylactic Antibiotic Selection[2]	313	96%	89%	90%	100%
Prophylactic Antibiotic Stopped[2,3]	315	30%	65%	72%	95%
Pregnancy Care					
Inpatient Neonatal Mortality	-	-	-	-	-
Third or Fourth Degree Laceration	-	-	3.58%	3.63%	3.27%

Petaluma Valley Hospital

400 N McDowell Boulevard
Petaluma, CA 94954
Phone: 707-778-1111
Fax: 707-778-9117
Ownership: Voluntary non-profit - Other
Accredited: Yes
Emergency Services: Yes
Licensed Beds: 80

Key Personnel:

CEO................................. Michael Glasberg
Chief of Medical Staff..................... Gary Greenfweit
Emergency Room .... Loren Fong
Manager Infection Control .... Connie Musser, RN
Manager Intensive Coronary .... Nancy Corda, RN
Manager Medical/Surgical .... Lynn Finley, RN
Director Respiratory...................... Dan Cress

Measure	Cases	This Hospital	State Average	U.S. Average	Top Hospital
Heart Attack Care					
ACE Inhibitor or ARB for LVSD[1]	4	50%	82%	82%	100%
Aspirin at Arrival	51	98%	95%	92%	100%
Aspirin at Discharge	27	96%	90%	90%	100%
Beta Blocker at Arrival	40	100%	89%	87%	100%
Beta Blocker at Discharge	25	100%	89%	90%	100%
Fibrinolytic Medication Timing[1]	11	55%	40%	31%	100%

NOTE: Hospital profiles are in alphabetical order by state, then city, then hospital within the city; Rankings are sorted by rate in descending order and exclude hospitals with less than 25 cases; (1) The number of cases is too small (n<25) for purposes of reliably predicting hospital performance; (2) Measure reflects the hospital's indication that its submission was based upon a sample of its relevant discharges; (3) Rate reflects fewer than the maximum possible quarters of data for the measure; (4) Inaccurate information submitted and suppressed for one or more quarters; (5) No data is available from the hospital for this measure; Please refer to the User's Guide for a full explanation of data

PCI Within 90 Minutes of Arrival	0	-	52%	54%	95%
Smoking Cessation Advice[1]	4	75%	87%	88%	100%
Heart Failure Care					
ACE Inhibitor or ARB for LVSD[1]	16	94%	84%	82%	100%
Discharge Instructions	56	59%	56%	61%	93%
Evaluation of LVS Function	82	91%	84%	83%	99%
Smoking Cessation Advice[1]	14	29%	82%	82%	100%
Pneumonia Care					
Appropriate Initial Antibiotic	95	74%	82%	83%	94%
Blood Culture Timing	45	80%	89%	90%	100%
Influenza Vaccine	28	79%	58%	70%	100%
Initial Antibiotic Timing	101	77%	75%	80%	93%
Oxygenation Assessment	139	100%	99%	99%	100%
Pneumococcal Vaccine	87	85%	58%	69%	94%
Smoking Cessation Advice[1]	24	62%	75%	80%	100%
Surgical Infection Prevention					
Prophylactic Antibiotic Given[2,3]	81	75%	74%	77%	95%
Prophylactic Antibiotic Selection[2]	30	87%	89%	90%	100%
Prophylactic Antibiotic Stopped[2,3]	81	69%	65%	72%	95%
Pregnancy Care					
Inpatient Neonatal Mortality	-	-	-	-	-
Third or Fourth Degree Laceration	-	-	3.58%	3.63%	3.27%

Placentia-Linda Hospital

1301 N Rose Drive
Placentia, CA 92870
URL: www.placentialinda.com
Ownership: Proprietary
Emergency Services: Yes

Phone: 714-993-2000
Fax: 714-961-8427
Accredited: Yes
Licensed Beds: 114

Key Personnel:

CEO. . . . . Kent Clayton
Chief Medical Staff. . . . . Paul Jordan, MD
Cardiac Lab . . . . Michael Babaeff, RPT
Emergency Room . . . . Bryan Hoynak, MD
Intensive/Coronary Care . . . . Vicki Shrock, RN
Medical Surgical Nursing . . . . Denise Gillette, RN
Respiratory/Cardiopulmonary. . . . . Michael Babaeff

Measure	Cases	This Hospital	State Average	U.S. Average	Top Hospital
Heart Attack Care					
ACE Inhibitor or ARB for LVSD[1]	7	57%	82%	82%	100%
Aspirin at Arrival	37	95%	95%	92%	100%
Aspirin at Discharge[1]	16	81%	90%	90%	100%
Beta Blocker at Arrival[1]	23	91%	89%	87%	100%
Beta Blocker at Discharge[1]	20	80%	89%	90%	100%
Fibrinolytic Medication Timing[1]	5	40%	40%	31%	100%
PCI Within 90 Minutes of Arrival	0	-	52%	54%	95%
Smoking Cessation Advice	0	-	87%	88%	100%
Heart Failure Care					
ACE Inhibitor or ARB for LVSD	36	72%	84%	82%	100%
Discharge Instructions	74	84%	56%	61%	93%
Evaluation of LVS Function	110	90%	84%	83%	99%
Smoking Cessation Advice[1]	3	100%	82%	82%	100%
Pneumonia Care					
Appropriate Initial Antibiotic	146	92%	82%	83%	94%
Blood Culture Timing	145	96%	89%	90%	100%
Influenza Vaccine	40	82%	58%	70%	100%
Initial Antibiotic Timing	187	91%	75%	80%	93%
Oxygenation Assessment	229	100%	99%	99%	100%
Pneumococcal Vaccine	164	80%	58%	69%	94%
Smoking Cessation Advice	30	77%	75%	80%	100%
Surgical Infection Prevention					
Prophylactic Antibiotic Given[2]	145	90%	74%	77%	95%
Prophylactic Antibiotic Selection[2]	41	85%	89%	90%	100%
Prophylactic Antibiotic Stopped[2]	139	84%	65%	72%	95%
Pregnancy Care					
Inpatient Neonatal Mortality	-	-	-	-	-
Third or Fourth Degree Laceration	-	-	3.58%	3.63%	3.27%

Marshall Medical Center

1100 Marshall Way
Placerville, CA 95667
URL: www.marshallmedical.org
Ownership: Voluntary non-profit - Other
Emergency Services: Yes

Phone: 530-626-2601
Fax: 530-622-7853
Accredited: Yes
Licensed Beds: 105

Key Personnel:

Chairman/CEO. . . . . James Whipple
President . . . . George Cook
Chief Medical Staff. . . . . Reginald Rice, Sr, MD
Cardiac Lab . . . . Melinda Head, RN
Catheterization Lab . . . . Melinda Head, RN
Manager Emergency Room . . . . Janice Weaver
Manager Emergency Room . . . . Carol Velasquez
Infection Control. . . . . Sue Deal, RN
ICU Supervising Nurse. . . . . Dennis Bietz
Manager CCU . . . . Dennis Bietz
Director Medical/Surgical Nursing . . . . Claire Pacific, RN
Surgical Services Manager . . . . Bonnie Line
Manager Respiratory Services. . . . . Joel Porter

Measure	Cases	This Hospital	State Average	U.S. Average	Top Hospital
Heart Attack Care					
ACE Inhibitor or ARB for LVSD[1]	8	62%	82%	82%	100%
Aspirin at Arrival	35	94%	95%	92%	100%
Aspirin at Discharge[1]	18	94%	90%	90%	100%
Beta Blocker at Arrival	32	94%	89%	87%	100%
Beta Blocker at Discharge[1]	24	92%	89%	90%	100%
Fibrinolytic Medication Timing[1]	5	40%	40%	31%	100%
PCI Within 90 Minutes of Arrival	0	-	52%	54%	95%
Smoking Cessation Advice[1]	4	75%	87%	88%	100%
Heart Failure Care					
ACE Inhibitor or ARB for LVSD	55	73%	84%	82%	100%
Discharge Instructions	137	37%	56%	61%	93%
Evaluation of LVS Function	171	89%	84%	83%	99%
Smoking Cessation Advice[1]	16	100%	82%	82%	100%
Pneumonia Care					
Appropriate Initial Antibiotic	111	84%	82%	83%	94%
Blood Culture Timing	120	95%	89%	90%	100%
Influenza Vaccine[4,5]	-	-	58%	70%	100%
Initial Antibiotic Timing	148	81%	75%	80%	93%
Oxygenation Assessment	182	100%	99%	99%	100%
Pneumococcal Vaccine	125	38%	58%	69%	94%
Smoking Cessation Advice	33	94%	75%	80%	100%
Surgical Infection Prevention					
Prophylactic Antibiotic Given[2,3]	197	90%	74%	77%	95%
Prophylactic Antibiotic Selection[2]	62	92%	89%	90%	100%
Prophylactic Antibiotic Stopped[2,3]	188	79%	65%	72%	95%
Pregnancy Care					
Inpatient Neonatal Mortality	-	-	-	-	-
Third or Fourth Degree Laceration	-	-	3.58%	3.63%	3.27%

Pomona Valley Hospital Medical Center

1798 N Garey Avenue
Pomona, CA 91767
URL: www.pvhmc.com
Ownership: Voluntary non-profit - Other
Emergency Services: Yes

Phone: 909-865-9500
Fax: 909-623-4021
Accredited: Yes
Licensed Beds: 446

Key Personnel:

President/CEO. . . . . Rich Yochum
Chief Medical Staff. . . . . Kenneth Nakamoto, MD
CCU Spvg. Nurse . . . . Karen Blessing
Director Medical/Surgical Nursing . . . . Darlene Scafiddi
Director Respiratory Therapy . . . . Jerry Choppi

Measure	Cases	This Hospital	State Average	U.S. Average	Top Hospital
Heart Attack Care					
ACE Inhibitor or ARB for LVSD	98	80%	82%	82%	100%
Aspirin at Arrival	259	93%	95%	92%	100%
Aspirin at Discharge	265	96%	90%	90%	100%
Beta Blocker at Arrival	164	87%	89%	87%	100%
Beta Blocker at Discharge	254	93%	89%	90%	100%
Fibrinolytic Medication Timing[1]	1	0%	40%	31%	100%

NOTE: Hospital profiles are in alphabetical order by state, then city, then hospital within the city; Rankings are sorted by rate in descending order and exclude hospitals with less than 25 cases; (1) The number of cases is too small (n<25) for purposes of reliably predicting hospital performance; (2) Measure reflects the hospital's indication that its submission was based upon a sample of its relevant discharges; (3) Rate reflects fewer than the maximum possible quarters of data for the measure; (4) Inaccurate information submitted and suppressed for one or more quarters; (5) No data is available from the hospital for this measure; Please refer to the User's Guide for a full explanation of data

PCI Within 90 Minutes of Arrival[1]	13	46%	52%	54%	95%
Smoking Cessation Advice	78	99%	87%	88%	100%
Heart Failure Care					
ACE Inhibitor or ARB for LVSD	261	89%	84%	82%	100%
Discharge Instructions	484	76%	56%	61%	93%
Evaluation of LVS Function	604	94%	84%	83%	99%
Smoking Cessation Advice	123	98%	82%	82%	100%
Pneumonia Care					
Appropriate Initial Antibiotic	180	91%	82%	83%	94%
Blood Culture Timing	198	84%	89%	90%	100%
Influenza Vaccine	68	66%	58%	70%	100%
Initial Antibiotic Timing	311	71%	75%	80%	93%
Oxygenation Assessment	406	100%	99%	99%	100%
Pneumococcal Vaccine	226	58%	58%	69%	94%
Smoking Cessation Advice	69	88%	75%	80%	100%
Surgical Infection Prevention					
Prophylactic Antibiotic Given	712	84%	74%	77%	95%
Prophylactic Antibiotic Selection	173	95%	89%	90%	100%
Prophylactic Antibiotic Stopped	683	45%	65%	72%	95%
Pregnancy Care					
Inpatient Neonatal Mortality[2]	1,007	0.20%	-	-	-
Third or Fourth Degree Laceration[2]	637	2.51%	3.58%	3.63%	3.27%

Sierra View District Hospital

465 W Putnam Avenue
Porterville, CA 93257
Phone: 559-784-1110
Fax: 559-788-6135
E-mail: webmaster@sierra-view.com
URL: www.sierra-view.com
Ownership: Govt - Hospital District or Authority
Accredited: No
Emergency Services: Yes
Licensed Beds: 163

Key Personnel:

President/CEO. . . . . Kelly C Morgan
Chief Medical Staff. . . . . Oscar Velasco, MD
Director Emergency Room. . . . . Brenda Jeffrey
Director Infection Control . . . . Betty Jones
Director Maternal & Child Health . . . . Joyce Crawford
Director Surgery. . . . . Roger McPhetridge
Director Radiology . . . . Onalu Shinn

Measure	Cases	This Hospital	State Average	U.S. Average	Top Hospital
Heart Attack Care					
ACE Inhibitor or ARB for LVSD[1]	11	91%	82%	82%	100%
Aspirin at Arrival	80	95%	95%	92%	100%
Aspirin at Discharge	44	93%	90%	90%	100%
Beta Blocker at Arrival	64	73%	89%	87%	100%
Beta Blocker at Discharge	40	95%	89%	90%	100%
Fibrinolytic Medication Timing[1]	16	50%	40%	31%	100%
PCI Within 90 Minutes of Arrival	0	-	52%	54%	95%
Smoking Cessation Advice[1]	17	100%	87%	88%	100%
Heart Failure Care					
ACE Inhibitor or ARB for LVSD	47	94%	84%	82%	100%
Discharge Instructions	174	73%	56%	61%	93%
Evaluation of LVS Function	227	67%	84%	83%	99%
Smoking Cessation Advice	36	92%	82%	82%	100%
Pneumonia Care					
Appropriate Initial Antibiotic	160	79%	82%	83%	94%
Blood Culture Timing	160	84%	89%	90%	100%
Influenza Vaccine	60	65%	58%	70%	100%
Initial Antibiotic Timing	240	63%	75%	80%	93%
Oxygenation Assessment	317	100%	99%	99%	100%
Pneumococcal Vaccine	169	66%	58%	69%	94%
Smoking Cessation Advice	57	93%	75%	80%	100%
Surgical Infection Prevention					
Prophylactic Antibiotic Given[3]	130	53%	74%	77%	95%
Prophylactic Antibiotic Selection	63	98%	89%	90%	100%
Prophylactic Antibiotic Stopped[3]	113	39%	65%	72%	95%
Pregnancy Care					
Inpatient Neonatal Mortality	-	-	-	-	-
Third or Fourth Degree Laceration	-	-	3.58%	3.63%	3.27%

Eastern Plumas Health Care

Alternate Name: Eastern Plumas District Hospital
500 First Avenue
Portola, CA 96122
Toll-Free: 800-571-3742
Phone: 530-832-6500
Fax: 530-832-4494
E-mail: info@ephc.org
URL: www.ephc.org
Ownership: Govt - Hospital District or Authority
Accredited: No
Emergency Services: Yes
Licensed Beds: 24

Key Personnel:

CEO. . . . . Charles R Guenther
Director Medical/Surgical Nursing . . . . Sharon Clarke
CNO. . . . . Maxine Flora
Chief Radiology . . . . Steven Bartok, MD
Director Respiratory Therapy . . . . David Rodriguez

Measure	Cases	This Hospital	State Average	U.S. Average	Top Hospital
Heart Attack Care					
ACE Inhibitor or ARB for LVSD[5]	-	-	82%	82%	100%
Aspirin at Arrival[5]	-	-	95%	92%	100%
Aspirin at Discharge[5]	-	-	90%	90%	100%
Beta Blocker at Arrival[5]	-	-	89%	87%	100%
Beta Blocker at Discharge[5]	-	-	89%	90%	100%
Fibrinolytic Medication Timing[5]	-	-	40%	31%	100%
PCI Within 90 Minutes of Arrival[5]	-	-	52%	54%	95%
Smoking Cessation Advice[5]	-	-	87%	88%	100%
Heart Failure Care					
ACE Inhibitor or ARB for LVSD[5]	-	-	84%	82%	100%
Discharge Instructions[5]	-	-	56%	61%	93%
Evaluation of LVS Function[5]	-	-	84%	83%	99%
Smoking Cessation Advice[5]	-	-	82%	82%	100%
Pneumonia Care					
Appropriate Initial Antibiotic[1,3]	1	100%	82%	83%	94%
Blood Culture Timing[1,3]	1	100%	89%	90%	100%
Influenza Vaccine[5]	-	-	58%	70%	100%
Initial Antibiotic Timing[3]	0	-	75%	80%	93%
Oxygenation Assessment[1,3]	2	100%	99%	99%	100%
Pneumococcal Vaccine[1,3]	2	0%	58%	69%	94%
Smoking Cessation Advice[3]	0	-	75%	80%	100%
Surgical Infection Prevention					
Prophylactic Antibiotic Given[5]	-	-	74%	77%	95%
Prophylactic Antibiotic Selection[5]	-	-	89%	90%	100%
Prophylactic Antibiotic Stopped[5]	-	-	65%	72%	95%
Pregnancy Care					
Inpatient Neonatal Mortality	-	-	-	-	-
Third or Fourth Degree Laceration	-	-	3.58%	3.63%	3.27%

Pomerado Hospital

15615 Pomerado Road
Poway, CA 92064
Phone: 858-613-4000
Fax: 858-675-5077
URL: www.pph.org
Ownership: Govt - Hospital District or Authority
Accredited: Yes
Emergency Services: Yes
Licensed Beds: 107

Key Personnel:

Interim CEO. . . . . Michael Covert
Chief Medical Staff. . . . . Paul Tornambe
Emergency Room . . . . Kim Colonnelli
Infection Control. . . . . Val Tesoro, MD
ICU . . . . Ellen McKissick
Medical Surgical Nursing . . . . Beth Gardner
OB/GYN/Women's Health . . . . Caroline Brown
Chief Radiology . . . . Kirk Burst
Director of Pulmonary/Respiratory Care. . . . . . . Ron Duncan

Measure	Cases	This Hospital	State Average	U.S. Average	Top Hospital
Heart Attack Care					
ACE Inhibitor or ARB for LVSD[1]	4	100%	82%	82%	100%
Aspirin at Arrival	54	100%	95%	92%	100%
Aspirin at Discharge	25	96%	90%	90%	100%
Beta Blocker at Arrival	50	100%	89%	87%	100%
Beta Blocker at Discharge	25	100%	89%	90%	100%
Fibrinolytic Medication Timing	0	-	40%	31%	100%
PCI Within 90 Minutes of Arrival	0	-	52%	54%	95%
Smoking Cessation Advice[1]	5	60%	87%	88%	100%
Heart Failure Care					

NOTE: Hospital profiles are in alphabetical order by state, then city, then hospital within the city; Rankings are sorted by rate in descending order and exclude hospitals with less than 25 cases; (1) The number of cases is too small (n<25) for purposes of reliably predicting hospital performance; (2) Measure reflects the hospital's indication that its submission was based upon a sample of its relevant discharges; (3) Rate reflects fewer than the maximum possible quarters of data for the measure; (4) Inaccurate information submitted and suppressed for one or more quarters; (5) No data is available from the hospital for this measure; Please refer to the User's Guide for a full explanation of data

Measure	Cases	This Hospital	State Average	U.S. Average	Top Hospital
ACE Inhibitor or ARB for LVSD	29	100%	84%	82%	100%
Discharge Instructions	122	81%	56%	61%	93%
Evaluation of LVS Function	133	98%	84%	83%	99%
Smoking Cessation Advice[1]	17	100%	82%	82%	100%
Pneumonia Care					
Appropriate Initial Antibiotic	155	90%	82%	83%	94%
Blood Culture Timing	140	89%	89%	90%	100%
Influenza Vaccine	35	49%	58%	70%	100%
Initial Antibiotic Timing	160	80%	75%	80%	93%
Oxygenation Assessment	206	100%	99%	99%	100%
Pneumococcal Vaccine	148	64%	58%	69%	94%
Smoking Cessation Advice	26	77%	75%	80%	100%
Surgical Infection Prevention					
Prophylactic Antibiotic Given[2,3]	146	76%	74%	77%	95%
Prophylactic Antibiotic Selection[2]	46	87%	89%	90%	100%
Prophylactic Antibiotic Stopped[2,3]	142	81%	65%	72%	95%
Pregnancy Care					
Inpatient Neonatal Mortality	-	-	-	-	-
Third or Fourth Degree Laceration	-	-	3.58%	3.63%	3.27%

Eisenhower Medical Center

Alternate Name: Betty Ford Center
39000 Bob Hope Drive — Phone: 760-340-3911
Rancho Mirage, CA 92270 — Fax: 760-773-1421
URL: www.emc.org
Ownership: Voluntary non-profit - Other — Accredited: Yes
Emergency Services: Yes — Licensed Beds: 253

Key Personnel:

CEO . . . . Aubrey Serfline
Medical Staff President . . . . Stephen Steele, DO
Emergency Room . . . . Ian Hart
Admin Director Med/Surg Services . . . . Mary Ann McLaughlin
Admin Director Surgical Services . . . . Lynn Hart
Cardiology Section Chief . . . . Damon Kelsay, MD

Measure	Cases	This Hospital	State Average	U.S. Average	Top Hospital
Heart Attack Care					
ACE Inhibitor or ARB for LVSD	100	80%	82%	82%	100%
Aspirin at Arrival	319	92%	95%	92%	100%
Aspirin at Discharge	317	91%	90%	90%	100%
Beta Blocker at Arrival	182	85%	89%	87%	100%
Beta Blocker at Discharge	354	92%	89%	90%	100%
Fibrinolytic Medication Timing	0	-	40%	31%	100%
PCI Within 90 Minutes of Arrival[1]	11	82%	52%	54%	95%
Smoking Cessation Advice	75	96%	87%	88%	100%
Heart Failure Care					
ACE Inhibitor or ARB for LVSD	310	86%	84%	82%	100%
Discharge Instructions	480	56%	56%	61%	93%
Evaluation of LVS Function	619	90%	84%	83%	99%
Smoking Cessation Advice	73	95%	82%	82%	100%
Pneumonia Care					
Appropriate Initial Antibiotic	359	77%	82%	83%	94%
Blood Culture Timing	197	79%	89%	90%	100%
Influenza Vaccine	96	71%	58%	70%	100%
Initial Antibiotic Timing	369	67%	75%	80%	93%
Oxygenation Assessment	455	100%	99%	99%	100%
Pneumococcal Vaccine	342	64%	58%	69%	94%
Smoking Cessation Advice	61	92%	75%	80%	100%
Surgical Infection Prevention					
Prophylactic Antibiotic Given[2,3]	666	86%	74%	77%	95%
Prophylactic Antibiotic Selection[2]	74	96%	89%	90%	100%
Prophylactic Antibiotic Stopped[2,3]	650	75%	65%	72%	95%
Pregnancy Care					
Inpatient Neonatal Mortality	-	-	-	-	-
Third or Fourth Degree Laceration	-	-	3.58%	3.63%	3.27%

Saint Elizabeth Community Hospital

2550 Sister Mary Columba Drive — Phone: 530-529-8000
Red Bluff, CA 96080 — Fax: 530-529-8033
URL: redbluff.mercy.org
Ownership: Voluntary non-profit - Church — Accredited: Yes
Emergency Services: Yes — Licensed Beds: 83

Key Personnel:

President . . . . Jon Halfhide
Emergency Room . . . . Penny Costa, RN
Director Medical/Surgical Nursing . . . . Joanne Heffner, RN
OB/GYN Womens Health. . . . . Lynn Springer, RN
Chief Radiology . . . . Jack Kure, MD
Director Respiratory Therapy . . . . Mary Gonzales

Measure	Cases	This Hospital	State Average	U.S. Average	Top Hospital
Heart Attack Care					
ACE Inhibitor or ARB for LVSD[1]	5	80%	82%	82%	100%
Aspirin at Arrival	40	92%	95%	92%	100%
Aspirin at Discharge[1]	23	78%	90%	90%	100%
Beta Blocker at Arrival	39	85%	89%	87%	100%
Beta Blocker at Discharge	25	76%	89%	90%	100%
Fibrinolytic Medication Timing[1]	1	0%	40%	31%	100%
PCI Within 90 Minutes of Arrival	0	-	52%	54%	95%
Smoking Cessation Advice[1]	7	100%	87%	88%	100%
Heart Failure Care					
ACE Inhibitor or ARB for LVSD[1]	17	88%	84%	82%	100%
Discharge Instructions	65	98%	56%	61%	93%
Evaluation of LVS Function	67	88%	84%	83%	99%
Smoking Cessation Advice[1]	13	100%	82%	82%	100%
Pneumonia Care					
Appropriate Initial Antibiotic	152	90%	82%	83%	94%
Blood Culture Timing	89	87%	89%	90%	100%
Influenza Vaccine	30	87%	58%	70%	100%
Initial Antibiotic Timing	168	89%	75%	80%	93%
Oxygenation Assessment	200	100%	99%	99%	100%
Pneumococcal Vaccine	121	95%	58%	69%	94%
Smoking Cessation Advice	48	100%	75%	80%	100%
Surgical Infection Prevention					
Prophylactic Antibiotic Given[2,3]	168	73%	74%	77%	95%
Prophylactic Antibiotic Selection[2]	54	67%	89%	90%	100%
Prophylactic Antibiotic Stopped[2,3]	164	77%	65%	72%	95%
Pregnancy Care					
Inpatient Neonatal Mortality	721	0.00%	-	-	-
Third or Fourth Degree Laceration	507	2.56%	3.58%	3.63%	3.27%

Mercy Medical Center-Redding

2175 Rosaline Avenue — Phone: 530-225-6000
Redding, CA 96049 — Fax: 530-225-6125
URL: www.redding.mercy.org
Ownership: Voluntary non-profit - Church — Accredited: Yes
Emergency Services: Yes — Licensed Beds: 256

Key Personnel:

CEO/President. . . . . Ray Barnet
Chief Medical Staff. . . . . William de Vlaming, MD
Director Infection/Disease Control . . . . Cathy Carl, RN
Manager Respiratory Therapy . . . . Michael Brown

Measure	Cases	This Hospital	State Average	U.S. Average	Top Hospital
Heart Attack Care					
ACE Inhibitor or ARB for LVSD	57	98%	82%	82%	100%
Aspirin at Arrival	173	100%	95%	92%	100%
Aspirin at Discharge	262	97%	90%	90%	100%
Beta Blocker at Arrival	131	98%	89%	87%	100%
Beta Blocker at Discharge	257	98%	89%	90%	100%
Fibrinolytic Medication Timing[1]	21	62%	40%	31%	100%
PCI Within 90 Minutes of Arrival[1]	7	29%	52%	54%	95%
Smoking Cessation Advice	116	100%	87%	88%	100%
Heart Failure Care					
ACE Inhibitor or ARB for LVSD	121	89%	84%	82%	100%
Discharge Instructions	221	72%	56%	61%	93%
Evaluation of LVS Function	276	92%	84%	83%	99%
Smoking Cessation Advice	65	100%	82%	82%	100%
Pneumonia Care					

NOTE: Hospital profiles are in alphabetical order by state, then city, then hospital within the city; Rankings are sorted by rate in descending order and exclude hospitals with less than 25 cases; (1) The number of cases is too small (n<25) for purposes of reliably predicting hospital performance; (2) Measure reflects the hospital's indication that its submission was based upon a sample of its relevant discharges; (3) Rate reflects fewer than the maximum possible quarters of data for the measure; (4) Inaccurate information submitted and suppressed for one or more quarters; (5) No data is available from the hospital for this measure; Please refer to the User's Guide for a full explanation of data

Appropriate Initial Antibiotic	274	89%	82%	83%	94%
Blood Culture Timing	180	88%	89%	90%	100%
Influenza Vaccine	66	80%	58%	70%	100%
Initial Antibiotic Timing	316	80%	75%	80%	93%
Oxygenation Assessment	410	100%	99%	99%	100%
Pneumococcal Vaccine	260	78%	58%	69%	94%
Smoking Cessation Advice	111	100%	75%	80%	100%
Surgical Infection Prevention					
Prophylactic Antibiotic Given[2,3]	274	89%	74%	77%	95%
Prophylactic Antibiotic Selection[2]	89	93%	89%	90%	100%
Prophylactic Antibiotic Stopped[2,3]	271	82%	65%	72%	95%
Pregnancy Care					
Inpatient Neonatal Mortality	2,239	0.04%	-	-	-
Third or Fourth Degree Laceration	1,482	2.09%	3.58%	3.63%	3.27%

Patients' Hospital of Redding

2900 Eureka Way
Redding, CA 96001
Phone: 530-225-8700
Ownership: Proprietary
Accredited: No
Emergency Services: No

Measure	Cases	This Hospital	State Average	U.S. Average	Top Hospital
Heart Attack Care					
ACE Inhibitor or ARB for LVSD[5]	-	-	82%	82%	100%
Aspirin at Arrival[5]	-	-	95%	92%	100%
Aspirin at Discharge[5]	-	-	90%	90%	100%
Beta Blocker at Arrival[5]	-	-	89%	87%	100%
Beta Blocker at Discharge[5]	-	-	89%	90%	100%
Fibrinolytic Medication Timing[5]	-	-	40%	31%	100%
PCI Within 90 Minutes of Arrival[5]	-	-	52%	54%	95%
Smoking Cessation Advice[5]	-	-	87%	88%	100%
Heart Failure Care					
ACE Inhibitor or ARB for LVSD[5]	-	-	84%	82%	100%
Discharge Instructions[5]	-	-	56%	61%	93%
Evaluation of LVS Function[5]	-	-	84%	83%	99%
Smoking Cessation Advice[5]	-	-	82%	82%	100%
Pneumonia Care					
Appropriate Initial Antibiotic[5]	-	-	82%	83%	94%
Blood Culture Timing[5]	-	-	89%	90%	100%
Influenza Vaccine[5]	-	-	58%	70%	100%
Initial Antibiotic Timing[5]	-	-	75%	80%	93%
Oxygenation Assessment[5]	-	-	99%	99%	100%
Pneumococcal Vaccine[5]	-	-	58%	69%	94%
Smoking Cessation Advice[5]	-	-	75%	80%	100%
Surgical Infection Prevention					
Prophylactic Antibiotic Given	79	90%	74%	77%	95%
Prophylactic Antibiotic Selection[1]	20	95%	89%	90%	100%
Prophylactic Antibiotic Stopped	78	100%	65%	72%	95%
Pregnancy Care					
Inpatient Neonatal Mortality	-	-	-	-	-
Third or Fourth Degree Laceration	-	-	3.58%	3.63%	3.27%

Shasta Regional Medical Center

1100 Butte Street
Redding, CA 96001
Toll-Free: 800-300-1450
Phone: 530-244-5400
Fax: 530-244-5384
E-mail: info@shastaregional.com
URL: www.shastaregional.com
Ownership: Proprietary
Accredited: Yes
Emergency Services: Yes
Licensed Beds: 246

Key Personnel:

CEO. . . . . Thomas Salren
Chief Medical Staff. . . . . Mark Nicholas
Head Emergency Room. . . . . Marry House
Director Respiratory Therapy . . . . Steve Buhler

Measure	Cases	This Hospital	State Average	U.S. Average	Top Hospital
Heart Attack Care					
ACE Inhibitor or ARB for LVSD	32	94%	82%	82%	100%
Aspirin at Arrival	94	99%	95%	92%	100%
Aspirin at Discharge	114	97%	90%	90%	100%
Beta Blocker at Arrival	69	97%	89%	87%	100%
Beta Blocker at Discharge	111	96%	89%	90%	100%
Fibrinolytic Medication Timing[1]	4	50%	40%	31%	100%
PCI Within 90 Minutes of Arrival[1]	4	25%	52%	54%	95%
Smoking Cessation Advice	47	98%	87%	88%	100%
Heart Failure Care					
ACE Inhibitor or ARB for LVSD	98	90%	84%	82%	100%
Discharge Instructions	176	66%	56%	61%	93%
Evaluation of LVS Function	216	95%	84%	83%	99%
Smoking Cessation Advice	61	100%	82%	82%	100%
Pneumonia Care					
Appropriate Initial Antibiotic	232	89%	82%	83%	94%
Blood Culture Timing	229	90%	89%	90%	100%
Influenza Vaccine	65	82%	58%	70%	100%
Initial Antibiotic Timing	313	81%	75%	80%	93%
Oxygenation Assessment	381	100%	99%	99%	100%
Pneumococcal Vaccine	241	80%	58%	69%	94%
Smoking Cessation Advice	153	95%	75%	80%	100%
Surgical Infection Prevention					
Prophylactic Antibiotic Given	736	92%	74%	77%	95%
Prophylactic Antibiotic Selection	189	94%	89%	90%	100%
Prophylactic Antibiotic Stopped	714	87%	65%	72%	95%
Pregnancy Care					
Inpatient Neonatal Mortality	-	-	-	-	-
Third or Fourth Degree Laceration	-	-	3.58%	3.63%	3.27%

Redlands Community Hospital

350 Terracina Boulevard
Redlands, CA 92373
Phone: 909-335-5500
Fax: 909-335-6497
URL: www.redlandshospital.com
Ownership: Voluntary non-profit - Other
Accredited: Yes
Emergency Services: Yes
Licensed Beds: 172

Key Personnel:

President/CEO. . . . . James R Holmes
Chief Medical Staff. . . . . Carolina Rosario

Measure	Cases	This Hospital	State Average	U.S. Average	Top Hospital
Heart Attack Care					
ACE Inhibitor or ARB for LVSD	30	80%	82%	82%	100%
Aspirin at Arrival	163	95%	95%	92%	100%
Aspirin at Discharge	88	92%	90%	90%	100%
Beta Blocker at Arrival	114	96%	89%	87%	100%
Beta Blocker at Discharge	91	92%	89%	90%	100%
Fibrinolytic Medication Timing[1,3]	1	100%	40%	31%	100%
PCI Within 90 Minutes of Arrival	0	-	52%	54%	95%
Smoking Cessation Advice[1,3]	1	100%	87%	88%	100%
Heart Failure Care					
ACE Inhibitor or ARB for LVSD	110	79%	84%	82%	100%
Discharge Instructions[3]	45	73%	56%	61%	93%
Evaluation of LVS Function	265	91%	84%	83%	99%
Smoking Cessation Advice[1,3]	7	100%	82%	82%	100%
Pneumonia Care					
Appropriate Initial Antibiotic[1,3]	22	82%	82%	83%	94%
Blood Culture Timing[3]	49	78%	89%	90%	100%
Influenza Vaccine[5]	-	-	58%	70%	100%
Initial Antibiotic Timing	216	75%	75%	80%	93%
Oxygenation Assessment	259	100%	99%	99%	100%
Pneumococcal Vaccine	177	67%	58%	69%	94%
Smoking Cessation Advice[1,3]	11	100%	75%	80%	100%
Surgical Infection Prevention					
Prophylactic Antibiotic Given[3]	144	84%	74%	77%	95%
Prophylactic Antibiotic Selection[5]	-	-	89%	90%	100%
Prophylactic Antibiotic Stopped[3]	140	56%	65%	72%	95%
Pregnancy Care					
Inpatient Neonatal Mortality[2]	583	1.03%	-	-	-
Third or Fourth Degree Laceration[2]	431	4.41%	3.58%	3.63%	3.27%

NOTE: Hospital profiles are in alphabetical order by state, then city, then hospital within the city; Rankings are sorted by rate in descending order and exclude hospitals with less than 25 cases; (1) The number of cases is too small (n<25) for purposes of reliably predicting hospital performance; (2) Measure reflects the hospital's indication that its submission was based upon a sample of its relevant discharges; (3) Rate reflects fewer than the maximum possible quarters of data for the measure; (4) Inaccurate information submitted and suppressed for one or more quarters; (5) No data is available from the hospital for this measure; Please refer to the User's Guide for a full explanation of data

Kaiser Redwood City Medical Center

1150 Veterans Boulevard
Redwood City, CA 94063
Ownership: Voluntary non-profit - Other
Emergency Services: Yes
Phone: 650-299-2000
Fax: 650-299-2421
Accredited: Yes
Licensed Beds: 171

Key Personnel:
Chief Medical Staff . . . . Henry Brodkin, MD
OB/GYN Womens Health. . . . . John Wood, MD
Chief Radiology . . . . Edward Talberth, MD

Measure	Cases	This Hospital	State Average	U.S. Average	Top Hospital
Heart Attack Care					
ACE Inhibitor or ARB for LVSD[1]	6	100%	82%	82%	100%
Aspirin at Arrival	104	100%	95%	92%	100%
Aspirin at Discharge	50	96%	90%	90%	100%
Beta Blocker at Arrival	98	100%	89%	87%	100%
Beta Blocker at Discharge	53	100%	89%	90%	100%
Fibrinolytic Medication Timing[1]	12	58%	40%	31%	100%
PCI Within 90 Minutes of Arrival	0	-	52%	54%	95%
Smoking Cessation Advice[1]	4	100%	87%	88%	100%
Heart Failure Care					
ACE Inhibitor or ARB for LVSD	37	97%	84%	82%	100%
Discharge Instructions	112	40%	56%	61%	93%
Evaluation of LVS Function	124	98%	84%	83%	99%
Smoking Cessation Advice[1]	9	78%	82%	82%	100%
Pneumonia Care					
Appropriate Initial Antibiotic	96	89%	82%	83%	94%
Blood Culture Timing	114	89%	89%	90%	100%
Influenza Vaccine	31	65%	58%	70%	100%
Initial Antibiotic Timing	137	84%	75%	80%	93%
Oxygenation Assessment	168	100%	99%	99%	100%
Pneumococcal Vaccine	119	81%	58%	69%	94%
Smoking Cessation Advice	26	73%	75%	80%	100%
Surgical Infection Prevention					
Prophylactic Antibiotic Given	367	82%	74%	77%	95%
Prophylactic Antibiotic Selection	82	95%	89%	90%	100%
Prophylactic Antibiotic Stopped	367	85%	65%	72%	95%
Pregnancy Care					
Inpatient Neonatal Mortality	1,430	0.42%	-	-	-
Third or Fourth Degree Laceration	1,131	3.01%	3.58%	3.63%	3.27%

Sequoia Hospital

170 Alameda De Las Pulgas
Redwood City, CA 94062
URL: www.sequoiahospital.org
Ownership: Govt - Hospital District or Authority
Emergency Services: Yes
Phone: 650-369-5811
Fax: 650-367-5100
Accredited: Yes

Measure	Cases	This Hospital	State Average	U.S. Average	Top Hospital
Heart Attack Care					
ACE Inhibitor or ARB for LVSD[1]	21	95%	82%	82%	100%
Aspirin at Arrival	82	99%	95%	92%	100%
Aspirin at Discharge	79	99%	90%	90%	100%
Beta Blocker at Arrival	51	96%	89%	87%	100%
Beta Blocker at Discharge	73	97%	89%	90%	100%
Fibrinolytic Medication Timing	0	-	40%	31%	100%
PCI Within 90 Minutes of Arrival[1]	4	100%	52%	54%	95%
Smoking Cessation Advice[1]	13	100%	87%	88%	100%
Heart Failure Care					
ACE Inhibitor or ARB for LVSD	95	91%	84%	82%	100%
Discharge Instructions	262	98%	56%	61%	93%
Evaluation of LVS Function	285	99%	84%	83%	99%
Smoking Cessation Advice[1]	17	100%	82%	82%	100%
Pneumonia Care					
Appropriate Initial Antibiotic	67	94%	82%	83%	94%
Blood Culture Timing	71	96%	89%	90%	100%
Influenza Vaccine	29	86%	58%	70%	100%
Initial Antibiotic Timing	92	93%	75%	80%	93%
Oxygenation Assessment	119	100%	99%	99%	100%
Pneumococcal Vaccine	98	86%	58%	69%	94%
Smoking Cessation Advice[1]	10	40%	75%	80%	100%
Surgical Infection Prevention					
Prophylactic Antibiotic Given[2,3]	248	88%	74%	77%	95%
Prophylactic Antibiotic Selection[2]	86	78%	89%	90%	100%
Prophylactic Antibiotic Stopped[2,3]	244	79%	65%	72%	95%
Pregnancy Care					
Inpatient Neonatal Mortality	1,088	0.00%	-	-	-
Third or Fourth Degree Laceration	817	3.30%	3.58%	3.63%	3.27%

Sierra Kings District Hospital

372 W Cypress Avenue
Reedley, CA 93654
URL: www.skdh.org
Ownership: Govt - Hospital District or Authority
Emergency Services: Yes
Phone: 559-638-8155
Fax: 559-637-7555
Accredited: Yes
Licensed Beds: 44

Key Personnel:
CEO. . . . . Melvyn Patashnick
Chief Medical Staff . . . . Calvin Schuster, MD
ER Manager. . . . . Paula Krahn, RN
Infection Control . . . . Lori Bray, RN
Chief Radiology . . . . Joe Torres, Jr
Director Respiratory Therapy . . . . Mark Willis

Measure	Cases	This Hospital	State Average	U.S. Average	Top Hospital
Heart Attack Care					
ACE Inhibitor or ARB for LVSD[3]	0	-	82%	82%	100%
Aspirin at Arrival[1,3]	1	100%	95%	92%	100%
Aspirin at Discharge[1,3]	1	0%	90%	90%	100%
Beta Blocker at Arrival[1,3]	1	0%	89%	87%	100%
Beta Blocker at Discharge[1,3]	1	100%	89%	90%	100%
Fibrinolytic Medication Timing[5]	-	-	40%	31%	100%
PCI Within 90 Minutes of Arrival[5]	-	-	52%	54%	95%
Smoking Cessation Advice[5]	-	-	87%	88%	100%
Heart Failure Care					
ACE Inhibitor or ARB for LVSD[1]	1	100%	84%	82%	100%
Discharge Instructions[1,3]	1	0%	56%	61%	93%
Evaluation of LVS Function	25	0%	84%	83%	99%
Smoking Cessation Advice[3]	0	-	82%	82%	100%
Pneumonia Care					
Appropriate Initial Antibiotic[1,3]	8	100%	82%	83%	94%
Blood Culture Timing[1,3]	8	75%	89%	90%	100%
Influenza Vaccine[5]	-	-	58%	70%	100%
Initial Antibiotic Timing	109	83%	75%	80%	93%
Oxygenation Assessment	128	100%	99%	99%	100%
Pneumococcal Vaccine	85	53%	58%	69%	94%
Smoking Cessation Advice[1,3]	1	100%	75%	80%	100%
Surgical Infection Prevention					
Prophylactic Antibiotic Given[1,3]	7	100%	74%	77%	95%
Prophylactic Antibiotic Selection[5]	-	-	89%	90%	100%
Prophylactic Antibiotic Stopped[1,3]	7	100%	65%	72%	95%
Pregnancy Care					
Inpatient Neonatal Mortality	1,118	0.00%	-	-	-
Third or Fourth Degree Laceration	690	2.61%	3.58%	3.63%	3.27%

Ridgecrest Regional Hospital

1081 N China Lake Boulevard
Ridgecrest, CA 93555
URL: www.rrh.org
Ownership: Voluntary non-profit - Private
Emergency Services: Yes
Phone: 760-446-3551
Fax: 760-499-3014
Accredited: Yes
Licensed Beds: 80

Key Personnel:
CEO. . . . . David Mechtenberg
Emergency Services Clinical Manager. . . . . Bridget Mosier
Surgery Coordinator. . . . . Sally Caruso
Medical/Surgical Clinical Manager . . . . Celia Mills
Cardiopulmonary Manager. . . . . Roger Berg

Measure	Cases	This Hospital	State Average	U.S. Average	Top Hospital
Heart Attack Care					
ACE Inhibitor or ARB for LVSD[1]	1	100%	82%	82%	100%
Aspirin at Arrival[1]	21	90%	95%	92%	100%
Aspirin at Discharge[1]	10	70%	90%	90%	100%
Beta Blocker at Arrival[1]	15	80%	89%	87%	100%
Beta Blocker at Discharge[1]	8	75%	89%	90%	100%
Fibrinolytic Medication Timing[1]	3	0%	40%	31%	100%

NOTE: Hospital profiles are in alphabetical order by state, then city, then hospital within the city; Rankings are sorted by rate in descending order and exclude hospitals with less than 25 cases; (1) The number of cases is too small (n<25) for purposes of reliably predicting hospital performance; (2) Measure reflects the hospital's indication that its submission was based upon a sample of its relevant discharges; (3) Rate reflects fewer than the maximum possible quarters of data for the measure; (4) Inaccurate information submitted and suppressed for one or more quarters; (5) No data is available from the hospital for this measure; Please refer to the User's Guide for a full explanation of data

Measure	Cases	This Hospital	State Average	U.S. Average	Top Hospital
PCI Within 90 Minutes of Arrival	0	-	52%	54%	95%
Smoking Cessation Advice[1]	4	75%	87%	88%	100%
Heart Failure Care					
ACE Inhibitor or ARB for LVSD	25	80%	84%	82%	100%
Discharge Instructions	74	77%	56%	61%	93%
Evaluation of LVS Function	82	87%	84%	83%	99%
Smoking Cessation Advice[1]	15	80%	82%	82%	100%
Pneumonia Care					
Appropriate Initial Antibiotic	97	81%	82%	83%	94%
Blood Culture Timing[1]	24	79%	89%	90%	100%
Influenza Vaccine[4,5]	-	-	58%	70%	100%
Initial Antibiotic Timing	121	68%	75%	80%	93%
Oxygenation Assessment	145	100%	99%	99%	100%
Pneumococcal Vaccine	80	59%	58%	69%	94%
Smoking Cessation Advice	46	63%	75%	80%	100%
Surgical Infection Prevention					
Prophylactic Antibiotic Given[3]	47	47%	74%	77%	95%
Prophylactic Antibiotic Selection[1]	18	61%	89%	90%	100%
Prophylactic Antibiotic Stopped[3]	46	76%	65%	72%	95%
Pregnancy Care					
Inpatient Neonatal Mortality	-	-	-	-	-
Third or Fourth Degree Laceration	-	-	3.58%	3.63%	3.27%

Kaiser Foundation Hospital-Riverside

10800 Magnolia Avenue Phone: 951-353-2000
Riverside, CA 92505
Ownership: Voluntary non-profit - Other Accredited: Yes
Emergency Services: Yes

Measure	Cases	This Hospital	State Average	U.S. Average	Top Hospital
Heart Attack Care					
ACE Inhibitor or ARB for LVSD[1]	20	90%	82%	82%	100%
Aspirin at Arrival	140	98%	95%	92%	100%
Aspirin at Discharge	80	91%	90%	90%	100%
Beta Blocker at Arrival	125	92%	89%	87%	100%
Beta Blocker at Discharge	90	92%	89%	90%	100%
Fibrinolytic Medication Timing	30	50%	40%	31%	100%
PCI Within 90 Minutes of Arrival	0	-	52%	54%	95%
Smoking Cessation Advice[1]	19	95%	87%	88%	100%
Heart Failure Care					
ACE Inhibitor or ARB for LVSD	126	93%	84%	82%	100%
Discharge Instructions	329	62%	56%	61%	93%
Evaluation of LVS Function	358	95%	84%	83%	99%
Smoking Cessation Advice	47	91%	82%	82%	100%
Pneumonia Care					
Appropriate Initial Antibiotic	86	85%	82%	83%	94%
Blood Culture Timing	51	82%	89%	90%	100%
Influenza Vaccine[1]	17	71%	58%	70%	100%
Initial Antibiotic Timing	94	56%	75%	80%	93%
Oxygenation Assessment	125	100%	99%	99%	100%
Pneumococcal Vaccine	79	96%	58%	69%	94%
Smoking Cessation Advice	25	64%	75%	80%	100%
Surgical Infection Prevention					
Prophylactic Antibiotic Given[3]	50	82%	74%	77%	95%
Prophylactic Antibiotic Selection	49	90%	89%	90%	100%
Prophylactic Antibiotic Stopped[3]	47	38%	65%	72%	95%
Pregnancy Care					
Inpatient Neonatal Mortality	3,785	0.05%	-	-	-
Third or Fourth Degree Laceration	2,733	2.38%	3.58%	3.63%	3.27%

Parkview Community Hospital

3865 Jackson Street Phone: 951-688-2211
Riverside, CA 92503 Fax: 951-352-5394
URL: www.pchmc.org
Ownership: Voluntary non-profit - Private Accredited: Yes
Emergency Services: Yes Licensed Beds: 193

Key Personnel:

CEO. . . . . Douglas Drumwright

Measure	Cases	This Hospital	State Average	U.S. Average	Top Hospital
Heart Attack Care					
ACE Inhibitor or ARB for LVSD[1]	5	80%	82%	82%	100%
Aspirin at Arrival	66	97%	95%	92%	100%
Aspirin at Discharge	35	91%	90%	90%	100%
Beta Blocker at Arrival	64	100%	89%	87%	100%
Beta Blocker at Discharge	37	95%	89%	90%	100%
Fibrinolytic Medication Timing[1]	9	22%	40%	31%	100%
PCI Within 90 Minutes of Arrival	0	-	52%	54%	95%
Smoking Cessation Advice[1]	9	89%	87%	88%	100%
Heart Failure Care					
ACE Inhibitor or ARB for LVSD	52	90%	84%	82%	100%
Discharge Instructions	159	49%	56%	61%	93%
Evaluation of LVS Function	204	78%	84%	83%	99%
Smoking Cessation Advice	29	90%	82%	82%	100%
Pneumonia Care					
Appropriate Initial Antibiotic	161	83%	82%	83%	94%
Blood Culture Timing	197	91%	89%	90%	100%
Influenza Vaccine	54	43%	58%	70%	100%
Initial Antibiotic Timing	332	82%	75%	80%	93%
Oxygenation Assessment	381	100%	99%	99%	100%
Pneumococcal Vaccine	217	30%	58%	69%	94%
Smoking Cessation Advice	52	94%	75%	80%	100%
Surgical Infection Prevention					
Prophylactic Antibiotic Given[3]	126	59%	74%	77%	95%
Prophylactic Antibiotic Selection	81	94%	89%	90%	100%
Prophylactic Antibiotic Stopped[3]	116	97%	65%	72%	95%
Pregnancy Care					
Inpatient Neonatal Mortality[2]	888	0.34%	-	-	-
Third or Fourth Degree Laceration[2]	584	3.25%	3.58%	3.63%	3.27%

Riverside Community Hospital

4445 Magnolia Avenue Phone: 951-788-3000
Riverside, CA 92501
Ownership: Voluntary non-profit - Other Accredited: Yes
Emergency Services: Yes

Measure	Cases	This Hospital	State Average	U.S. Average	Top Hospital
Heart Attack Care					
ACE Inhibitor or ARB for LVSD	85	84%	82%	82%	100%
Aspirin at Arrival	245	93%	95%	92%	100%
Aspirin at Discharge	358	93%	90%	90%	100%
Beta Blocker at Arrival	218	87%	89%	87%	100%
Beta Blocker at Discharge	346	85%	89%	90%	100%
Fibrinolytic Medication Timing[1]	1	0%	40%	31%	100%
PCI Within 90 Minutes of Arrival[1]	14	14%	52%	54%	95%
Smoking Cessation Advice	116	93%	87%	88%	100%
Heart Failure Care					
ACE Inhibitor or ARB for LVSD	193	81%	84%	82%	100%
Discharge Instructions	439	70%	56%	61%	93%
Evaluation of LVS Function	542	89%	84%	83%	99%
Smoking Cessation Advice	107	94%	82%	82%	100%
Pneumonia Care					
Appropriate Initial Antibiotic	261	90%	82%	83%	94%
Blood Culture Timing	308	83%	89%	90%	100%
Influenza Vaccine	90	66%	58%	70%	100%
Initial Antibiotic Timing	523	80%	75%	80%	93%
Oxygenation Assessment	618	100%	99%	99%	100%
Pneumococcal Vaccine	321	78%	58%	69%	94%
Smoking Cessation Advice	116	84%	75%	80%	100%
Surgical Infection Prevention					
Prophylactic Antibiotic Given[2,3]	284	55%	74%	77%	95%
Prophylactic Antibiotic Selection[2]	136	92%	89%	90%	100%
Prophylactic Antibiotic Stopped[2,3]	255	48%	65%	72%	95%
Pregnancy Care					
Inpatient Neonatal Mortality	-	-	-	-	-
Third or Fourth Degree Laceration	-	-	3.58%	3.63%	3.27%

NOTE: Hospital profiles are in alphabetical order by state, then city, then hospital within the city; Rankings are sorted by rate in descending order and exclude hospitals with less than 25 cases; (1) The number of cases is too small (n<25) for purposes of reliably predicting hospital performance; (2) Measure reflects the hospital's indication that its submission was based upon a sample of its relevant discharges; (3) Rate reflects fewer than the maximum possible quarters of data for the measure; (4) Inaccurate information submitted and suppressed for one or more quarters; (5) No data is available from the hospital for this measure; Please refer to the User's Guide for a full explanation of data

Sutter Roseville Medical Center

One Medical Plaza
Roseville, CA 95661

Toll-Free: 800-478-8837
Phone: 916-781-1000
Fax: 916-781-1605

URL: www.sutterroseville.org
Ownership: Voluntary non-profit - Other
Emergency Services: Yes

Accredited: Yes
Licensed Beds: 172

Key Personnel:
President/CEO . . . . Sarah Krevans
Administrator . . . . Patrick R Brady

Measure	Cases	This Hospital	State Average	U.S. Average	Top Hospital
Heart Attack Care					
ACE Inhibitor or ARB for LVSD	33	85%	82%	82%	100%
Aspirin at Arrival	201	99%	95%	92%	100%
Aspirin at Discharge	129	95%	90%	90%	100%
Beta Blocker at Arrival	159	97%	89%	87%	100%
Beta Blocker at Discharge	139	99%	89%	90%	100%
Fibrinolytic Medication Timing[1]	20	75%	40%	31%	100%
PCI Within 90 Minutes of Arrival[1]	1	100%	52%	54%	95%
Smoking Cessation Advice	31	97%	87%	88%	100%
Heart Failure Care					
ACE Inhibitor or ARB for LVSD[2]	94	80%	84%	82%	100%
Discharge Instructions[2]	222	84%	56%	61%	93%
Evaluation of LVS Function[2]	279	95%	84%	83%	99%
Smoking Cessation Advice[2]	32	94%	82%	82%	100%
Pneumonia Care					
Appropriate Initial Antibiotic[2]	119	86%	82%	83%	94%
Blood Culture Timing[2]	97	87%	89%	90%	100%
Influenza Vaccine[2]	31	87%	58%	70%	100%
Initial Antibiotic Timing[2]	159	70%	75%	80%	93%
Oxygenation Assessment[2]	200	100%	99%	99%	100%
Pneumococcal Vaccine[2]	142	82%	58%	69%	94%
Smoking Cessation Advice[2]	43	98%	75%	80%	100%
Surgical Infection Prevention					
Prophylactic Antibiotic Given[2]	228	92%	74%	77%	95%
Prophylactic Antibiotic Selection[2]	52	96%	89%	90%	100%
Prophylactic Antibiotic Stopped[2]	224	86%	65%	72%	95%
Pregnancy Care					
Inpatient Neonatal Mortality[2]	2,046	0.05%	-	-	-
Third or Fourth Degree Laceration[2]	1,554	1.74%	3.58%	3.63%	3.27%

Kaiser Foundation Hospital-South Sacramento

6600 Bruceville Road
Sacramento, CA 95823

Phone: 916-688-2000

Ownership: Voluntary non-profit - Other
Emergency Services: Yes

Accredited: Yes

Measure	Cases	This Hospital	State Average	U.S. Average	Top Hospital
Heart Attack Care					
ACE Inhibitor or ARB for LVSD	30	100%	82%	82%	100%
Aspirin at Arrival	246	100%	95%	92%	100%
Aspirin at Discharge	152	97%	90%	90%	100%
Beta Blocker at Arrival	207	97%	89%	87%	100%
Beta Blocker at Discharge	166	99%	89%	90%	100%
Fibrinolytic Medication Timing[1]	12	42%	40%	31%	100%
PCI Within 90 Minutes of Arrival	0	-	52%	54%	95%
Smoking Cessation Advice	30	90%	87%	88%	100%
Heart Failure Care					
ACE Inhibitor or ARB for LVSD	101	98%	84%	82%	100%
Discharge Instructions	255	83%	56%	61%	93%
Evaluation of LVS Function	285	99%	84%	83%	99%
Smoking Cessation Advice	46	96%	82%	82%	100%
Pneumonia Care					
Appropriate Initial Antibiotic	202	89%	82%	83%	94%
Blood Culture Timing	179	92%	89%	90%	100%
Influenza Vaccine	47	81%	58%	70%	100%
Initial Antibiotic Timing	210	80%	75%	80%	93%
Oxygenation Assessment	285	100%	99%	99%	100%
Pneumococcal Vaccine	189	89%	58%	69%	94%
Smoking Cessation Advice	50	98%	75%	80%	100%
Surgical Infection Prevention					
Prophylactic Antibiotic Given	735	90%	74%	77%	95%
Prophylactic Antibiotic Selection	177	93%	89%	90%	100%
Prophylactic Antibiotic Stopped	730	71%	65%	72%	95%
Pregnancy Care					
Inpatient Neonatal Mortality	3,606	0.03%	-	-	-
Third or Fourth Degree Laceration	2,866	3.98%	3.58%	3.63%	3.27%

Kaiser Permanente Sacramento Medical Center

2025 Morse Avenue
Sacramento, CA 95825

Phone: 916-973-5000

URL: www.kaiserpermanente.org
Ownership: Voluntary non-profit - Other
Emergency Services: Yes

Accredited: Yes
Licensed Beds: 340

Key Personnel:
CEO. . . . . Edd Glavis
OB/GYN Womens Health. . . . . Michael Maddox, MD
Chief Radiology . . . . William Brown, MD

Measure	Cases	This Hospital	State Average	U.S. Average	Top Hospital
Heart Attack Care					
ACE Inhibitor or ARB for LVSD	45	69%	82%	82%	100%
Aspirin at Arrival	337	95%	95%	92%	100%
Aspirin at Discharge	253	87%	90%	90%	100%
Beta Blocker at Arrival	287	93%	89%	87%	100%
Beta Blocker at Discharge	263	95%	89%	90%	100%
Fibrinolytic Medication Timing	39	26%	40%	31%	100%
PCI Within 90 Minutes of Arrival	0	-	52%	54%	95%
Smoking Cessation Advice	37	49%	87%	88%	100%
Heart Failure Care					
ACE Inhibitor or ARB for LVSD	235	73%	84%	82%	100%
Discharge Instructions	654	40%	56%	61%	93%
Evaluation of LVS Function	789	97%	84%	83%	99%
Smoking Cessation Advice	79	67%	82%	82%	100%
Pneumonia Care					
Appropriate Initial Antibiotic	298	89%	82%	83%	94%
Blood Culture Timing	338	90%	89%	90%	100%
Influenza Vaccine	108	58%	58%	70%	100%
Initial Antibiotic Timing	425	66%	75%	80%	93%
Oxygenation Assessment	573	100%	99%	99%	100%
Pneumococcal Vaccine	433	82%	58%	69%	94%
Smoking Cessation Advice	95	75%	75%	80%	100%
Surgical Infection Prevention					
Prophylactic Antibiotic Given	622	76%	74%	77%	95%
Prophylactic Antibiotic Selection	144	84%	89%	90%	100%
Prophylactic Antibiotic Stopped	614	72%	65%	72%	95%
Pregnancy Care					
Inpatient Neonatal Mortality	4,283	0.42%	-	-	-
Third or Fourth Degree Laceration	2,701	2.85%	3.58%	3.63%	3.27%

Mercy General Hospital

4001 J Street
Sacramento, CA 95819

Phone: 916-453-4545
Fax: 916-453-4587

URL: www.mercygeneral.org
Ownership: Voluntary non-profit - Church
Emergency Services: Yes

Accredited: Yes
Licensed Beds: 343

Key Personnel:
Chief Medical Staff. . . . . Richard Atkinson, MD
Cardiac Lab . . . . Jim Roxburgh
Catheterization Lab . . . . Jim Roxburgh
Emergency Room . . . . Mark Smedley, MD
Infection Control Coordinator . . . . Roberta Stultz
Medical/Surgical Nursing . . . . Page West
OB/GYN Womens Health. . . . . Gail Maduri
Respiratory Therapy Manager . . . . Jim Roxburgh

Measure	Cases	This Hospital	State Average	U.S. Average	Top Hospital
Heart Attack Care					
ACE Inhibitor or ARB for LVSD	165	85%	82%	82%	100%
Aspirin at Arrival	233	99%	95%	92%	100%
Aspirin at Discharge	966	99%	90%	90%	100%
Beta Blocker at Arrival	190	96%	89%	87%	100%
Beta Blocker at Discharge	997	98%	89%	90%	100%

NOTE: Hospital profiles are in alphabetical order by state, then city, then hospital within the city; Rankings are sorted by rate in descending order and exclude hospitals with less than 25 cases; (1) The number of cases is too small (n<25) for purposes of reliably predicting hospital performance; (2) Measure reflects the hospital's indication that its submission was based upon a sample of its relevant discharges; (3) Rate reflects fewer than the maximum possible quarters of data for the measure; (4) Inaccurate information submitted and suppressed for one or more quarters; (5) No data is available from the hospital for this measure; Please refer to the User's Guide for a full explanation of data

Measure	Cases	This Hospital	State Average	U.S. Average	Top Hospital
Fibrinolytic Medication Timing[1]	11	82%	40%	31%	100%
PCI Within 90 Minutes of Arrival[1]	14	71%	52%	54%	95%
Smoking Cessation Advice	329	99%	87%	88%	100%
Heart Failure Care					
ACE Inhibitor or ARB for LVSD	269	89%	84%	82%	100%
Discharge Instructions	511	91%	56%	61%	93%
Evaluation of LVS Function	562	96%	84%	83%	99%
Smoking Cessation Advice	127	99%	82%	82%	100%
Pneumonia Care					
Appropriate Initial Antibiotic	166	83%	82%	83%	94%
Blood Culture Timing	214	97%	89%	90%	100%
Influenza Vaccine	79	81%	58%	70%	100%
Initial Antibiotic Timing	365	89%	75%	80%	93%
Oxygenation Assessment	409	100%	99%	99%	100%
Pneumococcal Vaccine	286	83%	58%	69%	94%
Smoking Cessation Advice	64	98%	75%	80%	100%
Surgical Infection Prevention					
Prophylactic Antibiotic Given[2,3]	299	82%	74%	77%	95%
Prophylactic Antibiotic Selection[2]	104	90%	89%	90%	100%
Prophylactic Antibiotic Stopped[2,3]	285	69%	65%	72%	95%
Pregnancy Care					
Inpatient Neonatal Mortality	2,603	0.12%	-	-	-
Third or Fourth Degree Laceration	1,897	2.48%	3.58%	3.63%	3.27%

Methodist Hospital of Sacramento

7500 Hospital Drive
Sacramento, CA 95823
Phone: 916-423-3000
Fax: 916-689-7833
URL: www.methodistsacramento.org
Ownership: Voluntary non-profit - Other
Accredited: Yes
Emergency Services: Yes
Licensed Beds: 355

Key Personnel:

President . . . . Timothy Moran
Emergency Room . . . . Sindy Myas
Medical & Surgical Nursing Manager . . . . Laura Newman
OB/GYN Womens Health Manager . . . . Denise Cantrell
Respiratory Care Manager. . . . . Christ Findlay

Measure	Cases	This Hospital	State Average	U.S. Average	Top Hospital
Heart Attack Care					
ACE Inhibitor or ARB for LVSD[1]	5	100%	82%	82%	100%
Aspirin at Arrival	32	100%	95%	92%	100%
Aspirin at Discharge[1]	15	100%	90%	90%	100%
Beta Blocker at Arrival	28	96%	89%	87%	100%
Beta Blocker at Discharge[1]	13	92%	89%	90%	100%
Fibrinolytic Medication Timing[1]	2	50%	40%	31%	100%
PCI Within 90 Minutes of Arrival	0	-	52%	54%	95%
Smoking Cessation Advice[1]	3	100%	87%	88%	100%
Heart Failure Care					
ACE Inhibitor or ARB for LVSD	88	91%	84%	82%	100%
Discharge Instructions	249	69%	56%	61%	93%
Evaluation of LVS Function	276	92%	84%	83%	99%
Smoking Cessation Advice	50	100%	82%	82%	100%
Pneumonia Care					
Appropriate Initial Antibiotic	181	92%	82%	83%	94%
Blood Culture Timing	209	95%	89%	90%	100%
Influenza Vaccine	51	65%	58%	70%	100%
Initial Antibiotic Timing	255	80%	75%	80%	93%
Oxygenation Assessment	304	100%	99%	99%	100%
Pneumococcal Vaccine	182	60%	58%	69%	94%
Smoking Cessation Advice	38	97%	75%	80%	100%
Surgical Infection Prevention					
Prophylactic Antibiotic Given[2,3]	154	60%	74%	77%	95%
Prophylactic Antibiotic Selection[2]	47	94%	89%	90%	100%
Prophylactic Antibiotic Stopped[2,3]	154	52%	65%	72%	95%
Pregnancy Care					
Inpatient Neonatal Mortality	1,473	0.07%	-	-	-
Third or Fourth Degree Laceration	960	2.60%	3.58%	3.63%	3.27%

Sutter General Hospital

2801 L Street
Sacramento, CA 95816
Toll-Free: 800-478-8837
Phone: 916-454-2222
Fax: 916-733-8388
URL: www.suttermedicalcenter.org
Ownership: Voluntary non-profit - Other
Accredited: Yes
Emergency Services: Yes
Licensed Beds: 306

Key Personnel:

President/CEO. . . . . Sarah Krevans

Measure	Cases	This Hospital	State Average	U.S. Average	Top Hospital
Heart Attack Care					
ACE Inhibitor or ARB for LVSD	87	91%	82%	82%	100%
Aspirin at Arrival	205	98%	95%	92%	100%
Aspirin at Discharge	501	98%	90%	90%	100%
Beta Blocker at Arrival	183	93%	89%	87%	100%
Beta Blocker at Discharge	492	98%	89%	90%	100%
Fibrinolytic Medication Timing[1]	4	50%	40%	31%	100%
PCI Within 90 Minutes of Arrival[1]	1	0%	52%	54%	95%
Smoking Cessation Advice	152	99%	87%	88%	100%
Heart Failure Care					
ACE Inhibitor or ARB for LVSD[2]	124	94%	84%	82%	100%
Discharge Instructions[2]	248	85%	56%	61%	93%
Evaluation of LVS Function[2]	300	99%	84%	83%	99%
Smoking Cessation Advice[2]	53	100%	82%	82%	100%
Pneumonia Care					
Appropriate Initial Antibiotic[2]	111	90%	82%	83%	94%
Blood Culture Timing[2]	135	90%	89%	90%	100%
Influenza Vaccine[4,5]	-	-	58%	70%	100%
Initial Antibiotic Timing[2]	180	81%	75%	80%	93%
Oxygenation Assessment[2]	207	100%	99%	99%	100%
Pneumococcal Vaccine[2]	130	78%	58%	69%	94%
Smoking Cessation Advice[2]	50	98%	75%	80%	100%
Surgical Infection Prevention					
Prophylactic Antibiotic Given[2]	370	83%	74%	77%	95%
Prophylactic Antibiotic Selection[2]	88	80%	89%	90%	100%
Prophylactic Antibiotic Stopped[2]	356	72%	65%	72%	95%
Pregnancy Care					
Inpatient Neonatal Mortality	-	-	-	-	-
Third or Fourth Degree Laceration	-	-	3.58%	3.63%	3.27%

University of California Davis Health System

Alternate Name: University of California Davis Medical Center
2315 Stockton Boulevard
Sacramento, CA 95817
Phone: 916-734-2011
Fax: 916-734-8080
URL: www.ucdmc.ucdavis.edu
Ownership: Voluntary non-profit - Other
Accredited: Yes
Emergency Services: Yes
Licensed Beds: 528

Key Personnel:

CEO. . . . . Robert Chason
Chief Medical Staff. . . . . Gibbe Parsons, MD
Chief Emergency Medicine . . . . Robert Derlet, MD
Manager Infection Control . . . . Marsha Koopman
ICU . . . . Carol Robinson
Medical Surgical Nursing . . . . Carol Robinson
Manager Obstetrics/Gynecology . . . . Pamela Bigelow
Chief Respiratory . . . . Timothy Albertson, MD

Measure	Cases	This Hospital	State Average	U.S. Average	Top Hospital
Heart Attack Care					
ACE Inhibitor or ARB for LVSD[2]	67	75%	82%	82%	100%
Aspirin at Arrival[2]	191	98%	95%	92%	100%
Aspirin at Discharge[2]	220	99%	90%	90%	100%
Beta Blocker at Arrival[2]	151	95%	89%	87%	100%
Beta Blocker at Discharge[2]	247	98%	89%	90%	100%
Fibrinolytic Medication Timing[2]	0	-	40%	31%	100%
PCI Within 90 Minutes of Arrival[1,2]	9	44%	52%	54%	95%
Smoking Cessation Advice[2]	97	96%	87%	88%	100%
Heart Failure Care					
ACE Inhibitor or ARB for LVSD[2]	188	77%	84%	82%	100%
Discharge Instructions[2]	308	46%	56%	61%	93%
Evaluation of LVS Function[2]	329	99%	84%	83%	99%
Smoking Cessation Advice[2]	101	95%	82%	82%	100%

NOTE: Hospital profiles are in alphabetical order by state, then city, then hospital within the city; Rankings are sorted by rate in descending order and exclude hospitals with less than 25 cases; (1) The number of cases is too small (n<25) for purposes of reliably predicting hospital performance; (2) Measure reflects the hospital's indication that its submission was based upon a sample of its relevant discharges; (3) Rate reflects fewer than the maximum possible quarters of data for the measure; (4) Inaccurate information submitted and suppressed for one or more quarters; (5) No data is available from the hospital for this measure; Please refer to the User's Guide for a full explanation of data

Measure	Cases	This Hospital	State Average	U.S. Average	Top Hospital
Pneumonia Care					
Appropriate Initial Antibiotic[2]	105	85%	82%	83%	94%
Blood Culture Timing[2]	112	86%	89%	90%	100%
Influenza Vaccine[2]	27	74%	58%	70%	100%
Initial Antibiotic Timing[2]	169	55%	75%	80%	93%
Oxygenation Assessment[2]	200	100%	99%	99%	100%
Pneumococcal Vaccine[2]	90	69%	58%	69%	94%
Smoking Cessation Advice[2]	73	92%	75%	80%	100%
Surgical Infection Prevention					
Prophylactic Antibiotic Given[2]	536	94%	74%	77%	95%
Prophylactic Antibiotic Selection[2]	75	87%	89%	90%	100%
Prophylactic Antibiotic Stopped[2]	491	73%	65%	72%	95%
Pregnancy Care					
Inpatient Neonatal Mortality[2]	622	1.29%	-	-	-
Third or Fourth Degree Laceration	1,893	3.70%	3.58%	3.63%	3.27%

Saint Helena Hospital

10 Woodland Road — Phone: 707-963-3611
Deer Park, CA 94574 — Fax: 707-963-6461
URL: www.sthelenahospital.org
Ownership: Voluntary non-profit - Church — Accredited: Yes
Emergency Services: Yes — Licensed Beds: 181

Key Personnel:

President/CEO . . . . Joaline Olson
Chief Medical Staff . . . . Pam Lomar
Cardiology . . . . Dave Tilton
Emergency Room . . . . Maria Pana

Measure	Cases	This Hospital	State Average	U.S. Average	Top Hospital
Heart Attack Care					
ACE Inhibitor or ARB for LVSD[1]	17	94%	82%	82%	100%
Aspirin at Arrival[1]	20	100%	95%	92%	100%
Aspirin at Discharge	76	100%	90%	90%	100%
Beta Blocker at Arrival[1]	15	100%	89%	87%	100%
Beta Blocker at Discharge	67	97%	89%	90%	100%
Fibrinolytic Medication Timing	0	-	40%	31%	100%
PCI Within 90 Minutes of Arrival[1]	2	50%	52%	54%	95%
Smoking Cessation Advice	38	100%	87%	88%	100%
Heart Failure Care					
ACE Inhibitor or ARB for LVSD[1]	23	83%	84%	82%	100%
Discharge Instructions	67	90%	56%	61%	93%
Evaluation of LVS Function	82	98%	84%	83%	99%
Smoking Cessation Advice[1]	19	95%	82%	82%	100%
Pneumonia Care					
Appropriate Initial Antibiotic	27	96%	82%	83%	94%
Blood Culture Timing	27	100%	89%	90%	100%
Influenza Vaccine[1]	14	36%	58%	70%	100%
Initial Antibiotic Timing	42	93%	75%	80%	93%
Oxygenation Assessment	48	100%	99%	99%	100%
Pneumococcal Vaccine	46	50%	58%	69%	94%
Smoking Cessation Advice[1]	12	100%	75%	80%	100%
Surgical Infection Prevention					
Prophylactic Antibiotic Given	261	95%	74%	77%	95%
Prophylactic Antibiotic Selection	63	97%	89%	90%	100%
Prophylactic Antibiotic Stopped	256	80%	65%	72%	95%
Pregnancy Care					
Inpatient Neonatal Mortality	-	-	-	-	-
Third or Fourth Degree Laceration	-	-	3.58%	3.63%	3.27%

Natividad Medical Center

1441 Constitution Boulevard — Phone: 831-755-4111
Salinas, CA 93906 — Fax: 831-755-6254
URL: www.natividad.com
Ownership: Government - Local — Accredited: Yes
Emergency Services: Yes — Licensed Beds: 172

Key Personnel:

CEO . . . . Lionel Chadwick
Chief Medical Staff . . . . Leter Leeson
Emergency Room . . . . Steve Cox
Emergency Room . . . . Judy Jackson, RN
Director Medical/Surgical Nursing . . . . Mary Schapper, RN
Service Director OB/GYN . . . . Robert Park, MD
Director Radiology . . . . Joan Oakley
Director of Respiratory Therapy . . . . John Nevill

Measure	Cases	This Hospital	State Average	U.S. Average	Top Hospital
Heart Attack Care					
ACE Inhibitor or ARB for LVSD	0	-	82%	82%	100%
Aspirin at Arrival[1]	10	100%	95%	92%	100%
Aspirin at Discharge[1]	5	100%	90%	90%	100%
Beta Blocker at Arrival[1]	5	100%	89%	87%	100%
Beta Blocker at Discharge[1]	3	100%	89%	90%	100%
Fibrinolytic Medication Timing	0	-	40%	31%	100%
PCI Within 90 Minutes of Arrival	0	-	52%	54%	95%
Smoking Cessation Advice[1]	1	0%	87%	88%	100%
Heart Failure Care					
ACE Inhibitor or ARB for LVSD	28	100%	84%	82%	100%
Discharge Instructions	65	15%	56%	61%	93%
Evaluation of LVS Function	73	97%	84%	83%	99%
Smoking Cessation Advice[1]	16	38%	82%	82%	100%
Pneumonia Care					
Appropriate Initial Antibiotic	86	85%	82%	83%	94%
Blood Culture Timing	69	90%	89%	90%	100%
Influenza Vaccine[1]	11	36%	58%	70%	100%
Initial Antibiotic Timing	89	76%	75%	80%	93%
Oxygenation Assessment	118	100%	99%	99%	100%
Pneumococcal Vaccine	36	39%	58%	69%	94%
Smoking Cessation Advice	32	38%	75%	80%	100%
Surgical Infection Prevention					
Prophylactic Antibiotic Given[2,3]	50	74%	74%	77%	95%
Prophylactic Antibiotic Selection[1,2]	17	100%	89%	90%	100%
Prophylactic Antibiotic Stopped[2,3]	54	100%	65%	72%	95%
Pregnancy Care					
Inpatient Neonatal Mortality	2,607	0.31%	-	-	-
Third or Fourth Degree Laceration	1,853	4.21%	3.58%	3.63%	3.27%

Salinas Valley Memorial Health Care District

450 E Romie Lane — Phone: 831-757-4333
Salinas, CA 93901 — Fax: 831-753-6297
URL: www.svmh.com
Ownership: Govt - Hospital District or Authority — Accredited: Yes
Emergency Services: Yes — Licensed Beds: 266

Key Personnel:

President/CEO . . . . Samuel W Downing
Chief Medical Staff . . . . David Perrott, MD
Cardiology . . . . Lesley Turpin
Catheterization Lab . . . . Irene Neumeister
Emergency Room . . . . Nuala Rippere
Director Infection/Disease Control . . . . Wendy Oliva
Director Intensive/Coronary Care . . . . Annette Schuessler
Director Medical/Surgical Nursing . . . . Holly Cagle
OB/GYN Womens Health . . . . Judith Elk
Sr Admin Director Surgical Services . . . . Holly Cagle
Respiratory Therapy . . . . Marie Kasamatsu

Measure	Cases	This Hospital	State Average	U.S. Average	Top Hospital
Heart Attack Care					
ACE Inhibitor or ARB for LVSD	40	92%	82%	82%	100%
Aspirin at Arrival	137	95%	95%	92%	100%
Aspirin at Discharge	215	100%	90%	90%	100%
Beta Blocker at Arrival	74	97%	89%	87%	100%
Beta Blocker at Discharge	226	99%	89%	90%	100%
Fibrinolytic Medication Timing[3]	0	-	40%	31%	100%
PCI Within 90 Minutes of Arrival[1]	8	100%	52%	54%	95%
Smoking Cessation Advice[1,3]	18	94%	87%	88%	100%
Heart Failure Care					
ACE Inhibitor or ARB for LVSD	142	88%	84%	82%	100%
Discharge Instructions[3]	78	86%	56%	61%	93%
Evaluation of LVS Function	429	92%	84%	83%	99%
Smoking Cessation Advice[1,3]	6	100%	82%	82%	100%
Pneumonia Care					
Appropriate Initial Antibiotic[3]	26	85%	82%	83%	94%
Blood Culture Timing[3]	37	89%	89%	90%	100%
Influenza Vaccine[5]	-	-	58%	70%	100%
Initial Antibiotic Timing	280	67%	75%	80%	93%

NOTE: Hospital profiles are in alphabetical order by state, then city, then hospital within the city; Rankings are sorted by rate in descending order and exclude hospitals with less than 25 cases; (1) The number of cases is too small (n<25) for purposes of reliably predicting hospital performance; (2) Measure reflects the hospital's indication that its submission was based upon a sample of its relevant discharges; (3) Rate reflects fewer than the maximum possible quarters of data for the measure; (4) Inaccurate information submitted and suppressed for one or more quarters; (5) No data is available from the hospital for this measure; Please refer to the User's Guide for a full explanation of data

Measure	Cases	This Hospital	State Average	U.S. Average	Top Hospital
Oxygenation Assessment	296	99%	99%	99%	100%
Pneumococcal Vaccine	206	78%	58%	69%	94%
Smoking Cessation Advice[1,3]	11	82%	75%	80%	100%
Surgical Infection Prevention					
Prophylactic Antibiotic Given[3]	221	82%	74%	77%	95%
Prophylactic Antibiotic Selection[5]	-	-	89%	90%	100%
Prophylactic Antibiotic Stopped[3]	208	72%	65%	72%	95%
Pregnancy Care					
Inpatient Neonatal Mortality	-	-	-	-	-
Third or Fourth Degree Laceration	-	-	3.58%	3.63%	3.27%

Mark Twain Saint Joseph's Hospital

768 Mountain Ranch Road | Phone: 209-754-3521
San Andreas, CA 95249 | Fax: 209-754-2626
E-mail: lrussell@chw.edu
URL: www.chw.edu/sanandreas
Ownership: Voluntary non-profit - Other | Accredited: Yes
Emergency Services: Yes | Licensed Beds: 48

Key Personnel:
CEO. . . . . Michael Lawson
Chief Medical Staff. . . . . Peter Gierke, MD
Emergency Room Director. . . . . Marc Walter
Director Medical/Surgical Nursing . . . . Yvonne Dowdin, RN
OB/GYN Womens Health. . . . . Rodger Orman, MD
Chief Radiology . . . . William Griffin, MD
Manager Respiratory Therapy . . . . Dick James

Measure	Cases	This Hospital	State Average	U.S. Average	Top Hospital
Heart Attack Care					
ACE Inhibitor or ARB for LVSD[1]	1	100%	82%	82%	100%
Aspirin at Arrival[1]	11	100%	95%	92%	100%
Aspirin at Discharge[1]	1	100%	90%	90%	100%
Beta Blocker at Arrival[1]	10	100%	89%	87%	100%
Beta Blocker at Discharge[1]	3	100%	89%	90%	100%
Fibrinolytic Medication Timing[1,3]	1	0%	40%	31%	100%
PCI Within 90 Minutes of Arrival	0	-	52%	54%	95%
Smoking Cessation Advice	0	-	87%	88%	100%
Heart Failure Care					
ACE Inhibitor or ARB for LVSD[1]	13	100%	84%	82%	100%
Discharge Instructions	54	56%	56%	61%	93%
Evaluation of LVS Function	69	100%	84%	83%	99%
Smoking Cessation Advice[1]	13	85%	82%	82%	100%
Pneumonia Care					
Appropriate Initial Antibiotic	82	88%	82%	83%	94%
Blood Culture Timing	55	100%	89%	90%	100%
Influenza Vaccine[4,5]	-	-	58%	70%	100%
Initial Antibiotic Timing	89	76%	75%	80%	93%
Oxygenation Assessment	122	100%	99%	99%	100%
Pneumococcal Vaccine	79	72%	58%	69%	94%
Smoking Cessation Advice	25	100%	75%	80%	100%
Surgical Infection Prevention					
Prophylactic Antibiotic Given[2,3]	32	84%	74%	77%	95%
Prophylactic Antibiotic Selection[2]	32	100%	89%	90%	100%
Prophylactic Antibiotic Stopped[2,3]	31	94%	65%	72%	95%
Pregnancy Care					
Inpatient Neonatal Mortality	-	-	-	-	-
Third or Fourth Degree Laceration	-	-	3.58%	3.63%	3.27%

Community Hospital of San Bernardino

1805 Medical Center Drive | Phone: 909-887-6333
San Bernardino, CA 92411 | Fax: 909-887-6468
URL: www.chw.edu
Ownership: Voluntary non-profit - Other | Accredited: Yes
Emergency Services: Yes | Licensed Beds: 374

Key Personnel:
CEO. . . . . Bruce Satzger
Chief Medical Staff. . . . . Edward Puttre
OB/GYN Womens Health. . . . . Mary Black-Williams
Director Cardio-Pulmonary Services . . . . Phil Liang

Measure	Cases	This Hospital	State Average	U.S. Average	Top Hospital
Heart Attack Care					
ACE Inhibitor or ARB for LVSD[1]	8	100%	82%	82%	100%
Aspirin at Arrival	52	96%	95%	92%	100%
Aspirin at Discharge[1]	23	83%	90%	90%	100%
Beta Blocker at Arrival	35	91%	89%	87%	100%
Beta Blocker at Discharge[1]	18	83%	89%	90%	100%
Fibrinolytic Medication Timing[1]	8	38%	40%	31%	100%
PCI Within 90 Minutes of Arrival	0	-	52%	54%	95%
Smoking Cessation Advice[1]	7	100%	87%	88%	100%
Heart Failure Care					
ACE Inhibitor or ARB for LVSD	67	99%	84%	82%	100%
Discharge Instructions	227	93%	56%	61%	93%
Evaluation of LVS Function	247	94%	84%	83%	99%
Smoking Cessation Advice	68	99%	82%	82%	100%
Pneumonia Care					
Appropriate Initial Antibiotic	167	80%	82%	83%	94%
Blood Culture Timing	151	89%	89%	90%	100%
Influenza Vaccine[4,5]	-	-	58%	70%	100%
Initial Antibiotic Timing	212	74%	75%	80%	93%
Oxygenation Assessment	289	100%	99%	99%	100%
Pneumococcal Vaccine	134	85%	58%	69%	94%
Smoking Cessation Advice	65	95%	75%	80%	100%
Surgical Infection Prevention					
Prophylactic Antibiotic Given[2,3]	68	65%	74%	77%	95%
Prophylactic Antibiotic Selection[1,2]	18	94%	89%	90%	100%
Prophylactic Antibiotic Stopped[2,3]	64	39%	65%	72%	95%
Pregnancy Care					
Inpatient Neonatal Mortality	2,561	0.16%	-	-	-
Third or Fourth Degree Laceration	1,570	1.91%	3.58%	3.63%	3.27%

Saint Bernardine Medical Center

2101 N Waterman Avenue | Phone: 909-883-8711
San Bernardino, CA 92404 | Fax: 909-881-4481
URL: www.stbernardinemedicalcenter.com
Ownership: Voluntary non-profit - Church | Accredited: Yes
Emergency Services: Yes | Licensed Beds: 463

Key Personnel:
CEO. . . . . Steve Barron
Chief Medical Staff. . . . . John Udeh
Emergency Room . . . . Brian Bearie
Emergency Room . . . . Pierre Assaf, MD
Director Infection/Disease Control . . . . Bridget Connell
Cardiology Chief . . . . Aaron Jordan
OB/GYN Womens Health. . . . . Peter Yang
Respiratory Chief . . . . Thomas Hellwig

Measure	Cases	This Hospital	State Average	U.S. Average	Top Hospital
Heart Attack Care					
ACE Inhibitor or ARB for LVSD[2]	45	91%	82%	82%	100%
Aspirin at Arrival[2]	101	98%	95%	92%	100%
Aspirin at Discharge[2]	273	99%	90%	90%	100%
Beta Blocker at Arrival[2]	50	96%	89%	87%	100%
Beta Blocker at Discharge[2]	248	98%	89%	90%	100%
Fibrinolytic Medication Timing[1,2]	2	0%	40%	31%	100%
PCI Within 90 Minutes of Arrival[1,2]	5	20%	52%	54%	95%
Smoking Cessation Advice[2]	76	99%	87%	88%	100%
Heart Failure Care					
ACE Inhibitor or ARB for LVSD[2]	91	95%	84%	82%	100%
Discharge Instructions[2]	275	76%	56%	61%	93%
Evaluation of LVS Function[2]	310	95%	84%	83%	99%
Smoking Cessation Advice[2]	55	98%	82%	82%	100%
Pneumonia Care					
Appropriate Initial Antibiotic[2]	85	93%	82%	83%	94%
Blood Culture Timing[2]	72	85%	89%	90%	100%
Influenza Vaccine[1,2]	17	59%	58%	70%	100%
Initial Antibiotic Timing[2]	115	90%	75%	80%	93%
Oxygenation Assessment[2]	147	100%	99%	99%	100%
Pneumococcal Vaccine[2]	77	81%	58%	69%	94%
Smoking Cessation Advice[2]	29	83%	75%	80%	100%
Surgical Infection Prevention					
Prophylactic Antibiotic Given[2,3]	239	74%	74%	77%	95%
Prophylactic Antibiotic Selection[2]	80	69%	89%	90%	100%
Prophylactic Antibiotic Stopped[2,3]	235	55%	65%	72%	95%
Pregnancy Care					

NOTE: Hospital profiles are in alphabetical order by state, then city, then hospital within the city; Rankings are sorted by rate in descending order and exclude hospitals with less than 25 cases; (1) The number of cases is too small (n<25) for purposes of reliably predicting hospital performance; (2) Measure reflects the hospital's indication that its submission was based upon a sample of its relevant discharges; (3) Rate reflects fewer than the maximum possible quarters of data for the measure; (4) Inaccurate information submitted and suppressed for one or more quarters; (5) No data is available from the hospital for this measure; Please refer to the User's Guide for a full explanation of data

Inpatient Neonatal Mortality	-	-	-	-	-
Third or Fourth Degree Laceration	-	-	3.58%	3.63%	3.27%

Alvarado Hospital Medical Center

6655 Alvarado Road
San Diego, CA 92120
URL: www.alvaradohospital.com
Ownership: Proprietary
Emergency Services: No

Phone: 619-287-3270
Fax: 619-229-7020

Accredited: Yes
Licensed Beds: 231

Key Personnel:
Administrator . . . . B Weinbaum
CEO. . . . . Mark Palmer
Chief Medical Staff. . . . . Lauren Stephen-Porter

Measure	Cases	This Hospital	State Average	U.S. Average	Top Hospital
Heart Attack Care					
ACE Inhibitor or ARB for LVSD[5]	-	-	82%	82%	100%
Aspirin at Arrival[5]	-	-	95%	92%	100%
Aspirin at Discharge[5]	-	-	90%	90%	100%
Beta Blocker at Arrival[5]	-	-	89%	87%	100%
Beta Blocker at Discharge[5]	-	-	89%	90%	100%
Fibrinolytic Medication Timing[5]	-	-	40%	31%	100%
PCI Within 90 Minutes of Arrival[5]	-	-	52%	54%	95%
Smoking Cessation Advice[5]	-	-	87%	88%	100%
Heart Failure Care					
ACE Inhibitor or ARB for LVSD[5]	-	-	84%	82%	100%
Discharge Instructions[5]	-	-	56%	61%	93%
Evaluation of LVS Function[5]	-	-	84%	83%	99%
Smoking Cessation Advice[5]	-	-	82%	82%	100%
Pneumonia Care					
Appropriate Initial Antibiotic[5]	-	-	82%	83%	94%
Blood Culture Timing[5]	-	-	89%	90%	100%
Influenza Vaccine[5]	-	-	58%	70%	100%
Initial Antibiotic Timing[5]	-	-	75%	80%	93%
Oxygenation Assessment[5]	-	-	99%	99%	100%
Pneumococcal Vaccine[5]	-	-	58%	69%	94%
Smoking Cessation Advice[5]	-	-	75%	80%	100%
Surgical Infection Prevention					
Prophylactic Antibiotic Given[5]	-	-	74%	77%	95%
Prophylactic Antibiotic Selection[5]	-	-	89%	90%	100%
Prophylactic Antibiotic Stopped[5]	-	-	65%	72%	95%
Pregnancy Care					
Inpatient Neonatal Mortality	-	-	-	-	-
Third or Fourth Degree Laceration	-	-	3.58%	3.63%	3.27%

Kaiser Foundation Hospital-San Diego

4647 Zion Avenue
San Diego, CA 92120
URL: www.kaiserpermanente.org
Ownership: Voluntary non-profit - Other
Emergency Services: Yes

Phone: 619-528-5000
Fax: 626-405-3176

Accredited: Yes
Licensed Beds: 395

Key Personnel:
Chief Medical Staff. . . . . Daniel Anderson, MD
Emergency Department . . . . Raymond Poliakoff, MD
Chief OB/GYN . . . . Silverio Chavez, MD

Measure	Cases	This Hospital	State Average	U.S. Average	Top Hospital
Heart Attack Care					
ACE Inhibitor or ARB for LVSD	27	93%	82%	82%	100%
Aspirin at Arrival	235	92%	95%	92%	100%
Aspirin at Discharge	95	93%	90%	90%	100%
Beta Blocker at Arrival	215	95%	89%	87%	100%
Beta Blocker at Discharge	101	96%	89%	90%	100%
Fibrinolytic Medication Timing[1]	7	14%	40%	31%	100%
PCI Within 90 Minutes of Arrival	0	-	52%	54%	95%
Smoking Cessation Advice[1]	19	53%	87%	88%	100%
Heart Failure Care					
ACE Inhibitor or ARB for LVSD	242	86%	84%	82%	100%
Discharge Instructions	575	53%	56%	61%	93%
Evaluation of LVS Function	625	94%	84%	83%	99%
Smoking Cessation Advice	67	82%	82%	82%	100%
Pneumonia Care					
Appropriate Initial Antibiotic	94	36%	82%	83%	94%
Blood Culture Timing	71	85%	89%	90%	100%
Influenza Vaccine	29	69%	58%	70%	100%
Initial Antibiotic Timing	112	66%	75%	80%	93%
Oxygenation Assessment	144	100%	99%	99%	100%
Pneumococcal Vaccine	86	81%	58%	69%	94%
Smoking Cessation Advice[1]	17	65%	75%	80%	100%
Surgical Infection Prevention					
Prophylactic Antibiotic Given[3]	31	58%	74%	77%	95%
Prophylactic Antibiotic Selection	30	100%	89%	90%	100%
Prophylactic Antibiotic Stopped[3]	28	57%	65%	72%	95%
Pregnancy Care					
Inpatient Neonatal Mortality	3,983	0.40%	-	-	-
Third or Fourth Degree Laceration	2,640	3.94%	3.58%	3.63%	3.27%

Promise Hospital of San Diego

Alternate Name: Univeristy Community Medical Center
5550 University Avenue
San Diego, CA 92105
E-mail: cbrunner@tmisnet.com
URL: www.ucmedctr.com
Ownership: Voluntary non-profit - Other
Emergency Services: Yes

Phone: 619-582-3800
Fax: 619-286-2026

Accredited: Yes
Licensed Beds: 100

Key Personnel:
President/CEO . . . . Jim Patten
Infection Control . . . . Guylaine Robert, RN
ICU . . . . Arleneia Barongan
Med/Surg Nurse . . . . Arlene Barongan
Respiratory/Cardiopulmonary. . . . . Sue Henning

Measure	Cases	This Hospital	State Average	U.S. Average	Top Hospital
Heart Attack Care					
ACE Inhibitor or ARB for LVSD[5]	-	-	82%	82%	100%
Aspirin at Arrival[5]	-	-	95%	92%	100%
Aspirin at Discharge[5]	-	-	90%	90%	100%
Beta Blocker at Arrival[5]	-	-	89%	87%	100%
Beta Blocker at Discharge[5]	-	-	89%	90%	100%
Fibrinolytic Medication Timing[5]	-	-	40%	31%	100%
PCI Within 90 Minutes of Arrival[5]	-	-	52%	54%	95%
Smoking Cessation Advice[5]	-	-	87%	88%	100%
Heart Failure Care					
ACE Inhibitor or ARB for LVSD[3]	0	-	84%	82%	100%
Discharge Instructions[1,3]	2	50%	56%	61%	93%
Evaluation of LVS Function[1,3]	2	50%	84%	83%	99%
Smoking Cessation Advice[3]	0	-	82%	82%	100%
Pneumonia Care					
Appropriate Initial Antibiotic[1]	4	50%	82%	83%	94%
Blood Culture Timing[1]	1	100%	89%	90%	100%
Influenza Vaccine[1]	3	33%	58%	70%	100%
Initial Antibiotic Timing[1]	10	80%	75%	80%	93%
Oxygenation Assessment[1]	16	100%	99%	99%	100%
Pneumococcal Vaccine[1]	6	33%	58%	69%	94%
Smoking Cessation Advice[1]	4	75%	75%	80%	100%
Surgical Infection Prevention					
Prophylactic Antibiotic Given[5]	-	-	74%	77%	95%
Prophylactic Antibiotic Selection[5]	-	-	89%	90%	100%
Prophylactic Antibiotic Stopped[5]	-	-	65%	72%	95%
Pregnancy Care					
Inpatient Neonatal Mortality	-	-	-	-	-
Third or Fourth Degree Laceration	-	-	3.58%	3.63%	3.27%

San Diego Hospice & Palliative Care

4311 Third Ave
San Diego, CA 92103
Ownership: Voluntary non-profit - Other
Emergency Services: No

Phone: 619-688-1600

Accredited: No

Measure	Cases	This Hospital	State Average	U.S. Average	Top Hospital
Heart Attack Care					
ACE Inhibitor or ARB for LVSD[5]	-	-	82%	82%	100%
Aspirin at Arrival[5]	-	-	95%	92%	100%
Aspirin at Discharge[5]	-	-	90%	90%	100%

NOTE: Hospital profiles are in alphabetical order by state, then city, then hospital within the city; Rankings are sorted by rate in descending order and exclude hospitals with less than 25 cases; (1) The number of cases is too small (n<25) for purposes of reliably predicting hospital performance; (2) Measure reflects the hospital's indication that its submission was based upon a sample of its relevant discharges; (3) Rate reflects fewer than the maximum possible quarters of data for the measure; (4) Inaccurate information submitted and suppressed for one or more quarters; (5) No data is available from the hospital for this measure; Please refer to the User's Guide for a full explanation of data

Measure	Cases	This Hospital	State Average	U.S. Average	Top Hospital
Beta Blocker at Arrival[5]	-	-	89%	87%	100%
Beta Blocker at Discharge[5]	-	-	89%	90%	100%
Fibrinolytic Medication Timing[5]	-	-	40%	31%	100%
PCI Within 90 Minutes of Arrival[5]	-	-	52%	54%	95%
Smoking Cessation Advice[5]	-	-	87%	88%	100%
Heart Failure Care					
ACE Inhibitor or ARB for LVSD[5]	-	-	84%	82%	100%
Discharge Instructions[5]	-	-	56%	61%	93%
Evaluation of LVS Function[5]	-	-	84%	83%	99%
Smoking Cessation Advice[5]	-	-	82%	82%	100%
Pneumonia Care					
Appropriate Initial Antibiotic[5]	-	-	82%	83%	94%
Blood Culture Timing[5]	-	-	89%	90%	100%
Influenza Vaccine[5]	-	-	58%	70%	100%
Initial Antibiotic Timing[5]	-	-	75%	80%	93%
Oxygenation Assessment[5]	-	-	99%	99%	100%
Pneumococcal Vaccine[5]	-	-	58%	69%	94%
Smoking Cessation Advice[5]	-	-	75%	80%	100%
Surgical Infection Prevention					
Prophylactic Antibiotic Given[5]	-	-	74%	77%	95%
Prophylactic Antibiotic Selection[5]	-	-	89%	90%	100%
Prophylactic Antibiotic Stopped[5]	-	-	65%	72%	95%
Pregnancy Care					
Inpatient Neonatal Mortality	-	-	-	-	-
Third or Fourth Degree Laceration	-	-	3.58%	3.63%	3.27%

Scripps Mercy Hospital

4077 Fifth Avenue
San Diego, CA 92103
Phone: 619-294-8111
Fax: 619-686-3530
URL: www.scrippshealth.org
Ownership: Voluntary non-profit - Other
Accredited: Yes
Emergency Services: Yes
Licensed Beds: 700

Key Personnel:

CEO . . . . Tom Gammiere
Director Respiratory Therapy . . . . Kevin Glynn, MD

Measure	Cases	This Hospital	State Average	U.S. Average	Top Hospital
Heart Attack Care					
ACE Inhibitor or ARB for LVSD	55	95%	82%	82%	100%
Aspirin at Arrival	336	100%	95%	92%	100%
Aspirin at Discharge	307	98%	90%	90%	100%
Beta Blocker at Arrival	278	99%	89%	87%	100%
Beta Blocker at Discharge	313	97%	89%	90%	100%
Fibrinolytic Medication Timing[1]	4	0%	40%	31%	100%
PCI Within 90 Minutes of Arrival[1]	22	77%	52%	54%	95%
Smoking Cessation Advice	87	95%	87%	88%	100%
Heart Failure Care					
ACE Inhibitor or ARB for LVSD	287	86%	84%	82%	100%
Discharge Instructions	740	69%	56%	61%	93%
Evaluation of LVS Function	860	89%	84%	83%	99%
Smoking Cessation Advice	145	92%	82%	82%	100%
Pneumonia Care					
Appropriate Initial Antibiotic	406	70%	82%	83%	94%
Blood Culture Timing	400	88%	89%	90%	100%
Influenza Vaccine	132	11%	58%	70%	100%
Initial Antibiotic Timing	552	63%	75%	80%	93%
Oxygenation Assessment	685	100%	99%	99%	100%
Pneumococcal Vaccine	402	22%	58%	69%	94%
Smoking Cessation Advice	146	77%	75%	80%	100%
Surgical Infection Prevention					
Prophylactic Antibiotic Given[2,3]	155	79%	74%	77%	95%
Prophylactic Antibiotic Selection[2]	80	91%	89%	90%	100%
Prophylactic Antibiotic Stopped[2,3]	148	57%	65%	72%	95%
Pregnancy Care					
Inpatient Neonatal Mortality	4,352	0.07%	-	-	-
Third or Fourth Degree Laceration	2,984	3.49%	3.58%	3.63%	3.27%

Sharp Mary Birch Hospital for Women

3003 Health Center Drive
Phone: 858-541-3017
San Diego, CA 92123
Ownership: Voluntary non-profit - Private
Accredited: Yes
Emergency Services: No

Measure	Cases	This Hospital	State Average	U.S. Average	Top Hospital
Heart Attack Care					
ACE Inhibitor or ARB for LVSD[5]	-	-	82%	82%	100%
Aspirin at Arrival[5]	-	-	95%	92%	100%
Aspirin at Discharge[5]	-	-	90%	90%	100%
Beta Blocker at Arrival[5]	-	-	89%	87%	100%
Beta Blocker at Discharge[5]	-	-	89%	90%	100%
Fibrinolytic Medication Timing[5]	-	-	40%	31%	100%
PCI Within 90 Minutes of Arrival[5]	-	-	52%	54%	95%
Smoking Cessation Advice[5]	-	-	87%	88%	100%
Heart Failure Care					
ACE Inhibitor or ARB for LVSD[5]	-	-	84%	82%	100%
Discharge Instructions[5]	-	-	56%	61%	93%
Evaluation of LVS Function[5]	-	-	84%	83%	99%
Smoking Cessation Advice[5]	-	-	82%	82%	100%
Pneumonia Care					
Appropriate Initial Antibiotic[5]	-	-	82%	83%	94%
Blood Culture Timing[5]	-	-	89%	90%	100%
Influenza Vaccine[5]	-	-	58%	70%	100%
Initial Antibiotic Timing[5]	-	-	75%	80%	93%
Oxygenation Assessment[5]	-	-	99%	99%	100%
Pneumococcal Vaccine[5]	-	-	58%	69%	94%
Smoking Cessation Advice[5]	-	-	75%	80%	100%
Surgical Infection Prevention					
Prophylactic Antibiotic Given[2,3]	35	83%	74%	77%	95%
Prophylactic Antibiotic Selection[5]	-	-	89%	90%	100%
Prophylactic Antibiotic Stopped[2,3]	35	94%	65%	72%	95%
Pregnancy Care					
Inpatient Neonatal Mortality	8,388	0.46%	-	-	-
Third or Fourth Degree Laceration	5,165	4.59%	3.58%	3.63%	3.27%

Sharp Memorial Hospital

7901 Frost Street
San Diego, CA 92123
Toll-Free: 800-82-SHARP
Phone: 858-939-3400
Fax: 858-499-5938
E-mail: info@sharp.com
URL: www.sharp.com
Ownership: Voluntary non-profit - Other
Accredited: Yes
Emergency Services: Yes
Licensed Beds: 464

Key Personnel:

Director Infection/Disease Control . . . . Judy Vargo
Chief of Respiratory/Pulmonary Therapy . . . . . . Charles Kllanders

Measure	Cases	This Hospital	State Average	U.S. Average	Top Hospital
Heart Attack Care					
ACE Inhibitor or ARB for LVSD	56	91%	82%	82%	100%
Aspirin at Arrival	275	99%	95%	92%	100%
Aspirin at Discharge	298	100%	90%	90%	100%
Beta Blocker at Arrival	196	98%	89%	87%	100%
Beta Blocker at Discharge	307	99%	89%	90%	100%
Fibrinolytic Medication Timing[1]	2	0%	40%	31%	100%
PCI Within 90 Minutes of Arrival[1]	10	70%	52%	54%	95%
Smoking Cessation Advice	61	100%	87%	88%	100%
Heart Failure Care					
ACE Inhibitor or ARB for LVSD	161	84%	84%	82%	100%
Discharge Instructions	365	63%	56%	61%	93%
Evaluation of LVS Function	454	90%	84%	83%	99%
Smoking Cessation Advice	42	95%	82%	82%	100%
Pneumonia Care					
Appropriate Initial Antibiotic[2]	235	78%	82%	83%	94%
Blood Culture Timing[2]	216	91%	89%	90%	100%
Influenza Vaccine[2]	69	52%	58%	70%	100%
Initial Antibiotic Timing[2]	308	60%	75%	80%	93%
Oxygenation Assessment[2]	366	100%	99%	99%	100%
Pneumococcal Vaccine[2]	237	41%	58%	69%	94%
Smoking Cessation Advice[2]	55	89%	75%	80%	100%

NOTE: Hospital profiles are in alphabetical order by state, then city, then hospital within the city; Rankings are sorted by rate in descending order and exclude hospitals with less than 25 cases; (1) The number of cases is too small (n<25) for purposes of reliably predicting hospital performance; (2) Measure reflects the hospital's indication that its submission was based upon a sample of its relevant discharges; (3) Rate reflects fewer than the maximum possible quarters of data for the measure; (4) Inaccurate information submitted and suppressed for one or more quarters; (5) No data is available from the hospital for this measure; Please refer to the User's Guide for a full explanation of data

Measure	Cases	This Hospital	State Average	U.S. Average	Top Hospital
Surgical Infection Prevention					
Prophylactic Antibiotic Given[2,3]	461	87%	74%	77%	95%
Prophylactic Antibiotic Selection[2]	172	91%	89%	90%	100%
Prophylactic Antibiotic Stopped[2,3]	449	76%	65%	72%	95%
Pregnancy Care					
Inpatient Neonatal Mortality	-	-	-	-	-
Third or Fourth Degree Laceration	-	-	3.58%	3.63%	3.27%

University of California San Diego Med Ctr

200 W Arbor Drive Phone: 619-543-6222
San Diego, CA 92103 Fax: 619-543-5423
URL: www.health.ucsd.edu
Ownership: Government - State Accredited: Yes
Emergency Services: Yes Licensed Beds: 558

Key Personnel:

CEO. . . . . Richard Liekweg
Chief Medical Staff. . . . . Stephen I Wasserman
Emergency Room . . . . . Kevin Jones
Director Infection/Disease Control . . . . . S Spencer, MD
OB/GYN Womens Health. . . . . Homer Chin
Chief Radiology . . . . . George Leopold, MD
Director of Pulmonary . . . . . Lewis Rubin

Measure	Cases	This Hospital	State Average	U.S. Average	Top Hospital
Heart Attack Care					
ACE Inhibitor or ARB for LVSD[1]	19	63%	82%	82%	100%
Aspirin at Arrival	161	100%	95%	92%	100%
Aspirin at Discharge	208	100%	90%	90%	100%
Beta Blocker at Arrival	131	100%	89%	87%	100%
Beta Blocker at Discharge	199	99%	89%	90%	100%
Fibrinolytic Medication Timing	0	-	40%	31%	100%
PCI Within 90 Minutes of Arrival[1]	3	67%	52%	54%	95%
Smoking Cessation Advice	53	98%	87%	88%	100%
Heart Failure Care					
ACE Inhibitor or ARB for LVSD[2]	152	88%	84%	82%	100%
Discharge Instructions[2]	270	60%	56%	61%	93%
Evaluation of LVS Function[2]	305	96%	84%	83%	99%
Smoking Cessation Advice[2]	77	96%	82%	82%	100%
Pneumonia Care					
Appropriate Initial Antibiotic[2]	141	68%	82%	83%	94%
Blood Culture Timing[2]	153	95%	89%	90%	100%
Influenza Vaccine[2]	29	34%	58%	70%	100%
Initial Antibiotic Timing[2]	192	65%	75%	80%	93%
Oxygenation Assessment[2]	248	100%	99%	99%	100%
Pneumococcal Vaccine[2]	85	56%	58%	69%	94%
Smoking Cessation Advice[2]	72	97%	75%	80%	100%
Surgical Infection Prevention					
Prophylactic Antibiotic Given[2,3]	336	81%	74%	77%	95%
Prophylactic Antibiotic Selection[2]	65	89%	89%	90%	100%
Prophylactic Antibiotic Stopped[2,3]	318	53%	65%	72%	95%
Pregnancy Care					
Inpatient Neonatal Mortality	-	-	-	-	-
Third or Fourth Degree Laceration	-	-	3.58%	3.63%	3.27%

San Dimas Community Hospital

1350 W Covina Boulevard Phone: 909-599-6811
San Dimas, CA 91773 Fax: 909-305-5677
E-mail: ketsana.nobouphasavanh@tenethealth.com
URL: www.sandimashospital.com
Ownership: Proprietary Accredited: Yes
Emergency Services: Yes Licensed Beds: 93

Key Personnel:

CEO. . . . . Dan Bowers
Chief Medical Staff. . . . . Dinesh Samant
Emergency Room . . . . . James Pagano, MD
Emergency Room . . . . . Mary Dahl
Infection Control. . . . . Jean Rathod
ICU . . . . . Mary Dahl
OB/GYN/Women's Health . . . . . Diana Wolff
Respiratory/Cardiopulmonary. . . . . Felix Laryea

Measure	Cases	This Hospital	State Average	U.S. Average	Top Hospital
Heart Attack Care					
ACE Inhibitor or ARB for LVSD[1]	7	100%	82%	82%	100%
Aspirin at Arrival	31	100%	95%	92%	100%
Aspirin at Discharge[1]	21	100%	90%	90%	100%
Beta Blocker at Arrival	32	78%	89%	87%	100%
Beta Blocker at Discharge[1]	22	82%	89%	90%	100%
Fibrinolytic Medication Timing	0	-	40%	31%	100%
PCI Within 90 Minutes of Arrival	0	-	52%	54%	95%
Smoking Cessation Advice	0	-	87%	88%	100%
Heart Failure Care					
ACE Inhibitor or ARB for LVSD	43	74%	84%	82%	100%
Discharge Instructions	83	78%	56%	61%	93%
Evaluation of LVS Function	120	92%	84%	83%	99%
Smoking Cessation Advice[1]	12	92%	82%	82%	100%
Pneumonia Care					
Appropriate Initial Antibiotic	128	87%	82%	83%	94%
Blood Culture Timing	171	90%	89%	90%	100%
Influenza Vaccine	50	96%	58%	70%	100%
Initial Antibiotic Timing	185	90%	75%	80%	93%
Oxygenation Assessment	254	100%	99%	99%	100%
Pneumococcal Vaccine	158	92%	58%	69%	94%
Smoking Cessation Advice	26	100%	75%	80%	100%
Surgical Infection Prevention					
Prophylactic Antibiotic Given[2]	318	90%	74%	77%	95%
Prophylactic Antibiotic Selection[2]	74	96%	89%	90%	100%
Prophylactic Antibiotic Stopped[2]	308	44%	65%	72%	95%
Pregnancy Care					
Inpatient Neonatal Mortality	-	-	-	-	-
Third or Fourth Degree Laceration	-	-	3.58%	3.63%	3.27%

California Pacific Medical Center

Alternate Name: Pacific Campus Hospital
PO Box 7999 Phone: 415-600-6000
San Francisco, CA 94120 Fax: 415-600-2985
E-mail: cpmcadmin@sutterhealth.org
URL: www.cpmc.org
Ownership: Voluntary non-profit - Private Accredited: Yes
Emergency Services: Yes Licensed Beds: 341

Key Personnel:

Administrator/President . . . . . Martin Brotman
Department Chair Cardiac Surgery . . . . . Soon J Park, MD
Director Surgical Services . . . . . Diane Petruzzella, RN
Department Chair Obstetrics & Gynocology. . . . Elliot K Main, MD

Measure	Cases	This Hospital	State Average	U.S. Average	Top Hospital
Heart Attack Care					
ACE Inhibitor or ARB for LVSD	56	91%	82%	82%	100%
Aspirin at Arrival	147	99%	95%	92%	100%
Aspirin at Discharge	179	99%	90%	90%	100%
Beta Blocker at Arrival	108	96%	89%	87%	100%
Beta Blocker at Discharge	181	99%	89%	90%	100%
Fibrinolytic Medication Timing	0	-	40%	31%	100%
PCI Within 90 Minutes of Arrival[1]	8	75%	52%	54%	95%
Smoking Cessation Advice	46	93%	87%	88%	100%
Heart Failure Care					
ACE Inhibitor or ARB for LVSD	177	92%	84%	82%	100%
Discharge Instructions	384	47%	56%	61%	93%
Evaluation of LVS Function	457	98%	84%	83%	99%
Smoking Cessation Advice	57	88%	82%	82%	100%
Pneumonia Care					
Appropriate Initial Antibiotic[2]	84	85%	82%	83%	94%
Blood Culture Timing[2]	106	97%	89%	90%	100%
Influenza Vaccine[1]	21	29%	58%	70%	100%
Initial Antibiotic Timing[2]	133	78%	75%	80%	93%
Oxygenation Assessment[2]	178	100%	99%	99%	100%
Pneumococcal Vaccine[2]	119	72%	58%	69%	94%
Smoking Cessation Advice[1,2]	23	74%	75%	80%	100%
Surgical Infection Prevention					
Prophylactic Antibiotic Given[2,3]	244	92%	74%	77%	95%
Prophylactic Antibiotic Selection[2]	82	98%	89%	90%	100%
Prophylactic Antibiotic Stopped[2,3]	242	80%	65%	72%	95%
Pregnancy Care					
Inpatient Neonatal Mortality[2]	1,003	0.40%	-	-	-

NOTE: Hospital profiles are in alphabetical order by state, then city, then hospital within the city; Rankings are sorted by rate in descending order and exclude hospitals with less than 25 cases; (1) The number of cases is too small (n<25) for purposes of reliably predicting hospital performance; (2) Measure reflects the hospital's indication that its submission was based upon a sample of its relevant discharges; (3) Rate reflects fewer than the maximum possible quarters of data for the measure; (4) Inaccurate information submitted and suppressed for one or more quarters; (5) No data is available from the hospital for this measure; Please refer to the User's Guide for a full explanation of data

Third or Fourth Degree Laceration[2]	741	3.91%	3.58%	3.63%	3.27%

Chinese Hospital

845 Jackson Street
San Francisco, CA 94133
URL: www.chinesehospital-sf.org
Ownership: Voluntary non-profit - Other
Emergency Services: Yes

Phone: 415-982-2400
Fax: 415-217-4188
Accredited: Yes
Licensed Beds: 54

Key Personnel:

President . . . . Joe Chan
CEO. . . . . Brenda Yee
Chief Medical Staff. . . . . Joseph Woo, MD
Emergency Room . . . . Michael L Shafer, MD
Infection Control Coordinator . . . . Stuart Fong
Cardiopulmonary Unit Manager . . . . Elena Wong

Measure	Cases	This Hospital	State Average	U.S. Average	Top Hospital
Heart Attack Care					
ACE Inhibitor or ARB for LVSD[1]	1	0%	82%	82%	100%
Aspirin at Arrival[1]	22	95%	95%	92%	100%
Aspirin at Discharge[1]	8	75%	90%	90%	100%
Beta Blocker at Arrival[1]	20	85%	89%	87%	100%
Beta Blocker at Discharge[1]	7	57%	89%	90%	100%
Fibrinolytic Medication Timing	0	-	40%	31%	100%
PCI Within 90 Minutes of Arrival	0	-	52%	54%	95%
Smoking Cessation Advice[1]	1	100%	87%	88%	100%
Heart Failure Care					
ACE Inhibitor or ARB for LVSD[1]	20	75%	84%	82%	100%
Discharge Instructions	82	62%	56%	61%	93%
Evaluation of LVS Function	91	87%	84%	83%	99%
Smoking Cessation Advice[1]	2	50%	82%	82%	100%
Pneumonia Care					
Appropriate Initial Antibiotic	176	94%	82%	83%	94%
Blood Culture Timing	115	91%	89%	90%	100%
Influenza Vaccine	44	91%	58%	70%	100%
Initial Antibiotic Timing	170	86%	75%	80%	93%
Oxygenation Assessment	203	100%	99%	99%	100%
Pneumococcal Vaccine	178	88%	58%	69%	94%
Smoking Cessation Advice[1]	21	90%	75%	80%	100%
Surgical Infection Prevention					
Prophylactic Antibiotic Given[1,3]	18	100%	74%	77%	95%
Prophylactic Antibiotic Selection[1]	18	94%	89%	90%	100%
Prophylactic Antibiotic Stopped[1,3]	18	17%	65%	72%	95%
Pregnancy Care					
Inpatient Neonatal Mortality	-	-	-	-	-
Third or Fourth Degree Laceration	-	-	3.58%	3.63%	3.27%

Davies Medical Center

Castro at Duboce
San Francisco, CA 94114
Ownership: Voluntary non-profit - Other
Emergency Services: Yes

Phone: 415-600-6000
Accredited: Yes

Measure	Cases	This Hospital	State Average	U.S. Average	Top Hospital
Heart Attack Care					
ACE Inhibitor or ARB for LVSD[1,3]	2	100%	82%	82%	100%
Aspirin at Arrival[1,3]	9	100%	95%	92%	100%
Aspirin at Discharge[1,3]	4	100%	90%	90%	100%
Beta Blocker at Arrival[1,3]	7	86%	89%	87%	100%
Beta Blocker at Discharge[1,3]	5	100%	89%	90%	100%
Fibrinolytic Medication Timing[3]	0	-	40%	31%	100%
PCI Within 90 Minutes of Arrival[5]	-	-	52%	54%	95%
Smoking Cessation Advice[1,3]	1	0%	87%	88%	100%
Heart Failure Care					
ACE Inhibitor or ARB for LVSD[1]	20	90%	84%	82%	100%
Discharge Instructions	53	58%	56%	61%	93%
Evaluation of LVS Function	63	97%	84%	83%	99%
Smoking Cessation Advice[1]	14	86%	82%	82%	100%
Pneumonia Care					
Appropriate Initial Antibiotic	50	82%	82%	83%	94%
Blood Culture Timing	62	92%	89%	90%	100%
Influenza Vaccine[1]	15	20%	58%	70%	100%
Initial Antibiotic Timing	75	77%	75%	80%	93%
Oxygenation Assessment	101	100%	99%	99%	100%
Pneumococcal Vaccine	51	67%	58%	69%	94%
Smoking Cessation Advice	29	79%	75%	80%	100%
Surgical Infection Prevention					
Prophylactic Antibiotic Given[1,3]	21	90%	74%	77%	95%
Prophylactic Antibiotic Selection[1]	4	100%	89%	90%	100%
Prophylactic Antibiotic Stopped[1,3]	20	100%	65%	72%	95%
Pregnancy Care					
Inpatient Neonatal Mortality	-	-	-	-	-
Third or Fourth Degree Laceration	-	-	3.58%	3.63%	3.27%

Kaiser Permanente San Francisco Med Ctr

2425 Geary Blvd
San Francisco, CA 94115
URL: www.permanente.net
Ownership: Govt - Hospital District or Authority
Emergency Services: Yes

Toll-Free: 877-393-2332
Phone: 415-833-2000
Fax: 415-833-4567
Accredited: Yes
Licensed Beds: 620

Key Personnel:

President/CEO. . . . . Mary Ann Theodore
Chief Medical Staff. . . . . Paul Feigenbaum, MD
Chief Catheterization Laboratory . . . . Howard Lurra, MD
Emergency Room . . . . Steve Lauterbach, MD
Director Infection/Disease Control . . . . Barbara Lamberto
OB/GYN Womens Health. . . . . James Lewis, MD
Chief Radiology . . . . John Rego, MD
Chief of Respiratory Care. . . . . Keith Rasmussen

Measure	Cases	This Hospital	State Average	U.S. Average	Top Hospital
Heart Attack Care					
ACE Inhibitor or ARB for LVSD	69	96%	82%	82%	100%
Aspirin at Arrival	75	99%	95%	92%	100%
Aspirin at Discharge	429	98%	90%	90%	100%
Beta Blocker at Arrival	62	98%	89%	87%	100%
Beta Blocker at Discharge	494	99%	89%	90%	100%
Fibrinolytic Medication Timing	0	-	40%	31%	100%
PCI Within 90 Minutes of Arrival[1]	4	75%	52%	54%	95%
Smoking Cessation Advice	120	100%	87%	88%	100%
Heart Failure Care					
ACE Inhibitor or ARB for LVSD	134	97%	84%	82%	100%
Discharge Instructions	336	79%	56%	61%	93%
Evaluation of LVS Function	353	97%	84%	83%	99%
Smoking Cessation Advice	41	98%	82%	82%	100%
Pneumonia Care					
Appropriate Initial Antibiotic	118	93%	82%	83%	94%
Blood Culture Timing	190	95%	89%	90%	100%
Influenza Vaccine	41	63%	58%	70%	100%
Initial Antibiotic Timing	222	83%	75%	80%	93%
Oxygenation Assessment	263	100%	99%	99%	100%
Pneumococcal Vaccine	186	81%	58%	69%	94%
Smoking Cessation Advice	31	77%	75%	80%	100%
Surgical Infection Prevention					
Prophylactic Antibiotic Given	631	92%	74%	77%	95%
Prophylactic Antibiotic Selection	175	97%	89%	90%	100%
Prophylactic Antibiotic Stopped	605	86%	65%	72%	95%
Pregnancy Care					
Inpatient Neonatal Mortality	2,612	0.23%	-	-	-
Third or Fourth Degree Laceration	1,675	6.87%	3.58%	3.63%	3.27%

Laguna Honda Hospital and Rehab Center

375 Laguna Honda Boulevard
San Francisco, CA 94116
URL: www.dph.sf.ca.us/chn/LagunaHondaHosp
Ownership: Government - Local
Emergency Services: Yes

Phone: 415-759-2300
Fax: 415-759-2374
Accredited: No
Licensed Beds: 1,457

Key Personnel:

President/CEO. . . . . John Kanaley
Chief Medical Staff. . . . . Paul Isakson, MD
Director Infection/Disease Control . . . . Julio Pineda, MD
Chief Radiology . . . . Joe Robertson
Director Respiratory Therapy . . . . Claudell LeBlanc

NOTE: Hospital profiles are in alphabetical order by state, then city, then hospital within the city; Rankings are sorted by rate in descending order and exclude hospitals with less than 25 cases; (1) The number of cases is too small (n<25) for purposes of reliably predicting hospital performance; (2) Measure reflects the hospital's indication that its submission was based upon a sample of its relevant discharges; (3) Rate reflects fewer than the maximum possible quarters of data for the measure; (4) Inaccurate information submitted and suppressed for one or more quarters; (5) No data is available from the hospital for this measure; Please refer to the User's Guide for a full explanation of data

Measure	Cases	This Hospital	State Average	U.S. Average	Top Hospital
Heart Attack Care					
ACE Inhibitor or ARB for LVSD[3]	0	-	82%	82%	100%
Aspirin at Arrival[1,3]	1	100%	95%	92%	100%
Aspirin at Discharge[1,3]	1	100%	90%	90%	100%
Beta Blocker at Arrival[1,3]	2	100%	89%	87%	100%
Beta Blocker at Discharge[1,3]	2	100%	89%	90%	100%
Fibrinolytic Medication Timing[5]	-	-	40%	31%	100%
PCI Within 90 Minutes of Arrival[5]	-	-	52%	54%	95%
Smoking Cessation Advice[5]	-	-	87%	88%	100%
Heart Failure Care					
ACE Inhibitor or ARB for LVSD[1,3]	1	100%	84%	82%	100%
Discharge Instructions[3]	0	-	56%	61%	93%
Evaluation of LVS Function[1,3]	1	100%	84%	83%	99%
Smoking Cessation Advice[3]	0	-	82%	82%	100%
Pneumonia Care					
Appropriate Initial Antibiotic[2,3]	0	-	82%	83%	94%
Blood Culture Timing[1,2,3]	1	100%	89%	90%	100%
Influenza Vaccine[5]	-	-	58%	70%	100%
Initial Antibiotic Timing[1,2]	9	78%	75%	80%	93%
Oxygenation Assessment[1,2]	17	100%	99%	99%	100%
Pneumococcal Vaccine[1,2]	9	56%	58%	69%	94%
Smoking Cessation Advice[2,3]	0	-	75%	80%	100%
Surgical Infection Prevention					
Prophylactic Antibiotic Given[5]	-	-	74%	77%	95%
Prophylactic Antibiotic Selection[5]	-	-	89%	90%	100%
Prophylactic Antibiotic Stopped[5]	-	-	65%	72%	95%
Pregnancy Care					
Inpatient Neonatal Mortality	-	-	-	-	-
Third or Fourth Degree Laceration	-	-	3.58%	3.63%	3.27%

Saint Francis Memorial Hospital

900 Hyde Street
San Francisco, CA 94109
URL: www.saintfrancismemorial.org
Ownership: Voluntary non-profit - Private
Emergency Services: Yes

Phone: 415-353-6000
Fax: 415-353-6912
Accredited: Yes
Licensed Beds: 356

Key Personnel:
President/CEO. . . . . Cheryl A Fama
Chief Medical Staff. . . . . Roger R Smith, MD
Chief Catheterization Laboratory . . . . Collin Quock, MD
Emergency Room . . . . Leighe Durlacher, MD
Emergency Room . . . . Richard Naidus, MD
Coordinator Infection Control . . . . Fred Deneau
CCU Spvg. Nurse . . . . Nancy Carewe
Chief Radiology . . . . Frank Mainzer, MD

Measure	Cases	This Hospital	State Average	U.S. Average	Top Hospital
Heart Attack Care					
ACE Inhibitor or ARB for LVSD[1]	6	100%	82%	82%	100%
Aspirin at Arrival[1]	16	100%	95%	92%	100%
Aspirin at Discharge[1]	11	82%	90%	90%	100%
Beta Blocker at Arrival[1]	7	100%	89%	87%	100%
Beta Blocker at Discharge[1]	10	100%	89%	90%	100%
Fibrinolytic Medication Timing	0	-	40%	31%	100%
PCI Within 90 Minutes of Arrival	0	-	52%	54%	95%
Smoking Cessation Advice[1]	1	100%	87%	88%	100%
Heart Failure Care					
ACE Inhibitor or ARB for LVSD[1]	22	100%	84%	82%	100%
Discharge Instructions	56	84%	56%	61%	93%
Evaluation of LVS Function	71	97%	84%	83%	99%
Smoking Cessation Advice[1]	5	100%	82%	82%	100%
Pneumonia Care					
Appropriate Initial Antibiotic	38	82%	82%	83%	94%
Blood Culture Timing	44	95%	89%	90%	100%
Influenza Vaccine[1]	8	75%	58%	70%	100%
Initial Antibiotic Timing	56	91%	75%	80%	93%
Oxygenation Assessment	67	100%	99%	99%	100%
Pneumococcal Vaccine	36	89%	58%	69%	94%
Smoking Cessation Advice[1]	8	100%	75%	80%	100%
Surgical Infection Prevention					
Prophylactic Antibiotic Given[2,3]	118	97%	74%	77%	95%
Prophylactic Antibiotic Selection[2]	41	85%	89%	90%	100%
Prophylactic Antibiotic Stopped[2,3]	116	72%	65%	72%	95%
Pregnancy Care					
Inpatient Neonatal Mortality	-	-	-	-	-
Third or Fourth Degree Laceration	-	-	3.58%	3.63%	3.27%

Saint Luke's Hospital

3555 Cesar Chavez Street
San Francisco, CA 94110
E-mail: seidera@suuterhealth.org
URL: www.stlukes.sf.org
Ownership: Voluntary non-profit - Church
Emergency Services: Yes

Phone: 415-647-8600
Accredited: Yes
Licensed Beds: 260

Key Personnel:
CEO/President. . . . . Martin Brotman, MD
Emergency Room . . . . Tommye Farley, RN
Medical Director of Emergency Room . . . . Marc Synder, MD
ICU . . . . Tommye Farley, RN
Intensive Coronary. . . . . Tommye Farley, RN
Director Medical/Surgical Nursing . . . . Susan McCorquodale
OB/GYN Womens Health. . . . . Louise Todd, RNC

Measure	Cases	This Hospital	State Average	U.S. Average	Top Hospital
Heart Attack Care					
ACE Inhibitor or ARB for LVSD[1]	6	83%	82%	82%	100%
Aspirin at Arrival	43	100%	95%	92%	100%
Aspirin at Discharge[1]	22	95%	90%	90%	100%
Beta Blocker at Arrival	34	94%	89%	87%	100%
Beta Blocker at Discharge	25	100%	89%	90%	100%
Fibrinolytic Medication Timing	0	-	40%	31%	100%
PCI Within 90 Minutes of Arrival	0	-	52%	54%	95%
Smoking Cessation Advice[1]	6	83%	87%	88%	100%
Heart Failure Care					
ACE Inhibitor or ARB for LVSD	75	92%	84%	82%	100%
Discharge Instructions	160	52%	56%	61%	93%
Evaluation of LVS Function	191	88%	84%	83%	99%
Smoking Cessation Advice	44	93%	82%	82%	100%
Pneumonia Care					
Appropriate Initial Antibiotic	116	84%	82%	83%	94%
Blood Culture Timing	108	87%	89%	90%	100%
Influenza Vaccine	27	11%	58%	70%	100%
Initial Antibiotic Timing	148	76%	75%	80%	93%
Oxygenation Assessment	169	100%	99%	99%	100%
Pneumococcal Vaccine	102	23%	58%	69%	94%
Smoking Cessation Advice	46	76%	75%	80%	100%
Surgical Infection Prevention					
Prophylactic Antibiotic Given	136	51%	74%	77%	95%
Prophylactic Antibiotic Selection	33	94%	89%	90%	100%
Prophylactic Antibiotic Stopped	128	77%	65%	72%	95%
Pregnancy Care					
Inpatient Neonatal Mortality[2]	255	0.00%	-	-	-
Third or Fourth Degree Laceration[2]	376	5.05%	3.58%	3.63%	3.27%

Saint Mary's Medical Center

450 Stanyan Street
San Francisco, CA 94117
URL: www.stmarysmedicalcenter.org
Ownership: Voluntary non-profit - Church
Emergency Services: Yes

Phone: 415-668-1000
Fax: 415-668-4531
Accredited: Yes
Licensed Beds: 531

Key Personnel:
Director of Cardiology/Cardiac Lab. . . . . James Seene
Emergency Room . . . . Keith Loring
Emergency Room . . . . Robert Mueller
OB/GYN Womens Health. . . . . Ziyad Hannon
Chief Radiology . . . . James Gorder, MD

Measure	Cases	This Hospital	State Average	U.S. Average	Top Hospital
Heart Attack Care					
ACE Inhibitor or ARB for LVSD	32	97%	82%	82%	100%
Aspirin at Arrival	88	99%	95%	92%	100%
Aspirin at Discharge	133	100%	90%	90%	100%
Beta Blocker at Arrival	73	100%	89%	87%	100%

NOTE: Hospital profiles are in alphabetical order by state, then city, then hospital within the city; Rankings are sorted by rate in descending order and exclude hospitals with less than 25 cases; (1) The number of cases is too small (n<25) for purposes of reliably predicting hospital performance; (2) Measure reflects the hospital's indication that its submission was based upon a sample of its relevant discharges; (3) Rate reflects fewer than the maximum possible quarters of data for the measure; (4) Inaccurate information submitted and suppressed for one or more quarters; (5) No data is available from the hospital for this measure; Please refer to the User's Guide for a full explanation of data

Measure	Cases	This Hospital	State Average	U.S. Average	Top Hospital
Beta Blocker at Discharge	141	100%	89%	90%	100%
Fibrinolytic Medication Timing	0	-	40%	31%	100%
PCI Within 90 Minutes of Arrival[1]	3	0%	52%	54%	95%
Smoking Cessation Advice	29	86%	87%	88%	100%
Heart Failure Care					
ACE Inhibitor or ARB for LVSD	78	96%	84%	82%	100%
Discharge Instructions	151	89%	56%	61%	93%
Evaluation of LVS Function	199	99%	84%	83%	99%
Smoking Cessation Advice[1]	22	95%	82%	82%	100%
Pneumonia Care					
Appropriate Initial Antibiotic	116	91%	82%	83%	94%
Blood Culture Timing	147	97%	89%	90%	100%
Influenza Vaccine	36	42%	58%	70%	100%
Initial Antibiotic Timing	184	88%	75%	80%	93%
Oxygenation Assessment	229	100%	99%	99%	100%
Pneumococcal Vaccine	162	61%	58%	69%	94%
Smoking Cessation Advice	31	100%	75%	80%	100%
Surgical Infection Prevention					
Prophylactic Antibiotic Given[2,3]	173	83%	74%	77%	95%
Prophylactic Antibiotic Selection[2]	55	100%	89%	90%	100%
Prophylactic Antibiotic Stopped[2,3]	166	34%	65%	72%	95%
Pregnancy Care					
Inpatient Neonatal Mortality	-	-	-	-	-
Third or Fourth Degree Laceration	-	-	3.58%	3.63%	3.27%

San Francisco General Hospital Medical Center

1001 Potrero Avenue — Phone: 415-206-8000
San Francisco, CA 94110 — Fax: 415-206-3434
URL: www.dph.sf.ca.us/chn/sfgh/default.asp
Ownership: Government - Local — Accredited: Yes
Emergency Services: Yes — Licensed Beds: 639

Key Personnel:
President/CEO . . . . Gene O'Connell
Administrator . . . . Anthony G Wagner
Chief Medical Staff . . . . Valerie Ng, MD
Chief Emergency Services . . . . Alan Gelb, MD
Emergency Room . . . . Alan Gelb, MD
Director Infection/Disease Control . . . . Henry Chambers, MD
CCU Spvg. Nurse . . . . Rita Smith, RN
OB/GYN Womens Health . . . . Philip Darney, MD
Chief Radiology . . . . Mike Gotway, MD

Measure	Cases	This Hospital	State Average	U.S. Average	Top Hospital
Heart Attack Care					
ACE Inhibitor or ARB for LVSD[1]	16	88%	82%	82%	100%
Aspirin at Arrival	101	100%	95%	92%	100%
Aspirin at Discharge	67	99%	90%	90%	100%
Beta Blocker at Arrival	87	100%	89%	87%	100%
Beta Blocker at Discharge	63	100%	89%	90%	100%
Fibrinolytic Medication Timing[1]	1	0%	40%	31%	100%
PCI Within 90 Minutes of Arrival[1]	4	0%	52%	54%	95%
Smoking Cessation Advice	26	73%	87%	88%	100%
Heart Failure Care					
ACE Inhibitor or ARB for LVSD[2]	200	96%	84%	82%	100%
Discharge Instructions[2]	280	41%	56%	61%	93%
Evaluation of LVS Function[2]	294	99%	84%	83%	99%
Smoking Cessation Advice[2]	122	90%	82%	82%	100%
Pneumonia Care					
Appropriate Initial Antibiotic[2]	174	86%	82%	83%	94%
Blood Culture Timing[2]	176	79%	89%	90%	100%
Influenza Vaccine[2]	26	35%	58%	70%	100%
Initial Antibiotic Timing[2]	244	50%	75%	80%	93%
Oxygenation Assessment[2]	271	100%	99%	99%	100%
Pneumococcal Vaccine[2]	62	68%	58%	69%	94%
Smoking Cessation Advice[2]	128	81%	75%	80%	100%
Surgical Infection Prevention					
Prophylactic Antibiotic Given[2,3]	121	87%	74%	77%	95%
Prophylactic Antibiotic Selection[2]	36	64%	89%	90%	100%
Prophylactic Antibiotic Stopped[2,3]	113	77%	65%	72%	95%
Pregnancy Care					
Inpatient Neonatal Mortality	-	-	-	-	-
Third or Fourth Degree Laceration	-	-	3.58%	3.63%	3.27%

UCSF Medical Center

Alternate Name: University of California SF Medical Center
500 Parnassus Avenue — Toll-Free: 888-689-8273
San Francisco, CA 94143 — Phone: 415-476-1000
E-mail: referral.center@ucsfmedicalcenter.org
URL: www.ucsfhealth.org
Ownership: Voluntary non-profit - Other — Accredited: Yes
Emergency Services: Yes — Licensed Beds: 688

Key Personnel:
CEO . . . . Mark Laret
Chief Medical Staff . . . . Ronald Miller, MD
Cardiac Lab . . . . William Grossman
Emergency Room . . . . Michael Callaham, MD
Emergency Room . . . . Ellen Weber, MD
Infection Control . . . . Amy Nichols, MD
ICU . . . . Michael Gropper, MD
Medical Surgical Nursing . . . . Catherine Wittenberg, RN
OB/GYN/Women's Health . . . . Eugene Washington, MD
Manager Respiratory Therapy . . . . Julio Barba

Measure	Cases	This Hospital	State Average	U.S. Average	Top Hospital
Heart Attack Care					
ACE Inhibitor or ARB for LVSD[1,2]	18	72%	82%	82%	100%
Aspirin at Arrival[2]	138	99%	95%	92%	100%
Aspirin at Discharge[2]	149	99%	90%	90%	100%
Beta Blocker at Arrival[2]	96	96%	89%	87%	100%
Beta Blocker at Discharge[2]	158	98%	89%	90%	100%
Fibrinolytic Medication Timing[2]	0	-	40%	31%	100%
PCI Within 90 Minutes of Arrival[1,2]	4	50%	52%	54%	95%
Smoking Cessation Advice[2]	34	85%	87%	88%	100%
Heart Failure Care					
ACE Inhibitor or ARB for LVSD[2]	136	82%	84%	82%	100%
Discharge Instructions[2]	292	63%	56%	61%	93%
Evaluation of LVS Function[2]	318	99%	84%	83%	99%
Smoking Cessation Advice[2]	59	69%	82%	82%	100%
Pneumonia Care					
Appropriate Initial Antibiotic[2]	94	94%	82%	83%	94%
Blood Culture Timing[2]	141	90%	89%	90%	100%
Influenza Vaccine[2]	29	52%	58%	70%	100%
Initial Antibiotic Timing[2]	153	65%	75%	80%	93%
Oxygenation Assessment[2]	208	100%	99%	99%	100%
Pneumococcal Vaccine[2]	106	81%	58%	69%	94%
Smoking Cessation Advice[2]	39	82%	75%	80%	100%
Surgical Infection Prevention					
Prophylactic Antibiotic Given[2]	533	83%	74%	77%	95%
Prophylactic Antibiotic Selection[2]	81	99%	89%	90%	100%
Prophylactic Antibiotic Stopped[2]	466	86%	65%	72%	95%
Pregnancy Care					
Inpatient Neonatal Mortality	-	-	-	-	-
Third or Fourth Degree Laceration	-	-	3.58%	3.63%	3.27%

San Gabriel Valley Medical Center

Alternate Name: Community Hospital of San Gabriel
438 W Las Tunas Drive — Phone: 626-289-5454
San Gabriel, CA 91778 — Fax: 626-570-6555
URL: www.sangabrielvalleymedctr.org
Ownership: Voluntary non-profit - Other — Accredited: Yes
Emergency Services: Yes — Licensed Beds: 274

Key Personnel:
President . . . . Makato Nakayama
Chief Medical Staff . . . . Sergio Blesa, MD
Cardiac Lab . . . . Delia DelAngel
Emergency Room . . . . Janice Skiver
Emergency Room . . . . Geri Woessner, RN
Infection Control . . . . Susan Feliciano
OB/GYN Womens Health . . . . Dominique Doan, MD
Chief Radiology . . . . A Franklin Turner, MD
Director Respiratory Therapy . . . . Dee Del Angel

Measure	Cases	This Hospital	State Average	U.S. Average	Top Hospital
Heart Attack Care					
ACE Inhibitor or ARB for LVSD[1]	19	95%	82%	82%	100%
Aspirin at Arrival	88	98%	95%	92%	100%
Aspirin at Discharge	56	89%	90%	90%	100%

NOTE: Hospital profiles are in alphabetical order by state, then city, then hospital within the city; Rankings are sorted by rate in descending order and exclude hospitals with less than 25 cases; (1) The number of cases is too small (n<25) for purposes of reliably predicting hospital performance; (2) Measure reflects the hospital's indication that its submission was based upon a sample of its relevant discharges; (3) Rate reflects fewer than the maximum possible quarters of data for the measure; (4) Inaccurate information submitted and suppressed for one or more quarters; (5) No data is available from the hospital for this measure; Please refer to the User's Guide for a full explanation of data

Beta Blocker at Arrival	66	95%	89%	87%	100%
Beta Blocker at Discharge	49	98%	89%	90%	100%
Fibrinolytic Medication Timing[1]	2	0%	40%	31%	100%
PCI Within 90 Minutes of Arrival[1]	4	25%	52%	54%	95%
Smoking Cessation Advice[1]	7	86%	87%	88%	100%
Heart Failure Care					
ACE Inhibitor or ARB for LVSD	79	87%	84%	82%	100%
Discharge Instructions	188	73%	56%	61%	93%
Evaluation of LVS Function	272	94%	84%	83%	99%
Smoking Cessation Advice	36	94%	82%	82%	100%
Pneumonia Care					
Appropriate Initial Antibiotic	200	82%	82%	83%	94%
Blood Culture Timing	242	90%	89%	90%	100%
Influenza Vaccine	85	44%	58%	70%	100%
Initial Antibiotic Timing	398	78%	75%	80%	93%
Oxygenation Assessment	444	100%	99%	99%	100%
Pneumococcal Vaccine	327	68%	58%	69%	94%
Smoking Cessation Advice	39	95%	75%	80%	100%
Surgical Infection Prevention					
Prophylactic Antibiotic Given[2,3]	127	59%	74%	77%	95%
Prophylactic Antibiotic Selection[2]	34	82%	89%	90%	100%
Prophylactic Antibiotic Stopped[2,3]	126	40%	65%	72%	95%
Pregnancy Care					
Inpatient Neonatal Mortality	2,142	0.33%	-	-	-
Third or Fourth Degree Laceration	1,308	1.45%	3.58%	3.63%	3.27%

Good Samaritan Hospital

2425 Samaritan Drive
San Jose, CA 95124

Toll-Free: 800-265-8624
Phone: 408-559-2011
Fax: 408-559-2662

URL: www.goodsamsj.org
Ownership: Proprietary
Emergency Services: Yes

Accredited: Yes
Licensed Beds: 422

Key Personnel:
CEO. . . . . William Piche

Measure	Cases	This Hospital	State Average	U.S. Average	Top Hospital
Heart Attack Care					
ACE Inhibitor or ARB for LVSD	56	93%	82%	82%	100%
Aspirin at Arrival	166	99%	95%	92%	100%
Aspirin at Discharge	638	99%	90%	90%	100%
Beta Blocker at Arrival	131	98%	89%	87%	100%
Beta Blocker at Discharge	625	99%	89%	90%	100%
Fibrinolytic Medication Timing[1]	1	0%	40%	31%	100%
PCI Within 90 Minutes of Arrival[1]	6	50%	52%	54%	95%
Smoking Cessation Advice	133	99%	87%	88%	100%
Heart Failure Care					
ACE Inhibitor or ARB for LVSD	113	60%	84%	82%	100%
Discharge Instructions	273	67%	56%	61%	93%
Evaluation of LVS Function	368	91%	84%	83%	99%
Smoking Cessation Advice	29	86%	82%	82%	100%
Pneumonia Care					
Appropriate Initial Antibiotic	227	87%	82%	83%	94%
Blood Culture Timing	215	89%	89%	90%	100%
Influenza Vaccine	71	59%	58%	70%	100%
Initial Antibiotic Timing	253	72%	75%	80%	93%
Oxygenation Assessment	322	100%	99%	99%	100%
Pneumococcal Vaccine	237	46%	58%	69%	94%
Smoking Cessation Advice	42	79%	75%	80%	100%
Surgical Infection Prevention					
Prophylactic Antibiotic Given[2,3]	274	84%	74%	77%	95%
Prophylactic Antibiotic Selection[2]	129	60%	89%	90%	100%
Prophylactic Antibiotic Stopped[2,3]	259	70%	65%	72%	95%
Pregnancy Care					
Inpatient Neonatal Mortality	-	-	-	-	-
Third or Fourth Degree Laceration	-	-	3.58%	3.63%	3.27%

Kaiser Permanente Santa Teresa Comm Med Ctr

250 Hospital Parkway
San Jose, CA 95119

Toll-Free: 800-967-4677
Phone: 408-972-7000
Fax: 888-805-7562

Ownership: Voluntary non-profit - Private
Emergency Services: Yes

Accredited: Yes
Licensed Beds: 228

Key Personnel:
CEO. . . . . George Ajlverson
Chief Physician . . . . Raj Bhandari, MD
Director Emergency Department . . . . Robin Parsons, RN

Measure	Cases	This Hospital	State Average	U.S. Average	Top Hospital
Heart Attack Care					
ACE Inhibitor or ARB for LVSD	28	93%	82%	82%	100%
Aspirin at Arrival	204	99%	95%	92%	100%
Aspirin at Discharge	120	99%	90%	90%	100%
Beta Blocker at Arrival	171	98%	89%	87%	100%
Beta Blocker at Discharge	135	100%	89%	90%	100%
Fibrinolytic Medication Timing[1]	4	50%	40%	31%	100%
PCI Within 90 Minutes of Arrival[1]	10	70%	52%	54%	95%
Smoking Cessation Advice	39	100%	87%	88%	100%
Heart Failure Care					
ACE Inhibitor or ARB for LVSD	138	90%	84%	82%	100%
Discharge Instructions	346	76%	56%	61%	93%
Evaluation of LVS Function	373	99%	84%	83%	99%
Smoking Cessation Advice	49	100%	82%	82%	100%
Pneumonia Care					
Appropriate Initial Antibiotic	105	90%	82%	83%	94%
Blood Culture Timing	101	92%	89%	90%	100%
Influenza Vaccine	28	57%	58%	70%	100%
Initial Antibiotic Timing	130	72%	75%	80%	93%
Oxygenation Assessment	160	100%	99%	99%	100%
Pneumococcal Vaccine	111	78%	58%	69%	94%
Smoking Cessation Advice[1]	15	100%	75%	80%	100%
Surgical Infection Prevention					
Prophylactic Antibiotic Given	197	41%	74%	77%	95%
Prophylactic Antibiotic Selection	49	76%	89%	90%	100%
Prophylactic Antibiotic Stopped	183	74%	65%	72%	95%
Pregnancy Care					
Inpatient Neonatal Mortality[2]	510	0.00%	-	-	-
Third or Fourth Degree Laceration[2]	382	4.19%	3.58%	3.63%	3.27%

O'Connor Hospital

2105 Forest Avenue
San Jose, CA 95128
URL: www.oconnorhospital.org
Ownership: Voluntary non-profit - Church
Emergency Services: Yes

Phone: 408-947-2500
Fax: 408-283-7778

Accredited: Yes
Licensed Beds: 358

Key Personnel:
President/CEO. . . . . Rob Curry
Chief Medical Staff. . . . . Howard Davis
Medical Director ER . . . . Sami Jadallah, MD
Director Infection/Disease Control . . . . Rosalie Sheveland

Measure	Cases	This Hospital	State Average	U.S. Average	Top Hospital
Heart Attack Care					
ACE Inhibitor or ARB for LVSD	32	97%	82%	82%	100%
Aspirin at Arrival	149	98%	95%	92%	100%
Aspirin at Discharge	151	97%	90%	90%	100%
Beta Blocker at Arrival	119	96%	89%	87%	100%
Beta Blocker at Discharge	142	95%	89%	90%	100%
Fibrinolytic Medication Timing	0	-	40%	31%	100%
PCI Within 90 Minutes of Arrival[1]	4	25%	52%	54%	95%
Smoking Cessation Advice	35	91%	87%	88%	100%
Heart Failure Care					
ACE Inhibitor or ARB for LVSD	123	95%	84%	82%	100%
Discharge Instructions	378	54%	56%	61%	93%
Evaluation of LVS Function	471	88%	84%	83%	99%
Smoking Cessation Advice	29	69%	82%	82%	100%
Pneumonia Care					
Appropriate Initial Antibiotic	176	88%	82%	83%	94%
Blood Culture Timing	184	92%	89%	90%	100%

NOTE: Hospital profiles are in alphabetical order by state, then city, then hospital within the city; Rankings are sorted by rate in descending order and exclude hospitals with less than 25 cases; (1) The number of cases is too small (n<25) for purposes of reliably predicting hospital performance; (2) Measure reflects the hospital's indication that its submission was based upon a sample of its relevant discharges; (3) Rate reflects fewer than the maximum possible quarters of data for the measure; (4) Inaccurate information submitted and suppressed for one or more quarters; (5) No data is available from the hospital for this measure; Please refer to the User's Guide for a full explanation of data

Measure	Cases	This Hospital	State Average	U.S. Average	Top Hospital
Influenza Vaccine	54	69%	58%	70%	100%
Initial Antibiotic Timing	238	78%	75%	80%	93%
Oxygenation Assessment	313	100%	99%	99%	100%
Pneumococcal Vaccine	236	64%	58%	69%	94%
Smoking Cessation Advice	31	52%	75%	80%	100%
Surgical Infection Prevention					
Prophylactic Antibiotic Given[2,3]	186	89%	74%	77%	95%
Prophylactic Antibiotic Selection[2]	65	95%	89%	90%	100%
Prophylactic Antibiotic Stopped[2,3]	186	80%	65%	72%	95%
Pregnancy Care					
Inpatient Neonatal Mortality	-	-	-	-	-
Third or Fourth Degree Laceration	-	-	3.58%	3.63%	3.27%

Regional Medical Center of San Jose

Alternate Name: Alexian Brothers Hospital
225 N Jackson Avenue — Phone: 408-259-5000
San Jose, CA 95116 — Fax: 408-729-2884
URL: www.regionalmedicalsanjose.com
Ownership: Voluntary non-profit - Church — Accredited: Yes
Emergency Services: Yes — Licensed Beds: 204
Key Personnel:
CEO. . . . . William L Gilbert

Measure	Cases	This Hospital	State Average	U.S. Average	Top Hospital
Heart Attack Care					
ACE Inhibitor or ARB for LVSD[1]	23	87%	82%	82%	100%
Aspirin at Arrival	169	94%	95%	92%	100%
Aspirin at Discharge	138	92%	90%	90%	100%
Beta Blocker at Arrival	89	93%	89%	87%	100%
Beta Blocker at Discharge	124	94%	89%	90%	100%
Fibrinolytic Medication Timing[1]	4	25%	40%	31%	100%
PCI Within 90 Minutes of Arrival[1]	14	36%	52%	54%	95%
Smoking Cessation Advice	36	97%	87%	88%	100%
Heart Failure Care					
ACE Inhibitor or ARB for LVSD	113	92%	84%	82%	100%
Discharge Instructions	353	33%	56%	61%	93%
Evaluation of LVS Function	429	77%	84%	83%	99%
Smoking Cessation Advice	54	81%	82%	82%	100%
Pneumonia Care					
Appropriate Initial Antibiotic[2]	292	86%	82%	83%	94%
Blood Culture Timing[2]	346	95%	89%	90%	100%
Influenza Vaccine	100	45%	58%	70%	100%
Initial Antibiotic Timing[2]	417	76%	75%	80%	93%
Oxygenation Assessment[2]	483	100%	99%	99%	100%
Pneumococcal Vaccine[2]	349	28%	58%	69%	94%
Smoking Cessation Advice[2]	53	55%	75%	80%	100%
Surgical Infection Prevention					
Prophylactic Antibiotic Given[2,3]	127	76%	74%	77%	95%
Prophylactic Antibiotic Selection[2]	56	82%	89%	90%	100%
Prophylactic Antibiotic Stopped[2,3]	114	61%	65%	72%	95%
Pregnancy Care					
Inpatient Neonatal Mortality	-	-	-	-	-
Third or Fourth Degree Laceration	-	-	3.58%	3.63%	3.27%

Santa Clara Valley Medical Center

751 S Bascom Avenue — Phone: 408-885-5000
San Jose, CA 95128 — Fax: 408-885-6459
URL: www.scvmed.org
Ownership: Government - Local — Accredited: Yes
Emergency Services: Yes — Licensed Beds: 524

Measure	Cases	This Hospital	State Average	U.S. Average	Top Hospital
Heart Attack Care					
ACE Inhibitor or ARB for LVSD[1]	14	79%	82%	82%	100%
Aspirin at Arrival	131	98%	95%	92%	100%
Aspirin at Discharge	134	95%	90%	90%	100%
Beta Blocker at Arrival	122	91%	89%	87%	100%
Beta Blocker at Discharge	137	95%	89%	90%	100%
Fibrinolytic Medication Timing[1]	1	0%	40%	31%	100%
PCI Within 90 Minutes of Arrival[1]	9	67%	52%	54%	95%
Smoking Cessation Advice	50	80%	87%	88%	100%
Heart Failure Care					
ACE Inhibitor or ARB for LVSD	172	69%	84%	82%	100%
Discharge Instructions	308	40%	56%	61%	93%
Evaluation of LVS Function	329	96%	84%	83%	99%
Smoking Cessation Advice	112	77%	82%	82%	100%
Pneumonia Care					
Appropriate Initial Antibiotic	245	69%	82%	83%	94%
Blood Culture Timing	201	79%	89%	90%	100%
Influenza Vaccine[4,5]	-	-	58%	70%	100%
Initial Antibiotic Timing	217	56%	75%	80%	93%
Oxygenation Assessment	337	99%	99%	99%	100%
Pneumococcal Vaccine	138	18%	58%	69%	94%
Smoking Cessation Advice	122	47%	75%	80%	100%
Surgical Infection Prevention					
Prophylactic Antibiotic Given	422	85%	74%	77%	95%
Prophylactic Antibiotic Selection	101	72%	89%	90%	100%
Prophylactic Antibiotic Stopped	410	86%	65%	72%	95%
Pregnancy Care					
Inpatient Neonatal Mortality	6,066	0.43%	-	-	-
Third or Fourth Degree Laceration	4,627	3.85%	3.58%	3.63%	3.27%

San Leandro Hospital

Alternate Name: Eden Medical Center
13855 E 14th Street — Phone: 510-357-6500
San Leandro, CA 94578 — Fax: 510-667-4572
URL: www.edenmedcenter.org
Ownership: Proprietary — Accredited: Yes
Emergency Services: Yes — Licensed Beds: 122
Key Personnel:
Chief Medical Staff. . . . . Merrill Chandler, MD
Director Medical/Surgical Nursing . . . . Rose Del Rosario
Director Medical/Surgical Nursing . . . . Karren Lemelin
Chief Radiology . . . . Malcolm McKinn, MD
Director Respiratory Therapy . . . . Tim Winn

Measure	Cases	This Hospital	State Average	U.S. Average	Top Hospital
Heart Attack Care					
ACE Inhibitor or ARB for LVSD[1]	8	88%	82%	82%	100%
Aspirin at Arrival	49	98%	95%	92%	100%
Aspirin at Discharge	32	97%	90%	90%	100%
Beta Blocker at Arrival	28	100%	89%	87%	100%
Beta Blocker at Discharge	39	95%	89%	90%	100%
Fibrinolytic Medication Timing[1]	1	0%	40%	31%	100%
PCI Within 90 Minutes of Arrival	0	-	52%	54%	95%
Smoking Cessation Advice[1]	5	100%	87%	88%	100%
Heart Failure Care					
ACE Inhibitor or ARB for LVSD	102	87%	84%	82%	100%
Discharge Instructions	319	62%	56%	61%	93%
Evaluation of LVS Function	370	89%	84%	83%	99%
Smoking Cessation Advice	86	100%	82%	82%	100%
Pneumonia Care					
Appropriate Initial Antibiotic	114	94%	82%	83%	94%
Blood Culture Timing	111	92%	89%	90%	100%
Influenza Vaccine	32	69%	58%	70%	100%
Initial Antibiotic Timing	163	74%	75%	80%	93%
Oxygenation Assessment	193	100%	99%	99%	100%
Pneumococcal Vaccine	132	77%	58%	69%	94%
Smoking Cessation Advice	36	94%	75%	80%	100%
Surgical Infection Prevention					
Prophylactic Antibiotic Given[2]	196	86%	74%	77%	95%
Prophylactic Antibiotic Selection[2]	35	100%	89%	90%	100%
Prophylactic Antibiotic Stopped[2]	184	75%	65%	72%	95%
Pregnancy Care					
Inpatient Neonatal Mortality	-	-	-	-	-
Third or Fourth Degree Laceration	-	-	3.58%	3.63%	3.27%

French Hospital Medical Center

Alternate Name: French Hospital-San Luis Obispo

NOTE: Hospital profiles are in alphabetical order by state, then city, then hospital within the city; Rankings are sorted by rate in descending order and exclude hospitals with less than 25 cases; (1) The number of cases is too small (n<25) for purposes of reliably predicting hospital performance; (2) Measure reflects the hospital's indication that its submission was based upon a sample of its relevant discharges; (3) Rate reflects fewer than the maximum possible quarters of data for the measure; (4) Inaccurate information submitted and suppressed for one or more quarters; (5) No data is available from the hospital for this measure; Please refer to the User's Guide for a full explanation of data

1911 Johnson Avenue Phone: 805-543-5353
San Luis Obispo, CA 93401
URL: www.frenchmedicalcenter.org
Ownership: Voluntary non-profit - Other Accredited: Yes
Emergency Services: Yes Licensed Beds: 112
Key Personnel:
President . . . . Alan E Atiniuk
Chief of Medical Staff . . . . Mark Soll, MD
Cardiac Lab . . . . Charlie Tagawa
Emergency Room . . . . Dan Culhane, MD
Emergency Room . . . . Shara Smith
Infection Control . . . . Vicki Warnock
ICU . . . . Jacque Taylor
Medical Surgical Nursing . . . . Rose Martin
OB/GYN . . . . Charlie Ault
Respiratory Therapy . . . . Barbara West

Measure	Cases	This Hospital	State Average	U.S. Average	Top Hospital
Heart Attack Care					
ACE Inhibitor or ARB for LVSD[1]	12	100%	82%	82%	100%
Aspirin at Arrival	47	100%	95%	92%	100%
Aspirin at Discharge	117	97%	90%	90%	100%
Beta Blocker at Arrival	42	100%	89%	87%	100%
Beta Blocker at Discharge	123	98%	89%	90%	100%
Fibrinolytic Medication Timing	0	-	40%	31%	100%
PCI Within 90 Minutes of Arrival	0	-	52%	54%	95%
Smoking Cessation Advice	35	100%	87%	88%	100%
Heart Failure Care					
ACE Inhibitor or ARB for LVSD	42	95%	84%	82%	100%
Discharge Instructions	110	96%	56%	61%	93%
Evaluation of LVS Function	131	96%	84%	83%	99%
Smoking Cessation Advice[1]	16	100%	82%	82%	100%
Pneumonia Care					
Appropriate Initial Antibiotic	103	88%	82%	83%	94%
Blood Culture Timing	91	97%	89%	90%	100%
Influenza Vaccine[1]	19	89%	58%	70%	100%
Initial Antibiotic Timing	109	94%	75%	80%	93%
Oxygenation Assessment	129	100%	99%	99%	100%
Pneumococcal Vaccine	98	89%	58%	69%	94%
Smoking Cessation Advice[1]	7	86%	75%	80%	100%
Surgical Infection Prevention					
Prophylactic Antibiotic Given[2,3]	224	86%	74%	77%	95%
Prophylactic Antibiotic Selection[2]	75	97%	89%	90%	100%
Prophylactic Antibiotic Stopped[2,3]	217	89%	65%	72%	95%
Pregnancy Care					
Inpatient Neonatal Mortality	-	-	-	-	-
Third or Fourth Degree Laceration	-	-	3.58%	3.63%	3.27%

Sierra Vista Regional Medical Center

1010 Murray Avenue Phone: 805-546-7600
PO Box 1367 Fax: 805-546-7892
San Luis Obispo, CA 93405
URL: www.sierravistaregional.com
Ownership: Proprietary Accredited: Yes
Emergency Services: Yes Licensed Beds: 201
Key Personnel:
CEO/President . . . . Candy Markwith
Chief Medical Staff . . . . Patrick Vaughn, MD
Emergency Room . . . . Tauny Sexton
Director of Pulmonary/Respiratory Care . . . . Glenn Knowles

Measure	Cases	This Hospital	State Average	U.S. Average	Top Hospital
Heart Attack Care					
ACE Inhibitor or ARB for LVSD[1]	20	95%	82%	82%	100%
Aspirin at Arrival	60	97%	95%	92%	100%
Aspirin at Discharge	100	96%	90%	90%	100%
Beta Blocker at Arrival	53	98%	89%	87%	100%
Beta Blocker at Discharge	94	95%	89%	90%	100%
Fibrinolytic Medication Timing[1]	1	0%	40%	31%	100%
PCI Within 90 Minutes of Arrival[1]	5	40%	52%	54%	95%
Smoking Cessation Advice	31	97%	87%	88%	100%
Heart Failure Care					
ACE Inhibitor or ARB for LVSD	29	90%	84%	82%	100%
Discharge Instructions	64	91%	56%	61%	93%
Evaluation of LVS Function	78	91%	84%	83%	99%
Smoking Cessation Advice[1]	12	92%	82%	82%	100%
Pneumonia Care					
Appropriate Initial Antibiotic	85	85%	82%	83%	94%
Blood Culture Timing	79	96%	89%	90%	100%
Influenza Vaccine	26	85%	58%	70%	100%
Initial Antibiotic Timing	85	86%	75%	80%	93%
Oxygenation Assessment	124	100%	99%	99%	100%
Pneumococcal Vaccine	79	70%	58%	69%	94%
Smoking Cessation Advice[1]	19	84%	75%	80%	100%
Surgical Infection Prevention					
Prophylactic Antibiotic Given[2]	241	75%	74%	77%	95%
Prophylactic Antibiotic Selection[2]	57	98%	89%	90%	100%
Prophylactic Antibiotic Stopped[2]	232	71%	65%	72%	95%
Pregnancy Care					
Inpatient Neonatal Mortality	-	-	-	-	-
Third or Fourth Degree Laceration	-	-	3.58%	3.63%	3.27%

San Mateo Medical Center

222 W 39th Avenue Phone: 650-573-2222
San Mateo, CA 94403 Fax: 650-573-2950
URL: www.sanmateomedicalcenter.org
Ownership: Government - Local Accredited: Yes
Emergency Services: Yes Licensed Beds: 509
Key Personnel:
CEO . . . . Nancy Steiger
Chief Medical Staff . . . . Dr David Marcus, MD
Emergency Room . . . . Robert Spencer, MD
Infection Control . . . . Mary Webb
ICU/Intensive Coronary . . . . Jim Lonergan

Measure	Cases	This Hospital	State Average	U.S. Average	Top Hospital
Heart Attack Care					
ACE Inhibitor or ARB for LVSD	0	-	82%	82%	100%
Aspirin at Arrival[1]	16	100%	95%	92%	100%
Aspirin at Discharge[1]	6	100%	90%	90%	100%
Beta Blocker at Arrival[1]	16	100%	89%	87%	100%
Beta Blocker at Discharge[1]	9	100%	89%	90%	100%
Fibrinolytic Medication Timing	0	-	40%	31%	100%
PCI Within 90 Minutes of Arrival	0	-	52%	54%	95%
Smoking Cessation Advice[1]	4	100%	87%	88%	100%
Heart Failure Care					
ACE Inhibitor or ARB for LVSD	33	100%	84%	82%	100%
Discharge Instructions	59	100%	56%	61%	93%
Evaluation of LVS Function	68	100%	84%	83%	99%
Smoking Cessation Advice	28	100%	82%	82%	100%
Pneumonia Care					
Appropriate Initial Antibiotic	43	77%	82%	83%	94%
Blood Culture Timing	40	85%	89%	90%	100%
Influenza Vaccine[1]	9	89%	58%	70%	100%
Initial Antibiotic Timing	55	87%	75%	80%	93%
Oxygenation Assessment	66	100%	99%	99%	100%
Pneumococcal Vaccine	26	92%	58%	69%	94%
Smoking Cessation Advice[1]	12	100%	75%	80%	100%
Surgical Infection Prevention					
Prophylactic Antibiotic Given	92	85%	74%	77%	95%
Prophylactic Antibiotic Selection[1]	23	91%	89%	90%	100%
Prophylactic Antibiotic Stopped	90	79%	65%	72%	95%
Pregnancy Care					
Inpatient Neonatal Mortality	-	-	-	-	-
Third or Fourth Degree Laceration	-	-	3.58%	3.63%	3.27%

Doctor's Medical Center-San Pablo Campus

2000 vale Road Phone: 510-970-5000
San Pablo, CA 94806 Fax: 510-970-5730
URL: www.doctorsmedicalcenter.org
Ownership: Govt - Hospital District or Authority Accredited: Yes
Emergency Services: Yes Licensed Beds: 326
Key Personnel:
CEO . . . . Irwin Hansen
Chief Medical Staff . . . . Paul Ryan, MD
Catheterization Lab . . . . Christy Holt

NOTE: Hospital profiles are in alphabetical order by state, then city, then hospital within the city; Rankings are sorted by rate in descending order and exclude hospitals with less than 25 cases; (1) The number of cases is too small (n<25) for purposes of reliably predicting hospital performance; (2) Measure reflects the hospital's indication that its submission was based upon a sample of its relevant discharges; (3) Rate reflects fewer than the maximum possible quarters of data for the measure; (4) Inaccurate information submitted and suppressed for one or more quarters; (5) No data is available from the hospital for this measure; Please refer to the User's Guide for a full explanation of data

Emergency Room . . . . Susan Ancell, RN
Infection Control. . . . . Nayda Ramiro
ICU . . . . Ronica Shelton
Medical Surgical Nursing . . . . Martha Iwaihara

Measure	Cases	This Hospital	State Average	U.S. Average	Top Hospital
Heart Attack Care					
ACE Inhibitor or ARB for LVSD	63	78%	82%	82%	100%
Aspirin at Arrival	147	97%	95%	92%	100%
Aspirin at Discharge	171	99%	90%	90%	100%
Beta Blocker at Arrival	123	95%	89%	87%	100%
Beta Blocker at Discharge	160	94%	89%	90%	100%
Fibrinolytic Medication Timing[1]	2	0%	40%	31%	100%
PCI Within 90 Minutes of Arrival[1]	8	75%	52%	54%	95%
Smoking Cessation Advice	56	80%	87%	88%	100%
Heart Failure Care					
ACE Inhibitor or ARB for LVSD	213	78%	84%	82%	100%
Discharge Instructions	366	48%	56%	61%	93%
Evaluation of LVS Function	441	93%	84%	83%	99%
Smoking Cessation Advice	114	89%	82%	82%	100%
Pneumonia Care					
Appropriate Initial Antibiotic	205	90%	82%	83%	94%
Blood Culture Timing	224	96%	89%	90%	100%
Influenza Vaccine	65	43%	58%	70%	100%
Initial Antibiotic Timing	295	88%	75%	80%	93%
Oxygenation Assessment	344	100%	99%	99%	100%
Pneumococcal Vaccine	213	56%	58%	69%	94%
Smoking Cessation Advice	73	77%	75%	80%	100%
Surgical Infection Prevention					
Prophylactic Antibiotic Given	225	48%	74%	77%	95%
Prophylactic Antibiotic Selection	53	91%	89%	90%	100%
Prophylactic Antibiotic Stopped	216	54%	65%	72%	95%
Pregnancy Care					
Inpatient Neonatal Mortality	-	-	-	-	-
Third or Fourth Degree Laceration	-	-	3.58%	3.63%	3.27%

Little Company of Mary-San Pedro Hospital

1300 W 7th Street Phone: 310-832-3311
San Pedro, CA 90732 Fax: 310-514-5314
URL: www.lcmweb.org
Ownership: Voluntary non-profit - Private Accredited: Yes
Emergency Services: Yes Licensed Beds: 387

Key Personnel:

Administrator . . . . Nancy Carlson
Chief Medical Officer . . . . Laurence Eason, MD
Emergency Room . . . . Sameer Mistry
Emergency Room . . . . Miles Shaw, MD
OB/GYN Womens Health. . . . . Barry Tischler, MD
Chief Radiology . . . . Neil Chafetz, MD
Director Respiratory . . . . Henry Moreta

Measure	Cases	This Hospital	State Average	U.S. Average	Top Hospital
Heart Attack Care					
ACE Inhibitor or ARB for LVSD[1]	5	100%	82%	82%	100%
Aspirin at Arrival	47	98%	95%	92%	100%
Aspirin at Discharge	25	92%	90%	90%	100%
Beta Blocker at Arrival	36	97%	89%	87%	100%
Beta Blocker at Discharge	25	92%	89%	90%	100%
Fibrinolytic Medication Timing[1]	8	50%	40%	31%	100%
PCI Within 90 Minutes of Arrival	0	-	52%	54%	95%
Smoking Cessation Advice[1]	3	100%	87%	88%	100%
Heart Failure Care					
ACE Inhibitor or ARB for LVSD	50	90%	84%	82%	100%
Discharge Instructions	166	62%	56%	61%	93%
Evaluation of LVS Function	202	90%	84%	83%	99%
Smoking Cessation Advice[1]	20	95%	82%	82%	100%
Pneumonia Care					
Appropriate Initial Antibiotic	132	90%	82%	83%	94%
Blood Culture Timing	121	88%	89%	90%	100%
Influenza Vaccine	41	59%	58%	70%	100%
Initial Antibiotic Timing	174	87%	75%	80%	93%
Oxygenation Assessment	221	100%	99%	99%	100%
Pneumococcal Vaccine	142	65%	58%	69%	94%
Smoking Cessation Advice	33	97%	75%	80%	100%
Surgical Infection Prevention					
Prophylactic Antibiotic Given[2]	160	76%	74%	77%	95%
Prophylactic Antibiotic Selection[2]	40	95%	89%	90%	100%
Prophylactic Antibiotic Stopped[2]	149	37%	65%	72%	95%
Pregnancy Care					
Inpatient Neonatal Mortality	-	-	-	-	-
Third or Fourth Degree Laceration	-	-	3.58%	3.63%	3.27%

San Rafael Medical Center

99 Montecillo Road Phone: 415-444-2000
San Rafael, CA 94903 Fax: 415-444-2492
URL: www.kaisersanrafael.org
Ownership: Voluntary non-profit - Other Accredited: Yes
Emergency Services: Yes Licensed Beds: 120

Key Personnel:

President/CEO. . . . . Dan Leetz
Chief Medical Staff. . . . . James Martin
Head Emergency Room. . . . . Don Bennet
Director Medical/Surgical Nursing . . . . Carol Paz
OB/GYN Womens Health. . . . . Mark Glasser
Chief Radiology . . . . Gordon Manashil, MD
Director Respiratory Therapy . . . . Elizabeth Miller

Measure	Cases	This Hospital	State Average	U.S. Average	Top Hospital
Heart Attack Care					
ACE Inhibitor or ARB for LVSD[1]	10	90%	82%	82%	100%
Aspirin at Arrival	82	99%	95%	92%	100%
Aspirin at Discharge	45	93%	90%	90%	100%
Beta Blocker at Arrival	76	99%	89%	87%	100%
Beta Blocker at Discharge	56	100%	89%	90%	100%
Fibrinolytic Medication Timing[1]	6	67%	40%	31%	100%
PCI Within 90 Minutes of Arrival[1]	5	40%	52%	54%	95%
Smoking Cessation Advice[1]	9	100%	87%	88%	100%
Heart Failure Care					
ACE Inhibitor or ARB for LVSD	49	98%	84%	82%	100%
Discharge Instructions	156	75%	56%	61%	93%
Evaluation of LVS Function	173	97%	84%	83%	99%
Smoking Cessation Advice[1]	11	82%	82%	82%	100%
Pneumonia Care					
Appropriate Initial Antibiotic	135	97%	82%	83%	94%
Blood Culture Timing	169	91%	89%	90%	100%
Influenza Vaccine	61	92%	58%	70%	100%
Initial Antibiotic Timing	210	82%	75%	80%	93%
Oxygenation Assessment	249	100%	99%	99%	100%
Pneumococcal Vaccine	189	96%	58%	69%	94%
Smoking Cessation Advice	38	89%	75%	80%	100%
Surgical Infection Prevention					
Prophylactic Antibiotic Given	522	85%	74%	77%	95%
Prophylactic Antibiotic Selection	131	95%	89%	90%	100%
Prophylactic Antibiotic Stopped	519	82%	65%	72%	95%
Pregnancy Care					
Inpatient Neonatal Mortality	-	-	-	-	-
Third or Fourth Degree Laceration	-	-	3.58%	3.63%	3.27%

San Ramon Regional Medical Center

6001 Norris Canyon Road Phone: 925-275-9200
San Ramon, CA 94583 Fax: 925-275-0107
URL: www.sanramonmedCentercom
Ownership: Proprietary Accredited: Yes
Emergency Services: Yes Licensed Beds: 150

Key Personnel:

CEO. . . . . Gary Sloan
Supervisor Cardiology . . . . Candy Hogan
Director Emergency Room. . . . . Kathy Kelly
Manager Respiratory Care. . . . . Joyce Wilson

Measure	Cases	This Hospital	State Average	U.S. Average	Top Hospital
Heart Attack Care					
ACE Inhibitor or ARB for LVSD[1]	6	50%	82%	82%	100%
Aspirin at Arrival	60	98%	95%	92%	100%
Aspirin at Discharge	60	95%	90%	90%	100%

NOTE: Hospital profiles are in alphabetical order by state, then city, then hospital within the city; Rankings are sorted by rate in descending order and exclude hospitals with less than 25 cases; (1) The number of cases is too small (n<25) for purposes of reliably predicting hospital performance; (2) Measure reflects the hospital's indication that its submission was based upon a sample of its relevant discharges; (3) Rate reflects fewer than the maximum possible quarters of data for the measure; (4) Inaccurate information submitted and suppressed for one or more quarters; (5) No data is available from the hospital for this measure; Please refer to the User's Guide for a full explanation of data

Beta Blocker at Arrival	58	98%	89%	87%	100%
Beta Blocker at Discharge	55	91%	89%	90%	100%
Fibrinolytic Medication Timing	0	-	40%	31%	100%
PCI Within 90 Minutes of Arrival[1]	5	80%	52%	54%	95%
Smoking Cessation Advice[1]	16	100%	87%	88%	100%
Heart Failure Care					
ACE Inhibitor or ARB for LVSD	33	88%	84%	82%	100%
Discharge Instructions	80	82%	56%	61%	93%
Evaluation of LVS Function	106	97%	84%	83%	99%
Smoking Cessation Advice[1]	8	100%	82%	82%	100%
Pneumonia Care					
Appropriate Initial Antibiotic	118	97%	82%	83%	94%
Blood Culture Timing	54	98%	89%	90%	100%
Influenza Vaccine	35	77%	58%	70%	100%
Initial Antibiotic Timing	115	89%	75%	80%	93%
Oxygenation Assessment	143	100%	99%	99%	100%
Pneumococcal Vaccine	112	95%	58%	69%	94%
Smoking Cessation Advice[1]	17	82%	75%	80%	100%
Surgical Infection Prevention					
Prophylactic Antibiotic Given[2]	325	88%	74%	77%	95%
Prophylactic Antibiotic Selection[2]	79	100%	89%	90%	100%
Prophylactic Antibiotic Stopped[2]	313	52%	65%	72%	95%
Pregnancy Care					
Inpatient Neonatal Mortality	-	-	-	-	-
Third or Fourth Degree Laceration	-	-	3.58%	3.63%	3.27%

Coastal Communities Hospital

2701 S Bristol Street
Santa Ana, CA 92704
Phone: 714-754-5454
URL: www.coastalcommhospital.com
Ownership: Proprietary
Accredited: Yes
Emergency Services: Yes
Licensed Beds: 178

Key Personnel:

Administrator/CEO . . . . Craig Myers
Chief Medical Staff . . . . Michael Seim, MD
Emergency Room . . . . Carol Frank
Infection Control Director . . . . Victor Lange
Head Cardiology . . . . Viane Coy
Nurse Director Surgical Services . . . . Lisa Momna
Head of Respiratory . . . . Scott Stimke

Measure	Cases	This Hospital	State Average	U.S. Average	Top Hospital
Heart Attack Care					
ACE Inhibitor or ARB for LVSD[1]	3	33%	82%	82%	100%
Aspirin at Arrival[1]	21	95%	95%	92%	100%
Aspirin at Discharge[1]	13	85%	90%	90%	100%
Beta Blocker at Arrival[1]	20	90%	89%	87%	100%
Beta Blocker at Discharge[1]	13	92%	89%	90%	100%
Fibrinolytic Medication Timing[1]	4	75%	40%	31%	100%
PCI Within 90 Minutes of Arrival	0	-	52%	54%	95%
Smoking Cessation Advice[1]	4	100%	87%	88%	100%
Heart Failure Care					
ACE Inhibitor or ARB for LVSD[1]	17	65%	84%	82%	100%
Discharge Instructions	54	24%	56%	61%	93%
Evaluation of LVS Function	65	85%	84%	83%	99%
Smoking Cessation Advice[1]	4	25%	82%	82%	100%
Pneumonia Care					
Appropriate Initial Antibiotic	50	64%	82%	83%	94%
Blood Culture Timing	113	87%	89%	90%	100%
Influenza Vaccine[4,5]	-	-	58%	70%	100%
Initial Antibiotic Timing	105	87%	75%	80%	93%
Oxygenation Assessment	142	100%	99%	99%	100%
Pneumococcal Vaccine	69	43%	58%	69%	94%
Smoking Cessation Advice[1]	9	89%	75%	80%	100%
Surgical Infection Prevention					
Prophylactic Antibiotic Given	101	79%	74%	77%	95%
Prophylactic Antibiotic Selection	26	96%	89%	90%	100%
Prophylactic Antibiotic Stopped	99	69%	65%	72%	95%
Pregnancy Care					
Inpatient Neonatal Mortality	-	-	-	-	-
Third or Fourth Degree Laceration	-	-	3.58%	3.63%	3.27%

Western Medical Center

Alternate Name: Santa Ana Tustin Community Hospital
1001 N Tustin Avenue
Phone: 714-953-3500
Santa Ana, CA 92705
Fax: 714-953-3613
URL: www.westernmedicalcenter.com
Ownership: Proprietary
Accredited: Yes
Emergency Services: Yes
Licensed Beds: 280

Key Personnel:

CEO . . . . Daniel Brothman
Chief Medical Staff . . . . David Stanton, MD
Emergency Room . . . . S Jones, RN
Director Medical/Surgical Nursing . . . . Debra Bourgette
OB/GYN Womens Health . . . . Thinakorn Shennavasin
Chief Radiology . . . . Joseph Brogman, MD

Measure	Cases	This Hospital	State Average	U.S. Average	Top Hospital
Heart Attack Care					
ACE Inhibitor or ARB for LVSD	26	96%	82%	82%	100%
Aspirin at Arrival	86	100%	95%	92%	100%
Aspirin at Discharge	176	99%	90%	90%	100%
Beta Blocker at Arrival	79	96%	89%	87%	100%
Beta Blocker at Discharge	170	98%	89%	90%	100%
Fibrinolytic Medication Timing	0	-	40%	31%	100%
PCI Within 90 Minutes of Arrival[1]	6	67%	52%	54%	95%
Smoking Cessation Advice	47	79%	87%	88%	100%
Heart Failure Care					
ACE Inhibitor or ARB for LVSD	101	93%	84%	82%	100%
Discharge Instructions	222	64%	56%	61%	93%
Evaluation of LVS Function	283	84%	84%	83%	99%
Smoking Cessation Advice	47	64%	82%	82%	100%
Pneumonia Care					
Appropriate Initial Antibiotic	101	82%	82%	83%	94%
Blood Culture Timing	89	89%	89%	90%	100%
Influenza Vaccine	29	62%	58%	70%	100%
Initial Antibiotic Timing	129	84%	75%	80%	93%
Oxygenation Assessment	168	99%	99%	99%	100%
Pneumococcal Vaccine	111	59%	58%	69%	94%
Smoking Cessation Advice[1]	18	44%	75%	80%	100%
Surgical Infection Prevention					
Prophylactic Antibiotic Given[3]	33	70%	74%	77%	95%
Prophylactic Antibiotic Selection	34	65%	89%	90%	100%
Prophylactic Antibiotic Stopped[3]	32	56%	65%	72%	95%
Pregnancy Care					
Inpatient Neonatal Mortality	-	-	-	-	-
Third or Fourth Degree Laceration	-	-	3.58%	3.63%	3.27%

Goleta Valley Cottage Hospital

Alternate Name: Goleta Valley Community Hospital
351 S Patterson Avenue
Phone: 805-967-3411
Santa Barbara, CA 93111
Fax: 805-681-6437
URL: www.sbch.org
Ownership: Voluntary non-profit - Other
Accredited: Yes
Emergency Services: Yes
Licensed Beds: 122

Key Personnel:

Emergency Room . . . . Leslie Houston
Respiratory Therapy . . . . Jeff Alan

Measure	Cases	This Hospital	State Average	U.S. Average	Top Hospital
Heart Attack Care					
ACE Inhibitor or ARB for LVSD[3]	0	-	82%	82%	100%
Aspirin at Arrival[1,3]	3	100%	95%	92%	100%
Aspirin at Discharge[1,3]	1	100%	90%	90%	100%
Beta Blocker at Arrival[1,3]	3	100%	89%	87%	100%
Beta Blocker at Discharge[1,3]	1	100%	89%	90%	100%
Fibrinolytic Medication Timing[3]	0	-	40%	31%	100%
PCI Within 90 Minutes of Arrival	0	-	52%	54%	95%
Smoking Cessation Advice[3]	0	-	87%	88%	100%
Heart Failure Care					
ACE Inhibitor or ARB for LVSD[1]	5	80%	84%	82%	100%
Discharge Instructions[1]	19	42%	56%	61%	93%
Evaluation of LVS Function[1]	24	71%	84%	83%	99%
Smoking Cessation Advice[1]	2	100%	82%	82%	100%
Pneumonia Care					

NOTE: Hospital profiles are in alphabetical order by state, then city, then hospital within the city; Rankings are sorted by rate in descending order and exclude hospitals with less than 25 cases; (1) The number of cases is too small (n<25) for purposes of reliably predicting hospital performance; (2) Measure reflects the hospital's indication that its submission was based upon a sample of its relevant discharges; (3) Rate reflects fewer than the maximum possible quarters of data for the measure; (4) Inaccurate information submitted and suppressed for one or more quarters; (5) No data is available from the hospital for this measure; Please refer to the User's Guide for a full explanation of data

Measure	Cases	This Hospital	State Average	U.S. Average	Top Hospital
Appropriate Initial Antibiotic	36	78%	82%	83%	94%
Blood Culture Timing[1]	21	90%	89%	90%	100%
Influenza Vaccine[1]	4	50%	58%	70%	100%
Initial Antibiotic Timing	38	84%	75%	80%	93%
Oxygenation Assessment	48	100%	99%	99%	100%
Pneumococcal Vaccine	36	58%	58%	69%	94%
Smoking Cessation Advice[1]	9	89%	75%	80%	100%
Surgical Infection Prevention					
Prophylactic Antibiotic Given[2,3]	108	84%	74%	77%	95%
Prophylactic Antibiotic Selection[2]	40	62%	89%	90%	100%
Prophylactic Antibiotic Stopped[2,3]	102	65%	65%	72%	95%
Pregnancy Care					
Inpatient Neonatal Mortality	296	0.00%	-	-	-
Third or Fourth Degree Laceration	237	2.53%	3.58%	3.63%	3.27%

Santa Barbara Cottage Hospital

Pueblo at Bath Street
PO Box 689
Santa Barbara, CA 93105
E-mail: joneill@cottagehealthsystem.org
URL: www.cottagehealthsystem.org
Phone: 805-682-7111
Fax: 805-569-8368
Ownership: Voluntary non-profit - Other
Emergency Services: Yes
Accredited: Yes
Licensed Beds: 443

Key Personnel:
Emergency Room . . . . James Thomas, MD
Director Infection/Disease Control . . . . Seth Anderson, MD
Director Outpatient Surgery . . . . Douglas Etsell, MD
Chief Radiology . . . . Brian Schnier, MD

Measure	Cases	This Hospital	State Average	U.S. Average	Top Hospital
Heart Attack Care					
ACE Inhibitor or ARB for LVSD	47	70%	82%	82%	100%
Aspirin at Arrival	157	94%	95%	92%	100%
Aspirin at Discharge	229	96%	90%	90%	100%
Beta Blocker at Arrival	116	89%	89%	87%	100%
Beta Blocker at Discharge	212	90%	89%	90%	100%
Fibrinolytic Medication Timing	0	-	40%	31%	100%
PCI Within 90 Minutes of Arrival[1]	14	71%	52%	54%	95%
Smoking Cessation Advice	55	98%	87%	88%	100%
Heart Failure Care					
ACE Inhibitor or ARB for LVSD	147	77%	84%	82%	100%
Discharge Instructions	310	47%	56%	61%	93%
Evaluation of LVS Function	382	88%	84%	83%	99%
Smoking Cessation Advice	52	73%	82%	82%	100%
Pneumonia Care					
Appropriate Initial Antibiotic	191	82%	82%	83%	94%
Blood Culture Timing	185	92%	89%	90%	100%
Influenza Vaccine	72	54%	58%	70%	100%
Initial Antibiotic Timing	256	80%	75%	80%	93%
Oxygenation Assessment	338	100%	99%	99%	100%
Pneumococcal Vaccine	234	59%	58%	69%	94%
Smoking Cessation Advice	57	54%	75%	80%	100%
Surgical Infection Prevention					
Prophylactic Antibiotic Given[2,3]	254	52%	74%	77%	95%
Prophylactic Antibiotic Selection[2]	81	96%	89%	90%	100%
Prophylactic Antibiotic Stopped[2,3]	242	29%	65%	72%	95%
Pregnancy Care					
Inpatient Neonatal Mortality	-	-	-	-	-
Third or Fourth Degree Laceration	-	-	3.58%	3.63%	3.27%

Kaiser Permanente Santa Clara Medical Center

900 Kiely Blvd
Santa Clara, CA 95051
URL: www.kaisersantaclara.org
Phone: 408-236-6400
Fax: 888-805-7562
Ownership: Voluntary non-profit - Other
Emergency Services: Yes
Accredited: Yes
Licensed Beds: 386

Key Personnel:
Physician in Chief. . . . . Bernadette Loftus, MD
Director Emergency Room. . . . . Eric Koscove, MD
Infection Control. . . . . Mark Lillo, MD
OB/GYN Womens Health. . . . . Mary Petersen, RN

Measure	Cases	This Hospital	State Average	U.S. Average	Top Hospital
Heart Attack Care					
ACE Inhibitor or ARB for LVSD	29	72%	82%	82%	100%
Aspirin at Arrival	149	99%	95%	92%	100%
Aspirin at Discharge	90	97%	90%	90%	100%
Beta Blocker at Arrival	114	100%	89%	87%	100%
Beta Blocker at Discharge	94	100%	89%	90%	100%
Fibrinolytic Medication Timing[1]	21	33%	40%	31%	100%
PCI Within 90 Minutes of Arrival	0	-	52%	54%	95%
Smoking Cessation Advice[1]	14	86%	87%	88%	100%
Heart Failure Care					
ACE Inhibitor or ARB for LVSD	115	60%	84%	82%	100%
Discharge Instructions	397	69%	56%	61%	93%
Evaluation of LVS Function	467	99%	84%	83%	99%
Smoking Cessation Advice	27	78%	82%	82%	100%
Pneumonia Care					
Appropriate Initial Antibiotic	90	86%	82%	83%	94%
Blood Culture Timing	106	92%	89%	90%	100%
Influenza Vaccine	26	69%	58%	70%	100%
Initial Antibiotic Timing	132	71%	75%	80%	93%
Oxygenation Assessment	173	100%	99%	99%	100%
Pneumococcal Vaccine	128	91%	58%	69%	94%
Smoking Cessation Advice[1]	18	78%	75%	80%	100%
Surgical Infection Prevention					
Prophylactic Antibiotic Given	197	79%	74%	77%	95%
Prophylactic Antibiotic Selection	45	84%	89%	90%	100%
Prophylactic Antibiotic Stopped	193	74%	65%	72%	95%
Pregnancy Care					
Inpatient Neonatal Mortality[2]	725	0.14%	-	-	-
Third or Fourth Degree Laceration[2]	489	5.73%	3.58%	3.63%	3.27%

Dominican Hospital

1555 Soquel Drive
Santa Cruz, CA 95065
URL: www.dominicanhospital.org
Phone: 831-462-7700
Fax: 831-464-8813
Ownership: Voluntary non-profit - Church
Emergency Services: Yes
Accredited: Yes
Licensed Beds: 375

Key Personnel:
President/CEO. . . . . Julie Hyer
Chief Medical Staff. . . . . Dean Kashino, MD
Manager Catheterization Laboratory . . . . Maryann Dunlap
Emergency Room . . . . Linda Starn, RN
Director Infection/Disease Control . . . . Nanette Mickiewicz, MD
Nurse Manager CCU . . . . Alison Reason, RN
OB/GYN Womens Health. . . . . Lawrence Lenz, MD
Manager Radiology . . . . Richard Crescini
Manager Cardio-Pulmonary Services. . . . . Richard Crescini

Measure	Cases	This Hospital	State Average	U.S. Average	Top Hospital
Heart Attack Care					
ACE Inhibitor or ARB for LVSD	50	84%	82%	82%	100%
Aspirin at Arrival	157	99%	95%	92%	100%
Aspirin at Discharge	160	100%	90%	90%	100%
Beta Blocker at Arrival	142	99%	89%	87%	100%
Beta Blocker at Discharge	153	99%	89%	90%	100%
Fibrinolytic Medication Timing	0	-	40%	31%	100%
PCI Within 90 Minutes of Arrival[1]	8	62%	52%	54%	95%
Smoking Cessation Advice	39	100%	87%	88%	100%
Heart Failure Care					
ACE Inhibitor or ARB for LVSD	96	76%	84%	82%	100%
Discharge Instructions	259	56%	56%	61%	93%
Evaluation of LVS Function	342	90%	84%	83%	99%
Smoking Cessation Advice	47	87%	82%	82%	100%
Pneumonia Care					
Appropriate Initial Antibiotic	185	88%	82%	83%	94%
Blood Culture Timing	168	85%	89%	90%	100%
Influenza Vaccine	55	62%	58%	70%	100%
Initial Antibiotic Timing	242	75%	75%	80%	93%
Oxygenation Assessment	292	100%	99%	99%	100%
Pneumococcal Vaccine	194	70%	58%	69%	94%
Smoking Cessation Advice	39	74%	75%	80%	100%
Surgical Infection Prevention					
Prophylactic Antibiotic Given[2,3]	214	64%	74%	77%	95%

NOTE: Hospital profiles are in alphabetical order by state, then city, then hospital within the city; Rankings are sorted by rate in descending order and exclude hospitals with less than 25 cases; (1) The number of cases is too small (n<25) for purposes of reliably predicting hospital performance; (2) Measure reflects the hospital's indication that its submission was based upon a sample of its relevant discharges; (3) Rate reflects fewer than the maximum possible quarters of data for the measure; (4) Inaccurate information submitted and suppressed for one or more quarters; (5) No data is available from the hospital for this measure; Please refer to the User's Guide for a full explanation of data

Measure	Cases	This Hospital	State Average	U.S. Average	Top Hospital
Prophylactic Antibiotic Selection[2]	69	86%	89%	90%	100%
Prophylactic Antibiotic Stopped[2,3]	207	57%	65%	72%	95%
Pregnancy Care					
Inpatient Neonatal Mortality	-	-	-	-	-
Third or Fourth Degree Laceration	-	-	3.58%	3.63%	3.27%

Sutter Maternity and Surgery Center

2900 Chanticleer Avenue Phone: 831-477-2200
Santa Cruz, CA 95065
Ownership: Voluntary non-profit - Private Accredited: Yes
Emergency Services: No

Measure	Cases	This Hospital	State Average	U.S. Average	Top Hospital
Heart Attack Care					
ACE Inhibitor or ARB for LVSD[5]	-	-	82%	82%	100%
Aspirin at Arrival[5]	-	-	95%	92%	100%
Aspirin at Discharge[5]	-	-	90%	90%	100%
Beta Blocker at Arrival[5]	-	-	89%	87%	100%
Beta Blocker at Discharge[5]	-	-	89%	90%	100%
Fibrinolytic Medication Timing[5]	-	-	40%	31%	100%
PCI Within 90 Minutes of Arrival[5]	-	-	52%	54%	95%
Smoking Cessation Advice[5]	-	-	87%	88%	100%
Heart Failure Care					
ACE Inhibitor or ARB for LVSD[3]	0	-	84%	82%	100%
Discharge Instructions[3]	0	-	56%	61%	93%
Evaluation of LVS Function[1,3]	1	0%	84%	83%	99%
Smoking Cessation Advice[3]	0	-	82%	82%	100%
Pneumonia Care					
Appropriate Initial Antibiotic[1,3]	5	80%	82%	83%	94%
Blood Culture Timing[1,3]	2	100%	89%	90%	100%
Influenza Vaccine[1]	1	100%	58%	70%	100%
Initial Antibiotic Timing[1,3]	4	25%	75%	80%	93%
Oxygenation Assessment[1,3]	5	100%	99%	99%	100%
Pneumococcal Vaccine[1,3]	2	50%	58%	69%	94%
Smoking Cessation Advice[1,3]	1	100%	75%	80%	100%
Surgical Infection Prevention					
Prophylactic Antibiotic Given[2]	222	68%	74%	77%	95%
Prophylactic Antibiotic Selection[2]	37	89%	89%	90%	100%
Prophylactic Antibiotic Stopped[2]	218	84%	65%	72%	95%
Pregnancy Care					
Inpatient Neonatal Mortality	874	0.00%	-	-	-
Third or Fourth Degree Laceration	689	5.81%	3.58%	3.63%	3.27%

Marian Medical Center

1400 E Church Street Phone: 805-739-3000
Santa Maria, CA 93456 Fax: 805-739-3060
URL: www.marinmedicalcenter.org
Ownership: Voluntary non-profit - Church Accredited: Yes
Emergency Services: Yes Licensed Beds: 227

Key Personnel:

CEO. . . . . Charles Cova
Chief of Medical Staff. Todd Bailey, MD
Director Cardiology . . . . Joan Nowell
Emergency Room . . . . Ann Marselay
Infection Control. . . . . Leslie Anderson
Director Medical/Surgical Nursing . . . . Sandy Mugg, RN
OB/GYN Womens Health. . . . . Carol Karamitsos, MD
Chief Radiology . . . . Richard Siegel, MD
Director Respiratory Therapy . . . . Judy Hoffman

Measure	Cases	This Hospital	State Average	U.S. Average	Top Hospital
Heart Attack Care					
ACE Inhibitor or ARB for LVSD[1]	6	100%	82%	82%	100%
Aspirin at Arrival	141	99%	95%	92%	100%
Aspirin at Discharge	127	99%	90%	90%	100%
Beta Blocker at Arrival	88	100%	89%	87%	100%
Beta Blocker at Discharge	102	100%	89%	90%	100%
Fibrinolytic Medication Timing[1]	21	81%	40%	31%	100%
PCI Within 90 Minutes of Arrival[1]	1	100%	52%	54%	95%
Smoking Cessation Advice	35	100%	87%	88%	100%
Heart Failure Care					
ACE Inhibitor or ARB for LVSD	78	96%	84%	82%	100%
Discharge Instructions	223	97%	56%	61%	93%
Evaluation of LVS Function	254	100%	84%	83%	99%
Smoking Cessation Advice[1]	22	100%	82%	82%	100%
Pneumonia Care					
Appropriate Initial Antibiotic	185	93%	82%	83%	94%
Blood Culture Timing	172	93%	89%	90%	100%
Influenza Vaccine	69	72%	58%	70%	100%
Initial Antibiotic Timing	234	86%	75%	80%	93%
Oxygenation Assessment	307	100%	99%	99%	100%
Pneumococcal Vaccine	225	75%	58%	69%	94%
Smoking Cessation Advice	44	100%	75%	80%	100%
Surgical Infection Prevention					
Prophylactic Antibiotic Given[2,3]	493	96%	74%	77%	95%
Prophylactic Antibiotic Selection[2]	172	91%	89%	90%	100%
Prophylactic Antibiotic Stopped[2,3]	481	62%	65%	72%	95%
Pregnancy Care					
Inpatient Neonatal Mortality	-	-	-	-	-
Third or Fourth Degree Laceration	-	-	3.58%	3.63%	3.27%

Saint John's Health Center

1328 22nd Street Phone: 310-829-5511
Santa Monica, CA 90404 Fax: 310-829-8005
URL: www.stjohns.org
Ownership: Voluntary non-profit - Church Accredited: Yes
Emergency Services: Yes Licensed Beds: 237

Key Personnel:

President/CEO. . . . . Lourdes Lazatin
Chief Medical Staff. . . . . Charles Pietrasesa
Emergency Room . . . . Karen Peirce
Director Medical/Surgical Nursing . . . . Sonia Chovance
Director Respiratory Therapy . . . . Gary Foltz

Measure	Cases	This Hospital	State Average	U.S. Average	Top Hospital
Heart Attack Care					
ACE Inhibitor or ARB for LVSD	25	84%	82%	82%	100%
Aspirin at Arrival	153	99%	95%	92%	100%
Aspirin at Discharge	143	94%	90%	90%	100%
Beta Blocker at Arrival	145	91%	89%	87%	100%
Beta Blocker at Discharge	141	94%	89%	90%	100%
Fibrinolytic Medication Timing	0	-	40%	31%	100%
PCI Within 90 Minutes of Arrival[1]	3	33%	52%	54%	95%
Smoking Cessation Advice	29	93%	87%	88%	100%
Heart Failure Care					
ACE Inhibitor or ARB for LVSD	92	91%	84%	82%	100%
Discharge Instructions	197	44%	56%	61%	93%
Evaluation of LVS Function	232	81%	84%	83%	99%
Smoking Cessation Advice[1]	8	38%	82%	82%	100%
Pneumonia Care					
Appropriate Initial Antibiotic	175	78%	82%	83%	94%
Blood Culture Timing	162	90%	89%	90%	100%
Influenza Vaccine	49	2%	58%	70%	100%
Initial Antibiotic Timing	222	72%	75%	80%	93%
Oxygenation Assessment	290	100%	99%	99%	100%
Pneumococcal Vaccine	215	29%	58%	69%	94%
Smoking Cessation Advice[1]	14	71%	75%	80%	100%
Surgical Infection Prevention					
Prophylactic Antibiotic Given	1,293	71%	74%	77%	95%
Prophylactic Antibiotic Selection	355	91%	89%	90%	100%
Prophylactic Antibiotic Stopped	1,265	73%	65%	72%	95%
Pregnancy Care					
Inpatient Neonatal Mortality	915	0.22%	-	-	-
Third or Fourth Degree Laceration	1,288	6.13%	3.58%	3.63%	3.27%

Santa Monica-UCLA Medical Center

1250 16th Street Phone: 310-319-4000
Santa Monica, CA 90404 Fax: 310-319-4821
URL: www.healthcare.ucla.edu
Ownership: Government - State Accredited: Yes
Emergency Services: Yes Licensed Beds: 600

Key Personnel:

Administrator/President . . . . Michael Carve, MD
Chief Medical Staff. . . . . Stephen Ross, MD
Chief Catheterization Laboratory . . . . Arnold Nedelman

NOTE: Hospital profiles are in alphabetical order by state, then city, then hospital within the city; Rankings are sorted by rate in descending order and exclude hospitals with less than 25 cases; (1) The number of cases is too small (n<25) for purposes of reliably predicting hospital performance; (2) Measure reflects the hospital's indication that its submission was based upon a sample of its relevant discharges; (3) Rate reflects fewer than the maximum possible quarters of data for the measure; (4) Inaccurate information submitted and suppressed for one or more quarters; (5) No data is available from the hospital for this measure; Please refer to the User's Guide for a full explanation of data

Emergency Room . . . . Wally Ghurabi
Director Infection/Disease Control . . . . Laverne Kroemer
CCU Spvg. Nurse . . . . Therese Carrabine
Director Medical/Surgical Nursing . . . . Therese Carrabine
OB/GYN Womens Health. . . . . William Parker, MD
Chief Radiology . . . . Kevin Drake, MD
Director Respiratory Therapy . . . . Kathleen Hunt

Measure	Cases	This Hospital	State Average	U.S. Average	Top Hospital
Heart Attack Care					
ACE Inhibitor or ARB for LVSD[1]	21	95%	82%	82%	100%
Aspirin at Arrival	109	100%	95%	92%	100%
Aspirin at Discharge	103	99%	90%	90%	100%
Beta Blocker at Arrival	97	100%	89%	87%	100%
Beta Blocker at Discharge	103	98%	89%	90%	100%
Fibrinolytic Medication Timing	0	-	40%	31%	100%
PCI Within 90 Minutes of Arrival[1]	3	0%	52%	54%	95%
Smoking Cessation Advice[1]	17	82%	87%	88%	100%
Heart Failure Care					
ACE Inhibitor or ARB for LVSD[2]	68	81%	84%	82%	100%
Discharge Instructions[2]	176	24%	56%	61%	93%
Evaluation of LVS Function[2]	247	95%	84%	83%	99%
Smoking Cessation Advice[1,2]	24	71%	82%	82%	100%
Pneumonia Care					
Appropriate Initial Antibiotic[2]	74	77%	82%	83%	94%
Blood Culture Timing[2]	109	98%	89%	90%	100%
Influenza Vaccine[2]	32	34%	58%	70%	100%
Initial Antibiotic Timing[2]	160	76%	75%	80%	93%
Oxygenation Assessment[2]	186	100%	99%	99%	100%
Pneumococcal Vaccine[2]	134	13%	58%	69%	94%
Smoking Cessation Advice[1,2]	19	53%	75%	80%	100%
Surgical Infection Prevention					
Prophylactic Antibiotic Given[2]	285	93%	74%	77%	95%
Prophylactic Antibiotic Selection[2]	46	91%	89%	90%	100%
Prophylactic Antibiotic Stopped[2]	276	38%	65%	72%	95%
Pregnancy Care					
Inpatient Neonatal Mortality[2]	369	0.81%	-	-	-
Third or Fourth Degree Laceration	781	4.61%	3.58%	3.63%	3.27%

Kaiser Foundation Hospital-Santa Rosa

401 Bicentennial Way
Santa Rosa, CA 95403
Phone: 707-571-4000
Ownership: Voluntary non-profit - Other
Accredited: Yes
Emergency Services: Yes

Measure	Cases	This Hospital	State Average	U.S. Average	Top Hospital
Heart Attack Care					
ACE Inhibitor or ARB for LVSD[1]	17	94%	82%	82%	100%
Aspirin at Arrival	171	98%	95%	92%	100%
Aspirin at Discharge	121	89%	90%	90%	100%
Beta Blocker at Arrival	162	96%	89%	87%	100%
Beta Blocker at Discharge	123	98%	89%	90%	100%
Fibrinolytic Medication Timing[1]	10	50%	40%	31%	100%
PCI Within 90 Minutes of Arrival	0	-	52%	54%	95%
Smoking Cessation Advice	25	92%	87%	88%	100%
Heart Failure Care					
ACE Inhibitor or ARB for LVSD	48	85%	84%	82%	100%
Discharge Instructions	113	67%	56%	61%	93%
Evaluation of LVS Function	123	96%	84%	83%	99%
Smoking Cessation Advice	25	68%	82%	82%	100%
Pneumonia Care					
Appropriate Initial Antibiotic	135	87%	82%	83%	94%
Blood Culture Timing	110	96%	89%	90%	100%
Influenza Vaccine	38	58%	58%	70%	100%
Initial Antibiotic Timing	156	70%	75%	80%	93%
Oxygenation Assessment	190	100%	99%	99%	100%
Pneumococcal Vaccine	140	81%	58%	69%	94%
Smoking Cessation Advice[1]	17	53%	75%	80%	100%
Surgical Infection Prevention					
Prophylactic Antibiotic Given	313	86%	74%	77%	95%
Prophylactic Antibiotic Selection	102	87%	89%	90%	100%
Prophylactic Antibiotic Stopped	307	67%	65%	72%	95%

Pregnancy Care					
Inpatient Neonatal Mortality[2]	1,458	0.00%	-	-	-
Third or Fourth Degree Laceration[2]	959	5.01%	3.58%	3.63%	3.27%

Santa Rosa Memorial Hospital

1165 Montgomery Drive
Santa Rosa, CA 95405
Phone: 707-546-3210
Fax: 707-522-1522
URL: www.stjosephhealth.org
Ownership: Voluntary non-profit - Church
Accredited: Yes
Emergency Services: Yes
Licensed Beds: 209

Key Personnel:

Chief Medical Staff. . . . . Jan Fonander, MD
Emergency Room . . . . Kristy Gaub, Dir
OB/GYN Womens Health. . . . . Thomas McCarthy
Chief Radiology . . . . Daniel Doran, MD
Director Respiratory Therapy . . . . Pan Cress

Measure	Cases	This Hospital	State Average	U.S. Average	Top Hospital
Heart Attack Care					
ACE Inhibitor or ARB for LVSD[1]	24	83%	82%	82%	100%
Aspirin at Arrival	101	97%	95%	92%	100%
Aspirin at Discharge	119	99%	90%	90%	100%
Beta Blocker at Arrival	86	94%	89%	87%	100%
Beta Blocker at Discharge	120	97%	89%	90%	100%
Fibrinolytic Medication Timing	0	-	40%	31%	100%
PCI Within 90 Minutes of Arrival[1]	6	100%	52%	54%	95%
Smoking Cessation Advice[1]	22	95%	87%	88%	100%
Heart Failure Care					
ACE Inhibitor or ARB for LVSD[2]	98	89%	84%	82%	100%
Discharge Instructions[2]	223	75%	56%	61%	93%
Evaluation of LVS Function[2]	255	96%	84%	83%	99%
Smoking Cessation Advice[2]	37	97%	82%	82%	100%
Pneumonia Care					
Appropriate Initial Antibiotic	213	72%	82%	83%	94%
Blood Culture Timing	171	87%	89%	90%	100%
Influenza Vaccine	46	63%	58%	70%	100%
Initial Antibiotic Timing	268	82%	75%	80%	93%
Oxygenation Assessment	324	98%	99%	99%	100%
Pneumococcal Vaccine	195	65%	58%	69%	94%
Smoking Cessation Advice	64	84%	75%	80%	100%
Surgical Infection Prevention					
Prophylactic Antibiotic Given[2,3]	186	58%	74%	77%	95%
Prophylactic Antibiotic Selection[2]	57	82%	89%	90%	100%
Prophylactic Antibiotic Stopped[2,3]	174	54%	65%	72%	95%
Pregnancy Care					
Inpatient Neonatal Mortality	-	-	-	-	-
Third or Fourth Degree Laceration	-	-	3.58%	3.63%	3.27%

Sutter Medical Center of Santa Rosa

3325 Chanate Road
Santa Rosa, CA 95404
Phone: 707-576-4000
Fax: 707-576-4318
E-mail: srsutter@sutterhealth.org
URL: www.suttersantarosa.org
Ownership: Government - Local
Accredited: Yes
Emergency Services: Yes
Licensed Beds: 175

Key Personnel:

CEO. . . . . Michael J Cohill
Chief Catheterization Laboratory . . . . Joel Ericson, MD
Emergency Room . . . . Judy Jacoby
Director Infection/Disease Control . . . . Marion McDonald, RN
Chief Radiology . . . . Gail McAlpin

Measure	Cases	This Hospital	State Average	U.S. Average	Top Hospital
Heart Attack Care					
ACE Inhibitor or ARB for LVSD	53	91%	82%	82%	100%
Aspirin at Arrival	70	97%	95%	92%	100%
Aspirin at Discharge	177	99%	90%	90%	100%
Beta Blocker at Arrival	65	100%	89%	87%	100%
Beta Blocker at Discharge	171	96%	89%	90%	100%
Fibrinolytic Medication Timing	0	-	40%	31%	100%
PCI Within 90 Minutes of Arrival[1]	4	25%	52%	54%	95%
Smoking Cessation Advice	58	98%	87%	88%	100%

NOTE: Hospital profiles are in alphabetical order by state, then city, then hospital within the city; Rankings are sorted by rate in descending order and exclude hospitals with less than 25 cases; (1) The number of cases is too small (n<25) for purposes of reliably predicting hospital performance; (2) Measure reflects the hospital's indication that its submission was based upon a sample of its relevant discharges; (3) Rate reflects fewer than the maximum possible quarters of data for the measure; (4) Inaccurate information submitted and suppressed for one or more quarters; (5) No data is available from the hospital for this measure; Please refer to the User's Guide for a full explanation of data

Heart Failure Care					
ACE Inhibitor or ARB for LVSD	97	87%	84%	82%	100%
Discharge Instructions	183	70%	56%	61%	93%
Evaluation of LVS Function	208	84%	84%	83%	99%
Smoking Cessation Advice	43	81%	82%	82%	100%
Pneumonia Care					
Appropriate Initial Antibiotic	126	78%	82%	83%	94%
Blood Culture Timing	89	89%	89%	90%	100%
Influenza Vaccine	32	6%	58%	70%	100%
Initial Antibiotic Timing	120	67%	75%	80%	93%
Oxygenation Assessment	156	100%	99%	99%	100%
Pneumococcal Vaccine	75	23%	58%	69%	94%
Smoking Cessation Advice	56	73%	75%	80%	100%
Surgical Infection Prevention					
Prophylactic Antibiotic Given[2]	507	67%	74%	77%	95%
Prophylactic Antibiotic Selection[2]	122	71%	89%	90%	100%
Prophylactic Antibiotic Stopped[2]	473	61%	65%	72%	95%
Pregnancy Care					
Inpatient Neonatal Mortality[2]	818	0.37%	-	-	-
Third or Fourth Degree Laceration[2]	826	4.00%	3.58%	3.63%	3.27%

Palm Drive Hospital

501 Petaluma Avenue
Sebastopol, CA 95472
URL: www.palmdrivehospital.com
Ownership: Voluntary non-profit - Other
Emergency Services: No
Phone: 707-823-8511
Fax: 707-829-4178
Accredited: No
Licensed Beds: 53

Key Personnel:

CEO . . . . Glenn Minevrinivick
Chief of Medical Staff . . . . Sue Platts
Emergency Room . . . . Susanne Landy
Emergency Room . . . . Malissa Reinders, RN
Respiratory Therapy . . . . Francis Slimmer

Measure	Cases	This Hospital	State Average	U.S. Average	Top Hospital
Heart Attack Care					
ACE Inhibitor or ARB for LVSD[3]	0	-	82%	82%	100%
Aspirin at Arrival[1,3]	10	100%	95%	92%	100%
Aspirin at Discharge[1,3]	5	80%	90%	90%	100%
Beta Blocker at Arrival[1,3]	7	86%	89%	87%	100%
Beta Blocker at Discharge[1,3]	4	25%	89%	90%	100%
Fibrinolytic Medication Timing[5]	-	-	40%	31%	100%
PCI Within 90 Minutes of Arrival[5]	-	-	52%	54%	95%
Smoking Cessation Advice[5]	-	-	87%	88%	100%
Heart Failure Care					
ACE Inhibitor or ARB for LVSD[1]	9	33%	84%	82%	100%
Discharge Instructions[1,3]	4	100%	56%	61%	93%
Evaluation of LVS Function	31	74%	84%	83%	99%
Smoking Cessation Advice[3]	0	-	82%	82%	100%
Pneumonia Care					
Appropriate Initial Antibiotic[1,3]	7	57%	82%	83%	94%
Blood Culture Timing[1,3]	5	100%	89%	90%	100%
Influenza Vaccine[5]	-	-	58%	70%	100%
Initial Antibiotic Timing	35	77%	75%	80%	93%
Oxygenation Assessment	42	100%	99%	99%	100%
Pneumococcal Vaccine	29	52%	58%	69%	94%
Smoking Cessation Advice[1,3]	2	50%	75%	80%	100%
Surgical Infection Prevention					
Prophylactic Antibiotic Given[1,3]	19	95%	74%	77%	95%
Prophylactic Antibiotic Selection[5]	-	-	89%	90%	100%
Prophylactic Antibiotic Stopped[1,3]	19	100%	65%	72%	95%
Pregnancy Care					
Inpatient Neonatal Mortality	-	-	-	-	-
Third or Fourth Degree Laceration	-	-	3.58%	3.63%	3.27%

Sherman Oaks Hospital

4929 Van Nuys Boulevard
Sherman Oaks, CA 91403
E-mail: info@shermanoakshospital.com
URL: www.shermanoakshospital.com
Ownership: Proprietary
Emergency Services: No
Phone: 818-981-7111
Fax: 818-907-4539
Accredited: Yes
Licensed Beds: 153

Key Personnel:

President/CEO . . . . David Levinsohn

Measure	Cases	This Hospital	State Average	U.S. Average	Top Hospital
Heart Attack Care					
ACE Inhibitor or ARB for LVSD[3]	0	-	82%	82%	100%
Aspirin at Arrival[1,3]	14	100%	95%	92%	100%
Aspirin at Discharge[1,3]	6	100%	90%	90%	100%
Beta Blocker at Arrival[1,3]	12	100%	89%	87%	100%
Beta Blocker at Discharge[1,3]	7	100%	89%	90%	100%
Fibrinolytic Medication Timing[3]	0	-	40%	31%	100%
PCI Within 90 Minutes of Arrival	0	-	52%	54%	95%
Smoking Cessation Advice[1,3]	1	100%	87%	88%	100%
Heart Failure Care					
ACE Inhibitor or ARB for LVSD[1,3]	7	100%	84%	82%	100%
Discharge Instructions[3]	32	100%	56%	61%	93%
Evaluation of LVS Function[3]	72	99%	84%	83%	99%
Smoking Cessation Advice[1,3]	4	100%	82%	82%	100%
Pneumonia Care					
Appropriate Initial Antibiotic[1,3]	14	100%	82%	83%	94%
Blood Culture Timing[3]	26	92%	89%	90%	100%
Influenza Vaccine[5]	-	-	58%	70%	100%
Initial Antibiotic Timing[3]	43	98%	75%	80%	93%
Oxygenation Assessment[3]	56	100%	99%	99%	100%
Pneumococcal Vaccine[3]	32	91%	58%	69%	94%
Smoking Cessation Advice[1,3]	3	100%	75%	80%	100%
Surgical Infection Prevention					
Prophylactic Antibiotic Given[1,3]	17	94%	74%	77%	95%
Prophylactic Antibiotic Selection[5]	-	-	89%	90%	100%
Prophylactic Antibiotic Stopped[1,3]	17	82%	65%	72%	95%
Pregnancy Care					
Inpatient Neonatal Mortality	-	-	-	-	-
Third or Fourth Degree Laceration	-	-	3.58%	3.63%	3.27%

Simi Valley Hospital

2975 Sycamore Drive
Simi Valley, CA 93065
URL: www.simivalleyhospital.com
Ownership: Voluntary non-profit - Church
Emergency Services: Yes
Phone: 805-955-6000
Fax: 805-526-0837
Accredited: Yes
Licensed Beds: 185

Key Personnel:

President/CEO . . . . Gary Irish
Chief Medical Staff . . . . Jonathan Kurohara
Emergency Room . . . . Peter Cho, MD
Infection Control . . . . Ken Archulet
Medical Surgical Nursing . . . . Vicki Vander Toorn
Chief Radiology . . . . Monica Berlin, MD
Manager Respiratory/Cardiopulmonary . . . . Rob Cohen

Measure	Cases	This Hospital	State Average	U.S. Average	Top Hospital
Heart Attack Care					
ACE Inhibitor or ARB for LVSD[1]	5	60%	82%	82%	100%
Aspirin at Arrival	49	82%	95%	92%	100%
Aspirin at Discharge[1]	8	75%	90%	90%	100%
Beta Blocker at Arrival	36	86%	89%	87%	100%
Beta Blocker at Discharge[1]	12	83%	89%	90%	100%
Fibrinolytic Medication Timing[1]	5	80%	40%	31%	100%
PCI Within 90 Minutes of Arrival	0	-	52%	54%	95%
Smoking Cessation Advice[1]	2	100%	87%	88%	100%
Heart Failure Care					
ACE Inhibitor or ARB for LVSD	38	76%	84%	82%	100%
Discharge Instructions	90	20%	56%	61%	93%
Evaluation of LVS Function	133	84%	84%	83%	99%
Smoking Cessation Advice[1]	15	93%	82%	82%	100%
Pneumonia Care					
Appropriate Initial Antibiotic	105	90%	82%	83%	94%

NOTE: Hospital profiles are in alphabetical order by state, then city, then hospital within the city; Rankings are sorted by rate in descending order and exclude hospitals with less than 25 cases; (1) The number of cases is too small (n<25) for purposes of reliably predicting hospital performance; (2) Measure reflects the hospital's indication that its submission was based upon a sample of its relevant discharges; (3) Rate reflects fewer than the maximum possible quarters of data for the measure; (4) Inaccurate information submitted and suppressed for one or more quarters; (5) No data is available from the hospital for this measure; Please refer to the User's Guide for a full explanation of data

Measure	Cases	This Hospital	State Average	U.S. Average	Top Hospital
Blood Culture Timing	107	87%	89%	90%	100%
Influenza Vaccine	34	65%	58%	70%	100%
Initial Antibiotic Timing	122	84%	75%	80%	93%
Oxygenation Assessment	185	100%	99%	99%	100%
Pneumococcal Vaccine	106	65%	58%	69%	94%
Smoking Cessation Advice	35	97%	75%	80%	100%
Surgical Infection Prevention					
Prophylactic Antibiotic Given	193	80%	74%	77%	95%
Prophylactic Antibiotic Selection	38	71%	89%	90%	100%
Prophylactic Antibiotic Stopped	187	41%	65%	72%	95%
Pregnancy Care					
Inpatient Neonatal Mortality	-	-	-	-	-
Third or Fourth Degree Laceration	-	-	3.58%	3.63%	3.27%

Santa Ynez Valley Cottage Hospital

2050 Viborg Road
Solvang, CA 93463
E-mail: bkline@sbch.org
URL: www.cottagehealthsystem.org
Ownership: Voluntary non-profit - Other
Emergency Services: Yes
Phone: 805-688-6431
Fax: 805-686-5561
Accredited: Yes
Licensed Beds: 20

Key Personnel:
VP . . . . Wende Cappetta
Manager Infection Control . . . . Leslie Stanfield
Director Women's Services . . . . Linda Bacon

Measure	Cases	This Hospital	State Average	U.S. Average	Top Hospital
Heart Attack Care					
ACE Inhibitor or ARB for LVSD[3]	0	-	82%	82%	100%
Aspirin at Arrival[3]	0	-	95%	92%	100%
Aspirin at Discharge[3]	0	-	90%	90%	100%
Beta Blocker at Arrival[3]	0	-	89%	87%	100%
Beta Blocker at Discharge[3]	0	-	89%	90%	100%
Fibrinolytic Medication Timing[3]	0	-	40%	31%	100%
PCI Within 90 Minutes of Arrival	0	-	52%	54%	95%
Smoking Cessation Advice[3]	0	-	87%	88%	100%
Heart Failure Care					
ACE Inhibitor or ARB for LVSD[1]	5	60%	84%	82%	100%
Discharge Instructions[1]	19	58%	56%	61%	93%
Evaluation of LVS Function[1]	23	61%	84%	83%	99%
Smoking Cessation Advice[1]	2	50%	82%	82%	100%
Pneumonia Care					
Appropriate Initial Antibiotic[1]	20	90%	82%	83%	94%
Blood Culture Timing[1]	15	93%	89%	90%	100%
Influenza Vaccine[1]	6	50%	58%	70%	100%
Initial Antibiotic Timing	25	80%	75%	80%	93%
Oxygenation Assessment	32	100%	99%	99%	100%
Pneumococcal Vaccine	25	68%	58%	69%	94%
Smoking Cessation Advice[1]	2	50%	75%	80%	100%
Surgical Infection Prevention					
Prophylactic Antibiotic Given[5]	-	-	74%	77%	95%
Prophylactic Antibiotic Selection[5]	-	-	89%	90%	100%
Prophylactic Antibiotic Stopped[5]	-	-	65%	72%	95%
Pregnancy Care					
Inpatient Neonatal Mortality	-	-	-	-	-
Third or Fourth Degree Laceration	-	-	3.58%	3.63%	3.27%

Sonoma Valley Hospital

347 Andrieux Street
PO Box 600
Sonoma, CA 95476
E-mail: administration@svh.com.
URL: www.svh.com
Ownership: Govt - Hospital District or Authority
Emergency Services: Yes
Phone: 707-935-5000
Fax: 707-938-0166
Accredited: Yes
Licensed Beds: 49

Key Personnel:
President . . . . Michael Nugent
CEO. . . . . Robert Kowal

Measure	Cases	This Hospital	State Average	U.S. Average	Top Hospital
Heart Attack Care					
ACE Inhibitor or ARB for LVSD[1]	2	100%	82%	82%	100%
Aspirin at Arrival[1]	8	88%	95%	92%	100%
Aspirin at Discharge[1]	6	83%	90%	90%	100%
Beta Blocker at Arrival[1]	4	25%	89%	87%	100%
Beta Blocker at Discharge[1]	6	100%	89%	90%	100%
Fibrinolytic Medication Timing	0	-	40%	31%	100%
PCI Within 90 Minutes of Arrival	0	-	52%	54%	95%
Smoking Cessation Advice	0	-	87%	88%	100%
Heart Failure Care					
ACE Inhibitor or ARB for LVSD[1]	17	71%	84%	82%	100%
Discharge Instructions	32	25%	56%	61%	93%
Evaluation of LVS Function	53	92%	84%	83%	99%
Smoking Cessation Advice[1]	9	89%	82%	82%	100%
Pneumonia Care					
Appropriate Initial Antibiotic	34	94%	82%	83%	94%
Blood Culture Timing	33	97%	89%	90%	100%
Influenza Vaccine[1]	15	47%	58%	70%	100%
Initial Antibiotic Timing	44	82%	75%	80%	93%
Oxygenation Assessment	58	100%	99%	99%	100%
Pneumococcal Vaccine	49	24%	58%	69%	94%
Smoking Cessation Advice[1]	10	80%	75%	80%	100%
Surgical Infection Prevention					
Prophylactic Antibiotic Given	91	86%	74%	77%	95%
Prophylactic Antibiotic Selection[1]	20	95%	89%	90%	100%
Prophylactic Antibiotic Stopped	88	58%	65%	72%	95%
Pregnancy Care					
Inpatient Neonatal Mortality	-	-	-	-	-
Third or Fourth Degree Laceration	-	-	3.58%	3.63%	3.27%

Sonora Regional Medical Center

1000 Greenley Road
Sonora, CA 95370
URL: www.sonorahospital.org
Ownership: Voluntary non-profit - Church
Emergency Services: Yes
Phone: 209-532-5000
Fax: 209-536-3500
Accredited: Yes
Licensed Beds: 152

Key Personnel:
President/CEO. . . . . Lary A Davis
Chief Medical Staff. . . . . Danny Anderson, MD
Birth Center . . . . Mary Kellogg, RN
Cardio-Pulmonary . . . . Larry Warnick, RT
Emergency Department. Marguerite Pratt, RN
Med/Surg Manager . . . . Gretchen Walters, RN
Medical Staff . . . . Kathy Mutchler
Surgery . . . . Marylou Meersman

Measure	Cases	This Hospital	State Average	U.S. Average	Top Hospital
Heart Attack Care					
ACE Inhibitor or ARB for LVSD[1]	5	80%	82%	82%	100%
Aspirin at Arrival	47	94%	95%	92%	100%
Aspirin at Discharge[1]	20	70%	90%	90%	100%
Beta Blocker at Arrival	29	90%	89%	87%	100%
Beta Blocker at Discharge[1]	24	79%	89%	90%	100%
Fibrinolytic Medication Timing[1]	7	57%	40%	31%	100%
PCI Within 90 Minutes of Arrival	0	-	52%	54%	95%
Smoking Cessation Advice[1]	9	100%	87%	88%	100%
Heart Failure Care					
ACE Inhibitor or ARB for LVSD[1]	23	78%	84%	82%	100%
Discharge Instructions	80	70%	56%	61%	93%
Evaluation of LVS Function	93	84%	84%	83%	99%
Smoking Cessation Advice[1]	4	50%	82%	82%	100%
Pneumonia Care					
Appropriate Initial Antibiotic	113	92%	82%	83%	94%
Blood Culture Timing	74	93%	89%	90%	100%
Influenza Vaccine[1]	24	88%	58%	70%	100%
Initial Antibiotic Timing	149	90%	75%	80%	93%
Oxygenation Assessment	172	100%	99%	99%	100%
Pneumococcal Vaccine	140	80%	58%	69%	94%
Smoking Cessation Advice	39	85%	75%	80%	100%
Surgical Infection Prevention					
Prophylactic Antibiotic Given[3]	271	85%	74%	77%	95%
Prophylactic Antibiotic Selection	85	98%	89%	90%	100%
Prophylactic Antibiotic Stopped[3]	262	89%	65%	72%	95%
Pregnancy Care					

NOTE: Hospital profiles are in alphabetical order by state, then city, then hospital within the city; Rankings are sorted by rate in descending order and exclude hospitals with less than 25 cases; (1) The number of cases is too small (n<25) for purposes of reliably predicting hospital performance; (2) Measure reflects the hospital's indication that its submission was based upon a sample of its relevant discharges; (3) Rate reflects fewer than the maximum possible quarters of data for the measure; (4) Inaccurate information submitted and suppressed for one or more quarters; (5) No data is available from the hospital for this measure; Please refer to the User's Guide for a full explanation of data

Measure	Cases	This Hospital	State Average	U.S. Average	Top Hospital
Inpatient Neonatal Mortality	-	-	-	-	-
Third or Fourth Degree Laceration	-	-	3.58%	3.63%	3.27%

Tuolumne General Hospital

101 Hospital Road
Sonora, CA 95370
E-mail: tgh.comrel@mode.com
URL: www.tghospital.com
Ownership: Government - Local
Emergency Services: Yes
Phone: 209-533-7100
Fax: 209-533-7228
Accredited: Yes
Licensed Beds: 79

Key Personnel:

CEO. . . . . Barry Woerman
Head Nurse Medical Surgical Nursing . . . . Kim Diaz, RN
Respiratory Therapy. . . . . Colette Such

Measure	Cases	This Hospital	State Average	U.S. Average	Top Hospital
Heart Attack Care					
ACE Inhibitor or ARB for LVSD[1]	3	100%	82%	82%	100%
Aspirin at Arrival[1]	10	90%	95%	92%	100%
Aspirin at Discharge[1]	7	100%	90%	90%	100%
Beta Blocker at Arrival[1]	10	70%	89%	87%	100%
Beta Blocker at Discharge[1]	8	75%	89%	90%	100%
Fibrinolytic Medication Timing[3]	0	-	40%	31%	100%
PCI Within 90 Minutes of Arrival	0	-	52%	54%	95%
Smoking Cessation Advice[3]	0	-	87%	88%	100%
Heart Failure Care					
ACE Inhibitor or ARB for LVSD[1]	12	92%	84%	82%	100%
Discharge Instructions[1,3]	9	0%	56%	61%	93%
Evaluation of LVS Function	36	56%	84%	83%	99%
Smoking Cessation Advice[3]	0	-	82%	82%	100%
Pneumonia Care					
Appropriate Initial Antibiotic[1,3]	8	62%	82%	83%	94%
Blood Culture Timing[1,3]	4	100%	89%	90%	100%
Influenza Vaccine[5]	-	-	58%	70%	100%
Initial Antibiotic Timing	72	90%	75%	80%	93%
Oxygenation Assessment	80	99%	99%	99%	100%
Pneumococcal Vaccine	47	9%	58%	69%	94%
Smoking Cessation Advice[1,3]	2	50%	75%	80%	100%
Surgical Infection Prevention					
Prophylactic Antibiotic Given[5]	-	-	74%	77%	95%
Prophylactic Antibiotic Selection[5]	-	-	89%	90%	100%
Prophylactic Antibiotic Stopped[5]	-	-	65%	72%	95%
Pregnancy Care					
Inpatient Neonatal Mortality	-	-	-	-	-
Third or Fourth Degree Laceration	-	-	3.58%	3.63%	3.27%

Greater El Monte Community Hospital

1701 Santa Anita Avenue
South El Monte, CA 91733
URL: www.greaterelmonte.com
Ownership: Voluntary non-profit - Private
Emergency Services: No
Phone: 626-579-7777
Fax: 626-350-0368
Accredited: Yes
Licensed Beds: 117

Key Personnel:

CEO. . . . . Philip A Cohen

Measure	Cases	This Hospital	State Average	U.S. Average	Top Hospital
Heart Attack Care					
ACE Inhibitor or ARB for LVSD[1,2]	5	60%	82%	82%	100%
Aspirin at Arrival[2]	41	93%	95%	92%	100%
Aspirin at Discharge[1,2]	12	75%	90%	90%	100%
Beta Blocker at Arrival[2]	36	67%	89%	87%	100%
Beta Blocker at Discharge[1,2]	13	31%	89%	90%	100%
Fibrinolytic Medication Timing[1,2]	1	0%	40%	31%	100%
PCI Within 90 Minutes of Arrival[2]	0	-	52%	54%	95%
Smoking Cessation Advice[2]	0	-	87%	88%	100%
Heart Failure Care					
ACE Inhibitor or ARB for LVSD[1,2]	22	82%	84%	82%	100%
Discharge Instructions[2]	75	5%	56%	61%	93%
Evaluation of LVS Function[2]	95	75%	84%	83%	99%
Smoking Cessation Advice[1,2]	13	69%	82%	82%	100%
Pneumonia Care					
Appropriate Initial Antibiotic[2]	98	86%	82%	83%	94%
Blood Culture Timing[2]	134	97%	89%	90%	100%
Influenza Vaccine	33	18%	58%	70%	100%
Initial Antibiotic Timing[2]	206	74%	75%	80%	93%
Oxygenation Assessment[2]	247	100%	99%	99%	100%
Pneumococcal Vaccine[2]	150	9%	58%	69%	94%
Smoking Cessation Advice[1,2]	24	46%	75%	80%	100%
Surgical Infection Prevention					
Prophylactic Antibiotic Given[1,2]	14	50%	74%	77%	95%
Prophylactic Antibiotic Selection[1,2]	1	100%	89%	90%	100%
Prophylactic Antibiotic Stopped[1,2]	13	85%	65%	72%	95%
Pregnancy Care					
Inpatient Neonatal Mortality	-	-	-	-	-
Third or Fourth Degree Laceration	-	-	3.58%	3.63%	3.27%

Barton Memorial Hospital

PO Box 9578
2170 South Avenue
South Lake Tahoe, CA 96158
E-mail: publicrelations@bartonhealth.org
URL: www.bartonhealth.org
Ownership: Voluntary non-profit - Other
Emergency Services: Yes
Phone: 530-541-3420
Fax: 530-542-3740
Accredited: Yes
Licensed Beds: 75

Key Personnel:

CEO. . . . . William G Gordon
Chief Medical Staff. . . . . Mike Shanahan
Emergency Room . . . . Peter Chau, MD
Infection Control. . . . . Dawn Spicer
ICU . . . . Kenneth Harvey
Director Medical/Surgical Nursing . . . . Susan Fairley
Director Medical/Surgical Nursing . . . . Cynthia Warren
OB/GYN Womens Health. . . . . Thomas Goldenberg, MD
Director Respiratory Therapy . . . . Tony Crooks

Measure	Cases	This Hospital	State Average	U.S. Average	Top Hospital
Heart Attack Care					
ACE Inhibitor or ARB for LVSD[1]	1	100%	82%	82%	100%
Aspirin at Arrival[1]	7	86%	95%	92%	100%
Aspirin at Discharge[1]	3	100%	90%	90%	100%
Beta Blocker at Arrival[1]	6	83%	89%	87%	100%
Beta Blocker at Discharge[1]	3	100%	89%	90%	100%
Fibrinolytic Medication Timing	0	-	40%	31%	100%
PCI Within 90 Minutes of Arrival	0	-	52%	54%	95%
Smoking Cessation Advice	0	-	87%	88%	100%
Heart Failure Care					
ACE Inhibitor or ARB for LVSD[1]	18	94%	84%	82%	100%
Discharge Instructions	65	14%	56%	61%	93%
Evaluation of LVS Function	64	80%	84%	83%	99%
Smoking Cessation Advice[1]	20	65%	82%	82%	100%
Pneumonia Care					
Appropriate Initial Antibiotic	83	73%	82%	83%	94%
Blood Culture Timing	48	71%	89%	90%	100%
Influenza Vaccine[1]	14	57%	58%	70%	100%
Initial Antibiotic Timing	61	74%	75%	80%	93%
Oxygenation Assessment	90	100%	99%	99%	100%
Pneumococcal Vaccine	47	60%	58%	69%	94%
Smoking Cessation Advice[1]	24	46%	75%	80%	100%
Surgical Infection Prevention					
Prophylactic Antibiotic Given[3]	124	90%	74%	77%	95%
Prophylactic Antibiotic Selection	34	100%	89%	90%	100%
Prophylactic Antibiotic Stopped[3]	121	15%	65%	72%	95%
Pregnancy Care					
Inpatient Neonatal Mortality	560	0.00%	-	-	-
Third or Fourth Degree Laceration	390	3.59%	3.58%	3.63%	3.27%

S San Francisco Medical Center

Alternate Name: Kaiser Foundation Hospital-S San Francisco
1200 El Camino
S San Francisco, CA 94080
Ownership: Voluntary non-profit - Other
Emergency Services: No
Phone: 650-742-2000
Fax: 888-805-7562
Accredited: Yes
Licensed Beds: 127

Key Personnel:

Chief Medical Staff. . . . . Laurie Weisberg, MD
Director Infection/Disease Control . . . . Ronald Tempesta, MD

NOTE: Hospital profiles are in alphabetical order by state, then city, then hospital within the city; Rankings are sorted by rate in descending order and exclude hospitals with less than 25 cases; (1) The number of cases is too small (n<25) for purposes of reliably predicting hospital performance; (2) Measure reflects the hospital's indication that its submission was based upon a sample of its relevant discharges; (3) Rate reflects fewer than the maximum possible quarters of data for the measure; (4) Inaccurate information submitted and suppressed for one or more quarters; (5) No data is available from the hospital for this measure; Please refer to the User's Guide for a full explanation of data

Chief OB/GYN .... Vincent Fausone, MD
Chief Radiology .... Herbert Steinhardt, MD
Director Respiratory Therapy .... Phil Mendoga

Measure	Cases	This Hospital	State Average	U.S. Average	Top Hospital
Heart Attack Care					
ACE Inhibitor or ARB for LVSD[1]	14	86%	82%	82%	100%
Aspirin at Arrival	123	98%	95%	92%	100%
Aspirin at Discharge	38	97%	90%	90%	100%
Beta Blocker at Arrival	83	100%	89%	87%	100%
Beta Blocker at Discharge	39	100%	89%	90%	100%
Fibrinolytic Medication Timing[1]	17	88%	40%	31%	100%
PCI Within 90 Minutes of Arrival	0	-	52%	54%	95%
Smoking Cessation Advice[1]	2	100%	87%	88%	100%
Heart Failure Care					
ACE Inhibitor or ARB for LVSD	70	90%	84%	82%	100%
Discharge Instructions	210	64%	56%	61%	93%
Evaluation of LVS Function	232	99%	84%	83%	99%
Smoking Cessation Advice	48	77%	82%	82%	100%
Pneumonia Care					
Appropriate Initial Antibiotic	108	81%	82%	83%	94%
Blood Culture Timing	112	94%	89%	90%	100%
Influenza Vaccine	25	64%	58%	70%	100%
Initial Antibiotic Timing	142	84%	75%	80%	93%
Oxygenation Assessment	179	100%	99%	99%	100%
Pneumococcal Vaccine	134	90%	58%	69%	94%
Smoking Cessation Advice[1]	22	45%	75%	80%	100%
Surgical Infection Prevention					
Prophylactic Antibiotic Given	282	97%	74%	77%	95%
Prophylactic Antibiotic Selection	58	95%	89%	90%	100%
Prophylactic Antibiotic Stopped	274	89%	65%	72%	95%
Pregnancy Care					
Inpatient Neonatal Mortality	-	-	-	-	-
Third or Fourth Degree Laceration	-	-	3.58%	3.63%	3.27%

Stanford Hospital

300 Pasteur Drive
Stanford, CA 94305
Phone: 650-723-4000
Fax: 650-723-0074
URL: www.stanfordhospital.com
Ownership: Voluntary non-profit - Private
Accredited: Yes
Emergency Services: Yes
Licensed Beds: 613

Key Personnel:
President/CEO .... Martha Marsh
Chief Medical Staff .... Larry Shuer, MD

Measure	Cases	This Hospital	State Average	U.S. Average	Top Hospital
Heart Attack Care					
ACE Inhibitor or ARB for LVSD[2]	37	86%	82%	82%	100%
Aspirin at Arrival[2]	158	99%	95%	92%	100%
Aspirin at Discharge[2]	215	99%	90%	90%	100%
Beta Blocker at Arrival[2]	115	96%	89%	87%	100%
Beta Blocker at Discharge[2]	185	98%	89%	90%	100%
Fibrinolytic Medication Timing[2]	0	-	40%	31%	100%
PCI Within 90 Minutes of Arrival[1,2]	6	33%	52%	54%	95%
Smoking Cessation Advice[2]	33	94%	87%	88%	100%
Heart Failure Care					
ACE Inhibitor or ARB for LVSD	150	87%	84%	82%	100%
Discharge Instructions	288	83%	56%	61%	93%
Evaluation of LVS Function	339	99%	84%	83%	99%
Smoking Cessation Advice	25	72%	82%	82%	100%
Pneumonia Care					
Appropriate Initial Antibiotic	178	80%	82%	83%	94%
Blood Culture Timing	199	95%	89%	90%	100%
Influenza Vaccine	47	89%	58%	70%	100%
Initial Antibiotic Timing	259	68%	75%	80%	93%
Oxygenation Assessment	351	100%	99%	99%	100%
Pneumococcal Vaccine	223	80%	58%	69%	94%
Smoking Cessation Advice	29	83%	75%	80%	100%
Surgical Infection Prevention					
Prophylactic Antibiotic Given[2,3]	110	79%	74%	77%	95%
Prophylactic Antibiotic Selection[2]	68	99%	89%	90%	100%
Prophylactic Antibiotic Stopped[2,3]	102	67%	65%	72%	95%
Pregnancy Care					
Inpatient Neonatal Mortality	-	-	-	-	-
Third or Fourth Degree Laceration	-	-	3.58%	3.63%	3.27%

Dameron Hospital

525 West Acacia Street
Stockton, CA 95203
Phone: 209-944-5550
Fax: 209-461-7578
E-mail: info@dameronhospital.org
URL: www.dameronhospital.org
Ownership: Voluntary non-profit - Other
Accredited: Yes
Emergency Services: Yes
Licensed Beds: 188

Key Personnel:
President/CEO .... Christopher Arismendi, MD
Chief Medical Staff .... Robert Lawrence, MD
Catheterization Lab .... Chris Peterson
Director Emergency Room .... Kathy Tedford, RN
CCU Nurse Manager .... Pattia Rocero, RN
Nurse Manager Surgical .... Lynn Renwick, RN
Nurse Manager OB/GYN .... Sherry Rufert
Director Radiology .... Thomas Beck
Director Respiratory Therapy .... Joyce Barber

Measure	Cases	This Hospital	State Average	U.S. Average	Top Hospital
Heart Attack Care					
ACE Inhibitor or ARB for LVSD[1]	19	95%	82%	82%	100%
Aspirin at Arrival	148	98%	95%	92%	100%
Aspirin at Discharge	145	91%	90%	90%	100%
Beta Blocker at Arrival	48	94%	89%	87%	100%
Beta Blocker at Discharge	62	95%	89%	90%	100%
Fibrinolytic Medication Timing[1]	16	44%	40%	31%	100%
PCI Within 90 Minutes of Arrival[1]	1	0%	52%	54%	95%
Smoking Cessation Advice	58	91%	87%	88%	100%
Heart Failure Care					
ACE Inhibitor or ARB for LVSD	93	91%	84%	82%	100%
Discharge Instructions	238	82%	56%	61%	93%
Evaluation of LVS Function	297	85%	84%	83%	99%
Smoking Cessation Advice	47	87%	82%	82%	100%
Pneumonia Care					
Appropriate Initial Antibiotic	121	93%	82%	83%	94%
Blood Culture Timing	121	72%	89%	90%	100%
Influenza Vaccine	38	34%	58%	70%	100%
Initial Antibiotic Timing	201	82%	75%	80%	93%
Oxygenation Assessment	221	100%	99%	99%	100%
Pneumococcal Vaccine	138	33%	58%	69%	94%
Smoking Cessation Advice	31	81%	75%	80%	100%
Surgical Infection Prevention					
Prophylactic Antibiotic Given[3]	289	40%	74%	77%	95%
Prophylactic Antibiotic Selection	45	84%	89%	90%	100%
Prophylactic Antibiotic Stopped[3]	259	48%	65%	72%	95%
Pregnancy Care					
Inpatient Neonatal Mortality	-	-	-	-	-
Third or Fourth Degree Laceration	-	-	3.58%	3.63%	3.27%

Saint Joseph's Medical Center of Stockton

1800 N California Street
Stockton, CA 95204
Phone: 209-943-2000
Fax: 209-461-3299
URL: www.stjospehscares.org
Ownership: Voluntary non-profit - Church
Accredited: Yes
Emergency Services: Yes
Licensed Beds: 294

Key Personnel:
President .... Donald Wiley
Chief Medical Staff .... Masanobu Kamigaki, MD
OB/GYN Womens Health .... David Eibling, MD
Chief Radiology .... Jack Funamura, MD
Manager Respiratory Therapy .... Robert Wright

Measure	Cases	This Hospital	State Average	U.S. Average	Top Hospital
Heart Attack Care					
ACE Inhibitor or ARB for LVSD	48	94%	82%	82%	100%
Aspirin at Arrival	185	98%	95%	92%	100%
Aspirin at Discharge	270	99%	90%	90%	100%
Beta Blocker at Arrival	122	98%	89%	87%	100%
Beta Blocker at Discharge	261	99%	89%	90%	100%

NOTE: Hospital profiles are in alphabetical order by state, then city, then hospital within the city; Rankings are sorted by rate in descending order and exclude hospitals with less than 25 cases; (1) The number of cases is too small (n<25) for purposes of reliably predicting hospital performance; (2) Measure reflects the hospital's indication that its submission was based upon a sample of its relevant discharges; (3) Rate reflects fewer than the maximum possible quarters of data for the measure; (4) Inaccurate information submitted and suppressed for one or more quarters; (5) No data is available from the hospital for this measure; Please refer to the User's Guide for a full explanation of data

Fibrinolytic Medication Timing[1]	9	44%	40%	31%	100%
PCI Within 90 Minutes of Arrival[1]	9	78%	52%	54%	95%
Smoking Cessation Advice	106	99%	87%	88%	100%
Heart Failure Care					
ACE Inhibitor or ARB for LVSD[2]	119	96%	84%	82%	100%
Discharge Instructions[2]	216	74%	56%	61%	93%
Evaluation of LVS Function[2]	296	99%	84%	83%	99%
Smoking Cessation Advice[2]	43	100%	82%	82%	100%
Pneumonia Care					
Appropriate Initial Antibiotic[2]	126	94%	82%	83%	94%
Blood Culture Timing[2]	114	93%	89%	90%	100%
Influenza Vaccine[1,2]	24	79%	58%	70%	100%
Initial Antibiotic Timing[2]	154	77%	75%	80%	93%
Oxygenation Assessment[2]	186	100%	99%	99%	100%
Pneumococcal Vaccine[2]	118	91%	58%	69%	94%
Smoking Cessation Advice[2]	35	97%	75%	80%	100%
Surgical Infection Prevention					
Prophylactic Antibiotic Given[2,3]	189	95%	74%	77%	95%
Prophylactic Antibiotic Selection[2]	64	88%	89%	90%	100%
Prophylactic Antibiotic Stopped[2,3]	185	59%	65%	72%	95%
Pregnancy Care					
Inpatient Neonatal Mortality	-	-	-	-	-
Third or Fourth Degree Laceration	-	-	3.58%	3.63%	3.27%

Menifee Valley Medical Center

Alternate Name: Hemet Valley Hospital District
28400 McCall Boulevard — Phone: 951-679-8888
Sun City, CA 92585 — Fax: 951-672-7050
Ownership: Govt - Hospital District or Authority — Accredited: Yes
Emergency Services: Yes — Licensed Beds: 84

Key Personnel:

CEO . . . . Jerry Lane
Chief Medical Staff . . . . Ratan Tiwari
Emergency Room . . . . Linda Dekiewiet
Director Medical/Surgical Nursing . . . . Kim Eastman, RN
Chief Radiology . . . . Alan Mare, MD
Respiratory Chief . . . . Roy Miller

Measure	Cases	This Hospital	State Average	U.S. Average	Top Hospital
Heart Attack Care					
ACE Inhibitor or ARB for LVSD[1]	14	71%	82%	82%	100%
Aspirin at Arrival	150	93%	95%	92%	100%
Aspirin at Discharge	52	81%	90%	90%	100%
Beta Blocker at Arrival	143	87%	89%	87%	100%
Beta Blocker at Discharge	75	80%	89%	90%	100%
Fibrinolytic Medication Timing[1]	19	53%	40%	31%	100%
PCI Within 90 Minutes of Arrival	0	-	52%	54%	95%
Smoking Cessation Advice[1]	10	80%	87%	88%	100%
Heart Failure Care					
ACE Inhibitor or ARB for LVSD	76	71%	84%	82%	100%
Discharge Instructions	220	52%	56%	61%	93%
Evaluation of LVS Function	248	87%	84%	83%	99%
Smoking Cessation Advice	40	78%	82%	82%	100%
Pneumonia Care					
Appropriate Initial Antibiotic	158	78%	82%	83%	94%
Blood Culture Timing	142	87%	89%	90%	100%
Influenza Vaccine	52	52%	58%	70%	100%
Initial Antibiotic Timing	221	71%	75%	80%	93%
Oxygenation Assessment	295	100%	99%	99%	100%
Pneumococcal Vaccine	211	42%	58%	69%	94%
Smoking Cessation Advice	45	89%	75%	80%	100%
Surgical Infection Prevention					
Prophylactic Antibiotic Given[1,3]	18	67%	74%	77%	95%
Prophylactic Antibiotic Selection[1]	19	42%	89%	90%	100%
Prophylactic Antibiotic Stopped[1,3]	16	0%	65%	72%	95%
Pregnancy Care					
Inpatient Neonatal Mortality	-	-	-	-	-
Third or Fourth Degree Laceration	-	-	3.58%	3.63%	3.27%

Pacifica Hospital of the Valley

9449 San Fernando Road — Phone: 818-767-3310
Sun Valley, CA 91352 — Fax: 818-252-2439
URL: www.pacificahospital.com
Ownership: Proprietary — Accredited: Yes
Emergency Services: Yes — Licensed Beds: 248

Key Personnel:

CEO . . . . SK Durairaj
Chief Medical Staff . . . . Allison Cunning
Emergency Room . . . . Jannet Latto
Chief Radiology . . . . Alberto Salcedo, MD
Director Respiratory Therapy . . . . Nelly Escudero

Measure	Cases	This Hospital	State Average	U.S. Average	Top Hospital
Heart Attack Care					
ACE Inhibitor or ARB for LVSD[1]	2	100%	82%	82%	100%
Aspirin at Arrival	42	93%	95%	92%	100%
Aspirin at Discharge[1]	15	87%	90%	90%	100%
Beta Blocker at Arrival	36	86%	89%	87%	100%
Beta Blocker at Discharge[1]	15	80%	89%	90%	100%
Fibrinolytic Medication Timing[1,3]	3	67%	40%	31%	100%
PCI Within 90 Minutes of Arrival	0	-	52%	54%	95%
Smoking Cessation Advice[1,3]	1	100%	87%	88%	100%
Heart Failure Care					
ACE Inhibitor or ARB for LVSD[1,2]	11	91%	84%	82%	100%
Discharge Instructions[1,2,3]	13	46%	56%	61%	93%
Evaluation of LVS Function[2]	83	93%	84%	83%	99%
Smoking Cessation Advice[1,2,3]	4	75%	82%	82%	100%
Pneumonia Care					
Appropriate Initial Antibiotic[1,3]	8	62%	82%	83%	94%
Blood Culture Timing[1,3]	10	80%	89%	90%	100%
Influenza Vaccine[5]	-	-	58%	70%	100%
Initial Antibiotic Timing	98	73%	75%	80%	93%
Oxygenation Assessment	102	100%	99%	99%	100%
Pneumococcal Vaccine	47	28%	58%	69%	94%
Smoking Cessation Advice[1,3]	6	33%	75%	80%	100%
Surgical Infection Prevention					
Prophylactic Antibiotic Given[1,2,3]	19	89%	74%	77%	95%
Prophylactic Antibiotic Selection[5]	-	-	89%	90%	100%
Prophylactic Antibiotic Stopped[1,2,3]	18	100%	65%	72%	95%
Pregnancy Care					
Inpatient Neonatal Mortality	-	-	-	-	-
Third or Fourth Degree Laceration	-	-	3.58%	3.63%	3.27%

Banner Lassen Medical Center

1800 Spring Ridge Drive — Phone: 530-252-2000
Susanville, CA 96130
Ownership: Proprietary — Accredited: Yes
Emergency Services: Yes

Measure	Cases	This Hospital	State Average	U.S. Average	Top Hospital
Heart Attack Care					
ACE Inhibitor or ARB for LVSD[1,3]	2	100%	82%	82%	100%
Aspirin at Arrival[1,3]	4	100%	95%	92%	100%
Aspirin at Discharge[1,3]	2	100%	90%	90%	100%
Beta Blocker at Arrival[1,3]	4	75%	89%	87%	100%
Beta Blocker at Discharge[1,3]	3	100%	89%	90%	100%
Fibrinolytic Medication Timing[1,3]	1	0%	40%	31%	100%
PCI Within 90 Minutes of Arrival	0	-	52%	54%	95%
Smoking Cessation Advice[1,3]	1	100%	87%	88%	100%
Heart Failure Care					
ACE Inhibitor or ARB for LVSD[1]	12	100%	84%	82%	100%
Discharge Instructions[1]	15	100%	56%	61%	93%
Evaluation of LVS Function[1]	20	100%	84%	83%	99%
Smoking Cessation Advice[1]	2	100%	82%	82%	100%
Pneumonia Care					
Appropriate Initial Antibiotic	45	87%	82%	83%	94%
Blood Culture Timing[1]	6	100%	89%	90%	100%
Influenza Vaccine[1]	7	100%	58%	70%	100%
Initial Antibiotic Timing[1]	11	100%	75%	80%	93%
Oxygenation Assessment	46	100%	99%	99%	100%
Pneumococcal Vaccine[1]	22	95%	58%	69%	94%

NOTE: Hospital profiles are in alphabetical order by state, then city, then hospital within the city; Rankings are sorted by rate in descending order and exclude hospitals with less than 25 cases; (1) The number of cases is too small (n<25) for purposes of reliably predicting hospital performance; (2) Measure reflects the hospital's indication that its submission was based upon a sample of its relevant discharges; (3) Rate reflects fewer than the maximum possible quarters of data for the measure; (4) Inaccurate information submitted and suppressed for one or more quarters; (5) No data is available from the hospital for this measure; Please refer to the User's Guide for a full explanation of data

Smoking Cessation Advice[1]	12	100%	75%	80%	100%
Surgical Infection Prevention					
Prophylactic Antibiotic Given[1,3]	10	50%	74%	77%	95%
Prophylactic Antibiotic Selection[1]	1	100%	89%	90%	100%
Prophylactic Antibiotic Stopped[1,3]	9	67%	65%	72%	95%
Pregnancy Care					
Inpatient Neonatal Mortality	-	-	-	-	-
Third or Fourth Degree Laceration	-	-	3.58%	3.63%	3.27%

Olive View-UCLA Medical Center

14445 Olive View Drive
San Fernando, CA 91342
Phone: 818-364-1555
Fax: 818-364-4206
URL: www.ladhs.org
Ownership: Government - Local
Accredited: Yes
Emergency Services: Yes
Licensed Beds: 377

Key Personnel:

Interim CEO . . . . Gretchen McGinley
Chief Medical Staff. . . . . Irwin Ziment, MD
Emergency Room . . . . David Talan, MD
Director Infection/Disease Control . . . . Glenn Mathison, MD
OB/GYN Womens Health. . . . . Howard L Judd, MD
Chief Radiology . . . . Ramesh Verma, MD

Measure	Cases	This Hospital	State Average	U.S. Average	Top Hospital
Heart Attack Care					
ACE Inhibitor or ARB for LVSD[1]	8	100%	82%	82%	100%
Aspirin at Arrival	104	99%	95%	92%	100%
Aspirin at Discharge	27	96%	90%	90%	100%
Beta Blocker at Arrival	90	98%	89%	87%	100%
Beta Blocker at Discharge	25	92%	89%	90%	100%
Fibrinolytic Medication Timing[1,3]	1	0%	40%	31%	100%
PCI Within 90 Minutes of Arrival	0	-	52%	54%	95%
Smoking Cessation Advice[1,3]	1	0%	87%	88%	100%
Heart Failure Care					
ACE Inhibitor or ARB for LVSD[2]	147	97%	84%	82%	100%
Discharge Instructions[2,3]	58	43%	56%	61%	93%
Evaluation of LVS Function[2]	297	99%	84%	83%	99%
Smoking Cessation Advice[1,2,3]	18	50%	82%	82%	100%
Pneumonia Care					
Appropriate Initial Antibiotic[1,2,3]	21	71%	82%	83%	94%
Blood Culture Timing[2,3]	30	63%	89%	90%	100%
Influenza Vaccine[5]	-	-	58%	70%	100%
Initial Antibiotic Timing[2]	158	61%	75%	80%	93%
Oxygenation Assessment[2]	178	100%	99%	99%	100%
Pneumococcal Vaccine[2]	70	33%	58%	69%	94%
Smoking Cessation Advice[1,2,3]	7	57%	75%	80%	100%
Surgical Infection Prevention					
Prophylactic Antibiotic Given[1,2,3]	22	82%	74%	77%	95%
Prophylactic Antibiotic Selection[5]	-	-	89%	90%	100%
Prophylactic Antibiotic Stopped[1,2,3]	22	91%	65%	72%	95%
Pregnancy Care					
Inpatient Neonatal Mortality	-	-	-	-	-
Third or Fourth Degree Laceration	-	-	3.58%	3.63%	3.27%

Encino-Tarzana Regional Medical Center

18321 Clark Street
Tarzana, CA 91356
Phone: 818-881-0800
Fax: 818-708-5565
E-mail: ETRMCPublicRelations@tenethealth.com
URL: www.encino-tarzana.com
Ownership: Proprietary
Accredited: Yes
Emergency Services: Yes
Licensed Beds: 396

Key Personnel:

CEO. . . . . Dale Surowitz
Chief Medical Officer . . . . Dr Jennifer Daly
VP Medical/Surgical Nursing . . . . Katie Walter, RN
OB/GYN Womens Health. . . . . Eugene Y Gootnick, MD
Chief Radiology . . . . Leroy Clark, MD
Director Respiratory Therapy . . . . George Torres

Measure	Cases	This Hospital	State Average	U.S. Average	Top Hospital
Heart Attack Care					
ACE Inhibitor or ARB for LVSD	47	89%	82%	82%	100%
Aspirin at Arrival	179	94%	95%	92%	100%
Aspirin at Discharge	209	88%	90%	90%	100%
Beta Blocker at Arrival	158	86%	89%	87%	100%
Beta Blocker at Discharge	206	85%	89%	90%	100%
Fibrinolytic Medication Timing	0	-	40%	31%	100%
PCI Within 90 Minutes of Arrival[1]	11	36%	52%	54%	95%
Smoking Cessation Advice	41	93%	87%	88%	100%
Heart Failure Care					
ACE Inhibitor or ARB for LVSD	130	82%	84%	82%	100%
Discharge Instructions	281	68%	56%	61%	93%
Evaluation of LVS Function	326	93%	84%	83%	99%
Smoking Cessation Advice[1]	16	75%	82%	82%	100%
Pneumonia Care					
Appropriate Initial Antibiotic	200	88%	82%	83%	94%
Blood Culture Timing	218	81%	89%	90%	100%
Influenza Vaccine	75	55%	58%	70%	100%
Initial Antibiotic Timing	246	83%	75%	80%	93%
Oxygenation Assessment	344	100%	99%	99%	100%
Pneumococcal Vaccine	246	55%	58%	69%	94%
Smoking Cessation Advice[1]	14	57%	75%	80%	100%
Surgical Infection Prevention					
Prophylactic Antibiotic Given[2]	152	73%	74%	77%	95%
Prophylactic Antibiotic Selection[2]	56	80%	89%	90%	100%
Prophylactic Antibiotic Stopped[2]	146	56%	65%	72%	95%
Pregnancy Care					
Inpatient Neonatal Mortality	-	-	-	-	-
Third or Fourth Degree Laceration	-	-	3.58%	3.63%	3.27%

Tehachapi Valley Healthcare District

Alternate Name: Tehachapi Hospital
115 W E Street
PO Box 1900
Tehachapi, CA 93581
Phone: 661-823-3000
Fax: 661-823-3081
E-mail: LMizumoto@tvhd.org
URL: www.tvhd.org
Ownership: Govt - Hospital District or Authority
Accredited: No
Emergency Services: Yes
Licensed Beds: 28

Key Personnel:

President . . . . Sam Conklin, MD
CEO. . . . . Robert Duncan
Respiratory Therapy. . . . . Sherman Croiset, RRT

Measure	Cases	This Hospital	State Average	U.S. Average	Top Hospital
Heart Attack Care					
ACE Inhibitor or ARB for LVSD[5]	-	-	82%	82%	100%
Aspirin at Arrival[5]	-	-	95%	92%	100%
Aspirin at Discharge[5]	-	-	90%	90%	100%
Beta Blocker at Arrival[5]	-	-	89%	87%	100%
Beta Blocker at Discharge[5]	-	-	89%	90%	100%
Fibrinolytic Medication Timing[5]	-	-	40%	31%	100%
PCI Within 90 Minutes of Arrival[5]	-	-	52%	54%	95%
Smoking Cessation Advice[5]	-	-	87%	88%	100%
Heart Failure Care					
ACE Inhibitor or ARB for LVSD[3]	0	-	84%	82%	100%
Discharge Instructions[1,3]	1	0%	56%	61%	93%
Evaluation of LVS Function[1,3]	1	0%	84%	83%	99%
Smoking Cessation Advice[3]	0	-	82%	82%	100%
Pneumonia Care					
Appropriate Initial Antibiotic[1,3]	12	92%	82%	83%	94%
Blood Culture Timing[1,3]	2	50%	89%	90%	100%
Influenza Vaccine	0	-	58%	70%	100%
Initial Antibiotic Timing[1,3]	9	100%	75%	80%	93%
Oxygenation Assessment[1,3]	13	100%	99%	99%	100%
Pneumococcal Vaccine[1,3]	7	14%	58%	69%	94%
Smoking Cessation Advice[1,3]	1	0%	75%	80%	100%
Surgical Infection Prevention					
Prophylactic Antibiotic Given[5]	-	-	74%	77%	95%
Prophylactic Antibiotic Selection[5]	-	-	89%	90%	100%
Prophylactic Antibiotic Stopped[5]	-	-	65%	72%	95%
Pregnancy Care					
Inpatient Neonatal Mortality	-	-	-	-	-
Third or Fourth Degree Laceration	-	-	3.58%	3.63%	3.27%

NOTE: Hospital profiles are in alphabetical order by state, then city, then hospital within the city; Rankings are sorted by rate in descending order and exclude hospitals with less than 25 cases; (1) The number of cases is too small (n<25) for purposes of reliably predicting hospital performance; (2) Measure reflects the hospital's indication that its submission was based upon a sample of its relevant discharges; (3) Rate reflects fewer than the maximum possible quarters of data for the measure; (4) Inaccurate information submitted and suppressed for one or more quarters; (5) No data is available from the hospital for this measure; Please refer to the User's Guide for a full explanation of data

Twin Cities Community Hospital

1100 Las Tablas Road
Templeton, CA 93465
URL: www.twincitieshospital.com
Ownership: Proprietary
Emergency Services: Yes
Phone: 805-434-3500
Fax: 805-434-2913
Accredited: Yes
Licensed Beds: 84

Key Personnel:
CEO . . . . . Richard D Lyons
Chief Medical Staff . . . . . Keven Colton
Catheterization Lab . . . . . Charlie Tagawa
Emergency Room . . . . . Beth Haberkern, RN
Infection Control . . . . . Jeanette Tosh
ICU . . . . . Doris Warren, RN
Medical/Surgical Nursing . . . . . Robert Cook, RN
OB/GYN/Womens Health . . . . . Ann Miller
Respiratory Therapy Director . . . . . Brad Kilavease

Measure	Cases	This Hospital	State Average	U.S. Average	Top Hospital
Heart Attack Care					
ACE Inhibitor or ARB for LVSD[1]	5	80%	82%	82%	100%
Aspirin at Arrival	35	97%	95%	92%	100%
Aspirin at Discharge[1]	19	95%	90%	90%	100%
Beta Blocker at Arrival	33	88%	89%	87%	100%
Beta Blocker at Discharge[1]	20	90%	89%	90%	100%
Fibrinolytic Medication Timing	0	-	40%	31%	100%
PCI Within 90 Minutes of Arrival	0	-	52%	54%	95%
Smoking Cessation Advice	0	-	87%	88%	100%
Heart Failure Care					
ACE Inhibitor or ARB for LVSD	41	83%	84%	82%	100%
Discharge Instructions	123	93%	56%	61%	93%
Evaluation of LVS Function	142	97%	84%	83%	99%
Smoking Cessation Advice[1]	10	100%	82%	82%	100%
Pneumonia Care					
Appropriate Initial Antibiotic	100	90%	82%	83%	94%
Blood Culture Timing	100	94%	89%	90%	100%
Influenza Vaccine	30	100%	58%	70%	100%
Initial Antibiotic Timing	153	90%	75%	80%	93%
Oxygenation Assessment	176	99%	99%	99%	100%
Pneumococcal Vaccine	130	98%	58%	69%	94%
Smoking Cessation Advice	35	94%	75%	80%	100%
Surgical Infection Prevention					
Prophylactic Antibiotic Given[2]	375	83%	74%	77%	95%
Prophylactic Antibiotic Selection[2]	86	93%	89%	90%	100%
Prophylactic Antibiotic Stopped[2]	351	91%	65%	72%	95%
Pregnancy Care					
Inpatient Neonatal Mortality	-	-	-	-	-
Third or Fourth Degree Laceration	-	-	3.58%	3.63%	3.27%

Los Robles Regional Medical Center

215 West Janss Road
Thousand Oaks, CA 91360
URL: www.losrobleshospital.com
Ownership: Proprietary
Emergency Services: Yes
Phone: 805-497-2727
Fax: 805-370-4813
Accredited: Yes
Licensed Beds: 265

Key Personnel:
CEO . . . . . Robert Shaw
Chief Medical Staff . . . . . David Newman, MD
Emergency Room . . . . . Ellen Connors
Infection Control . . . . . Diane Duff, RN
Intensive Coronary . . . . . Lisa Shaper, RN
OB/GYN Women's Health . . . . . Ronald dela Pena, MD
Chief Radiology . . . . . TJ Turkat, MD
Director Respiratory Therapy . . . . . Verne Arnold

Measure	Cases	This Hospital	State Average	U.S. Average	Top Hospital
Heart Attack Care					
ACE Inhibitor or ARB for LVSD	53	77%	82%	82%	100%
Aspirin at Arrival	202	89%	95%	92%	100%
Aspirin at Discharge	212	90%	90%	90%	100%
Beta Blocker at Arrival	147	80%	89%	87%	100%
Beta Blocker at Discharge	207	88%	89%	90%	100%
Fibrinolytic Medication Timing	0	-	40%	31%	100%
PCI Within 90 Minutes of Arrival[1]	16	56%	52%	54%	95%
Smoking Cessation Advice	48	94%	87%	88%	100%
Heart Failure Care					
ACE Inhibitor or ARB for LVSD	89	74%	84%	82%	100%
Discharge Instructions	205	64%	56%	61%	93%
Evaluation of LVS Function	232	91%	84%	83%	99%
Smoking Cessation Advice	27	85%	82%	82%	100%
Pneumonia Care					
Appropriate Initial Antibiotic	189	84%	82%	83%	94%
Blood Culture Timing	205	86%	89%	90%	100%
Influenza Vaccine	82	33%	58%	70%	100%
Initial Antibiotic Timing	270	69%	75%	80%	93%
Oxygenation Assessment	350	100%	99%	99%	100%
Pneumococcal Vaccine	233	40%	58%	69%	94%
Smoking Cessation Advice	44	68%	75%	80%	100%
Surgical Infection Prevention					
Prophylactic Antibiotic Given[2,3]	254	66%	74%	77%	95%
Prophylactic Antibiotic Selection[2]	115	95%	89%	90%	100%
Prophylactic Antibiotic Stopped[2,3]	245	67%	65%	72%	95%
Pregnancy Care					
Inpatient Neonatal Mortality	-	-	-	-	-
Third or Fourth Degree Laceration	-	-	3.58%	3.63%	3.27%

Thousand Oaks Surgical Hospital

401 Rolling Oaks Drive
Thousand Oaks, CA 91361
Ownership: Proprietary
Emergency Services: No
Phone: 805-777-7750
Accredited: No

Measure	Cases	This Hospital	State Average	U.S. Average	Top Hospital
Heart Attack Care					
ACE Inhibitor or ARB for LVSD[5]	-	-	82%	82%	100%
Aspirin at Arrival[5]	-	-	95%	92%	100%
Aspirin at Discharge[5]	-	-	90%	90%	100%
Beta Blocker at Arrival[5]	-	-	89%	87%	100%
Beta Blocker at Discharge[5]	-	-	89%	90%	100%
Fibrinolytic Medication Timing[5]	-	-	40%	31%	100%
PCI Within 90 Minutes of Arrival[5]	-	-	52%	54%	95%
Smoking Cessation Advice[5]	-	-	87%	88%	100%
Heart Failure Care					
ACE Inhibitor or ARB for LVSD[5]	-	-	84%	82%	100%
Discharge Instructions[5]	-	-	56%	61%	93%
Evaluation of LVS Function[5]	-	-	84%	83%	99%
Smoking Cessation Advice[5]	-	-	82%	82%	100%
Pneumonia Care					
Appropriate Initial Antibiotic[5]	-	-	82%	83%	94%
Blood Culture Timing[5]	-	-	89%	90%	100%
Influenza Vaccine[5]	-	-	58%	70%	100%
Initial Antibiotic Timing[5]	-	-	75%	80%	93%
Oxygenation Assessment[5]	-	-	99%	99%	100%
Pneumococcal Vaccine[5]	-	-	58%	69%	94%
Smoking Cessation Advice[5]	-	-	75%	80%	100%
Surgical Infection Prevention					
Prophylactic Antibiotic Given[2,3]	55	56%	74%	77%	95%
Prophylactic Antibiotic Selection[2]	44	91%	89%	90%	100%
Prophylactic Antibiotic Stopped[2,3]	53	87%	65%	72%	95%
Pregnancy Care					
Inpatient Neonatal Mortality	-	-	-	-	-
Third or Fourth Degree Laceration	-	-	3.58%	3.63%	3.27%

Little Company of Mary Hospital

4101 Torrance Boulevard
Torrance, CA 90503
URL: www.lcmhs.org
Ownership: Voluntary non-profit - Church
Emergency Services: Yes
Phone: 310-540-7676
Fax: 310-540-8408
Accredited: Yes

Key Personnel:
Administrator . . . . . Michael Hunn
Director Medical/Surgical Nursing . . . . . Kathy Harren
OB/GYN Womens Health . . . . . Ricardo Huete
Chief Radiology . . . . . Lee Secrist
Director Respiratory Therapy . . . . . Pam Michael

NOTE: Hospital profiles are in alphabetical order by state, then city, then hospital within the city; Rankings are sorted by rate in descending order and exclude hospitals with less than 25 cases; (1) The number of cases is too small (n<25) for purposes of reliably predicting hospital performance; (2) Measure reflects the hospital's indication that its submission was based upon a sample of its relevant discharges; (3) Rate reflects fewer than the maximum possible quarters of data for the measure; (4) Inaccurate information submitted and suppressed for one or more quarters; (5) No data is available from the hospital for this measure; Please refer to the User's Guide for a full explanation of data

Measure	Cases	This Hospital	State Average	U.S. Average	Top Hospital
Heart Attack Care					
ACE Inhibitor or ARB for LVSD	43	93%	82%	82%	100%
Aspirin at Arrival	246	100%	95%	92%	100%
Aspirin at Discharge	268	99%	90%	90%	100%
Beta Blocker at Arrival	209	99%	89%	87%	100%
Beta Blocker at Discharge	260	99%	89%	90%	100%
Fibrinolytic Medication Timing	0	-	40%	31%	100%
PCI Within 90 Minutes of Arrival[1]	11	45%	52%	54%	95%
Smoking Cessation Advice	66	98%	87%	88%	100%
Heart Failure Care					
ACE Inhibitor or ARB for LVSD	169	88%	84%	82%	100%
Discharge Instructions	349	87%	56%	61%	93%
Evaluation of LVS Function	501	95%	84%	83%	99%
Smoking Cessation Advice	42	100%	82%	82%	100%
Pneumonia Care					
Appropriate Initial Antibiotic	172	86%	82%	83%	94%
Blood Culture Timing	239	95%	89%	90%	100%
Influenza Vaccine	67	85%	58%	70%	100%
Initial Antibiotic Timing	290	82%	75%	80%	93%
Oxygenation Assessment	411	100%	99%	99%	100%
Pneumococcal Vaccine	285	86%	58%	69%	94%
Smoking Cessation Advice	51	98%	75%	80%	100%
Surgical Infection Prevention					
Prophylactic Antibiotic Given[2]	644	90%	74%	77%	95%
Prophylactic Antibiotic Selection[2]	157	92%	89%	90%	100%
Prophylactic Antibiotic Stopped[2]	618	65%	65%	72%	95%
Pregnancy Care					
Inpatient Neonatal Mortality	-	-	-	-	-
Third or Fourth Degree Laceration	-	-	3.58%	3.63%	3.27%

Los Angeles County Harbor-UCLA Medical Center

1000 W Carson Street
Torrance, CA 90509
Phone: 310-222-2345
Fax: 310-328-8450
URL: www.harbor-ucla.org
Ownership: Government - Local
Accredited: Yes
Emergency Services: Yes
Licensed Beds: 553

Key Personnel:

CEO. . . . . Tecla A Mickoseff
Chairman Emergency Room . . . . Robert Hockberger, MD
Director Infection Control . . . . Joel Ward, MD
Chairman OB/GYN Department. . . . . Michael Ross, MD
Director Respiratory Therapy . . . . David Adams

Measure	Cases	This Hospital	State Average	U.S. Average	Top Hospital
Heart Attack Care					
ACE Inhibitor or ARB for LVSD	39	67%	82%	82%	100%
Aspirin at Arrival	145	97%	95%	92%	100%
Aspirin at Discharge	161	98%	90%	90%	100%
Beta Blocker at Arrival	130	96%	89%	87%	100%
Beta Blocker at Discharge	157	98%	89%	90%	100%
Fibrinolytic Medication Timing[1]	22	36%	40%	31%	100%
PCI Within 90 Minutes of Arrival[1]	7	14%	52%	54%	95%
Smoking Cessation Advice	68	87%	87%	88%	100%
Heart Failure Care					
ACE Inhibitor or ARB for LVSD[2]	198	83%	84%	82%	100%
Discharge Instructions[2]	323	69%	56%	61%	93%
Evaluation of LVS Function[2]	332	95%	84%	83%	99%
Smoking Cessation Advice[2]	111	89%	82%	82%	100%
Pneumonia Care					
Appropriate Initial Antibiotic[2]	132	82%	82%	83%	94%
Blood Culture Timing[2]	129	81%	89%	90%	100%
Influenza Vaccine[2]	28	71%	58%	70%	100%
Initial Antibiotic Timing[2]	175	54%	75%	80%	93%
Oxygenation Assessment[2]	205	100%	99%	99%	100%
Pneumococcal Vaccine[2]	72	61%	58%	69%	94%
Smoking Cessation Advice[2]	45	73%	75%	80%	100%
Surgical Infection Prevention					
Prophylactic Antibiotic Given[2,3]	232	88%	74%	77%	95%
Prophylactic Antibiotic Selection[2]	53	91%	89%	90%	100%
Prophylactic Antibiotic Stopped[2,3]	225	40%	65%	72%	95%
Pregnancy Care					
Inpatient Neonatal Mortality[2]	285	1.40%	-	-	-
Third or Fourth Degree Laceration	694	1.87%	3.58%	3.63%	3.27%

Torrance Memorial Medical Center

3330 Lomita Boulevard
Torrance, CA 90505
Phone: 310-325-9110
Fax: 310-784-4801
URL: www.torrancememorial.org
Ownership: Voluntary non-profit - Other
Accredited: Yes
Emergency Services: Yes
Licensed Beds: 335

Key Personnel:

CEO. . . . . George W Graham
Chief Medical Staff. . . . . William Averill, MD
Director Cardiology . . . . Peggy Gould
Emergency Room . . . . Judy Retter
OB/GYN Womens Health. . . . . Beni Naghi
Chief Radiology . . . . Richard Krauthamer, MD
Director Respiratory Therapy . . . . Debbie Lasseter

Measure	Cases	This Hospital	State Average	U.S. Average	Top Hospital
Heart Attack Care					
ACE Inhibitor or ARB for LVSD	58	76%	82%	82%	100%
Aspirin at Arrival	296	98%	95%	92%	100%
Aspirin at Discharge	287	93%	90%	90%	100%
Beta Blocker at Arrival	252	88%	89%	87%	100%
Beta Blocker at Discharge	283	92%	89%	90%	100%
Fibrinolytic Medication Timing[1]	1	0%	40%	31%	100%
PCI Within 90 Minutes of Arrival[1]	17	82%	52%	54%	95%
Smoking Cessation Advice	55	91%	87%	88%	100%
Heart Failure Care					
ACE Inhibitor or ARB for LVSD	279	83%	84%	82%	100%
Discharge Instructions	467	76%	56%	61%	93%
Evaluation of LVS Function	600	97%	84%	83%	99%
Smoking Cessation Advice	63	89%	82%	82%	100%
Pneumonia Care					
Appropriate Initial Antibiotic[2]	201	86%	82%	83%	94%
Blood Culture Timing[2]	181	93%	89%	90%	100%
Influenza Vaccine	86	5%	58%	70%	100%
Initial Antibiotic Timing[2]	299	83%	75%	80%	93%
Oxygenation Assessment[2]	394	100%	99%	99%	100%
Pneumococcal Vaccine[2]	282	37%	58%	69%	94%
Smoking Cessation Advice[2]	48	67%	75%	80%	100%
Surgical Infection Prevention					
Prophylactic Antibiotic Given[2,3]	225	91%	74%	77%	95%
Prophylactic Antibiotic Selection[2]	81	93%	89%	90%	100%
Prophylactic Antibiotic Stopped[2,3]	225	75%	65%	72%	95%
Pregnancy Care					
Inpatient Neonatal Mortality	-	-	-	-	-
Third or Fourth Degree Laceration	-	-	3.58%	3.63%	3.27%

Sutter Tracy Community Hospital

1420 N Tracy Boulevard
Tracy, CA 95376
Phone: 209-835-1500
Fax: 209-832-6091
E-mail: alonzot@sutterhealth.org
URL: www.suttertracy.org
Ownership: Voluntary non-profit - Other
Accredited: Yes
Emergency Services: Yes
Licensed Beds: 79

Key Personnel:

CEO. . . . . David M Thompson
Chief of Medical Staff. . . . . Janice Crawford, MD
Director of Cardiology/Cardiac Lab. . . . . Bill Preegan
Emergency Room . . . . Denise Drewry, RN
Director Medical/Surgical Nursing . . . . Kim Bailey, RN
OB/GYN Womens Health. . . . . Helene Novesteras, MD
Chief Radiology . . . . H Walt Pepper, MD
Director Respiratory Therapy . . . . Mina Whyle, RN

Measure	Cases	This Hospital	State Average	U.S. Average	Top Hospital
Heart Attack Care					
ACE Inhibitor or ARB for LVSD[1]	3	100%	82%	82%	100%
Aspirin at Arrival[1]	24	96%	95%	92%	100%
Aspirin at Discharge[1]	8	100%	90%	90%	100%
Beta Blocker at Arrival[1]	20	95%	89%	87%	100%
Beta Blocker at Discharge[1]	9	100%	89%	90%	100%

NOTE: Hospital profiles are in alphabetical order by state, then city, then hospital within the city; Rankings are sorted by rate in descending order and exclude hospitals with less than 25 cases; (1) The number of cases is too small (n<25) for purposes of reliably predicting hospital performance; (2) Measure reflects the hospital's indication that its submission was based upon a sample of its relevant discharges; (3) Rate reflects fewer than the maximum possible quarters of data for the measure; (4) Inaccurate information submitted and suppressed for one or more quarters; (5) No data is available from the hospital for this measure; Please refer to the User's Guide for a full explanation of data

Measure	Cases	This Hospital	State Average	U.S. Average	Top Hospital
Fibrinolytic Medication Timing	0	-	40%	31%	100%
PCI Within 90 Minutes of Arrival	0	-	52%	54%	95%
Smoking Cessation Advice[1]	1	100%	87%	88%	100%
Heart Failure Care					
ACE Inhibitor or ARB for LVSD	26	100%	84%	82%	100%
Discharge Instructions	100	72%	56%	61%	93%
Evaluation of LVS Function	115	93%	84%	83%	99%
Smoking Cessation Advice[1]	22	91%	82%	82%	100%
Pneumonia Care					
Appropriate Initial Antibiotic	106	81%	82%	83%	94%
Blood Culture Timing	57	93%	89%	90%	100%
Influenza Vaccine	38	63%	58%	70%	100%
Initial Antibiotic Timing	101	82%	75%	80%	93%
Oxygenation Assessment	146	100%	99%	99%	100%
Pneumococcal Vaccine	75	61%	58%	69%	94%
Smoking Cessation Advice	25	84%	75%	80%	100%
Surgical Infection Prevention					
Prophylactic Antibiotic Given[2]	130	82%	74%	77%	95%
Prophylactic Antibiotic Selection[2]	29	100%	89%	90%	100%
Prophylactic Antibiotic Stopped[2]	123	60%	65%	72%	95%
Pregnancy Care					
Inpatient Neonatal Mortality	-	-	-	-	-
Third or Fourth Degree Laceration	-	-	3.58%	3.63%	3.27%

Tahoe Forest Hospital

10121 Pine Avenue
PO Box 759
Truckee, CA 96160
Phone: 530-587-6011
Fax: 530-587-2532
E-mail: information@tfhd.com
URL: www.tfhd.com
Ownership: Govt - Hospital District or Authority
Accredited: No
Emergency Services: Yes
Licensed Beds: 72

Key Personnel:

CEO. . . . . Robert A Schapper
Emergency Department Head . . . . Bev Brink
Infection Control. . . . . Laurel Holmer, RN
Director Medical/Surgery . . . . Ann Holmes DelForge
OB/GYN Women's Health . . . . Ann Delforge
Surgical Services . . . . Linda Harman
Respiratory Therapy. . . . . Bob Tilton

Measure	Cases	This Hospital	State Average	U.S. Average	Top Hospital
Heart Attack Care					
ACE Inhibitor or ARB for LVSD	0	-	82%	82%	100%
Aspirin at Arrival[1]	3	100%	95%	92%	100%
Aspirin at Discharge[1]	1	100%	90%	90%	100%
Beta Blocker at Arrival[1]	3	100%	89%	87%	100%
Beta Blocker at Discharge[1]	1	100%	89%	90%	100%
Fibrinolytic Medication Timing[1,3]	1	100%	40%	31%	100%
PCI Within 90 Minutes of Arrival	0	-	52%	54%	95%
Smoking Cessation Advice[3]	0	-	87%	88%	100%
Heart Failure Care					
ACE Inhibitor or ARB for LVSD[1]	9	89%	84%	82%	100%
Discharge Instructions[1,3]	6	0%	56%	61%	93%
Evaluation of LVS Function	26	65%	84%	83%	99%
Smoking Cessation Advice[3]	0	-	82%	82%	100%
Pneumonia Care					
Appropriate Initial Antibiotic[1,3]	6	67%	82%	83%	94%
Blood Culture Timing[1,3]	3	100%	89%	90%	100%
Influenza Vaccine[5]	-	-	58%	70%	100%
Initial Antibiotic Timing[1]	11	91%	75%	80%	93%
Oxygenation Assessment	29	97%	99%	99%	100%
Pneumococcal Vaccine[1]	19	21%	58%	69%	94%
Smoking Cessation Advice[1,3]	2	0%	75%	80%	100%
Surgical Infection Prevention					
Prophylactic Antibiotic Given[5]	-	-	74%	77%	95%
Prophylactic Antibiotic Selection[5]	-	-	89%	90%	100%
Prophylactic Antibiotic Stopped[5]	-	-	65%	72%	95%
Pregnancy Care					
Inpatient Neonatal Mortality	-	-	-	-	-
Third or Fourth Degree Laceration	-	-	3.58%	3.63%	3.27%

Tulare District Hospital

869 Cherry Street
Tulare, CA 93274
Phone: 559-688-0821
Fax: 559-685-3875
Ownership: Govt - Hospital District or Authority
Accredited: Yes
Emergency Services: Yes

Key Personnel:

CEO. . . . . Robert Montain
Chief of Medical Staff. . . . . Denise Cerry
Director Respiratory Therapy . . . . Stephanie Moen

Measure	Cases	This Hospital	State Average	U.S. Average	Top Hospital
Heart Attack Care					
ACE Inhibitor or ARB for LVSD[1]	4	100%	82%	82%	100%
Aspirin at Arrival	55	100%	95%	92%	100%
Aspirin at Discharge[1]	19	100%	90%	90%	100%
Beta Blocker at Arrival	50	94%	89%	87%	100%
Beta Blocker at Discharge[1]	21	95%	89%	90%	100%
Fibrinolytic Medication Timing[1]	2	50%	40%	31%	100%
PCI Within 90 Minutes of Arrival	0	-	52%	54%	95%
Smoking Cessation Advice[1]	10	100%	87%	88%	100%
Heart Failure Care					
ACE Inhibitor or ARB for LVSD	59	97%	84%	82%	100%
Discharge Instructions	124	81%	56%	61%	93%
Evaluation of LVS Function	144	99%	84%	83%	99%
Smoking Cessation Advice[1]	21	100%	82%	82%	100%
Pneumonia Care					
Appropriate Initial Antibiotic	128	88%	82%	83%	94%
Blood Culture Timing	74	95%	89%	90%	100%
Influenza Vaccine	36	83%	58%	70%	100%
Initial Antibiotic Timing	158	76%	75%	80%	93%
Oxygenation Assessment	197	100%	99%	99%	100%
Pneumococcal Vaccine	113	88%	58%	69%	94%
Smoking Cessation Advice	35	94%	75%	80%	100%
Surgical Infection Prevention					
Prophylactic Antibiotic Given[3]	35	77%	74%	77%	95%
Prophylactic Antibiotic Selection	35	100%	89%	90%	100%
Prophylactic Antibiotic Stopped[3]	35	91%	65%	72%	95%
Pregnancy Care					
Inpatient Neonatal Mortality	1,005	0.30%	-	-	-
Third or Fourth Degree Laceration	611	3.27%	3.58%	3.63%	3.27%

Emanuel Medical Center

825 Delbon Avenue
Turlock, CA 95382
Phone: 209-667-4200
Fax: 209-669-2372
URL: www.emanuelmedicalcenter.org
Ownership: Voluntary non-profit - Church
Accredited: Yes
Emergency Services: Yes
Licensed Beds: 150

Key Personnel:

President/CEO. . . . . John Sigsbury
Chief Medical Staff. . . . . Gordon Alldrin, MD
Director Respiratory Therapy . . . . Toni Jardine

Measure	Cases	This Hospital	State Average	U.S. Average	Top Hospital
Heart Attack Care					
ACE Inhibitor or ARB for LVSD[1]	10	80%	82%	82%	100%
Aspirin at Arrival	100	94%	95%	92%	100%
Aspirin at Discharge	43	93%	90%	90%	100%
Beta Blocker at Arrival	89	90%	89%	87%	100%
Beta Blocker at Discharge	42	74%	89%	90%	100%
Fibrinolytic Medication Timing[1]	15	27%	40%	31%	100%
PCI Within 90 Minutes of Arrival	0	-	52%	54%	95%
Smoking Cessation Advice[1]	8	75%	87%	88%	100%
Heart Failure Care					
ACE Inhibitor or ARB for LVSD	78	92%	84%	82%	100%
Discharge Instructions	213	80%	56%	61%	93%
Evaluation of LVS Function	263	90%	84%	83%	99%
Smoking Cessation Advice	33	70%	82%	82%	100%
Pneumonia Care					
Appropriate Initial Antibiotic	162	91%	82%	83%	94%
Blood Culture Timing	151	86%	89%	90%	100%
Influenza Vaccine	36	75%	58%	70%	100%
Initial Antibiotic Timing	232	77%	75%	80%	93%

NOTE: Hospital profiles are in alphabetical order by state, then city, then hospital within the city; Rankings are sorted by rate in descending order and exclude hospitals with less than 25 cases; (1) The number of cases is too small (n<25) for purposes of reliably predicting hospital performance; (2) Measure reflects the hospital's indication that its submission was based upon a sample of its relevant discharges; (3) Rate reflects fewer than the maximum possible quarters of data for the measure; (4) Inaccurate information submitted and suppressed for one or more quarters; (5) No data is available from the hospital for this measure; Please refer to the User's Guide for a full explanation of data

Measure	Cases	This Hospital	State Average	U.S. Average	Top Hospital
Oxygenation Assessment	259	100%	99%	99%	100%
Pneumococcal Vaccine	170	78%	58%	69%	94%
Smoking Cessation Advice	44	68%	75%	80%	100%
Surgical Infection Prevention					
Prophylactic Antibiotic Given	290	83%	74%	77%	95%
Prophylactic Antibiotic Selection	76	89%	89%	90%	100%
Prophylactic Antibiotic Stopped	287	51%	65%	72%	95%
Pregnancy Care					
Inpatient Neonatal Mortality	-	-	-	-	-
Third or Fourth Degree Laceration	-	-	3.58%	3.63%	3.27%

Tustin Hospital and Medical Center

14662 Newport Avenue
Tustin, CA 92780
Phone: 714-838-9600
Fax: 714-669-2087
E-mail: info@tustinhospital.com
URL: www.tustinhospital.com
Ownership: Proprietary
Accredited: Yes
Emergency Services: No
Licensed Beds: 177

Key Personnel:

CEO. . . . . R Michael Hartman
Chief Medical Staff. . . . . Charles Marcos
Chief Cardiology . . . . Debbie Lopez
Emergency Department. . . . . Pyekel Chez

Measure	Cases	This Hospital	State Average	U.S. Average	Top Hospital
Heart Attack Care					
ACE Inhibitor or ARB for LVSD[3]	0	-	82%	82%	100%
Aspirin at Arrival[1,3]	1	100%	95%	92%	100%
Aspirin at Discharge[3]	0	-	90%	90%	100%
Beta Blocker at Arrival[1,3]	1	100%	89%	87%	100%
Beta Blocker at Discharge[3]	0	-	89%	90%	100%
Fibrinolytic Medication Timing[5]	-	-	40%	31%	100%
PCI Within 90 Minutes of Arrival[5]	-	-	52%	54%	95%
Smoking Cessation Advice[5]	-	-	87%	88%	100%
Heart Failure Care					
ACE Inhibitor or ARB for LVSD[1,3]	2	100%	84%	82%	100%
Discharge Instructions[1,3]	2	0%	56%	61%	93%
Evaluation of LVS Function[1,3]	10	40%	84%	83%	99%
Smoking Cessation Advice[1,3]	2	100%	82%	82%	100%
Pneumonia Care					
Appropriate Initial Antibiotic[1,3]	3	33%	82%	83%	94%
Blood Culture Timing[1,3]	4	100%	89%	90%	100%
Influenza Vaccine[5]	-	-	58%	70%	100%
Initial Antibiotic Timing	26	58%	75%	80%	93%
Oxygenation Assessment	41	100%	99%	99%	100%
Pneumococcal Vaccine[1]	7	14%	58%	69%	94%
Smoking Cessation Advice[1,3]	3	33%	75%	80%	100%
Surgical Infection Prevention					
Prophylactic Antibiotic Given[5]	-	-	74%	77%	95%
Prophylactic Antibiotic Selection[5]	-	-	89%	90%	100%
Prophylactic Antibiotic Stopped[5]	-	-	65%	72%	95%
Pregnancy Care					
Inpatient Neonatal Mortality	-	-	-	-	-
Third or Fourth Degree Laceration	-	-	3.58%	3.63%	3.27%

Ukiah Valley Medical Center

275 Hospital Drive
Ukiah, CA 95482
Phone: 707-463-7360
Fax: 707-463-7384
URL: www.uvmc.org
Ownership: Voluntary non-profit - Other
Accredited: Yes
Emergency Services: Yes
Licensed Beds: 101

Key Personnel:

Administrator . . . . Mark Larose
Chief Medical Staff. . . . . Geoffrey Esselman, MD
Cardiac Lab . . . . Jill Bartolomie, RN
Catheterization Lab . . . . Jill Bartolomie, RN
Emergency Room . . . . Timon Rohan, RN
Emergency Room . . . . Mark Luoto
Director Infection/Disease Control . . . . Sue Mason, RN
Intensive/Coronary Care . . . . Jill Bartolomie, RN
Medical/Surgical Nursing . . . . Lesa McArdle, RN
OB/GYN Womens Health. . . . . Karen Stewart, RN
Director Respiratory Therapy . . . . Diana Lane

Measure	Cases	This Hospital	State Average	U.S. Average	Top Hospital
Heart Attack Care					
ACE Inhibitor or ARB for LVSD	0	-	82%	82%	100%
Aspirin at Arrival[1]	24	100%	95%	92%	100%
Aspirin at Discharge[1]	8	100%	90%	90%	100%
Beta Blocker at Arrival[1]	20	85%	89%	87%	100%
Beta Blocker at Discharge[1]	8	75%	89%	90%	100%
Fibrinolytic Medication Timing[1]	3	33%	40%	31%	100%
PCI Within 90 Minutes of Arrival	0	-	52%	54%	95%
Smoking Cessation Advice[1]	3	100%	87%	88%	100%
Heart Failure Care					
ACE Inhibitor or ARB for LVSD	26	96%	84%	82%	100%
Discharge Instructions	70	69%	56%	61%	93%
Evaluation of LVS Function	84	77%	84%	83%	99%
Smoking Cessation Advice[1]	14	86%	82%	82%	100%
Pneumonia Care					
Appropriate Initial Antibiotic	102	88%	82%	83%	94%
Blood Culture Timing	32	84%	89%	90%	100%
Influenza Vaccine	25	76%	58%	70%	100%
Initial Antibiotic Timing	128	85%	75%	80%	93%
Oxygenation Assessment	150	100%	99%	99%	100%
Pneumococcal Vaccine	91	91%	58%	69%	94%
Smoking Cessation Advice	37	62%	75%	80%	100%
Surgical Infection Prevention					
Prophylactic Antibiotic Given	173	65%	74%	77%	95%
Prophylactic Antibiotic Selection	40	92%	89%	90%	100%
Prophylactic Antibiotic Stopped	170	65%	65%	72%	95%
Pregnancy Care					
Inpatient Neonatal Mortality	-	-	-	-	-
Third or Fourth Degree Laceration	-	-	3.58%	3.63%	3.27%

San Antonio Community Hospital

999 San Bernardino Road
Upland, CA 91786
Phone: 909-985-2811
Fax: 909-920-6357
URL: www.sach.org
Ownership: Voluntary non-profit - Other
Accredited: Yes
Emergency Services: Yes
Licensed Beds: 329

Key Personnel:

President/CEO. . . . . Steven C Moreau
Emergency Room . . . . Debbie Poore
Infection Control. . . . . Karen Drinkwine

Measure	Cases	This Hospital	State Average	U.S. Average	Top Hospital
Heart Attack Care					
ACE Inhibitor or ARB for LVSD	54	83%	82%	82%	100%
Aspirin at Arrival	227	98%	95%	92%	100%
Aspirin at Discharge	219	98%	90%	90%	100%
Beta Blocker at Arrival	153	95%	89%	87%	100%
Beta Blocker at Discharge	209	98%	89%	90%	100%
Fibrinolytic Medication Timing[1]	11	27%	40%	31%	100%
PCI Within 90 Minutes of Arrival[1]	7	57%	52%	54%	95%
Smoking Cessation Advice	70	100%	87%	88%	100%
Heart Failure Care					
ACE Inhibitor or ARB for LVSD	207	81%	84%	82%	100%
Discharge Instructions	380	49%	56%	61%	93%
Evaluation of LVS Function	487	88%	84%	83%	99%
Smoking Cessation Advice	70	100%	82%	82%	100%
Pneumonia Care					
Appropriate Initial Antibiotic	338	84%	82%	83%	94%
Blood Culture Timing	306	86%	89%	90%	100%
Influenza Vaccine	92	26%	58%	70%	100%
Initial Antibiotic Timing	427	67%	75%	80%	93%
Oxygenation Assessment	551	99%	99%	99%	100%
Pneumococcal Vaccine	331	37%	58%	69%	94%
Smoking Cessation Advice	89	96%	75%	80%	100%
Surgical Infection Prevention					
Prophylactic Antibiotic Given[3]	694	82%	74%	77%	95%
Prophylactic Antibiotic Selection	241	92%	89%	90%	100%
Prophylactic Antibiotic Stopped[3]	680	69%	65%	72%	95%
Pregnancy Care					
Inpatient Neonatal Mortality	2,247	0.76%	-	-	-

NOTE: Hospital profiles are in alphabetical order by state, then city, then hospital within the city; Rankings are sorted by rate in descending order and exclude hospitals with less than 25 cases; (1) The number of cases is too small (n<25) for purposes of reliably predicting hospital performance; (2) Measure reflects the hospital's indication that its submission was based upon a sample of its relevant discharges; (3) Rate reflects fewer than the maximum possible quarters of data for the measure; (4) Inaccurate information submitted and suppressed for one or more quarters; (5) No data is available from the hospital for this measure; Please refer to the User's Guide for a full explanation of data

Third or Fourth Degree Laceration	1,302	3.46%	3.58%	3.63%	3.27%

VacaValley Hospital

1000 Nut Tree Road
Vacaville, CA 95687
URL: www.northbay.org
Ownership: Voluntary non-profit - Private
Emergency Services: Yes
Phone: 707-446-4000
Fax: 707-449-3742
Accredited: Yes
Licensed Beds: 50

Key Personnel:

President/CEO . . . . Deborah Sugiyama
Chief of Medical Staff . . . . M Johnson
Emergency Room . . . . Ed Ballerini
Director Medical/Surgical Nursing . . . . Mary Doherty
Director Radiology . . . . Russ Suey
Director Respiratory Therapy . . . . Coletta Ciacarelli

Measure	Cases	This Hospital	State Average	U.S. Average	Top Hospital
Heart Attack Care					
ACE Inhibitor or ARB for LVSD[1]	5	60%	82%	82%	100%
Aspirin at Arrival	55	93%	95%	92%	100%
Aspirin at Discharge[1]	17	94%	90%	90%	100%
Beta Blocker at Arrival	42	88%	89%	87%	100%
Beta Blocker at Discharge[1]	18	100%	89%	90%	100%
Fibrinolytic Medication Timing[1]	12	42%	40%	31%	100%
PCI Within 90 Minutes of Arrival	0	-	52%	54%	95%
Smoking Cessation Advice[1]	6	83%	87%	88%	100%
Heart Failure Care					
ACE Inhibitor or ARB for LVSD	39	79%	84%	82%	100%
Discharge Instructions	107	50%	56%	61%	93%
Evaluation of LVS Function	120	92%	84%	83%	99%
Smoking Cessation Advice	25	92%	82%	82%	100%
Pneumonia Care					
Appropriate Initial Antibiotic	138	93%	82%	83%	94%
Blood Culture Timing	160	94%	89%	90%	100%
Influenza Vaccine	31	39%	58%	70%	100%
Initial Antibiotic Timing	186	89%	75%	80%	93%
Oxygenation Assessment	221	100%	99%	99%	100%
Pneumococcal Vaccine	141	61%	58%	69%	94%
Smoking Cessation Advice	50	92%	75%	80%	100%
Surgical Infection Prevention					
Prophylactic Antibiotic Given	86	80%	74%	77%	95%
Prophylactic Antibiotic Selection[1]	18	100%	89%	90%	100%
Prophylactic Antibiotic Stopped	85	71%	65%	72%	95%
Pregnancy Care					
Inpatient Neonatal Mortality	-	-	-	-	-
Third or Fourth Degree Laceration	-	-	3.58%	3.63%	3.27%

Henry Mayo Newhall Memorial Hospital

23845 McBean Parkway
Valencia, CA 91355
URL: www.henrymayo.com
Ownership: Voluntary non-profit - Private
Emergency Services: Yes
Phone: 661-253-8000
Fax: 661-253-8142
Accredited: Yes
Licensed Beds: 217

Key Personnel:

CEO . . . . James Yoshikora
Chief Medical Staff . . . . Chand Khanna, MD
OB/GYN Womens Health . . . . Ajit Kittur, MD
Chief Radiology . . . . Patsy Desimone, MD
Director Respiratory Therapy . . . . Karen Bostwick

Measure	Cases	This Hospital	State Average	U.S. Average	Top Hospital
Heart Attack Care					
ACE Inhibitor or ARB for LVSD[1]	6	83%	82%	82%	100%
Aspirin at Arrival	113	98%	95%	92%	100%
Aspirin at Discharge	37	89%	90%	90%	100%
Beta Blocker at Arrival	95	96%	89%	87%	100%
Beta Blocker at Discharge	30	93%	89%	90%	100%
Fibrinolytic Medication Timing[1]	8	50%	40%	31%	100%
PCI Within 90 Minutes of Arrival	0	-	52%	54%	95%
Smoking Cessation Advice[1]	3	33%	87%	88%	100%
Heart Failure Care					
ACE Inhibitor or ARB for LVSD	69	75%	84%	82%	100%
Discharge Instructions	238	36%	56%	61%	93%
Evaluation of LVS Function	275	89%	84%	83%	99%
Smoking Cessation Advice[1]	19	47%	82%	82%	100%
Pneumonia Care					
Appropriate Initial Antibiotic	185	75%	82%	83%	94%
Blood Culture Timing	142	84%	89%	90%	100%
Influenza Vaccine[4,5]	-	-	58%	70%	100%
Initial Antibiotic Timing	234	75%	75%	80%	93%
Oxygenation Assessment	287	100%	99%	99%	100%
Pneumococcal Vaccine	182	14%	58%	69%	94%
Smoking Cessation Advice	32	25%	75%	80%	100%
Surgical Infection Prevention					
Prophylactic Antibiotic Given[3]	147	82%	74%	77%	95%
Prophylactic Antibiotic Selection	68	93%	89%	90%	100%
Prophylactic Antibiotic Stopped[3]	145	51%	65%	72%	95%
Pregnancy Care					
Inpatient Neonatal Mortality	-	-	-	-	-
Third or Fourth Degree Laceration	-	-	3.58%	3.63%	3.27%

Kaiser Foundation Hospital-Vallejo

975 Sereno Dr
Vallejo, CA 94590
Ownership: Voluntary non-profit - Other
Emergency Services: Yes
Phone: 707-651-1000
Accredited: Yes

Measure	Cases	This Hospital	State Average	U.S. Average	Top Hospital
Heart Attack Care					
ACE Inhibitor or ARB for LVSD[1]	23	87%	82%	82%	100%
Aspirin at Arrival	217	100%	95%	92%	100%
Aspirin at Discharge	97	99%	90%	90%	100%
Beta Blocker at Arrival	208	100%	89%	87%	100%
Beta Blocker at Discharge	103	100%	89%	90%	100%
Fibrinolytic Medication Timing[1]	17	41%	40%	31%	100%
PCI Within 90 Minutes of Arrival	0	-	52%	54%	95%
Smoking Cessation Advice[1]	11	100%	87%	88%	100%
Heart Failure Care					
ACE Inhibitor or ARB for LVSD	83	82%	84%	82%	100%
Discharge Instructions	267	49%	56%	61%	93%
Evaluation of LVS Function	303	97%	84%	83%	99%
Smoking Cessation Advice	43	86%	82%	82%	100%
Pneumonia Care					
Appropriate Initial Antibiotic	118	93%	82%	83%	94%
Blood Culture Timing	116	96%	89%	90%	100%
Influenza Vaccine	32	47%	58%	70%	100%
Initial Antibiotic Timing	137	85%	75%	80%	93%
Oxygenation Assessment	171	100%	99%	99%	100%
Pneumococcal Vaccine	106	82%	58%	69%	94%
Smoking Cessation Advice	27	85%	75%	80%	100%
Surgical Infection Prevention					
Prophylactic Antibiotic Given	192	92%	74%	77%	95%
Prophylactic Antibiotic Selection	46	91%	89%	90%	100%
Prophylactic Antibiotic Stopped	180	91%	65%	72%	95%
Pregnancy Care					
Inpatient Neonatal Mortality	2,510	0.24%	-	-	-
Third or Fourth Degree Laceration	1,750	3.71%	3.58%	3.63%	3.27%

Sutter Solano Medical Center

300 Hospital Drive
Vallejo, CA 94589
URL: www.suttersolano.org
Ownership: Voluntary non-profit - Other
Emergency Services: Yes
Phone: 707-554-4444
Fax: 707-648-3227
Accredited: Yes
Licensed Beds: 111

Key Personnel:

Chief of Medical Staff . . . . Gregory Coe
Director Medical/Surgical Nursing . . . . Polly Walker
OB/GYN Womens Health . . . . Jesus Baldonedo, MD

Measure	Cases	This Hospital	State Average	U.S. Average	Top Hospital
Heart Attack Care					
ACE Inhibitor or ARB for LVSD[1]	9	44%	82%	82%	100%
Aspirin at Arrival	69	91%	95%	92%	100%
Aspirin at Discharge	34	53%	90%	90%	100%
Beta Blocker at Arrival	63	86%	89%	87%	100%

NOTE: Hospital profiles are in alphabetical order by state, then city, then hospital within the city; Rankings are sorted by rate in descending order and exclude hospitals with less than 25 cases; (1) The number of cases is too small (n<25) for purposes of reliably predicting hospital performance; (2) Measure reflects the hospital's indication that its submission was based upon a sample of its relevant discharges; (3) Rate reflects fewer than the maximum possible quarters of data for the measure; (4) Inaccurate information submitted and suppressed for one or more quarters; (5) No data is available from the hospital for this measure; Please refer to the User's Guide for a full explanation of data

Beta Blocker at Discharge	32	59%	89%	90%	100%
Fibrinolytic Medication Timing[1]	12	33%	40%	31%	100%
PCI Within 90 Minutes of Arrival	0	-	52%	54%	95%
Smoking Cessation Advice[1]	10	70%	87%	88%	100%
Heart Failure Care					
ACE Inhibitor or ARB for LVSD	80	81%	84%	82%	100%
Discharge Instructions	313	71%	56%	61%	93%
Evaluation of LVS Function	328	82%	84%	83%	99%
Smoking Cessation Advice	106	79%	82%	82%	100%
Pneumonia Care					
Appropriate Initial Antibiotic	96	86%	82%	83%	94%
Blood Culture Timing	55	78%	89%	90%	100%
Influenza Vaccine	30	53%	58%	70%	100%
Initial Antibiotic Timing	131	63%	75%	80%	93%
Oxygenation Assessment	167	100%	99%	99%	100%
Pneumococcal Vaccine	73	68%	58%	69%	94%
Smoking Cessation Advice	53	89%	75%	80%	100%
Surgical Infection Prevention					
Prophylactic Antibiotic Given[2]	182	58%	74%	77%	95%
Prophylactic Antibiotic Selection[1,2]	10	90%	89%	90%	100%
Prophylactic Antibiotic Stopped[2]	169	78%	65%	72%	95%
Pregnancy Care					
Inpatient Neonatal Mortality	-	-	-	-	-
Third or Fourth Degree Laceration	-	-	3.58%	3.63%	3.27%

Valley Presbyterian Hospital

15107 Vanowen Street
Van Nuys, CA 91405
URL: www.valleypres.org
Phone: 818-782-6600
Fax: 818-902-3949
Ownership: Voluntary non-profit - Other
Emergency Services: Yes
Accredited: Yes
Licensed Beds: 290

Key Personnel:

CEO. . . . . Robert C Bills
Chief Cardiology . . . . David Aliabadi
Emergency Department. . . . . Ken Wong
Chief Pulmonary Therapy. . . . . Leonard Adelson

Measure	Cases	This Hospital	State Average	U.S. Average	Top Hospital
Heart Attack Care					
ACE Inhibitor or ARB for LVSD	34	76%	82%	82%	100%
Aspirin at Arrival	119	97%	95%	92%	100%
Aspirin at Discharge	138	95%	90%	90%	100%
Beta Blocker at Arrival	79	94%	89%	87%	100%
Beta Blocker at Discharge	142	96%	89%	90%	100%
Fibrinolytic Medication Timing[3]	0	-	40%	31%	100%
PCI Within 90 Minutes of Arrival[1]	7	43%	52%	54%	95%
Smoking Cessation Advice[1,3]	15	80%	87%	88%	100%
Heart Failure Care					
ACE Inhibitor or ARB for LVSD	52	71%	84%	82%	100%
Discharge Instructions[3]	43	0%	56%	61%	93%
Evaluation of LVS Function	214	88%	84%	83%	99%
Smoking Cessation Advice[1,3]	11	64%	82%	82%	100%
Pneumonia Care					
Appropriate Initial Antibiotic[1,3]	10	90%	82%	83%	94%
Blood Culture Timing[3]	32	88%	89%	90%	100%
Influenza Vaccine[5]	-	-	58%	70%	100%
Initial Antibiotic Timing	199	59%	75%	80%	93%
Oxygenation Assessment	236	100%	99%	99%	100%
Pneumococcal Vaccine	141	15%	58%	69%	94%
Smoking Cessation Advice[1,3]	2	50%	75%	80%	100%
Surgical Infection Prevention					
Prophylactic Antibiotic Given[2,3]	95	35%	74%	77%	95%
Prophylactic Antibiotic Selection[5]	-	-	89%	90%	100%
Prophylactic Antibiotic Stopped[2,3]	94	41%	65%	72%	95%
Pregnancy Care					
Inpatient Neonatal Mortality	-	-	-	-	-
Third or Fourth Degree Laceration	-	-	3.58%	3.63%	3.27%

Community Memorial Hospital Ventura

147 N Brent Street
Ventura, CA 93003
E-mail: jmasterson@cmhhospital.org
URL: www.cmhhospital.org
Phone: 805-652-5011
Fax: 805-643-7554
Ownership: Voluntary non-profit - Private
Emergency Services: Yes
Accredited: Yes
Licensed Beds: 240

Key Personnel:

President & CEO . . . . Gary Wilde
Chief Medical Staff. . . . . Peter Gaal
Cardiac Lab . . . . Carolyn Estrada
Catheterization Lab . . . . Carolyn Estrada
Emergency Room . . . . Dede Utley
Emergency Room . . . . Alex Kowblansky
Director Infection/Disease Control . . . . Chris Ouellette
ICU . . . . Carolyn Estrada
OB/GYN Womens Health. . . . . Vicki Beaver
Respiratory/Cardiopulmonary. . . . . Mary Stewart

Measure	Cases	This Hospital	State Average	U.S. Average	Top Hospital
Heart Attack Care					
ACE Inhibitor or ARB for LVSD	37	92%	82%	82%	100%
Aspirin at Arrival	181	97%	95%	92%	100%
Aspirin at Discharge	226	100%	90%	90%	100%
Beta Blocker at Arrival	165	92%	89%	87%	100%
Beta Blocker at Discharge	220	94%	89%	90%	100%
Fibrinolytic Medication Timing	0	-	40%	31%	100%
PCI Within 90 Minutes of Arrival[1]	8	62%	52%	54%	95%
Smoking Cessation Advice	53	91%	87%	88%	100%
Heart Failure Care					
ACE Inhibitor or ARB for LVSD	73	97%	84%	82%	100%
Discharge Instructions	206	33%	56%	61%	93%
Evaluation of LVS Function	253	95%	84%	83%	99%
Smoking Cessation Advice[1]	24	62%	82%	82%	100%
Pneumonia Care					
Appropriate Initial Antibiotic	181	83%	82%	83%	94%
Blood Culture Timing	231	87%	89%	90%	100%
Influenza Vaccine	60	57%	58%	70%	100%
Initial Antibiotic Timing	292	82%	75%	80%	93%
Oxygenation Assessment	375	100%	99%	99%	100%
Pneumococcal Vaccine	266	29%	58%	69%	94%
Smoking Cessation Advice	58	69%	75%	80%	100%
Surgical Infection Prevention					
Prophylactic Antibiotic Given[2,3]	127	34%	74%	77%	95%
Prophylactic Antibiotic Selection[2]	114	96%	89%	90%	100%
Prophylactic Antibiotic Stopped[2,3]	124	50%	65%	72%	95%
Pregnancy Care					
Inpatient Neonatal Mortality	-	-	-	-	-
Third or Fourth Degree Laceration	-	-	3.58%	3.63%	3.27%

Ventura County Medical Center

3291 Loma Vista Road
Ventura, CA 93003
URL: www.vchca.org
Phone: 805-652-6062
Fax: 805-652-6169
Ownership: Government - Local
Emergency Services: Yes
Accredited: Yes
Licensed Beds: 208

Key Personnel:

Administrator . . . . Pierre Durand
Associate Administrator . . . . Samuel Edwards
Emergency Room . . . . Sylvanna Guidotti, MD
Emergency Room . . . . Cyndie Cole, MD
Infection Control. . . . . Denise Bleak
Chief Cardiology . . . . Daniel Clark, MD
OB/GYN Womens Health. . . . . Cindy Cole
Manager Radiology . . . . Gerry Russell
Director Respiratory Therapy . . . . Deborah Robertson

Measure	Cases	This Hospital	State Average	U.S. Average	Top Hospital
Heart Attack Care					
ACE Inhibitor or ARB for LVSD[1]	7	100%	82%	82%	100%
Aspirin at Arrival	25	100%	95%	92%	100%
Aspirin at Discharge[1]	19	100%	90%	90%	100%
Beta Blocker at Arrival[1]	19	95%	89%	87%	100%

NOTE: Hospital profiles are in alphabetical order by state, then city, then hospital within the city; Rankings are sorted by rate in descending order and exclude hospitals with less than 25 cases; (1) The number of cases is too small (n<25) for purposes of reliably predicting hospital performance; (2) Measure reflects the hospital's indication that its submission was based upon a sample of its relevant discharges; (3) Rate reflects fewer than the maximum possible quarters of data for the measure; (4) Inaccurate information submitted and suppressed for one or more quarters; (5) No data is available from the hospital for this measure; Please refer to the User's Guide for a full explanation of data

Measure	Cases	This Hospital	State Average	U.S. Average	Top Hospital
Beta Blocker at Discharge[1]	17	100%	89%	90%	100%
Fibrinolytic Medication Timing	0	-	40%	31%	100%
PCI Within 90 Minutes of Arrival	0	-	52%	54%	95%
Smoking Cessation Advice[1]	6	100%	87%	88%	100%
Heart Failure Care					
ACE Inhibitor or ARB for LVSD	39	100%	84%	82%	100%
Discharge Instructions	88	93%	56%	61%	93%
Evaluation of LVS Function	102	98%	84%	83%	99%
Smoking Cessation Advice[1]	17	100%	82%	82%	100%
Pneumonia Care					
Appropriate Initial Antibiotic	87	86%	82%	83%	94%
Blood Culture Timing	71	90%	89%	90%	100%
Influenza Vaccine[1]	14	64%	58%	70%	100%
Initial Antibiotic Timing	73	81%	75%	80%	93%
Oxygenation Assessment	105	100%	99%	99%	100%
Pneumococcal Vaccine	39	69%	58%	69%	94%
Smoking Cessation Advice	28	96%	75%	80%	100%
Surgical Infection Prevention					
Prophylactic Antibiotic Given[1,3]	17	76%	74%	77%	95%
Prophylactic Antibiotic Selection[1]	16	100%	89%	90%	100%
Prophylactic Antibiotic Stopped[1,3]	16	62%	65%	72%	95%
Pregnancy Care					
Inpatient Neonatal Mortality	3,315	0.18%	-	-	-
Third or Fourth Degree Laceration	2,412	2.82%	3.58%	3.63%	3.27%

Desert Valley Hospital

16850 Bear Valley Road
Victorville, CA 92392
Phone: 760-241-8000
Fax: 760-245-0156
URL: www.dvmc.com
Ownership: Voluntary non-profit - Other
Accredited: Yes
Emergency Services: Yes

Key Personnel:

President/CEO. . . . . Lex Reddy

Measure	Cases	This Hospital	State Average	U.S. Average	Top Hospital
Heart Attack Care					
ACE Inhibitor or ARB for LVSD[1]	10	100%	82%	82%	100%
Aspirin at Arrival	106	99%	95%	92%	100%
Aspirin at Discharge	86	98%	90%	90%	100%
Beta Blocker at Arrival	102	99%	89%	87%	100%
Beta Blocker at Discharge	90	98%	89%	90%	100%
Fibrinolytic Medication Timing[1,3]	3	100%	40%	31%	100%
PCI Within 90 Minutes of Arrival	0	-	52%	54%	95%
Smoking Cessation Advice	29	100%	87%	88%	100%
Heart Failure Care					
ACE Inhibitor or ARB for LVSD[2]	64	100%	84%	82%	100%
Discharge Instructions[2,3]	118	98%	56%	61%	93%
Evaluation of LVS Function[2]	257	96%	84%	83%	99%
Smoking Cessation Advice[2]	54	100%	82%	82%	100%
Pneumonia Care					
Appropriate Initial Antibiotic[1,3]	14	86%	82%	83%	94%
Blood Culture Timing	134	95%	89%	90%	100%
Influenza Vaccine[5]	-	-	58%	70%	100%
Initial Antibiotic Timing	140	90%	75%	80%	93%
Oxygenation Assessment	185	100%	99%	99%	100%
Pneumococcal Vaccine	107	91%	58%	69%	94%
Smoking Cessation Advice	41	100%	75%	80%	100%
Surgical Infection Prevention					
Prophylactic Antibiotic Given[1,3]	23	65%	74%	77%	95%
Prophylactic Antibiotic Selection[1]	22	100%	89%	90%	100%
Prophylactic Antibiotic Stopped[1,3]	16	56%	65%	72%	95%
Pregnancy Care					
Inpatient Neonatal Mortality	-	-	-	-	-
Third or Fourth Degree Laceration	-	-	3.58%	3.63%	3.27%

Victor Valley Community Hospital

15248 11th Street East
Victorville, CA 92392
Phone: 760-245-8691
Fax: 760-952-1461
E-mail: hr@vvch.org
URL: www.vvch.org
Ownership: Voluntary non-profit - Other
Accredited: Yes
Emergency Services: Yes
Licensed Beds: 119

Key Personnel:

CEO. . . . . Margaret E Peterson, PhD
Catheterization Lab . . . . Jenny Hicks
Emergency Room . . . . Marian Peterson
Infection Control. . . . . Darcel Black, RN
Medical/Surgical Nursing Director . . . . Shandra Goldsmith
OB/GYN Womens Health. . . . . Vijay Arora, MD
Respiratory Therapy Director. . . . . Lori Burns

Measure	Cases	This Hospital	State Average	U.S. Average	Top Hospital
Heart Attack Care					
ACE Inhibitor or ARB for LVSD[1]	6	67%	82%	82%	100%
Aspirin at Arrival	63	81%	95%	92%	100%
Aspirin at Discharge	40	55%	90%	90%	100%
Beta Blocker at Arrival	64	64%	89%	87%	100%
Beta Blocker at Discharge	43	49%	89%	90%	100%
Fibrinolytic Medication Timing[3]	0	-	40%	31%	100%
PCI Within 90 Minutes of Arrival	0	-	52%	54%	95%
Smoking Cessation Advice[3]	0	-	87%	88%	100%
Heart Failure Care					
ACE Inhibitor or ARB for LVSD	35	66%	84%	82%	100%
Discharge Instructions[1,3]	23	35%	56%	61%	93%
Evaluation of LVS Function	171	57%	84%	83%	99%
Smoking Cessation Advice[1,3]	9	56%	82%	82%	100%
Pneumonia Care					
Appropriate Initial Antibiotic[1,3]	12	100%	82%	83%	94%
Blood Culture Timing[1,3]	13	77%	89%	90%	100%
Influenza Vaccine[5]	-	-	58%	70%	100%
Initial Antibiotic Timing	168	49%	75%	80%	93%
Oxygenation Assessment	201	99%	99%	99%	100%
Pneumococcal Vaccine	107	21%	58%	69%	94%
Smoking Cessation Advice[1,3]	5	60%	75%	80%	100%
Surgical Infection Prevention					
Prophylactic Antibiotic Given[3]	38	47%	74%	77%	95%
Prophylactic Antibiotic Selection[5]	-	-	89%	90%	100%
Prophylactic Antibiotic Stopped[3]	29	66%	65%	72%	95%
Pregnancy Care					
Inpatient Neonatal Mortality	-	-	-	-	-
Third or Fourth Degree Laceration	-	-	3.58%	3.63%	3.27%

Kaweah Delta Health Care District

Alternate Name: Kaweah Delta District Hospital
400 W Mineral King Street
Visalia, CA 93291
Phone: 559-624-2276
Fax: 559-635-4021
URL: www.kaweah.org
Ownership: Govt - Hospital District or Authority
Accredited: Yes
Emergency Services: Yes

Key Personnel:

Chief Medical Staff. . . . . Omesy Said
Director Infection/Disease Control . . . . Paul L Williams, MD
Chief OB/GYN . . . . Harlow Snoot
Chief Radiology . . . . Richard Anderson, MD
Director Respiratory Therapy . . . . Bill Dejainet

Measure	Cases	This Hospital	State Average	U.S. Average	Top Hospital
Heart Attack Care					
ACE Inhibitor or ARB for LVSD[2]	57	96%	82%	82%	100%
Aspirin at Arrival[2]	231	98%	95%	92%	100%
Aspirin at Discharge[2]	310	96%	90%	90%	100%
Beta Blocker at Arrival[2]	196	93%	89%	87%	100%
Beta Blocker at Discharge[2]	304	91%	89%	90%	100%
Fibrinolytic Medication Timing[1,2]	1	0%	40%	31%	100%
PCI Within 90 Minutes of Arrival[1,2]	12	58%	52%	54%	95%
Smoking Cessation Advice[2]	91	96%	87%	88%	100%
Heart Failure Care					
ACE Inhibitor or ARB for LVSD[2]	160	77%	84%	82%	100%

NOTE: Hospital profiles are in alphabetical order by state, then city, then hospital within the city; Rankings are sorted by rate in descending order and exclude hospitals with less than 25 cases; (1) The number of cases is too small (n<25) for purposes of reliably predicting hospital performance; (2) Measure reflects the hospital's indication that its submission was based upon a sample of its relevant discharges; (3) Rate reflects fewer than the maximum possible quarters of data for the measure; (4) Inaccurate information submitted and suppressed for one or more quarters; (5) No data is available from the hospital for this measure; Please refer to the User's Guide for a full explanation of data

Measure	Cases	This Hospital	State Average	U.S. Average	Top Hospital
Discharge Instructions[2]	329	46%	56%	61%	93%
Evaluation of LVS Function[2]	399	87%	84%	83%	99%
Smoking Cessation Advice[2]	59	86%	82%	82%	100%
Pneumonia Care					
Appropriate Initial Antibiotic[2]	446	87%	82%	83%	94%
Blood Culture Timing[2]	247	82%	89%	90%	100%
Influenza Vaccine[4,5]	-	-	58%	70%	100%
Initial Antibiotic Timing[2]	485	74%	75%	80%	93%
Oxygenation Assessment[2]	618	100%	99%	99%	100%
Pneumococcal Vaccine[2]	370	65%	58%	69%	94%
Smoking Cessation Advice[2]	134	66%	75%	80%	100%
Surgical Infection Prevention					
Prophylactic Antibiotic Given[2,3]	68	82%	74%	77%	95%
Prophylactic Antibiotic Selection[2]	70	89%	89%	90%	100%
Prophylactic Antibiotic Stopped[2,3]	65	35%	65%	72%	95%
Pregnancy Care					
Inpatient Neonatal Mortality	-	-	-	-	-
Third or Fourth Degree Laceration	-	-	3.58%	3.63%	3.27%

John Muir Medical Center

1601 Ygnacio Valley Road
Walnut Creek, CA 94598
URL: www.jmmdhs.com
Ownership: Voluntary non-profit - Private
Emergency Services: Yes

Phone: 925-939-3000
Fax: 925-947-4497

Accredited: Yes
Licensed Beds: 321

Key Personnel:
President/Chief Administrative Officer . . . . Kenneth L Meehan
Chief of Medical Staff . . . . Sally Davis

Measure	Cases	This Hospital	State Average	U.S. Average	Top Hospital
Heart Attack Care					
ACE Inhibitor or ARB for LVSD	26	88%	82%	82%	100%
Aspirin at Arrival	157	100%	95%	92%	100%
Aspirin at Discharge	133	100%	90%	90%	100%
Beta Blocker at Arrival	123	97%	89%	87%	100%
Beta Blocker at Discharge	126	100%	89%	90%	100%
Fibrinolytic Medication Timing	0	-	40%	31%	100%
PCI Within 90 Minutes of Arrival[1]	9	33%	52%	54%	95%
Smoking Cessation Advice	25	100%	87%	88%	100%
Heart Failure Care					
ACE Inhibitor or ARB for LVSD[2]	88	98%	84%	82%	100%
Discharge Instructions[2]	225	92%	56%	61%	93%
Evaluation of LVS Function[2]	272	96%	84%	83%	99%
Smoking Cessation Advice[1,2]	22	100%	82%	82%	100%
Pneumonia Care					
Appropriate Initial Antibiotic[2]	121	92%	82%	83%	94%
Blood Culture Timing[2]	132	99%	89%	90%	100%
Influenza Vaccine[2]	28	96%	58%	70%	100%
Initial Antibiotic Timing[2]	162	78%	75%	80%	93%
Oxygenation Assessment[2]	207	100%	99%	99%	100%
Pneumococcal Vaccine[2]	152	80%	58%	69%	94%
Smoking Cessation Advice[1,2]	21	95%	75%	80%	100%
Surgical Infection Prevention					
Prophylactic Antibiotic Given[2,3]	181	81%	74%	77%	95%
Prophylactic Antibiotic Selection[2]	55	62%	89%	90%	100%
Prophylactic Antibiotic Stopped[2,3]	171	53%	65%	72%	95%
Pregnancy Care					
Inpatient Neonatal Mortality[2]	620	0.16%	-	-	-
Third or Fourth Degree Laceration[2]	679	6.19%	3.58%	3.63%	3.27%

Kaiser Foundation Hospital-Walnut Creek

1425 S Main St
Walnut Creek, CA 94596
Ownership: Voluntary non-profit - Other
Emergency Services: Yes

Phone: 925-295-4000

Accredited: Yes

Measure	Cases	This Hospital	State Average	U.S. Average	Top Hospital
Heart Attack Care					
ACE Inhibitor or ARB for LVSD[1]	17	100%	82%	82%	100%
Aspirin at Arrival	225	96%	95%	92%	100%
Aspirin at Discharge	86	97%	90%	90%	100%
Beta Blocker at Arrival	197	99%	89%	87%	100%
Beta Blocker at Discharge	97	100%	89%	90%	100%
Fibrinolytic Medication Timing[1]	22	41%	40%	31%	100%
PCI Within 90 Minutes of Arrival	0	-	52%	54%	95%
Smoking Cessation Advice[1]	9	89%	87%	88%	100%
Heart Failure Care					
ACE Inhibitor or ARB for LVSD	41	93%	84%	82%	100%
Discharge Instructions	188	60%	56%	61%	93%
Evaluation of LVS Function	216	98%	84%	83%	99%
Smoking Cessation Advice[1]	16	94%	82%	82%	100%
Pneumonia Care					
Appropriate Initial Antibiotic	108	88%	82%	83%	94%
Blood Culture Timing	113	73%	89%	90%	100%
Influenza Vaccine	29	66%	58%	70%	100%
Initial Antibiotic Timing	115	66%	75%	80%	93%
Oxygenation Assessment	168	100%	99%	99%	100%
Pneumococcal Vaccine	124	86%	58%	69%	94%
Smoking Cessation Advice[1]	19	79%	75%	80%	100%
Surgical Infection Prevention					
Prophylactic Antibiotic Given	322	90%	74%	77%	95%
Prophylactic Antibiotic Selection	53	91%	89%	90%	100%
Prophylactic Antibiotic Stopped	313	81%	65%	72%	95%
Pregnancy Care					
Inpatient Neonatal Mortality	4,654	0.24%	-	-	-
Third or Fourth Degree Laceration	3,228	3.75%	3.58%	3.63%	3.27%

Watsonville Community Hospital

75 Nielsen Street
Watsonville, CA 95076
URL: www.watsonvillehospital.com
Ownership: Proprietary
Emergency Services: Yes

Phone: 831-724-4741
Fax: 831-728-4758

Accredited: Yes
Licensed Beds: 106

Key Personnel:
CEO . . . . Kaylor Shemberger
Chief Medical Staff . . . . Frank Rivago, MD

Measure	Cases	This Hospital	State Average	U.S. Average	Top Hospital
Heart Attack Care					
ACE Inhibitor or ARB for LVSD[1]	2	0%	82%	82%	100%
Aspirin at Arrival	30	97%	95%	92%	100%
Aspirin at Discharge[1]	22	91%	90%	90%	100%
Beta Blocker at Arrival[1]	21	86%	89%	87%	100%
Beta Blocker at Discharge[1]	20	85%	89%	90%	100%
Fibrinolytic Medication Timing[1]	2	100%	40%	31%	100%
PCI Within 90 Minutes of Arrival	0	-	52%	54%	95%
Smoking Cessation Advice[1]	3	100%	87%	88%	100%
Heart Failure Care					
ACE Inhibitor or ARB for LVSD	36	75%	84%	82%	100%
Discharge Instructions	156	78%	56%	61%	93%
Evaluation of LVS Function	177	72%	84%	83%	99%
Smoking Cessation Advice	27	63%	82%	82%	100%
Pneumonia Care					
Appropriate Initial Antibiotic	110	76%	82%	83%	94%
Blood Culture Timing	92	96%	89%	90%	100%
Influenza Vaccine	30	43%	58%	70%	100%
Initial Antibiotic Timing	151	69%	75%	80%	93%
Oxygenation Assessment	163	100%	99%	99%	100%
Pneumococcal Vaccine	100	32%	58%	69%	94%
Smoking Cessation Advice[1]	24	71%	75%	80%	100%
Surgical Infection Prevention					
Prophylactic Antibiotic Given[2,3]	126	72%	74%	77%	95%
Prophylactic Antibiotic Selection[2]	35	89%	89%	90%	100%
Prophylactic Antibiotic Stopped[2,3]	112	79%	65%	72%	95%
Pregnancy Care					
Inpatient Neonatal Mortality	-	-	-	-	-
Third or Fourth Degree Laceration	-	-	3.58%	3.63%	3.27%

NOTE: Hospital profiles are in alphabetical order by state, then city, then hospital within the city; Rankings are sorted by rate in descending order and exclude hospitals with less than 25 cases; (1) The number of cases is too small (n<25) for purposes of reliably predicting hospital performance; (2) Measure reflects the hospital's indication that its submission was based upon a sample of its relevant discharges; (3) Rate reflects fewer than the maximum possible quarters of data for the measure; (4) Inaccurate information submitted and suppressed for one or more quarters; (5) No data is available from the hospital for this measure; Please refer to the User's Guide for a full explanation of data

Mountain Community Medical Services

410 N Taylor St
Weaverville, CA 96093
E-mail: rcoe@trinitycounty.org
URL: www.trinitycounty.org
Ownership: Government - Local
Emergency Services: Yes
Phone: 530-623-5541
Fax: 530-623-6421
Accredited: No
Licensed Beds: 65

Key Personnel:
Interim CEO . . . . . Stan Oppegard
Chief Medical Staff . . . . . Jeanne Silvers
Infection Control . . . . . Judy Nondlund
Director Radiology . . . . . Vicky Williams
Respiratory/Cardiopulmonary . . . . . Taune Ruke

Measure	Cases	This Hospital	State Average	U.S. Average	Top Hospital
Heart Attack Care					
ACE Inhibitor or ARB for LVSD[5]	-	-	82%	82%	100%
Aspirin at Arrival[5]	-	-	95%	92%	100%
Aspirin at Discharge[5]	-	-	90%	90%	100%
Beta Blocker at Arrival[5]	-	-	89%	87%	100%
Beta Blocker at Discharge[5]	-	-	89%	90%	100%
Fibrinolytic Medication Timing[5]	-	-	40%	31%	100%
PCI Within 90 Minutes of Arrival[5]	-	-	52%	54%	95%
Smoking Cessation Advice[5]	-	-	87%	88%	100%
Heart Failure Care					
ACE Inhibitor or ARB for LVSD[5]	-	-	84%	82%	100%
Discharge Instructions[5]	-	-	56%	61%	93%
Evaluation of LVS Function[5]	-	-	84%	83%	99%
Smoking Cessation Advice[5]	-	-	82%	82%	100%
Pneumonia Care					
Appropriate Initial Antibiotic[1,3]	7	100%	82%	83%	94%
Blood Culture Timing[1,3]	4	100%	89%	90%	100%
Influenza Vaccine[5]	-	-	58%	70%	100%
Initial Antibiotic Timing[1,3]	7	86%	75%	80%	93%
Oxygenation Assessment[1,3]	9	100%	99%	99%	100%
Pneumococcal Vaccine[1,3]	3	0%	58%	69%	94%
Smoking Cessation Advice[1,3]	2	0%	75%	80%	100%
Surgical Infection Prevention					
Prophylactic Antibiotic Given[5]	-	-	74%	77%	95%
Prophylactic Antibiotic Selection[5]	-	-	89%	90%	100%
Prophylactic Antibiotic Stopped[5]	-	-	65%	72%	95%
Pregnancy Care					
Inpatient Neonatal Mortality	-	-	-	-	-
Third or Fourth Degree Laceration	-	-	3.58%	3.63%	3.27%

Citrus Valley Med Ctr Queen Valley Campus

1115 S Sunset Avenue
West Covina, CA 91790
URL: www.cvhp.org
Ownership: Voluntary non-profit - Other
Emergency Services: Yes
Phone: 626-962-4011
Fax: 626-858-8506
Accredited: Yes
Licensed Beds: 547

Key Personnel:
CEO/Administrator . . . . . Elvia Foulke
Chief Cardiology . . . . . Myhan Mguyen
Emergency Department . . . . . Jan Taylor
Chief Pulmonary Therapy . . . . . Fred Lopez

Measure	Cases	This Hospital	State Average	U.S. Average	Top Hospital
Heart Attack Care					
ACE Inhibitor or ARB for LVSD[1]	12	67%	82%	82%	100%
Aspirin at Arrival	62	90%	95%	92%	100%
Aspirin at Discharge	32	78%	90%	90%	100%
Beta Blocker at Arrival	41	95%	89%	87%	100%
Beta Blocker at Discharge	43	72%	89%	90%	100%
Fibrinolytic Medication Timing[1]	1	0%	40%	31%	100%
PCI Within 90 Minutes of Arrival	0	-	52%	54%	95%
Smoking Cessation Advice[1]	6	83%	87%	88%	100%
Heart Failure Care					
ACE Inhibitor or ARB for LVSD	154	78%	84%	82%	100%
Discharge Instructions	317	19%	56%	61%	93%
Evaluation of LVS Function	388	88%	84%	83%	99%
Smoking Cessation Advice	50	72%	82%	82%	100%
Pneumonia Care					
Appropriate Initial Antibiotic	207	84%	82%	83%	94%
Blood Culture Timing	205	67%	89%	90%	100%
Influenza Vaccine	64	23%	58%	70%	100%
Initial Antibiotic Timing	300	62%	75%	80%	93%
Oxygenation Assessment	378	99%	99%	99%	100%
Pneumococcal Vaccine	207	11%	58%	69%	94%
Smoking Cessation Advice	51	67%	75%	80%	100%
Surgical Infection Prevention					
Prophylactic Antibiotic Given[2,3]	314	73%	74%	77%	95%
Prophylactic Antibiotic Selection[2]	105	63%	89%	90%	100%
Prophylactic Antibiotic Stopped[2,3]	296	41%	65%	72%	95%
Pregnancy Care					
Inpatient Neonatal Mortality	-	-	-	-	-
Third or Fourth Degree Laceration	-	-	3.58%	3.63%	3.27%

Doctors Hospital of West Covina

725 S Orange Avenue
West Covina, CA 91790
Ownership: Proprietary
Emergency Services: No
Phone: 626-338-8481
Fax: 626-960-9178
Accredited: Yes
Licensed Beds: 51

Key Personnel:
Administrator . . . . . Gerald Wallman
Chief Medical Staff . . . . . Nashat Ateia, MD
Infection Control . . . . . Milad Shokair
Surgery Supervisor . . . . . Lisa Torres
Chief Radiology . . . . . John Raabe
Respiratory Therapy Supervisor . . . . . Charles Dunn

Measure	Cases	This Hospital	State Average	U.S. Average	Top Hospital
Heart Attack Care					
ACE Inhibitor or ARB for LVSD[5]	-	-	82%	82%	100%
Aspirin at Arrival[5]	-	-	95%	92%	100%
Aspirin at Discharge[5]	-	-	90%	90%	100%
Beta Blocker at Arrival[5]	-	-	89%	87%	100%
Beta Blocker at Discharge[5]	-	-	89%	90%	100%
Fibrinolytic Medication Timing[5]	-	-	40%	31%	100%
PCI Within 90 Minutes of Arrival[5]	-	-	52%	54%	95%
Smoking Cessation Advice[5]	-	-	87%	88%	100%
Heart Failure Care					
ACE Inhibitor or ARB for LVSD[3]	0	-	84%	82%	100%
Discharge Instructions[1,3]	4	0%	56%	61%	93%
Evaluation of LVS Function[1,3]	4	25%	84%	83%	99%
Smoking Cessation Advice[3]	0	-	82%	82%	100%
Pneumonia Care					
Appropriate Initial Antibiotic[1,3]	2	100%	82%	83%	94%
Blood Culture Timing[3]	0	-	89%	90%	100%
Influenza Vaccine[1]	1	100%	58%	70%	100%
Initial Antibiotic Timing[1,3]	2	0%	75%	80%	93%
Oxygenation Assessment[1,3]	3	100%	99%	99%	100%
Pneumococcal Vaccine[1,3]	2	50%	58%	69%	94%
Smoking Cessation Advice[1,3]	1	0%	75%	80%	100%
Surgical Infection Prevention					
Prophylactic Antibiotic Given[1,2,3]	12	67%	74%	77%	95%
Prophylactic Antibiotic Selection[1,2]	12	83%	89%	90%	100%
Prophylactic Antibiotic Stopped[1,2,3]	12	92%	65%	72%	95%
Pregnancy Care					
Inpatient Neonatal Mortality	-	-	-	-	-
Third or Fourth Degree Laceration	-	-	3.58%	3.63%	3.27%

West Hills Hospital and Medical Center

7300 Medical Center Drive
West Hills, CA 91307
URL: www.westhillshospital.com
Ownership: Proprietary
Emergency Services: Yes
Phone: 818-676-4000
Fax: 818-347-4519
Accredited: Yes
Licensed Beds: 236

Key Personnel:
President/CEO . . . . . Beverly Gilmore
President Medical Staff . . . . . Alan Kuban, MD

Measure	Cases	This Hospital	State Average	U.S. Average	Top Hospital
Heart Attack Care					
ACE Inhibitor or ARB for LVSD[1]	17	82%	82%	82%	100%

NOTE: Hospital profiles are in alphabetical order by state, then city, then hospital within the city; Rankings are sorted by rate in descending order and exclude hospitals with less than 25 cases; (1) The number of cases is too small (n<25) for purposes of reliably predicting hospital performance; (2) Measure reflects the hospital's indication that its submission was based upon a sample of its relevant discharges; (3) Rate reflects fewer than the maximum possible quarters of data for the measure; (4) Inaccurate information submitted and suppressed for one or more quarters; (5) No data is available from the hospital for this measure; Please refer to the User's Guide for a full explanation of data

Aspirin at Arrival	92	95%	95%	92%	100%
Aspirin at Discharge	91	90%	90%	90%	100%
Beta Blocker at Arrival	75	93%	89%	87%	100%
Beta Blocker at Discharge	88	95%	89%	90%	100%
Fibrinolytic Medication Timing[1]	6	33%	40%	31%	100%
PCI Within 90 Minutes of Arrival[1]	5	20%	52%	54%	95%
Smoking Cessation Advice[1]	17	94%	87%	88%	100%
Heart Failure Care					
ACE Inhibitor or ARB for LVSD	49	90%	84%	82%	100%
Discharge Instructions	138	26%	56%	61%	93%
Evaluation of LVS Function	201	78%	84%	83%	99%
Smoking Cessation Advice[1]	14	79%	82%	82%	100%
Pneumonia Care					
Appropriate Initial Antibiotic	210	66%	82%	83%	94%
Blood Culture Timing	264	94%	89%	90%	100%
Influenza Vaccine	80	61%	58%	70%	100%
Initial Antibiotic Timing	339	73%	75%	80%	93%
Oxygenation Assessment	446	99%	99%	99%	100%
Pneumococcal Vaccine	292	49%	58%	69%	94%
Smoking Cessation Advice	36	92%	75%	80%	100%
Surgical Infection Prevention					
Prophylactic Antibiotic Given[2,3]	211	80%	74%	77%	95%
Prophylactic Antibiotic Selection[2]	95	91%	89%	90%	100%
Prophylactic Antibiotic Stopped[2,3]	204	48%	65%	72%	95%
Pregnancy Care					
Inpatient Neonatal Mortality	-	-	-	-	-
Third or Fourth Degree Laceration	-	-	3.58%	3.63%	3.27%

Presbyterian Intercommunity Hospital

12401 Washington Boulevard — Phone: 562-698-0811
Whittier, CA 90602 — Fax: 562-945-6854
URL: www.whittierpres.com
Ownership: Voluntary non-profit - Private — Accredited: Yes
Emergency Services: Yes — Licensed Beds: 356

Key Personnel:

President/CEO . . . . Daniel F Adams
Chief Medical Staff . . . . Bharat Patel, MD
Emergency Room . . . . Stanley Combs, MD
Director Infection/Disease Control . . . . Patty Poynter
CCU Spvg. Nurse . . . . Reanna Thompson
OB/GYN Womens Health . . . . John Sanchez, MD
Chief Radiology . . . . William Shanahan, MD
Director Respiratory Therapy . . . . Hal Herlong

Measure	Cases	This Hospital	State Average	U.S. Average	Top Hospital
Heart Attack Care					
ACE Inhibitor or ARB for LVSD[2]	28	89%	82%	82%	100%
Aspirin at Arrival[2]	204	100%	95%	92%	100%
Aspirin at Discharge[2]	196	98%	90%	90%	100%
Beta Blocker at Arrival[2]	194	99%	89%	87%	100%
Beta Blocker at Discharge[2]	188	95%	89%	90%	100%
Fibrinolytic Medication Timing[1,2]	22	64%	40%	31%	100%
PCI Within 90 Minutes of Arrival[1,2]	2	0%	52%	54%	95%
Smoking Cessation Advice[2]	37	97%	87%	88%	100%
Heart Failure Care					
ACE Inhibitor or ARB for LVSD[2]	76	93%	84%	82%	100%
Discharge Instructions[2]	218	86%	56%	61%	93%
Evaluation of LVS Function[2]	255	97%	84%	83%	99%
Smoking Cessation Advice[2]	33	97%	82%	82%	100%
Pneumonia Care					
Appropriate Initial Antibiotic[2]	96	78%	82%	83%	94%
Blood Culture Timing[2]	101	92%	89%	90%	100%
Influenza Vaccine[1,2]	22	36%	58%	70%	100%
Initial Antibiotic Timing[2]	125	78%	75%	80%	93%
Oxygenation Assessment[2]	156	100%	99%	99%	100%
Pneumococcal Vaccine[2]	100	51%	58%	69%	94%
Smoking Cessation Advice[1,2]	12	83%	75%	80%	100%
Surgical Infection Prevention					
Prophylactic Antibiotic Given[2]	237	91%	74%	77%	95%
Prophylactic Antibiotic Selection[2]	64	94%	89%	90%	100%
Prophylactic Antibiotic Stopped[2]	225	64%	65%	72%	95%
Pregnancy Care					
Inpatient Neonatal Mortality	-	-	-	-	-
Third or Fourth Degree Laceration	-	-	3.58%	3.63%	3.27%

Whittier Hospital Medical Center

9080 Colima Road — Phone: 562-945-3561
Whittier, CA 90605 — Fax: 562-693-6811
URL: www.whittierhospital.com
Ownership: Proprietary — Accredited: Yes
Emergency Services: No — Licensed Beds: 181

Key Personnel:

CEO . . . . Howard Ternes
Cardiology Director . . . . Ernie Matsuo
Emergency Room . . . . Patrick Sargent
Infection Control . . . . Kym Lengyel
ICU . . . . Sandra Alderman
OB/GYN Womens Health . . . . Michael Grisanti
Director Respiratory Therapy . . . . Ernie Matsuo

Measure	Cases	This Hospital	State Average	U.S. Average	Top Hospital
Heart Attack Care					
ACE Inhibitor or ARB for LVSD[1,2]	6	67%	82%	82%	100%
Aspirin at Arrival[2]	122	98%	95%	92%	100%
Aspirin at Discharge[2]	38	89%	90%	90%	100%
Beta Blocker at Arrival[2]	101	91%	89%	87%	100%
Beta Blocker at Discharge[2]	50	90%	89%	90%	100%
Fibrinolytic Medication Timing[1,2]	16	38%	40%	31%	100%
PCI Within 90 Minutes of Arrival[2]	0	-	52%	54%	95%
Smoking Cessation Advice[1,2]	9	100%	87%	88%	100%
Heart Failure Care					
ACE Inhibitor or ARB for LVSD[2]	52	92%	84%	82%	100%
Discharge Instructions[2]	182	95%	56%	61%	93%
Evaluation of LVS Function[2]	251	96%	84%	83%	99%
Smoking Cessation Advice[1,2]	23	96%	82%	82%	100%
Pneumonia Care					
Appropriate Initial Antibiotic[2]	191	88%	82%	83%	94%
Blood Culture Timing[2]	219	93%	89%	90%	100%
Influenza Vaccine	66	79%	58%	70%	100%
Initial Antibiotic Timing[2]	292	77%	75%	80%	93%
Oxygenation Assessment[2]	353	100%	99%	99%	100%
Pneumococcal Vaccine[2]	229	78%	58%	69%	94%
Smoking Cessation Advice[2]	26	96%	75%	80%	100%
Surgical Infection Prevention					
Prophylactic Antibiotic Given[2]	272	88%	74%	77%	95%
Prophylactic Antibiotic Selection[2]	69	83%	89%	90%	100%
Prophylactic Antibiotic Stopped[2]	266	38%	65%	72%	95%
Pregnancy Care					
Inpatient Neonatal Mortality	-	-	-	-	-
Third or Fourth Degree Laceration	-	-	3.58%	3.63%	3.27%

Frank R Howard Memorial Hospital

One Madrone Street — Phone: 707-459-6801
Willits, CA 95490 — Fax: 707-459-9486
URL: www.howardhospital.com
Ownership: Voluntary non-profit - Church — Accredited: Yes
Emergency Services: Yes — Licensed Beds: 38

Key Personnel:

CEO . . . . Kevin Erich
Chief Medical Staff . . . . Carla Longthamp
Emergency Room . . . . Marilyn Depew
Director Respiratory Therapy . . . . John White

Measure	Cases	This Hospital	State Average	U.S. Average	Top Hospital
Heart Attack Care					
ACE Inhibitor or ARB for LVSD	0	-	82%	82%	100%
Aspirin at Arrival[1]	2	100%	95%	92%	100%
Aspirin at Discharge	0	-	90%	90%	100%
Beta Blocker at Arrival[1]	2	100%	89%	87%	100%
Beta Blocker at Discharge	0	-	89%	90%	100%
Fibrinolytic Medication Timing	0	-	40%	31%	100%
PCI Within 90 Minutes of Arrival	0	-	52%	54%	95%
Smoking Cessation Advice	0	-	87%	88%	100%
Heart Failure Care					
ACE Inhibitor or ARB for LVSD[1]	4	100%	84%	82%	100%

NOTE: Hospital profiles are in alphabetical order by state, then city, then hospital within the city; Rankings are sorted by rate in descending order and exclude hospitals with less than 25 cases; (1) The number of cases is too small (n<25) for purposes of reliably predicting hospital performance; (2) Measure reflects the hospital's indication that its submission was based upon a sample of its relevant discharges; (3) Rate reflects fewer than the maximum possible quarters of data for the measure; (4) Inaccurate information submitted and suppressed for one or more quarters; (5) No data is available from the hospital for this measure; Please refer to the User's Guide for a full explanation of data

Discharge Instructions[1]	14	50%	56%	61%	93%
Evaluation of LVS Function[1]	17	94%	84%	83%	99%
Smoking Cessation Advice[1]	3	33%	82%	82%	100%
Pneumonia Care					
Appropriate Initial Antibiotic	40	80%	82%	83%	94%
Blood Culture Timing[1]	21	90%	89%	90%	100%
Influenza Vaccine[1]	8	88%	58%	70%	100%
Initial Antibiotic Timing	47	91%	75%	80%	93%
Oxygenation Assessment	60	100%	99%	99%	100%
Pneumococcal Vaccine	34	68%	58%	69%	94%
Smoking Cessation Advice[1]	22	95%	75%	80%	100%
Surgical Infection Prevention					
Prophylactic Antibiotic Given[2,3]	25	100%	74%	77%	95%
Prophylactic Antibiotic Selection[2]	26	96%	89%	90%	100%
Prophylactic Antibiotic Stopped[2,3]	25	84%	65%	72%	95%
Pregnancy Care					
Inpatient Neonatal Mortality	-	-	-	-	-
Third or Fourth Degree Laceration	-	-	3.58%	3.63%	3.27%

Glenn Medical Center

1133 W Sycamore St
Willows, CA 95988
Phone: 530-934-1818
Ownership: Voluntary non-profit - Private
Accredited: No
Emergency Services: Yes

Measure	Cases	This Hospital	State Average	U.S. Average	Top Hospital
Heart Attack Care					
ACE Inhibitor or ARB for LVSD[5]	-	-	82%	82%	100%
Aspirin at Arrival[5]	-	-	95%	92%	100%
Aspirin at Discharge[5]	-	-	90%	90%	100%
Beta Blocker at Arrival[5]	-	-	89%	87%	100%
Beta Blocker at Discharge[5]	-	-	89%	90%	100%
Fibrinolytic Medication Timing[5]	-	-	40%	31%	100%
PCI Within 90 Minutes of Arrival[5]	-	-	52%	54%	95%
Smoking Cessation Advice[5]	-	-	87%	88%	100%
Heart Failure Care					
ACE Inhibitor or ARB for LVSD[5]	-	-	84%	82%	100%
Discharge Instructions[5]	-	-	56%	61%	93%
Evaluation of LVS Function[5]	-	-	84%	83%	99%
Smoking Cessation Advice[5]	-	-	82%	82%	100%
Pneumonia Care					
Appropriate Initial Antibiotic[1,3]	4	75%	82%	83%	94%
Blood Culture Timing[1,3]	3	100%	89%	90%	100%
Influenza Vaccine[5]	-	-	58%	70%	100%
Initial Antibiotic Timing[1,3]	7	86%	75%	80%	93%
Oxygenation Assessment[1,3]	7	100%	99%	99%	100%
Pneumococcal Vaccine[1,3]	2	100%	58%	69%	94%
Smoking Cessation Advice[1,3]	3	67%	75%	80%	100%
Surgical Infection Prevention					
Prophylactic Antibiotic Given[5]	-	-	74%	77%	95%
Prophylactic Antibiotic Selection[5]	-	-	89%	90%	100%
Prophylactic Antibiotic Stopped[5]	-	-	65%	72%	95%
Pregnancy Care					
Inpatient Neonatal Mortality	-	-	-	-	-
Third or Fourth Degree Laceration	-	-	3.58%	3.63%	3.27%

Woodland Healthcare

Alternate Name: Woodland Memorial Hospital
1325 Cottonwood Street
Woodland, CA 95695
Phone: 530-662-3961
Fax: 530-666-7948
URL: www.woodlandhealthcare.org
Ownership: Voluntary non-profit - Other
Accredited: Yes
Emergency Services: Yes
Licensed Beds: 103

Key Personnel:

President/CEO. . . . . Kevin Vazri
Director Medical/Surgical Nursing . . . . Debbie Kinney
OB/GYN Womens Health. . . . . George Wong, MD
Chief Radiology . . . . Steven Liston, MD

Measure	Cases	This Hospital	State Average	U.S. Average	Top Hospital
Heart Attack Care					
ACE Inhibitor or ARB for LVSD[1]	1	100%	82%	82%	100%
Aspirin at Arrival[1]	21	100%	95%	92%	100%
Aspirin at Discharge[1]	7	71%	90%	90%	100%
Beta Blocker at Arrival[1]	20	100%	89%	87%	100%
Beta Blocker at Discharge[1]	6	100%	89%	90%	100%
Fibrinolytic Medication Timing[1]	5	40%	40%	31%	100%
PCI Within 90 Minutes of Arrival	0	-	52%	54%	95%
Smoking Cessation Advice[1]	1	0%	87%	88%	100%
Heart Failure Care					
ACE Inhibitor or ARB for LVSD	34	94%	84%	82%	100%
Discharge Instructions	81	81%	56%	61%	93%
Evaluation of LVS Function	99	97%	84%	83%	99%
Smoking Cessation Advice[1]	16	100%	82%	82%	100%
Pneumonia Care					
Appropriate Initial Antibiotic	62	81%	82%	83%	94%
Blood Culture Timing	65	97%	89%	90%	100%
Influenza Vaccine[1]	24	62%	58%	70%	100%
Initial Antibiotic Timing	88	91%	75%	80%	93%
Oxygenation Assessment	104	100%	99%	99%	100%
Pneumococcal Vaccine	65	91%	58%	69%	94%
Smoking Cessation Advice[1]	21	76%	75%	80%	100%
Surgical Infection Prevention					
Prophylactic Antibiotic Given[2,3]	117	82%	74%	77%	95%
Prophylactic Antibiotic Selection[2]	46	96%	89%	90%	100%
Prophylactic Antibiotic Stopped[2,3]	113	91%	65%	72%	95%
Pregnancy Care					
Inpatient Neonatal Mortality	771	0.13%	-	-	-
Third or Fourth Degree Laceration	566	1.41%	3.58%	3.63%	3.27%

Kaiser Foundation Hospital

5601 De Soto
Woodland Hills, CA 91367
Phone: 818-719-3800
Ownership: Voluntary non-profit - Private
Accredited: Yes
Emergency Services: Yes

Measure	Cases	This Hospital	State Average	U.S. Average	Top Hospital
Heart Attack Care					
ACE Inhibitor or ARB for LVSD[1]	15	100%	82%	82%	100%
Aspirin at Arrival	100	94%	95%	92%	100%
Aspirin at Discharge	80	89%	90%	90%	100%
Beta Blocker at Arrival	100	95%	89%	87%	100%
Beta Blocker at Discharge	87	99%	89%	90%	100%
Fibrinolytic Medication Timing[1]	16	81%	40%	31%	100%
PCI Within 90 Minutes of Arrival	0	-	52%	54%	95%
Smoking Cessation Advice[1]	12	92%	87%	88%	100%
Heart Failure Care					
ACE Inhibitor or ARB for LVSD	92	85%	84%	82%	100%
Discharge Instructions	282	68%	56%	61%	93%
Evaluation of LVS Function	299	96%	84%	83%	99%
Smoking Cessation Advice[1]	20	75%	82%	82%	100%
Pneumonia Care					
Appropriate Initial Antibiotic	76	37%	82%	83%	94%
Blood Culture Timing	69	77%	89%	90%	100%
Influenza Vaccine	30	77%	58%	70%	100%
Initial Antibiotic Timing	99	47%	75%	80%	93%
Oxygenation Assessment	124	100%	99%	99%	100%
Pneumococcal Vaccine	96	70%	58%	69%	94%
Smoking Cessation Advice[1]	18	72%	75%	80%	100%
Surgical Infection Prevention					
Prophylactic Antibiotic Given[3]	49	84%	74%	77%	95%
Prophylactic Antibiotic Selection	49	86%	89%	90%	100%
Prophylactic Antibiotic Stopped[3]	48	73%	65%	72%	95%
Pregnancy Care					
Inpatient Neonatal Mortality	1,761	0.28%	-	-	-
Third or Fourth Degree Laceration	1,219	3.77%	3.58%	3.63%	3.27%

NOTE: Hospital profiles are in alphabetical order by state, then city, then hospital within the city; Rankings are sorted by rate in descending order and exclude hospitals with less than 25 cases; (1) The number of cases is too small (n<25) for purposes of reliably predicting hospital performance; (2) Measure reflects the hospital's indication that its submission was based upon a sample of its relevant discharges; (3) Rate reflects fewer than the maximum possible quarters of data for the measure; (4) Inaccurate information submitted and suppressed for one or more quarters; (5) No data is available from the hospital for this measure; Please refer to the User's Guide for a full explanation of data

Motion Picture & Television Hospital

23388 Mulholland Drive
Woodland Hills, CA 91364
URL: www.mptvfund.org
Ownership: Voluntary non-profit - Other
Emergency Services: No
Phone: 818-876-1888
Fax: 818-876-1079
Accredited: Yes
Licensed Beds: 256

Key Personnel:

President/CEO. . . . . David Tillman, MD
Chief of Medical Staff. . . . . Saeed Humaun
Director Medical/Surgical Nursing . . . . . Nancy Ramirez, RN
Chief Radiology . . . . . Bruce Shragg, MD
Director Respiratory Therapy . . . . . John Palean

Measure	Cases	This Hospital	State Average	U.S. Average	Top Hospital
Heart Attack Care					
ACE Inhibitor or ARB for LVSD[3]	0	-	82%	82%	100%
Aspirin at Arrival[1,3]	5	100%	95%	92%	100%
Aspirin at Discharge[3]	0	-	90%	90%	100%
Beta Blocker at Arrival[1,3]	3	67%	89%	87%	100%
Beta Blocker at Discharge[3]	0	-	89%	90%	100%
Fibrinolytic Medication Timing[3]	0	-	40%	31%	100%
PCI Within 90 Minutes of Arrival[5]	-	-	52%	54%	95%
Smoking Cessation Advice[1,3]	1	100%	87%	88%	100%
Heart Failure Care					
ACE Inhibitor or ARB for LVSD[1]	15	80%	84%	82%	100%
Discharge Instructions	36	58%	56%	61%	93%
Evaluation of LVS Function	49	96%	84%	83%	99%
Smoking Cessation Advice[1]	5	20%	82%	82%	100%
Pneumonia Care					
Appropriate Initial Antibiotic[1]	18	72%	82%	83%	94%
Blood Culture Timing[1]	2	100%	89%	90%	100%
Influenza Vaccine[1]	8	25%	58%	70%	100%
Initial Antibiotic Timing[1]	22	73%	75%	80%	93%
Oxygenation Assessment	29	100%	99%	99%	100%
Pneumococcal Vaccine[1]	16	69%	58%	69%	94%
Smoking Cessation Advice[1]	4	25%	75%	80%	100%
Surgical Infection Prevention					
Prophylactic Antibiotic Given[3]	26	69%	74%	77%	95%
Prophylactic Antibiotic Selection[1]	2	50%	89%	90%	100%
Prophylactic Antibiotic Stopped[1,3]	19	79%	65%	72%	95%
Pregnancy Care					
Inpatient Neonatal Mortality	-	-	-	-	-
Third or Fourth Degree Laceration	-	-	3.58%	3.63%	3.27%

Veterans Home of California

100 California Drive
Yountville, CA 94599
Ownership: Government - State
Emergency Services: No
Phone: 707-944-4600
Fax: 707-944-5005
Accredited: No
Licensed Beds: 824

Key Personnel:

Administrator . . . . . Marcella M McCormack
Chief Medical Staff. . . . . Paul B Chin, MD
Director Infection/Disease Control . . . . . Sandra Foley

Measure	Cases	This Hospital	State Average	U.S. Average	Top Hospital
Heart Attack Care					
ACE Inhibitor or ARB for LVSD[3]	0	-	82%	82%	100%
Aspirin at Arrival[1,3]	1	100%	95%	92%	100%
Aspirin at Discharge[1,3]	1	100%	90%	90%	100%
Beta Blocker at Arrival[1,3]	1	100%	89%	87%	100%
Beta Blocker at Discharge[1,3]	1	0%	89%	90%	100%
Fibrinolytic Medication Timing[3]	0	-	40%	31%	100%
PCI Within 90 Minutes of Arrival[5]	-	-	52%	54%	95%
Smoking Cessation Advice[3]	0	-	87%	88%	100%
Heart Failure Care					
ACE Inhibitor or ARB for LVSD[3]	0	-	84%	82%	100%
Discharge Instructions[3]	0	-	56%	61%	93%
Evaluation of LVS Function[1,3]	6	0%	84%	83%	99%
Smoking Cessation Advice[3]	0	-	82%	82%	100%
Pneumonia Care					
Appropriate Initial Antibiotic[1]	13	92%	82%	83%	94%
Blood Culture Timing[1]	1	100%	89%	90%	100%
Influenza Vaccine[1]	4	75%	58%	70%	100%
Initial Antibiotic Timing[1]	17	94%	75%	80%	93%
Oxygenation Assessment[1]	20	100%	99%	99%	100%
Pneumococcal Vaccine[1]	18	94%	58%	69%	94%
Smoking Cessation Advice[1]	4	75%	75%	80%	100%
Surgical Infection Prevention					
Prophylactic Antibiotic Given[5]	-	-	74%	77%	95%
Prophylactic Antibiotic Selection[5]	-	-	89%	90%	100%
Prophylactic Antibiotic Stopped[5]	-	-	65%	72%	95%
Pregnancy Care					
Inpatient Neonatal Mortality	-	-	-	-	-
Third or Fourth Degree Laceration	-	-	3.58%	3.63%	3.27%

Fairchild Medical Center

444 Bruce Street
Yreka, CA 96097
E-mail: inquiries@fairchildmed.org
URL: www.fairchildmed.org
Ownership: Voluntary non-profit - Other
Emergency Services: Yes
Phone: 530-842-4121
Fax: 530-841-0913
Accredited: Yes
Licensed Beds: 25

Key Personnel:

CEO. . . . . Dwayne Jones

Measure	Cases	This Hospital	State Average	U.S. Average	Top Hospital
Heart Attack Care					
ACE Inhibitor or ARB for LVSD[5]	-	-	82%	82%	100%
Aspirin at Arrival[5]	-	-	95%	92%	100%
Aspirin at Discharge[5]	-	-	90%	90%	100%
Beta Blocker at Arrival[5]	-	-	89%	87%	100%
Beta Blocker at Discharge[5]	-	-	89%	90%	100%
Fibrinolytic Medication Timing[5]	-	-	40%	31%	100%
PCI Within 90 Minutes of Arrival[5]	-	-	52%	54%	95%
Smoking Cessation Advice[5]	-	-	87%	88%	100%
Heart Failure Care					
ACE Inhibitor or ARB for LVSD[5]	-	-	84%	82%	100%
Discharge Instructions[5]	-	-	56%	61%	93%
Evaluation of LVS Function[5]	-	-	84%	83%	99%
Smoking Cessation Advice[5]	-	-	82%	82%	100%
Pneumonia Care					
Appropriate Initial Antibiotic[5]	-	-	82%	83%	94%
Blood Culture Timing[5]	-	-	89%	90%	100%
Influenza Vaccine[4,5]	-	-	58%	70%	100%
Initial Antibiotic Timing[5]	-	-	75%	80%	93%
Oxygenation Assessment[5]	-	-	99%	99%	100%
Pneumococcal Vaccine[5]	-	-	58%	69%	94%
Smoking Cessation Advice[5]	-	-	75%	80%	100%
Surgical Infection Prevention					
Prophylactic Antibiotic Given[5]	-	-	74%	77%	95%
Prophylactic Antibiotic Selection[5]	-	-	89%	90%	100%
Prophylactic Antibiotic Stopped[5]	-	-	65%	72%	95%
Pregnancy Care					
Inpatient Neonatal Mortality	-	-	-	-	-
Third or Fourth Degree Laceration	-	-	3.58%	3.63%	3.27%

NOTE: Hospital profiles are in alphabetical order by state, then city, then hospital within the city; Rankings are sorted by rate in descending order and exclude hospitals with less than 25 cases; (1) The number of cases is too small (n<25) for purposes of reliably predicting hospital performance; (2) Measure reflects the hospital's indication that its submission was based upon a sample of its relevant discharges; (3) Rate reflects fewer than the maximum possible quarters of data for the measure; (4) Inaccurate information submitted and suppressed for one or more quarters; (5) No data is available from the hospital for this measure; Please refer to the User's Guide for a full explanation of data

Heart Attack Care

1. ACE Inhibitor or ARB for LVSD

Hospital Name	City	Rate	Cases
Parkview Medical Center	Pueblo	100%	47
Saint Anthony Central Hospital	Denver	100%	58
Memorial Hospital	Colorado Springs	98%	50
North Colorado Medical Center	Greeley	96%	46
Swedish Medical Center	Englewood	92%	38
Saint Mary's Hospital & Medical Center	Grand Junction	91%	67
Medical Center of Aurora	Aurora	90%	42
Penrose Saint Francis Health Services	Colorado Springs	88%	74
Porter Adventist Hospital	Denver	88%	25
Poudre Valley Hospital	Fort Collins	88%	89
Exempla Saint Joseph Hospital	Denver	85%	34
University of Colorado Hospital	Denver	85%	27
Exempla Lutheran Medical Center	Wheat Ridge	78%	36

2. Aspirin at Arrival

Hospital Name	City	Rate	Cases
Avista Adventist Hospital	Louisville	100%	26
Boulder Community Hospital	Boulder	100%	69
Exempla Lutheran Medical Center	Wheat Ridge	100%	270
Littleton Adventist Hospital	Littleton	100%	106
Medical Center of Aurora	Aurora	100%	278
Montrose Memorial Hospital	Montrose	100%	33
North Suburban Medical Center	Thornton	100%	106
Parkview Medical Center	Pueblo	100%	117
Presbyterian-Saint Luke's Medical Center	Denver	100%	39
Rose Medical Center	Denver	100%	137
Saint Anthony Central Hospital	Denver	100%	182
Saint Anthony North Hospital	Westminster	100%	104
Saint Mary-Corwin Medical Center	Pueblo	100%	80
Sky Ridge Medical Center	Lone Tree	100%	63
Exempla Saint Joseph Hospital	Denver	99%	182
Memorial Hospital	Colorado Springs	99%	318
Parker Adventist Hospital	Parker	99%	74
Penrose Saint Francis Health Services	Colorado Springs	99%	293
Poudre Valley Hospital	Fort Collins	99%	226
University of Colorado Hospital	Denver	99%	115
Exempla Good Samaritan Medical Center	Lafayette	98%	126
Mercy Regional Medical Center	Durango	98%	49
North Colorado Medical Center	Greeley	98%	157
Saint Mary's Hospital & Medical Center	Grand Junction	98%	167
Swedish Medical Center	Englewood	98%	176
Denver Health Medical Center	Denver	97%	79
McKee Medical Center	Loveland	97%	62
Porter Adventist Hospital	Denver	97%	97
Longmont United Hospital	Longmont	95%	78
Delta County Memorial Hospital	Delta	89%	38

3. Aspirin at Discharge

Hospital Name	City	Rate	Cases
Boulder Community Hospital	Boulder	100%	88
Exempla Saint Joseph Hospital	Denver	100%	204
McKee Medical Center	Loveland	100%	46
Mercy Regional Medical Center	Durango	100%	66
North Suburban Medical Center	Thornton	100%	89
Presbyterian-Saint Luke's Medical Center	Denver	100%	115
Rose Medical Center	Denver	100%	132
Saint Anthony Central Hospital	Denver	100%	270
Saint Mary's Hospital & Medical Center	Grand Junction	100%	305
Sky Ridge Medical Center	Lone Tree	100%	54
Medical Center of Aurora	Aurora	99%	350
North Colorado Medical Center	Greeley	99%	216
Parkview Medical Center	Pueblo	99%	186
Poudre Valley Hospital	Fort Collins	99%	361
Saint Anthony North Hospital	Westminster	99%	86
University of Colorado Hospital	Denver	99%	137
Exempla Lutheran Medical Center	Wheat Ridge	98%	240
Memorial Hospital	Colorado Springs	98%	363
Porter Adventist Hospital	Denver	98%	91
Denver Health Medical Center	Denver	97%	59
Exempla Good Samaritan Medical Center	Lafayette	97%	110
Littleton Adventist Hospital	Littleton	97%	75
Longmont United Hospital	Longmont	97%	64
Montrose Memorial Hospital	Montrose	97%	33
Parker Adventist Hospital	Parker	97%	67
Penrose Saint Francis Health Services	Colorado Springs	97%	316
Saint Mary-Corwin Medical Center	Pueblo	97%	96
Swedish Medical Center	Englewood	96%	142
Delta County Memorial Hospital	Delta	85%	26

4. Beta Blocker at Arrival

Hospital Name	City	Rate	Cases
Mercy Regional Medical Center	Durango	100%	36
Montrose Memorial Hospital	Montrose	100%	28
North Suburban Medical Center	Thornton	100%	74
Presbyterian-Saint Luke's Medical Center	Denver	100%	25
Rose Medical Center	Denver	100%	100
Saint Mary-Corwin Medical Center	Pueblo	100%	76
Littleton Adventist Hospital	Littleton	99%	77
Parkview Medical Center	Pueblo	99%	91
Saint Anthony North Hospital	Westminster	99%	96
Exempla Good Samaritan Medical Center	Lafayette	98%	95
McKee Medical Center	Loveland	98%	48
Medical Center of Aurora	Aurora	98%	211
Memorial Hospital	Colorado Springs	98%	245
Parker Adventist Hospital	Parker	98%	63
Swedish Medical Center	Englewood	98%	138
Saint Anthony Central Hospital	Denver	97%	154
Saint Mary's Hospital & Medical Center	Grand Junction	97%	104
Exempla Saint Joseph Hospital	Denver	96%	133
North Colorado Medical Center	Greeley	96%	129
Porter Adventist Hospital	Denver	96%	80
Poudre Valley Hospital	Fort Collins	96%	168
University of Colorado Hospital	Denver	96%	84
Boulder Community Hospital	Boulder	95%	66
Delta County Memorial Hospital	Delta	95%	39
Denver Health Medical Center	Denver	95%	62
Sky Ridge Medical Center	Lone Tree	95%	41
Penrose Saint Francis Health Services	Colorado Springs	93%	227
Exempla Lutheran Medical Center	Wheat Ridge	92%	169
Longmont United Hospital	Longmont	85%	62

5. Beta Blocker at Discharge

Hospital Name	City	Rate	Cases
Exempla Saint Joseph Hospital	Denver	100%	255
Montrose Memorial Hospital	Montrose	100%	33
Parkview Medical Center	Pueblo	100%	193
Rose Medical Center	Denver	100%	130
Saint Anthony Central Hospital	Denver	100%	252
Saint Anthony North Hospital	Westminster	100%	82
Memorial Hospital	Colorado Springs	99%	347
North Suburban Medical Center	Thornton	99%	74
Presbyterian-Saint Luke's Medical Center	Denver	99%	135
Saint Mary's Hospital & Medical Center	Grand Junction	99%	293
University of Colorado Hospital	Denver	99%	161
Exempla Good Samaritan Medical Center	Lafayette	98%	133
Exempla Lutheran Medical Center	Wheat Ridge	98%	230
Littleton Adventist Hospital	Littleton	98%	92
McKee Medical Center	Loveland	98%	48
Medical Center of Aurora	Aurora	98%	369
North Colorado Medical Center	Greeley	98%	208
Porter Adventist Hospital	Denver	98%	117
Poudre Valley Hospital	Fort Collins	98%	450
Sky Ridge Medical Center	Lone Tree	98%	61
Boulder Community Hospital	Boulder	97%	87
Denver Health Medical Center	Denver	97%	59
Parker Adventist Hospital	Parker	97%	70
Saint Mary-Corwin Medical Center	Pueblo	97%	94
Swedish Medical Center	Englewood	97%	188
Longmont United Hospital	Longmont	95%	78
Mercy Regional Medical Center	Durango	95%	63
Penrose Saint Francis Health Services	Colorado Springs	95%	346
Delta County Memorial Hospital	Delta	86%	29

7. PCI Within 90 Minutes of Arrival

Hospital Name	City	Rate	Cases
Poudre Valley Hospital	Fort Collins	68%	28

8. Smoking Cessation Advice

Hospital Name	City	Rate	Cases
Memorial Hospital	Colorado Springs	100%	137
North Suburban Medical Center	Thornton	100%	50
Parkview Medical Center	Pueblo	100%	62
Penrose Saint Francis Health Services	Colorado Springs	100%	120
Presbyterian-Saint Luke's Medical Center	Denver	100%	40
Saint Anthony Central Hospital	Denver	100%	102
Saint Anthony North Hospital	Westminster	100%	28
Saint Mary's Hospital & Medical Center	Grand Junction	100%	107
University of Colorado Hospital	Denver	100%	67
Exempla Lutheran Medical Center	Wheat Ridge	99%	89
Swedish Medical Center	Englewood	99%	70
North Colorado Medical Center	Greeley	98%	56

NOTE: Hospital profiles are in alphabetical order by state, then city, then hospital within the city; Rankings are sorted by rate in descending order and exclude hospitals with less than 25 cases; (1) The number of cases is too small (n<25) for purposes of reliably predicting hospital performance; (2) Measure reflects the hospital's indication that its submission was based upon a sample of its relevant discharges; (3) Rate reflects fewer than the maximum possible quarters of data for the measure; (4) Inaccurate information submitted and suppressed for one or more quarters; (5) No data is available from the hospital for this measure; Please refer to the User's Guide for a full explanation of data

Hospital Name	City	Rate	Cases
Porter Adventist Hospital	Denver	98%	40
Saint Mary-Corwin Medical Center	Pueblo	98%	53
Exempla Good Samaritan Medical Center	Lafayette	97%	38
Exempla Saint Joseph Hospital	Denver	97%	74
Rose Medical Center	Denver	97%	39
Longmont United Hospital	Longmont	96%	28
Poudre Valley Hospital	Fort Collins	96%	163
Medical Center of Aurora	Aurora	95%	132
Denver Health Medical Center	Denver	90%	41

Heart Failure Care

9. ACE Inhibitor or ARB for LVSD

Hospital Name	City	Rate	Cases
North Suburban Medical Center	Thornton	100%	26
Parkview Medical Center	Pueblo	100%	84
North Colorado Medical Center	Greeley	95%	109
Presbyterian-Saint Luke's Medical Center	Denver	95%	66
Saint Anthony North Hospital	Westminster	94%	47
McKee Medical Center	Loveland	93%	29
Medical Center of Aurora	Aurora	92%	119
Mercy Regional Medical Center	Durango	92%	25
Exempla Lutheran Medical Center	Wheat Ridge	90%	94
Memorial Hospital	Colorado Springs	90%	207
Saint Mary-Corwin Medical Center	Pueblo	90%	40
Denver Health Medical Center	Denver	89%	159
Saint Anthony Central Hospital	Denver	89%	76
University of Colorado Hospital	Denver	89%	150
Porter Adventist Hospital	Denver	88%	49
Rose Medical Center	Denver	86%	70
Penrose Saint Francis Health Services	Colorado Springs	85%	194
Saint Mary's Hospital & Medical Center	Grand Junction	85%	74
Exempla Saint Joseph Hospital	Denver	84%	92
Swedish Medical Center	Englewood	82%	93
Littleton Adventist Hospital	Littleton	79%	38
Sky Ridge Medical Center	Lone Tree	79%	29
Exempla Good Samaritan Medical Center	Lafayette	76%	62
Poudre Valley Hospital	Fort Collins	76%	85
Boulder Community Hospital	Boulder	73%	71
Longmont United Hospital	Longmont	69%	62

10. Discharge Instructions

Hospital Name	City	Rate	Cases
Parkview Medical Center	Pueblo	100%	183
Exempla Lutheran Medical Center	Wheat Ridge	95%	190
North Suburban Medical Center	Thornton	92%	61
Saint Mary-Corwin Medical Center	Pueblo	92%	120
Exempla Saint Joseph Hospital	Denver	91%	223
Exempla Good Samaritan Medical Center	Lafayette	87%	201
McKee Medical Center	Loveland	87%	63
University of Colorado Hospital	Denver	86%	277
Presbyterian-Saint Luke's Medical Center	Denver	84%	142
Penrose Saint Francis Health Services	Colorado Springs	83%	318
Community Hospital	Grand Junction	82%	34
Valley View Hospital	Glenwood Springs	82%	28
Swedish Medical Center	Englewood	75%	216
Mercy Regional Medical Center	Durango	73%	56
Memorial Hospital	Colorado Springs	72%	414
Littleton Adventist Hospital	Littleton	70%	73
Platte Valley Medical Center	Brighton	68%	40
Porter Adventist Hospital	Denver	67%	166
Rose Medical Center	Denver	65%	160
Denver Health Medical Center	Denver	64%	247
Poudre Valley Hospital	Fort Collins	64%	181
Colorado Plains Medical Center	Fort Morgan	62%	26
Saint Anthony North Hospital	Westminster	62%	130
Medical Center of Aurora	Aurora	61%	273
North Colorado Medical Center	Greeley	59%	211
Saint Anthony Central Hospital	Denver	59%	150
Saint Mary's Hospital & Medical Center	Grand Junction	54%	155
Arkansas Valley Regional Medical Center	La Junta	49%	51
Delta County Memorial Hospital	Delta	49%	47
Boulder Community Hospital	Boulder	46%	127
Sterling Regional MedCenter	Sterling	43%	30
Parker Adventist Hospital	Parker	41%	51
Longmont United Hospital	Longmont	35%	122
Sky Ridge Medical Center	Lone Tree	29%	70
Montrose Memorial Hospital	Montrose	15%	33
Saint Thomas More Hospital	Canon City	10%	31
Prowers Medical Center	Lamar	0%	25

11. Evaluation of LVS Function

Hospital Name	City	Rate	Cases
Mercy Regional Medical Center	Durango	100%	61
North Suburban Medical Center	Thornton	100%	87
Parkview Medical Center	Pueblo	100%	223
Denver Health Medical Center	Denver	98%	259
Presbyterian-Saint Luke's Medical Center	Denver	98%	165
Rose Medical Center	Denver	98%	205
Sky Ridge Medical Center	Lone Tree	98%	92
Exempla Lutheran Medical Center	Wheat Ridge	97%	260
Saint Anthony North Hospital	Westminster	97%	162
Saint Mary's Hospital & Medical Center	Grand Junction	97%	189
University of Colorado Hospital	Denver	97%	308
Valley View Hospital	Glenwood Springs	97%	33
McKee Medical Center	Loveland	96%	90
Porter Adventist Hospital	Denver	96%	201
Exempla Saint Joseph Hospital	Denver	95%	278
Saint Anthony Central Hospital	Denver	95%	187
Exempla Good Samaritan Medical Center	Lafayette	94%	232
Penrose Saint Francis Health Services	Colorado Springs	94%	394
Swedish Medical Center	Englewood	94%	287
Medical Center of Aurora	Aurora	93%	341
Memorial Hospital	Colorado Springs	93%	476
Saint Mary-Corwin Medical Center	Pueblo	93%	140
Littleton Adventist Hospital	Littleton	92%	108
Parker Adventist Hospital	Parker	91%	64
Poudre Valley Hospital	Fort Collins	90%	241
Boulder Community Hospital	Boulder	89%	158
North Colorado Medical Center	Greeley	89%	266
Longmont United Hospital	Longmont	86%	182
Delta County Memorial Hospital	Delta	83%	63
Platte Valley Medical Center	Brighton	82%	50
Community Hospital	Grand Junction	81%	48
Sterling Regional MedCenter	Sterling	81%	47
Avista Adventist Hospital	Louisville	77%	26
Colorado Plains Medical Center	Fort Morgan	76%	41
San Luis Valley Regional Medical Center	Alamosa	72%	25
Arkansas Valley Regional Medical Center	La Junta	69%	70
Memorial Hospital	Craig	68%	25
Saint Thomas More Hospital	Canon City	62%	39
Montrose Memorial Hospital	Montrose	60%	48
Prowers Medical Center	Lamar	50%	28

12. Smoking Cessation Advice

Hospital Name	City	Rate	Cases
Exempla Lutheran Medical Center	Wheat Ridge	100%	37
Parkview Medical Center	Pueblo	100%	35
Saint Anthony Central Hospital	Denver	100%	40
Saint Mary-Corwin Medical Center	Pueblo	100%	26
Memorial Hospital	Colorado Springs	99%	90
University of Colorado Hospital	Denver	99%	81
Exempla Saint Joseph Hospital	Denver	97%	31
Penrose Saint Francis Health Services	Colorado Springs	97%	58
Presbyterian-Saint Luke's Medical Center	Denver	97%	31
Medical Center of Aurora	Aurora	94%	64
Poudre Valley Hospital	Fort Collins	93%	58
Porter Adventist Hospital	Denver	92%	36
Exempla Good Samaritan Medical Center	Lafayette	91%	33
North Colorado Medical Center	Greeley	91%	47
Saint Mary's Hospital & Medical Center	Grand Junction	89%	35
Denver Health Medical Center	Denver	79%	117
Swedish Medical Center	Englewood	77%	39

Pneumonia Care

13. Appropriate Initial Antibiotic

Hospital Name	City	Rate	Cases
Mercy Regional Medical Center	Durango	97%	58
East Morgan County Hospital	Brush	96%	28
Parker Adventist Hospital	Parker	94%	79
Rose Medical Center	Denver	94%	141
Exempla Lutheran Medical Center	Wheat Ridge	93%	113
North Suburban Medical Center	Thornton	93%	97
Saint Mary's Hospital & Medical Center	Grand Junction	92%	158
Swedish Medical Center	Englewood	92%	170
McKee Medical Center	Loveland	91%	88
Community Hospital	Grand Junction	90%	39
Delta County Memorial Hospital	Delta	90%	90
Grand River Hospital District	Rifle	90%	29
Yampa Valley Medical Center	Steamboat Springs	89%	46
Exempla Good Samaritan Medical Center	Lafayette	88%	101
Littleton Adventist Hospital	Littleton	88%	163
Medical Center of Aurora	Aurora	88%	212

NOTE: Hospital profiles are in alphabetical order by state, then city, then hospital within the city; Rankings are sorted by rate in descending order and exclude hospitals with less than 25 cases; (1) The number of cases is too small (n<25) for purposes of reliably predicting hospital performance; (2) Measure reflects the hospital's indication that its submission was based upon a sample of its relevant discharges; (3) Rate reflects fewer than the maximum possible quarters of data for the measure; (4) Inaccurate information submitted and suppressed for one or more quarters; (5) No data is available from the hospital for this measure; Please refer to the User's Guide for a full explanation of data

Hospital Name	City	Rate	Cases
North Colorado Medical Center	Greeley	88%	134
Parkview Medical Center	Pueblo	88%	186
Penrose Saint Francis Health Services	Colorado Springs	88%	354
Colorado Plains Medical Center	Fort Morgan	87%	61
Denver Health Medical Center	Denver	87%	127
Exempla Saint Joseph Hospital	Denver	87%	83
Porter Adventist Hospital	Denver	87%	137
Saint Mary-Corwin Medical Center	Pueblo	87%	119
Arkansas Valley Regional Medical Center	La Junta	86%	117
Platte Valley Medical Center	Brighton	86%	65
Saint Anthony North Hospital	Westminster	85%	135
Saint Thomas More Hospital	Canon City	85%	67
Memorial Hospital	Craig	84%	25
Poudre Valley Hospital	Fort Collins	84%	177
Saint Anthony Central Hospital	Denver	84%	103
Longmont United Hospital	Longmont	83%	90
Memorial Hospital	Colorado Springs	83%	270
Sky Ridge Medical Center	Lone Tree	83%	78
University of Colorado Hospital	Denver	83%	89
Avista Adventist Hospital	Louisville	81%	58
Boulder Community Hospital	Boulder	81%	101
Presbyterian-Saint Luke's Medical Center	Denver	80%	55
Sterling Regional MedCenter	Sterling	79%	34
Montrose Memorial Hospital	Montrose	77%	69
Prowers Medical Center	Lamar	73%	45
Valley View Hospital	Glenwood Springs	68%	40

14. Blood Culture Timing

Hospital Name	City	Rate	Cases
Prowers Medical Center	Lamar	100%	27
McKee Medical Center	Loveland	97%	68
Porter Adventist Hospital	Denver	97%	144
Rose Medical Center	Denver	97%	125
Sterling Regional MedCenter	Sterling	97%	30
Swedish Medical Center	Englewood	97%	150
Valley View Hospital	Glenwood Springs	97%	34
Boulder Community Hospital	Boulder	96%	83
Parker Adventist Hospital	Parker	96%	78
Parkview Medical Center	Pueblo	96%	183
Exempla Lutheran Medical Center	Wheat Ridge	95%	96
Poudre Valley Hospital	Fort Collins	95%	104
Presbyterian-Saint Luke's Medical Center	Denver	95%	59
Medical Center of Aurora	Aurora	94%	215
Mercy Regional Medical Center	Durango	94%	71
Saint Mary-Corwin Medical Center	Pueblo	94%	79
Longmont United Hospital	Longmont	93%	46
Saint Mary's Hospital & Medical Center	Grand Junction	93%	132
Arkansas Valley Regional Medical Center	La Junta	92%	74
Exempla Saint Joseph Hospital	Denver	92%	87
Littleton Adventist Hospital	Littleton	92%	167
North Suburban Medical Center	Thornton	92%	120
Avista Adventist Hospital	Louisville	91%	45
North Colorado Medical Center	Greeley	91%	89
Penrose Saint Francis Health Services	Colorado Springs	91%	275
Denver Health Medical Center	Denver	90%	79
Montrose Memorial Hospital	Montrose	90%	51
Platte Valley Medical Center	Brighton	90%	31
Saint Anthony Central Hospital	Denver	90%	124
Delta County Memorial Hospital	Delta	89%	73
Saint Thomas More Hospital	Canon City	89%	46
Colorado Plains Medical Center	Fort Morgan	88%	60
Saint Anthony North Hospital	Westminster	86%	112
Exempla Good Samaritan Medical Center	Lafayette	85%	75
Sky Ridge Medical Center	Lone Tree	85%	60
Community Hospital	Grand Junction	84%	31
University of Colorado Hospital	Denver	83%	115
Memorial Hospital	Colorado Springs	82%	168

15. Influenza Vaccine

Hospital Name	City	Rate	Cases
North Suburban Medical Center	Thornton	97%	29
Parkview Medical Center	Pueblo	93%	55
Saint Thomas More Hospital	Canon City	92%	26
McKee Medical Center	Loveland	91%	32
Delta County Memorial Hospital	Delta	90%	30
Saint Anthony Central Hospital	Denver	84%	31
Saint Mary's Hospital & Medical Center	Grand Junction	84%	38
Rose Medical Center	Denver	79%	29
Longmont United Hospital	Longmont	78%	27
Medical Center of Aurora	Aurora	75%	73
Swedish Medical Center	Englewood	74%	53
North Colorado Medical Center	Greeley	71%	31
Poudre Valley Hospital	Fort Collins	71%	42
Arkansas Valley Regional Medical Center	La Junta	64%	44
Saint Anthony North Hospital	Westminster	58%	36
Penrose Saint Francis Health Services	Colorado Springs	45%	97
Littleton Adventist Hospital	Littleton	35%	51
Porter Adventist Hospital	Denver	14%	43

16. Initial Antibiotic Timing

Hospital Name	City	Rate	Cases
East Morgan County Hospital	Brush	97%	34
Spanish Peaks Regional Health Center	Walsenburg	96%	27
Colorado Plains Medical Center	Fort Morgan	92%	99
Porter Adventist Hospital	Denver	92%	207
Saint Mary's Hospital & Medical Center	Grand Junction	92%	201
Mercy Regional Medical Center	Durango	91%	88
Rose Medical Center	Denver	91%	180
Delta County Memorial Hospital	Delta	89%	114
Littleton Adventist Hospital	Littleton	89%	202
Memorial Hospital	Craig	89%	28
Saint Mary-Corwin Medical Center	Pueblo	89%	131
Saint Thomas More Hospital	Canon City	89%	89
Sterling Regional MedCenter	Sterling	89%	47
Avista Adventist Hospital	Louisville	88%	66
North Suburban Medical Center	Thornton	88%	157
Longmont United Hospital	Longmont	87%	127
Montrose Memorial Hospital	Montrose	87%	82
Parker Adventist Hospital	Parker	87%	89
Parkview Medical Center	Pueblo	87%	211
San Luis Valley Regional Medical Center	Alamosa	87%	53
Yampa Valley Medical Center	Steamboat Springs	87%	52
Sky Ridge Medical Center	Lone Tree	86%	93
Exempla Saint Joseph Hospital	Denver	85%	115
Arkansas Valley Regional Medical Center	La Junta	84%	146
Platte Valley Medical Center	Brighton	84%	74
McKee Medical Center	Loveland	83%	119
Penrose Saint Francis Health Services	Colorado Springs	83%	463
Southwest Memorial Hospital	Cortez	83%	66
Saint Anthony North Hospital	Westminster	81%	189
Swedish Medical Center	Englewood	80%	240
Community Hospital	Grand Junction	79%	48
Exempla Lutheran Medical Center	Wheat Ridge	79%	150
Medical Center of Aurora	Aurora	79%	295
Saint Anthony Central Hospital	Denver	78%	194
Boulder Community Hospital	Boulder	77%	145
Presbyterian-Saint Luke's Medical Center	Denver	76%	94
North Colorado Medical Center	Greeley	73%	198
Denver Health Medical Center	Denver	72%	162
Grand River Hospital District	Rifle	71%	41
Poudre Valley Hospital	Fort Collins	71%	232
Exempla Good Samaritan Medical Center	Lafayette	70%	109
University of Colorado Hospital	Denver	69%	151
Valley View Hospital	Glenwood Springs	68%	41
Memorial Hospital	Colorado Springs	65%	309
Prowers Medical Center	Lamar	55%	47

17. Oxygenation Assessment

Hospital Name	City	Rate	Cases
Aspen Valley Hospital	Aspen	100%	27
Avista Adventist Hospital	Louisville	100%	88
Boulder Community Hospital	Boulder	100%	191
Colorado Plains Medical Center	Fort Morgan	100%	110
Community Hospital	Grand Junction	100%	55
Delta County Memorial Hospital	Delta	100%	140
Denver Health Medical Center	Denver	100%	184
East Morgan County Hospital	Brush	100%	39
Exempla Good Samaritan Medical Center	Lafayette	100%	148
Exempla Lutheran Medical Center	Wheat Ridge	100%	180
Exempla Saint Joseph Hospital	Denver	100%	146
Grand River Hospital District	Rifle	100%	43
Littleton Adventist Hospital	Littleton	100%	255
Longmont United Hospital	Longmont	100%	143
McKee Medical Center	Loveland	100%	142
Medical Center of Aurora	Aurora	100%	350
Memorial Hospital	Colorado Springs	100%	363
Mercy Regional Medical Center	Durango	100%	103
Montrose Memorial Hospital	Montrose	100%	96
North Colorado Medical Center	Greeley	100%	215
North Suburban Medical Center	Thornton	100%	205
Parker Adventist Hospital	Parker	100%	109
Parkview Medical Center	Pueblo	100%	300
Penrose Saint Francis Health Services	Colorado Springs	100%	545
Platte Valley Medical Center	Brighton	100%	94
Porter Adventist Hospital	Denver	100%	234
Poudre Valley Hospital	Fort Collins	100%	299
Presbyterian-Saint Luke's Medical Center	Denver	100%	115
Prowers Medical Center	Lamar	100%	62

NOTE: Hospital profiles are in alphabetical order by state, then city, then hospital within the city; Rankings are sorted by rate in descending order and exclude hospitals with less than 25 cases; (1) The number of cases is too small (n<25) for purposes of reliably predicting hospital performance; (2) Measure reflects the hospital's indication that its submission was based upon a sample of its relevant discharges; (3) Rate reflects fewer than the maximum possible quarters of data for the measure; (4) Inaccurate information submitted and suppressed for one or more quarters; (5) No data is available from the hospital for this measure; Please refer to the User's Guide for a full explanation of data

Hospital Name	City	Rate	Cases
Rose Medical Center	Denver	100%	216
Saint Anthony Central Hospital	Denver	100%	213
Saint Anthony North Hospital	Westminster	100%	205
Saint Mary's Hospital & Medical Center	Grand Junction	100%	258
Saint Mary-Corwin Medical Center	Pueblo	100%	167
Saint Thomas More Hospital	Canon City	100%	111
San Luis Valley Regional Medical Center	Alamosa	100%	58
Sky Ridge Medical Center	Lone Tree	100%	115
Southwest Memorial Hospital	Cortez	100%	87
Spanish Peaks Regional Health Center	Walsenburg	100%	30
Sterling Regional MedCenter	Sterling	100%	59
Swedish Medical Center	Englewood	100%	318
University of Colorado Hospital	Denver	100%	186
Valley View Hospital	Glenwood Spgs	100%	55
Yampa Valley Medical Center	Steamboat Spgs	100%	55
Arkansas Valley Regional Medical Center	La Junta	99%	175
Memorial Hospital	Craig	97%	34

18. Pneumococcal Vaccine

Hospital Name	City	Rate	Cases
Parkview Medical Center	Pueblo	98%	172
Saint Anthony Central Hospital	Denver	95%	135
Community Hospital	Grand Junction	92%	36
Penrose Saint Francis Health Services	Colorado Springs	91%	341
Sterling Regional MedCenter	Sterling	91%	35
North Suburban Medical Center	Thornton	90%	89
Saint Thomas More Hospital	Canon City	88%	56
Medical Center of Aurora	Aurora	87%	173
Rose Medical Center	Denver	86%	136
Saint Mary-Corwin Medical Center	Pueblo	86%	118
Saint Mary's Hospital & Medical Center	Grand Junction	85%	160
Denver Health Medical Center	Denver	83%	53
Exempla Good Samaritan Medical Center	Lafayette	83%	109
Littleton Adventist Hospital	Littleton	82%	167
McKee Medical Center	Loveland	82%	107
Saint Anthony North Hospital	Westminster	81%	131
Exempla Lutheran Medical Center	Wheat Ridge	79%	99
Platte Valley Medical Center	Brighton	79%	47
Valley View Hospital	Glenwood Spgs	78%	32
Colorado Plains Medical Center	Fort Morgan	76%	84
Avista Adventist Hospital	Louisville	75%	48
Delta County Memorial Hospital	Delta	75%	91
Parker Adventist Hospital	Parker	75%	63
Longmont United Hospital	Longmont	74%	86
North Colorado Medical Center	Greeley	74%	141
East Morgan County Hospital	Brush	71%	28
Arkansas Valley Regional Medical Center	La Junta	69%	116
Boulder Community Hospital	Boulder	68%	114
Swedish Medical Center	Englewood	68%	175
Sky Ridge Medical Center	Lone Tree	67%	52
Memorial Hospital	Colorado Springs	66%	214
Mercy Regional Medical Center	Durango	66%	73
Exempla Saint Joseph Hospital	Denver	65%	97
Porter Adventist Hospital	Denver	65%	160
Presbyterian-Saint Luke's Medical Center	Denver	64%	64
Poudre Valley Hospital	Fort Collins	63%	191
Montrose Memorial Hospital	Montrose	57%	61
Southwest Memorial Hospital	Cortez	54%	54
San Luis Valley Regional Medical Center	Alamosa	48%	40
Yampa Valley Medical Center	Steamboat Spgs	40%	25
University of Colorado Hospital	Denver	30%	70
Prowers Medical Center	Lamar	10%	41

19. Smoking Cessation Advice

Hospital Name	City	Rate	Cases
Memorial Hospital	Colorado Springs	100%	113
Mercy Regional Medical Center	Durango	100%	26
North Suburban Medical Center	Thornton	100%	74
Parkview Medical Center	Pueblo	100%	93
Saint Anthony Central Hospital	Denver	100%	61
Sky Ridge Medical Center	Lone Tree	100%	26
Saint Anthony North Hospital	Westminster	99%	71
Saint Mary's Hospital & Medical Center	Grand Junction	98%	63
Exempla Lutheran Medical Center	Wheat Ridge	97%	35
Medical Center of Aurora	Aurora	96%	91
University of Colorado Hospital	Denver	96%	69
Poudre Valley Hospital	Fort Collins	95%	66
Saint Mary-Corwin Medical Center	Pueblo	95%	44
Boulder Community Hospital	Boulder	94%	31
Parker Adventist Hospital	Parker	93%	27
Penrose Saint Francis Health Services	Colorado Springs	92%	132
Littleton Adventist Hospital	Littleton	91%	32
Longmont United Hospital	Longmont	89%	28
Rose Medical Center	Denver	87%	47
Arkansas Valley Regional Medical Center	La Junta	86%	37
Exempla Saint Joseph Hospital	Denver	84%	37
Exempla Good Samaritan Medical Center	Lafayette	83%	36
Delta County Memorial Hospital	Delta	82%	33
Denver Health Medical Center	Denver	80%	104
North Colorado Medical Center	Greeley	78%	51
Saint Thomas More Hospital	Canon City	78%	32
Porter Adventist Hospital	Denver	74%	43
McKee Medical Center	Loveland	70%	30
Swedish Medical Center	Englewood	64%	72
Presbyterian-Saint Luke's Medical Center	Denver	62%	32

Surgical Infection Prevention

20. Prophylactic Antibiotic Given

Hospital Name	City	Rate	Cases
Yampa Valley Medical Center	Steamboat Spgs	98%	46
Mercy Regional Medical Center	Durango	96%	247
Saint Mary's Hospital & Medical Center	Grand Junction	96%	1047
Exempla Good Samaritan Medical Center	Lafayette	94%	171
Exempla Saint Joseph Hospital	Denver	94%	307
McKee Medical Center	Loveland	93%	45
Memorial Hospital	Colorado Springs	93%	412
Valley View Hospital	Glenwood Spgs	93%	208
Animas Surgical Hospital	Durango	92%	25
Penrose Saint Francis Health Services	Colorado Springs	92%	573
Vail Valley Medical Center	Vail	92%	25
Exempla Lutheran Medical Center	Wheat Ridge	90%	297
Platte Valley Medical Center	Brighton	90%	197
Colorado Plains Medical Center	Fort Morgan	89%	83
Parkview Medical Center	Pueblo	89%	264
Saint Thomas More Hospital	Canon City	89%	168
Poudre Valley Hospital	Fort Collins	88%	219
Community Hospital	Grand Junction	87%	134
Delta County Memorial Hospital	Delta	87%	143
Saint Mary-Corwin Medical Center	Pueblo	86%	315
Avista Adventist Hospital	Louisville	85%	158
Sky Ridge Medical Center	Lone Tree	85%	176
Swedish Medical Center	Englewood	85%	233
Denver Health Medical Center	Denver	84%	200
Porter Adventist Hospital	Denver	84%	349
Saint Anthony Central Hospital	Denver	84%	363
Parker Adventist Hospital	Parker	83%	236
Littleton Adventist Hospital	Littleton	81%	325
North Suburban Medical Center	Thornton	81%	129
Boulder Community Hospital	Boulder	80%	246
University of Colorado Hospital	Denver	78%	335
Southwest Memorial Hospital	Cortez	76%	33
Longmont United Hospital	Longmont	75%	352
Saint Anthony North Hospital	Westminster	75%	165
Presbyterian-Saint Luke's Medical Center	Denver	72%	218
Sterling Regional MedCenter	Sterling	72%	25
Saint Anthony Summit Medical Center	Frisco	71%	28
Medical Center of Aurora	Aurora	68%	247
San Luis Valley Regional Medical Center	Alamosa	68%	41
Montrose Memorial Hospital	Montrose	63%	274
North Colorado Medical Center	Greeley	62%	125
Rose Medical Center	Denver	56%	211

21. Prophylactic Antibiotic Selection

Hospital Name	City	Rate	Cases
Avista Adventist Hospital	Louisville	100%	48
Platte Valley Medical Center	Brighton	100%	41
Saint Anthony North Hospital	Westminster	100%	40
Yampa Valley Medical Center	Steamboat Spgs	100%	47
Exempla Lutheran Medical Center	Wheat Ridge	99%	70
Delta County Memorial Hospital	Delta	98%	55
Memorial Hospital	Colorado Springs	98%	135
Rose Medical Center	Denver	98%	99
Exempla Saint Joseph Hospital	Denver	97%	72
Longmont United Hospital	Longmont	97%	116
Mercy Regional Medical Center	Durango	97%	69
Parkview Medical Center	Pueblo	97%	116
Saint Anthony Central Hospital	Denver	97%	115
Exempla Good Samaritan Medical Center	Lafayette	95%	42
Boulder Community Hospital	Boulder	94%	65
North Suburban Medical Center	Thornton	94%	49
Penrose Saint Francis Health Services	Colorado Springs	94%	155
Porter Adventist Hospital	Denver	94%	122
Saint Mary's Hospital & Medical Center	Grand Junction	94%	235
Poudre Valley Hospital	Fort Collins	93%	73
Saint Mary-Corwin Medical Center	Pueblo	93%	76
Parker Adventist Hospital	Parker	92%	65
Saint Thomas More Hospital	Canon City	92%	51

NOTE: Hospital profiles are in alphabetical order by state, then city, then hospital within the city; Rankings are sorted by rate in descending order and exclude hospitals with less than 25 cases; (1) The number of cases is too small (n<25) for purposes of reliably predicting hospital performance; (2) Measure reflects the hospital's indication that its submission was based upon a sample of its relevant discharges; (3) Rate reflects fewer than the maximum possible quarters of data for the measure; (4) Inaccurate information submitted and suppressed for one or more quarters; (5) No data is available from the hospital for this measure; Please refer to the User's Guide for a full explanation of data

Sky Ridge Medical Center	Lone Tree	92%	74
Sterling Regional MedCenter	Sterling	92%	25
Community Hospital	Grand Junction	91%	46
North Colorado Medical Center	Greeley	91%	117
Swedish Medical Center	Englewood	91%	92
Littleton Adventist Hospital	Littleton	89%	131
Montrose Memorial Hospital	Montrose	89%	63
Medical Center of Aurora	Aurora	88%	115
Valley View Hospital	Glenwood Spgs	88%	51
Denver Health Medical Center	Denver	85%	48
Vail Valley Medical Center	Vail	84%	25
University of Colorado Hospital	Denver	78%	68
Presbyterian-Saint Luke's Medical Center	Denver	73%	90
McKee Medical Center	Loveland	42%	45

22. Prophylactic Antibiotic Stopped

Hospital Name	City	Rate	Cases
San Luis Valley Regional Medical Center	Alamosa	100%	39
Vail Valley Medical Center	Vail	100%	25
Southwest Memorial Hospital	Cortez	94%	31
Saint Mary's Hospital & Medical Center	Grand Junction	92%	1005
Avista Adventist Hospital	Louisville	88%	155
Valley View Hospital	Glenwood Spgs	86%	206
Littleton Adventist Hospital	Littleton	84%	312
Memorial Hospital	Colorado Springs	84%	399
Mercy Regional Medical Center	Durango	82%	243
Parker Adventist Hospital	Parker	82%	228
Penrose Saint Francis Health Services	Colorado Springs	82%	559
University of Colorado Hospital	Denver	82%	337
Delta County Memorial Hospital	Delta	81%	140
Saint Anthony Central Hospital	Denver	81%	341
Porter Adventist Hospital	Denver	80%	338
Saint Thomas More Hospital	Canon City	78%	161
Community Hospital	Grand Junction	77%	133
Rose Medical Center	Denver	76%	214
Swedish Medical Center	Englewood	76%	223
Exempla Lutheran Medical Center	Wheat Ridge	75%	288
Parkview Medical Center	Pueblo	74%	257
Saint Mary-Corwin Medical Center	Pueblo	74%	303
Exempla Saint Joseph Hospital	Denver	73%	300
Platte Valley Medical Center	Brighton	72%	188
Denver Health Medical Center	Denver	70%	191
Sky Ridge Medical Center	Lone Tree	70%	174
Presbyterian-Saint Luke's Medical Center	Denver	61%	203
Saint Anthony North Hospital	Westminster	61%	149
Exempla Good Samaritan Medical Center	Lafayette	59%	168
Longmont United Hospital	Longmont	59%	330
Montrose Memorial Hospital	Montrose	57%	265
Animas Surgical Hospital	Durango	56%	25
Poudre Valley Hospital	Fort Collins	56%	211
Yampa Valley Medical Center	Steamboat Spgs	54%	46
McKee Medical Center	Loveland	52%	44
Medical Center of Aurora	Aurora	49%	237
Boulder Community Hospital	Boulder	47%	231
North Suburban Medical Center	Thornton	45%	121
North Colorado Medical Center	Greeley	42%	115
Colorado Plains Medical Center	Fort Morgan	36%	80
Saint Anthony Summit Medical Center	Frisco	31%	26

Pregnancy Care

23. Inpatient Neonatal Mortality

Hospital Name	City	Rate	Cases
Avista Adventist Hospital	Louisville	0.00%	2645
Vail Valley Medical Center	Vail	0.00%	603
Sky Ridge Medical Center	Lone Tree	0.07%	3024
Medical Center of Aurora	Aurora	0.12%	2570
Longmont United Hospital	Longmont	0.13%	1505
North Suburban Medical Center	Thornton	0.15%	1948
Poudre Valley Hospital	Fort Collins	0.21%	2818
Rose Medical Center	Denver	0.23%	3846
Parker Adventist Hospital	Parker	0.32%	1262
Saint Mary's Hospital & Medical Center	Grand Junction	0.38%	2338
Littleton Adventist Hospital	Littleton	0.46%	1737
University of Colorado Hospital	Denver	1.05%	666
Presbyterian-Saint Luke's Medical Center	Denver	3.62%	1656

24. Third or Fourth Degree Laceration

Hospital Name	City	Rate	Cases
Saint Mary's Hospital & Medical Center	Grand Junction	1.97%	1676
University of Colorado Hospital	Denver	2.89%	2280
Presbyterian-Saint Luke's Medical Center	Denver	3.24%	863
Medical Center of Aurora	Aurora	3.34%	1917
Longmont United Hospital	Longmont	3.77%	1113
Parker Adventist Hospital	Parker	4.15%	891
Littleton Adventist Hospital	Littleton	4.27%	1266
Avista Adventist Hospital	Louisville	4.84%	2003
Rose Medical Center	Denver	4.85%	2434
Poudre Valley Hospital	Fort Collins	5.01%	1938
North Suburban Medical Center	Thornton	5.27%	1461
Sky Ridge Medical Center	Lone Tree	5.70%	2105
Vail Valley Medical Center	Vail	6.63%	362

NOTE: Hospital profiles are in alphabetical order by state, then city, then hospital within the city; Rankings are sorted by rate in descending order and exclude hospitals with less than 25 cases; (1) The number of cases is too small (n<25) for purposes of reliably predicting hospital performance; (2) Measure reflects the hospital's indication that its submission was based upon a sample of its relevant discharges; (3) Rate reflects fewer than the maximum possible quarters of data for the measure; (4) Inaccurate information submitted and suppressed for one or more quarters; (5) No data is available from the hospital for this measure; Please refer to the User's Guide for a full explanation of data

San Luis Valley Regional Medical Center

106 Blanca Avenue
Alamosa, CO 81101
URL: www.slvrmc.org
Ownership: Voluntary non-profit - Private
Emergency Services: No

Phone: 719-589-2511
Fax: 719-587-1372

Accredited: Yes
Licensed Beds: 85

Key Personnel:
CEO. . . . . Larry Pochardt
Director Infection/Disease Control . . . . Leonard Snow
Director Medical/Surgical Nursing . . . . Kathy Pachelli
Chief Radiology . . . . Fred Casanova

Measure	Cases	This Hospital	State Average	U.S. Average	Top Hospital
Heart Attack Care					
ACE Inhibitor or ARB for LVSD	0	-	91%	82%	100%
Aspirin at Arrival[1]	3	100%	95%	92%	100%
Aspirin at Discharge[1]	1	100%	97%	90%	100%
Beta Blocker at Arrival[1]	5	80%	93%	87%	100%
Beta Blocker at Discharge[1]	3	67%	93%	90%	100%
Fibrinolytic Medication Timing[3]	0	-	31%	31%	100%
PCI Within 90 Minutes of Arrival	0	-	69%	54%	95%
Smoking Cessation Advice[1,3]	1	100%	91%	88%	100%
Heart Failure Care					
ACE Inhibitor or ARB for LVSD[1]	4	100%	84%	82%	100%
Discharge Instructions[1,3]	9	0%	53%	61%	93%
Evaluation of LVS Function	25	72%	81%	83%	99%
Smoking Cessation Advice[3]	0	-	79%	82%	100%
Pneumonia Care					
Appropriate Initial Antibiotic[1,3]	8	50%	85%	83%	94%
Blood Culture Timing[1,3]	10	80%	91%	90%	100%
Influenza Vaccine[5]	-	-	70%	70%	100%
Initial Antibiotic Timing	53	87%	83%	80%	93%
Oxygenation Assessment	58	100%	100%	99%	100%
Pneumococcal Vaccine	40	48%	72%	69%	94%
Smoking Cessation Advice[1,3]	3	100%	78%	80%	100%
Surgical Infection Prevention					
Prophylactic Antibiotic Given[3]	41	68%	83%	77%	95%
Prophylactic Antibiotic Selection[5]	-	-	92%	90%	100%
Prophylactic Antibiotic Stopped[3]	39	100%	70%	72%	95%
Pregnancy Care					
Inpatient Neonatal Mortality	-	-	-	-	-
Third or Fourth Degree Laceration	-	-	4.02%	3.63%	3.27%

Aspen Valley Hospital

0401 Castle Creek Road
Aspen, CO 81611
URL: www.avhaspen.org
Ownership: Govt - Hospital District or Authority
Emergency Services: Yes

Phone: 970-925-1120
Fax: 970-544-1585

Accredited: Yes
Licensed Beds: 25

Key Personnel:
CEO. . . . . Dave Ressler
Chief Medical Staff. . . . . Kim Scheuer, MD
Director Emergency Department . . . . Steve Knowles
Infection Control Nurse. . . . . Kathy Gibbard, RN
CNO. . . . . Natalie Booker, RN
Chief Radiology . . . . David Hollander, MD
Director Respiratory Therapy . . . . Kathy Schneider, RT

Measure	Cases	This Hospital	State Average	U.S. Average	Top Hospital
Heart Attack Care					
ACE Inhibitor or ARB for LVSD[1]	2	100%	91%	82%	100%
Aspirin at Arrival[1]	6	100%	95%	92%	100%
Aspirin at Discharge[1]	5	100%	97%	90%	100%
Beta Blocker at Arrival[1]	5	100%	93%	87%	100%
Beta Blocker at Discharge[1]	4	100%	93%	90%	100%
Fibrinolytic Medication Timing	0	-	31%	31%	100%
PCI Within 90 Minutes of Arrival	0	-	69%	54%	95%
Smoking Cessation Advice[1]	1	0%	91%	88%	100%
Heart Failure Care					
ACE Inhibitor or ARB for LVSD	0	-	84%	82%	100%
Discharge Instructions[1]	11	9%	53%	61%	93%
Evaluation of LVS Function[1]	12	100%	81%	83%	99%
Smoking Cessation Advice[1]	1	0%	79%	82%	100%
Pneumonia Care					
Appropriate Initial Antibiotic[1]	19	100%	85%	83%	94%
Blood Culture Timing[1]	16	94%	91%	90%	100%
Influenza Vaccine[4,5]	-	-	70%	70%	100%
Initial Antibiotic Timing[1]	19	74%	83%	80%	93%
Oxygenation Assessment	27	100%	100%	99%	100%
Pneumococcal Vaccine[1]	16	38%	72%	69%	94%
Smoking Cessation Advice[1]	1	0%	78%	80%	100%
Surgical Infection Prevention					
Prophylactic Antibiotic Given[5]	-	-	83%	77%	95%
Prophylactic Antibiotic Selection[5]	-	-	92%	90%	100%
Prophylactic Antibiotic Stopped[5]	-	-	70%	72%	95%
Pregnancy Care					
Inpatient Neonatal Mortality	-	-	-	-	-
Third or Fourth Degree Laceration	-	-	4.02%	3.63%	3.27%

Medical Center of Aurora

1501 South Potomac Street
Aurora, CO 80012
URL: www.auroramed.com
Ownership: Proprietary
Emergency Services: Yes

Phone: 303-695-2600
Fax: 303-873-5682

Accredited: Yes
Licensed Beds: 372

Key Personnel:
President/CEO. . . . . John G Hill
OB/GYN Womens Health. . . . . Mark Saunders, MD

Measure	Cases	This Hospital	State Average	U.S. Average	Top Hospital
Heart Attack Care					
ACE Inhibitor or ARB for LVSD	42	90%	91%	82%	100%
Aspirin at Arrival	278	100%	95%	92%	100%
Aspirin at Discharge	350	99%	97%	90%	100%
Beta Blocker at Arrival	211	98%	93%	87%	100%
Beta Blocker at Discharge	369	98%	93%	90%	100%
Fibrinolytic Medication Timing	0	-	31%	31%	100%
PCI Within 90 Minutes of Arrival[1]	21	52%	69%	54%	95%
Smoking Cessation Advice	132	95%	91%	88%	100%
Heart Failure Care					
ACE Inhibitor or ARB for LVSD	119	92%	84%	82%	100%
Discharge Instructions	273	61%	53%	61%	93%
Evaluation of LVS Function	341	93%	81%	83%	99%
Smoking Cessation Advice	64	94%	79%	82%	100%
Pneumonia Care					
Appropriate Initial Antibiotic	212	88%	85%	83%	94%
Blood Culture Timing	215	94%	91%	90%	100%
Influenza Vaccine	73	75%	70%	70%	100%
Initial Antibiotic Timing	295	79%	83%	80%	93%
Oxygenation Assessment	350	100%	100%	99%	100%
Pneumococcal Vaccine	173	87%	72%	69%	94%
Smoking Cessation Advice	91	96%	78%	80%	100%
Surgical Infection Prevention					
Prophylactic Antibiotic Given[2,3]	247	68%	83%	77%	95%
Prophylactic Antibiotic Selection[2]	115	88%	92%	90%	100%
Prophylactic Antibiotic Stopped[2,3]	237	49%	70%	72%	95%
Pregnancy Care					
Inpatient Neonatal Mortality	2,570	0.12%	-	-	-
Third or Fourth Degree Laceration	1,917	3.34%	4.02%	3.63%	3.27%

Boulder Community Hospital

1100 Balsam Avenue
PO Box 9019
Boulder, CO 80301
E-mail: pr@bch.org
URL: www.bch.org
Ownership: Voluntary non-profit - Other
Emergency Services: Yes

Phone: 303-440-2273
Fax: 303-441-0478

Accredited: Yes
Licensed Beds: 265

Key Personnel:
President/CEO. . . . . David P Gehant
Chief Medical Staff. . . . . Patrick Moran
Director Cardiac Lab . . . . Darryl Brown
Director Emergency Room. . . . . Holly Pederson
Infection Control. . . . . Betty Sutton
ICU . . . . Holly Pederson
Director Womens/Family Services . . . . Laure Lisk

NOTE: Hospital profiles are in alphabetical order by state, then city, then hospital within the city; Rankings are sorted by rate in descending order and exclude hospitals with less than 25 cases; (1) The number of cases is too small (n<25) for purposes of reliably predicting hospital performance; (2) Measure reflects the hospital's indication that its submission was based upon a sample of its relevant discharges; (3) Rate reflects fewer than the maximum possible quarters of data for the measure; (4) Inaccurate information submitted and suppressed for one or more quarters; (5) No data is available from the hospital for this measure; Please refer to the User's Guide for a full explanation of data

Respiratory/Cardiopulmonary. . . . . Darryl Brown

Measure	Cases	This Hospital	State Average	U.S. Average	Top Hospital
Heart Attack Care					
ACE Inhibitor or ARB for LVSD[1]	17	82%	91%	82%	100%
Aspirin at Arrival	69	100%	95%	92%	100%
Aspirin at Discharge	88	100%	97%	90%	100%
Beta Blocker at Arrival	66	95%	93%	87%	100%
Beta Blocker at Discharge	87	97%	93%	90%	100%
Fibrinolytic Medication Timing	0	-	31%	31%	100%
PCI Within 90 Minutes of Arrival[1]	5	60%	69%	54%	95%
Smoking Cessation Advice[1]	21	100%	91%	88%	100%
Heart Failure Care					
ACE Inhibitor or ARB for LVSD	71	73%	84%	82%	100%
Discharge Instructions	127	46%	53%	61%	93%
Evaluation of LVS Function	158	89%	81%	83%	99%
Smoking Cessation Advice[1]	22	95%	79%	82%	100%
Pneumonia Care					
Appropriate Initial Antibiotic	101	81%	85%	83%	94%
Blood Culture Timing	83	96%	91%	90%	100%
Influenza Vaccine[4,5]	-	-	70%	70%	100%
Initial Antibiotic Timing	145	77%	83%	80%	93%
Oxygenation Assessment	191	100%	100%	99%	100%
Pneumococcal Vaccine	114	68%	72%	69%	94%
Smoking Cessation Advice	31	94%	78%	80%	100%
Surgical Infection Prevention					
Prophylactic Antibiotic Given	246	80%	83%	77%	95%
Prophylactic Antibiotic Selection	65	94%	92%	90%	100%
Prophylactic Antibiotic Stopped	231	47%	70%	72%	95%
Pregnancy Care					
Inpatient Neonatal Mortality	-	-	-	-	-
Third or Fourth Degree Laceration	-	-	4.02%	3.63%	3.27%

Platte Valley Medical Center

1850 Egbert Street
Brighton, CO 80601
URL: www.pvmc.org
Ownership: Voluntary non-profit - Private
Emergency Services: Yes

Phone: 303-659-1531
Fax: 303-659-6401
Accredited: Yes
Licensed Beds: 58

Key Personnel:

CEO. . . . . John Hicks
Infection Control. . . . . Diane Jaeger, RN
Surgical Services Director . . . . Jo Jordan, RN
Chief Radiology . . . . Karen Swanson, MD
Respiratory . . . . Ryan Hamblin

Measure	Cases	This Hospital	State Average	U.S. Average	Top Hospital
Heart Attack Care					
ACE Inhibitor or ARB for LVSD[1]	1	100%	91%	82%	100%
Aspirin at Arrival[1]	18	94%	95%	92%	100%
Aspirin at Discharge[1]	8	88%	97%	90%	100%
Beta Blocker at Arrival[1]	16	94%	93%	87%	100%
Beta Blocker at Discharge[1]	7	71%	93%	90%	100%
Fibrinolytic Medication Timing	0	-	31%	31%	100%
PCI Within 90 Minutes of Arrival	0	-	69%	54%	95%
Smoking Cessation Advice[1]	1	0%	91%	88%	100%
Heart Failure Care					
ACE Inhibitor or ARB for LVSD[1]	20	85%	84%	82%	100%
Discharge Instructions	40	68%	53%	61%	93%
Evaluation of LVS Function	50	82%	81%	83%	99%
Smoking Cessation Advice[1]	11	100%	79%	82%	100%
Pneumonia Care					
Appropriate Initial Antibiotic	65	86%	85%	83%	94%
Blood Culture Timing	31	90%	91%	90%	100%
Influenza Vaccine[1]	14	64%	70%	70%	100%
Initial Antibiotic Timing	74	84%	83%	80%	93%
Oxygenation Assessment	94	100%	100%	99%	100%
Pneumococcal Vaccine	47	79%	72%	69%	94%
Smoking Cessation Advice[1]	18	83%	78%	80%	100%
Surgical Infection Prevention					
Prophylactic Antibiotic Given	197	90%	83%	77%	95%
Prophylactic Antibiotic Selection	41	100%	92%	90%	100%
Prophylactic Antibiotic Stopped	188	72%	70%	72%	95%
Pregnancy Care					
Inpatient Neonatal Mortality	-	-	-	-	-
Third or Fourth Degree Laceration	-	-	4.02%	3.63%	3.27%

East Morgan County Hospital

2400 West Edison
Brush, CO 80723
URL: www.emchbrush.com or www.bannerhealth.com
Ownership: Voluntary non-profit - Other
Emergency Services: Yes

Phone: 970-842-6200
Fax: 970-842-4827
Accredited: No
Licensed Beds: 25

Key Personnel:

President/CEO. . . . . Anne Platt
Emergency Room . . . . Linda Schneider
Infection Control. . . . . Kelly Plessman

Measure	Cases	This Hospital	State Average	U.S. Average	Top Hospital
Heart Attack Care					
ACE Inhibitor or ARB for LVSD[3]	0	-	91%	82%	100%
Aspirin at Arrival[1,3]	1	0%	95%	92%	100%
Aspirin at Discharge[1,3]	1	100%	97%	90%	100%
Beta Blocker at Arrival[1,3]	1	100%	93%	87%	100%
Beta Blocker at Discharge[1,3]	2	100%	93%	90%	100%
Fibrinolytic Medication Timing[3]	0	-	31%	31%	100%
PCI Within 90 Minutes of Arrival	0	-	69%	54%	95%
Smoking Cessation Advice[3]	0	-	91%	88%	100%
Heart Failure Care					
ACE Inhibitor or ARB for LVSD[1]	1	100%	84%	82%	100%
Discharge Instructions[1]	6	67%	53%	61%	93%
Evaluation of LVS Function[1]	14	86%	81%	83%	99%
Smoking Cessation Advice[1]	2	100%	79%	82%	100%
Pneumonia Care					
Appropriate Initial Antibiotic	28	96%	85%	83%	94%
Blood Culture Timing[1]	15	87%	91%	90%	100%
Influenza Vaccine[4,5]	-	-	70%	70%	100%
Initial Antibiotic Timing	34	97%	83%	80%	93%
Oxygenation Assessment	39	100%	100%	99%	100%
Pneumococcal Vaccine	28	71%	72%	69%	94%
Smoking Cessation Advice[1]	4	50%	78%	80%	100%
Surgical Infection Prevention					
Prophylactic Antibiotic Given[1,3]	2	100%	83%	77%	95%
Prophylactic Antibiotic Selection[1]	2	100%	92%	90%	100%
Prophylactic Antibiotic Stopped[1,3]	2	0%	70%	72%	95%
Pregnancy Care					
Inpatient Neonatal Mortality	-	-	-	-	-
Third or Fourth Degree Laceration	-	-	4.02%	3.63%	3.27%

Kit Carson County Memorial Hospital

Alternate Name: Kit Carson County Health Service District
286 16th Street
Burlington, CO 80807
URL: www.kccmh.org
Ownership: Govt - Hospital District or Authority
Emergency Services: No

Phone: 719-346-5311
Fax: 719-346-5252
Accredited: No
Licensed Beds: 25

Key Personnel:

CEO. . . . . James H Jordan
Chief Medical Staff. . . . . Sacremento Pimentel, MD
Supervisor Cardiac Lab . . . . Tonda Scott, RN
Emergency Room . . . . Vicki Cox, DON
Director Medical/Surgical Nursing . . . . Vicki Cox, RN
Director Respiratory Therapy . . . . Justeen Judson

Measure	Cases	This Hospital	State Average	U.S. Average	Top Hospital
Heart Attack Care					
ACE Inhibitor or ARB for LVSD[5]	-	-	91%	82%	100%
Aspirin at Arrival[5]	-	-	95%	92%	100%
Aspirin at Discharge[5]	-	-	97%	90%	100%
Beta Blocker at Arrival[5]	-	-	93%	87%	100%
Beta Blocker at Discharge[5]	-	-	93%	90%	100%
Fibrinolytic Medication Timing[5]	-	-	31%	31%	100%
PCI Within 90 Minutes of Arrival[5]	-	-	69%	54%	95%
Smoking Cessation Advice[5]	-	-	91%	88%	100%

NOTE: Hospital profiles are in alphabetical order by state, then city, then hospital within the city; Rankings are sorted by rate in descending order and exclude hospitals with less than 25 cases; (1) The number of cases is too small (n<25) for purposes of reliably predicting hospital performance; (2) Measure reflects the hospital's indication that its submission was based upon a sample of its relevant discharges; (3) Rate reflects fewer than the maximum possible quarters of data for the measure; (4) Inaccurate information submitted and suppressed for one or more quarters; (5) No data is available from the hospital for this measure; Please refer to the User's Guide for a full explanation of data

Measure	Cases	This Hospital	State Average	U.S. Average	Top Hospital
Heart Failure Care					
ACE Inhibitor or ARB for LVSD[5]	-	-	84%	82%	100%
Discharge Instructions[5]	-	-	53%	61%	93%
Evaluation of LVS Function[5]	-	-	81%	83%	99%
Smoking Cessation Advice[5]	-	-	79%	82%	100%
Pneumonia Care					
Appropriate Initial Antibiotic[5]	-	-	85%	83%	94%
Blood Culture Timing[5]	-	-	91%	90%	100%
Influenza Vaccine[5]	-	-	70%	70%	100%
Initial Antibiotic Timing[5]	-	-	83%	80%	93%
Oxygenation Assessment[5]	-	-	100%	99%	100%
Pneumococcal Vaccine[5]	-	-	72%	69%	94%
Smoking Cessation Advice[5]	-	-	78%	80%	100%
Surgical Infection Prevention					
Prophylactic Antibiotic Given[5]	-	-	83%	77%	95%
Prophylactic Antibiotic Selection[5]	-	-	92%	90%	100%
Prophylactic Antibiotic Stopped[5]	-	-	70%	72%	95%
Pregnancy Care					
Inpatient Neonatal Mortality	-	-	-	-	-
Third or Fourth Degree Laceration	-	-	4.02%	3.63%	3.27%

Saint Thomas More Hospital

1338 Phay Avenue
Canon City, CO 81212
URL: www.stthomasmorehosp.org
Ownership: Voluntary non-profit - Church
Emergency Services: Yes

Phone: 719-285-2000
Fax: 719-285-2016
Accredited: Yes
Licensed Beds: 55

Key Personnel:

CEO. . . . . Nathan Olson
Director Infection Control . . . . Pam Galkowski
CNO. . . . . Diane Swagger, MSN
Director Respiratory Therapy . . . . Rick Kamerzell

Measure	Cases	This Hospital	State Average	U.S. Average	Top Hospital
Heart Attack Care					
ACE Inhibitor or ARB for LVSD[1,2]	3	100%	91%	82%	100%
Aspirin at Arrival[1,2]	19	89%	95%	92%	100%
Aspirin at Discharge[1,2]	7	86%	97%	90%	100%
Beta Blocker at Arrival[1,2]	13	85%	93%	87%	100%
Beta Blocker at Discharge[1,2]	6	83%	93%	90%	100%
Fibrinolytic Medication Timing[1,2]	2	0%	31%	31%	100%
PCI Within 90 Minutes of Arrival[2]	0	-	69%	54%	95%
Smoking Cessation Advice[2]	0	-	91%	88%	100%
Heart Failure Care					
ACE Inhibitor or ARB for LVSD[1,2]	5	100%	84%	82%	100%
Discharge Instructions[2]	31	10%	53%	61%	93%
Evaluation of LVS Function[2]	39	62%	81%	83%	99%
Smoking Cessation Advice[1,2]	6	50%	79%	82%	100%
Pneumonia Care					
Appropriate Initial Antibiotic[2]	67	85%	85%	83%	94%
Blood Culture Timing[2]	46	89%	91%	90%	100%
Influenza Vaccine[2]	26	92%	70%	70%	100%
Initial Antibiotic Timing[2]	89	89%	83%	80%	93%
Oxygenation Assessment[2]	111	100%	100%	99%	100%
Pneumococcal Vaccine[2]	56	88%	72%	69%	94%
Smoking Cessation Advice[2]	32	78%	78%	80%	100%
Surgical Infection Prevention					
Prophylactic Antibiotic Given[2,3]	168	89%	83%	77%	95%
Prophylactic Antibiotic Selection[2]	51	92%	92%	90%	100%
Prophylactic Antibiotic Stopped[2,3]	161	78%	70%	72%	95%
Pregnancy Care					
Inpatient Neonatal Mortality	-	-	-	-	-
Third or Fourth Degree Laceration	-	-	4.02%	3.63%	3.27%

Keefe Memorial Hospital

Alternate Name: Cheyenne County Hospital
602 N 6th Street W
Cheyenne Wells, CO 80810
Ownership: Government - Local
Emergency Services: Yes

Phone: 719-767-5661
Fax: 719-767-8042
Accredited: No
Licensed Beds: 32

Key Personnel:

CEO/President. . . . . Curtis Hawkinson
Chief of Medical Staff . . . . Saied Ahmad Pour
Director Medical/Surgical Nursing . . . . Sue Kern
Director of Pulmonary/Respiratory Care. . . . . . . Kathy Donnelly

Measure	Cases	This Hospital	State Average	U.S. Average	Top Hospital
Heart Attack Care					
ACE Inhibitor or ARB for LVSD[3]	0	-	91%	82%	100%
Aspirin at Arrival[1,3]	1	100%	95%	92%	100%
Aspirin at Discharge[3]	0	-	97%	90%	100%
Beta Blocker at Arrival[1,3]	1	0%	93%	87%	100%
Beta Blocker at Discharge[3]	0	-	93%	90%	100%
Fibrinolytic Medication Timing[1,3]	1	0%	31%	31%	100%
PCI Within 90 Minutes of Arrival[5]	-	-	69%	54%	95%
Smoking Cessation Advice[3]	0	-	91%	88%	100%
Heart Failure Care					
ACE Inhibitor or ARB for LVSD[5]	-	-	84%	82%	100%
Discharge Instructions[5]	-	-	53%	61%	93%
Evaluation of LVS Function[5]	-	-	81%	83%	99%
Smoking Cessation Advice[5]	-	-	79%	82%	100%
Pneumonia Care					
Appropriate Initial Antibiotic[1]	13	69%	85%	83%	94%
Blood Culture Timing[1]	3	100%	91%	90%	100%
Influenza Vaccine[1]	6	100%	70%	70%	100%
Initial Antibiotic Timing[1]	16	94%	83%	80%	93%
Oxygenation Assessment[1]	16	100%	100%	99%	100%
Pneumococcal Vaccine[1]	12	92%	72%	69%	94%
Smoking Cessation Advice[1]	2	100%	78%	80%	100%
Surgical Infection Prevention					
Prophylactic Antibiotic Given[5]	-	-	83%	77%	95%
Prophylactic Antibiotic Selection[5]	-	-	92%	90%	100%
Prophylactic Antibiotic Stopped[5]	-	-	70%	72%	95%
Pregnancy Care					
Inpatient Neonatal Mortality	-	-	-	-	-
Third or Fourth Degree Laceration	-	-	4.02%	3.63%	3.27%

Memorial Hospital

1400 E Boulder Street
Colorado Springs, CO 80909

Toll-Free: 800-826-4889
Phone: 719-365-5000
Fax: 719-365-2472

E-mail: info@memorialhealthsystem.com
URL: www.memorialhospital.com
Ownership: Government - Local
Emergency Services: Yes

Accredited: Yes
Licensed Beds: 386

Key Personnel:

President/CEO. . . . . Michael Schrader
Associate Administrator . . . . Donna Lastra
Chief of Medical Staff. John Flack, MD
Emergency Room . . . . Donna Young, RN
Director Infection/Disease Control . . . . Joan Walker, RN
Director Medical/Surgical Nursing . . . . Pat McClendon
OB/GYN Womens Health. . . . . June Chan, RN
Director Radiology . . . . Sandy Anderson
Director Respiratory Therapy . . . . Pat Shepperdson

Measure	Cases	This Hospital	State Average	U.S. Average	Top Hospital
Heart Attack Care					
ACE Inhibitor or ARB for LVSD	50	98%	91%	82%	100%
Aspirin at Arrival	318	99%	95%	92%	100%
Aspirin at Discharge	363	98%	97%	90%	100%
Beta Blocker at Arrival	245	98%	93%	87%	100%
Beta Blocker at Discharge	347	99%	93%	90%	100%
Fibrinolytic Medication Timing[1]	2	0%	31%	31%	100%
PCI Within 90 Minutes of Arrival[1]	7	71%	69%	54%	95%
Smoking Cessation Advice	137	100%	91%	88%	100%
Heart Failure Care					
ACE Inhibitor or ARB for LVSD	207	90%	84%	82%	100%
Discharge Instructions	414	72%	53%	61%	93%
Evaluation of LVS Function	476	93%	81%	83%	99%
Smoking Cessation Advice	90	99%	79%	82%	100%
Pneumonia Care					
Appropriate Initial Antibiotic	270	83%	85%	83%	94%
Blood Culture Timing	168	82%	91%	90%	100%
Influenza Vaccine[4,5]	-	-	70%	70%	100%
Initial Antibiotic Timing	309	65%	83%	80%	93%

NOTE: Hospital profiles are in alphabetical order by state, then city, then hospital within the city; Rankings are sorted by rate in descending order and exclude hospitals with less than 25 cases; (1) The number of cases is too small (n<25) for purposes of reliably predicting hospital performance; (2) Measure reflects the hospital's indication that its submission was based upon a sample of its relevant discharges; (3) Rate reflects fewer than the maximum possible quarters of data for the measure; (4) Inaccurate information submitted and suppressed for one or more quarters; (5) No data is available from the hospital for this measure; Please refer to the User's Guide for a full explanation of data

Oxygenation Assessment	363	100%	100%	99%	100%
Pneumococcal Vaccine	214	66%	72%	69%	94%
Smoking Cessation Advice	113	100%	78%	80%	100%
Surgical Infection Prevention					
Prophylactic Antibiotic Given[2,3]	412	93%	83%	77%	95%
Prophylactic Antibiotic Selection[2]	135	98%	92%	90%	100%
Prophylactic Antibiotic Stopped[2,3]	399	84%	70%	72%	95%
Pregnancy Care					
Inpatient Neonatal Mortality	-	-	-	-	-
Third or Fourth Degree Laceration	-	-	4.02%	3.63%	3.27%

Penrose Saint Francis Health Services

Alternate Name: Centura Health-St. Francis Hospital Systems
825 E Pikes Peak Avenue — Phone: 719-776-5000
Colorado Springs, CO 80903 — Fax: 719-776-2770
URL: www.centurahealth.com
Ownership: Voluntary non-profit - Church — Accredited: Yes
Emergency Services: Yes — Licensed Beds: 522

Key Personnel:
President/CEO . . . . Rick O'Connell
Chief Medical Staff. . . . . Tom Davis
Cardiac Lab . . . . Keathe Hanley
Emergency Room . . . . Kate McCord
Infection Control. . . . . Marie Lucero
ICU . . . . Trilby McDonald
Intensive/Coronary Care . . . . Kate McCord
Medical/Surgical Nursing . . . . Charlotte Schyler
OB/GYN Womens Health. . . . . Geri Towndron
Respiratory/Cardiopulmonary. . . . . Keathe Hanley

Measure	Cases	This Hospital	State Average	U.S. Average	Top Hospital
Heart Attack Care					
ACE Inhibitor or ARB for LVSD[2]	74	88%	91%	82%	100%
Aspirin at Arrival[2]	293	99%	95%	92%	100%
Aspirin at Discharge[2]	316	97%	97%	90%	100%
Beta Blocker at Arrival[2]	227	93%	93%	87%	100%
Beta Blocker at Discharge[2]	346	95%	93%	90%	100%
Fibrinolytic Medication Timing[1,2]	14	50%	31%	31%	100%
PCI Within 90 Minutes of Arrival[1,2]	16	56%	69%	54%	95%
Smoking Cessation Advice[2]	120	100%	91%	88%	100%
Heart Failure Care					
ACE Inhibitor or ARB for LVSD[2]	194	85%	84%	82%	100%
Discharge Instructions[2]	318	83%	53%	61%	93%
Evaluation of LVS Function[2]	394	94%	81%	83%	99%
Smoking Cessation Advice[2]	58	97%	79%	82%	100%
Pneumonia Care					
Appropriate Initial Antibiotic[2]	354	88%	85%	83%	94%
Blood Culture Timing[2]	275	91%	91%	90%	100%
Influenza Vaccine[2]	97	45%	70%	70%	100%
Initial Antibiotic Timing[2]	463	83%	83%	80%	93%
Oxygenation Assessment[2]	545	100%	100%	99%	100%
Pneumococcal Vaccine[2]	341	91%	72%	69%	94%
Smoking Cessation Advice[2]	132	92%	78%	80%	100%
Surgical Infection Prevention					
Prophylactic Antibiotic Given[2,3]	573	92%	83%	77%	95%
Prophylactic Antibiotic Selection[2]	155	94%	92%	90%	100%
Prophylactic Antibiotic Stopped[2,3]	559	82%	70%	72%	95%
Pregnancy Care					
Inpatient Neonatal Mortality	-	-	-	-	-
Third or Fourth Degree Laceration	-	-	4.02%	3.63%	3.27%

Southwest Memorial Hospital

1311 N Mildred Road — Phone: 970-565-6666
Cortez, CO 81321 — Fax: 970-564-2403
URL: www.swhealth.org
Ownership: Voluntary non-profit - Private — Accredited: Yes
Emergency Services: Yes — Licensed Beds: 61

Key Personnel:
CEO. . . . . Chuck Bill
Emergency Room . . . . Liz Sellers
OB/GYN Womens Health. . . . . Emily Sutcliffe, MD

Measure	Cases	This Hospital	State Average	U.S. Average	Top Hospital
Heart Attack Care					
ACE Inhibitor or ARB for LVSD[1]	3	67%	91%	82%	100%
Aspirin at Arrival[1]	10	70%	95%	92%	100%
Aspirin at Discharge[1]	10	90%	97%	90%	100%
Beta Blocker at Arrival[1]	12	67%	93%	87%	100%
Beta Blocker at Discharge[1]	10	90%	93%	90%	100%
Fibrinolytic Medication Timing[3]	0	-	31%	31%	100%
PCI Within 90 Minutes of Arrival	0	-	69%	54%	95%
Smoking Cessation Advice[3]	0	-	91%	88%	100%
Heart Failure Care					
ACE Inhibitor or ARB for LVSD[1]	4	50%	84%	82%	100%
Discharge Instructions[1,3]	5	60%	53%	61%	93%
Evaluation of LVS Function[1]	22	68%	81%	83%	99%
Smoking Cessation Advice[1,3]	1	100%	79%	82%	100%
Pneumonia Care					
Appropriate Initial Antibiotic[1,3]	7	86%	85%	83%	94%
Blood Culture Timing[1,3]	5	80%	91%	90%	100%
Influenza Vaccine[5]	-	-	70%	70%	100%
Initial Antibiotic Timing	66	83%	83%	80%	93%
Oxygenation Assessment	87	100%	100%	99%	100%
Pneumococcal Vaccine	54	54%	72%	69%	94%
Smoking Cessation Advice[1,3]	4	100%	78%	80%	100%
Surgical Infection Prevention					
Prophylactic Antibiotic Given[3]	33	76%	83%	77%	95%
Prophylactic Antibiotic Selection[5]	-	-	92%	90%	100%
Prophylactic Antibiotic Stopped[3]	31	94%	70%	72%	95%
Pregnancy Care					
Inpatient Neonatal Mortality	-	-	-	-	-
Third or Fourth Degree Laceration	-	-	4.02%	3.63%	3.27%

Memorial Hospital

785 Russell Street — Phone: 970-824-9411
Craig, CO 81625 — Fax: 970-824-2235
URL: www.thememorialhospital.com
Ownership: Government - Local — Accredited: Yes
Emergency Services: Yes — Licensed Beds: 29

Key Personnel:
Administrator . . . . M Randell Phelps
Cardiac Lab . . . . Chris Evans
Emergency Room . . . . Marle Kettle
Director Infection/Disease Control . . . . Beka Warren
CNO. . . . . Suzanne Frappier
Medical/Surgical Nursing . . . . Dale Bergstrom
Respiratory/Cardiopulmonary. . . . . Chris Evans

Measure	Cases	This Hospital	State Average	U.S. Average	Top Hospital
Heart Attack Care					
ACE Inhibitor or ARB for LVSD	0	-	91%	82%	100%
Aspirin at Arrival[1]	6	100%	95%	92%	100%
Aspirin at Discharge[1]	5	100%	97%	90%	100%
Beta Blocker at Arrival[1]	5	100%	93%	87%	100%
Beta Blocker at Discharge[1]	6	100%	93%	90%	100%
Fibrinolytic Medication Timing	0	-	31%	31%	100%
PCI Within 90 Minutes of Arrival	0	-	69%	54%	95%
Smoking Cessation Advice[1]	1	100%	91%	88%	100%
Heart Failure Care					
ACE Inhibitor or ARB for LVSD[1]	4	75%	84%	82%	100%
Discharge Instructions[1]	19	47%	53%	61%	93%
Evaluation of LVS Function	25	68%	81%	83%	99%
Smoking Cessation Advice[1]	7	86%	79%	82%	100%
Pneumonia Care					
Appropriate Initial Antibiotic	25	84%	85%	83%	94%
Blood Culture Timing[1]	14	86%	91%	90%	100%
Influenza Vaccine[1]	6	100%	70%	70%	100%
Initial Antibiotic Timing	28	89%	83%	80%	93%
Oxygenation Assessment	34	97%	100%	99%	100%
Pneumococcal Vaccine[1]	20	95%	72%	69%	94%
Smoking Cessation Advice[1]	6	83%	78%	80%	100%
Surgical Infection Prevention					
Prophylactic Antibiotic Given[1]	21	86%	83%	77%	95%
Prophylactic Antibiotic Selection[1]	4	100%	92%	90%	100%
Prophylactic Antibiotic Stopped[1]	21	29%	70%	72%	95%

NOTE: Hospital profiles are in alphabetical order by state, then city, then hospital within the city; Rankings are sorted by rate in descending order and exclude hospitals with less than 25 cases; (1) The number of cases is too small (n<25) for purposes of reliably predicting hospital performance; (2) Measure reflects the hospital's indication that its submission was based upon a sample of its relevant discharges; (3) Rate reflects fewer than the maximum possible quarters of data for the measure; (4) Inaccurate information submitted and suppressed for one or more quarters; (5) No data is available from the hospital for this measure; Please refer to the User's Guide for a full explanation of data

Pregnancy Care					
Inpatient Neonatal Mortality	-	-	-	-	-
Third or Fourth Degree Laceration	-	-	4.02%	3.63%	3.27%

Delta County Memorial Hospital

100 Stafford Lane
Delta, CO 81416
E-mail: info@deltahospital.org
URL: www.deltahospital.org
Ownership: Govt - Hospital District or Authority
Emergency Services: Yes
Phone: 970-874-7681
Fax: 970-874-2204
Accredited: Yes

Key Personnel:
President/CEO . . . . Tom Mingen
Emergency Room . . . . Paula Holman

Measure	Cases	This Hospital	State Average	U.S. Average	Top Hospital
Heart Attack Care					
ACE Inhibitor or ARB for LVSD[1]	4	100%	91%	82%	100%
Aspirin at Arrival	38	89%	95%	92%	100%
Aspirin at Discharge	26	85%	97%	90%	100%
Beta Blocker at Arrival	39	95%	93%	87%	100%
Beta Blocker at Discharge	29	86%	93%	90%	100%
Fibrinolytic Medication Timing[1]	3	33%	31%	31%	100%
PCI Within 90 Minutes of Arrival	0	-	69%	54%	95%
Smoking Cessation Advice[1]	4	100%	91%	88%	100%
Heart Failure Care					
ACE Inhibitor or ARB for LVSD[1]	15	87%	84%	82%	100%
Discharge Instructions	47	49%	53%	61%	93%
Evaluation of LVS Function	63	83%	81%	83%	99%
Smoking Cessation Advice[1]	7	100%	79%	82%	100%
Pneumonia Care					
Appropriate Initial Antibiotic	90	90%	85%	83%	94%
Blood Culture Timing	73	89%	91%	90%	100%
Influenza Vaccine	30	90%	70%	70%	100%
Initial Antibiotic Timing	114	89%	83%	80%	93%
Oxygenation Assessment	140	100%	100%	99%	100%
Pneumococcal Vaccine	91	75%	72%	69%	94%
Smoking Cessation Advice	33	82%	78%	80%	100%
Surgical Infection Prevention					
Prophylactic Antibiotic Given[3]	143	87%	83%	77%	95%
Prophylactic Antibiotic Selection	55	98%	92%	90%	100%
Prophylactic Antibiotic Stopped[3]	140	81%	70%	72%	95%
Pregnancy Care					
Inpatient Neonatal Mortality	-	-	-	-	-
Third or Fourth Degree Laceration	-	-	4.02%	3.63%	3.27%

Denver Health Medical Center

777 Bannock Street
Denver, CO 80204
Ownership: Govt - Hospital District or Authority
Emergency Services: Yes
Phone: 303-436-6000
Fax: 303-436-7159
Accredited: Yes
Licensed Beds: 398

Key Personnel:
CEO/Medical Director . . . . Patricia A Gabow, MD

Measure	Cases	This Hospital	State Average	U.S. Average	Top Hospital
Heart Attack Care					
ACE Inhibitor or ARB for LVSD[1]	15	80%	91%	82%	100%
Aspirin at Arrival	79	97%	95%	92%	100%
Aspirin at Discharge	59	97%	97%	90%	100%
Beta Blocker at Arrival	62	95%	93%	87%	100%
Beta Blocker at Discharge	59	97%	93%	90%	100%
Fibrinolytic Medication Timing	0	-	31%	31%	100%
PCI Within 90 Minutes of Arrival	0	-	69%	54%	95%
Smoking Cessation Advice	41	90%	91%	88%	100%
Heart Failure Care					
ACE Inhibitor or ARB for LVSD[2]	159	89%	84%	82%	100%
Discharge Instructions[2]	247	64%	53%	61%	93%
Evaluation of LVS Function[2]	259	98%	81%	83%	99%
Smoking Cessation Advice[2]	117	79%	79%	82%	100%
Pneumonia Care					
Appropriate Initial Antibiotic[2]	127	87%	85%	83%	94%
Blood Culture Timing[2]	79	90%	91%	90%	100%
Influenza Vaccine[1,2]	23	87%	70%	70%	100%
Initial Antibiotic Timing[2]	162	72%	83%	80%	93%
Oxygenation Assessment[2]	184	100%	100%	99%	100%
Pneumococcal Vaccine[2]	53	83%	72%	69%	94%
Smoking Cessation Advice[2]	104	80%	78%	80%	100%
Surgical Infection Prevention					
Prophylactic Antibiotic Given[2,3]	200	84%	83%	77%	95%
Prophylactic Antibiotic Selection[2]	48	85%	92%	90%	100%
Prophylactic Antibiotic Stopped[2,3]	191	70%	70%	72%	95%
Pregnancy Care					
Inpatient Neonatal Mortality	-	-	-	-	-
Third or Fourth Degree Laceration	-	-	4.02%	3.63%	3.27%

Exempla Saint Joseph Hospital

1835 Franklin Street
Denver, CO 80218
URL: www.exempla.org
Ownership: Voluntary non-profit - Private
Emergency Services: Yes
Phone: 303-837-7111
Fax: 303-318-2115
Accredited: Yes
Licensed Beds: 565

Key Personnel:
CEO. . . . . Robert Minkin
President of Medical Staff . . . . Debra J Parsons, MD

Measure	Cases	This Hospital	State Average	U.S. Average	Top Hospital
Heart Attack Care					
ACE Inhibitor or ARB for LVSD[2]	34	85%	91%	82%	100%
Aspirin at Arrival[2]	182	99%	95%	92%	100%
Aspirin at Discharge[2]	204	100%	97%	90%	100%
Beta Blocker at Arrival[2]	133	96%	93%	87%	100%
Beta Blocker at Discharge[2]	255	100%	93%	90%	100%
Fibrinolytic Medication Timing[2]	0	-	31%	31%	100%
PCI Within 90 Minutes of Arrival[1,2]	14	79%	69%	54%	95%
Smoking Cessation Advice[2]	74	97%	91%	88%	100%
Heart Failure Care					
ACE Inhibitor or ARB for LVSD[2]	92	84%	84%	82%	100%
Discharge Instructions[2]	223	91%	53%	61%	93%
Evaluation of LVS Function[2]	278	95%	81%	83%	99%
Smoking Cessation Advice[2]	31	97%	79%	82%	100%
Pneumonia Care					
Appropriate Initial Antibiotic[2]	83	87%	85%	83%	94%
Blood Culture Timing[2]	87	92%	91%	90%	100%
Influenza Vaccine[1,2]	23	83%	70%	70%	100%
Initial Antibiotic Timing[2]	115	85%	83%	80%	93%
Oxygenation Assessment[2]	146	100%	100%	99%	100%
Pneumococcal Vaccine[2]	97	65%	72%	69%	94%
Smoking Cessation Advice[2]	37	84%	78%	80%	100%
Surgical Infection Prevention					
Prophylactic Antibiotic Given[2]	307	94%	83%	77%	95%
Prophylactic Antibiotic Selection[2]	72	97%	92%	90%	100%
Prophylactic Antibiotic Stopped[2]	300	73%	70%	72%	95%
Pregnancy Care					
Inpatient Neonatal Mortality	-	-	-	-	-
Third or Fourth Degree Laceration	-	-	4.02%	3.63%	3.27%

National Jewish Medical and Research Center

1400 Jackson Street
Denver, CO 80206
E-mail: lungline@njc.org
URL: www.njc.org
Ownership: Voluntary non-profit - Private
Emergency Services: No
Toll-Free: 800-222-5864
Phone: 303-388-4461
Fax: 303-270-2165
Accredited: Yes
Licensed Beds: 46

Key Personnel:
President/CEO. . . . . Michael Salem, MD

Measure	Cases	This Hospital	State Average	U.S. Average	Top Hospital
Heart Attack Care					
ACE Inhibitor or ARB for LVSD[5]	-	-	91%	82%	100%
Aspirin at Arrival[5]	-	-	95%	92%	100%
Aspirin at Discharge[5]	-	-	97%	90%	100%
Beta Blocker at Arrival[5]	-	-	93%	87%	100%
Beta Blocker at Discharge[5]	-	-	93%	90%	100%

NOTE: Hospital profiles are in alphabetical order by state, then city, then hospital within the city; Rankings are sorted by rate in descending order and exclude hospitals with less than 25 cases; (1) The number of cases is too small (n<25) for purposes of reliably predicting hospital performance; (2) Measure reflects the hospital's indication that its submission was based upon a sample of its relevant discharges; (3) Rate reflects fewer than the maximum possible quarters of data for the measure; (4) Inaccurate information submitted and suppressed for one or more quarters; (5) No data is available from the hospital for this measure; Please refer to the User's Guide for a full explanation of data

Measure	Cases	This Hospital	State Average	U.S. Average	Top Hospital
Fibrinolytic Medication Timing[5]	-	-	31%	31%	100%
PCI Within 90 Minutes of Arrival[5]	-	-	69%	54%	95%
Smoking Cessation Advice[5]	-	-	91%	88%	100%
Heart Failure Care					
ACE Inhibitor or ARB for LVSD[5]	-	-	84%	82%	100%
Discharge Instructions[5]	-	-	53%	61%	93%
Evaluation of LVS Function[5]	-	-	81%	83%	99%
Smoking Cessation Advice[5]	-	-	79%	82%	100%
Pneumonia Care					
Appropriate Initial Antibiotic[5]	-	-	85%	83%	94%
Blood Culture Timing[5]	-	-	91%	90%	100%
Influenza Vaccine[5]	-	-	70%	70%	100%
Initial Antibiotic Timing[5]	-	-	83%	80%	93%
Oxygenation Assessment[5]	-	-	100%	99%	100%
Pneumococcal Vaccine[5]	-	-	72%	69%	94%
Smoking Cessation Advice[5]	-	-	78%	80%	100%
Surgical Infection Prevention					
Prophylactic Antibiotic Given[5]	-	-	83%	77%	95%
Prophylactic Antibiotic Selection[5]	-	-	92%	90%	100%
Prophylactic Antibiotic Stopped[5]	-	-	70%	72%	95%
Pregnancy Care					
Inpatient Neonatal Mortality	-	-	-	-	-
Third or Fourth Degree Laceration	-	-	4.02%	3.63%	3.27%

Porter Adventist Hospital

2525 S Downing Street — Phone: 303-778-1955
Denver, CO 80210 — Fax: 303-778-5252
URL: www.centura.org
Ownership: Voluntary non-profit - Church — Accredited: Yes
Emergency Services: Yes — Licensed Beds: 368

Key Personnel:

- President/CEO . . . . Ruthia Fike
- Chief Medical Staff . . . . Carol Landry
- Cardiac Lab . . . . Jane Broaten
- Catheterization Lab . . . . Lorraine Wotking
- Emergency Room . . . . Pat Keller
- Emergency Room . . . . Curt Johnson
- Infection Control . . . . Cindy Thistel
- ICU . . . . Lynn Motthias
- Intensive/Coronary Care . . . . Karolyn Scheneman
- Medical/Surgical Nursing . . . . Chris Hartwick
- Respiratory/Cardiopulmonary . . . . Mindy Lemons

Measure	Cases	This Hospital	State Average	U.S. Average	Top Hospital
Heart Attack Care					
ACE Inhibitor or ARB for LVSD[2]	25	88%	91%	82%	100%
Aspirin at Arrival[2]	97	97%	95%	92%	100%
Aspirin at Discharge[2]	91	98%	97%	90%	100%
Beta Blocker at Arrival[2]	80	96%	93%	87%	100%
Beta Blocker at Discharge[2]	117	98%	93%	90%	100%
Fibrinolytic Medication Timing[2]	0	-	31%	31%	100%
PCI Within 90 Minutes of Arrival[1,2]	5	60%	69%	54%	95%
Smoking Cessation Advice[2]	40	98%	91%	88%	100%
Heart Failure Care					
ACE Inhibitor or ARB for LVSD[2]	49	88%	84%	82%	100%
Discharge Instructions[2]	166	67%	53%	61%	93%
Evaluation of LVS Function[2]	201	96%	81%	83%	99%
Smoking Cessation Advice[2]	36	92%	79%	82%	100%
Pneumonia Care					
Appropriate Initial Antibiotic[2]	137	87%	85%	83%	94%
Blood Culture Timing[2]	144	97%	91%	90%	100%
Influenza Vaccine[2]	43	14%	70%	70%	100%
Initial Antibiotic Timing[2]	207	92%	83%	80%	93%
Oxygenation Assessment[2]	234	100%	100%	99%	100%
Pneumococcal Vaccine[2]	160	65%	72%	69%	94%
Smoking Cessation Advice[2]	43	74%	78%	80%	100%
Surgical Infection Prevention					
Prophylactic Antibiotic Given[2,3]	349	84%	83%	77%	95%
Prophylactic Antibiotic Selection[2]	122	94%	92%	90%	100%
Prophylactic Antibiotic Stopped[2,3]	338	80%	70%	72%	95%
Pregnancy Care					
Inpatient Neonatal Mortality	-	-	-	-	-
Third or Fourth Degree Laceration	-	-	4.02%	3.63%	3.27%

Presbyterian-Saint Luke's Medical Center

1719 East 19th Avenue — Phone: 303-839-6000
Denver, CO 80218 — Fax: 303-839-7294
E-mail: paula.cooper@healthonecares.com
URL: www.pslmc.com
Ownership: Government - State — Accredited: Yes
Emergency Services: Yes — Licensed Beds: 680

Key Personnel:

- President/CEO . . . . Madeleine Roberson
- Chief Medical Staff . . . . Katherine Fitting, MD
- Cardiac Lab . . . . Tammy Woolley
- Emergency Room . . . . Stan Siefer, MD
- Emergency Room . . . . Don Myers
- ICU . . . . Rocky Billups
- Medical/Surgical Nursing . . . . Ginnie Ferraro
- OB/GYN Womens Health . . . . Richard P Porrecot, MD
- Respiratory Therapy . . . . Rocky Billups

Measure	Cases	This Hospital	State Average	U.S. Average	Top Hospital
Heart Attack Care					
ACE Inhibitor or ARB for LVSD[1]	13	100%	91%	82%	100%
Aspirin at Arrival	39	100%	95%	92%	100%
Aspirin at Discharge	115	100%	97%	90%	100%
Beta Blocker at Arrival	25	100%	93%	87%	100%
Beta Blocker at Discharge	135	99%	93%	90%	100%
Fibrinolytic Medication Timing	0	-	31%	31%	100%
PCI Within 90 Minutes of Arrival	0	-	69%	54%	95%
Smoking Cessation Advice	40	100%	91%	88%	100%
Heart Failure Care					
ACE Inhibitor or ARB for LVSD	66	95%	84%	82%	100%
Discharge Instructions	142	84%	53%	61%	93%
Evaluation of LVS Function	165	98%	81%	83%	99%
Smoking Cessation Advice	31	97%	79%	82%	100%
Pneumonia Care					
Appropriate Initial Antibiotic	55	80%	85%	83%	94%
Blood Culture Timing	59	95%	91%	90%	100%
Influenza Vaccine[1]	21	57%	70%	70%	100%
Initial Antibiotic Timing	94	76%	83%	80%	93%
Oxygenation Assessment	115	100%	100%	99%	100%
Pneumococcal Vaccine	64	64%	72%	69%	94%
Smoking Cessation Advice	32	62%	78%	80%	100%
Surgical Infection Prevention					
Prophylactic Antibiotic Given[2,3]	218	72%	83%	77%	95%
Prophylactic Antibiotic Selection[2]	90	73%	92%	90%	100%
Prophylactic Antibiotic Stopped[2,3]	203	61%	70%	72%	95%
Pregnancy Care					
Inpatient Neonatal Mortality	1,656	3.62%	-	-	-
Third or Fourth Degree Laceration	863	3.24%	4.02%	3.63%	3.27%

Rose Medical Center

4567 E 9th Avenue — Phone: 303-320-2121
Denver, CO 80220 — Fax: 303-320-2200
URL: www.rosemed.com
Ownership: Proprietary — Accredited: Yes
Emergency Services: Yes — Licensed Beds: 420

Key Personnel:

- President/CEO . . . . Kenneth H Feiler
- Medical Staff President . . . . Donald J Lefkowits
- Emergency Room . . . . Donald J Lefkowits
- Emergency Room . . . . Brenda Cox
- Chairman OB/GYN . . . . Gerald Zarlengo, MD

Measure	Cases	This Hospital	State Average	U.S. Average	Top Hospital
Heart Attack Care					
ACE Inhibitor or ARB for LVSD[1]	17	76%	91%	82%	100%
Aspirin at Arrival	137	100%	95%	92%	100%
Aspirin at Discharge	132	100%	97%	90%	100%
Beta Blocker at Arrival	100	100%	93%	87%	100%
Beta Blocker at Discharge	130	100%	93%	90%	100%
Fibrinolytic Medication Timing	0	-	31%	31%	100%
PCI Within 90 Minutes of Arrival[1]	5	80%	69%	54%	95%
Smoking Cessation Advice	39	97%	91%	88%	100%
Heart Failure Care					

NOTE: Hospital profiles are in alphabetical order by state, then city, then hospital within the city; Rankings are sorted by rate in descending order and exclude hospitals with less than 25 cases; (1) The number of cases is too small (n<25) for purposes of reliably predicting hospital performance; (2) Measure reflects the hospital's indication that its submission was based upon a sample of its relevant discharges; (3) Rate reflects fewer than the maximum possible quarters of data for the measure; (4) Inaccurate information submitted and suppressed for one or more quarters; (5) No data is available from the hospital for this measure; Please refer to the User's Guide for a full explanation of data

ACE Inhibitor or ARB for LVSD	70	86%	84%	82%	100%
Discharge Instructions	160	65%	53%	61%	93%
Evaluation of LVS Function	205	98%	81%	83%	99%
Smoking Cessation Advice[1]	20	90%	79%	82%	100%
Pneumonia Care					
Appropriate Initial Antibiotic	141	94%	85%	83%	94%
Blood Culture Timing	125	97%	91%	90%	100%
Influenza Vaccine	29	79%	70%	70%	100%
Initial Antibiotic Timing	180	91%	83%	80%	93%
Oxygenation Assessment	216	100%	100%	99%	100%
Pneumococcal Vaccine	136	86%	72%	69%	94%
Smoking Cessation Advice	47	87%	78%	80%	100%
Surgical Infection Prevention					
Prophylactic Antibiotic Given[2,3]	211	56%	83%	77%	95%
Prophylactic Antibiotic Selection[2]	99	98%	92%	90%	100%
Prophylactic Antibiotic Stopped[2,3]	214	76%	70%	72%	95%
Pregnancy Care					
Inpatient Neonatal Mortality	3,846	0.23%	-	-	-
Third or Fourth Degree Laceration	2,434	4.85%	4.02%	3.63%	3.27%

Saint Anthony Central Hospital

Alternate Name: Centura Health
4231 W 16th Avenue — Phone: 303-629-3511
Denver, CO 80204 — Fax: 303-629-2318
URL: www.stanthonyhosp.org
Ownership: Voluntary non-profit - Church — Accredited: Yes
Emergency Services: Yes — Licensed Beds: 498

Key Personnel:
CEO. . . . . George A Zara

Measure	Cases	This Hospital	State Average	U.S. Average	Top Hospital
Heart Attack Care					
ACE Inhibitor or ARB for LVSD[2]	58	100%	91%	82%	100%
Aspirin at Arrival[2]	182	100%	95%	92%	100%
Aspirin at Discharge[2]	270	100%	97%	90%	100%
Beta Blocker at Arrival[2]	154	97%	93%	87%	100%
Beta Blocker at Discharge[2]	252	100%	93%	90%	100%
Fibrinolytic Medication Timing[2]	0	-	31%	31%	100%
PCI Within 90 Minutes of Arrival[1,2]	12	100%	69%	54%	95%
Smoking Cessation Advice[2]	102	100%	91%	88%	100%
Heart Failure Care					
ACE Inhibitor or ARB for LVSD[2]	76	89%	84%	82%	100%
Discharge Instructions[2]	150	59%	53%	61%	93%
Evaluation of LVS Function[2]	187	95%	81%	83%	99%
Smoking Cessation Advice[2]	40	100%	79%	82%	100%
Pneumonia Care					
Appropriate Initial Antibiotic[2]	103	84%	85%	83%	94%
Blood Culture Timing[2]	124	90%	91%	90%	100%
Influenza Vaccine[2]	31	84%	70%	70%	100%
Initial Antibiotic Timing[2]	194	78%	83%	80%	93%
Oxygenation Assessment[2]	213	100%	100%	99%	100%
Pneumococcal Vaccine[2]	135	95%	72%	69%	94%
Smoking Cessation Advice[2]	61	100%	78%	80%	100%
Surgical Infection Prevention					
Prophylactic Antibiotic Given[2,3]	363	84%	83%	77%	95%
Prophylactic Antibiotic Selection[2]	115	97%	92%	90%	100%
Prophylactic Antibiotic Stopped[2,3]	341	81%	70%	72%	95%
Pregnancy Care					
Inpatient Neonatal Mortality	-	-	-	-	-
Third or Fourth Degree Laceration	-	-	4.02%	3.63%	3.27%

University of Colorado Hospital

4200 E Ninth Avenue — Phone: 303-372-0000
Campus Box FA12 — Fax: 303-372-5344
Denver, CO 80262
URL: www.uch.edu
Ownership: Govt - Hospital District or Authority — Accredited: Yes
Emergency Services: Yes — Licensed Beds: 373

Key Personnel:
CEO. . . . . Joy Cashman
Chief Medical Staff. . . . . Gregory Stiegmann, MD
Director of Cardiology Department. . . . . Sue Bromini
Director of Emergency Room. . . . . Lorna Prutzman
Director of Pulmonary/Respiratory Care. . . . . . . Allen Wentworth

Measure	Cases	This Hospital	State Average	U.S. Average	Top Hospital
Heart Attack Care					
ACE Inhibitor or ARB for LVSD	27	85%	91%	82%	100%
Aspirin at Arrival	115	99%	95%	92%	100%
Aspirin at Discharge	137	99%	97%	90%	100%
Beta Blocker at Arrival	84	96%	93%	87%	100%
Beta Blocker at Discharge	161	99%	93%	90%	100%
Fibrinolytic Medication Timing	0	-	31%	31%	100%
PCI Within 90 Minutes of Arrival[1]	16	75%	69%	54%	95%
Smoking Cessation Advice	67	100%	91%	88%	100%
Heart Failure Care					
ACE Inhibitor or ARB for LVSD[2]	150	89%	84%	82%	100%
Discharge Instructions[2]	277	86%	53%	61%	93%
Evaluation of LVS Function[2]	308	97%	81%	83%	99%
Smoking Cessation Advice[2]	81	99%	79%	82%	100%
Pneumonia Care					
Appropriate Initial Antibiotic[2]	89	83%	85%	83%	94%
Blood Culture Timing[2]	115	83%	91%	90%	100%
Influenza Vaccine[1,2]	23	26%	70%	70%	100%
Initial Antibiotic Timing[2]	151	69%	83%	80%	93%
Oxygenation Assessment[2]	186	100%	100%	99%	100%
Pneumococcal Vaccine[2]	70	30%	72%	69%	94%
Smoking Cessation Advice[2]	69	96%	78%	80%	100%
Surgical Infection Prevention					
Prophylactic Antibiotic Given[2,3]	335	78%	83%	77%	95%
Prophylactic Antibiotic Selection[2]	68	78%	92%	90%	100%
Prophylactic Antibiotic Stopped[2,3]	337	82%	70%	72%	95%
Pregnancy Care					
Inpatient Neonatal Mortality[2]	666	1.05%	-	-	-
Third or Fourth Degree Laceration	2,280	2.89%	4.02%	3.63%	3.27%

Animas Surgical Hospital

575 Rivergate Lane — Phone: 970-247-3537
Durango, CO 81301
Ownership: Proprietary — Accredited: No
Emergency Services: Yes

Key Personnel:
Cardiology . . . . Bruce Andrea, MD
OBGYN . . . . Elizabeth Baca, MD

Measure	Cases	This Hospital	State Average	U.S. Average	Top Hospital
Heart Attack Care					
ACE Inhibitor or ARB for LVSD[5]	-	-	91%	82%	100%
Aspirin at Arrival[5]	-	-	95%	92%	100%
Aspirin at Discharge[5]	-	-	97%	90%	100%
Beta Blocker at Arrival[5]	-	-	93%	87%	100%
Beta Blocker at Discharge[5]	-	-	93%	90%	100%
Fibrinolytic Medication Timing[5]	-	-	31%	31%	100%
PCI Within 90 Minutes of Arrival[5]	-	-	69%	54%	95%
Smoking Cessation Advice[5]	-	-	91%	88%	100%
Heart Failure Care					
ACE Inhibitor or ARB for LVSD[5]	-	-	84%	82%	100%
Discharge Instructions[5]	-	-	53%	61%	93%
Evaluation of LVS Function[5]	-	-	81%	83%	99%
Smoking Cessation Advice[5]	-	-	79%	82%	100%
Pneumonia Care					
Appropriate Initial Antibiotic[5]	-	-	85%	83%	94%
Blood Culture Timing[5]	-	-	91%	90%	100%
Influenza Vaccine[5]	-	-	70%	70%	100%
Initial Antibiotic Timing[5]	-	-	83%	80%	93%
Oxygenation Assessment[5]	-	-	100%	99%	100%
Pneumococcal Vaccine[5]	-	-	72%	69%	94%
Smoking Cessation Advice[5]	-	-	78%	80%	100%
Surgical Infection Prevention					
Prophylactic Antibiotic Given[2,3]	25	92%	83%	77%	95%
Prophylactic Antibiotic Selection[5]	-	-	92%	90%	100%
Prophylactic Antibiotic Stopped[2,3]	25	56%	70%	72%	95%
Pregnancy Care					
Inpatient Neonatal Mortality	-	-	-	-	-
Third or Fourth Degree Laceration	-	-	4.02%	3.63%	3.27%

NOTE: Hospital profiles are in alphabetical order by state, then city, then hospital within the city; Rankings are sorted by rate in descending order and exclude hospitals with less than 25 cases; (1) The number of cases is too small (n<25) for purposes of reliably predicting hospital performance; (2) Measure reflects the hospital's indication that its submission was based upon a sample of its relevant discharges; (3) Rate reflects fewer than the maximum possible quarters of data for the measure; (4) Inaccurate information submitted and suppressed for one or more quarters; (5) No data is available from the hospital for this measure; Please refer to the User's Guide for a full explanation of data

Mercy Regional Medical Center

1010 Three Springs Boulevard
Durango, CO 81301

Toll-Free: 800-345-2516
Phone: 970-247-4311
Fax: 970-764-3759

URL: www.mercydurango.org
Ownership: Voluntary non-profit - Church
Emergency Services: Yes

Accredited: Yes
Licensed Beds: 110

Key Personnel:

President/CEO . . . . . Kirk Dignum
Chief of Medical Staff . . . . . John Boyde
Cardiac Lab . . . . . Amry Elliott
Catheterization Lab . . . . . Mary Elliott
Head Emergency Room . . . . . Pat Wilson
ICU . . . . . Linda Riggle
Chief Respiratory Care . . . . . Jim Bagwell

Measure	Cases	This Hospital	State Average	U.S. Average	Top Hospital
Heart Attack Care					
ACE Inhibitor or ARB for LVSD[1]	7	100%	91%	82%	100%
Aspirin at Arrival	49	98%	95%	92%	100%
Aspirin at Discharge	66	100%	97%	90%	100%
Beta Blocker at Arrival	36	100%	93%	87%	100%
Beta Blocker at Discharge	63	95%	93%	90%	100%
Fibrinolytic Medication Timing	0	-	31%	31%	100%
PCI Within 90 Minutes of Arrival[1]	2	50%	69%	54%	95%
Smoking Cessation Advice[1]	16	100%	91%	88%	100%
Heart Failure Care					
ACE Inhibitor or ARB for LVSD	25	92%	84%	82%	100%
Discharge Instructions	56	73%	53%	61%	93%
Evaluation of LVS Function	61	100%	81%	83%	99%
Smoking Cessation Advice[1]	7	86%	79%	82%	100%
Pneumonia Care					
Appropriate Initial Antibiotic	58	97%	85%	83%	94%
Blood Culture Timing	71	94%	91%	90%	100%
Influenza Vaccine[1]	23	83%	70%	70%	100%
Initial Antibiotic Timing	88	91%	83%	80%	93%
Oxygenation Assessment	103	100%	100%	99%	100%
Pneumococcal Vaccine	73	66%	72%	69%	94%
Smoking Cessation Advice	26	100%	78%	80%	100%
Surgical Infection Prevention					
Prophylactic Antibiotic Given	247	96%	83%	77%	95%
Prophylactic Antibiotic Selection	69	97%	92%	90%	100%
Prophylactic Antibiotic Stopped	243	82%	70%	72%	95%
Pregnancy Care					
Inpatient Neonatal Mortality	-	-	-	-	-
Third or Fourth Degree Laceration	-	-	4.02%	3.63%	3.27%

Swedish Medical Center

501 East Hampden Avenue
Englewood, CO 80113

Phone: 303-788-5000
Fax: 303-788-6029

E-mail: Maria.Isquierdo@HealthONEcares.com
URL: www.swedishhospital.com/Default.asp
Ownership: Proprietary
Emergency Services: Yes

Accredited: Yes
Licensed Beds: 368

Key Personnel:

President/CEO . . . . . Mary M White
Chief Medical Staff . . . . . Jeanneld Siebert, MD
Catheterization Lab . . . . . Ann Randall
Emergency Room . . . . . Vicki Owens

Measure	Cases	This Hospital	State Average	U.S. Average	Top Hospital
Heart Attack Care					
ACE Inhibitor or ARB for LVSD	38	92%	91%	82%	100%
Aspirin at Arrival	176	98%	95%	92%	100%
Aspirin at Discharge	142	96%	97%	90%	100%
Beta Blocker at Arrival	138	98%	93%	87%	100%
Beta Blocker at Discharge	188	97%	93%	90%	100%
Fibrinolytic Medication Timing	0	-	31%	31%	100%
PCI Within 90 Minutes of Arrival[1]	23	70%	69%	54%	95%
Smoking Cessation Advice	70	99%	91%	88%	100%
Heart Failure Care					
ACE Inhibitor or ARB for LVSD	93	82%	84%	82%	100%
Discharge Instructions	216	75%	53%	61%	93%
Evaluation of LVS Function	287	94%	81%	83%	99%
Smoking Cessation Advice	39	77%	79%	82%	100%
Pneumonia Care					
Appropriate Initial Antibiotic[2]	170	92%	85%	83%	94%
Blood Culture Timing[2]	150	97%	91%	90%	100%
Influenza Vaccine	53	74%	70%	70%	100%
Initial Antibiotic Timing[2]	240	80%	83%	80%	93%
Oxygenation Assessment[2]	318	100%	100%	99%	100%
Pneumococcal Vaccine[2]	175	68%	72%	69%	94%
Smoking Cessation Advice[2]	72	64%	78%	80%	100%
Surgical Infection Prevention					
Prophylactic Antibiotic Given[2,3]	233	85%	83%	77%	95%
Prophylactic Antibiotic Selection[2]	92	91%	92%	90%	100%
Prophylactic Antibiotic Stopped[2,3]	223	76%	70%	72%	95%
Pregnancy Care					
Inpatient Neonatal Mortality	-	-	-	-	-
Third or Fourth Degree Laceration	-	-	4.02%	3.63%	3.27%

Estes Park Medical Center

555 Prospect Avenue
PO Box 2740
Estes Park, CO 80517

Phone: 970-586-2317
Fax: 970-586-0109

E-mail: info@epmedcenter.com
URL: www.epmedcenter.com
Ownership: Govt - Hospital District or Authority
Emergency Services: Yes

Accredited: No
Licensed Beds: 15

Key Personnel:

President/CEO . . . . . Andrew Wills
Chief Medical Staff . . . . . Martin Koschnitzke, MD
Emergency Room . . . . . Jeff Hemstreet, MD
Emergency Room . . . . . Cindy Bauinghatt, RN
Medical/Surgical Nursing . . . . . Mary Leonard
OB/GYN Womens Health . . . . . Brenda Taylor

Measure	Cases	This Hospital	State Average	U.S. Average	Top Hospital
Heart Attack Care					
ACE Inhibitor or ARB for LVSD[5]	-	-	91%	82%	100%
Aspirin at Arrival[5]	-	-	95%	92%	100%
Aspirin at Discharge[5]	-	-	97%	90%	100%
Beta Blocker at Arrival[5]	-	-	93%	87%	100%
Beta Blocker at Discharge[5]	-	-	93%	90%	100%
Fibrinolytic Medication Timing[5]	-	-	31%	31%	100%
PCI Within 90 Minutes of Arrival[5]	-	-	69%	54%	95%
Smoking Cessation Advice[5]	-	-	91%	88%	100%
Heart Failure Care					
ACE Inhibitor or ARB for LVSD[3]	0	-	84%	82%	100%
Discharge Instructions[1,3]	3	0%	53%	61%	93%
Evaluation of LVS Function[1,3]	4	50%	81%	83%	99%
Smoking Cessation Advice[3]	0	-	79%	82%	100%
Pneumonia Care					
Appropriate Initial Antibiotic[1,3]	15	53%	85%	83%	94%
Blood Culture Timing[1,3]	6	83%	91%	90%	100%
Influenza Vaccine[5]	-	-	70%	70%	100%
Initial Antibiotic Timing[1,3]	16	75%	83%	80%	93%
Oxygenation Assessment[1,3]	20	100%	100%	99%	100%
Pneumococcal Vaccine[1,3]	14	79%	72%	69%	94%
Smoking Cessation Advice[1,3]	6	33%	78%	80%	100%
Surgical Infection Prevention					
Prophylactic Antibiotic Given[1,3]	12	92%	83%	77%	95%
Prophylactic Antibiotic Selection[1]	1	100%	92%	90%	100%
Prophylactic Antibiotic Stopped[1,3]	11	100%	70%	72%	95%
Pregnancy Care					
Inpatient Neonatal Mortality	-	-	-	-	-
Third or Fourth Degree Laceration	-	-	4.02%	3.63%	3.27%

NOTE: Hospital profiles are in alphabetical order by state, then city, then hospital within the city; Rankings are sorted by rate in descending order and exclude hospitals with less than 25 cases; (1) The number of cases is too small (n<25) for purposes of reliably predicting hospital performance; (2) Measure reflects the hospital's indication that its submission was based upon a sample of its relevant discharges; (3) Rate reflects fewer than the maximum possible quarters of data for the measure; (4) Inaccurate information submitted and suppressed for one or more quarters; (5) No data is available from the hospital for this measure; Please refer to the User's Guide for a full explanation of data

Poudre Valley Hospital

1024 S Lemay Avenue
Fort Collins, CO 80524
E-mail: PVHS@pvh.org
URL: www.pvhs.org
Ownership: Voluntary non-profit - Private
Emergency Services: Yes
Phone: 970-495-7000
Fax: 970-495-7600
Accredited: Yes
Licensed Beds: 235

Key Personnel:
President/CEO. . . . . Kevin Unger
Chief Medical Staff. . . . . William Miller, MD
OB/GYN Womens Health. . . . . Norma Stiglich, MD
Director Respiratory Therapy . . . . Paul Cocking

Measure	Cases	This Hospital	State Average	U.S. Average	Top Hospital
Heart Attack Care					
ACE Inhibitor or ARB for LVSD	89	88%	91%	82%	100%
Aspirin at Arrival	226	99%	95%	92%	100%
Aspirin at Discharge	361	99%	97%	90%	100%
Beta Blocker at Arrival	168	96%	93%	87%	100%
Beta Blocker at Discharge	450	98%	93%	90%	100%
Fibrinolytic Medication Timing	0	-	31%	31%	100%
PCI Within 90 Minutes of Arrival	28	68%	69%	54%	95%
Smoking Cessation Advice	163	96%	91%	88%	100%
Heart Failure Care					
ACE Inhibitor or ARB for LVSD	85	76%	84%	82%	100%
Discharge Instructions	181	64%	53%	61%	93%
Evaluation of LVS Function	241	90%	81%	83%	99%
Smoking Cessation Advice	58	93%	79%	82%	100%
Pneumonia Care					
Appropriate Initial Antibiotic	177	84%	85%	83%	94%
Blood Culture Timing	104	95%	91%	90%	100%
Influenza Vaccine	42	71%	70%	70%	100%
Initial Antibiotic Timing	232	71%	83%	80%	93%
Oxygenation Assessment	299	100%	100%	99%	100%
Pneumococcal Vaccine	191	63%	72%	69%	94%
Smoking Cessation Advice	66	95%	78%	80%	100%
Surgical Infection Prevention					
Prophylactic Antibiotic Given[3]	219	88%	83%	77%	95%
Prophylactic Antibiotic Selection	73	93%	92%	90%	100%
Prophylactic Antibiotic Stopped[3]	211	56%	70%	72%	95%
Pregnancy Care					
Inpatient Neonatal Mortality	2,818	0.21%	-	-	-
Third or Fourth Degree Laceration	1,938	5.01%	4.02%	3.63%	3.27%

Colorado Plains Medical Center

1000 Lincoln Street
CS 4200
Fort Morgan, CO 80701
URL: www.prhc.net
Ownership: Voluntary non-profit - Other
Emergency Services: Yes
Phone: 970-867-3391
Fax: 970-542-4352
Accredited: Yes
Licensed Beds: 50

Key Personnel:
CEO. . . . . Michael A Anayar Sr

Measure	Cases	This Hospital	State Average	U.S. Average	Top Hospital
Heart Attack Care					
ACE Inhibitor or ARB for LVSD	0	-	91%	82%	100%
Aspirin at Arrival[1]	8	88%	95%	92%	100%
Aspirin at Discharge[1]	3	67%	97%	90%	100%
Beta Blocker at Arrival[1]	4	75%	93%	87%	100%
Beta Blocker at Discharge[1]	1	0%	93%	90%	100%
Fibrinolytic Medication Timing[1]	1	0%	31%	31%	100%
PCI Within 90 Minutes of Arrival	0	-	69%	54%	95%
Smoking Cessation Advice[1]	1	100%	91%	88%	100%
Heart Failure Care					
ACE Inhibitor or ARB for LVSD[1]	14	86%	84%	82%	100%
Discharge Instructions	26	62%	53%	61%	93%
Evaluation of LVS Function	41	76%	81%	83%	99%
Smoking Cessation Advice[1]	7	86%	79%	82%	100%
Pneumonia Care					
Appropriate Initial Antibiotic	61	87%	85%	83%	94%
Blood Culture Timing	60	88%	91%	90%	100%
Influenza Vaccine[4,5]	-	-	70%	70%	100%
Initial Antibiotic Timing	99	92%	83%	80%	93%
Oxygenation Assessment	110	100%	100%	99%	100%
Pneumococcal Vaccine	84	76%	72%	69%	94%
Smoking Cessation Advice[1]	20	70%	78%	80%	100%
Surgical Infection Prevention					
Prophylactic Antibiotic Given	83	89%	83%	77%	95%
Prophylactic Antibiotic Selection[1]	23	100%	92%	90%	100%
Prophylactic Antibiotic Stopped	80	36%	70%	72%	95%
Pregnancy Care					
Inpatient Neonatal Mortality	-	-	-	-	-
Third or Fourth Degree Laceration	-	-	4.02%	3.63%	3.27%

Saint Anthony Summit Medical Center

340 Peak One Drive
Frisco, CO 80443
Ownership: Voluntary non-profit - Church
Emergency Services: Yes
Phone: 970-668-3300
Fax: 970-668-1517
Accredited: Yes
Licensed Beds: 9

Key Personnel:
CEO. . . . . Carol Turrin
Emergency Room . . . . Lory Profota, RN
Director Medical/Surgical Nursing . . . . Carol Turrin

Measure	Cases	This Hospital	State Average	U.S. Average	Top Hospital
Heart Attack Care					
ACE Inhibitor or ARB for LVSD[5]	-	-	91%	82%	100%
Aspirin at Arrival[5]	-	-	95%	92%	100%
Aspirin at Discharge[5]	-	-	97%	90%	100%
Beta Blocker at Arrival[5]	-	-	93%	87%	100%
Beta Blocker at Discharge[5]	-	-	93%	90%	100%
Fibrinolytic Medication Timing[5]	-	-	31%	31%	100%
PCI Within 90 Minutes of Arrival[5]	-	-	69%	54%	95%
Smoking Cessation Advice[5]	-	-	91%	88%	100%
Heart Failure Care					
ACE Inhibitor or ARB for LVSD[2,3]	0	-	84%	82%	100%
Discharge Instructions[1,2,3]	5	40%	53%	61%	93%
Evaluation of LVS Function[1,2,3]	5	80%	81%	83%	99%
Smoking Cessation Advice[1,2,3]	1	100%	79%	82%	100%
Pneumonia Care					
Appropriate Initial Antibiotic[1,2,3]	14	79%	85%	83%	94%
Blood Culture Timing[1,2]	13	92%	91%	90%	100%
Influenza Vaccine[1,2]	3	100%	70%	70%	100%
Initial Antibiotic Timing[1,2,3]	11	91%	83%	80%	93%
Oxygenation Assessment[1,2,3]	16	100%	100%	99%	100%
Pneumococcal Vaccine[1,2,3]	8	75%	72%	69%	94%
Smoking Cessation Advice[1,2,3]	2	100%	78%	80%	100%
Surgical Infection Prevention					
Prophylactic Antibiotic Given[2,3]	28	71%	83%	77%	95%
Prophylactic Antibiotic Selection[1,2]	12	75%	92%	90%	100%
Prophylactic Antibiotic Stopped[2,3]	26	31%	70%	72%	95%
Pregnancy Care					
Inpatient Neonatal Mortality	-	-	-	-	-
Third or Fourth Degree Laceration	-	-	4.02%	3.63%	3.27%

Valley View Hospital

1906 Blake Avenue
Glenwood Springs, CO 81602
E-mail: vvhadmin@ruralhealth.org
Ownership: Government - Local
Emergency Services: Yes
Phone: 970-945-6535
Fax: 970-945-2073
Accredited: Yes
Licensed Beds: 80

Key Personnel:
CEO. . . . . Gary Brewer
Chief Medical Staff. . . . . Rob Macaulay
Emergency Room . . . . Vickie Smith
Infection Control. . . . . Trish Cerise
Director Radiology . . . . Jeff Vickick, MD
Manager Respiratory Therapy . . . . Claudia Piccione

Measure	Cases	This Hospital	State Average	U.S. Average	Top Hospital
Heart Attack Care					
ACE Inhibitor or ARB for LVSD[1]	2	100%	91%	82%	100%
Aspirin at Arrival[1]	18	100%	95%	92%	100%
Aspirin at Discharge[1]	11	82%	97%	90%	100%

NOTE: Hospital profiles are in alphabetical order by state, then city, then hospital within the city; Rankings are sorted by rate in descending order and exclude hospitals with less than 25 cases; (1) The number of cases is too small (n<25) for purposes of reliably predicting hospital performance; (2) Measure reflects the hospital's indication that its submission was based upon a sample of its relevant discharges; (3) Rate reflects fewer than the maximum possible quarters of data for the measure; (4) Inaccurate information submitted and suppressed for one or more quarters; (5) No data is available from the hospital for this measure; Please refer to the User's Guide for a full explanation of data

Beta Blocker at Arrival[1]	13	100%	93%	87%	100%
Beta Blocker at Discharge[1]	10	100%	93%	90%	100%
Fibrinolytic Medication Timing[1]	2	50%	31%	31%	100%
PCI Within 90 Minutes of Arrival	0	-	69%	54%	95%
Smoking Cessation Advice[1]	3	100%	91%	88%	100%
Heart Failure Care					
ACE Inhibitor or ARB for LVSD[1]	10	90%	84%	82%	100%
Discharge Instructions	28	82%	53%	61%	93%
Evaluation of LVS Function	33	97%	81%	83%	99%
Smoking Cessation Advice[1]	7	100%	79%	82%	100%
Pneumonia Care					
Appropriate Initial Antibiotic	40	68%	85%	83%	94%
Blood Culture Timing	34	97%	91%	90%	100%
Influenza Vaccine[1]	12	58%	70%	70%	100%
Initial Antibiotic Timing	41	68%	83%	80%	93%
Oxygenation Assessment	55	100%	100%	99%	100%
Pneumococcal Vaccine	32	78%	72%	69%	94%
Smoking Cessation Advice[1]	9	89%	78%	80%	100%
Surgical Infection Prevention					
Prophylactic Antibiotic Given[2]	208	93%	83%	77%	95%
Prophylactic Antibiotic Selection[2]	51	88%	92%	90%	100%
Prophylactic Antibiotic Stopped[2]	206	86%	70%	72%	95%
Pregnancy Care					
Inpatient Neonatal Mortality	-	-	-	-	-
Third or Fourth Degree Laceration	-	-	4.02%	3.63%	3.27%

Community Hospital

2021 N 12th Street
Grand Junction, CO 81501

Toll-Free: 800-621-0926
Phone: 970-242-0920
Fax: 970-256-6510

E-mail: bjessen@gjhosp.org
URL: www.gjhosp.org
Ownership: Voluntary non-profit - Private
Emergency Services: Yes
Accredited: Yes
Licensed Beds: 78

Key Personnel:

CEO. . . . . Mark Francis
Chief of Medical Staff. . . . . Mann Mariekjosa
Director Radiology . . . . Cheryl Heuschkel
Director Respiratory Therapy . . . . Steve Crow

Measure	Cases	This Hospital	State Average	U.S. Average	Top Hospital
Heart Attack Care					
ACE Inhibitor or ARB for LVSD[1]	1	100%	91%	82%	100%
Aspirin at Arrival[1]	13	85%	95%	92%	100%
Aspirin at Discharge[1]	7	100%	97%	90%	100%
Beta Blocker at Arrival[1]	11	91%	93%	87%	100%
Beta Blocker at Discharge[1]	7	86%	93%	90%	100%
Fibrinolytic Medication Timing	0	-	31%	31%	100%
PCI Within 90 Minutes of Arrival	0	-	69%	54%	95%
Smoking Cessation Advice[1]	2	50%	91%	88%	100%
Heart Failure Care					
ACE Inhibitor or ARB for LVSD[1]	9	89%	84%	82%	100%
Discharge Instructions	34	82%	53%	61%	93%
Evaluation of LVS Function	48	81%	81%	83%	99%
Smoking Cessation Advice[1]	8	88%	79%	82%	100%
Pneumonia Care					
Appropriate Initial Antibiotic	39	90%	85%	83%	94%
Blood Culture Timing	31	84%	91%	90%	100%
Influenza Vaccine[1]	13	92%	70%	70%	100%
Initial Antibiotic Timing	48	79%	83%	80%	93%
Oxygenation Assessment	55	100%	100%	99%	100%
Pneumococcal Vaccine	36	92%	72%	69%	94%
Smoking Cessation Advice[1]	14	86%	78%	80%	100%
Surgical Infection Prevention					
Prophylactic Antibiotic Given[3]	134	87%	83%	77%	95%
Prophylactic Antibiotic Selection	46	91%	92%	90%	100%
Prophylactic Antibiotic Stopped[3]	133	77%	70%	72%	95%
Pregnancy Care					
Inpatient Neonatal Mortality	-	-	-	-	-
Third or Fourth Degree Laceration	-	-	4.02%	3.63%	3.27%

Saint Mary's Hospital & Medical Center

Alternate Name: Hilltop Rehabilitation Hospital
2635 N 7th Street
PO Box 1628
Grand Junction, CO 81502
URL: www.stmarygj.com
Ownership: Voluntary non-profit - Church
Emergency Services: Yes

Toll-Free: 800-458-3888
Phone: 970-244-2273
Fax: 970-244-7510
Accredited: Yes
Licensed Beds: 346

Key Personnel:

CEO. . . . . Robert Landanburger
Chief Medical Staff. . . . . Robert Halpenny, MD
Chief Catheterization Laboratory . . . . Doug Jones
Emergency Room . . . . Roy Cromer, MD
Director Infection/Disease Control . . . . William Cobb, MD
Director Medical/Surgical Nursing . . . . Vickie Batson, RN
Chief Radiology . . . . Richard Fulton, MD
Director Respiratory Therapy . . . . Jane Wild

Measure	Cases	This Hospital	State Average	U.S. Average	Top Hospital
Heart Attack Care					
ACE Inhibitor or ARB for LVSD	67	91%	91%	82%	100%
Aspirin at Arrival	167	98%	95%	92%	100%
Aspirin at Discharge	305	100%	97%	90%	100%
Beta Blocker at Arrival	104	97%	93%	87%	100%
Beta Blocker at Discharge	293	99%	93%	90%	100%
Fibrinolytic Medication Timing[1]	1	0%	31%	31%	100%
PCI Within 90 Minutes of Arrival[1]	8	62%	69%	54%	95%
Smoking Cessation Advice	107	100%	91%	88%	100%
Heart Failure Care					
ACE Inhibitor or ARB for LVSD	74	85%	84%	82%	100%
Discharge Instructions	155	54%	53%	61%	93%
Evaluation of LVS Function	189	97%	81%	83%	99%
Smoking Cessation Advice	35	89%	79%	82%	100%
Pneumonia Care					
Appropriate Initial Antibiotic	158	92%	85%	83%	94%
Blood Culture Timing	132	93%	91%	90%	100%
Influenza Vaccine	38	84%	70%	70%	100%
Initial Antibiotic Timing	201	92%	83%	80%	93%
Oxygenation Assessment	258	100%	100%	99%	100%
Pneumococcal Vaccine	160	85%	72%	69%	94%
Smoking Cessation Advice	63	98%	78%	80%	100%
Surgical Infection Prevention					
Prophylactic Antibiotic Given	1,047	96%	83%	77%	95%
Prophylactic Antibiotic Selection	235	94%	92%	90%	100%
Prophylactic Antibiotic Stopped	1,005	92%	70%	72%	95%
Pregnancy Care					
Inpatient Neonatal Mortality	2,338	0.38%	-	-	-
Third or Fourth Degree Laceration	1,676	1.97%	4.02%	3.63%	3.27%

North Colorado Medical Center

1801 16th Street
Greeley, CO 80631
URL: www.bannerhealth.com
Ownership: Voluntary non-profit - Private
Emergency Services: Yes

Phone: 970-352-4121
Fax: 970-350-6114
Accredited: No
Licensed Beds: 326

Key Personnel:

CEO. . . . . John Sewell
Head of Emergency Room. . . . . April Asdury
Director of Pulmonary . . . . Ed Amend

Measure	Cases	This Hospital	State Average	U.S. Average	Top Hospital
Heart Attack Care					
ACE Inhibitor or ARB for LVSD[2]	46	96%	91%	82%	100%
Aspirin at Arrival[2]	157	98%	95%	92%	100%
Aspirin at Discharge[2]	216	99%	97%	90%	100%
Beta Blocker at Arrival[2]	129	96%	93%	87%	100%
Beta Blocker at Discharge[2]	208	98%	93%	90%	100%
Fibrinolytic Medication Timing[2]	0	-	31%	31%	100%
PCI Within 90 Minutes of Arrival[1,2]	12	75%	69%	54%	95%
Smoking Cessation Advice[2]	56	98%	91%	88%	100%
Heart Failure Care					
ACE Inhibitor or ARB for LVSD[2]	109	95%	84%	82%	100%
Discharge Instructions[2]	211	59%	53%	61%	93%

NOTE: Hospital profiles are in alphabetical order by state, then city, then hospital within the city; Rankings are sorted by rate in descending order and exclude hospitals with less than 25 cases; (1) The number of cases is too small (n<25) for purposes of reliably predicting hospital performance; (2) Measure reflects the hospital's indication that its submission was based upon a sample of its relevant discharges; (3) Rate reflects fewer than the maximum possible quarters of data for the measure; (4) Inaccurate information submitted and suppressed for one or more quarters; (5) No data is available from the hospital for this measure; Please refer to the User's Guide for a full explanation of data

Measure	Cases	This Hospital	State Average	U.S. Average	Top Hospital
Evaluation of LVS Function[2]	266	89%	81%	83%	99%
Smoking Cessation Advice[2]	47	91%	79%	82%	100%
Pneumonia Care					
Appropriate Initial Antibiotic[2]	134	88%	85%	83%	94%
Blood Culture Timing[2]	89	91%	91%	90%	100%
Influenza Vaccine[2]	31	71%	70%	70%	100%
Initial Antibiotic Timing[2]	198	73%	83%	80%	93%
Oxygenation Assessment[2]	215	100%	100%	99%	100%
Pneumococcal Vaccine[2]	141	74%	72%	69%	94%
Smoking Cessation Advice[2]	51	78%	78%	80%	100%
Surgical Infection Prevention					
Prophylactic Antibiotic Given[3]	125	62%	83%	77%	95%
Prophylactic Antibiotic Selection	117	91%	92%	90%	100%
Prophylactic Antibiotic Stopped[3]	115	42%	70%	72%	95%
Pregnancy Care					
Inpatient Neonatal Mortality	-	-	-	-	-
Third or Fourth Degree Laceration	-	-	4.02%	3.63%	3.27%

Gunnison Valley Hospital

711 N Taylor Street
PO Box 759
Gunnison, CO 81230
URL: www.gvh-colorado.org
Phone: 970-641-1456
Fax: 970-641-4461
Ownership: Government - Local
Emergency Services: Yes
Accredited: No
Licensed Beds: 21

Key Personnel:

CEO. . . . . Randy Phelps
Chief Medical Staff. . . . . John Tarr, MD
Emergency Room . . . . Kirstie Pike, RN
Medical Surgical Nursing . . . . Barb Hammond, RN
Respiratory/Cardiopulmonary. . . . . Chris Anastacio

Measure	Cases	This Hospital	State Average	U.S. Average	Top Hospital
Heart Attack Care					
ACE Inhibitor or ARB for LVSD[3]	0	-	91%	82%	100%
Aspirin at Arrival[1,3]	1	100%	95%	92%	100%
Aspirin at Discharge[1,3]	1	100%	97%	90%	100%
Beta Blocker at Arrival[3]	0	-	93%	87%	100%
Beta Blocker at Discharge[3]	0	-	93%	90%	100%
Fibrinolytic Medication Timing[3]	0	-	31%	31%	100%
PCI Within 90 Minutes of Arrival[5]	-	-	69%	54%	95%
Smoking Cessation Advice[3]	0	-	91%	88%	100%
Heart Failure Care					
ACE Inhibitor or ARB for LVSD[1,3]	1	100%	84%	82%	100%
Discharge Instructions[1,3]	11	0%	53%	61%	93%
Evaluation of LVS Function[1,3]	12	25%	81%	83%	99%
Smoking Cessation Advice[1,3]	1	0%	79%	82%	100%
Pneumonia Care					
Appropriate Initial Antibiotic[1]	16	44%	85%	83%	94%
Blood Culture Timing[1]	2	100%	91%	90%	100%
Influenza Vaccine[1]	1	100%	70%	70%	100%
Initial Antibiotic Timing[1]	14	79%	83%	80%	93%
Oxygenation Assessment[1]	19	95%	100%	99%	100%
Pneumococcal Vaccine[1]	10	70%	72%	69%	94%
Smoking Cessation Advice[1]	3	67%	78%	80%	100%
Surgical Infection Prevention					
Prophylactic Antibiotic Given[1]	21	71%	83%	77%	95%
Prophylactic Antibiotic Selection[1]	4	100%	92%	90%	100%
Prophylactic Antibiotic Stopped[1]	21	90%	70%	72%	95%
Pregnancy Care					
Inpatient Neonatal Mortality	-	-	-	-	-
Third or Fourth Degree Laceration	-	-	4.02%	3.63%	3.27%

Melissa Memorial Hospital

505 S Baxter Avenue
Holyoke, CO 80734
E-mail: arlene.harms@bannerhealth.com
URL: www.melissamemorial.org
Phone: 970-854-2241
Fax: 970-854-3821
Ownership: Govt - Hospital District or Authority
Emergency Services: Yes
Accredited: No
Licensed Beds: 25

Key Personnel:

CEO. . . . . Arlene Harms
Chief Medical Staff. . . . . Dennis Jelden, MD
Infection Control. . . . . Marla Smith

Measure	Cases	This Hospital	State Average	U.S. Average	Top Hospital
Heart Attack Care					
ACE Inhibitor or ARB for LVSD[3]	0	-	91%	82%	100%
Aspirin at Arrival[3]	0	-	95%	92%	100%
Aspirin at Discharge[1,3]	1	100%	97%	90%	100%
Beta Blocker at Arrival[3]	0	-	93%	87%	100%
Beta Blocker at Discharge[3]	0	-	93%	90%	100%
Fibrinolytic Medication Timing[3]	0	-	31%	31%	100%
PCI Within 90 Minutes of Arrival[5]	-	-	69%	54%	95%
Smoking Cessation Advice[3]	0	-	91%	88%	100%
Heart Failure Care					
ACE Inhibitor or ARB for LVSD[1,2]	1	100%	84%	82%	100%
Discharge Instructions[1,2]	8	62%	53%	61%	93%
Evaluation of LVS Function[1,2]	12	92%	81%	83%	99%
Smoking Cessation Advice[1,2]	1	100%	79%	82%	100%
Pneumonia Care					
Appropriate Initial Antibiotic[1,3]	5	100%	85%	83%	94%
Blood Culture Timing[1,3]	2	50%	91%	90%	100%
Influenza Vaccine[1]	2	100%	70%	70%	100%
Initial Antibiotic Timing[1,3]	5	100%	83%	80%	93%
Oxygenation Assessment[1,3]	9	100%	100%	99%	100%
Pneumococcal Vaccine[1,3]	6	67%	72%	69%	94%
Smoking Cessation Advice[3]	0	-	78%	80%	100%
Surgical Infection Prevention					
Prophylactic Antibiotic Given[5]	-	-	83%	77%	95%
Prophylactic Antibiotic Selection[5]	-	-	92%	90%	100%
Prophylactic Antibiotic Stopped[5]	-	-	70%	72%	95%
Pregnancy Care					
Inpatient Neonatal Mortality	-	-	-	-	-
Third or Fourth Degree Laceration	-	-	4.02%	3.63%	3.27%

Arkansas Valley Regional Medical Center

1100 Carson Avenue
La Junta, CO 81050
URL: www.avrmc.org
Phone: 719-384-5412
Fax: 719-383-6005
Ownership: Voluntary non-profit - Private
Emergency Services: Yes
Accredited: Yes
Licensed Beds: 203

Key Personnel:

Administrator/CEO. . . . . Lynn Crowell
Chief Medical Staff. . . . . Brad Bruckermd
Director Surgical Services . . . . Tonya Kersey
Emergency Room . . . . Bryan Hynes
Director Medical/Surgical Nursing . . . . Barbara Westbrook
OB/GYN Women's Health . . . . Sheila Clodfelter
Director Surgical Services . . . . Sandra Price
Director of Pulmonary . . . . Ronald Reodicamd

Measure	Cases	This Hospital	State Average	U.S. Average	Top Hospital
Heart Attack Care					
ACE Inhibitor or ARB for LVSD	0	-	91%	82%	100%
Aspirin at Arrival[1]	14	100%	95%	92%	100%
Aspirin at Discharge[1]	3	100%	97%	90%	100%
Beta Blocker at Arrival[1]	17	82%	93%	87%	100%
Beta Blocker at Discharge[1]	7	71%	93%	90%	100%
Fibrinolytic Medication Timing[1]	3	33%	31%	31%	100%
PCI Within 90 Minutes of Arrival	0	-	69%	54%	95%
Smoking Cessation Advice[1]	1	100%	91%	88%	100%
Heart Failure Care					
ACE Inhibitor or ARB for LVSD[1]	14	86%	84%	82%	100%
Discharge Instructions	51	49%	53%	61%	93%
Evaluation of LVS Function	70	69%	81%	83%	99%
Smoking Cessation Advice[1]	11	64%	79%	82%	100%
Pneumonia Care					
Appropriate Initial Antibiotic	117	86%	85%	83%	94%
Blood Culture Timing	74	92%	91%	90%	100%
Influenza Vaccine	44	64%	70%	70%	100%
Initial Antibiotic Timing	146	84%	83%	80%	93%
Oxygenation Assessment	175	99%	100%	99%	100%
Pneumococcal Vaccine	116	69%	72%	69%	94%
Smoking Cessation Advice	37	86%	78%	80%	100%

NOTE: Hospital profiles are in alphabetical order by state, then city, then hospital within the city; Rankings are sorted by rate in descending order and exclude hospitals with less than 25 cases; (1) The number of cases is too small (n<25) for purposes of reliably predicting hospital performance; (2) Measure reflects the hospital's indication that its submission was based upon a sample of its relevant discharges; (3) Rate reflects fewer than the maximum possible quarters of data for the measure; (4) Inaccurate information submitted and suppressed for one or more quarters; (5) No data is available from the hospital for this measure; Please refer to the User's Guide for a full explanation of data

Measure	Cases	This Hospital	State Average	U.S. Average	Top Hospital
Surgical Infection Prevention					
Prophylactic Antibiotic Given[1]	13	62%	83%	77%	95%
Prophylactic Antibiotic Selection[1]	3	67%	92%	90%	100%
Prophylactic Antibiotic Stopped[1]	11	91%	70%	72%	95%
Pregnancy Care					
Inpatient Neonatal Mortality	-	-	-	-	-
Third or Fourth Degree Laceration	-	-	4.02%	3.63%	3.27%

Exempla Good Samaritan Medical Center

200 Exempla Circle
Lafayette, CO 80026
Phone: 303-689-4000
Ownership: Voluntary non-profit - Private
Accredited: Yes
Emergency Services: Yes

Measure	Cases	This Hospital	State Average	U.S. Average	Top Hospital
Heart Attack Care					
ACE Inhibitor or ARB for LVSD[1]	22	95%	91%	82%	100%
Aspirin at Arrival	126	98%	95%	92%	100%
Aspirin at Discharge	110	97%	97%	90%	100%
Beta Blocker at Arrival	95	98%	93%	87%	100%
Beta Blocker at Discharge	133	98%	93%	90%	100%
Fibrinolytic Medication Timing	0	-	31%	31%	100%
PCI Within 90 Minutes of Arrival[1]	8	88%	69%	54%	95%
Smoking Cessation Advice	38	97%	91%	88%	100%
Heart Failure Care					
ACE Inhibitor or ARB for LVSD[2]	62	76%	84%	82%	100%
Discharge Instructions[2]	201	87%	53%	61%	93%
Evaluation of LVS Function[2]	232	94%	81%	83%	99%
Smoking Cessation Advice[2]	33	91%	79%	82%	100%
Pneumonia Care					
Appropriate Initial Antibiotic[2]	101	88%	85%	83%	94%
Blood Culture Timing[2]	75	85%	91%	90%	100%
Influenza Vaccine[1,2]	21	81%	70%	70%	100%
Initial Antibiotic Timing[2]	109	70%	83%	80%	93%
Oxygenation Assessment[2]	148	100%	100%	99%	100%
Pneumococcal Vaccine[2]	109	83%	72%	69%	94%
Smoking Cessation Advice[2]	36	83%	78%	80%	100%
Surgical Infection Prevention					
Prophylactic Antibiotic Given[2]	171	94%	83%	77%	95%
Prophylactic Antibiotic Selection[2]	42	95%	92%	90%	100%
Prophylactic Antibiotic Stopped[2]	168	59%	70%	72%	95%
Pregnancy Care					
Inpatient Neonatal Mortality	-	-	-	-	-
Third or Fourth Degree Laceration	-	-	4.02%	3.63%	3.27%

Prowers Medical Center

401 Kendall Drive
Lamar, CO 81052
Phone: 719-336-4343
Fax: 719-336-3805
E-mail: shawnah@lpmc.org
URL: www.prowersmedical.com
Ownership: Govt - Hospital District or Authority
Accredited: No
Emergency Services: Yes
Licensed Beds: 28

Key Personnel:

CEO . . . . Greg G Gerard
Chief Medical Staff . . . . Sam Downing
Emergency Room . . . . Marge Campbell, RN
Emergency Room . . . . John Abbott, DO
Infection Control . . . . Martha Thompson
ICU . . . . Nikki Hamilton
Medical/Surgical Nursing . . . . Nikki Hamilton
Respiratory/Cardiopulmonary . . . . George Chambers

Measure	Cases	This Hospital	State Average	U.S. Average	Top Hospital
Heart Attack Care					
ACE Inhibitor or ARB for LVSD[3]	0	-	91%	82%	100%
Aspirin at Arrival[3]	0	-	95%	92%	100%
Aspirin at Discharge[3]	0	-	97%	90%	100%
Beta Blocker at Arrival[3]	0	-	93%	87%	100%
Beta Blocker at Discharge[3]	0	-	93%	90%	100%
Fibrinolytic Medication Timing[3]	0	-	31%	31%	100%
PCI Within 90 Minutes of Arrival[5]	-	-	69%	54%	95%
Smoking Cessation Advice[3]	0	-	91%	88%	100%
Heart Failure Care					
ACE Inhibitor or ARB for LVSD[1,3]	2	50%	84%	82%	100%
Discharge Instructions[3]	25	0%	53%	61%	93%
Evaluation of LVS Function[3]	28	50%	81%	83%	99%
Smoking Cessation Advice[3]	0	-	79%	82%	100%
Pneumonia Care					
Appropriate Initial Antibiotic[3]	45	73%	85%	83%	94%
Blood Culture Timing[3]	27	100%	91%	90%	100%
Influenza Vaccine[1]	12	0%	70%	70%	100%
Initial Antibiotic Timing[3]	47	55%	83%	80%	93%
Oxygenation Assessment[3]	62	100%	100%	99%	100%
Pneumococcal Vaccine[3]	41	10%	72%	69%	94%
Smoking Cessation Advice[1,3]	14	7%	78%	80%	100%
Surgical Infection Prevention					
Prophylactic Antibiotic Given[5]	-	-	83%	77%	95%
Prophylactic Antibiotic Selection[5]	-	-	92%	90%	100%
Prophylactic Antibiotic Stopped[5]	-	-	70%	72%	95%
Pregnancy Care					
Inpatient Neonatal Mortality	-	-	-	-	-
Third or Fourth Degree Laceration	-	-	4.02%	3.63%	3.27%

Saint Vincent General Hospital

822 W 4th Street
Leadville, CO 80461
Phone: 719-486-0230
Fax: 719-486-1077
E-mail: info@svghd.org
URL: www.svghd.org
Ownership: Govt - Hospital District or Authority
Accredited: No
Emergency Services: Yes
Licensed Beds: 25

Key Personnel:

President . . . . Charleen Smith
CEO . . . . Joan Fretz, RN, DON
Chief Staff . . . . Lisa Zwerdlinger, MD
Emergency Room . . . . Jone Fretz
Education/Infection Control . . . . Sarah Martin
Medical Surgical Nursing . . . . Bettyann Hazell, DON/COO
Chief Radiology . . . . Susan Kissell
Director Respiratory Therapy . . . . Michael Blackford

Measure	Cases	This Hospital	State Average	U.S. Average	Top Hospital
Heart Attack Care					
ACE Inhibitor or ARB for LVSD[5]	-	-	91%	82%	100%
Aspirin at Arrival[5]	-	-	95%	92%	100%
Aspirin at Discharge[5]	-	-	97%	90%	100%
Beta Blocker at Arrival[5]	-	-	93%	87%	100%
Beta Blocker at Discharge[5]	-	-	93%	90%	100%
Fibrinolytic Medication Timing[5]	-	-	31%	31%	100%
PCI Within 90 Minutes of Arrival[5]	-	-	69%	54%	95%
Smoking Cessation Advice[5]	-	-	91%	88%	100%
Heart Failure Care					
ACE Inhibitor or ARB for LVSD[5]	-	-	84%	82%	100%
Discharge Instructions[5]	-	-	53%	61%	93%
Evaluation of LVS Function[5]	-	-	81%	83%	99%
Smoking Cessation Advice[5]	-	-	79%	82%	100%
Pneumonia Care					
Appropriate Initial Antibiotic[5]	-	-	85%	83%	94%
Blood Culture Timing[5]	-	-	91%	90%	100%
Influenza Vaccine[5]	-	-	70%	70%	100%
Initial Antibiotic Timing[5]	-	-	83%	80%	93%
Oxygenation Assessment[5]	-	-	100%	99%	100%
Pneumococcal Vaccine[5]	-	-	72%	69%	94%
Smoking Cessation Advice[5]	-	-	78%	80%	100%
Surgical Infection Prevention					
Prophylactic Antibiotic Given[5]	-	-	83%	77%	95%
Prophylactic Antibiotic Selection[5]	-	-	92%	90%	100%
Prophylactic Antibiotic Stopped[5]	-	-	70%	72%	95%
Pregnancy Care					
Inpatient Neonatal Mortality	-	-	-	-	-
Third or Fourth Degree Laceration	-	-	4.02%	3.63%	3.27%

NOTE: Hospital profiles are in alphabetical order by state, then city, then hospital within the city; Rankings are sorted by rate in descending order and exclude hospitals with less than 25 cases; (1) The number of cases is too small (n<25) for purposes of reliably predicting hospital performance; (2) Measure reflects the hospital's indication that its submission was based upon a sample of its relevant discharges; (3) Rate reflects fewer than the maximum possible quarters of data for the measure; (4) Inaccurate information submitted and suppressed for one or more quarters; (5) No data is available from the hospital for this measure; Please refer to the User's Guide for a full explanation of data

Littleton Adventist Hospital

7700 South Broadway
Littleton, CO 80122
URL: www.centura.org
Ownership: Voluntary non-profit - Church
Emergency Services: Yes
Phone: 303-730-8900
Fax: 303-738-2688
Accredited: Yes
Licensed Beds: 134

Key Personnel:

President/CEO . . . . David Crane
Chief Cardiology . . . . J Kern Buckner
Emergency Department . . . . Stephen C Altmin
Chief Pulmonary Therapy . . . . David R Ladd

Measure	Cases	This Hospital	State Average	U.S. Average	Top Hospital
Heart Attack Care					
ACE Inhibitor or ARB for LVSD[1,2]	10	80%	91%	82%	100%
Aspirin at Arrival[2]	106	100%	95%	92%	100%
Aspirin at Discharge[2]	75	97%	97%	90%	100%
Beta Blocker at Arrival[2]	77	99%	93%	87%	100%
Beta Blocker at Discharge[2]	92	98%	93%	90%	100%
Fibrinolytic Medication Timing[2]	0	-	31%	31%	100%
PCI Within 90 Minutes of Arrival[1,2]	14	93%	69%	54%	95%
Smoking Cessation Advice[1,2]	20	80%	91%	88%	100%
Heart Failure Care					
ACE Inhibitor or ARB for LVSD[2]	38	79%	84%	82%	100%
Discharge Instructions[2]	73	70%	53%	61%	93%
Evaluation of LVS Function[2]	108	92%	81%	83%	99%
Smoking Cessation Advice[1,2]	18	83%	79%	82%	100%
Pneumonia Care					
Appropriate Initial Antibiotic[2]	163	88%	85%	83%	94%
Blood Culture Timing[2]	167	92%	91%	90%	100%
Influenza Vaccine[2]	51	35%	70%	70%	100%
Initial Antibiotic Timing[2]	202	89%	83%	80%	93%
Oxygenation Assessment[2]	255	100%	100%	99%	100%
Pneumococcal Vaccine[2]	167	82%	72%	69%	94%
Smoking Cessation Advice[2]	32	91%	78%	80%	100%
Surgical Infection Prevention					
Prophylactic Antibiotic Given[2,3]	325	81%	83%	77%	95%
Prophylactic Antibiotic Selection[2]	131	89%	92%	90%	100%
Prophylactic Antibiotic Stopped[2,3]	312	84%	70%	72%	95%
Pregnancy Care					
Inpatient Neonatal Mortality[2]	1,737	0.46%	-	-	-
Third or Fourth Degree Laceration[2]	1,266	4.27%	4.02%	3.63%	3.27%

Sky Ridge Medical Center

10101 Ridge Gate Parkway
Lone Tree, CO 80124
URL: www.skyridgemedicalcenter.com
Ownership: Proprietary
Emergency Services: Yes
Phone: 720-225-1000
Fax: 720-225-1029
Accredited: Yes
Licensed Beds: 138

Key Personnel:

CEO . . . . Maureen Tarrant
President Medical Staff . . . . Stephen M Heinz, MD

Measure	Cases	This Hospital	State Average	U.S. Average	Top Hospital
Heart Attack Care					
ACE Inhibitor or ARB for LVSD[1]	10	90%	91%	82%	100%
Aspirin at Arrival	63	100%	95%	92%	100%
Aspirin at Discharge	54	100%	97%	90%	100%
Beta Blocker at Arrival	41	95%	93%	87%	100%
Beta Blocker at Discharge	61	98%	93%	90%	100%
Fibrinolytic Medication Timing	0	-	31%	31%	100%
PCI Within 90 Minutes of Arrival[1]	8	88%	69%	54%	95%
Smoking Cessation Advice[1]	21	95%	91%	88%	100%
Heart Failure Care					
ACE Inhibitor or ARB for LVSD	29	79%	84%	82%	100%
Discharge Instructions	70	29%	53%	61%	93%
Evaluation of LVS Function	92	98%	81%	83%	99%
Smoking Cessation Advice[1]	8	75%	79%	82%	100%
Pneumonia Care					
Appropriate Initial Antibiotic	78	83%	85%	83%	94%
Blood Culture Timing	60	85%	91%	90%	100%
Influenza Vaccine[1]	14	57%	70%	70%	100%
Initial Antibiotic Timing	93	86%	83%	80%	93%
Oxygenation Assessment	115	100%	100%	99%	100%
Pneumococcal Vaccine	52	67%	72%	69%	94%
Smoking Cessation Advice	26	100%	78%	80%	100%
Surgical Infection Prevention					
Prophylactic Antibiotic Given[2,3]	176	85%	83%	77%	95%
Prophylactic Antibiotic Selection[2]	74	92%	92%	90%	100%
Prophylactic Antibiotic Stopped[2,3]	174	70%	70%	72%	95%
Pregnancy Care					
Inpatient Neonatal Mortality	3,024	0.07%	-	-	-
Third or Fourth Degree Laceration	2,105	5.70%	4.02%	3.63%	3.27%

Longmont United Hospital

1950 W Mountain View Avenue
Longmont, CO 80501
Ownership: Voluntary non-profit - Other
Emergency Services: Yes
Phone: 303-651-5111
Fax: 303-678-4050
Accredited: Yes
Licensed Beds: 143

Key Personnel:

CEO . . . . Ken Huey
Manager Cardio-Pulmonary Services . . . . Jenifer Manuel

Measure	Cases	This Hospital	State Average	U.S. Average	Top Hospital
Heart Attack Care					
ACE Inhibitor or ARB for LVSD[1]	10	70%	91%	82%	100%
Aspirin at Arrival	78	95%	95%	92%	100%
Aspirin at Discharge	64	97%	97%	90%	100%
Beta Blocker at Arrival	62	85%	93%	87%	100%
Beta Blocker at Discharge	78	95%	93%	90%	100%
Fibrinolytic Medication Timing	0	-	31%	31%	100%
PCI Within 90 Minutes of Arrival[1]	7	57%	69%	54%	95%
Smoking Cessation Advice	28	96%	91%	88%	100%
Heart Failure Care					
ACE Inhibitor or ARB for LVSD	62	69%	84%	82%	100%
Discharge Instructions	122	35%	53%	61%	93%
Evaluation of LVS Function	182	86%	81%	83%	99%
Smoking Cessation Advice[1]	11	91%	79%	82%	100%
Pneumonia Care					
Appropriate Initial Antibiotic	90	83%	85%	83%	94%
Blood Culture Timing	46	93%	91%	90%	100%
Influenza Vaccine	27	78%	70%	70%	100%
Initial Antibiotic Timing	127	87%	83%	80%	93%
Oxygenation Assessment	143	100%	100%	99%	100%
Pneumococcal Vaccine	86	74%	72%	69%	94%
Smoking Cessation Advice	28	89%	78%	80%	100%
Surgical Infection Prevention					
Prophylactic Antibiotic Given[2,3]	352	75%	83%	77%	95%
Prophylactic Antibiotic Selection[2]	116	97%	92%	90%	100%
Prophylactic Antibiotic Stopped[2,3]	330	59%	70%	72%	95%
Pregnancy Care					
Inpatient Neonatal Mortality	1,505	0.13%	-	-	-
Third or Fourth Degree Laceration	1,113	3.77%	4.02%	3.63%	3.27%

Avista Adventist Hospital

100 Health Park Drive
Louisville, CO 80027
URL: www.avistaadventist.org
Ownership: Voluntary non-profit - Church
Emergency Services: Yes
Phone: 303-673-1000
Fax: 303-673-1283
Accredited: Yes
Licensed Beds: 99

Key Personnel:

CEO . . . . John Sackett

Measure	Cases	This Hospital	State Average	U.S. Average	Top Hospital
Heart Attack Care					
ACE Inhibitor or ARB for LVSD[1,2]	6	100%	91%	82%	100%
Aspirin at Arrival[2]	26	100%	95%	92%	100%
Aspirin at Discharge[1,2]	23	96%	97%	90%	100%
Beta Blocker at Arrival[1,2]	21	95%	93%	87%	100%
Beta Blocker at Discharge[1,2]	22	86%	93%	90%	100%
Fibrinolytic Medication Timing[2]	0	-	31%	31%	100%
PCI Within 90 Minutes of Arrival[1,2]	2	0%	69%	54%	95%
Smoking Cessation Advice[1,2]	4	100%	91%	88%	100%
Heart Failure Care					

NOTE: Hospital profiles are in alphabetical order by state, then city, then hospital within the city; Rankings are sorted by rate in descending order and exclude hospitals with less than 25 cases; (1) The number of cases is too small (n<25) for purposes of reliably predicting hospital performance; (2) Measure reflects the hospital's indication that its submission was based upon a sample of its relevant discharges; (3) Rate reflects fewer than the maximum possible quarters of data for the measure; (4) Inaccurate information submitted and suppressed for one or more quarters; (5) No data is available from the hospital for this measure; Please refer to the User's Guide for a full explanation of data

ACE Inhibitor or ARB for LVSD[1,2]	7	43%	84%	82%	100%
Discharge Instructions[1,2]	23	26%	53%	61%	93%
Evaluation of LVS Function[2]	26	77%	81%	83%	99%
Smoking Cessation Advice[1,2]	2	50%	79%	82%	100%
Pneumonia Care					
Appropriate Initial Antibiotic[2]	58	81%	85%	83%	94%
Blood Culture Timing[2]	45	91%	91%	90%	100%
Influenza Vaccine[1,2]	20	70%	70%	70%	100%
Initial Antibiotic Timing[2]	66	88%	83%	80%	93%
Oxygenation Assessment[2]	88	100%	100%	99%	100%
Pneumococcal Vaccine[2]	48	75%	72%	69%	94%
Smoking Cessation Advice[1,2]	19	79%	78%	80%	100%
Surgical Infection Prevention					
Prophylactic Antibiotic Given[2,3]	158	85%	83%	77%	95%
Prophylactic Antibiotic Selection[2]	48	100%	92%	90%	100%
Prophylactic Antibiotic Stopped[2,3]	155	88%	70%	72%	95%
Pregnancy Care					
Inpatient Neonatal Mortality[2]	2,645	0.00%	-	-	-
Third or Fourth Degree Laceration[2]	2,003	4.84%	4.02%	3.63%	3.27%

McKee Medical Center

Alternate Name: Banner Health McKee Medical Center
2000 Boise Avenue — Phone: 970-669-4640
Loveland, CO 80538 — Fax: 970-635-4066
URL: www.bannerhealth.com
Ownership: Voluntary non-profit - Private — Accredited: Yes
Emergency Services: Yes — Licensed Beds: 132

Key Personnel:

CEO. . . . . Richard O Sutton
Associate Administrator . . . . Marilyn Schock
Emergency Room Director. . . . . Jayne Brundage
Emergency Room . . . . Teri Huffman
Infection Control Director . . . . Joan Strauch
Medical/Surgical Nursing Director . . . . . Donlyn Foster
Director OB/GYN . . . . Glenda Skaggs
Director Radiology . . . . Cherlene Goodle
Respiratory Director . . . . Charlie Schneider

Measure	Cases	This Hospital	State Average	U.S. Average	Top Hospital
Heart Attack Care					
ACE Inhibitor or ARB for LVSD[1]	14	93%	91%	82%	100%
Aspirin at Arrival	62	97%	95%	92%	100%
Aspirin at Discharge	46	100%	97%	90%	100%
Beta Blocker at Arrival	48	98%	93%	87%	100%
Beta Blocker at Discharge	48	98%	93%	90%	100%
Fibrinolytic Medication Timing	0	-	31%	31%	100%
PCI Within 90 Minutes of Arrival	0	-	69%	54%	95%
Smoking Cessation Advice[1]	10	90%	91%	88%	100%
Heart Failure Care					
ACE Inhibitor or ARB for LVSD	29	93%	84%	82%	100%
Discharge Instructions	63	87%	53%	61%	93%
Evaluation of LVS Function	90	96%	81%	83%	99%
Smoking Cessation Advice[1]	8	100%	79%	82%	100%
Pneumonia Care					
Appropriate Initial Antibiotic	88	91%	85%	83%	94%
Blood Culture Timing	68	97%	91%	90%	100%
Influenza Vaccine	32	91%	70%	70%	100%
Initial Antibiotic Timing	119	83%	83%	80%	93%
Oxygenation Assessment	142	100%	100%	99%	100%
Pneumococcal Vaccine	107	82%	72%	69%	94%
Smoking Cessation Advice	30	70%	78%	80%	100%
Surgical Infection Prevention					
Prophylactic Antibiotic Given[3]	45	93%	83%	77%	95%
Prophylactic Antibiotic Selection	45	42%	92%	90%	100%
Prophylactic Antibiotic Stopped[3]	44	52%	70%	72%	95%
Pregnancy Care					
Inpatient Neonatal Mortality	-	-	-	-	-
Third or Fourth Degree Laceration	-	-	4.02%	3.63%	3.27%

Pioneers Hospital of Rio Blanco County

Alternate Name: Pioneers Medical Center
345 Cleveland — Phone: 970-878-5047
Meeker, CO 81641 — Fax: 970-878-3285
E-mail: tmorgan@pioneershospital.com
URL: www.pioneershospital.org
Ownership: Government - Local — Accredited: No
Emergency Services: Yes — Licensed Beds: 15

Key Personnel:

CEO. . . . . Robert Omer
Chief Medical Staff. . . . . Victor Mihal, DO
Emergency Room . . . . Drew Varland
Infection Control. . . . . Amy May, RN
Director Medical/Surgical Nursing . . . . . Mary Jayne Kitchens
Director Radiology . . . . John Kapushion
Manager Respiratory Therapy . . . . Marnell Bradfield

Measure	Cases	This Hospital	State Average	U.S. Average	Top Hospital
Heart Attack Care					
ACE Inhibitor or ARB for LVSD[3]	0	-	91%	82%	100%
Aspirin at Arrival[1,3]	2	100%	95%	92%	100%
Aspirin at Discharge[1,3]	1	100%	97%	90%	100%
Beta Blocker at Arrival[1,3]	2	100%	93%	87%	100%
Beta Blocker at Discharge[1,3]	1	100%	93%	90%	100%
Fibrinolytic Medication Timing[3]	0	-	31%	31%	100%
PCI Within 90 Minutes of Arrival[5]	-	-	69%	54%	95%
Smoking Cessation Advice[3]	0	-	91%	88%	100%
Heart Failure Care					
ACE Inhibitor or ARB for LVSD[1]	2	0%	84%	82%	100%
Discharge Instructions[1]	12	0%	53%	61%	93%
Evaluation of LVS Function[1]	15	13%	81%	83%	99%
Smoking Cessation Advice[1]	4	25%	79%	82%	100%
Pneumonia Care					
Appropriate Initial Antibiotic[1]	16	75%	85%	83%	94%
Blood Culture Timing[1]	2	100%	91%	90%	100%
Influenza Vaccine[1]	4	0%	70%	70%	100%
Initial Antibiotic Timing[1]	19	89%	83%	80%	93%
Oxygenation Assessment[1]	20	100%	100%	99%	100%
Pneumococcal Vaccine[1]	16	6%	72%	69%	94%
Smoking Cessation Advice[1]	5	20%	78%	80%	100%
Surgical Infection Prevention					
Prophylactic Antibiotic Given[5]	-	-	83%	77%	95%
Prophylactic Antibiotic Selection[5]	-	-	92%	90%	100%
Prophylactic Antibiotic Stopped[5]	-	-	70%	72%	95%
Pregnancy Care					
Inpatient Neonatal Mortality	-	-	-	-	-
Third or Fourth Degree Laceration	-	-	4.02%	3.63%	3.27%

Montrose Memorial Hospital

800 South Third Street — Phone: 970-249-2211
Montrose, CO 81401 — Fax: 970-240-7350
URL: www.montrosehospital.com
Ownership: Government - Local — Accredited: Yes
Emergency Services: Yes — Licensed Beds: 75

Key Personnel:

CEO. . . . . Kenneth Platou
Chief Medical Staff. . . . . Michael Brezinsky, MD
Cardiac Lab . . . . Larry Peeters
Emergency Room . . . . Sharon Holbrook, RN
Infection Control. . . . . Bert Hatter, RN
ICU . . . . Jeri Rea
Director Medical/Surgical Nursing . . . . . Susan Smith, RN
OB/GYN Womens Health. . . . . Coral Ann Hackett, RN
Chief Radiology . . . . Paula Krull
Director Respiratory Therapy . . . . Duke Richardson

Measure	Cases	This Hospital	State Average	U.S. Average	Top Hospital
Heart Attack Care					
ACE Inhibitor or ARB for LVSD[1]	10	80%	91%	82%	100%
Aspirin at Arrival	33	100%	95%	92%	100%
Aspirin at Discharge	33	97%	97%	90%	100%
Beta Blocker at Arrival	28	100%	93%	87%	100%
Beta Blocker at Discharge	33	100%	93%	90%	100%
Fibrinolytic Medication Timing[1]	1	100%	31%	31%	100%
PCI Within 90 Minutes of Arrival[1]	3	33%	69%	54%	95%

NOTE: Hospital profiles are in alphabetical order by state, then city, then hospital within the city; Rankings are sorted by rate in descending order and exclude hospitals with less than 25 cases; (1) The number of cases is too small (n<25) for purposes of reliably predicting hospital performance; (2) Measure reflects the hospital's indication that its submission was based upon a sample of its relevant discharges; (3) Rate reflects fewer than the maximum possible quarters of data for the measure; (4) Inaccurate information submitted and suppressed for one or more quarters; (5) No data is available from the hospital for this measure; Please refer to the User's Guide for a full explanation of data

Smoking Cessation Advice[1]	11	91%	91%	88%	100%
Heart Failure Care					
ACE Inhibitor or ARB for LVSD[1]	19	84%	84%	82%	100%
Discharge Instructions	33	15%	53%	61%	93%
Evaluation of LVS Function	48	60%	81%	83%	99%
Smoking Cessation Advice[1]	10	40%	79%	82%	100%
Pneumonia Care					
Appropriate Initial Antibiotic	69	77%	85%	83%	94%
Blood Culture Timing	51	90%	91%	90%	100%
Influenza Vaccine[1]	15	40%	70%	70%	100%
Initial Antibiotic Timing	82	87%	83%	80%	93%
Oxygenation Assessment	96	100%	100%	99%	100%
Pneumococcal Vaccine	61	57%	72%	69%	94%
Smoking Cessation Advice[1]	17	65%	78%	80%	100%
Surgical Infection Prevention					
Prophylactic Antibiotic Given[2]	274	63%	83%	77%	95%
Prophylactic Antibiotic Selection[2]	63	89%	92%	90%	100%
Prophylactic Antibiotic Stopped[2]	265	57%	70%	72%	95%
Pregnancy Care					
Inpatient Neonatal Mortality	-	-	-	-	-
Third or Fourth Degree Laceration	-	-	4.02%	3.63%	3.27%

Parker Adventist Hospital

9395 Crown Crest Boulevard
Parker, CO 80138
URL: www.parkerhospital.org
Ownership: Voluntary non-profit - Church
Emergency Services: Yes
Phone: 303-269-4000
Fax: 303-269-4031
Accredited: Yes
Licensed Beds: 100

Key Personnel:
CEO. . . . . Ken Bacon

Measure	Cases	This Hospital	State Average	U.S. Average	Top Hospital
Heart Attack Care					
ACE Inhibitor or ARB for LVSD[1,2]	8	100%	91%	82%	100%
Aspirin at Arrival[2]	74	99%	95%	92%	100%
Aspirin at Discharge[2]	67	97%	97%	90%	100%
Beta Blocker at Arrival[2]	63	98%	93%	87%	100%
Beta Blocker at Discharge[2]	70	97%	93%	90%	100%
Fibrinolytic Medication Timing[2]	0	-	31%	31%	100%
PCI Within 90 Minutes of Arrival[1,2]	11	91%	69%	54%	95%
Smoking Cessation Advice[1,2]	20	90%	91%	88%	100%
Heart Failure Care					
ACE Inhibitor or ARB for LVSD[1,2]	14	93%	84%	82%	100%
Discharge Instructions[2]	51	41%	53%	61%	93%
Evaluation of LVS Function[2]	64	91%	81%	83%	99%
Smoking Cessation Advice[1,2]	7	86%	79%	82%	100%
Pneumonia Care					
Appropriate Initial Antibiotic[2]	79	94%	85%	83%	94%
Blood Culture Timing[2]	78	96%	91%	90%	100%
Influenza Vaccine[1,2]	24	88%	70%	70%	100%
Initial Antibiotic Timing[2]	89	87%	83%	80%	93%
Oxygenation Assessment[2]	109	100%	100%	99%	100%
Pneumococcal Vaccine[2]	63	75%	72%	69%	94%
Smoking Cessation Advice[2]	27	93%	78%	80%	100%
Surgical Infection Prevention					
Prophylactic Antibiotic Given[2]	236	83%	83%	77%	95%
Prophylactic Antibiotic Selection[2]	65	92%	92%	90%	100%
Prophylactic Antibiotic Stopped[2]	228	82%	70%	72%	95%
Pregnancy Care					
Inpatient Neonatal Mortality[2]	1,262	0.32%	-	-	-
Third or Fourth Degree Laceration[2]	891	4.15%	4.02%	3.63%	3.27%

Colorado Mental Health Institute-Pueblo

1600 W 24th Street
Pueblo, CO 81003
Ownership: Government - State
Emergency Services: No
Phone: 719-546-4000
Fax: 719-546-4484
Accredited: Yes
Licensed Beds: 841

Key Personnel:
Infection Control. . . . . Karen Baker, RN
Director Medical Surgical Nursing . . . . Sharon Gilbert, RN
Respiratory/Cardiopulmonary. . . . . Dan Kirkland

Measure	Cases	This Hospital	State Average	U.S. Average	Top Hospital
Heart Attack Care					
ACE Inhibitor or ARB for LVSD[5]	-	-	91%	82%	100%
Aspirin at Arrival[5]	-	-	95%	92%	100%
Aspirin at Discharge[5]	-	-	97%	90%	100%
Beta Blocker at Arrival[5]	-	-	93%	87%	100%
Beta Blocker at Discharge[5]	-	-	93%	90%	100%
Fibrinolytic Medication Timing[5]	-	-	31%	31%	100%
PCI Within 90 Minutes of Arrival[5]	-	-	69%	54%	95%
Smoking Cessation Advice[5]	-	-	91%	88%	100%
Heart Failure Care					
ACE Inhibitor or ARB for LVSD[5]	-	-	84%	82%	100%
Discharge Instructions[5]	-	-	53%	61%	93%
Evaluation of LVS Function[5]	-	-	81%	83%	99%
Smoking Cessation Advice[5]	-	-	79%	82%	100%
Pneumonia Care					
Appropriate Initial Antibiotic[5]	-	-	85%	83%	94%
Blood Culture Timing[5]	-	-	91%	90%	100%
Influenza Vaccine[5]	-	-	70%	70%	100%
Initial Antibiotic Timing[5]	-	-	83%	80%	93%
Oxygenation Assessment[5]	-	-	100%	99%	100%
Pneumococcal Vaccine[5]	-	-	72%	69%	94%
Smoking Cessation Advice[5]	-	-	78%	80%	100%
Surgical Infection Prevention					
Prophylactic Antibiotic Given[5]	-	-	83%	77%	95%
Prophylactic Antibiotic Selection[5]	-	-	92%	90%	100%
Prophylactic Antibiotic Stopped[5]	-	-	70%	72%	95%
Pregnancy Care					
Inpatient Neonatal Mortality	-	-	-	-	-
Third or Fourth Degree Laceration	-	-	4.02%	3.63%	3.27%

Parkview Medical Center

400 West 16th Street
Pueblo, CO 81003
E-mail: info@parkviewmc.org
URL: www.parkviewmc.com
Ownership: Voluntary non-profit - Private
Emergency Services: Yes
Phone: 719-584-4000
Fax: 719-544-6663
Accredited: Yes
Licensed Beds: 219

Measure	Cases	This Hospital	State Average	U.S. Average	Top Hospital
Heart Attack Care					
ACE Inhibitor or ARB for LVSD	47	100%	91%	82%	100%
Aspirin at Arrival	117	100%	95%	92%	100%
Aspirin at Discharge	186	99%	97%	90%	100%
Beta Blocker at Arrival	91	99%	93%	87%	100%
Beta Blocker at Discharge	193	100%	93%	90%	100%
Fibrinolytic Medication Timing	0	-	31%	31%	100%
PCI Within 90 Minutes of Arrival[1]	6	17%	69%	54%	95%
Smoking Cessation Advice	62	100%	91%	88%	100%
Heart Failure Care					
ACE Inhibitor or ARB for LVSD	84	100%	84%	82%	100%
Discharge Instructions	183	100%	53%	61%	93%
Evaluation of LVS Function	223	100%	81%	83%	99%
Smoking Cessation Advice	35	100%	79%	82%	100%
Pneumonia Care					
Appropriate Initial Antibiotic[2]	186	88%	85%	83%	94%
Blood Culture Timing[2]	183	96%	91%	90%	100%
Influenza Vaccine[2]	55	93%	70%	70%	100%
Initial Antibiotic Timing[2]	211	87%	83%	80%	93%
Oxygenation Assessment[2]	300	100%	100%	99%	100%
Pneumococcal Vaccine[2]	172	98%	72%	69%	94%
Smoking Cessation Advice[2]	93	100%	78%	80%	100%
Surgical Infection Prevention					
Prophylactic Antibiotic Given[2,3]	264	89%	83%	77%	95%
Prophylactic Antibiotic Selection[2]	116	97%	92%	90%	100%
Prophylactic Antibiotic Stopped[2,3]	257	74%	70%	72%	95%
Pregnancy Care					
Inpatient Neonatal Mortality	-	-	-	-	-
Third or Fourth Degree Laceration	-	-	4.02%	3.63%	3.27%

NOTE: Hospital profiles are in alphabetical order by state, then city, then hospital within the city; Rankings are sorted by rate in descending order and exclude hospitals with less than 25 cases; (1) The number of cases is too small (n<25) for purposes of reliably predicting hospital performance; (2) Measure reflects the hospital's indication that its submission was based upon a sample of its relevant discharges; (3) Rate reflects fewer than the maximum possible quarters of data for the measure; (4) Inaccurate information submitted and suppressed for one or more quarters; (5) No data is available from the hospital for this measure; Please refer to the User's Guide for a full explanation of data

Saint Mary-Corwin Medical Center

1008 Minnequa Avenue
Pueblo, CO 81004
Toll-Free: 800-228-4039
Phone: 719-557-4000
Fax: 719-557-5950

URL: www.stmarycorwin.org
Ownership: Voluntary non-profit - Church
Emergency Services: Yes
Accredited: Yes
Licensed Beds: 408

Key Personnel:
CEO. . . . . Tom Anderson
Chief Medical Officer . . . . Dr Steve Brown
Manager Emergency Services . . . . Charley Romero
Coordinator Infection Control . . . . Sandra Gallegos
Intensive Coronary Care . . . . Jodee Trainor
Director Women's Services . . . . Paulette Mapes
Director Respiratory Therapy . . . . Tom Trujillo

Measure	Cases	This Hospital	State Average	U.S. Average	Top Hospital
Heart Attack Care					
ACE Inhibitor or ARB for LVSD[1,2]	16	88%	91%	82%	100%
Aspirin at Arrival[2]	80	100%	95%	92%	100%
Aspirin at Discharge[2]	96	97%	97%	90%	100%
Beta Blocker at Arrival[2]	76	100%	93%	87%	100%
Beta Blocker at Discharge[2]	94	97%	93%	90%	100%
Fibrinolytic Medication Timing[2]	0	-	31%	31%	100%
PCI Within 90 Minutes of Arrival[1,2]	2	100%	69%	54%	95%
Smoking Cessation Advice[2]	53	98%	91%	88%	100%
Heart Failure Care					
ACE Inhibitor or ARB for LVSD[2]	40	90%	84%	82%	100%
Discharge Instructions[2]	120	92%	53%	61%	93%
Evaluation of LVS Function[2]	140	93%	81%	83%	99%
Smoking Cessation Advice[2]	26	100%	79%	82%	100%
Pneumonia Care					
Appropriate Initial Antibiotic[2]	119	87%	85%	83%	94%
Blood Culture Timing[2]	79	94%	91%	90%	100%
Influenza Vaccine[4,5]	-	-	70%	70%	100%
Initial Antibiotic Timing[2]	131	89%	83%	80%	93%
Oxygenation Assessment[2]	167	100%	100%	99%	100%
Pneumococcal Vaccine[2]	118	86%	72%	69%	94%
Smoking Cessation Advice[2]	44	95%	78%	80%	100%
Surgical Infection Prevention					
Prophylactic Antibiotic Given[2]	315	86%	83%	77%	95%
Prophylactic Antibiotic Selection[2]	76	93%	92%	90%	100%
Prophylactic Antibiotic Stopped[2]	303	74%	70%	72%	95%
Pregnancy Care					
Inpatient Neonatal Mortality	-	-	-	-	-
Third or Fourth Degree Laceration	-	-	4.02%	3.63%	3.27%

Rangely District Hospital

511 S White Avenue
Rangely, CO 81648
Phone: 970-675-5011
Fax: 970-675-5224
URL: www.rangelyhospital.com
Ownership: Govt - Hospital District or Authority
Emergency Services: Yes
Accredited: No
Licensed Beds: 25

Key Personnel:
CEO. . . . . Michael C Boyles
Director Radiology . . . . Nancy Droste

Measure	Cases	This Hospital	State Average	U.S. Average	Top Hospital
Heart Attack Care					
ACE Inhibitor or ARB for LVSD[5]	-	-	91%	82%	100%
Aspirin at Arrival[5]	-	-	95%	92%	100%
Aspirin at Discharge[5]	-	-	97%	90%	100%
Beta Blocker at Arrival[5]	-	-	93%	87%	100%
Beta Blocker at Discharge[5]	-	-	93%	90%	100%
Fibrinolytic Medication Timing[5]	-	-	31%	31%	100%
PCI Within 90 Minutes of Arrival[5]	-	-	69%	54%	95%
Smoking Cessation Advice[5]	-	-	91%	88%	100%
Heart Failure Care					
ACE Inhibitor or ARB for LVSD[3]	0	-	84%	82%	100%
Discharge Instructions[1,3]	1	0%	53%	61%	93%
Evaluation of LVS Function[1,3]	1	0%	81%	83%	99%
Smoking Cessation Advice[3]	0	-	79%	82%	100%
Pneumonia Care					
Appropriate Initial Antibiotic[5]	-	-	85%	83%	94%
Blood Culture Timing[5]	-	-	91%	90%	100%
Influenza Vaccine[5]	-	-	70%	70%	100%
Initial Antibiotic Timing[5]	-	-	83%	80%	93%
Oxygenation Assessment[5]	-	-	100%	99%	100%
Pneumococcal Vaccine[5]	-	-	72%	69%	94%
Smoking Cessation Advice[5]	-	-	78%	80%	100%
Surgical Infection Prevention					
Prophylactic Antibiotic Given[5]	-	-	83%	77%	95%
Prophylactic Antibiotic Selection[5]	-	-	92%	90%	100%
Prophylactic Antibiotic Stopped[5]	-	-	70%	72%	95%
Pregnancy Care					
Inpatient Neonatal Mortality	-	-	-	-	-
Third or Fourth Degree Laceration	-	-	4.02%	3.63%	3.27%

Grand River Hospital District

501 Airport Road
Rifle, CO 81650
Phone: 970-625-1510
Fax: 970-625-6486
URL: www.grhd.org
Ownership: Govt - Hospital District or Authority
Emergency Services: Yes
Accredited: No
Licensed Beds: 25

Key Personnel:
CEO. . . . . Martie Wisdom
President Medical Staff . . . . Deborah Brown, MD
Emergency Room Manager . . . . Cleo Castle, RN
Infection Control. . . . . Sara Jacobson
Director of Respiratory/Cardiopulmonary . . . . . . Spencer Aikin

Measure	Cases	This Hospital	State Average	U.S. Average	Top Hospital
Heart Attack Care					
ACE Inhibitor or ARB for LVSD[5]	-	-	91%	82%	100%
Aspirin at Arrival[5]	-	-	95%	92%	100%
Aspirin at Discharge[5]	-	-	97%	90%	100%
Beta Blocker at Arrival[5]	-	-	93%	87%	100%
Beta Blocker at Discharge[5]	-	-	93%	90%	100%
Fibrinolytic Medication Timing[5]	-	-	31%	31%	100%
PCI Within 90 Minutes of Arrival[5]	-	-	69%	54%	95%
Smoking Cessation Advice[5]	-	-	91%	88%	100%
Heart Failure Care					
ACE Inhibitor or ARB for LVSD[1]	1	100%	84%	82%	100%
Discharge Instructions[1]	14	29%	53%	61%	93%
Evaluation of LVS Function[1]	19	63%	81%	83%	99%
Smoking Cessation Advice[1]	3	67%	79%	82%	100%
Pneumonia Care					
Appropriate Initial Antibiotic	29	90%	85%	83%	94%
Blood Culture Timing[1]	18	94%	91%	90%	100%
Influenza Vaccine[1]	5	80%	70%	70%	100%
Initial Antibiotic Timing	41	71%	83%	80%	93%
Oxygenation Assessment	43	100%	100%	99%	100%
Pneumococcal Vaccine[1]	23	87%	72%	69%	94%
Smoking Cessation Advice[1]	10	20%	78%	80%	100%
Surgical Infection Prevention					
Prophylactic Antibiotic Given[5]	-	-	83%	77%	95%
Prophylactic Antibiotic Selection[5]	-	-	92%	90%	100%
Prophylactic Antibiotic Stopped[5]	-	-	70%	72%	95%
Pregnancy Care					
Inpatient Neonatal Mortality	-	-	-	-	-
Third or Fourth Degree Laceration	-	-	4.02%	3.63%	3.27%

Yampa Valley Medical Center

Alternate Name: Routt Memorial Hospital
1024 Central Park Drive
Steamboat Springs, CO 80487
Phone: 970-879-1322
Fax: 970-870-1223
URL: www.yvmc.org
Ownership: Voluntary non-profit - Private
Emergency Services: Yes
Accredited: Yes
Licensed Beds: 29

Key Personnel:
CEO. . . . . Karl Gill
Chief Medical Staff. . . . . G Edward Kimm, MD
Director Medical/Surgical Nursing . . . . Sandra Spiegal
OB/GYN Womens Health. . . . . David Schaller, MD
Chief Radiology . . . . Fred Jones, MD
Director Respiratory Therapy . . . . Ann Heselbach

NOTE: Hospital profiles are in alphabetical order by state, then city, then hospital within the city; Rankings are sorted by rate in descending order and exclude hospitals with less than 25 cases; (1) The number of cases is too small (n<25) for purposes of reliably predicting hospital performance; (2) Measure reflects the hospital's indication that its submission was based upon a sample of its relevant discharges; (3) Rate reflects fewer than the maximum possible quarters of data for the measure; (4) Inaccurate information submitted and suppressed for one or more quarters; (5) No data is available from the hospital for this measure; Please refer to the User's Guide for a full explanation of data

Measure	Cases	This Hospital	State Average	U.S. Average	Top Hospital
Heart Attack Care					
ACE Inhibitor or ARB for LVSD[1]	1	100%	91%	82%	100%
Aspirin at Arrival[1]	1	100%	95%	92%	100%
Aspirin at Discharge[1]	1	100%	97%	90%	100%
Beta Blocker at Arrival[1]	1	100%	93%	87%	100%
Beta Blocker at Discharge[1]	1	100%	93%	90%	100%
Fibrinolytic Medication Timing[1]	3	33%	31%	31%	100%
PCI Within 90 Minutes of Arrival	0	-	69%	54%	95%
Smoking Cessation Advice	0	-	91%	88%	100%
Heart Failure Care					
ACE Inhibitor or ARB for LVSD[1]	7	100%	84%	82%	100%
Discharge Instructions[1]	11	100%	53%	61%	93%
Evaluation of LVS Function[1]	12	100%	81%	83%	99%
Smoking Cessation Advice[1]	1	100%	79%	82%	100%
Pneumonia Care					
Appropriate Initial Antibiotic	46	89%	85%	83%	94%
Blood Culture Timing[1]	9	100%	91%	90%	100%
Influenza Vaccine[1]	6	33%	70%	70%	100%
Initial Antibiotic Timing	52	87%	83%	80%	93%
Oxygenation Assessment	55	100%	100%	99%	100%
Pneumococcal Vaccine	25	40%	72%	69%	94%
Smoking Cessation Advice[1]	11	45%	78%	80%	100%
Surgical Infection Prevention					
Prophylactic Antibiotic Given[3]	46	98%	83%	77%	95%
Prophylactic Antibiotic Selection	47	100%	92%	90%	100%
Prophylactic Antibiotic Stopped[3]	46	54%	70%	72%	95%
Pregnancy Care					
Inpatient Neonatal Mortality	-	-	-	-	-
Third or Fourth Degree Laceration	-	-	4.02%	3.63%	3.27%

Sterling Regional MedCenter

615 Fairhurst
PO Box 3500
Sterling, CO 80751
URL: www.wphn.com/srmc_frm.htm
Ownership: Voluntary non-profit - Private
Emergency Services: Yes
Phone: 970-522-0122
Fax: 970-522-8532
Accredited: Yes
Licensed Beds: 36

Key Personnel:

CEO. . . . . Michael J Gillen
Chief Medical Staff. . . . . Dan Elliff, MD
Emergency Room . . . . Jeanne Schuppe, RN
Infection Control. . . . . Janet Conner
Director Medical/Surgical Nursing . . . . Katie Olme, RN
OB/GYN Womens Health. . . . . Curtis Clark, MD
Respiratory Therapy. . . . . Nancy Zwirn

Measure	Cases	This Hospital	State Average	U.S. Average	Top Hospital
Heart Attack Care					
ACE Inhibitor or ARB for LVSD	0	-	91%	82%	100%
Aspirin at Arrival[1]	10	100%	95%	92%	100%
Aspirin at Discharge[1]	5	100%	97%	90%	100%
Beta Blocker at Arrival[1]	5	100%	93%	87%	100%
Beta Blocker at Discharge[1]	5	80%	93%	90%	100%
Fibrinolytic Medication Timing	0	-	31%	31%	100%
PCI Within 90 Minutes of Arrival	0	-	69%	54%	95%
Smoking Cessation Advice	0	-	91%	88%	100%
Heart Failure Care					
ACE Inhibitor or ARB for LVSD[1]	11	91%	84%	82%	100%
Discharge Instructions	30	43%	53%	61%	93%
Evaluation of LVS Function	47	81%	81%	83%	99%
Smoking Cessation Advice[1]	7	57%	79%	82%	100%
Pneumonia Care					
Appropriate Initial Antibiotic	34	79%	85%	83%	94%
Blood Culture Timing	30	97%	91%	90%	100%
Influenza Vaccine[1]	15	87%	70%	70%	100%
Initial Antibiotic Timing	47	89%	83%	80%	93%
Oxygenation Assessment	59	100%	100%	99%	100%
Pneumococcal Vaccine	35	91%	72%	69%	94%
Smoking Cessation Advice[1]	15	73%	78%	80%	100%
Surgical Infection Prevention					
Prophylactic Antibiotic Given[3]	25	72%	83%	77%	95%
Prophylactic Antibiotic Selection	25	92%	92%	90%	100%
Prophylactic Antibiotic Stopped[1,3]	23	78%	70%	72%	95%
Pregnancy Care					
Inpatient Neonatal Mortality	-	-	-	-	-
Third or Fourth Degree Laceration	-	-	4.02%	3.63%	3.27%

North Suburban Medical Center

9191 Grant Street
Thornton, CO 80229
URL: www.northsuburban.com
Ownership: Voluntary non-profit - Private
Emergency Services: Yes
Phone: 303-451-7800
Fax: 303-450-4458
Accredited: Yes
Licensed Beds: 157

Measure	Cases	This Hospital	State Average	U.S. Average	Top Hospital
Heart Attack Care					
ACE Inhibitor or ARB for LVSD[1]	6	100%	91%	82%	100%
Aspirin at Arrival	106	100%	95%	92%	100%
Aspirin at Discharge	89	100%	97%	90%	100%
Beta Blocker at Arrival	74	100%	93%	87%	100%
Beta Blocker at Discharge	74	99%	93%	90%	100%
Fibrinolytic Medication Timing[1]	1	100%	31%	31%	100%
PCI Within 90 Minutes of Arrival[1]	5	100%	69%	54%	95%
Smoking Cessation Advice	50	100%	91%	88%	100%
Heart Failure Care					
ACE Inhibitor or ARB for LVSD	26	100%	84%	82%	100%
Discharge Instructions	61	92%	53%	61%	93%
Evaluation of LVS Function	87	100%	81%	83%	99%
Smoking Cessation Advice[1]	11	100%	79%	82%	100%
Pneumonia Care					
Appropriate Initial Antibiotic	97	93%	85%	83%	94%
Blood Culture Timing	120	92%	91%	90%	100%
Influenza Vaccine	29	97%	70%	70%	100%
Initial Antibiotic Timing	157	88%	83%	80%	93%
Oxygenation Assessment	205	100%	100%	99%	100%
Pneumococcal Vaccine	89	90%	72%	69%	94%
Smoking Cessation Advice	74	100%	78%	80%	100%
Surgical Infection Prevention					
Prophylactic Antibiotic Given[2,3]	129	81%	83%	77%	95%
Prophylactic Antibiotic Selection[2]	49	94%	92%	90%	100%
Prophylactic Antibiotic Stopped[2,3]	121	45%	70%	72%	95%
Pregnancy Care					
Inpatient Neonatal Mortality	1,948	0.15%	-	-	-
Third or Fourth Degree Laceration	1,461	5.27%	4.02%	3.63%	3.27%

Vail Valley Medical Center

181 W Meadow Drive
Vail, CO 81657
URL: www.vvmc.com
Ownership: Voluntary non-profit - Other
Emergency Services: Yes
Phone: 970-476-2451
Fax: 970-479-7192
Accredited: Yes
Licensed Beds: 58

Key Personnel:

CEO. . . . . Greg Repetti
Emergency Room . . . . Joyce Morgan, RN
Director of Respiratory . . . . Christi Clymo

Measure	Cases	This Hospital	State Average	U.S. Average	Top Hospital
Heart Attack Care					
ACE Inhibitor or ARB for LVSD[3]	0	-	91%	82%	100%
Aspirin at Arrival[3]	0	-	95%	92%	100%
Aspirin at Discharge[3]	0	-	97%	90%	100%
Beta Blocker at Arrival[1,3]	1	100%	93%	87%	100%
Beta Blocker at Discharge[1,3]	1	100%	93%	90%	100%
Fibrinolytic Medication Timing[3]	0	-	31%	31%	100%
PCI Within 90 Minutes of Arrival	0	-	69%	54%	95%
Smoking Cessation Advice[3]	0	-	91%	88%	100%
Heart Failure Care					
ACE Inhibitor or ARB for LVSD[1]	3	67%	84%	82%	100%
Discharge Instructions[1]	9	11%	53%	61%	93%
Evaluation of LVS Function[1]	8	50%	81%	83%	99%
Smoking Cessation Advice[1]	1	0%	79%	82%	100%
Pneumonia Care					
Appropriate Initial Antibiotic[1]	9	89%	85%	83%	94%

NOTE: Hospital profiles are in alphabetical order by state, then city, then hospital within the city; Rankings are sorted by rate in descending order and exclude hospitals with less than 25 cases; (1) The number of cases is too small (n<25) for purposes of reliably predicting hospital performance; (2) Measure reflects the hospital's indication that its submission was based upon a sample of its relevant discharges; (3) Rate reflects fewer than the maximum possible quarters of data for the measure; (4) Inaccurate information submitted and suppressed for one or more quarters; (5) No data is available from the hospital for this measure; Please refer to the User's Guide for a full explanation of data

Measure	Cases	This Hospital	State Average	U.S. Average	Top Hospital
Blood Culture Timing[1]	6	100%	91%	90%	100%
Influenza Vaccine[1]	4	25%	70%	70%	100%
Initial Antibiotic Timing[1]	6	67%	83%	80%	93%
Oxygenation Assessment[1]	10	100%	100%	99%	100%
Pneumococcal Vaccine[1]	5	60%	72%	69%	94%
Smoking Cessation Advice[1]	2	50%	78%	80%	100%
Surgical Infection Prevention					
Prophylactic Antibiotic Given[3]	25	92%	83%	77%	95%
Prophylactic Antibiotic Selection	25	84%	92%	90%	100%
Prophylactic Antibiotic Stopped[3]	25	100%	70%	72%	95%
Pregnancy Care					
Inpatient Neonatal Mortality	603	0.00%	-	-	-
Third or Fourth Degree Laceration	362	6.63%	4.02%	3.63%	3.27%

Spanish Peaks Regional Health Center

23500 Us Hwy 160 Phone: 719-738-5100
Walsenburg, CO 81089
Ownership: Govt - Hospital District or Authority Accredited: No
Emergency Services: Yes

Measure	Cases	This Hospital	State Average	U.S. Average	Top Hospital
Heart Attack Care					
ACE Inhibitor or ARB for LVSD[5]	-	-	91%	82%	100%
Aspirin at Arrival[5]	-	-	95%	92%	100%
Aspirin at Discharge[5]	-	-	97%	90%	100%
Beta Blocker at Arrival[5]	-	-	93%	87%	100%
Beta Blocker at Discharge[5]	-	-	93%	90%	100%
Fibrinolytic Medication Timing[5]	-	-	31%	31%	100%
PCI Within 90 Minutes of Arrival[5]	-	-	69%	54%	95%
Smoking Cessation Advice[5]	-	-	91%	88%	100%
Heart Failure Care					
ACE Inhibitor or ARB for LVSD[3]	0	-	84%	82%	100%
Discharge Instructions[1,3]	12	42%	53%	61%	93%
Evaluation of LVS Function[1,3]	15	53%	81%	83%	99%
Smoking Cessation Advice[1,3]	1	0%	79%	82%	100%
Pneumonia Care					
Appropriate Initial Antibiotic[1,3]	16	94%	85%	83%	94%
Blood Culture Timing[1,3]	8	88%	91%	90%	100%
Influenza Vaccine[1]	4	100%	70%	70%	100%
Initial Antibiotic Timing[3]	27	96%	83%	80%	93%
Oxygenation Assessment[3]	30	100%	100%	99%	100%
Pneumococcal Vaccine[1,3]	23	96%	72%	69%	94%
Smoking Cessation Advice[1,3]	7	100%	78%	80%	100%
Surgical Infection Prevention					
Prophylactic Antibiotic Given[5]	-	-	83%	77%	95%
Prophylactic Antibiotic Selection[5]	-	-	92%	90%	100%
Prophylactic Antibiotic Stopped[5]	-	-	70%	72%	95%
Pregnancy Care					
Inpatient Neonatal Mortality	-	-	-	-	-
Third or Fourth Degree Laceration	-	-	4.02%	3.63%	3.27%

Saint Anthony North Hospital

2551 W 84th Avenue Phone: 303-426-2151
Westminster, CO 80031 Fax: 303-426-2155
URL: www.stanthonyhosp.org
Ownership: Voluntary non-profit - Church Accredited: No
Emergency Services: Yes Licensed Beds: 196

Key Personnel:

President/CEO . . . . James Dover
Chief Medical Staff . . . . Jodi Chambers
Emergency Room . . . . Garland Crowell
Infection Control . . . . Chris Baumann
ICU . . . . Cathy Laguardia
Intensive/Coronary Care . . . . Cathy Laguardia
Medical Surgical Nursing . . . . Jeff Birch
OB/GYN . . . . Deb Mordecai
Respiratory/Cardiopulmonary . . . . Scott Reistad

Measure	Cases	This Hospital	State Average	U.S. Average	Top Hospital
Heart Attack Care					
ACE Inhibitor or ARB for LVSD[1,2]	10	90%	91%	82%	100%
Aspirin at Arrival[2]	104	100%	95%	92%	100%
Aspirin at Discharge[2]	86	99%	97%	90%	100%
Beta Blocker at Arrival[2]	96	99%	93%	87%	100%
Beta Blocker at Discharge[2]	82	100%	93%	90%	100%
Fibrinolytic Medication Timing[2]	0	-	31%	31%	100%
PCI Within 90 Minutes of Arrival[1,2]	12	100%	69%	54%	95%
Smoking Cessation Advice[2]	28	100%	91%	88%	100%
Heart Failure Care					
ACE Inhibitor or ARB for LVSD[2]	47	94%	84%	82%	100%
Discharge Instructions[2]	130	62%	53%	61%	93%
Evaluation of LVS Function[2]	162	97%	81%	83%	99%
Smoking Cessation Advice[1,2]	23	100%	79%	82%	100%
Pneumonia Care					
Appropriate Initial Antibiotic[2]	135	85%	85%	83%	94%
Blood Culture Timing[2]	112	86%	91%	90%	100%
Influenza Vaccine[2]	36	58%	70%	70%	100%
Initial Antibiotic Timing[2]	189	81%	83%	80%	93%
Oxygenation Assessment[2]	205	100%	100%	99%	100%
Pneumococcal Vaccine[2]	131	81%	72%	69%	94%
Smoking Cessation Advice[2]	71	99%	78%	80%	100%
Surgical Infection Prevention					
Prophylactic Antibiotic Given[2,3]	165	75%	83%	77%	95%
Prophylactic Antibiotic Selection[2]	40	100%	92%	90%	100%
Prophylactic Antibiotic Stopped[2,3]	149	61%	70%	72%	95%
Pregnancy Care					
Inpatient Neonatal Mortality	-	-	-	-	-
Third or Fourth Degree Laceration	-	-	4.02%	3.63%	3.27%

Exempla Lutheran Medical Center

Alternate Name: Lutheran Medical Center
8300 W 38th Avenue Phone: 303-425-4500
Wheat Ridge, CO 80033 Fax: 303-425-8198
URL: www.exemlpa.org
Ownership: Voluntary non-profit - Private Accredited: Yes
Emergency Services: Yes Licensed Beds: 382

Key Personnel:

Emergency Room . . . . Dr. Jim Thompson

Measure	Cases	This Hospital	State Average	U.S. Average	Top Hospital
Heart Attack Care					
ACE Inhibitor or ARB for LVSD[2]	36	78%	91%	82%	100%
Aspirin at Arrival[2]	270	100%	95%	92%	100%
Aspirin at Discharge[2]	240	98%	97%	90%	100%
Beta Blocker at Arrival[2]	169	92%	93%	87%	100%
Beta Blocker at Discharge[2]	230	98%	93%	90%	100%
Fibrinolytic Medication Timing[2]	0	-	31%	31%	100%
PCI Within 90 Minutes of Arrival[1,2]	8	62%	69%	54%	95%
Smoking Cessation Advice[2]	89	99%	91%	88%	100%
Heart Failure Care					
ACE Inhibitor or ARB for LVSD[2]	94	90%	84%	82%	100%
Discharge Instructions[2]	190	95%	53%	61%	93%
Evaluation of LVS Function[2]	260	97%	81%	83%	99%
Smoking Cessation Advice[2]	37	100%	79%	82%	100%
Pneumonia Care					
Appropriate Initial Antibiotic[2]	113	93%	85%	83%	94%
Blood Culture Timing[2]	96	95%	91%	90%	100%
Influenza Vaccine[1,2]	23	48%	70%	70%	100%
Initial Antibiotic Timing[2]	150	79%	83%	80%	93%
Oxygenation Assessment[2]	180	100%	100%	99%	100%
Pneumococcal Vaccine[2]	99	79%	72%	69%	94%
Smoking Cessation Advice[2]	35	97%	78%	80%	100%
Surgical Infection Prevention					
Prophylactic Antibiotic Given[2]	297	90%	83%	77%	95%
Prophylactic Antibiotic Selection[2]	70	99%	92%	90%	100%
Prophylactic Antibiotic Stopped[2]	288	75%	70%	72%	95%
Pregnancy Care					
Inpatient Neonatal Mortality	-	-	-	-	-
Third or Fourth Degree Laceration	-	-	4.02%	3.63%	3.27%

NOTE: Hospital profiles are in alphabetical order by state, then city, then hospital within the city; Rankings are sorted by rate in descending order and exclude hospitals with less than 25 cases; (1) The number of cases is too small (n<25) for purposes of reliably predicting hospital performance; (2) Measure reflects the hospital's indication that its submission was based upon a sample of its relevant discharges; (3) Rate reflects fewer than the maximum possible quarters of data for the measure; (4) Inaccurate information submitted and suppressed for one or more quarters; (5) No data is available from the hospital for this measure; Please refer to the User's Guide for a full explanation of data

Wray Community Hospital

340 Birch Street
Wray, CO 80758
URL: www.wphn.com/wray_frm.htm
Ownership: Voluntary non-profit - Other
Emergency Services: Yes

Phone: 970-332-4811
Fax: 970-332-4017

Accredited: No
Licensed Beds: 15

Key Personnel:

President/CEO. . . . . Ed Finley
Chief Medical Staff. . . . . Robert Loyd, MD
Emergency Room . . . . Christine Wall
Infection Control. . . . . Kathy Bard
Respiratory/Cardiopulmonary. . . . . Jennifer Shultz

Measure	Cases	This Hospital	State Average	U.S. Average	Top Hospital
Heart Attack Care					
ACE Inhibitor or ARB for LVSD	0	-	91%	82%	100%
Aspirin at Arrival[1]	6	100%	95%	92%	100%
Aspirin at Discharge[1]	3	100%	97%	90%	100%
Beta Blocker at Arrival[1]	7	86%	93%	87%	100%
Beta Blocker at Discharge[1]	4	100%	93%	90%	100%
Fibrinolytic Medication Timing[1]	2	0%	31%	31%	100%
PCI Within 90 Minutes of Arrival	0	-	69%	54%	95%
Smoking Cessation Advice	0	-	91%	88%	100%
Heart Failure Care					
ACE Inhibitor or ARB for LVSD[1]	1	100%	84%	82%	100%
Discharge Instructions[1]	6	0%	53%	61%	93%
Evaluation of LVS Function[1]	11	64%	81%	83%	99%
Smoking Cessation Advice[1]	3	33%	79%	82%	100%
Pneumonia Care					
Appropriate Initial Antibiotic[1]	16	100%	85%	83%	94%
Blood Culture Timing[1]	3	100%	91%	90%	100%
Influenza Vaccine[1]	5	80%	70%	70%	100%
Initial Antibiotic Timing[1]	21	86%	83%	80%	93%
Oxygenation Assessment[1]	24	100%	100%	99%	100%
Pneumococcal Vaccine[1]	19	74%	72%	69%	94%
Smoking Cessation Advice[1]	7	57%	78%	80%	100%
Surgical Infection Prevention					
Prophylactic Antibiotic Given[1]	15	80%	83%	77%	95%
Prophylactic Antibiotic Selection[1]	3	100%	92%	90%	100%
Prophylactic Antibiotic Stopped[1]	15	93%	70%	72%	95%
Pregnancy Care					
Inpatient Neonatal Mortality	-	-	-	-	-
Third or Fourth Degree Laceration	-	-	4.02%	3.63%	3.27%

NOTE: Hospital profiles are in alphabetical order by state, then city, then hospital within the city; Rankings are sorted by rate in descending order and exclude hospitals with less than 25 cases; (1) The number of cases is too small (n<25) for purposes of reliably predicting hospital performance; (2) Measure reflects the hospital's indication that its submission was based upon a sample of its relevant discharges; (3) Rate reflects fewer than the maximum possible quarters of data for the measure; (4) Inaccurate information submitted and suppressed for one or more quarters; (5) No data is available from the hospital for this measure; Please refer to the User's Guide for a full explanation of data

Heart Attack Care

1. ACE Inhibitor or ARB for LVSD

Hospital Name	City	Rate	Cases
Maui Memorial Hospital	Wailuku	88%	25
The Queen's Medical Center	Honolulu	86%	88
Moanalua Medical Center and Clinic	Honolulu	85%	68
Hilo Medical Center	Hilo	84%	31
Hawaii Medical Center East	Honolulu	66%	32
Straub Clinic and Hospital	Honolulu	62%	69

2. Aspirin at Arrival

Hospital Name	City	Rate	Cases
Kapiolani Health at Pali Momi	Aiea	100%	68
Castle Medical Center	Kailua	98%	130
Moanalua Medical Center and Clinic	Honolulu	97%	173
Straub Clinic and Hospital	Honolulu	97%	158
Hawaii Medical Center East	Honolulu	95%	86
Maui Memorial Hospital	Wailuku	95%	135
The Queen's Medical Center	Honolulu	95%	242
Wilcox Memorial Hospital	Lihue	94%	34
Hilo Medical Center	Hilo	93%	203
Kona Community Hospital	Kealakekua	93%	29
Kuakini Medical Center	Honolulu	93%	73
Hawaii Medical Center West	Ewa Beach	91%	68
North Hawaii Community Hospital	Kamuela	88%	25

3. Aspirin at Discharge

Hospital Name	City	Rate	Cases
Kapiolani Health at Pali Momi	Aiea	100%	32
Moanalua Medical Center and Clinic	Honolulu	97%	293
Castle Medical Center	Kailua	96%	104
The Queen's Medical Center	Honolulu	96%	400
Hawaii Medical Center East	Honolulu	95%	169
Kuakini Medical Center	Honolulu	94%	106
Maui Memorial Hospital	Wailuku	94%	68
Straub Clinic and Hospital	Honolulu	94%	277
Hilo Medical Center	Hilo	88%	165
Hawaii Medical Center West	Ewa Beach	72%	25

4. Beta Blocker at Arrival

Hospital Name	City	Rate	Cases
Kapiolani Health at Pali Momi	Aiea	100%	57
The Queen's Medical Center	Honolulu	98%	173
Straub Clinic and Hospital	Honolulu	97%	137
Moanalua Medical Center and Clinic	Honolulu	96%	160
Castle Medical Center	Kailua	95%	85
Hilo Medical Center	Hilo	95%	221
Maui Memorial Hospital	Wailuku	93%	118
Kuakini Medical Center	Honolulu	89%	53
Wilcox Memorial Hospital	Lihue	86%	29
North Hawaii Community Hospital	Kamuela	85%	26
Hawaii Medical Center East	Honolulu	84%	75
Hawaii Medical Center West	Ewa Beach	84%	56
Kona Community Hospital	Kealakekua	69%	29

5. Beta Blocker at Discharge

Hospital Name	City	Rate	Cases
Kapiolani Health at Pali Momi	Aiea	100%	36
The Queen's Medical Center	Honolulu	98%	390
Moanalua Medical Center and Clinic	Honolulu	97%	292
Castle Medical Center	Kailua	95%	108
Hawaii Medical Center East	Honolulu	95%	171
Kuakini Medical Center	Honolulu	95%	126
Straub Clinic and Hospital	Honolulu	94%	267
Maui Memorial Hospital	Wailuku	91%	69
Hilo Medical Center	Hilo	90%	180
Hawaii Medical Center West	Ewa Beach	85%	26

8. Smoking Cessation Advice

Hospital Name	City	Rate	Cases
Hilo Medical Center	Hilo	92%	62
Moanalua Medical Center and Clinic	Honolulu	92%	65
The Queen's Medical Center	Honolulu	92%	131
Castle Medical Center	Kailua	91%	32
Straub Clinic and Hospital	Honolulu	84%	73
Kuakini Medical Center	Honolulu	82%	33
Hawaii Medical Center East	Honolulu	59%	58

Heart Failure Care

9. ACE Inhibitor or ARB for LVSD

Hospital Name	City	Rate	Cases
Kapiolani Health at Pali Momi	Aiea	96%	106
Kuakini Medical Center	Honolulu	88%	75
Moanalua Medical Center and Clinic	Honolulu	88%	114
The Queen's Medical Center	Honolulu	88%	293
Hawaii Medical Center East	Honolulu	86%	71
Hawaii Medical Center West	Ewa Beach	82%	78
Maui Memorial Hospital	Wailuku	82%	143
Hilo Medical Center	Hilo	78%	50
Wilcox Memorial Hospital	Lihue	77%	56
Castle Medical Center	Kailua	76%	54
Straub Clinic and Hospital	Honolulu	72%	107
Kona Community Hospital	Kealakekua	68%	25

10. Discharge Instructions

Hospital Name	City	Rate	Cases
Castle Medical Center	Kailua	86%	249
Hilo Medical Center	Hilo	79%	205
The Queen's Medical Center	Honolulu	78%	482
Wahiawa General Hospital	Wahiawa	71%	79
Kapiolani Health at Pali Momi	Aiea	70%	253
Maui Memorial Hospital	Wailuku	43%	277
Moanalua Medical Center and Clinic	Honolulu	38%	270
Straub Clinic and Hospital	Honolulu	36%	207
Wilcox Memorial Hospital	Lihue	34%	92
Kuakini Medical Center	Honolulu	31%	159
Hawaii Medical Center West	Ewa Beach	25%	213
Hawaii Medical Center East	Honolulu	24%	211
North Hawaii Community Hospital	Kamuela	23%	61
Kona Community Hospital	Kealakekua	21%	70

11. Evaluation of LVS Function

Hospital Name	City	Rate	Cases
Moanalua Medical Center and Clinic	Honolulu	96%	275
Kuakini Medical Center	Honolulu	94%	172
The Queen's Medical Center	Honolulu	93%	515
Straub Clinic and Hospital	Honolulu	91%	229
Kapiolani Health at Pali Momi	Aiea	89%	240
Hawaii Medical Center East	Honolulu	86%	234
Castle Medical Center	Kailua	85%	256
Maui Memorial Hospital	Wailuku	85%	283
Wilcox Memorial Hospital	Lihue	85%	95
North Hawaii Community Hospital	Kamuela	77%	53
Hilo Medical Center	Hilo	72%	226
Wahiawa General Hospital	Wahiawa	70%	81
Hawaii Medical Center West	Ewa Beach	67%	228
Kona Community Hospital	Kealakekua	64%	80

12. Smoking Cessation Advice

Hospital Name	City	Rate	Cases
Moanalua Medical Center and Clinic	Honolulu	95%	41
The Queen's Medical Center	Honolulu	94%	113
Hilo Medical Center	Hilo	90%	50
Kapiolani Health at Pali Momi	Aiea	89%	45
Castle Medical Center	Kailua	86%	43
Kuakini Medical Center	Honolulu	81%	26
Maui Memorial Hospital	Wailuku	68%	44
Hawaii Medical Center West	Ewa Beach	52%	65
Hawaii Medical Center East	Honolulu	44%	45

Pneumonia Care

13. Appropriate Initial Antibiotic

Hospital Name	City	Rate	Cases
Kona Community Hospital	Kealakekua	94%	95
Kapiolani Health at Pali Momi	Aiea	89%	139
Kuakini Medical Center	Honolulu	89%	105
Wahiawa General Hospital	Wahiawa	88%	42
Hawaii Medical Center West	Ewa Beach	84%	132
Moanalua Medical Center and Clinic	Honolulu	83%	269
The Queen's Medical Center	Honolulu	83%	245
Castle Medical Center	Kailua	81%	119
Maui Memorial Hospital	Wailuku	79%	148
Hawaii Medical Center East	Honolulu	77%	94
Wilcox Memorial Hospital	Lihue	76%	75
Hilo Medical Center	Hilo	73%	119
Straub Clinic and Hospital	Honolulu	61%	131
North Hawaii Community Hospital	Kamuela	52%	56

NOTE: Hospital profiles are in alphabetical order by state, then city, then hospital within the city; Rankings are sorted by rate in descending order and exclude hospitals with less than 25 cases; (1) The number of cases is too small (n<25) for purposes of reliably predicting hospital performance; (2) Measure reflects the hospital's indication that its submission was based upon a sample of its relevant discharges; (3) Rate reflects fewer than the maximum possible quarters of data for the measure; (4) Inaccurate information submitted and suppressed for one or more quarters; (5) No data is available from the hospital for this measure; Please refer to the User's Guide for a full explanation of data

14. Blood Culture Timing

Hospital Name	City	Rate	Cases
Castle Medical Center	Kailua	95%	128
Kapiolani Health at Pali Momi	Aiea	94%	225
Kona Community Hospital	Kealakekua	94%	70
Kuakini Medical Center	Honolulu	94%	95
Moanalua Medical Center and Clinic	Honolulu	93%	193
Hawaii Medical Center West	Ewa Beach	92%	155
North Hawaii Community Hospital	Kamuela	91%	35
Straub Clinic and Hospital	Honolulu	91%	152
Hilo Medical Center	Hilo	90%	91
Maui Memorial Hospital	Wailuku	90%	101
Hawaii Medical Center East	Honolulu	85%	96
The Queen's Medical Center	Honolulu	83%	262
Wilcox Memorial Hospital	Lihue	80%	59
Wahiawa General Hospital	Wahiawa	69%	35

15. Influenza Vaccine

Hospital Name	City	Rate	Cases
Kapiolani Health at Pali Momi	Aiea	86%	64
Straub Clinic and Hospital	Honolulu	82%	38
Hawaii Medical Center East	Honolulu	75%	40
Castle Medical Center	Kailua	68%	34
Maui Memorial Hospital	Wailuku	65%	31
Moanalua Medical Center and Clinic	Honolulu	64%	56
Kuakini Medical Center	Honolulu	58%	33
The Queen's Medical Center	Honolulu	53%	75
Hawaii Medical Center West	Ewa Beach	51%	41
Hilo Medical Center	Hilo	29%	28

16. Initial Antibiotic Timing

Hospital Name	City	Rate	Cases
Maui Memorial Hospital	Wailuku	88%	185
Wahiawa General Hospital	Wahiawa	87%	46
Hawaii Medical Center West	Ewa Beach	85%	241
Kapiolani Health at Pali Momi	Aiea	85%	288
Castle Medical Center	Kailua	82%	147
Kona Community Hospital	Kealakekua	81%	88
Kuakini Medical Center	Honolulu	80%	142
Hawaii Medical Center East	Honolulu	77%	158
Moanalua Medical Center and Clinic	Honolulu	77%	266
The Queen's Medical Center	Honolulu	73%	319
North Hawaii Community Hospital	Kamuela	72%	50
Straub Clinic and Hospital	Honolulu	71%	182
Wilcox Memorial Hospital	Lihue	71%	80
Hilo Medical Center	Hilo	66%	112

17. Oxygenation Assessment

Hospital Name	City	Rate	Cases
Hawaii Medical Center East	Honolulu	100%	204
Hawaii Medical Center West	Ewa Beach	100%	264
Kapiolani Health at Pali Momi	Aiea	100%	345
Kona Community Hospital	Kealakekua	100%	130
Kuakini Medical Center	Honolulu	100%	167
Maui Memorial Hospital	Wailuku	100%	227
Moanalua Medical Center and Clinic	Honolulu	100%	362
North Hawaii Community Hospital	Kamuela	100%	65
Straub Clinic and Hospital	Honolulu	100%	223
The Queen's Medical Center	Honolulu	100%	413
Wahiawa General Hospital	Wahiawa	100%	55
Wilcox Memorial Hospital	Lihue	100%	109
Castle Medical Center	Kailua	99%	178
Hilo Medical Center	Hilo	99%	197

18. Pneumococcal Vaccine

Hospital Name	City	Rate	Cases
Moanalua Medical Center and Clinic	Honolulu	89%	251
Kapiolani Health at Pali Momi	Aiea	76%	218
Castle Medical Center	Kailua	75%	95
Straub Clinic and Hospital	Honolulu	62%	156
Wilcox Memorial Hospital	Lihue	59%	68
The Queen's Medical Center	Honolulu	58%	234
Kuakini Medical Center	Honolulu	53%	124
Hawaii Medical Center East	Honolulu	49%	136
Maui Memorial Hospital	Wailuku	47%	154
Hilo Medical Center	Hilo	34%	109
Hawaii Medical Center West	Ewa Beach	30%	161
Kona Community Hospital	Kealakekua	26%	69
North Hawaii Community Hospital	Kamuela	24%	41
Wahiawa General Hospital	Wahiawa	15%	33

19. Smoking Cessation Advice

Hospital Name	City	Rate	Cases
Maui Memorial Hospital	Wailuku	96%	45
Castle Medical Center	Kailua	95%	37
Kapiolani Health at Pali Momi	Aiea	92%	39
Hilo Medical Center	Hilo	83%	48
The Queen's Medical Center	Honolulu	77%	81
Moanalua Medical Center and Clinic	Honolulu	60%	47
Hawaii Medical Center East	Honolulu	53%	30
Hawaii Medical Center West	Ewa Beach	47%	49

Surgical Infection Prevention

20. Prophylactic Antibiotic Given

Hospital Name	City	Rate	Cases
Castle Medical Center	Kailua	93%	100
Kona Community Hospital	Kealakekua	90%	49
Kuakini Medical Center	Honolulu	88%	152
Straub Clinic and Hospital	Honolulu	88%	125
The Queen's Medical Center	Honolulu	88%	1018
North Hawaii Community Hospital	Kamuela	84%	38
Kapiolani Health at Pali Momi	Aiea	81%	226
Moanalua Medical Center and Clinic	Honolulu	80%	537
Hawaii Medical Center East	Honolulu	79%	261
Hilo Medical Center	Hilo	75%	126
Maui Memorial Hospital	Wailuku	71%	249
Wilcox Memorial Hospital	Lihue	53%	30
Hawaii Medical Center West	Ewa Beach	48%	50

21. Prophylactic Antibiotic Selection

Hospital Name	City	Rate	Cases
Moanalua Medical Center and Clinic	Honolulu	99%	147
Kapiolani Health at Pali Momi	Aiea	98%	84
The Queen's Medical Center	Honolulu	97%	373
Straub Clinic and Hospital	Honolulu	96%	77
Maui Memorial Hospital	Wailuku	93%	54
Castle Medical Center	Kailua	92%	39
Kuakini Medical Center	Honolulu	91%	46
Wilcox Memorial Hospital	Lihue	90%	29
Hawaii Medical Center East	Honolulu	86%	50
Hilo Medical Center	Hilo	75%	36

22. Prophylactic Antibiotic Stopped

Hospital Name	City	Rate	Cases
Wilcox Memorial Hospital	Lihue	100%	29
Kona Community Hospital	Kealakekua	89%	28
Straub Clinic and Hospital	Honolulu	87%	119
The Queen's Medical Center	Honolulu	85%	993
Hawaii Medical Center West	Ewa Beach	83%	47
Castle Medical Center	Kailua	76%	100
North Hawaii Community Hospital	Kamuela	69%	35
Kuakini Medical Center	Honolulu	66%	150
Maui Memorial Hospital	Wailuku	61%	240
Hilo Medical Center	Hilo	57%	123
Moanalua Medical Center and Clinic	Honolulu	49%	521
Hawaii Medical Center East	Honolulu	42%	239
Kapiolani Health at Pali Momi	Aiea	41%	219

Pregnancy Care

23. Inpatient Neonatal Mortality

Hospital Name	City	Rate	Cases
The Queen's Medical Center	Honolulu	0.04%	2275
Moanalua Medical Center and Clinic	Honolulu	0.67%	1931

24. Third or Fourth Degree Laceration

Hospital Name	City	Rate	Cases
Moanalua Medical Center and Clinic	Honolulu	4.81%	1435
The Queen's Medical Center	Honolulu	5.45%	1744

NOTE: Hospital profiles are in alphabetical order by state, then city, then hospital within the city; Rankings are sorted by rate in descending order and exclude hospitals with less than 25 cases; (1) The number of cases is too small (n<25) for purposes of reliably predicting hospital performance; (2) Measure reflects the hospital's indication that its submission was based upon a sample of its relevant discharges; (3) Rate reflects fewer than the maximum possible quarters of data for the measure; (4) Inaccurate information submitted and suppressed for one or more quarters; (5) No data is available from the hospital for this measure; Please refer to the User's Guide for a full explanation of data

Kapiolani Health at Pali Momi

98-1079 Moanalua Road
Aiea, HI 96701
URL: www.kapiolani.org
Ownership: Proprietary
Emergency Services: Yes
Phone: 808-486-6000
Fax: 808-485-4400
Accredited: Yes
Licensed Beds: 116

Key Personnel:
Chief Medical Officer . . . . Kenneth Nakamura, MD
Director Radiology . . . . Alice Deppe

Measure	Cases	This Hospital	State Average	U.S. Average	Top Hospital
Heart Attack Care					
ACE Inhibitor or ARB for LVSD[1]	10	100%	76%	82%	100%
Aspirin at Arrival	68	100%	94%	92%	100%
Aspirin at Discharge	32	100%	90%	90%	100%
Beta Blocker at Arrival	57	100%	89%	87%	100%
Beta Blocker at Discharge	36	100%	89%	90%	100%
Fibrinolytic Medication Timing[1]	2	100%	40%	31%	100%
PCI Within 90 Minutes of Arrival	0	-	45%	54%	95%
Smoking Cessation Advice[1]	8	100%	79%	88%	100%
Heart Failure Care					
ACE Inhibitor or ARB for LVSD	106	96%	83%	82%	100%
Discharge Instructions	253	70%	44%	61%	93%
Evaluation of LVS Function	240	89%	77%	83%	99%
Smoking Cessation Advice	45	89%	74%	82%	100%
Pneumonia Care					
Appropriate Initial Antibiotic	139	89%	79%	83%	94%
Blood Culture Timing	225	94%	89%	90%	100%
Influenza Vaccine	64	86%	60%	70%	100%
Initial Antibiotic Timing	288	85%	78%	80%	93%
Oxygenation Assessment	345	100%	100%	99%	100%
Pneumococcal Vaccine	218	76%	50%	69%	94%
Smoking Cessation Advice	39	92%	63%	80%	100%
Surgical Infection Prevention					
Prophylactic Antibiotic Given[3]	226	81%	73%	77%	95%
Prophylactic Antibiotic Selection	84	98%	90%	90%	100%
Prophylactic Antibiotic Stopped[3]	219	41%	71%	72%	95%
Pregnancy Care					
Inpatient Neonatal Mortality	-	-	-	-	-
Third or Fourth Degree Laceration	-	-	-	3.63%	3.27%

Hawaii Medical Center West

91-2141 Fort Weaver Road
Ewa Beach, HI 96706
Ownership: Voluntary non-profit - Church
Emergency Services: Yes
Phone: 808-678-7000
Accredited: Yes

Measure	Cases	This Hospital	State Average	U.S. Average	Top Hospital
Heart Attack Care					
ACE Inhibitor or ARB for LVSD[1]	10	70%	76%	82%	100%
Aspirin at Arrival	68	91%	94%	92%	100%
Aspirin at Discharge	25	72%	90%	90%	100%
Beta Blocker at Arrival	56	84%	89%	87%	100%
Beta Blocker at Discharge	26	85%	89%	90%	100%
Fibrinolytic Medication Timing[1]	6	50%	40%	31%	100%
PCI Within 90 Minutes of Arrival	0	-	45%	54%	95%
Smoking Cessation Advice[1]	4	75%	79%	88%	100%
Heart Failure Care					
ACE Inhibitor or ARB for LVSD	78	82%	83%	82%	100%
Discharge Instructions	213	25%	44%	61%	93%
Evaluation of LVS Function	228	67%	77%	83%	99%
Smoking Cessation Advice	65	52%	74%	82%	100%
Pneumonia Care					
Appropriate Initial Antibiotic[2]	132	84%	79%	83%	94%
Blood Culture Timing[2]	155	92%	89%	90%	100%
Influenza Vaccine	41	51%	60%	70%	100%
Initial Antibiotic Timing[2]	241	85%	78%	80%	93%
Oxygenation Assessment[2]	264	100%	100%	99%	100%
Pneumococcal Vaccine[2]	161	30%	50%	69%	94%
Smoking Cessation Advice[2]	49	47%	63%	80%	100%
Surgical Infection Prevention					
Prophylactic Antibiotic Given	50	48%	73%	77%	95%
Prophylactic Antibiotic Selection[1]	13	77%	90%	90%	100%
Prophylactic Antibiotic Stopped	47	83%	71%	72%	95%
Pregnancy Care					
Inpatient Neonatal Mortality	-	-	-	-	-
Third or Fourth Degree Laceration	-	-	-	3.63%	3.27%

Hilo Medical Center

Alternate Name: Hilo Hospital
1190 Waianuenue Avenue
Hilo, HI 96720
E-mail: hhsc@hhsc.org
URL: www.hhsc.org
Ownership: Government - State
Emergency Services: Yes
Phone: 808-974-4700
Fax: 808-974-4746
Accredited: Yes
Licensed Beds: 275

Key Personnel:
President/CEO. . . . . Ronald Schurra
Chief of Medical Staff. . . . . Buddy Festerly
Infection Control. . . . . John Halloran, RN
Medical Surgery Nurse Manager . . . . Susan Poai, RN
Respiratory Therapy Manager . . . . Darrel Mosher

Measure	Cases	This Hospital	State Average	U.S. Average	Top Hospital
Heart Attack Care					
ACE Inhibitor or ARB for LVSD	31	84%	76%	82%	100%
Aspirin at Arrival	203	93%	94%	92%	100%
Aspirin at Discharge	165	88%	90%	90%	100%
Beta Blocker at Arrival	221	95%	89%	87%	100%
Beta Blocker at Discharge	180	90%	89%	90%	100%
Fibrinolytic Medication Timing[1]	8	38%	40%	31%	100%
PCI Within 90 Minutes of Arrival	0	-	45%	54%	95%
Smoking Cessation Advice	62	92%	79%	88%	100%
Heart Failure Care					
ACE Inhibitor or ARB for LVSD	50	78%	83%	82%	100%
Discharge Instructions	205	79%	44%	61%	93%
Evaluation of LVS Function	226	72%	77%	83%	99%
Smoking Cessation Advice	50	90%	74%	82%	100%
Pneumonia Care					
Appropriate Initial Antibiotic	119	73%	79%	83%	94%
Blood Culture Timing	91	90%	89%	90%	100%
Influenza Vaccine	28	29%	60%	70%	100%
Initial Antibiotic Timing	112	66%	78%	80%	93%
Oxygenation Assessment	197	99%	100%	99%	100%
Pneumococcal Vaccine	109	34%	50%	69%	94%
Smoking Cessation Advice	48	83%	63%	80%	100%
Surgical Infection Prevention					
Prophylactic Antibiotic Given[2]	126	75%	73%	77%	95%
Prophylactic Antibiotic Selection[2]	36	75%	90%	90%	100%
Prophylactic Antibiotic Stopped[2]	123	57%	71%	72%	95%
Pregnancy Care					
Inpatient Neonatal Mortality	-	-	-	-	-
Third or Fourth Degree Laceration	-	-	-	3.63%	3.27%

Hawaii Medical Center East

2230 Liliha Street
Honolulu, HI 96817
Ownership: Voluntary non-profit - Church
Emergency Services: Yes
Phone: 808-547-6011
Fax: 808-547-6611
Accredited: Yes
Licensed Beds: 308

Key Personnel:
CEO. . . . . Sr Beatrice Tom
Chief Medical Staff. . . . . Eugene Wong, MD
Cardiac Lab . . . . Kathy Nekomoto
Catheterization Lab . . . . Terri Burden
Emergency Room . . . . Lonni Matsusaka
Emergency Room . . . . Douglas Ostman, MD
Infection Control. . . . . Jim Reisen
Medical/Surgical Nursing . . . . Pat Kalua
Chief Radiology . . . . Lansdale Lau, MD
Director Respiratory Therapy . . . . Frank Rincon

Measure	Cases	This Hospital	State Average	U.S. Average	Top Hospital
Heart Attack Care					
ACE Inhibitor or ARB for LVSD	32	66%	76%	82%	100%
Aspirin at Arrival	86	95%	94%	92%	100%

NOTE: Hospital profiles are in alphabetical order by state, then city, then hospital within the city; Rankings are sorted by rate in descending order and exclude hospitals with less than 25 cases; (1) The number of cases is too small (n<25) for purposes of reliably predicting hospital performance; (2) Measure reflects the hospital's indication that its submission was based upon a sample of its relevant discharges; (3) Rate reflects fewer than the maximum possible quarters of data for the measure; (4) Inaccurate information submitted and suppressed for one or more quarters; (5) No data is available from the hospital for this measure; Please refer to the User's Guide for a full explanation of data

Measure	Cases	This Hospital	State Average	U.S. Average	Top Hospital
Aspirin at Discharge	169	95%	90%	90%	100%
Beta Blocker at Arrival	75	84%	89%	87%	100%
Beta Blocker at Discharge	171	95%	89%	90%	100%
Fibrinolytic Medication Timing[1]	2	50%	40%	31%	100%
PCI Within 90 Minutes of Arrival	0	-	45%	54%	95%
Smoking Cessation Advice	58	59%	79%	88%	100%
Heart Failure Care					
ACE Inhibitor or ARB for LVSD	71	86%	83%	82%	100%
Discharge Instructions	211	24%	44%	61%	93%
Evaluation of LVS Function	234	86%	77%	83%	99%
Smoking Cessation Advice	45	44%	74%	82%	100%
Pneumonia Care					
Appropriate Initial Antibiotic	94	77%	79%	83%	94%
Blood Culture Timing	96	85%	89%	90%	100%
Influenza Vaccine	40	75%	60%	70%	100%
Initial Antibiotic Timing	158	77%	78%	80%	93%
Oxygenation Assessment	204	100%	100%	99%	100%
Pneumococcal Vaccine	136	49%	50%	69%	94%
Smoking Cessation Advice	30	53%	63%	80%	100%
Surgical Infection Prevention					
Prophylactic Antibiotic Given[2]	261	79%	73%	77%	95%
Prophylactic Antibiotic Selection[2]	50	86%	90%	90%	100%
Prophylactic Antibiotic Stopped[2]	239	42%	71%	72%	95%
Pregnancy Care					
Inpatient Neonatal Mortality	-	-	-	-	-
Third or Fourth Degree Laceration	-	-	-	3.63%	3.27%

Kuakini Medical Center

347 North Kuakini Street
Honolulu, HI 96817
E-mail: pr@kuakini.org
URL: www.kuakini.org
Ownership: Voluntary non-profit - Private
Emergency Services: Yes
Phone: 808-536-2236
Fax: 808-547-9547
Accredited: Yes
Licensed Beds: 250

Key Personnel:
President/CEO . . . . Gary K Kajiwara

Measure	Cases	This Hospital	State Average	U.S. Average	Top Hospital
Heart Attack Care					
ACE Inhibitor or ARB for LVSD[1]	19	74%	76%	82%	100%
Aspirin at Arrival	73	93%	94%	92%	100%
Aspirin at Discharge	106	94%	90%	90%	100%
Beta Blocker at Arrival	53	89%	89%	87%	100%
Beta Blocker at Discharge	126	95%	89%	90%	100%
Fibrinolytic Medication Timing	0	-	40%	31%	100%
PCI Within 90 Minutes of Arrival[1]	2	50%	45%	54%	95%
Smoking Cessation Advice	33	82%	79%	88%	100%
Heart Failure Care					
ACE Inhibitor or ARB for LVSD	75	88%	83%	82%	100%
Discharge Instructions	159	31%	44%	61%	93%
Evaluation of LVS Function	172	94%	77%	83%	99%
Smoking Cessation Advice	26	81%	74%	82%	100%
Pneumonia Care					
Appropriate Initial Antibiotic[2]	105	89%	79%	83%	94%
Blood Culture Timing[2]	95	94%	89%	90%	100%
Influenza Vaccine	33	58%	60%	70%	100%
Initial Antibiotic Timing[2]	142	80%	78%	80%	93%
Oxygenation Assessment[2]	167	100%	100%	99%	100%
Pneumococcal Vaccine[2]	124	53%	50%	69%	94%
Smoking Cessation Advice[1,2]	16	62%	63%	80%	100%
Surgical Infection Prevention					
Prophylactic Antibiotic Given[2,3]	152	88%	73%	77%	95%
Prophylactic Antibiotic Selection[2]	46	91%	90%	90%	100%
Prophylactic Antibiotic Stopped[2,3]	150	66%	71%	72%	95%
Pregnancy Care					
Inpatient Neonatal Mortality	-	-	-	-	-
Third or Fourth Degree Laceration	-	-	-	3.63%	3.27%

Moanalua Medical Center and Clinic

3288 Moanalua Road
Honolulu, HI 96819
URL: www.kaiserpermanente.com
Ownership: Voluntary non-profit - Private
Emergency Services: Yes
Phone: 808-432-0000
Fax: 808-432-7736
Accredited: Yes
Licensed Beds: 202

Key Personnel:
Chief Medical Staff . . . . Martin Leftik, MD
CCU Spvg. Nurse . . . . Hazel Villegas
Director Medical/Surgical Nursing . . . . Paula Zencen
Chief OB/GYN . . . . Joyce Nakamura, MD
Chief Radiology . . . . Thomas Smith, MD
Director Respiratory Therapy . . . . Judy Morrell

Measure	Cases	This Hospital	State Average	U.S. Average	Top Hospital
Heart Attack Care					
ACE Inhibitor or ARB for LVSD	68	85%	76%	82%	100%
Aspirin at Arrival	173	97%	94%	92%	100%
Aspirin at Discharge	293	97%	90%	90%	100%
Beta Blocker at Arrival	160	96%	89%	87%	100%
Beta Blocker at Discharge	292	97%	89%	90%	100%
Fibrinolytic Medication Timing	0	-	40%	31%	100%
PCI Within 90 Minutes of Arrival[1]	4	100%	45%	54%	95%
Smoking Cessation Advice	65	92%	79%	88%	100%
Heart Failure Care					
ACE Inhibitor or ARB for LVSD	114	88%	83%	82%	100%
Discharge Instructions	270	38%	44%	61%	93%
Evaluation of LVS Function	275	96%	77%	83%	99%
Smoking Cessation Advice	41	95%	74%	82%	100%
Pneumonia Care					
Appropriate Initial Antibiotic	269	83%	79%	83%	94%
Blood Culture Timing	193	93%	89%	90%	100%
Influenza Vaccine	56	64%	60%	70%	100%
Initial Antibiotic Timing	266	77%	78%	80%	93%
Oxygenation Assessment	362	100%	100%	99%	100%
Pneumococcal Vaccine	251	89%	50%	69%	94%
Smoking Cessation Advice	47	60%	63%	80%	100%
Surgical Infection Prevention					
Prophylactic Antibiotic Given	537	80%	73%	77%	95%
Prophylactic Antibiotic Selection	147	99%	90%	90%	100%
Prophylactic Antibiotic Stopped	521	49%	71%	72%	95%
Pregnancy Care					
Inpatient Neonatal Mortality	1,931	0.67%	-	-	-
Third or Fourth Degree Laceration	1,435	4.81%	-	3.63%	3.27%

Straub Clinic and Hospital

888 S King Street
Honolulu, HI 96813
Ownership: Proprietary
Emergency Services: Yes
Phone: 808-522-4000
Fax: 808-522-4111
Accredited: Yes
Licensed Beds: 159

Key Personnel:
CEO . . . . Ray Vara
Chief of Medical Staff . . . . George McPheeters, MD
Cardiology . . . . Kym Kaohi
Emergency Room . . . . Sally Kamai, MD
Infection Control . . . . Diadema Bonnell
Director Medical/Surgical Nursing . . . . Marianne Yoshida, RN
OB/GYN Womens Health . . . . Simon Chang
Surgical Services . . . . Clara McIntosh, RN
Chief Radiology . . . . Robert May, MD
Respiratory . . . . Glenda Kaalakea

Measure	Cases	This Hospital	State Average	U.S. Average	Top Hospital
Heart Attack Care					
ACE Inhibitor or ARB for LVSD	69	62%	76%	82%	100%
Aspirin at Arrival	158	97%	94%	92%	100%
Aspirin at Discharge	277	94%	90%	90%	100%
Beta Blocker at Arrival	137	97%	89%	87%	100%
Beta Blocker at Discharge	267	94%	89%	90%	100%
Fibrinolytic Medication Timing[1]	6	67%	40%	31%	100%
PCI Within 90 Minutes of Arrival[1]	4	50%	45%	54%	95%
Smoking Cessation Advice	73	84%	79%	88%	100%
Heart Failure Care					

NOTE: Hospital profiles are in alphabetical order by state, then city, then hospital within the city; Rankings are sorted by rate in descending order and exclude hospitals with less than 25 cases; (1) The number of cases is too small (n<25) for purposes of reliably predicting hospital performance; (2) Measure reflects the hospital's indication that its submission was based upon a sample of its relevant discharges; (3) Rate reflects fewer than the maximum possible quarters of data for the measure; (4) Inaccurate information submitted and suppressed for one or more quarters; (5) No data is available from the hospital for this measure; Please refer to the User's Guide for a full explanation of data

Measure	Cases	This Hospital	State Average	U.S. Average	Top Hospital
ACE Inhibitor or ARB for LVSD	107	72%	83%	82%	100%
Discharge Instructions	207	36%	44%	61%	93%
Evaluation of LVS Function	229	91%	77%	83%	99%
Smoking Cessation Advice[1]	24	58%	74%	82%	100%
Pneumonia Care					
Appropriate Initial Antibiotic[2]	131	61%	79%	83%	94%
Blood Culture Timing[2]	152	91%	89%	90%	100%
Influenza Vaccine[2]	38	82%	60%	70%	100%
Initial Antibiotic Timing[2]	182	71%	78%	80%	93%
Oxygenation Assessment[2]	223	100%	100%	99%	100%
Pneumococcal Vaccine[2]	156	62%	50%	69%	94%
Smoking Cessation Advice[1,2]	20	30%	63%	80%	100%
Surgical Infection Prevention					
Prophylactic Antibiotic Given[2,3]	125	88%	73%	77%	95%
Prophylactic Antibiotic Selection[2]	77	96%	90%	90%	100%
Prophylactic Antibiotic Stopped[2,3]	119	87%	71%	72%	95%
Pregnancy Care					
Inpatient Neonatal Mortality	-	-	-	-	-
Third or Fourth Degree Laceration	-	-	-	3.63%	3.27%

The Queen's Medical Center

1301 Punchbowl Street
Honolulu, HI 96813
URL: www.queens.org
Ownership: Voluntary non-profit - Other
Emergency Services: Yes
Phone: 808-538-9011
Fax: 808-537-7887
Accredited: Yes
Licensed Beds: 505

Key Personnel:
President/CEO. . . . . Arthur A Ushijima

Measure	Cases	This Hospital	State Average	U.S. Average	Top Hospital
Heart Attack Care					
ACE Inhibitor or ARB for LVSD	88	86%	76%	82%	100%
Aspirin at Arrival	242	95%	94%	92%	100%
Aspirin at Discharge	400	96%	90%	90%	100%
Beta Blocker at Arrival	173	98%	89%	87%	100%
Beta Blocker at Discharge	390	98%	89%	90%	100%
Fibrinolytic Medication Timing[1]	4	25%	40%	31%	100%
PCI Within 90 Minutes of Arrival[1]	13	23%	45%	54%	95%
Smoking Cessation Advice	131	92%	79%	88%	100%
Heart Failure Care					
ACE Inhibitor or ARB for LVSD[2]	293	88%	83%	82%	100%
Discharge Instructions[2]	482	78%	44%	61%	93%
Evaluation of LVS Function[2]	515	93%	77%	83%	99%
Smoking Cessation Advice[2]	113	94%	74%	82%	100%
Pneumonia Care					
Appropriate Initial Antibiotic	245	83%	79%	83%	94%
Blood Culture Timing	262	83%	89%	90%	100%
Influenza Vaccine	75	53%	60%	70%	100%
Initial Antibiotic Timing	319	73%	78%	80%	93%
Oxygenation Assessment	413	100%	100%	99%	100%
Pneumococcal Vaccine	234	58%	50%	69%	94%
Smoking Cessation Advice	81	77%	63%	80%	100%
Surgical Infection Prevention					
Prophylactic Antibiotic Given[2,3]	1,018	88%	73%	77%	95%
Prophylactic Antibiotic Selection[2]	373	97%	90%	90%	100%
Prophylactic Antibiotic Stopped[2,3]	993	85%	71%	72%	95%
Pregnancy Care					
Inpatient Neonatal Mortality	2,275	0.04%	-	-	-
Third or Fourth Degree Laceration	1,744	5.45%	-	3.63%	3.27%

Castle Medical Center

640 Ulukahiki Street
Kailua, HI 96734
URL: www.castlemed.com
Ownership: Voluntary non-profit - Church
Emergency Services: Yes
Phone: 808-263-5500
Fax: 808-263-5123
Accredited: Yes
Licensed Beds: 160

Key Personnel:
President/CEO. . . . . Kevin A Roberts, FACHE
Director Medical/Surgical Nursing . . . . Donna Awana, RN
Director Cardio-Pulmonary Services . . . . Ron Sanderson

Measure	Cases	This Hospital	State Average	U.S. Average	Top Hospital
Heart Attack Care					
ACE Inhibitor or ARB for LVSD[1]	15	67%	76%	82%	100%
Aspirin at Arrival	130	98%	94%	92%	100%
Aspirin at Discharge	104	96%	90%	90%	100%
Beta Blocker at Arrival	85	95%	89%	87%	100%
Beta Blocker at Discharge	108	95%	89%	90%	100%
Fibrinolytic Medication Timing	0	-	40%	31%	100%
PCI Within 90 Minutes of Arrival[1]	2	0%	45%	54%	95%
Smoking Cessation Advice	32	91%	79%	88%	100%
Heart Failure Care					
ACE Inhibitor or ARB for LVSD	54	76%	83%	82%	100%
Discharge Instructions	249	86%	44%	61%	93%
Evaluation of LVS Function	256	85%	77%	83%	99%
Smoking Cessation Advice	43	86%	74%	82%	100%
Pneumonia Care					
Appropriate Initial Antibiotic	119	81%	79%	83%	94%
Blood Culture Timing	128	95%	89%	90%	100%
Influenza Vaccine	34	68%	60%	70%	100%
Initial Antibiotic Timing	147	82%	78%	80%	93%
Oxygenation Assessment	178	99%	100%	99%	100%
Pneumococcal Vaccine	95	75%	50%	69%	94%
Smoking Cessation Advice	37	95%	63%	80%	100%
Surgical Infection Prevention					
Prophylactic Antibiotic Given[2,3]	100	93%	73%	77%	95%
Prophylactic Antibiotic Selection[2]	39	92%	90%	90%	100%
Prophylactic Antibiotic Stopped[2,3]	100	76%	71%	72%	95%
Pregnancy Care					
Inpatient Neonatal Mortality	-	-	-	-	-
Third or Fourth Degree Laceration	-	-	-	3.63%	3.27%

North Hawaii Community Hospital

67-125 Mamalohoa Highway
Kamuela, HI 96743
URL: www.northhawaiicommunityhospital.org
Ownership: Voluntary non-profit - Private
Emergency Services: Yes
Phone: 808-885-4444
Fax: 808-881-4415
Accredited: Yes
Licensed Beds: 40

Key Personnel:
CEO. . . . . Stan Berry

Measure	Cases	This Hospital	State Average	U.S. Average	Top Hospital
Heart Attack Care					
ACE Inhibitor or ARB for LVSD[1]	2	50%	76%	82%	100%
Aspirin at Arrival	25	88%	94%	92%	100%
Aspirin at Discharge[1]	11	73%	90%	90%	100%
Beta Blocker at Arrival	26	85%	89%	87%	100%
Beta Blocker at Discharge[1]	12	83%	89%	90%	100%
Fibrinolytic Medication Timing[1]	5	40%	40%	31%	100%
PCI Within 90 Minutes of Arrival	0	-	45%	54%	95%
Smoking Cessation Advice[1]	2	0%	79%	88%	100%
Heart Failure Care					
ACE Inhibitor or ARB for LVSD[1]	16	100%	83%	82%	100%
Discharge Instructions	61	23%	44%	61%	93%
Evaluation of LVS Function	53	77%	77%	83%	99%
Smoking Cessation Advice[1]	10	50%	74%	82%	100%
Pneumonia Care					
Appropriate Initial Antibiotic	56	52%	79%	83%	94%
Blood Culture Timing	35	91%	89%	90%	100%
Influenza Vaccine[1]	18	28%	60%	70%	100%
Initial Antibiotic Timing	50	72%	78%	80%	93%
Oxygenation Assessment	65	100%	100%	99%	100%
Pneumococcal Vaccine	41	24%	50%	69%	94%
Smoking Cessation Advice[1]	11	45%	63%	80%	100%
Surgical Infection Prevention					
Prophylactic Antibiotic Given[3]	38	84%	73%	77%	95%
Prophylactic Antibiotic Selection[1]	18	89%	90%	90%	100%
Prophylactic Antibiotic Stopped[3]	35	69%	71%	72%	95%
Pregnancy Care					
Inpatient Neonatal Mortality	-	-	-	-	-
Third or Fourth Degree Laceration	-	-	-	3.63%	3.27%

Kona Community Hospital

Alternate Name: Kona Hospital

NOTE: Hospital profiles are in alphabetical order by state, then city, then hospital within the city; Rankings are sorted by rate in descending order and exclude hospitals with less than 25 cases; (1) The number of cases is too small (n<25) for purposes of reliably predicting hospital performance; (2) Measure reflects the hospital's indication that its submission was based upon a sample of its relevant discharges; (3) Rate reflects fewer than the maximum possible quarters of data for the measure; (4) Inaccurate information submitted and suppressed for one or more quarters; (5) No data is available from the hospital for this measure; Please refer to the User's Guide for a full explanation of data

79-1019 Haukapila Street
Kealakekua, HI 96750
URL: www.kch.hhsc.org
Ownership: Government - State
Emergency Services: Yes

Phone: 808-322-9311
Fax: 808-322-4488
Accredited: Yes
Licensed Beds: 94

Key Personnel:

CEO. . . . . Donald Lewis
Chief of Medical Staff. . . . . Lawrence Peebles
Emergency Room . . . . Richard McDowell, MD
Surgical Services Nurse Manager . . . . Dawn Brewer

Measure	Cases	This Hospital	State Average	U.S. Average	Top Hospital
Heart Attack Care					
ACE Inhibitor or ARB for LVSD	0	-	76%	82%	100%
Aspirin at Arrival	29	93%	94%	92%	100%
Aspirin at Discharge[1]	13	92%	90%	90%	100%
Beta Blocker at Arrival	29	69%	89%	87%	100%
Beta Blocker at Discharge[1]	13	62%	89%	90%	100%
Fibrinolytic Medication Timing[1]	1	0%	40%	31%	100%
PCI Within 90 Minutes of Arrival	0	-	45%	54%	95%
Smoking Cessation Advice	0	-	79%	88%	100%
Heart Failure Care					
ACE Inhibitor or ARB for LVSD	25	68%	83%	82%	100%
Discharge Instructions	70	21%	44%	61%	93%
Evaluation of LVS Function	80	64%	77%	83%	99%
Smoking Cessation Advice[1]	10	50%	74%	82%	100%
Pneumonia Care					
Appropriate Initial Antibiotic	95	94%	79%	83%	94%
Blood Culture Timing	70	94%	89%	90%	100%
Influenza Vaccine[1]	14	43%	60%	70%	100%
Initial Antibiotic Timing	88	81%	78%	80%	93%
Oxygenation Assessment	130	100%	100%	99%	100%
Pneumococcal Vaccine	69	26%	50%	69%	94%
Smoking Cessation Advice[1]	22	32%	63%	80%	100%
Surgical Infection Prevention					
Prophylactic Antibiotic Given[3]	49	90%	73%	77%	95%
Prophylactic Antibiotic Selection[1]	18	100%	90%	90%	100%
Prophylactic Antibiotic Stopped[3]	28	89%	71%	72%	95%
Pregnancy Care					
Inpatient Neonatal Mortality	-	-	-	-	-
Third or Fourth Degree Laceration	-	-	-	3.63%	3.27%

Kula Hospital

100 Keokea Place
Kula, HI 96790
Ownership: Proprietary
Emergency Services: Yes

Phone: 808-878-1221
Fax: 808-878-1791
Accredited: No
Licensed Beds: 110

Key Personnel:

CEO. . . . . John Schaumburg
Chief Medical Staff. . . . . Albert Yazawa, MD

Measure	Cases	This Hospital	State Average	U.S. Average	Top Hospital
Heart Attack Care					
ACE Inhibitor or ARB for LVSD[5]	-	-	76%	82%	100%
Aspirin at Arrival[5]	-	-	94%	92%	100%
Aspirin at Discharge[5]	-	-	90%	90%	100%
Beta Blocker at Arrival[5]	-	-	89%	87%	100%
Beta Blocker at Discharge[5]	-	-	89%	90%	100%
Fibrinolytic Medication Timing[5]	-	-	40%	31%	100%
PCI Within 90 Minutes of Arrival[5]	-	-	45%	54%	95%
Smoking Cessation Advice[5]	-	-	79%	88%	100%
Heart Failure Care					
ACE Inhibitor or ARB for LVSD[3]	0	-	83%	82%	100%
Discharge Instructions[1,3]	1	0%	44%	61%	93%
Evaluation of LVS Function[1,3]	1	0%	77%	83%	99%
Smoking Cessation Advice[3]	0	-	74%	82%	100%
Pneumonia Care					
Appropriate Initial Antibiotic[5]	-	-	79%	83%	94%
Blood Culture Timing[5]	-	-	89%	90%	100%
Influenza Vaccine[5]	-	-	60%	70%	100%
Initial Antibiotic Timing[5]	-	-	78%	80%	93%
Oxygenation Assessment[5]	-	-	100%	99%	100%
Pneumococcal Vaccine[5]	-	-	50%	69%	94%
Smoking Cessation Advice[5]	-	-	63%	80%	100%
Surgical Infection Prevention					
Prophylactic Antibiotic Given[5]	-	-	73%	77%	95%
Prophylactic Antibiotic Selection[5]	-	-	90%	90%	100%
Prophylactic Antibiotic Stopped[5]	-	-	71%	72%	95%
Pregnancy Care					
Inpatient Neonatal Mortality	-	-	-	-	-
Third or Fourth Degree Laceration	-	-	-	3.63%	3.27%

Wilcox Memorial Hospital

3-3420 Kuhio Highway
Lihue, HI 96766
URL: www.wilcoxhealth.org
Ownership: Government - Federal
Emergency Services: Yes

Phone: 808-245-1100
Fax: 808-245-1211
Accredited: Yes
Licensed Beds: 86

Key Personnel:

EVP/Chief Medical Officer . . . . Kenneth B Robbins, MD
Emergency Room . . . . Linda Leavitt, RN
Director Medical/Surgical Nursing . . . . C Michele Ferguson, RN
Director Radiology . . . . Larry R Wampler, MD

Measure	Cases	This Hospital	State Average	U.S. Average	Top Hospital
Heart Attack Care					
ACE Inhibitor or ARB for LVSD[1]	8	88%	76%	82%	100%
Aspirin at Arrival	34	94%	94%	92%	100%
Aspirin at Discharge[1]	11	100%	90%	90%	100%
Beta Blocker at Arrival	29	86%	89%	87%	100%
Beta Blocker at Discharge[1]	14	86%	89%	90%	100%
Fibrinolytic Medication Timing[1]	6	17%	40%	31%	100%
PCI Within 90 Minutes of Arrival	0	-	45%	54%	95%
Smoking Cessation Advice[1]	1	100%	79%	88%	100%
Heart Failure Care					
ACE Inhibitor or ARB for LVSD	56	77%	83%	82%	100%
Discharge Instructions	92	34%	44%	61%	93%
Evaluation of LVS Function	95	85%	77%	83%	99%
Smoking Cessation Advice[1]	21	90%	74%	82%	100%
Pneumonia Care					
Appropriate Initial Antibiotic	75	76%	79%	83%	94%
Blood Culture Timing	59	80%	89%	90%	100%
Influenza Vaccine[1]	19	84%	60%	70%	100%
Initial Antibiotic Timing	80	71%	78%	80%	93%
Oxygenation Assessment	109	100%	100%	99%	100%
Pneumococcal Vaccine	68	59%	50%	69%	94%
Smoking Cessation Advice[1]	20	85%	63%	80%	100%
Surgical Infection Prevention					
Prophylactic Antibiotic Given[2,3]	30	53%	73%	77%	95%
Prophylactic Antibiotic Selection[2]	29	90%	90%	90%	100%
Prophylactic Antibiotic Stopped[2,3]	29	100%	71%	72%	95%
Pregnancy Care					
Inpatient Neonatal Mortality	-	-	-	-	-
Third or Fourth Degree Laceration	-	-	-	3.63%	3.27%

Wahiawa General Hospital

128 Lehua Street
Wahiawa, HI 96786
E-mail: ContactUs@wahiawageneral.org
URL: www.wahiawageneral.org
Ownership: Voluntary non-profit - Private
Emergency Services: Yes

Phone: 808-621-8411
Fax: 808-621-4451
Accredited: Yes
Licensed Beds: 162

Key Personnel:

CEO. . . . . Jack Julius
Chief Medical Staff. . . . . Dan Tamashiro, MD
Chief Medical Staff. . . . . Leo Pastua
OB/GYN Womens Health. . . . . Sheryl Gardner, MD

Measure	Cases	This Hospital	State Average	U.S. Average	Top Hospital
Heart Attack Care					
ACE Inhibitor or ARB for LVSD[1]	4	75%	76%	82%	100%
Aspirin at Arrival[1]	24	88%	94%	92%	100%
Aspirin at Discharge[1]	12	67%	90%	90%	100%
Beta Blocker at Arrival[1]	23	70%	89%	87%	100%

NOTE: Hospital profiles are in alphabetical order by state, then city, then hospital within the city; Rankings are sorted by rate in descending order and exclude hospitals with less than 25 cases; (1) The number of cases is too small (n<25) for purposes of reliably predicting hospital performance; (2) Measure reflects the hospital's indication that its submission was based upon a sample of its relevant discharges; (3) Rate reflects fewer than the maximum possible quarters of data for the measure; (4) Inaccurate information submitted and suppressed for one or more quarters; (5) No data is available from the hospital for this measure; Please refer to the User's Guide for a full explanation of data

Beta Blocker at Discharge[1]	12	75%	89%	90%	100%
Fibrinolytic Medication Timing[1]	1	0%	40%	31%	100%
PCI Within 90 Minutes of Arrival	0	-	45%	54%	95%
Smoking Cessation Advice[1]	4	100%	79%	88%	100%
Heart Failure Care					
ACE Inhibitor or ARB for LVSD[1]	20	85%	83%	82%	100%
Discharge Instructions	79	71%	44%	61%	93%
Evaluation of LVS Function	81	70%	77%	83%	99%
Smoking Cessation Advice[1]	13	85%	74%	82%	100%
Pneumonia Care					
Appropriate Initial Antibiotic	42	88%	79%	83%	94%
Blood Culture Timing	35	69%	89%	90%	100%
Influenza Vaccine[1]	8	50%	60%	70%	100%
Initial Antibiotic Timing	46	87%	78%	80%	93%
Oxygenation Assessment	55	100%	100%	99%	100%
Pneumococcal Vaccine	33	15%	50%	69%	94%
Smoking Cessation Advice[1]	7	29%	63%	80%	100%
Surgical Infection Prevention					
Prophylactic Antibiotic Given[1,3]	11	9%	73%	77%	95%
Prophylactic Antibiotic Selection[1]	4	75%	90%	90%	100%
Prophylactic Antibiotic Stopped[1,3]	10	90%	71%	72%	95%
Pregnancy Care					
Inpatient Neonatal Mortality	-	-	-	-	-
Third or Fourth Degree Laceration	-	-	-	3.63%	3.27%

Maui Memorial Hospital

221 Mahalani Street
Wailuku, HI 96793
Ownership: Government - State
Emergency Services: Yes

Phone: 808-244-9056
Fax: 808-243-4628
Accredited: Yes
Licensed Beds: 191

Key Personnel:

CEO. . . . . Wesley Lo
Chief Medical Staff. . . . . Darren Egamia, MD
Director of Cardiology/Cardiac Lab. . . . . Mark Schwak, MD
Emergency Room . . . . EmiLou Alves
OB/GYN Womens Health. . . . . Nancy Rogers, MD
Chief Radiology . . . . Leerge Miyasato
Director Respiratory Therapy . . . . Sandra Saiki

Measure	Cases	This Hospital	State Average	U.S. Average	Top Hospital
Heart Attack Care					
ACE Inhibitor or ARB for LVSD	25	88%	76%	82%	100%
Aspirin at Arrival	135	95%	94%	92%	100%
Aspirin at Discharge	68	94%	90%	90%	100%
Beta Blocker at Arrival	118	93%	89%	87%	100%
Beta Blocker at Discharge	69	91%	89%	90%	100%
Fibrinolytic Medication Timing[1]	18	50%	40%	31%	100%
PCI Within 90 Minutes of Arrival	0	-	45%	54%	95%
Smoking Cessation Advice[1]	8	62%	79%	88%	100%
Heart Failure Care					
ACE Inhibitor or ARB for LVSD	143	82%	83%	82%	100%
Discharge Instructions	277	43%	44%	61%	93%
Evaluation of LVS Function	283	85%	77%	83%	99%
Smoking Cessation Advice	44	68%	74%	82%	100%
Pneumonia Care					
Appropriate Initial Antibiotic	148	79%	79%	83%	94%
Blood Culture Timing	101	90%	89%	90%	100%
Influenza Vaccine	31	65%	60%	70%	100%
Initial Antibiotic Timing	185	88%	78%	80%	93%
Oxygenation Assessment	227	100%	100%	99%	100%
Pneumococcal Vaccine	154	47%	50%	69%	94%
Smoking Cessation Advice	45	96%	63%	80%	100%
Surgical Infection Prevention					
Prophylactic Antibiotic Given	249	71%	73%	77%	95%
Prophylactic Antibiotic Selection	54	93%	90%	90%	100%
Prophylactic Antibiotic Stopped	240	61%	71%	72%	95%
Pregnancy Care					
Inpatient Neonatal Mortality	-	-	-	-	-
Third or Fourth Degree Laceration	-	-	-	3.63%	3.27%

NOTE: Hospital profiles are in alphabetical order by state, then city, then hospital within the city; Rankings are sorted by rate in descending order and exclude hospitals with less than 25 cases; (1) The number of cases is too small (n<25) for purposes of reliably predicting hospital performance; (2) Measure reflects the hospital's indication that its submission was based upon a sample of its relevant discharges; (3) Rate reflects fewer than the maximum possible quarters of data for the measure; (4) Inaccurate information submitted and suppressed for one or more quarters; (5) No data is available from the hospital for this measure; Please refer to the User's Guide for a full explanation of data

Heart Attack Care

1. ACE Inhibitor or ARB for LVSD

Hospital Name	City	Rate	Cases
Kootenai Medical Center	Coeur d'Alene	100%	26
Saint Alphonsus Regional Medical Center	Boise	100%	31
Magic Valley Regional Medical Center	Twin Falls	95%	38
Saint Luke's Regional Medical Center	Boise	95%	58
Portneuf Medical Center	Pocatello	65%	26

2. Aspirin at Arrival

Hospital Name	City	Rate	Cases
Mercy Medical Center	Nampa	100%	95
Kootenai Medical Center	Coeur d'Alene	99%	171
Saint Alphonsus Regional Medical Center	Boise	99%	151
Saint Luke's Regional Medical Center	Boise	99%	144
Eastern Idaho Regional Medical Center	Idaho Falls	98%	109
Portneuf Medical Center	Pocatello	97%	98
Magic Valley Regional Medical Center	Twin Falls	96%	101
West Valley Medical Center	Caldwell	89%	27

3. Aspirin at Discharge

Hospital Name	City	Rate	Cases
Kootenai Medical Center	Coeur d'Alene	100%	222
Mercy Medical Center	Nampa	100%	87
Saint Luke's Regional Medical Center	Boise	100%	387
Saint Alphonsus Regional Medical Center	Boise	99%	285
Eastern Idaho Regional Medical Center	Idaho Falls	98%	205
Portneuf Medical Center	Pocatello	98%	120
Magic Valley Regional Medical Center	Twin Falls	97%	109

4. Beta Blocker at Arrival

Hospital Name	City	Rate	Cases
Mercy Medical Center	Nampa	100%	85
Saint Luke's Regional Medical Center	Boise	100%	136
Saint Alphonsus Regional Medical Center	Boise	99%	137
Magic Valley Regional Medical Center	Twin Falls	97%	86
Eastern Idaho Regional Medical Center	Idaho Falls	95%	78
Kootenai Medical Center	Coeur d'Alene	94%	125
Portneuf Medical Center	Pocatello	93%	69
West Valley Medical Center	Caldwell	75%	28

5. Beta Blocker at Discharge

Hospital Name	City	Rate	Cases
Mercy Medical Center	Nampa	100%	81
Saint Luke's Regional Medical Center	Boise	100%	373
Saint Alphonsus Regional Medical Center	Boise	99%	276
Eastern Idaho Regional Medical Center	Idaho Falls	98%	205
Kootenai Medical Center	Coeur d'Alene	98%	189
Magic Valley Regional Medical Center	Twin Falls	98%	135
Portneuf Medical Center	Pocatello	94%	109

8. Smoking Cessation Advice

Hospital Name	City	Rate	Cases
Kootenai Medical Center	Coeur d'Alene	100%	80
Mercy Medical Center	Nampa	100%	32
Saint Luke's Regional Medical Center	Boise	100%	141
Saint Alphonsus Regional Medical Center	Boise	99%	92
Magic Valley Regional Medical Center	Twin Falls	96%	28
Eastern Idaho Regional Medical Center	Idaho Falls	93%	69
Portneuf Medical Center	Pocatello	92%	38

Heart Failure Care

9. ACE Inhibitor or ARB for LVSD

Hospital Name	City	Rate	Cases
Kootenai Medical Center	Coeur d'Alene	98%	46
Saint Alphonsus Regional Medical Center	Boise	95%	87
Magic Valley Regional Medical Center	Twin Falls	91%	32
Saint Luke's Regional Medical Center	Boise	88%	148
Saint Joseph Regional Medical Center	Lewiston	78%	32
West Valley Medical Center	Caldwell	76%	25
Eastern Idaho Regional Medical Center	Idaho Falls	74%	46
Portneuf Medical Center	Pocatello	71%	58

10. Discharge Instructions

Hospital Name	City	Rate	Cases
Mercy Medical Center	Nampa	94%	72
Saint Luke's Regional Medical Center	Boise	90%	284
Saint Alphonsus Regional Medical Center	Boise	85%	184
Eastern Idaho Regional Medical Center	Idaho Falls	81%	139
Kootenai Medical Center	Coeur d'Alene	75%	158
Cassia Regional Medical Center	Burley	72%	65
Magic Valley Regional Medical Center	Twin Falls	69%	58
Saint Joseph Regional Medical Center	Lewiston	67%	55
West Valley Medical Center	Caldwell	62%	80
Bonner General Hospital	Sandpoint	60%	35
Madison Memorial Hospital	Rexburg	36%	25
Portneuf Medical Center	Pocatello	12%	150

11. Evaluation of LVS Function

Hospital Name	City	Rate	Cases
Saint Alphonsus Regional Medical Center	Boise	98%	228
Kootenai Medical Center	Coeur d'Alene	97%	201
Mercy Medical Center	Nampa	96%	96
Saint Luke's Regional Medical Center	Boise	96%	345
Magic Valley Regional Medical Center	Twin Falls	92%	120
West Valley Medical Center	Caldwell	92%	98
Bonner General Hospital	Sandpoint	91%	43
Saint Joseph Regional Medical Center	Lewiston	86%	81
Eastern Idaho Regional Medical Center	Idaho Falls	81%	177
Portneuf Medical Center	Pocatello	76%	169
Cassia Regional Medical Center	Burley	70%	81
Madison Memorial Hospital	Rexburg	55%	33

12. Smoking Cessation Advice

Hospital Name	City	Rate	Cases
Kootenai Medical Center	Coeur d'Alene	97%	39
Saint Luke's Regional Medical Center	Boise	94%	52
Eastern Idaho Regional Medical Center	Idaho Falls	93%	27
Saint Alphonsus Regional Medical Center	Boise	88%	25
Portneuf Medical Center	Pocatello	76%	29
West Valley Medical Center	Caldwell	76%	29

Pneumonia Care

13. Appropriate Initial Antibiotic

Hospital Name	City	Rate	Cases
Magic Valley Regional Medical Center	Twin Falls	96%	27
Kootenai Medical Center	Coeur d'Alene	92%	185
Saint Luke's Medical Center	Ketchum	92%	25
Mercy Medical Center	Nampa	91%	151
Saint Alphonsus Regional Medical Center	Boise	91%	108
Saint Luke's Regional Medical Center	Boise	91%	270
Madison Memorial Hospital	Rexburg	89%	54
Saint Joseph Regional Medical Center	Lewiston	89%	66
Eastern Idaho Regional Medical Center	Idaho Falls	86%	160
Cassia Regional Medical Center	Burley	85%	65
Portneuf Medical Center	Pocatello	85%	136
West Valley Medical Center	Caldwell	84%	103
Bonner General Hospital	Sandpoint	68%	31

14. Blood Culture Timing

Hospital Name	City	Rate	Cases
Cassia Regional Medical Center	Burley	96%	45
Magic Valley Regional Medical Center	Twin Falls	96%	188
Mercy Medical Center	Nampa	96%	114
Saint Joseph Regional Medical Center	Lewiston	95%	83
Portneuf Medical Center	Pocatello	94%	145
Kootenai Medical Center	Coeur d'Alene	92%	117
Saint Luke's Regional Medical Center	Boise	91%	245
West Valley Medical Center	Caldwell	89%	55
Saint Alphonsus Regional Medical Center	Boise	88%	116
Eastern Idaho Regional Medical Center	Idaho Falls	87%	121

15. Influenza Vaccine

Hospital Name	City	Rate	Cases
Mercy Medical Center	Nampa	97%	38
Eastern Idaho Regional Medical Center	Idaho Falls	89%	45
Saint Joseph Regional Medical Center	Lewiston	75%	28
Portneuf Medical Center	Pocatello	66%	32
West Valley Medical Center	Caldwell	57%	28
Saint Luke's Regional Medical Center	Boise	54%	74
Kootenai Medical Center	Coeur d'Alene	53%	49

16. Initial Antibiotic Timing

Hospital Name	City	Rate	Cases
Madison Memorial Hospital	Rexburg	98%	49
Magic Valley Regional Medical Center	Twin Falls	93%	282
Kootenai Medical Center	Coeur d'Alene	91%	267
Saint Alphonsus Regional Medical Center	Boise	91%	187

NOTE: Hospital profiles are in alphabetical order by state, then city, then hospital within the city; Rankings are sorted by rate in descending order and exclude hospitals with less than 25 cases; (1) The number of cases is too small (n<25) for purposes of reliably predicting hospital performance; (2) Measure reflects the hospital's indication that its submission was based upon a sample of its relevant discharges; (3) Rate reflects fewer than the maximum possible quarters of data for the measure; (4) Inaccurate information submitted and suppressed for one or more quarters; (5) No data is available from the hospital for this measure; Please refer to the User's Guide for a full explanation of data

Hospital Name	City	Rate	Cases
Saint Luke's Regional Medical Center	Boise	88%	328
West Valley Medical Center	Caldwell	87%	128
Mercy Medical Center	Nampa	83%	183
Saint Joseph Regional Medical Center	Lewiston	78%	92
Eastern Idaho Regional Medical Center	Idaho Falls	77%	230
Bonner General Hospital	Sandpoint	76%	34
Cassia Regional Medical Center	Burley	66%	67
Portneuf Medical Center	Pocatello	59%	212

17. Oxygenation Assessment

Hospital Name	City	Rate	Cases
Bonner General Hospital	Sandpoint	100%	44
Cassia Regional Medical Center	Burley	100%	86
Eastern Idaho Regional Medical Center	Idaho Falls	100%	299
Kootenai Medical Center	Coeur d'Alene	100%	330
Madison Memorial Hospital	Rexburg	100%	62
Magic Valley Regional Medical Center	Twin Falls	100%	333
Mercy Medical Center	Nampa	100%	215
Portneuf Medical Center	Pocatello	100%	246
Saint Alphonsus Regional Medical Center	Boise	100%	237
Saint Luke's Medical Center	Ketchum	100%	32
Saint Luke's Regional Medical Center	Boise	100%	403
West Valley Medical Center	Caldwell	100%	145
Saint Joseph Regional Medical Center	Lewiston	99%	148

18. Pneumococcal Vaccine

Hospital Name	City	Rate	Cases
Mercy Medical Center	Nampa	92%	122
Saint Alphonsus Regional Medical Center	Boise	91%	153
West Valley Medical Center	Caldwell	85%	104
Eastern Idaho Regional Medical Center	Idaho Falls	83%	183
Madison Memorial Hospital	Rexburg	83%	36
Magic Valley Regional Medical Center	Twin Falls	76%	210
Cassia Regional Medical Center	Burley	73%	60
Kootenai Medical Center	Coeur d'Alene	73%	226
Saint Luke's Regional Medical Center	Boise	67%	280
Bonner General Hospital	Sandpoint	62%	29
Portneuf Medical Center	Pocatello	60%	150
Saint Joseph Regional Medical Center	Lewiston	43%	95

19. Smoking Cessation Advice

Hospital Name	City	Rate	Cases
Mercy Medical Center	Nampa	98%	52
Kootenai Medical Center	Coeur d'Alene	93%	74
Saint Alphonsus Regional Medical Center	Boise	92%	76
Magic Valley Regional Medical Center	Twin Falls	91%	64
Portneuf Medical Center	Pocatello	88%	73
Saint Luke's Regional Medical Center	Boise	85%	102
Saint Joseph Regional Medical Center	Lewiston	67%	27
Eastern Idaho Regional Medical Center	Idaho Falls	61%	79
West Valley Medical Center	Caldwell	60%	48

Surgical Infection Prevention

20. Prophylactic Antibiotic Given

Hospital Name	City	Rate	Cases
Healthsouth Treasure Valley Hospital	Boise	100%	49
Eastern Idaho Regional Medical Center	Idaho Falls	93%	208
Mercy Medical Center	Nampa	93%	190
Saint Alphonsus Regional Medical Center	Boise	91%	358
Saint Luke's Regional Medical Center	Boise	91%	518
Northwest Specialty Hospital	Post Falls	89%	103
Bonner General Hospital	Sandpoint	88%	93
Saint Joseph Regional Medical Center	Lewiston	86%	429
Kootenai Medical Center	Coeur d'Alene	85%	866
Portneuf Medical Center	Pocatello	83%	510
West Valley Medical Center	Caldwell	80%	117
Cassia Regional Medical Center	Burley	79%	175
Madison Memorial Hospital	Rexburg	76%	177
Magic Valley Regional Medical Center	Twin Falls	66%	53
Mountain View Hospital	Idaho Falls	52%	33

21. Prophylactic Antibiotic Selection

Hospital Name	City	Rate	Cases
Bonner General Hospital	Sandpoint	100%	34
Mercy Medical Center	Nampa	98%	57
Mountain View Hospital	Idaho Falls	97%	33
Saint Luke's Regional Medical Center	Boise	96%	522
Cassia Regional Medical Center	Burley	95%	42
Eastern Idaho Regional Medical Center	Idaho Falls	95%	86
Kootenai Medical Center	Coeur d'Alene	95%	203
Saint Joseph Regional Medical Center	Lewiston	95%	101
West Valley Medical Center	Caldwell	95%	41
Portneuf Medical Center	Pocatello	93%	123
Saint Alphonsus Regional Medical Center	Boise	92%	113
Magic Valley Regional Medical Center	Twin Falls	91%	54
Madison Memorial Hospital	Rexburg	84%	50

22. Prophylactic Antibiotic Stopped

Hospital Name	City	Rate	Cases
Healthsouth Treasure Valley Hospital	Boise	92%	49
Saint Luke's Regional Medical Center	Boise	92%	505
Bonner General Hospital	Sandpoint	85%	91
Saint Alphonsus Regional Medical Center	Boise	81%	350
Magic Valley Regional Medical Center	Twin Falls	80%	54
Kootenai Medical Center	Coeur d'Alene	79%	820
Saint Joseph Regional Medical Center	Lewiston	78%	418
Madison Memorial Hospital	Rexburg	67%	174
West Valley Medical Center	Caldwell	67%	112
Mercy Medical Center	Nampa	60%	191
Eastern Idaho Regional Medical Center	Idaho Falls	54%	178
Portneuf Medical Center	Pocatello	51%	485
Cassia Regional Medical Center	Burley	36%	172
Mountain View Hospital	Idaho Falls	33%	33
Northwest Specialty Hospital	Post Falls	24%	102

Pregnancy Care

23. Inpatient Neonatal Mortality

Hospital Name	City	Rate	Cases
Mercy Medical Center	Nampa	0.34%	1478

24. Third or Fourth Degree Laceration

Hospital Name	City	Rate	Cases
Mercy Medical Center	Nampa	3.34%	1257

NOTE: Hospital profiles are in alphabetical order by state, then city, then hospital within the city; Rankings are sorted by rate in descending order and exclude hospitals with less than 25 cases; (1) The number of cases is too small (n<25) for purposes of reliably predicting hospital performance; (2) Measure reflects the hospital's indication that its submission was based upon a sample of its relevant discharges; (3) Rate reflects fewer than the maximum possible quarters of data for the measure; (4) Inaccurate information submitted and suppressed for one or more quarters; (5) No data is available from the hospital for this measure; Please refer to the User's Guide for a full explanation of data

Idaho Doctors Hospital

350 North Meridian Street
Blackfoot, ID 83221
Ownership: Proprietary
Emergency Services: Yes

Phone: 208-782-0300
Accredited: No

Measure	Cases	This Hospital	State Average	U.S. Average	Top Hospital
Heart Attack Care					
ACE Inhibitor or ARB for LVSD[5]	-	-	84%	82%	100%
Aspirin at Arrival[5]	-	-	96%	92%	100%
Aspirin at Discharge[5]	-	-	95%	90%	100%
Beta Blocker at Arrival[5]	-	-	92%	87%	100%
Beta Blocker at Discharge[5]	-	-	88%	90%	100%
Fibrinolytic Medication Timing[5]	-	-	11%	31%	100%
PCI Within 90 Minutes of Arrival[5]	-	-	76%	54%	95%
Smoking Cessation Advice[5]	-	-	96%	88%	100%
Heart Failure Care					
ACE Inhibitor or ARB for LVSD[5]	-	-	72%	82%	100%
Discharge Instructions[5]	-	-	66%	61%	93%
Evaluation of LVS Function[5]	-	-	86%	83%	99%
Smoking Cessation Advice[5]	-	-	82%	82%	100%
Pneumonia Care					
Appropriate Initial Antibiotic[5]	-	-	88%	83%	94%
Blood Culture Timing[5]	-	-	93%	90%	100%
Influenza Vaccine[5]	-	-	72%	70%	100%
Initial Antibiotic Timing[5]	-	-	82%	80%	93%
Oxygenation Assessment[5]	-	-	100%	99%	100%
Pneumococcal Vaccine[5]	-	-	75%	69%	94%
Smoking Cessation Advice[5]	-	-	70%	80%	100%
Surgical Infection Prevention					
Prophylactic Antibiotic Given[5]	-	-	83%	77%	95%
Prophylactic Antibiotic Selection[5]	-	-	93%	90%	100%
Prophylactic Antibiotic Stopped[5]	-	-	65%	72%	95%
Pregnancy Care					
Inpatient Neonatal Mortality	-	-	-	-	-
Third or Fourth Degree Laceration	-	-	-	3.63%	3.27%

Healthsouth Treasure Valley Hospital

8800 West Emerald Street
Boise, ID 83704
Ownership: Proprietary
Emergency Services: No

Phone: 208-373-5000
Accredited: Yes

Key Personnel:
President/CEO. . . . . Jay Grinney
Executive VP/CFO. . . . . John L Workman

Measure	Cases	This Hospital	State Average	U.S. Average	Top Hospital
Heart Attack Care					
ACE Inhibitor or ARB for LVSD[5]	-	-	84%	82%	100%
Aspirin at Arrival[5]	-	-	96%	92%	100%
Aspirin at Discharge[5]	-	-	95%	90%	100%
Beta Blocker at Arrival[5]	-	-	92%	87%	100%
Beta Blocker at Discharge[5]	-	-	88%	90%	100%
Fibrinolytic Medication Timing[5]	-	-	11%	31%	100%
PCI Within 90 Minutes of Arrival[5]	-	-	76%	54%	95%
Smoking Cessation Advice[5]	-	-	96%	88%	100%
Heart Failure Care					
ACE Inhibitor or ARB for LVSD[5]	-	-	72%	82%	100%
Discharge Instructions[5]	-	-	66%	61%	93%
Evaluation of LVS Function[5]	-	-	86%	83%	99%
Smoking Cessation Advice[5]	-	-	82%	82%	100%
Pneumonia Care					
Appropriate Initial Antibiotic[5]	-	-	88%	83%	94%
Blood Culture Timing[5]	-	-	93%	90%	100%
Influenza Vaccine[5]	-	-	72%	70%	100%
Initial Antibiotic Timing[5]	-	-	82%	80%	93%
Oxygenation Assessment[5]	-	-	100%	99%	100%
Pneumococcal Vaccine[5]	-	-	75%	69%	94%
Smoking Cessation Advice[5]	-	-	70%	80%	100%
Surgical Infection Prevention					
Prophylactic Antibiotic Given	49	100%	83%	77%	95%
Prophylactic Antibiotic Selection[1]	8	88%	93%	90%	100%
Prophylactic Antibiotic Stopped	49	92%	65%	72%	95%
Pregnancy Care					
Inpatient Neonatal Mortality	-	-	-	-	-
Third or Fourth Degree Laceration	-	-	-	3.63%	3.27%

Saint Alphonsus Regional Medical Center

1055 N Curtis Road
Boise, ID 83706
E-mail: inquiries@sarmc.org
URL: www.saintalphonsus.org
Ownership: Voluntary non-profit - Church
Emergency Services: Yes

Phone: 208-367-2121
Fax: 208-367-3123
Accredited: Yes
Licensed Beds: 381

Key Personnel:
President/CEO. . . . . Sandra Bennett Bruce

Measure	Cases	This Hospital	State Average	U.S. Average	Top Hospital
Heart Attack Care					
ACE Inhibitor or ARB for LVSD	31	100%	84%	82%	100%
Aspirin at Arrival	151	99%	96%	92%	100%
Aspirin at Discharge	285	99%	95%	90%	100%
Beta Blocker at Arrival	137	99%	92%	87%	100%
Beta Blocker at Discharge	276	99%	88%	90%	100%
Fibrinolytic Medication Timing[1]	1	0%	11%	31%	100%
PCI Within 90 Minutes of Arrival[1]	11	45%	76%	54%	95%
Smoking Cessation Advice	92	99%	96%	88%	100%
Heart Failure Care					
ACE Inhibitor or ARB for LVSD	87	95%	72%	82%	100%
Discharge Instructions	184	85%	66%	61%	93%
Evaluation of LVS Function	228	98%	86%	83%	99%
Smoking Cessation Advice	25	88%	82%	82%	100%
Pneumonia Care					
Appropriate Initial Antibiotic	108	91%	88%	83%	94%
Blood Culture Timing	116	88%	93%	90%	100%
Influenza Vaccine[4,5]	-	-	72%	70%	100%
Initial Antibiotic Timing	187	91%	82%	80%	93%
Oxygenation Assessment	237	100%	100%	99%	100%
Pneumococcal Vaccine	153	91%	75%	69%	94%
Smoking Cessation Advice	76	92%	70%	80%	100%
Surgical Infection Prevention					
Prophylactic Antibiotic Given[2]	358	91%	83%	77%	95%
Prophylactic Antibiotic Selection[2]	113	92%	93%	90%	100%
Prophylactic Antibiotic Stopped[2]	350	81%	65%	72%	95%
Pregnancy Care					
Inpatient Neonatal Mortality	-	-	-	-	-
Third or Fourth Degree Laceration	-	-	-	3.63%	3.27%

Saint Luke's Regional Medical Center

Alternate Name: Saint Luke's Health System
190 E Bannock Street
Boise, ID 83712
URL: www.slrmc.org
Ownership: Voluntary non-profit - Other
Emergency Services: Yes

Phone: 208-381-1200
Fax: 208-381-2861
Accredited: Yes
Licensed Beds: 369

Key Personnel:
CEO. . . . . Gary Fletcher
Chief Medical Staff. . . . . Peter Livers
Director Medical/Surgical Nursing . . . . Mary Ellen Grobe
Chief Radiology . . . . Peter Langhus, MD
Director Respiratory Therapy . . . . Dave Shuldes

Measure	Cases	This Hospital	State Average	U.S. Average	Top Hospital
Heart Attack Care					
ACE Inhibitor or ARB for LVSD	58	95%	84%	82%	100%
Aspirin at Arrival	144	99%	96%	92%	100%
Aspirin at Discharge	387	100%	95%	90%	100%
Beta Blocker at Arrival	136	100%	92%	87%	100%
Beta Blocker at Discharge	373	100%	88%	90%	100%
Fibrinolytic Medication Timing	0	-	11%	31%	100%
PCI Within 90 Minutes of Arrival[1]	14	100%	76%	54%	95%
Smoking Cessation Advice	141	100%	96%	88%	100%
Heart Failure Care					
ACE Inhibitor or ARB for LVSD	148	88%	72%	82%	100%

NOTE: Hospital profiles are in alphabetical order by state, then city, then hospital within the city; Rankings are sorted by rate in descending order and exclude hospitals with less than 25 cases; (1) The number of cases is too small (n<25) for purposes of reliably predicting hospital performance; (2) Measure reflects the hospital's indication that its submission was based upon a sample of its relevant discharges; (3) Rate reflects fewer than the maximum possible quarters of data for the measure; (4) Inaccurate information submitted and suppressed for one or more quarters; (5) No data is available from the hospital for this measure; Please refer to the User's Guide for a full explanation of data

Discharge Instructions	284	90%	66%	61%	93%
Evaluation of LVS Function	345	96%	86%	83%	99%
Smoking Cessation Advice	52	94%	82%	82%	100%
Pneumonia Care					
Appropriate Initial Antibiotic	270	91%	88%	83%	94%
Blood Culture Timing	245	91%	93%	90%	100%
Influenza Vaccine	74	54%	72%	70%	100%
Initial Antibiotic Timing	328	88%	82%	80%	93%
Oxygenation Assessment	403	100%	100%	99%	100%
Pneumococcal Vaccine	280	67%	75%	69%	94%
Smoking Cessation Advice	102	85%	70%	80%	100%
Surgical Infection Prevention					
Prophylactic Antibiotic Given[3]	518	91%	83%	77%	95%
Prophylactic Antibiotic Selection	522	96%	93%	90%	100%
Prophylactic Antibiotic Stopped[3]	505	92%	65%	72%	95%
Pregnancy Care					
Inpatient Neonatal Mortality	-	-	-	-	-
Third or Fourth Degree Laceration	-	-	-	3.63%	3.27%

Cassia Regional Medical Center

Alternate Name: Cassia Memorial Hospital
1501 Hiland Avenue — Phone: 208-678-4444
Burley, ID 83318 — Fax: 208-677-6555
URL: www.ihc.com
Ownership: Voluntary non-profit - Other — Accredited: Yes
Emergency Services: Yes — Licensed Beds: 25

Key Personnel:

Administrator . . . . Ken Harmon
Head of Emergency Room. . . . . Maria Hoggan
Director Medical/Surgical Nursing . . . . Marilyn King, RN
OB/GYN Womens Health. . . . . Mark Dowdle, MD
Chief Radiology . . . . Eric Hoffman, MD
Chief of Pulmonary. . . . . Shauna Reater

Measure	Cases	This Hospital	State Average	U.S. Average	Top Hospital
Heart Attack Care					
ACE Inhibitor or ARB for LVSD	0	-	84%	82%	100%
Aspirin at Arrival[1]	7	71%	96%	92%	100%
Aspirin at Discharge[1]	5	60%	95%	90%	100%
Beta Blocker at Arrival[1]	7	57%	92%	87%	100%
Beta Blocker at Discharge[1]	5	60%	88%	90%	100%
Fibrinolytic Medication Timing	0	-	11%	31%	100%
PCI Within 90 Minutes of Arrival	0	-	76%	54%	95%
Smoking Cessation Advice[1]	1	100%	96%	88%	100%
Heart Failure Care					
ACE Inhibitor or ARB for LVSD[1]	14	71%	72%	82%	100%
Discharge Instructions	65	72%	66%	61%	93%
Evaluation of LVS Function	81	70%	86%	83%	99%
Smoking Cessation Advice[1]	6	83%	82%	82%	100%
Pneumonia Care					
Appropriate Initial Antibiotic	65	85%	88%	83%	94%
Blood Culture Timing	45	96%	93%	90%	100%
Influenza Vaccine[1]	19	63%	72%	70%	100%
Initial Antibiotic Timing	67	66%	82%	80%	93%
Oxygenation Assessment	86	100%	100%	99%	100%
Pneumococcal Vaccine	60	73%	75%	69%	94%
Smoking Cessation Advice[1]	12	42%	70%	80%	100%
Surgical Infection Prevention					
Prophylactic Antibiotic Given	175	79%	83%	77%	95%
Prophylactic Antibiotic Selection	42	95%	93%	90%	100%
Prophylactic Antibiotic Stopped	172	36%	65%	72%	95%
Pregnancy Care					
Inpatient Neonatal Mortality	-	-	-	-	-
Third or Fourth Degree Laceration	-	-	-	3.63%	3.27%

West Valley Medical Center

Alternate Name: West Valley Medical Center
1717 Arlington — Phone: 208-459-4641
Caldwell, ID 83605 — Fax: 208-455-3717
Ownership: Proprietary — Accredited: Yes
Emergency Services: Yes — Licensed Beds: 150

Key Personnel:

CEO. . . . . Kathy D Moore
Emergency Room . . . . J Mullins, MD
Director Medical/Surgical Nursing . . . . Mary Ellen Kelly

Measure	Cases	This Hospital	State Average	U.S. Average	Top Hospital
Heart Attack Care					
ACE Inhibitor or ARB for LVSD[1]	5	60%	84%	82%	100%
Aspirin at Arrival	27	89%	96%	92%	100%
Aspirin at Discharge[1]	12	83%	95%	90%	100%
Beta Blocker at Arrival	28	75%	92%	87%	100%
Beta Blocker at Discharge[1]	20	100%	88%	90%	100%
Fibrinolytic Medication Timing	0	-	11%	31%	100%
PCI Within 90 Minutes of Arrival	0	-	76%	54%	95%
Smoking Cessation Advice[1]	1	100%	96%	88%	100%
Heart Failure Care					
ACE Inhibitor or ARB for LVSD	25	76%	72%	82%	100%
Discharge Instructions	80	62%	66%	61%	93%
Evaluation of LVS Function	98	92%	86%	83%	99%
Smoking Cessation Advice	29	76%	82%	82%	100%
Pneumonia Care					
Appropriate Initial Antibiotic	103	84%	88%	83%	94%
Blood Culture Timing	55	89%	93%	90%	100%
Influenza Vaccine	28	57%	72%	70%	100%
Initial Antibiotic Timing	128	87%	82%	80%	93%
Oxygenation Assessment	145	100%	100%	99%	100%
Pneumococcal Vaccine	104	85%	75%	69%	94%
Smoking Cessation Advice	48	60%	70%	80%	100%
Surgical Infection Prevention					
Prophylactic Antibiotic Given[2,3]	117	80%	83%	77%	95%
Prophylactic Antibiotic Selection[2]	41	95%	93%	90%	100%
Prophylactic Antibiotic Stopped[2,3]	112	67%	65%	72%	95%
Pregnancy Care					
Inpatient Neonatal Mortality	-	-	-	-	-
Third or Fourth Degree Laceration	-	-	-	3.63%	3.27%

Kootenai Medical Center

2003 Lincoln Way — Phone: 208-666-2000
Coeur d'Alene, ID 83814 — Fax: 208-666-3299
URL: www.kmc.org
Ownership: Govt - Hospital District or Authority — Accredited: Yes
Emergency Services: Yes — Licensed Beds: 225

Key Personnel:

President . . . . James Y Lea
Chief Medical Staff. . . . . Charles Britt, MD
Director Emergency Department . . . . Roger Evans
Director Infection Control . . . . Marty Fallon
Director Medical/Surgical Nursing . . . . Mary Ramsrud
OB/GYN Womens Health. . . . . Tony Henneberg, MD
Director Respiratory Therapy . . . . Jan Moseley

Measure	Cases	This Hospital	State Average	U.S. Average	Top Hospital
Heart Attack Care					
ACE Inhibitor or ARB for LVSD	26	100%	84%	82%	100%
Aspirin at Arrival	171	99%	96%	92%	100%
Aspirin at Discharge	222	100%	95%	90%	100%
Beta Blocker at Arrival	125	94%	92%	87%	100%
Beta Blocker at Discharge	189	98%	88%	90%	100%
Fibrinolytic Medication Timing	0	-	11%	31%	100%
PCI Within 90 Minutes of Arrival[1]	20	95%	76%	54%	95%
Smoking Cessation Advice	80	100%	96%	88%	100%
Heart Failure Care					
ACE Inhibitor or ARB for LVSD	46	98%	72%	82%	100%
Discharge Instructions	158	75%	66%	61%	93%
Evaluation of LVS Function	201	97%	86%	83%	99%
Smoking Cessation Advice	39	97%	82%	82%	100%
Pneumonia Care					
Appropriate Initial Antibiotic	185	92%	88%	83%	94%
Blood Culture Timing	117	92%	93%	90%	100%
Influenza Vaccine	49	53%	72%	70%	100%
Initial Antibiotic Timing	267	91%	82%	80%	93%
Oxygenation Assessment	330	100%	100%	99%	100%
Pneumococcal Vaccine	226	73%	75%	69%	94%
Smoking Cessation Advice	74	93%	70%	80%	100%

NOTE: Hospital profiles are in alphabetical order by state, then city, then hospital within the city; Rankings are sorted by rate in descending order and exclude hospitals with less than 25 cases; (1) The number of cases is too small (n<25) for purposes of reliably predicting hospital performance; (2) Measure reflects the hospital's indication that its submission was based upon a sample of its relevant discharges; (3) Rate reflects fewer than the maximum possible quarters of data for the measure; (4) Inaccurate information submitted and suppressed for one or more quarters; (5) No data is available from the hospital for this measure; Please refer to the User's Guide for a full explanation of data

Surgical Infection Prevention					
Prophylactic Antibiotic Given	866	85%	83%	77%	95%
Prophylactic Antibiotic Selection	203	95%	93%	90%	100%
Prophylactic Antibiotic Stopped	820	79%	65%	72%	95%
Pregnancy Care					
Inpatient Neonatal Mortality	-	-	-	-	-
Third or Fourth Degree Laceration	-	-	-	3.63%	3.27%

Eastern Idaho Regional Medical Center

3100 Channing Way
Idaho Falls, ID 83404
URL: www.eirmc.org
Ownership: Proprietary
Emergency Services: Yes

Phone: 208-529-6111
Fax: 208-529-7021
Accredited: Yes
Licensed Beds: 336

Key Personnel:
CEO. . . . . Doug Crabtree
President Medical Staff . . . . Michael H Denyer, MD
Director Cardiology Services . . . . Elizabeth Later
Director Emergency Department . . . . Lynette Sharp
Manager Emergency Department . . . . Brad Hobbs
Coordinator Infection Control . . . . Jan Griffin
Executive Director ICU/IMC/Cardiology . . . . Elizabeth Later
Manager Medical/Surgical Unit. . . . . Dorothy Watson
CNO. . . . . Edith Irving
Director Women's Services . . . . Darla Miller
Director Surgical Services . . . . Byron Burlingame

Measure	Cases	This Hospital	State Average	U.S. Average	Top Hospital
Heart Attack Care					
ACE Inhibitor or ARB for LVSD[1]	23	52%	84%	82%	100%
Aspirin at Arrival	109	98%	96%	92%	100%
Aspirin at Discharge	205	98%	95%	90%	100%
Beta Blocker at Arrival	78	95%	92%	87%	100%
Beta Blocker at Discharge	205	98%	88%	90%	100%
Fibrinolytic Medication Timing	0	-	11%	31%	100%
PCI Within 90 Minutes of Arrival[1]	13	77%	76%	54%	95%
Smoking Cessation Advice	69	93%	96%	88%	100%
Heart Failure Care					
ACE Inhibitor or ARB for LVSD	46	74%	72%	82%	100%
Discharge Instructions	139	81%	66%	61%	93%
Evaluation of LVS Function	177	81%	86%	83%	99%
Smoking Cessation Advice	27	93%	82%	82%	100%
Pneumonia Care					
Appropriate Initial Antibiotic[2]	160	86%	88%	83%	94%
Blood Culture Timing[2]	121	87%	93%	90%	100%
Influenza Vaccine	45	89%	72%	70%	100%
Initial Antibiotic Timing[2]	230	77%	82%	80%	93%
Oxygenation Assessment[2]	299	100%	100%	99%	100%
Pneumococcal Vaccine[2]	183	83%	75%	69%	94%
Smoking Cessation Advice[2]	79	61%	70%	80%	100%
Surgical Infection Prevention					
Prophylactic Antibiotic Given[2,3]	208	93%	83%	77%	95%
Prophylactic Antibiotic Selection[2]	86	95%	93%	90%	100%
Prophylactic Antibiotic Stopped[2,3]	178	54%	65%	72%	95%
Pregnancy Care					
Inpatient Neonatal Mortality	-	-	-	-	-
Third or Fourth Degree Laceration	-	-	-	3.63%	3.27%

Idaho Falls Recovery Center

1957 East 17th Street
Idaho Falls, ID 83404
Ownership: Voluntary non-profit - Private
Emergency Services: No

Phone: 208-529-5285
Accredited: No

Measure	Cases	This Hospital	State Average	U.S. Average	Top Hospital
Heart Attack Care					
ACE Inhibitor or ARB for LVSD[5]	-	-	84%	82%	100%
Aspirin at Arrival[5]	-	-	96%	92%	100%
Aspirin at Discharge[5]	-	-	95%	90%	100%
Beta Blocker at Arrival[5]	-	-	92%	87%	100%
Beta Blocker at Discharge[5]	-	-	88%	90%	100%
Fibrinolytic Medication Timing[5]	-	-	11%	31%	100%
PCI Within 90 Minutes of Arrival[5]	-	-	76%	54%	95%
Smoking Cessation Advice[5]	-	-	96%	88%	100%
Heart Failure Care					
ACE Inhibitor or ARB for LVSD[5]	-	-	72%	82%	100%
Discharge Instructions[5]	-	-	66%	61%	93%
Evaluation of LVS Function[5]	-	-	86%	83%	99%
Smoking Cessation Advice[5]	-	-	82%	82%	100%
Pneumonia Care					
Appropriate Initial Antibiotic[5]	-	-	88%	83%	94%
Blood Culture Timing[5]	-	-	93%	90%	100%
Influenza Vaccine[5]	-	-	72%	70%	100%
Initial Antibiotic Timing[5]	-	-	82%	80%	93%
Oxygenation Assessment[5]	-	-	100%	99%	100%
Pneumococcal Vaccine[5]	-	-	75%	69%	94%
Smoking Cessation Advice[5]	-	-	70%	80%	100%
Surgical Infection Prevention					
Prophylactic Antibiotic Given[5]	-	-	83%	77%	95%
Prophylactic Antibiotic Selection[5]	-	-	93%	90%	100%
Prophylactic Antibiotic Stopped[5]	-	-	65%	72%	95%
Pregnancy Care					
Inpatient Neonatal Mortality	-	-	-	-	-
Third or Fourth Degree Laceration	-	-	-	3.63%	3.27%

Mountain View Hospital

2325 Coronado Street
Idaho Falls, ID 83404
Ownership: Government - Federal
Emergency Services: No

Phone: 208-557-2700
Accredited: No

Measure	Cases	This Hospital	State Average	U.S. Average	Top Hospital
Heart Attack Care					
ACE Inhibitor or ARB for LVSD[5]	-	-	84%	82%	100%
Aspirin at Arrival[5]	-	-	96%	92%	100%
Aspirin at Discharge[5]	-	-	95%	90%	100%
Beta Blocker at Arrival[5]	-	-	92%	87%	100%
Beta Blocker at Discharge[5]	-	-	88%	90%	100%
Fibrinolytic Medication Timing[5]	-	-	11%	31%	100%
PCI Within 90 Minutes of Arrival[5]	-	-	76%	54%	95%
Smoking Cessation Advice[5]	-	-	96%	88%	100%
Heart Failure Care					
ACE Inhibitor or ARB for LVSD[5]	-	-	72%	82%	100%
Discharge Instructions[5]	-	-	66%	61%	93%
Evaluation of LVS Function[5]	-	-	86%	83%	99%
Smoking Cessation Advice[5]	-	-	82%	82%	100%
Pneumonia Care					
Appropriate Initial Antibiotic[5]	-	-	88%	83%	94%
Blood Culture Timing[5]	-	-	93%	90%	100%
Influenza Vaccine[5]	-	-	72%	70%	100%
Initial Antibiotic Timing[5]	-	-	82%	80%	93%
Oxygenation Assessment[5]	-	-	100%	99%	100%
Pneumococcal Vaccine[5]	-	-	75%	69%	94%
Smoking Cessation Advice[5]	-	-	70%	80%	100%
Surgical Infection Prevention					
Prophylactic Antibiotic Given[2,3]	33	52%	83%	77%	95%
Prophylactic Antibiotic Selection[2]	33	97%	93%	90%	100%
Prophylactic Antibiotic Stopped[2,3]	33	33%	65%	72%	95%
Pregnancy Care					
Inpatient Neonatal Mortality	-	-	-	-	-
Third or Fourth Degree Laceration	-	-	-	3.63%	3.27%

Saint Luke's Medical Center

100 Hospital Drive
PO Box 100
Ketchum, ID 83340
Ownership: Voluntary non-profit - Private
Emergency Services: Yes

Phone: 208-727-8800
Fax: 208-727-8412
Accredited: Yes
Licensed Beds: 39

Key Personnel:
CEO. . . . . Bruce Jensen
Chief Medical Staff. . . . . Dr. Herb Alexander
Emergency Room . . . . Keith Sivertson
Infection Control. . . . . Jodie Alverson
Chief Radiology . . . . Dennis Davis, MD
Director Respiratory Therapy . . . . Scott Tracey

NOTE: Hospital profiles are in alphabetical order by state, then city, then hospital within the city; Rankings are sorted by rate in descending order and exclude hospitals with less than 25 cases; (1) The number of cases is too small (n<25) for purposes of reliably predicting hospital performance; (2) Measure reflects the hospital's indication that its submission was based upon a sample of its relevant discharges; (3) Rate reflects fewer than the maximum possible quarters of data for the measure; (4) Inaccurate information submitted and suppressed for one or more quarters; (5) No data is available from the hospital for this measure; Please refer to the User's Guide for a full explanation of data

Measure	Cases	This Hospital	State Average	U.S. Average	Top Hospital
Heart Attack Care					
ACE Inhibitor or ARB for LVSD[3]	0	-	84%	82%	100%
Aspirin at Arrival[1,3]	2	100%	96%	92%	100%
Aspirin at Discharge[1,3]	1	100%	95%	90%	100%
Beta Blocker at Arrival[1,3]	2	100%	92%	87%	100%
Beta Blocker at Discharge[1,3]	1	100%	88%	90%	100%
Fibrinolytic Medication Timing[3]	0	-	11%	31%	100%
PCI Within 90 Minutes of Arrival[5]	-	-	76%	54%	95%
Smoking Cessation Advice[3]	0	-	96%	88%	100%
Heart Failure Care					
ACE Inhibitor or ARB for LVSD[1]	1	0%	72%	82%	100%
Discharge Instructions[1]	13	54%	66%	61%	93%
Evaluation of LVS Function[1]	14	86%	86%	83%	99%
Smoking Cessation Advice	0	-	82%	82%	100%
Pneumonia Care					
Appropriate Initial Antibiotic	25	92%	88%	83%	94%
Blood Culture Timing[1]	10	100%	93%	90%	100%
Influenza Vaccine[1]	4	75%	72%	70%	100%
Initial Antibiotic Timing[1]	23	74%	82%	80%	93%
Oxygenation Assessment	32	100%	100%	99%	100%
Pneumococcal Vaccine[1]	24	83%	75%	69%	94%
Smoking Cessation Advice[1]	4	50%	70%	80%	100%
Surgical Infection Prevention					
Prophylactic Antibiotic Given[5]	-	-	83%	77%	95%
Prophylactic Antibiotic Selection[5]	-	-	93%	90%	100%
Prophylactic Antibiotic Stopped[5]	-	-	65%	72%	95%
Pregnancy Care					
Inpatient Neonatal Mortality	-	-	-	-	-
Third or Fourth Degree Laceration	-	-	-	3.63%	3.27%

Saint Joseph Regional Medical Center

415 6th Street
PO Box 816
Lewiston, ID 83501
URL: www.sjrmc.org
Ownership: Voluntary non-profit - Church
Emergency Services: Yes
Phone: 208-743-2511
Fax: 208-799-6508
Accredited: Yes
Licensed Beds: 125

Key Personnel:

CEO. . . . . Howard A Hayes
Emergency Room . . . . Paula Hornbeck
Director Surgical Nursing . . . . Coralee Gash
Director Outpatient Surgery . . . . Rodney Sanders
Director Radiology . . . . Bob Jones
Director Respiratory Therapy . . . . Barbara Rosselle

Measure	Cases	This Hospital	State Average	U.S. Average	Top Hospital
Heart Attack Care					
ACE Inhibitor or ARB for LVSD[1]	5	80%	84%	82%	100%
Aspirin at Arrival[1]	11	100%	96%	92%	100%
Aspirin at Discharge[1]	10	100%	95%	90%	100%
Beta Blocker at Arrival[1]	8	88%	92%	87%	100%
Beta Blocker at Discharge[1]	10	70%	88%	90%	100%
Fibrinolytic Medication Timing	0	-	11%	31%	100%
PCI Within 90 Minutes of Arrival	0	-	76%	54%	95%
Smoking Cessation Advice[1]	4	75%	96%	88%	100%
Heart Failure Care					
ACE Inhibitor or ARB for LVSD	32	78%	72%	82%	100%
Discharge Instructions	55	67%	66%	61%	93%
Evaluation of LVS Function	81	86%	86%	83%	99%
Smoking Cessation Advice[1]	22	73%	82%	82%	100%
Pneumonia Care					
Appropriate Initial Antibiotic	66	89%	88%	83%	94%
Blood Culture Timing	83	95%	93%	90%	100%
Influenza Vaccine	28	75%	72%	70%	100%
Initial Antibiotic Timing	92	78%	82%	80%	93%
Oxygenation Assessment	148	99%	100%	99%	100%
Pneumococcal Vaccine	95	43%	75%	69%	94%
Smoking Cessation Advice	27	67%	70%	80%	100%
Surgical Infection Prevention					
Prophylactic Antibiotic Given[2]	429	86%	83%	77%	95%
Prophylactic Antibiotic Selection[2]	101	95%	93%	90%	100%
Prophylactic Antibiotic Stopped[2]	418	78%	65%	72%	95%
Pregnancy Care					
Inpatient Neonatal Mortality	-	-	-	-	-
Third or Fourth Degree Laceration	-	-	-	3.63%	3.27%

Mercy Medical Center

1512 12th Avenue Road
Nampa, ID 83686
URL: www.mercyoftoday.com
Ownership: Voluntary non-profit - Church
Emergency Services: Yes
Phone: 208-463-5000
Fax: 208-463-5775
Accredited: Yes
Licensed Beds: 104

Key Personnel:

President/CEO. . . . . Joseph Messmer
Chief Medical Staff. . . . . Joseph Kronz, MD
Infection Control. . . . . Karen Otter
ICU . . . . Kathy Grzeskiewicz
OB/GYN Womens Health. . . . . Diane Markus

Measure	Cases	This Hospital	State Average	U.S. Average	Top Hospital
Heart Attack Care					
ACE Inhibitor or ARB for LVSD[1]	18	94%	84%	82%	100%
Aspirin at Arrival	95	100%	96%	92%	100%
Aspirin at Discharge	87	100%	95%	90%	100%
Beta Blocker at Arrival	85	100%	92%	87%	100%
Beta Blocker at Discharge	81	100%	88%	90%	100%
Fibrinolytic Medication Timing	0	-	11%	31%	100%
PCI Within 90 Minutes of Arrival[1]	10	80%	76%	54%	95%
Smoking Cessation Advice	32	100%	96%	88%	100%
Heart Failure Care					
ACE Inhibitor or ARB for LVSD[1]	20	95%	72%	82%	100%
Discharge Instructions	72	94%	66%	61%	93%
Evaluation of LVS Function	96	96%	86%	83%	99%
Smoking Cessation Advice[1]	14	86%	82%	82%	100%
Pneumonia Care					
Appropriate Initial Antibiotic	151	91%	88%	83%	94%
Blood Culture Timing	114	96%	93%	90%	100%
Influenza Vaccine	38	97%	72%	70%	100%
Initial Antibiotic Timing	183	83%	82%	80%	93%
Oxygenation Assessment	215	100%	100%	99%	100%
Pneumococcal Vaccine	122	92%	75%	69%	94%
Smoking Cessation Advice	52	98%	70%	80%	100%
Surgical Infection Prevention					
Prophylactic Antibiotic Given[3]	190	93%	83%	77%	95%
Prophylactic Antibiotic Selection	57	98%	93%	90%	100%
Prophylactic Antibiotic Stopped[3]	191	60%	65%	72%	95%
Pregnancy Care					
Inpatient Neonatal Mortality	1,478	0.34%	-	-	-
Third or Fourth Degree Laceration	1,257	3.34%	-	3.63%	3.27%

Portneuf Medical Center

651 Memorial Drive
Pocatello, ID 83201
URL: www.portmed.org
Ownership: Government - Local
Emergency Services: Yes
Phone: 208-239-1000
Fax: 208-239-1993
Accredited: Yes
Licensed Beds: 274

Key Personnel:

CEO. . . . . Patrick M Hermanson
Director Medical/Surgical Nursing . . . . Terry Elquist, RN
OB/GYN Womens Health. . . . . DA Dyer, MD
Chief Radiology . . . . George Stephens, MD

Measure	Cases	This Hospital	State Average	U.S. Average	Top Hospital
Heart Attack Care					
ACE Inhibitor or ARB for LVSD	26	65%	84%	82%	100%
Aspirin at Arrival	98	97%	96%	92%	100%
Aspirin at Discharge	120	98%	95%	90%	100%
Beta Blocker at Arrival	69	93%	92%	87%	100%
Beta Blocker at Discharge	109	94%	88%	90%	100%
Fibrinolytic Medication Timing[1]	12	33%	11%	31%	100%
PCI Within 90 Minutes of Arrival[1]	4	50%	76%	54%	95%
Smoking Cessation Advice	38	92%	96%	88%	100%
Heart Failure Care					

NOTE: Hospital profiles are in alphabetical order by state, then city, then hospital within the city; Rankings are sorted by rate in descending order and exclude hospitals with less than 25 cases; (1) The number of cases is too small (n<25) for purposes of reliably predicting hospital performance; (2) Measure reflects the hospital's indication that its submission was based upon a sample of its relevant discharges; (3) Rate reflects fewer than the maximum possible quarters of data for the measure; (4) Inaccurate information submitted and suppressed for one or more quarters; (5) No data is available from the hospital for this measure; Please refer to the User's Guide for a full explanation of data

ACE Inhibitor or ARB for LVSD	58	71%	72%	82%	100%
Discharge Instructions	150	12%	66%	61%	93%
Evaluation of LVS Function	169	76%	86%	83%	99%
Smoking Cessation Advice	29	76%	82%	82%	100%
Pneumonia Care					
Appropriate Initial Antibiotic	136	85%	88%	83%	94%
Blood Culture Timing	145	94%	93%	90%	100%
Influenza Vaccine	32	66%	72%	70%	100%
Initial Antibiotic Timing	212	59%	82%	80%	93%
Oxygenation Assessment	246	100%	100%	99%	100%
Pneumococcal Vaccine	150	60%	75%	69%	94%
Smoking Cessation Advice	73	88%	70%	80%	100%
Surgical Infection Prevention					
Prophylactic Antibiotic Given	510	83%	83%	77%	95%
Prophylactic Antibiotic Selection	123	93%	93%	90%	100%
Prophylactic Antibiotic Stopped	485	51%	65%	72%	95%
Pregnancy Care					
Inpatient Neonatal Mortality	-	-	-	-	-
Third or Fourth Degree Laceration	-	-	-	3.63%	3.27%

Northwest Specialty Hospital

1593 East Polston Avenue
Post Falls, ID 83854
Phone: 208-262-2300
Ownership: Proprietary
Accredited: No
Emergency Services: No

Key Personnel:

CEO. . . . . Nick Genna

Measure	Cases	This Hospital	State Average	U.S. Average	Top Hospital
Heart Attack Care					
ACE Inhibitor or ARB for LVSD[5]	-	-	84%	82%	100%
Aspirin at Arrival[5]	-	-	96%	92%	100%
Aspirin at Discharge[5]	-	-	95%	90%	100%
Beta Blocker at Arrival[5]	-	-	92%	87%	100%
Beta Blocker at Discharge[5]	-	-	88%	90%	100%
Fibrinolytic Medication Timing[5]	-	-	11%	31%	100%
PCI Within 90 Minutes of Arrival[5]	-	-	76%	54%	95%
Smoking Cessation Advice[5]	-	-	96%	88%	100%
Heart Failure Care					
ACE Inhibitor or ARB for LVSD[5]	-	-	72%	82%	100%
Discharge Instructions[5]	-	-	66%	61%	93%
Evaluation of LVS Function[5]	-	-	86%	83%	99%
Smoking Cessation Advice[5]	-	-	82%	82%	100%
Pneumonia Care					
Appropriate Initial Antibiotic[5]	-	-	88%	83%	94%
Blood Culture Timing[5]	-	-	93%	90%	100%
Influenza Vaccine[5]	-	-	72%	70%	100%
Initial Antibiotic Timing[5]	-	-	82%	80%	93%
Oxygenation Assessment[5]	-	-	100%	99%	100%
Pneumococcal Vaccine[5]	-	-	75%	69%	94%
Smoking Cessation Advice[5]	-	-	70%	80%	100%
Surgical Infection Prevention					
Prophylactic Antibiotic Given	103	89%	83%	77%	95%
Prophylactic Antibiotic Selection[1]	18	89%	93%	90%	100%
Prophylactic Antibiotic Stopped	102	24%	65%	72%	95%
Pregnancy Care					
Inpatient Neonatal Mortality	-	-	-	-	-
Third or Fourth Degree Laceration	-	-	-	3.63%	3.27%

Madison Memorial Hospital

450 E Main Street
PO Box 310
Rexburg, ID 83440
Phone: 208-356-3691
Fax: 208-359-6454
URL: www.madisonhospital.org
Ownership: Government - Local
Accredited: No
Emergency Services: Yes
Licensed Beds: 49

Key Personnel:

CEO. . . . . Keith M Steiner
Chief Medical Staff. . . . . David V Hansen, MD
Cardiac Lab . . . . Kirt Crittenden
Emergency Room . . . . Mary Zollinger, RN
Infection Control. . . . . Chris Hobbs
Respiratory/Cardiopulmonary. . . . . Rod Cleverley

Measure	Cases	This Hospital	State Average	U.S. Average	Top Hospital
Heart Attack Care					
ACE Inhibitor or ARB for LVSD[1]	1	100%	84%	82%	100%
Aspirin at Arrival[1]	6	100%	96%	92%	100%
Aspirin at Discharge[1]	1	100%	95%	90%	100%
Beta Blocker at Arrival[1]	5	100%	92%	87%	100%
Beta Blocker at Discharge[1]	2	50%	88%	90%	100%
Fibrinolytic Medication Timing[1]	1	0%	11%	31%	100%
PCI Within 90 Minutes of Arrival	0	-	76%	54%	95%
Smoking Cessation Advice	0	-	96%	88%	100%
Heart Failure Care					
ACE Inhibitor or ARB for LVSD[1,2]	3	0%	72%	82%	100%
Discharge Instructions[2]	25	36%	66%	61%	93%
Evaluation of LVS Function[2]	33	55%	86%	83%	99%
Smoking Cessation Advice[1,2]	3	33%	82%	82%	100%
Pneumonia Care					
Appropriate Initial Antibiotic	54	89%	88%	83%	94%
Blood Culture Timing[1]	6	83%	93%	90%	100%
Influenza Vaccine[1]	9	89%	72%	70%	100%
Initial Antibiotic Timing	49	98%	82%	80%	93%
Oxygenation Assessment	62	100%	100%	99%	100%
Pneumococcal Vaccine	36	83%	75%	69%	94%
Smoking Cessation Advice[1]	13	85%	70%	80%	100%
Surgical Infection Prevention					
Prophylactic Antibiotic Given	177	76%	83%	77%	95%
Prophylactic Antibiotic Selection	50	84%	93%	90%	100%
Prophylactic Antibiotic Stopped	174	67%	65%	72%	95%
Pregnancy Care					
Inpatient Neonatal Mortality	-	-	-	-	-
Third or Fourth Degree Laceration	-	-	-	3.63%	3.27%

Bonner General Hospital

520 North Third Avenue
PO Box 1448
Sandpoint, ID 83864
Phone: 208-263-1441
Fax: 208-265-1277
E-mail: infosyst@bonnergen.org
URL: www.bonnergen.org
Ownership: Voluntary non-profit - Private
Accredited: Yes
Emergency Services: Yes
Licensed Beds: 48

Key Personnel:

President/CEO. . . . . Gene Tomt
Chief Medical Staff. . . . . Mark Weber, MD
Infection Control. . . . . Lauren Chaiet, RN
ICU . . . . Linda Rammler, RN
Intensive/Coronary Care . . . . Linda Rammler, RN
Medical/Surgical Nursing . . . . Dorothy Bailey, RN
OB/GYN Women's Health . . . . Margaret Maisel, RN
Respiratory/Cardiopulmonary. . . . . Steve Foord

Measure	Cases	This Hospital	State Average	U.S. Average	Top Hospital
Heart Attack Care					
ACE Inhibitor or ARB for LVSD[3]	0	-	84%	82%	100%
Aspirin at Arrival[1,3]	6	100%	96%	92%	100%
Aspirin at Discharge[1,3]	6	100%	95%	90%	100%
Beta Blocker at Arrival[1,3]	5	100%	92%	87%	100%
Beta Blocker at Discharge[1,3]	4	75%	88%	90%	100%
Fibrinolytic Medication Timing[3]	0	-	11%	31%	100%
PCI Within 90 Minutes of Arrival	0	-	76%	54%	95%
Smoking Cessation Advice[3]	0	-	96%	88%	100%
Heart Failure Care					
ACE Inhibitor or ARB for LVSD[1]	17	100%	72%	82%	100%
Discharge Instructions	35	60%	66%	61%	93%
Evaluation of LVS Function	43	91%	86%	83%	99%
Smoking Cessation Advice[1]	6	83%	82%	82%	100%
Pneumonia Care					
Appropriate Initial Antibiotic	31	68%	88%	83%	94%
Blood Culture Timing[1]	9	100%	93%	90%	100%
Influenza Vaccine[1]	7	71%	72%	70%	100%
Initial Antibiotic Timing	34	76%	82%	80%	93%
Oxygenation Assessment	44	100%	100%	99%	100%
Pneumococcal Vaccine	29	62%	75%	69%	94%
Smoking Cessation Advice[1]	10	0%	70%	80%	100%

NOTE: Hospital profiles are in alphabetical order by state, then city, then hospital within the city; Rankings are sorted by rate in descending order and exclude hospitals with less than 25 cases; (1) The number of cases is too small (n<25) for purposes of reliably predicting hospital performance; (2) Measure reflects the hospital's indication that its submission was based upon a sample of its relevant discharges; (3) Rate reflects fewer than the maximum possible quarters of data for the measure; (4) Inaccurate information submitted and suppressed for one or more quarters; (5) No data is available from the hospital for this measure; Please refer to the User's Guide for a full explanation of data

Surgical Infection Prevention					
Prophylactic Antibiotic Given[3]	93	88%	83%	77%	95%
Prophylactic Antibiotic Selection	34	100%	93%	90%	100%
Prophylactic Antibiotic Stopped[3]	91	85%	65%	72%	95%
Pregnancy Care					
Inpatient Neonatal Mortality	-	-	-	-	-
Third or Fourth Degree Laceration	-	-	-	3.63%	3.27%

Magic Valley Regional Medical Center

650 Addison Avenue W
Twin Falls, ID 83301

Toll-Free: 800-947-4852
Phone: 208-737-2000
Fax: 208-737-2786

URL: www.stlukesonline.org/magic_valley
Ownership: Government - Local
Emergency Services: Yes

Accredited: Yes
Licensed Beds: 173

Key Personnel:

CEO. . . . . John Kee
CNO. . . . . Anne Erickson
Emergency Room . . . . Marlys Massey
Director Medical/Surgical Nursing . . . . Anne Erickson
OB/GYN Womens Health. . . . . Monte Crandall, MD
Director Radiology . . . . Gary Andrews
Director of Pulmonary . . . . Dave Kissinger

Measure	Cases	This Hospital	State Average	U.S. Average	Top Hospital
Heart Attack Care					
ACE Inhibitor or ARB for LVSD	38	95%	84%	82%	100%
Aspirin at Arrival	101	96%	96%	92%	100%
Aspirin at Discharge	109	97%	95%	90%	100%
Beta Blocker at Arrival	86	97%	92%	87%	100%
Beta Blocker at Discharge	135	98%	88%	90%	100%
Fibrinolytic Medication Timing[3]	0	-	11%	31%	100%
PCI Within 90 Minutes of Arrival[1]	12	83%	76%	54%	95%
Smoking Cessation Advice[3]	28	96%	96%	88%	100%
Heart Failure Care					
ACE Inhibitor or ARB for LVSD	32	91%	72%	82%	100%
Discharge Instructions[3]	58	69%	66%	61%	93%
Evaluation of LVS Function	120	92%	86%	83%	99%
Smoking Cessation Advice[1,3]	15	100%	82%	82%	100%
Pneumonia Care					
Appropriate Initial Antibiotic[3]	27	96%	88%	83%	94%
Blood Culture Timing	188	96%	93%	90%	100%
Influenza Vaccine[5]	-	-	72%	70%	100%
Initial Antibiotic Timing	282	93%	82%	80%	93%
Oxygenation Assessment	333	100%	100%	99%	100%
Pneumococcal Vaccine	210	76%	75%	69%	94%
Smoking Cessation Advice[3]	64	91%	70%	80%	100%
Surgical Infection Prevention					
Prophylactic Antibiotic Given[3]	53	66%	83%	77%	95%
Prophylactic Antibiotic Selection	54	91%	93%	90%	100%
Prophylactic Antibiotic Stopped[3]	54	80%	65%	72%	95%
Pregnancy Care					
Inpatient Neonatal Mortality	-	-	-	-	-
Third or Fourth Degree Laceration	-	-	-	3.63%	3.27%

NOTE: Hospital profiles are in alphabetical order by state, then city, then hospital within the city; Rankings are sorted by rate in descending order and exclude hospitals with less than 25 cases; (1) The number of cases is too small (n<25) for purposes of reliably predicting hospital performance; (2) Measure reflects the hospital's indication that its submission was based upon a sample of its relevant discharges; (3) Rate reflects fewer than the maximum possible quarters of data for the measure; (4) Inaccurate information submitted and suppressed for one or more quarters; (5) No data is available from the hospital for this measure; Please refer to the User's Guide for a full explanation of data

Heart Attack Care

1. ACE Inhibitor or ARB for LVSD

Hospital Name	City	Rate	Cases
Billings Clinic	Billings	98%	53
Saint Patrick Hosp and Health Sci Ctr	Missoula	96%	50
Saint Vincent Healthcare	Billings	69%	81

2. Aspirin at Arrival

Hospital Name	City	Rate	Cases
Bozeman Deaconess Hospital	Bozeman	100%	82
Community Medical Center	Missoula	100%	49
Benefis Healthcare	Great Falls	99%	94
Billings Clinic	Billings	99%	157
Kalispell Regional Medical Center	Kalispell	99%	151
Saint Patrick Hosp and Health Sci Ctr	Missoula	99%	125
Saint Peter's Hospital	Helena	99%	75
Saint James Community Hospital	Butte	96%	67
Saint Vincent Healthcare	Billings	95%	151

3. Aspirin at Discharge

Hospital Name	City	Rate	Cases
Saint Patrick Hosp and Health Sci Ctr	Missoula	100%	284
Benefis Healthcare	Great Falls	99%	136
Billings Clinic	Billings	98%	311
Kalispell Regional Medical Center	Kalispell	98%	198
Saint Vincent Healthcare	Billings	98%	302
Community Medical Center	Missoula	97%	87
Bozeman Deaconess Hospital	Bozeman	96%	68
Saint Peter's Hospital	Helena	96%	71
Saint James Community Hospital	Butte	94%	50

4. Beta Blocker at Arrival

Hospital Name	City	Rate	Cases
Saint Peter's Hospital	Helena	100%	59
Kalispell Regional Medical Center	Kalispell	99%	134
Saint Patrick Hosp and Health Sci Ctr	Missoula	99%	111
Community Medical Center	Missoula	98%	45
Bozeman Deaconess Hospital	Bozeman	97%	68
Billings Clinic	Billings	96%	130
Benefis Healthcare	Great Falls	95%	77
Saint James Community Hospital	Butte	90%	50
Saint Vincent Healthcare	Billings	90%	145

5. Beta Blocker at Discharge

Hospital Name	City	Rate	Cases
Benefis Healthcare	Great Falls	99%	136
Billings Clinic	Billings	99%	302
Community Medical Center	Missoula	99%	85
Saint Patrick Hosp and Health Sci Ctr	Missoula	99%	273
Saint Peter's Hospital	Helena	98%	66
Bozeman Deaconess Hospital	Bozeman	97%	71
Kalispell Regional Medical Center	Kalispell	96%	191
Saint Vincent Healthcare	Billings	90%	294
Saint James Community Hospital	Butte	81%	54

8. Smoking Cessation Advice

Hospital Name	City	Rate	Cases
Billings Clinic	Billings	100%	114
Saint Patrick Hosp and Health Sci Ctr	Missoula	100%	85
Saint Vincent Healthcare	Billings	99%	94
Benefis Healthcare	Great Falls	98%	45
Saint James Community Hospital	Butte	94%	34
Community Medical Center	Missoula	92%	37
Kalispell Regional Medical Center	Kalispell	88%	69

Heart Failure Care

9. ACE Inhibitor or ARB for LVSD

Hospital Name	City	Rate	Cases
Saint Patrick Hosp and Health Sci Ctr	Missoula	97%	115
Billings Clinic	Billings	96%	121
Benefis Healthcare	Great Falls	92%	78
Saint Vincent Healthcare	Billings	92%	86
Kalispell Regional Medical Center	Kalispell	89%	47
Bozeman Deaconess Hospital	Bozeman	81%	36

10. Discharge Instructions

Hospital Name	City	Rate	Cases
Billings Clinic	Billings	90%	215
Benefis Healthcare	Great Falls	82%	175
Holy Rosary Health Care	Miles City	82%	34
Saint Vincent Healthcare	Billings	78%	200
Community Medical Center	Missoula	75%	68
Saint Patrick Hosp and Health Sci Ctr	Missoula	69%	189
Kalispell Regional Medical Center	Kalispell	66%	105
Saint Peter's Hospital	Helena	66%	56
Livingston Memorial Hospital	Livingston	63%	27
Sidney Health Center	Sidney	50%	28
Saint James Community Hospital	Butte	48%	75
Bozeman Deaconess Hospital	Bozeman	42%	131
Northern Montana Hospital	Havre	41%	39
Trinity Hospital	Wolf Point	41%	32

11. Evaluation of LVS Function

Hospital Name	City	Rate	Cases
Saint Patrick Hosp and Health Sci Ctr	Missoula	100%	220
Billings Clinic	Billings	99%	249
Benefis Healthcare	Great Falls	97%	221
Community Medical Center	Missoula	94%	89
Saint Peter's Hospital	Helena	94%	71
Bozeman Deaconess Hospital	Bozeman	93%	143
Kalispell Regional Medical Center	Kalispell	91%	139
Saint Vincent Healthcare	Billings	89%	242
Livingston Memorial Hospital	Livingston	88%	33
Northern Montana Hospital	Havre	87%	45
Saint James Community Hospital	Butte	85%	102
Sidney Health Center	Sidney	78%	37
Holy Rosary Health Care	Miles City	64%	50
Saint Luke Community Hospital	Ronan	64%	25
Trinity Hospital	Wolf Point	63%	35
Roundup Memorial Hospital & Nursing Home	Roundup	44%	27
PHS Indian Hospital-Browning	Browning	41%	27

12. Smoking Cessation Advice

Hospital Name	City	Rate	Cases
Benefis Healthcare	Great Falls	100%	30
Billings Clinic	Billings	100%	27
Saint Patrick Hosp and Health Sci Ctr	Missoula	100%	35
Saint Vincent Healthcare	Billings	88%	43

Pneumonia Care

13. Appropriate Initial Antibiotic

Hospital Name	City	Rate	Cases
Barrett Hospital	Dillon	100%	42
Saint Luke Community Hospital	Ronan	95%	43
Community Hosp and Nursing Home of Anaconda	Anaconda	94%	34
Saint Peter's Hospital	Helena	94%	95
Benefis Healthcare	Great Falls	93%	179
Community Medical Center	Missoula	90%	68
Billings Clinic	Billings	88%	109
Holy Rosary Health Care	Miles City	88%	81
Saint Vincent Healthcare	Billings	87%	209
Northern Montana Hospital	Havre	86%	57
Saint James Community Hospital	Butte	85%	91
Central Montana Medical Center	Lewistown	82%	34
Kalispell Regional Medical Center	Kalispell	82%	121
Marcus Daly Memorial Hospital	Hamilton	82%	28
Bozeman Deaconess Hospital	Bozeman	80%	76
Saint Patrick Hosp and Health Sci Ctr	Missoula	79%	92
Glendive Medical Center	Glendive	78%	40
Livingston Memorial Hospital	Livingston	78%	50
Saint Joseph Hospital	Polson	75%	32
North Valley Hospital	Whitefish	72%	43

14. Blood Culture Timing

Hospital Name	City	Rate	Cases
Holy Rosary Health Care	Miles City	97%	38
Saint James Community Hospital	Butte	97%	72
Bozeman Deaconess Hospital	Bozeman	96%	57
Glendive Medical Center	Glendive	96%	26
Saint Peter's Hospital	Helena	96%	74
Northern Montana Hospital	Havre	95%	43
Saint Patrick Hosp and Health Sci Ctr	Missoula	94%	93
Benefis Healthcare	Great Falls	93%	125
Community Medical Center	Missoula	90%	59
Kalispell Regional Medical Center	Kalispell	90%	119
Livingston Memorial Hospital	Livingston	90%	30
North Valley Hospital	Whitefish	90%	31
Saint Vincent Healthcare	Billings	90%	132
Billings Clinic	Billings	88%	132

NOTE: Hospital profiles are in alphabetical order by state, then city, then hospital within the city; Rankings are sorted by rate in descending order and exclude hospitals with less than 25 cases; (1) The number of cases is too small (n<25) for purposes of reliably predicting hospital performance; (2) Measure reflects the hospital's indication that its submission was based upon a sample of its relevant discharges; (3) Rate reflects fewer than the maximum possible quarters of data for the measure; (4) Inaccurate information submitted and suppressed for one or more quarters; (5) No data is available from the hospital for this measure; Please refer to the User's Guide for a full explanation of data

Hospital Name	City	Rate	Cases
Saint Luke Community Hospital	Ronan	80%	30

15. Influenza Vaccine

Hospital Name	City	Rate	Cases
Billings Clinic	Billings	100%	32
Saint Vincent Healthcare	Billings	100%	39
Saint Peter's Hospital	Helena	96%	27
Benefis Healthcare	Great Falls	60%	43

16. Initial Antibiotic Timing

Hospital Name	City	Rate	Cases
Community Hosp and Nursing Home of Anaconda	Anaconda	96%	50
Holy Rosary Health Care	Miles City	95%	76
North Valley Hospital	Whitefish	94%	51
Kalispell Regional Medical Center	Kalispell	93%	155
Saint Joseph Hospital	Polson	93%	27
Central Montana Medical Center	Lewistown	92%	39
Bozeman Deaconess Hospital	Bozeman	90%	93
Billings Clinic	Billings	89%	154
Livingston Memorial Hospital	Livingston	89%	57
Saint James Community Hospital	Butte	89%	105
Saint Peter's Hospital	Helena	89%	122
Roundup Memorial Hospital & Nursing Home	Roundup	88%	34
Saint Patrick Hosp and Health Sci Ctr	Missoula	88%	131
Barrett Hospital	Dillon	86%	43
PHS Indian Hospital-Browning	Browning	85%	47
Glendive Medical Center	Glendive	84%	56
Marcus Daly Memorial Hospital	Hamilton	84%	38
Saint Luke Community Hospital	Ronan	83%	53
Saint Vincent Healthcare	Billings	83%	215
Benefis Healthcare	Great Falls	82%	231
Community Medical Center	Missoula	78%	82
Northeast Montana Healthcare Poplar Hospital	Poplar	77%	31
Northern Montana Hospital	Havre	77%	69
Trinity Hospital	Wolf Point	70%	27

17. Oxygenation Assessment

Hospital Name	City	Rate	Cases
Barrett Hospital	Dillon	100%	47
Billings Clinic	Billings	100%	207
Bozeman Deaconess Hospital	Bozeman	100%	119
Central Montana Medical Center	Lewistown	100%	42
Community Hosp and Nursing Home of Anaconda	Anaconda	100%	56
Community Medical Center	Missoula	100%	98
Frances Mahon Deaconess Hospital	Glasgow	100%	26
Glendive Medical Center	Glendive	100%	60
Holy Rosary Health Care	Miles City	100%	95
Kalispell Regional Medical Center	Kalispell	100%	195
Livingston Memorial Hospital	Livingston	100%	67
Marcus Daly Memorial Hospital	Hamilton	100%	44
Marias Medical Center	Shelby	100%	29
North Valley Hospital	Whitefish	100%	60
Northeast Montana Healthcare Poplar Hospital	Poplar	100%	32
Northern Montana Hospital	Havre	100%	85
PHS Indian Hospital-Browning	Browning	100%	57
Roundup Memorial Hospital & Nursing Home	Roundup	100%	38
Saint James Community Hospital	Butte	100%	130
Saint Joseph Hospital	Polson	100%	33
Saint Luke Community Hospital	Ronan	100%	61
Saint Patrick Hosp and Health Sci Ctr	Missoula	100%	159
Saint Peter's Hospital	Helena	100%	159
Saint Vincent Healthcare	Billings	100%	260
Trinity Hospital	Wolf Point	100%	31
Benefis Healthcare	Great Falls	99%	309

18. Pneumococcal Vaccine

Hospital Name	City	Rate	Cases
Barrett Hospital	Dillon	100%	32
Community Hosp and Nursing Home of Anaconda	Anaconda	100%	37
Marcus Daly Memorial Hospital	Hamilton	100%	28
Billings Clinic	Billings	98%	128
Saint Peter's Hospital	Helena	96%	102
Holy Rosary Health Care	Miles City	94%	72
Livingston Memorial Hospital	Livingston	94%	47
Saint Patrick Hosp and Health Sci Ctr	Missoula	91%	105
Community Medical Center	Missoula	90%	58
Bozeman Deaconess Hospital	Bozeman	89%	71
Glendive Medical Center	Glendive	88%	40
North Valley Hospital	Whitefish	88%	40
PHS Indian Hospital-Browning	Browning	88%	34
Benefis Healthcare	Great Falls	87%	199
Central Montana Medical Center	Lewistown	84%	31
Saint Vincent Healthcare	Billings	81%	154
Saint Luke Community Hospital	Ronan	79%	28
Saint James Community Hospital	Butte	74%	72
Northern Montana Hospital	Havre	59%	51
Kalispell Regional Medical Center	Kalispell	58%	126

19. Smoking Cessation Advice

Hospital Name	City	Rate	Cases
Billings Clinic	Billings	100%	59
Saint Patrick Hosp and Health Sci Ctr	Missoula	95%	41
Community Medical Center	Missoula	92%	39
Benefis Healthcare	Great Falls	91%	87
Saint Vincent Healthcare	Billings	85%	86
Saint Peter's Hospital	Helena	84%	32
Saint James Community Hospital	Butte	78%	36
Kalispell Regional Medical Center	Kalispell	69%	55

Surgical Infection Prevention

20. Prophylactic Antibiotic Given

Hospital Name	City	Rate	Cases
Benefis Healthcare	Great Falls	98%	200
Saint James Community Hospital	Butte	97%	346
Billings Clinic	Billings	96%	1171
Marcus Daly Memorial Hospital	Hamilton	96%	47
Sidney Health Center	Sidney	96%	53
Saint Peter's Hospital	Helena	95%	237
Bozeman Deaconess Hospital	Bozeman	94%	241
Saint Vincent Healthcare	Billings	94%	1334
Community Medical Center	Missoula	93%	621
Saint Patrick Hosp and Health Sci Ctr	Missoula	93%	402
Northern Montana Hospital	Havre	90%	89
Holy Rosary Health Care	Miles City	89%	56
Glendive Medical Center	Glendive	81%	73
Livingston Memorial Hospital	Livingston	81%	74
Saint Joseph Hospital	Polson	81%	36
Kalispell Regional Medical Center	Kalispell	77%	502
North Valley Hospital	Whitefish	74%	95
Barrett Hospital	Dillon	73%	26
Health Center Northwest	Kalispell	73%	239
Central Montana Medical Center	Lewistown	67%	48

21. Prophylactic Antibiotic Selection

Hospital Name	City	Rate	Cases
Saint Peter's Hospital	Helena	100%	59
Benefis Healthcare	Great Falls	99%	68
Billings Clinic	Billings	99%	278
Saint Patrick Hosp and Health Sci Ctr	Missoula	98%	152
Health Center Northwest	Kalispell	96%	25
Saint Vincent Healthcare	Billings	93%	295
Community Medical Center	Missoula	92%	50
Kalispell Regional Medical Center	Kalispell	92%	108
Bozeman Deaconess Hospital	Bozeman	90%	49
Saint James Community Hospital	Butte	79%	72

22. Prophylactic Antibiotic Stopped

Hospital Name	City	Rate	Cases
North Valley Hospital	Whitefish	98%	80
Livingston Memorial Hospital	Livingston	96%	72
Billings Clinic	Billings	94%	1150
Bozeman Deaconess Hospital	Bozeman	92%	230
Saint Patrick Hosp and Health Sci Ctr	Missoula	92%	391
Glendive Medical Center	Glendive	91%	70
Saint Peter's Hospital	Helena	91%	229
Central Montana Medical Center	Lewistown	90%	48
Holy Rosary Health Care	Miles City	89%	56
Saint Vincent Healthcare	Billings	89%	1317
Barrett Hospital	Dillon	88%	25
Saint Joseph Hospital	Polson	88%	34
Community Medical Center	Missoula	87%	612
Northern Montana Hospital	Havre	84%	87
Sidney Health Center	Sidney	81%	53
Health Center Northwest	Kalispell	80%	232
Saint James Community Hospital	Butte	75%	334
Marcus Daly Memorial Hospital	Hamilton	72%	46
Benefis Healthcare	Great Falls	67%	189
Kalispell Regional Medical Center	Kalispell	53%	491

Pregnancy Care

23. Inpatient Neonatal Mortality

Hospital Name	City	Rate	Cases
Kalispell Regional Medical Center	Kalispell	0.00%	572

NOTE: Hospital profiles are in alphabetical order by state, then city, then hospital within the city; Rankings are sorted by rate in descending order and exclude hospitals with less than 25 cases; (1) The number of cases is too small (n<25) for purposes of reliably predicting hospital performance; (2) Measure reflects the hospital's indication that its submission was based upon a sample of its relevant discharges; (3) Rate reflects fewer than the maximum possible quarters of data for the measure; (4) Inaccurate information submitted and suppressed for one or more quarters; (5) No data is available from the hospital for this measure; Please refer to the User's Guide for a full explanation of data

Saint James Community Hospital	Butte	0.00%	525
Saint Peter's Hospital	Helena	0.00%	875

24. Third or Fourth Degree Laceration

Hospital Name	City	Rate	Cases
Saint Peter's Hospital	Helena	3.54%	594
Saint James Community Hospital	Butte	3.82%	393
Kalispell Regional Medical Center	Kalispell	4.88%	430

NOTE: Hospital profiles are in alphabetical order by state, then city, then hospital within the city; Rankings are sorted by rate in descending order and exclude hospitals with less than 25 cases; (1) The number of cases is too small (n<25) for purposes of reliably predicting hospital performance; (2) Measure reflects the hospital's indication that its submission was based upon a sample of its relevant discharges; (3) Rate reflects fewer than the maximum possible quarters of data for the measure; (4) Inaccurate information submitted and suppressed for one or more quarters; (5) No data is available from the hospital for this measure; Please refer to the User's Guide for a full explanation of data

Community Hosp and Nursing Home of Anaconda

401 W Pennsylvania Avenue — Phone: 406-563-8500
Anaconda, MT 59711 — Fax: 406-563-8565
Ownership: Voluntary non-profit - Private — Accredited: No
Emergency Services: Yes — Licensed Beds: 40

Key Personnel:

CEO . . . . Steve McNeece
Chief of Medical Staff . . . . Michael Rafferty
Emergency Room . . . . Meg Bryan
Respiratory Care . . . . Jim Bleile

Measure	Cases	This Hospital	State Average	U.S. Average	Top Hospital
Heart Attack Care					
ACE Inhibitor or ARB for LVSD	0	-	78%	82%	100%
Aspirin at Arrival[1]	11	100%	96%	92%	100%
Aspirin at Discharge[1]	3	100%	85%	90%	100%
Beta Blocker at Arrival[1]	7	100%	81%	87%	100%
Beta Blocker at Discharge[1]	3	100%	80%	90%	100%
Fibrinolytic Medication Timing[1]	1	100%	32%	31%	100%
PCI Within 90 Minutes of Arrival	0	-	73%	54%	95%
Smoking Cessation Advice[1]	1	100%	87%	88%	100%
Heart Failure Care					
ACE Inhibitor or ARB for LVSD[1]	2	100%	83%	82%	100%
Discharge Instructions[1]	13	92%	47%	61%	93%
Evaluation of LVS Function[1]	20	95%	73%	83%	99%
Smoking Cessation Advice[1]	3	100%	74%	82%	100%
Pneumonia Care					
Appropriate Initial Antibiotic	34	94%	81%	83%	94%
Blood Culture Timing[1]	17	94%	93%	90%	100%
Influenza Vaccine[1]	10	100%	83%	70%	100%
Initial Antibiotic Timing	50	96%	87%	80%	93%
Oxygenation Assessment	56	100%	97%	99%	100%
Pneumococcal Vaccine	37	100%	79%	69%	94%
Smoking Cessation Advice[1]	11	100%	69%	80%	100%
Surgical Infection Prevention					
Prophylactic Antibiotic Given[1]	15	100%	86%	77%	95%
Prophylactic Antibiotic Selection[1]	5	100%	94%	90%	100%
Prophylactic Antibiotic Stopped[1]	15	100%	87%	72%	95%
Pregnancy Care					
Inpatient Neonatal Mortality	-	-	-	-	-
Third or Fourth Degree Laceration	-	-	-	3.63%	3.27%

Pioneer Medical Center

301 W 7th Ave — Phone: 406-932-4603
Big Timber, MT 59011
Ownership: Government - Local — Accredited: No
Emergency Services: Yes

Measure	Cases	This Hospital	State Average	U.S. Average	Top Hospital
Heart Attack Care					
ACE Inhibitor or ARB for LVSD[1,3]	1	100%	78%	82%	100%
Aspirin at Arrival[1,3]	1	100%	96%	92%	100%
Aspirin at Discharge[1,3]	1	0%	85%	90%	100%
Beta Blocker at Arrival[1,3]	1	100%	81%	87%	100%
Beta Blocker at Discharge[1,3]	1	100%	80%	90%	100%
Fibrinolytic Medication Timing[3]	0	-	32%	31%	100%
PCI Within 90 Minutes of Arrival	0	-	73%	54%	95%
Smoking Cessation Advice[3]	0	-	87%	88%	100%
Heart Failure Care					
ACE Inhibitor or ARB for LVSD[1]	4	100%	83%	82%	100%
Discharge Instructions[1]	4	0%	47%	61%	93%
Evaluation of LVS Function[1]	9	56%	73%	83%	99%
Smoking Cessation Advice[1]	1	100%	74%	82%	100%
Pneumonia Care					
Appropriate Initial Antibiotic[1]	13	92%	81%	83%	94%
Blood Culture Timing[1]	2	100%	93%	90%	100%
Influenza Vaccine[1]	5	100%	83%	70%	100%
Initial Antibiotic Timing[1]	22	95%	87%	80%	93%
Oxygenation Assessment[1]	24	100%	97%	99%	100%
Pneumococcal Vaccine[1]	16	94%	79%	69%	94%
Smoking Cessation Advice[1]	1	0%	69%	80%	100%
Surgical Infection Prevention					
Prophylactic Antibiotic Given[5]	-	-	86%	77%	95%
Prophylactic Antibiotic Selection[5]	-	-	94%	90%	100%
Prophylactic Antibiotic Stopped[5]	-	-	87%	72%	95%
Pregnancy Care					
Inpatient Neonatal Mortality	-	-	-	-	-
Third or Fourth Degree Laceration	-	-	-	3.63%	3.27%

Billings Clinic

2800 10th Avenue North — Phone: 406-657-4000
PO Box 37000 — Fax: 406-238-2355
Billings, MT 59107
URL: www.billngsclinic.com
Ownership: Voluntary non-profit - Private — Accredited: Yes
Emergency Services: Yes — Licensed Beds: 272

Key Personnel:

President & CEO . . . . Nicholas J Wolter, MD
CNO . . . . Alice Gordon
Pulmonary & Critical Care Medicine . . . . Robert K Merchant, MD

Measure	Cases	This Hospital	State Average	U.S. Average	Top Hospital
Heart Attack Care					
ACE Inhibitor or ARB for LVSD	53	98%	78%	82%	100%
Aspirin at Arrival	157	99%	96%	92%	100%
Aspirin at Discharge	311	98%	85%	90%	100%
Beta Blocker at Arrival	130	96%	81%	87%	100%
Beta Blocker at Discharge	302	99%	80%	90%	100%
Fibrinolytic Medication Timing	0	-	32%	31%	100%
PCI Within 90 Minutes of Arrival[1]	8	75%	73%	54%	95%
Smoking Cessation Advice	114	100%	87%	88%	100%
Heart Failure Care					
ACE Inhibitor or ARB for LVSD	121	96%	83%	82%	100%
Discharge Instructions	215	90%	47%	61%	93%
Evaluation of LVS Function	249	99%	73%	83%	99%
Smoking Cessation Advice	27	100%	74%	82%	100%
Pneumonia Care					
Appropriate Initial Antibiotic	109	88%	81%	83%	94%
Blood Culture Timing	132	88%	93%	90%	100%
Influenza Vaccine	32	100%	83%	70%	100%
Initial Antibiotic Timing	154	89%	87%	80%	93%
Oxygenation Assessment	207	100%	97%	99%	100%
Pneumococcal Vaccine	128	98%	79%	69%	94%
Smoking Cessation Advice	59	100%	69%	80%	100%
Surgical Infection Prevention					
Prophylactic Antibiotic Given[2]	1,171	96%	86%	77%	95%
Prophylactic Antibiotic Selection[2]	278	99%	94%	90%	100%
Prophylactic Antibiotic Stopped[2]	1,150	94%	87%	72%	95%
Pregnancy Care					
Inpatient Neonatal Mortality	-	-	-	-	-
Third or Fourth Degree Laceration	-	-	-	3.63%	3.27%

Saint Vincent Healthcare

1233 N 30th Street — Phone: 406-657-7000
Billings, MT 59107 — Fax: 406-237-3078
E-mail: web-rn@svh-mt.org
URL: www.svh-mt.org
Ownership: Voluntary non-profit - Private — Accredited: Yes
Emergency Services: Yes — Licensed Beds: 300

Key Personnel:

Manager Respiratory Therapy . . . . Paula Dowdle

Measure	Cases	This Hospital	State Average	U.S. Average	Top Hospital
Heart Attack Care					
ACE Inhibitor or ARB for LVSD	81	69%	78%	82%	100%
Aspirin at Arrival	151	95%	96%	92%	100%
Aspirin at Discharge	302	98%	85%	90%	100%
Beta Blocker at Arrival	145	90%	81%	87%	100%
Beta Blocker at Discharge	294	90%	80%	90%	100%
Fibrinolytic Medication Timing	0	-	32%	31%	100%
PCI Within 90 Minutes of Arrival[1]	8	62%	73%	54%	95%
Smoking Cessation Advice	94	99%	87%	88%	100%
Heart Failure Care					
ACE Inhibitor or ARB for LVSD	86	92%	83%	82%	100%

NOTE: Hospital profiles are in alphabetical order by state, then city, then hospital within the city; Rankings are sorted by rate in descending order and exclude hospitals with less than 25 cases; (1) The number of cases is too small (n<25) for purposes of reliably predicting hospital performance; (2) Measure reflects the hospital's indication that its submission was based upon a sample of its relevant discharges; (3) Rate reflects fewer than the maximum possible quarters of data for the measure; (4) Inaccurate information submitted and suppressed for one or more quarters; (5) No data is available from the hospital for this measure; Please refer to the User's Guide for a full explanation of data

Measure	Cases	This Hospital	State Average	U.S. Average	Top Hospital
Discharge Instructions	200	78%	47%	61%	93%
Evaluation of LVS Function	242	89%	73%	83%	99%
Smoking Cessation Advice	43	88%	74%	82%	100%
Pneumonia Care					
Appropriate Initial Antibiotic	209	87%	81%	83%	94%
Blood Culture Timing	132	90%	93%	90%	100%
Influenza Vaccine	39	100%	83%	70%	100%
Initial Antibiotic Timing	215	83%	87%	80%	93%
Oxygenation Assessment	260	100%	97%	99%	100%
Pneumococcal Vaccine	154	81%	79%	69%	94%
Smoking Cessation Advice	86	85%	69%	80%	100%
Surgical Infection Prevention					
Prophylactic Antibiotic Given	1,334	94%	86%	77%	95%
Prophylactic Antibiotic Selection	295	93%	94%	90%	100%
Prophylactic Antibiotic Stopped	1,317	89%	87%	72%	95%
Pregnancy Care					
Inpatient Neonatal Mortality	-	-	-	-	-
Third or Fourth Degree Laceration	-	-	-	3.63%	3.27%

Bozeman Deaconess Hospital

915 Highland Boulevard
Bozeman, MT 59715
Ownership: Voluntary non-profit - Private
Emergency Services: Yes
Phone: 406-585-5000
Fax: 406-585-1071
Accredited: No
Licensed Beds: 86

Key Personnel:
President/CEO. . . . . John Nordwick
Chief Medical Staff. . . . . Dr. Stephen Ley

Measure	Cases	This Hospital	State Average	U.S. Average	Top Hospital
Heart Attack Care					
ACE Inhibitor or ARB for LVSD[1]	9	100%	78%	82%	100%
Aspirin at Arrival	82	100%	96%	92%	100%
Aspirin at Discharge	68	96%	85%	90%	100%
Beta Blocker at Arrival	68	97%	81%	87%	100%
Beta Blocker at Discharge	71	97%	80%	90%	100%
Fibrinolytic Medication Timing	0	-	32%	31%	100%
PCI Within 90 Minutes of Arrival[1]	8	88%	73%	54%	95%
Smoking Cessation Advice[1]	16	100%	87%	88%	100%
Heart Failure Care					
ACE Inhibitor or ARB for LVSD	36	81%	83%	82%	100%
Discharge Instructions	131	42%	47%	61%	93%
Evaluation of LVS Function	143	93%	73%	83%	99%
Smoking Cessation Advice[1]	15	67%	74%	82%	100%
Pneumonia Care					
Appropriate Initial Antibiotic	76	80%	81%	83%	94%
Blood Culture Timing	57	96%	93%	90%	100%
Influenza Vaccine[1]	13	100%	83%	70%	100%
Initial Antibiotic Timing	93	90%	87%	80%	93%
Oxygenation Assessment	119	100%	97%	99%	100%
Pneumococcal Vaccine	71	89%	79%	69%	94%
Smoking Cessation Advice[1]	11	73%	69%	80%	100%
Surgical Infection Prevention					
Prophylactic Antibiotic Given[2]	241	94%	86%	77%	95%
Prophylactic Antibiotic Selection[2]	49	90%	94%	90%	100%
Prophylactic Antibiotic Stopped[2]	230	92%	87%	72%	95%
Pregnancy Care					
Inpatient Neonatal Mortality	-	-	-	-	-
Third or Fourth Degree Laceration	-	-	-	3.63%	3.27%

PHS Indian Hospital-Browning

PO Box 760
Browning, MT 59417
Ownership: Government - Federal
Emergency Services: Yes
Phone: 406-338-6157
Accredited: Yes

Measure	Cases	This Hospital	State Average	U.S. Average	Top Hospital
Heart Attack Care					
ACE Inhibitor or ARB for LVSD[5]	-	-	78%	82%	100%
Aspirin at Arrival[5]	-	-	96%	92%	100%
Aspirin at Discharge[5]	-	-	85%	90%	100%
Beta Blocker at Arrival[5]	-	-	81%	87%	100%
Beta Blocker at Discharge[5]	-	-	80%	90%	100%
Fibrinolytic Medication Timing[5]	-	-	32%	31%	100%
PCI Within 90 Minutes of Arrival[5]	-	-	73%	54%	95%
Smoking Cessation Advice[5]	-	-	87%	88%	100%
Heart Failure Care					
ACE Inhibitor or ARB for LVSD[1,2]	2	100%	83%	82%	100%
Discharge Instructions[1,2,3]	5	60%	47%	61%	93%
Evaluation of LVS Function[2]	27	41%	73%	83%	99%
Smoking Cessation Advice[1,2,3]	1	100%	74%	82%	100%
Pneumonia Care					
Appropriate Initial Antibiotic[1,3]	2	0%	81%	83%	94%
Blood Culture Timing[1,3]	5	60%	93%	90%	100%
Influenza Vaccine[5]	-	-	83%	70%	100%
Initial Antibiotic Timing	47	85%	87%	80%	93%
Oxygenation Assessment	57	100%	97%	99%	100%
Pneumococcal Vaccine	34	88%	79%	69%	94%
Smoking Cessation Advice[1,3]	4	75%	69%	80%	100%
Surgical Infection Prevention					
Prophylactic Antibiotic Given[5]	-	-	86%	77%	95%
Prophylactic Antibiotic Selection[5]	-	-	94%	90%	100%
Prophylactic Antibiotic Stopped[5]	-	-	87%	72%	95%
Pregnancy Care					
Inpatient Neonatal Mortality	-	-	-	-	-
Third or Fourth Degree Laceration	-	-	-	3.63%	3.27%

Saint James Community Hospital

400 S Clark Street
Butte, MT 59701
E-mail: info@sjch.org
URL: www.stjameshealthcare.org
Ownership: Voluntary non-profit - Church
Emergency Services: Yes
Phone: 406-723-2500
Fax: 406-723-2534
Accredited: Yes
Licensed Beds: 164

Key Personnel:
CEO/President. . . . . James Kiscer
Chief Medical Staff. . . . . Keith J Popovich, MD
Head of Emergency Room. . . . . Judie Williams
Emergency Room . . . . Richard Thorne
Director Medical/Surgical Nursing . . . . Susan Kerschen, RN
OB/GYN Womens Health. . . . . Andrew D Jamieson, MD
Chief Radiology . . . . J Michael Driscoll, MD
Director of Respiratory Therapy . . . . Christie George

Measure	Cases	This Hospital	State Average	U.S. Average	Top Hospital
Heart Attack Care					
ACE Inhibitor or ARB for LVSD[1]	13	69%	78%	82%	100%
Aspirin at Arrival	67	96%	96%	92%	100%
Aspirin at Discharge	50	94%	85%	90%	100%
Beta Blocker at Arrival	50	90%	81%	87%	100%
Beta Blocker at Discharge	54	81%	80%	90%	100%
Fibrinolytic Medication Timing[1]	2	50%	32%	31%	100%
PCI Within 90 Minutes of Arrival[1]	2	100%	73%	54%	95%
Smoking Cessation Advice	34	94%	87%	88%	100%
Heart Failure Care					
ACE Inhibitor or ARB for LVSD[1]	20	65%	83%	82%	100%
Discharge Instructions	75	48%	47%	61%	93%
Evaluation of LVS Function	102	85%	73%	83%	99%
Smoking Cessation Advice[1]	15	100%	74%	82%	100%
Pneumonia Care					
Appropriate Initial Antibiotic	91	85%	81%	83%	94%
Blood Culture Timing	72	97%	93%	90%	100%
Influenza Vaccine[1]	20	95%	83%	70%	100%
Initial Antibiotic Timing	105	89%	87%	80%	93%
Oxygenation Assessment	130	100%	97%	99%	100%
Pneumococcal Vaccine	72	74%	79%	69%	94%
Smoking Cessation Advice	36	78%	69%	80%	100%
Surgical Infection Prevention					
Prophylactic Antibiotic Given	346	97%	86%	77%	95%
Prophylactic Antibiotic Selection	72	79%	94%	90%	100%
Prophylactic Antibiotic Stopped	334	75%	87%	72%	95%
Pregnancy Care					
Inpatient Neonatal Mortality	525	0.00%	-	-	-
Third or Fourth Degree Laceration	393	3.82%	-	3.63%	3.27%

NOTE: Hospital profiles are in alphabetical order by state, then city, then hospital within the city; Rankings are sorted by rate in descending order and exclude hospitals with less than 25 cases; (1) The number of cases is too small (n<25) for purposes of reliably predicting hospital performance; (2) Measure reflects the hospital's indication that its submission was based upon a sample of its relevant discharges; (3) Rate reflects fewer than the maximum possible quarters of data for the measure; (4) Inaccurate information submitted and suppressed for one or more quarters; (5) No data is available from the hospital for this measure; Please refer to the User's Guide for a full explanation of data

Teton Medical Center

915 4th Street NW Phone: 406-466-5763
Choteau, MT 59422 Fax: 406-466-5852
E-mail: tetonmc@tetonmedicalcenter.net
URL: www.tetonmedicalcenter.net
Ownership: Govt - Hospital District or Authority Accredited: No
Emergency Services: Yes Licensed Beds: 7

Key Personnel:
Administrator/CEO . . . . H Ray Gibbons
Chief Medical Staff . . . . Laura Shelton, MD
Manager Radiology . . . . Susan Murphy, RHIT

Measure	Cases	This Hospital	State Average	U.S. Average	Top Hospital
Heart Attack Care					
ACE Inhibitor or ARB for LVSD[5]	-	-	78%	82%	100%
Aspirin at Arrival[5]	-	-	96%	92%	100%
Aspirin at Discharge[5]	-	-	85%	90%	100%
Beta Blocker at Arrival[5]	-	-	81%	87%	100%
Beta Blocker at Discharge[5]	-	-	80%	90%	100%
Fibrinolytic Medication Timing[5]	-	-	32%	31%	100%
PCI Within 90 Minutes of Arrival[5]	-	-	73%	54%	95%
Smoking Cessation Advice[5]	-	-	87%	88%	100%
Heart Failure Care					
ACE Inhibitor or ARB for LVSD[5]	-	-	83%	82%	100%
Discharge Instructions[5]	-	-	47%	61%	93%
Evaluation of LVS Function[5]	-	-	73%	83%	99%
Smoking Cessation Advice[5]	-	-	74%	82%	100%
Pneumonia Care					
Appropriate Initial Antibiotic[5]	-	-	81%	83%	94%
Blood Culture Timing[5]	-	-	93%	90%	100%
Influenza Vaccine[5]	-	-	83%	70%	100%
Initial Antibiotic Timing[5]	-	-	87%	80%	93%
Oxygenation Assessment[5]	-	-	97%	99%	100%
Pneumococcal Vaccine[5]	-	-	79%	69%	94%
Smoking Cessation Advice[5]	-	-	69%	80%	100%
Surgical Infection Prevention					
Prophylactic Antibiotic Given[5]	-	-	86%	77%	95%
Prophylactic Antibiotic Selection[5]	-	-	94%	90%	100%
Prophylactic Antibiotic Stopped[5]	-	-	87%	72%	95%
Pregnancy Care					
Inpatient Neonatal Mortality	-	-	-	-	-
Third or Fourth Degree Laceration	-	-	-	3.63%	3.27%

Mccone County Health Center

605 Sullivan Ave Phone: 406-485-3381
Circle, MT 59215
Ownership: Government - Local Accredited: No
Emergency Services: No

Measure	Cases	This Hospital	State Average	U.S. Average	Top Hospital
Heart Attack Care					
ACE Inhibitor or ARB for LVSD[5]	-	-	78%	82%	100%
Aspirin at Arrival[5]	-	-	96%	92%	100%
Aspirin at Discharge[5]	-	-	85%	90%	100%
Beta Blocker at Arrival[5]	-	-	81%	87%	100%
Beta Blocker at Discharge[5]	-	-	80%	90%	100%
Fibrinolytic Medication Timing[5]	-	-	32%	31%	100%
PCI Within 90 Minutes of Arrival[5]	-	-	73%	54%	95%
Smoking Cessation Advice[5]	-	-	87%	88%	100%
Heart Failure Care					
ACE Inhibitor or ARB for LVSD[3]	0	-	83%	82%	100%
Discharge Instructions[1,3]	2	0%	47%	61%	93%
Evaluation of LVS Function[1,3]	5	0%	73%	83%	99%
Smoking Cessation Advice[1,3]	1	0%	74%	82%	100%
Pneumonia Care					
Appropriate Initial Antibiotic[1,3]	2	50%	81%	83%	94%
Blood Culture Timing[3]	0	-	93%	90%	100%
Influenza Vaccine	0	-	83%	70%	100%
Initial Antibiotic Timing[1,3]	2	50%	87%	80%	93%
Oxygenation Assessment[1,3]	2	100%	97%	99%	100%
Pneumococcal Vaccine[1,3]	2	50%	79%	69%	94%
Smoking Cessation Advice[3]	0	-	69%	80%	100%
Surgical Infection Prevention					
Prophylactic Antibiotic Given[5]	-	-	86%	77%	95%
Prophylactic Antibiotic Selection[5]	-	-	94%	90%	100%
Prophylactic Antibiotic Stopped[5]	-	-	87%	72%	95%
Pregnancy Care					
Inpatient Neonatal Mortality	-	-	-	-	-
Third or Fourth Degree Laceration	-	-	-	3.63%	3.27%

Stillwater Community Hospital

44 W 4th Avenue N Phone: 406-322-5316
PO Box 969 Fax: 406-322-5207
Columbus, MT 59019
Ownership: Voluntary non-profit - Private Accredited: No
Emergency Services: Yes Licensed Beds: 23

Key Personnel:
Administrator . . . . Tim Russell
Infection Control . . . . Denise Donohue

Measure	Cases	This Hospital	State Average	U.S. Average	Top Hospital
Heart Attack Care					
ACE Inhibitor or ARB for LVSD[5]	-	-	78%	82%	100%
Aspirin at Arrival[5]	-	-	96%	92%	100%
Aspirin at Discharge[5]	-	-	85%	90%	100%
Beta Blocker at Arrival[5]	-	-	81%	87%	100%
Beta Blocker at Discharge[5]	-	-	80%	90%	100%
Fibrinolytic Medication Timing[5]	-	-	32%	31%	100%
PCI Within 90 Minutes of Arrival[5]	-	-	73%	54%	95%
Smoking Cessation Advice[5]	-	-	87%	88%	100%
Heart Failure Care					
ACE Inhibitor or ARB for LVSD[5]	-	-	83%	82%	100%
Discharge Instructions[5]	-	-	47%	61%	93%
Evaluation of LVS Function[5]	-	-	73%	83%	99%
Smoking Cessation Advice[5]	-	-	74%	82%	100%
Pneumonia Care					
Appropriate Initial Antibiotic[5]	-	-	81%	83%	94%
Blood Culture Timing[5]	-	-	93%	90%	100%
Influenza Vaccine[5]	-	-	83%	70%	100%
Initial Antibiotic Timing[5]	-	-	87%	80%	93%
Oxygenation Assessment[5]	-	-	97%	99%	100%
Pneumococcal Vaccine[5]	-	-	79%	69%	94%
Smoking Cessation Advice[5]	-	-	69%	80%	100%
Surgical Infection Prevention					
Prophylactic Antibiotic Given[5]	-	-	86%	77%	95%
Prophylactic Antibiotic Selection[5]	-	-	94%	90%	100%
Prophylactic Antibiotic Stopped[5]	-	-	87%	72%	95%
Pregnancy Care					
Inpatient Neonatal Mortality	-	-	-	-	-
Third or Fourth Degree Laceration	-	-	-	3.63%	3.27%

Pondera Medical Center

805 Sunset Boulevard Phone: 406-271-3211
Conrad, MT 59425 Fax: 406-271-3917
URL: www.ourpmc.com
Ownership: Proprietary Accredited: No
Emergency Services: Yes Licensed Beds: 20

Key Personnel:
CEO . . . . C James Christensen

Measure	Cases	This Hospital	State Average	U.S. Average	Top Hospital
Heart Attack Care					
ACE Inhibitor or ARB for LVSD[5]	-	-	78%	82%	100%
Aspirin at Arrival[5]	-	-	96%	92%	100%
Aspirin at Discharge[5]	-	-	85%	90%	100%
Beta Blocker at Arrival[5]	-	-	81%	87%	100%
Beta Blocker at Discharge[5]	-	-	80%	90%	100%
Fibrinolytic Medication Timing[5]	-	-	32%	31%	100%
PCI Within 90 Minutes of Arrival[5]	-	-	73%	54%	95%
Smoking Cessation Advice[5]	-	-	87%	88%	100%
Heart Failure Care					
ACE Inhibitor or ARB for LVSD[1]	2	100%	83%	82%	100%
Discharge Instructions[1]	7	86%	47%	61%	93%
Evaluation of LVS Function[1]	8	100%	73%	83%	99%

NOTE: Hospital profiles are in alphabetical order by state, then city, then hospital within the city; Rankings are sorted by rate in descending order and exclude hospitals with less than 25 cases; (1) The number of cases is too small (n<25) for purposes of reliably predicting hospital performance; (2) Measure reflects the hospital's indication that its submission was based upon a sample of its relevant discharges; (3) Rate reflects fewer than the maximum possible quarters of data for the measure; (4) Inaccurate information submitted and suppressed for one or more quarters; (5) No data is available from the hospital for this measure; Please refer to the User's Guide for a full explanation of data

Smoking Cessation Advice[1]	1	100%	74%	82%	100%
Pneumonia Care					
Appropriate Initial Antibiotic[1]	5	80%	81%	83%	94%
Blood Culture Timing[1]	1	100%	93%	90%	100%
Influenza Vaccine[1]	1	100%	83%	70%	100%
Initial Antibiotic Timing[1]	6	67%	87%	80%	93%
Oxygenation Assessment[1]	6	83%	97%	99%	100%
Pneumococcal Vaccine[1]	5	80%	79%	69%	94%
Smoking Cessation Advice	0	-	69%	80%	100%
Surgical Infection Prevention					
Prophylactic Antibiotic Given[5]	-	-	86%	77%	95%
Prophylactic Antibiotic Selection[5]	-	-	94%	90%	100%
Prophylactic Antibiotic Stopped[5]	-	-	87%	72%	95%
Pregnancy Care					
Inpatient Neonatal Mortality	-	-	-	-	-
Third or Fourth Degree Laceration	-	-	-	3.63%	3.27%

Crow/Northern Cheyenne Hospital

Alternate Name: PHS Indian Hospital Crow
PO Box 9 Phone: 406-638-3461
Crow Agency, MT 59002 Fax: 406-638-3569
Ownership: Government - Federal Accredited: Yes
Emergency Services: Yes Licensed Beds: 24

Key Personnel:
CEO.................................. Kevin Ftiffarm
Chief Medical Staff........................ Dr. Leonard Thomas
Chief Medical Staff........................ David Mark
Emergency Room .... Joseph Keel
Emergency Room .... Dr. Clayton Bunt

Measure	Cases	This Hospital	State Average	U.S. Average	Top Hospital
Heart Attack Care					
ACE Inhibitor or ARB for LVSD[3]	0	-	78%	82%	100%
Aspirin at Arrival[3]	0	-	96%	92%	100%
Aspirin at Discharge[3]	0	-	85%	90%	100%
Beta Blocker at Arrival[3]	0	-	81%	87%	100%
Beta Blocker at Discharge[3]	0	-	80%	90%	100%
Fibrinolytic Medication Timing[3]	0	-	32%	31%	100%
PCI Within 90 Minutes of Arrival[5]	-	-	73%	54%	95%
Smoking Cessation Advice[3]	0	-	87%	88%	100%
Heart Failure Care					
ACE Inhibitor or ARB for LVSD[1]	5	100%	83%	82%	100%
Discharge Instructions[1]	8	25%	47%	61%	93%
Evaluation of LVS Function[1]	16	88%	73%	83%	99%
Smoking Cessation Advice[1]	2	50%	74%	82%	100%
Pneumonia Care					
Appropriate Initial Antibiotic[1]	21	71%	81%	83%	94%
Blood Culture Timing[1]	12	83%	93%	90%	100%
Influenza Vaccine[1]	6	67%	83%	70%	100%
Initial Antibiotic Timing[1]	19	100%	87%	80%	93%
Oxygenation Assessment[1]	24	100%	97%	99%	100%
Pneumococcal Vaccine[1]	15	100%	79%	69%	94%
Smoking Cessation Advice[1]	5	40%	69%	80%	100%
Surgical Infection Prevention					
Prophylactic Antibiotic Given[1]	8	50%	86%	77%	95%
Prophylactic Antibiotic Selection[1]	2	100%	94%	90%	100%
Prophylactic Antibiotic Stopped[1]	6	100%	87%	72%	95%
Pregnancy Care					
Inpatient Neonatal Mortality	-	-	-	-	-
Third or Fourth Degree Laceration	-	-	-	3.63%	3.27%

Barrett Hospital

90 Highway 91 South Phone: 406-683-3000
Dillon, MT 59725 Fax: 406-683-3011
URL: www.barretthospital.org
Ownership: Govt - Hospital District or Authority Accredited: No
Emergency Services: Yes Licensed Beds: 20

Key Personnel:
CEO.................................. John M Mootry
Chief Medical Staff........................ Karen Weed, MD

Measure	Cases	This Hospital	State Average	U.S. Average	Top Hospital
Heart Attack Care					
ACE Inhibitor or ARB for LVSD	0	-	78%	82%	100%
Aspirin at Arrival[1]	3	100%	96%	92%	100%
Aspirin at Discharge[1]	1	100%	85%	90%	100%
Beta Blocker at Arrival[1]	3	67%	81%	87%	100%
Beta Blocker at Discharge[1]	1	100%	80%	90%	100%
Fibrinolytic Medication Timing[1]	4	50%	32%	31%	100%
PCI Within 90 Minutes of Arrival	0	-	73%	54%	95%
Smoking Cessation Advice	0	-	87%	88%	100%
Heart Failure Care					
ACE Inhibitor or ARB for LVSD[1]	6	100%	83%	82%	100%
Discharge Instructions[1]	13	92%	47%	61%	93%
Evaluation of LVS Function[1]	14	93%	73%	83%	99%
Smoking Cessation Advice	0	-	74%	82%	100%
Pneumonia Care					
Appropriate Initial Antibiotic	42	100%	81%	83%	94%
Blood Culture Timing[1]	18	94%	93%	90%	100%
Influenza Vaccine[1]	13	100%	83%	70%	100%
Initial Antibiotic Timing	43	86%	87%	80%	93%
Oxygenation Assessment	47	100%	97%	99%	100%
Pneumococcal Vaccine	32	100%	79%	69%	94%
Smoking Cessation Advice[1]	5	100%	69%	80%	100%
Surgical Infection Prevention					
Prophylactic Antibiotic Given	26	73%	86%	77%	95%
Prophylactic Antibiotic Selection[1]	4	100%	94%	90%	100%
Prophylactic Antibiotic Stopped	25	88%	87%	72%	95%
Pregnancy Care					
Inpatient Neonatal Mortality	-	-	-	-	-
Third or Fourth Degree Laceration	-	-	-	3.63%	3.27%

Missouri River Medical Center

1501 Saint Charles Phone: 406-622-3331
PO Box 249 Fax: 406-622-5670
Fort Benton, MT 59442
E-mail: mrmc@mtintouch.net
URL: www.mrmcfb.org
Ownership: Voluntary non-profit - Other Accredited: No
Emergency Services: Yes Licensed Beds: 52

Key Personnel:
Administrator .... Jay Pottenger, MSA CHE
Chief Medical Staff........................ Mark Buck, MD

Measure	Cases	This Hospital	State Average	U.S. Average	Top Hospital
Heart Attack Care					
ACE Inhibitor or ARB for LVSD[5]	-	-	78%	82%	100%
Aspirin at Arrival[5]	-	-	96%	92%	100%
Aspirin at Discharge[5]	-	-	85%	90%	100%
Beta Blocker at Arrival[5]	-	-	81%	87%	100%
Beta Blocker at Discharge[5]	-	-	80%	90%	100%
Fibrinolytic Medication Timing[5]	-	-	32%	31%	100%
PCI Within 90 Minutes of Arrival[5]	-	-	73%	54%	95%
Smoking Cessation Advice[5]	-	-	87%	88%	100%
Heart Failure Care					
ACE Inhibitor or ARB for LVSD[5]	-	-	83%	82%	100%
Discharge Instructions[1,3]	4	0%	47%	61%	93%
Evaluation of LVS Function[5]	-	-	73%	83%	99%
Smoking Cessation Advice[3]	0	-	74%	82%	100%
Pneumonia Care					
Appropriate Initial Antibiotic[1,3]	5	60%	81%	83%	94%
Blood Culture Timing[1,3]	1	100%	93%	90%	100%
Influenza Vaccine[1]	2	50%	83%	70%	100%
Initial Antibiotic Timing[1,3]	4	100%	87%	80%	93%
Oxygenation Assessment[1,3]	6	100%	97%	99%	100%
Pneumococcal Vaccine[1,3]	7	43%	79%	69%	94%
Smoking Cessation Advice[1,3]	1	100%	69%	80%	100%
Surgical Infection Prevention					
Prophylactic Antibiotic Given[5]	-	-	86%	77%	95%
Prophylactic Antibiotic Selection[5]	-	-	94%	90%	100%
Prophylactic Antibiotic Stopped[5]	-	-	87%	72%	95%
Pregnancy Care					
Inpatient Neonatal Mortality	-	-	-	-	-
Third or Fourth Degree Laceration	-	-	-	3.63%	3.27%

NOTE: Hospital profiles are in alphabetical order by state, then city, then hospital within the city; Rankings are sorted by rate in descending order and exclude hospitals with less than 25 cases; (1) The number of cases is too small (n<25) for purposes of reliably predicting hospital performance; (2) Measure reflects the hospital's indication that its submission was based upon a sample of its relevant discharges; (3) Rate reflects fewer than the maximum possible quarters of data for the measure; (4) Inaccurate information submitted and suppressed for one or more quarters; (5) No data is available from the hospital for this measure; Please refer to the User's Guide for a full explanation of data

Frances Mahon Deaconess Hospital

621 3rd Street S
Glasgow, MT 59230
Phone: 406-228-3500
Fax: 406-228-3535
Ownership: Proprietary
Accredited: Yes
Emergency Services: Yes
Licensed Beds: 25

Key Personnel:

President/CEO . . . . Randall G Holom
Chief Medical Staff . . . . Lawrence Palazzo, MD
Cardiac Lab . . . . Bev Falcon
Emergency Room . . . . Brenda Koessl, RN
Infection Control . . . . Rose Scuville
ICU . . . . Jan Jacobson, RN
Medical Surgical Nursing . . . . Joy De Puydt, RN

Measure	Cases	This Hospital	State Average	U.S. Average	Top Hospital
Heart Attack Care					
ACE Inhibitor or ARB for LVSD[3]	0	-	78%	82%	100%
Aspirin at Arrival[1,3]	1	100%	96%	92%	100%
Aspirin at Discharge[3]	0	-	85%	90%	100%
Beta Blocker at Arrival[1,3]	1	100%	81%	87%	100%
Beta Blocker at Discharge[1,3]	1	100%	80%	90%	100%
Fibrinolytic Medication Timing[1,3]	1	0%	32%	31%	100%
PCI Within 90 Minutes of Arrival	0	-	73%	54%	95%
Smoking Cessation Advice[3]	0	-	87%	88%	100%
Heart Failure Care					
ACE Inhibitor or ARB for LVSD[1]	3	100%	83%	82%	100%
Discharge Instructions[1]	18	61%	47%	61%	93%
Evaluation of LVS Function[1]	18	67%	73%	83%	99%
Smoking Cessation Advice[1]	8	100%	74%	82%	100%
Pneumonia Care					
Appropriate Initial Antibiotic[1]	19	89%	81%	83%	94%
Blood Culture Timing[3]	0	-	93%	90%	100%
Influenza Vaccine[1]	10	100%	83%	70%	100%
Initial Antibiotic Timing[1]	23	83%	87%	80%	93%
Oxygenation Assessment	26	100%	97%	99%	100%
Pneumococcal Vaccine[1]	19	89%	79%	69%	94%
Smoking Cessation Advice[1]	6	100%	69%	80%	100%
Surgical Infection Prevention					
Prophylactic Antibiotic Given[1,2]	14	93%	86%	77%	95%
Prophylactic Antibiotic Selection[1,2]	3	100%	94%	90%	100%
Prophylactic Antibiotic Stopped[1,2]	14	100%	87%	72%	95%
Pregnancy Care					
Inpatient Neonatal Mortality	-	-	-	-	-
Third or Fourth Degree Laceration	-	-	-	3.63%	3.27%

Glendive Medical Center

202 Prospect Drive
Glendive, MT 59330
Toll-Free: 800-660-4325
Phone: 406-345-3306
Fax: 406-345-3358
URL: www.gmc.org
Ownership: Voluntary non-profit - Private
Accredited: No
Emergency Services: Yes
Licensed Beds: 46

Key Personnel:

CEO . . . . Scott A Duke
Chief Medical Staff . . . . Bruce Fwarny
Surgical/Anesthesia Services Exec Dir. . . . . Judy Courtney
Infection Control Coordinator . . . . Nina Helvik
Surgery Manager . . . . Shawna Dorwart
Respiratory Therapy Manager . . . . Sheila Stedman

Measure	Cases	This Hospital	State Average	U.S. Average	Top Hospital
Heart Attack Care					
ACE Inhibitor or ARB for LVSD[1]	1	100%	78%	82%	100%
Aspirin at Arrival[1]	9	78%	96%	92%	100%
Aspirin at Discharge[1]	5	40%	85%	90%	100%
Beta Blocker at Arrival[1]	8	88%	81%	87%	100%
Beta Blocker at Discharge[1]	4	100%	80%	90%	100%
Fibrinolytic Medication Timing	0	-	32%	31%	100%
PCI Within 90 Minutes of Arrival	0	-	73%	54%	95%
Smoking Cessation Advice	0	-	87%	88%	100%
Heart Failure Care					
ACE Inhibitor or ARB for LVSD[1]	6	83%	83%	82%	100%
Discharge Instructions[1]	14	57%	47%	61%	93%
Evaluation of LVS Function[1]	20	60%	73%	83%	99%
Smoking Cessation Advice[1]	5	80%	74%	82%	100%
Pneumonia Care					
Appropriate Initial Antibiotic	40	78%	81%	83%	94%
Blood Culture Timing	26	96%	93%	90%	100%
Influenza Vaccine[1]	9	89%	83%	70%	100%
Initial Antibiotic Timing	56	84%	87%	80%	93%
Oxygenation Assessment	60	100%	97%	99%	100%
Pneumococcal Vaccine	40	88%	79%	69%	94%
Smoking Cessation Advice[1]	9	67%	69%	80%	100%
Surgical Infection Prevention					
Prophylactic Antibiotic Given	73	81%	86%	77%	95%
Prophylactic Antibiotic Selection[1]	13	92%	94%	90%	100%
Prophylactic Antibiotic Stopped	70	91%	87%	72%	95%
Pregnancy Care					
Inpatient Neonatal Mortality	-	-	-	-	-
Third or Fourth Degree Laceration	-	-	-	3.63%	3.27%

Benefis Healthcare

1101 26th Street S
Great Falls, MT 59405
Phone: 406-761-1200
Fax: 406-455-4995
E-mail: benefis@benefis.org
URL: www.benefis.org
Ownership: Proprietary
Accredited: Yes
Emergency Services: Yes
Licensed Beds: 326

Key Personnel:

President . . . . Laura Goldhahn
CEO . . . . John Goodnow
VP/Chief Medical Officer . . . . Paul Dolan

Measure	Cases	This Hospital	State Average	U.S. Average	Top Hospital
Heart Attack Care					
ACE Inhibitor or ARB for LVSD[1]	22	77%	78%	82%	100%
Aspirin at Arrival	94	99%	96%	92%	100%
Aspirin at Discharge	136	99%	85%	90%	100%
Beta Blocker at Arrival	77	95%	81%	87%	100%
Beta Blocker at Discharge	136	99%	80%	90%	100%
Fibrinolytic Medication Timing[1]	1	0%	32%	31%	100%
PCI Within 90 Minutes of Arrival[1]	8	88%	73%	54%	95%
Smoking Cessation Advice	45	98%	87%	88%	100%
Heart Failure Care					
ACE Inhibitor or ARB for LVSD	78	92%	83%	82%	100%
Discharge Instructions	175	82%	47%	61%	93%
Evaluation of LVS Function	221	97%	73%	83%	99%
Smoking Cessation Advice	30	100%	74%	82%	100%
Pneumonia Care					
Appropriate Initial Antibiotic	179	93%	81%	83%	94%
Blood Culture Timing	125	93%	93%	90%	100%
Influenza Vaccine	43	60%	83%	70%	100%
Initial Antibiotic Timing	231	82%	87%	80%	93%
Oxygenation Assessment	309	99%	97%	99%	100%
Pneumococcal Vaccine	199	87%	79%	69%	94%
Smoking Cessation Advice	87	91%	69%	80%	100%
Surgical Infection Prevention					
Prophylactic Antibiotic Given[2,3]	200	98%	86%	77%	95%
Prophylactic Antibiotic Selection[2]	68	99%	94%	90%	100%
Prophylactic Antibiotic Stopped[2,3]	189	67%	87%	72%	95%
Pregnancy Care					
Inpatient Neonatal Mortality	-	-	-	-	-
Third or Fourth Degree Laceration	-	-	-	3.63%	3.27%

Central Montana Surgical Hospital

1411 9th Saint S
Great Falls, MT 59405
Phone: 406-727-5577
Ownership: Proprietary
Accredited: No
Emergency Services: No

Measure	Cases	This Hospital	State Average	U.S. Average	Top Hospital
Heart Attack Care					
ACE Inhibitor or ARB for LVSD[5]	-	-	78%	82%	100%
Aspirin at Arrival[5]	-	-	96%	92%	100%
Aspirin at Discharge[5]	-	-	85%	90%	100%

NOTE: Hospital profiles are in alphabetical order by state, then city, then hospital within the city; Rankings are sorted by rate in descending order and exclude hospitals with less than 25 cases; (1) The number of cases is too small (n<25) for purposes of reliably predicting hospital performance; (2) Measure reflects the hospital's indication that its submission was based upon a sample of its relevant discharges; (3) Rate reflects fewer than the maximum possible quarters of data for the measure; (4) Inaccurate information submitted and suppressed for one or more quarters; (5) No data is available from the hospital for this measure; Please refer to the User's Guide for a full explanation of data

Measure	Cases	This Hospital	State Average	U.S. Average	Top Hospital
Beta Blocker at Arrival[5]	-	-	81%	87%	100%
Beta Blocker at Discharge[5]	-	-	80%	90%	100%
Fibrinolytic Medication Timing[5]	-	-	32%	31%	100%
PCI Within 90 Minutes of Arrival[5]	-	-	73%	54%	95%
Smoking Cessation Advice[5]	-	-	87%	88%	100%
Heart Failure Care					
ACE Inhibitor or ARB for LVSD[3]	0	-	83%	82%	100%
Discharge Instructions[3]	0	-	47%	61%	93%
Evaluation of LVS Function[3]	0	-	73%	83%	99%
Smoking Cessation Advice[3]	0	-	74%	82%	100%
Pneumonia Care					
Appropriate Initial Antibiotic[5]	-	-	81%	83%	94%
Blood Culture Timing[5]	-	-	93%	90%	100%
Influenza Vaccine[5]	-	-	83%	70%	100%
Initial Antibiotic Timing[5]	-	-	87%	80%	93%
Oxygenation Assessment[5]	-	-	97%	99%	100%
Pneumococcal Vaccine[5]	-	-	79%	69%	94%
Smoking Cessation Advice[5]	-	-	69%	80%	100%
Surgical Infection Prevention					
Prophylactic Antibiotic Given[1,3]	10	90%	86%	77%	95%
Prophylactic Antibiotic Selection[5]	-	-	94%	90%	100%
Prophylactic Antibiotic Stopped[1,3]	10	100%	87%	72%	95%
Pregnancy Care					
Inpatient Neonatal Mortality	-	-	-	-	-
Third or Fourth Degree Laceration	-	-	-	3.63%	3.27%

Marcus Daly Memorial Hospital

1200 Westwood Drive — Phone: 406-363-2211
Hamilton, MT 59840 — Fax: 406-363-6536
E-mail: info@mdmh.org
URL: www.mdmh.org
Ownership: Government - Local — Accredited: No
Emergency Services: Yes — Licensed Beds: 48

Key Personnel:
CEO. . . . . John Bartos
Chief of Medical Staff. . . . . Marshall White, Jr, MD
Chief Medical Officer . . . . Mark Jergens, MD, MHA
Emergency Room . . . . James Hansen, MD

Measure	Cases	This Hospital	State Average	U.S. Average	Top Hospital
Heart Attack Care					
ACE Inhibitor or ARB for LVSD[3]	0	-	78%	82%	100%
Aspirin at Arrival[1,3]	4	75%	96%	92%	100%
Aspirin at Discharge[1,3]	2	50%	85%	90%	100%
Beta Blocker at Arrival[1,3]	4	50%	81%	87%	100%
Beta Blocker at Discharge[1,3]	2	0%	80%	90%	100%
Fibrinolytic Medication Timing[3]	0	-	32%	31%	100%
PCI Within 90 Minutes of Arrival	0	-	73%	54%	95%
Smoking Cessation Advice[3]	0	-	87%	88%	100%
Heart Failure Care					
ACE Inhibitor or ARB for LVSD[1,3]	2	50%	83%	82%	100%
Discharge Instructions[1,3]	15	20%	47%	61%	93%
Evaluation of LVS Function[1,3]	17	65%	73%	83%	99%
Smoking Cessation Advice[1,3]	1	0%	74%	82%	100%
Pneumonia Care					
Appropriate Initial Antibiotic[3]	28	82%	81%	83%	94%
Blood Culture Timing[1,3]	10	80%	93%	90%	100%
Influenza Vaccine[5]	-	-	83%	70%	100%
Initial Antibiotic Timing[3]	38	84%	87%	80%	93%
Oxygenation Assessment[3]	44	100%	97%	99%	100%
Pneumococcal Vaccine[3]	28	100%	79%	69%	94%
Smoking Cessation Advice[1,3]	9	22%	69%	80%	100%
Surgical Infection Prevention					
Prophylactic Antibiotic Given[3]	47	96%	86%	77%	95%
Prophylactic Antibiotic Selection[1]	13	69%	94%	90%	100%
Prophylactic Antibiotic Stopped[3]	46	72%	87%	72%	95%
Pregnancy Care					
Inpatient Neonatal Mortality	-	-	-	-	-
Third or Fourth Degree Laceration	-	-	-	3.63%	3.27%

Northern Montana Hospital

PO Box 1231 — Phone: 406-265-2211
Havre, MT 59501 — Fax: 406-265-1651
URL: www.nmhcare.com
Ownership: Voluntary non-profit - Private — Accredited: No
Emergency Services: Yes — Licensed Beds: 49

Key Personnel:
President/CEO. . . . . David C Henry
Chief Medical Staff. . . . . Frank Miller, MD
Emergency Room . . . . Riki Hanstede
Director of Pulmonary . . . . Mark Kelly

Measure	Cases	This Hospital	State Average	U.S. Average	Top Hospital
Heart Attack Care					
ACE Inhibitor or ARB for LVSD[1,3]	2	100%	78%	82%	100%
Aspirin at Arrival[1,3]	2	100%	96%	92%	100%
Aspirin at Discharge[1,3]	1	100%	85%	90%	100%
Beta Blocker at Arrival[1,3]	4	75%	81%	87%	100%
Beta Blocker at Discharge[1,3]	2	100%	80%	90%	100%
Fibrinolytic Medication Timing[1,3]	2	50%	32%	31%	100%
PCI Within 90 Minutes of Arrival	0	-	73%	54%	95%
Smoking Cessation Advice[3]	0	-	87%	88%	100%
Heart Failure Care					
ACE Inhibitor or ARB for LVSD[1]	6	83%	83%	82%	100%
Discharge Instructions	39	41%	47%	61%	93%
Evaluation of LVS Function	45	87%	73%	83%	99%
Smoking Cessation Advice[1]	8	88%	74%	82%	100%
Pneumonia Care					
Appropriate Initial Antibiotic	57	86%	81%	83%	94%
Blood Culture Timing	43	95%	93%	90%	100%
Influenza Vaccine[1]	14	57%	83%	70%	100%
Initial Antibiotic Timing	69	77%	87%	80%	93%
Oxygenation Assessment	85	100%	97%	99%	100%
Pneumococcal Vaccine	51	59%	79%	69%	94%
Smoking Cessation Advice[1]	23	83%	69%	80%	100%
Surgical Infection Prevention					
Prophylactic Antibiotic Given[2]	89	90%	86%	77%	95%
Prophylactic Antibiotic Selection[1,2]	15	100%	94%	90%	100%
Prophylactic Antibiotic Stopped[2]	87	84%	87%	72%	95%
Pregnancy Care					
Inpatient Neonatal Mortality	-	-	-	-	-
Third or Fourth Degree Laceration	-	-	-	3.63%	3.27%

Saint Peter's Hospital

Alternate Name: Saint Peter's Community Hospital
2475 Broadway — Phone: 406-442-2480
Helena, MT 59601 — Fax: 406-444-2389
Ownership: Voluntary non-profit - Private — Accredited: Yes
Emergency Services: Yes — Licensed Beds: 99

Key Personnel:
President/CEO. . . . . John Solheim

Measure	Cases	This Hospital	State Average	U.S. Average	Top Hospital
Heart Attack Care					
ACE Inhibitor or ARB for LVSD[1]	14	100%	78%	82%	100%
Aspirin at Arrival	75	99%	96%	92%	100%
Aspirin at Discharge	71	96%	85%	90%	100%
Beta Blocker at Arrival	59	100%	81%	87%	100%
Beta Blocker at Discharge	66	98%	80%	90%	100%
Fibrinolytic Medication Timing	0	-	32%	31%	100%
PCI Within 90 Minutes of Arrival[1]	2	0%	73%	54%	95%
Smoking Cessation Advice[1]	22	86%	87%	88%	100%
Heart Failure Care					
ACE Inhibitor or ARB for LVSD[1]	16	88%	83%	82%	100%
Discharge Instructions	56	66%	47%	61%	93%
Evaluation of LVS Function	71	94%	73%	83%	99%
Smoking Cessation Advice[1]	11	100%	74%	82%	100%
Pneumonia Care					
Appropriate Initial Antibiotic	95	94%	81%	83%	94%
Blood Culture Timing	74	96%	93%	90%	100%
Influenza Vaccine	27	96%	83%	70%	100%
Initial Antibiotic Timing	122	89%	87%	80%	93%

NOTE: Hospital profiles are in alphabetical order by state, then city, then hospital within the city; Rankings are sorted by rate in descending order and exclude hospitals with less than 25 cases; (1) The number of cases is too small (n<25) for purposes of reliably predicting hospital performance; (2) Measure reflects the hospital's indication that its submission was based upon a sample of its relevant discharges; (3) Rate reflects fewer than the maximum possible quarters of data for the measure; (4) Inaccurate information submitted and suppressed for one or more quarters; (5) No data is available from the hospital for this measure; Please refer to the User's Guide for a full explanation of data

Oxygenation Assessment	159	100%	97%	99%	100%
Pneumococcal Vaccine	102	96%	79%	69%	94%
Smoking Cessation Advice	32	84%	69%	80%	100%
Surgical Infection Prevention					
Prophylactic Antibiotic Given	237	95%	86%	77%	95%
Prophylactic Antibiotic Selection	59	100%	94%	90%	100%
Prophylactic Antibiotic Stopped	229	91%	87%	72%	95%
Pregnancy Care					
Inpatient Neonatal Mortality	875	0.00%	-	-	-
Third or Fourth Degree Laceration	594	3.54%	-	3.63%	3.27%

Garfield County Health Center

PO Box 389 Phone: 406-557-2500
Jordan, MT 59337
Ownership: Government - Federal Accredited: No
Emergency Services: Yes

Measure	Cases	This Hospital	State Average	U.S. Average	Top Hospital
Heart Attack Care					
ACE Inhibitor or ARB for LVSD[5]	-	-	78%	82%	100%
Aspirin at Arrival[5]	-	-	96%	92%	100%
Aspirin at Discharge[5]	-	-	85%	90%	100%
Beta Blocker at Arrival[5]	-	-	81%	87%	100%
Beta Blocker at Discharge[5]	-	-	80%	90%	100%
Fibrinolytic Medication Timing[5]	-	-	32%	31%	100%
PCI Within 90 Minutes of Arrival[5]	-	-	73%	54%	95%
Smoking Cessation Advice[5]	-	-	87%	88%	100%
Heart Failure Care					
ACE Inhibitor or ARB for LVSD[5]	-	-	83%	82%	100%
Discharge Instructions[5]	-	-	47%	61%	93%
Evaluation of LVS Function[5]	-	-	73%	83%	99%
Smoking Cessation Advice[5]	-	-	74%	82%	100%
Pneumonia Care					
Appropriate Initial Antibiotic[5]	-	-	81%	83%	94%
Blood Culture Timing[5]	-	-	93%	90%	100%
Influenza Vaccine[5]	-	-	83%	70%	100%
Initial Antibiotic Timing[5]	-	-	87%	80%	93%
Oxygenation Assessment[5]	-	-	97%	99%	100%
Pneumococcal Vaccine[5]	-	-	79%	69%	94%
Smoking Cessation Advice[5]	-	-	69%	80%	100%
Surgical Infection Prevention					
Prophylactic Antibiotic Given[5]	-	-	86%	77%	95%
Prophylactic Antibiotic Selection[5]	-	-	94%	90%	100%
Prophylactic Antibiotic Stopped[5]	-	-	87%	72%	95%
Pregnancy Care					
Inpatient Neonatal Mortality	-	-	-	-	-
Third or Fourth Degree Laceration	-	-	-	3.63%	3.27%

Health Center Northwest

320 Sunnyview Lane Phone: 406-751-1724
Kalispell, MT 59901
Ownership: Proprietary Accredited: No
Emergency Services: No

Measure	Cases	This Hospital	State Average	U.S. Average	Top Hospital
Heart Attack Care					
ACE Inhibitor or ARB for LVSD[3]	0	-	78%	82%	100%
Aspirin at Arrival[3]	0	-	96%	92%	100%
Aspirin at Discharge[3]	0	-	85%	90%	100%
Beta Blocker at Arrival[1,3]	1	0%	81%	87%	100%
Beta Blocker at Discharge[1,3]	1	0%	80%	90%	100%
Fibrinolytic Medication Timing[3]	0	-	32%	31%	100%
PCI Within 90 Minutes of Arrival	0	-	73%	54%	95%
Smoking Cessation Advice[3]	0	-	87%	88%	100%
Heart Failure Care					
ACE Inhibitor or ARB for LVSD[3]	0	-	83%	82%	100%
Discharge Instructions[1,3]	2	0%	47%	61%	93%
Evaluation of LVS Function[1,3]	3	67%	73%	83%	99%
Smoking Cessation Advice[3]	0	-	74%	82%	100%
Pneumonia Care					
Appropriate Initial Antibiotic[1]	5	100%	81%	83%	94%
Blood Culture Timing[1]	1	100%	93%	90%	100%
Influenza Vaccine[1]	2	50%	83%	70%	100%
Initial Antibiotic Timing[1]	3	100%	87%	80%	93%
Oxygenation Assessment[1]	6	100%	97%	99%	100%
Pneumococcal Vaccine[1]	16	38%	79%	69%	94%
Smoking Cessation Advice[1]	7	71%	69%	80%	100%
Surgical Infection Prevention					
Prophylactic Antibiotic Given[2]	239	73%	86%	77%	95%
Prophylactic Antibiotic Selection[2]	25	96%	94%	90%	100%
Prophylactic Antibiotic Stopped[2]	232	80%	87%	72%	95%
Pregnancy Care					
Inpatient Neonatal Mortality	-	-	-	-	-
Third or Fourth Degree Laceration	-	-	-	3.63%	3.27%

Kalispell Regional Medical Center

Alternate Name: Kalispell Regional Hospital
310 Sunnyview Lane Phone: 406-752-5111
Kalispell, MT 59901 Fax: 406-756-2703
E-mail: jolive@krmc.orgrg
URL: www.krmc.org
Ownership: Voluntary non-profit - Private Accredited: Yes
Emergency Services: Yes Licensed Beds: 143

Key Personnel:

President/CEO. . . . . Velinda Stevens
Chief Medical Staff. . . . . Keith Lara
Cardiac Lab . . . . Renae Solum
Emergency Room . . . . Allison Meilicke
Infection Control. . . . . Tereal Dammell
ICU . . . . Karen Lee
OB/GYN/Women's Health . . . . Nancy Greer

Measure	Cases	This Hospital	State Average	U.S. Average	Top Hospital
Heart Attack Care					
ACE Inhibitor or ARB for LVSD[1]	24	92%	78%	82%	100%
Aspirin at Arrival	151	99%	96%	92%	100%
Aspirin at Discharge	198	98%	85%	90%	100%
Beta Blocker at Arrival	134	99%	81%	87%	100%
Beta Blocker at Discharge	191	96%	80%	90%	100%
Fibrinolytic Medication Timing	0	-	32%	31%	100%
PCI Within 90 Minutes of Arrival[1]	12	83%	73%	54%	95%
Smoking Cessation Advice	69	88%	87%	88%	100%
Heart Failure Care					
ACE Inhibitor or ARB for LVSD	47	89%	83%	82%	100%
Discharge Instructions	105	66%	47%	61%	93%
Evaluation of LVS Function	139	91%	73%	83%	99%
Smoking Cessation Advice[1]	18	89%	74%	82%	100%
Pneumonia Care					
Appropriate Initial Antibiotic	121	82%	81%	83%	94%
Blood Culture Timing	119	90%	93%	90%	100%
Influenza Vaccine[1]	23	57%	83%	70%	100%
Initial Antibiotic Timing	155	93%	87%	80%	93%
Oxygenation Assessment	195	100%	97%	99%	100%
Pneumococcal Vaccine	126	58%	79%	69%	94%
Smoking Cessation Advice	55	69%	69%	80%	100%
Surgical Infection Prevention					
Prophylactic Antibiotic Given[2]	502	77%	86%	77%	95%
Prophylactic Antibiotic Selection[2]	108	92%	94%	90%	100%
Prophylactic Antibiotic Stopped[2]	491	53%	87%	72%	95%
Pregnancy Care					
Inpatient Neonatal Mortality[2]	572	0.00%	-	-	-
Third or Fourth Degree Laceration[2]	430	4.88%	-	3.63%	3.27%

Central Montana Medical Center

408 Wendell Avenue Phone: 406-538-7711
Lewistown, MT 59457 Fax: 406-538-6392
URL: www.cmmccares.com
Ownership: Voluntary non-profit - Private Accredited: No
Emergency Services: Yes Licensed Beds: 47

Key Personnel:

President/CEO. . . . . David Faulkner
Chief Medical Staff. . . . . Thomas Troop, MD
Cardiac Rehabilitation . . . . Debbie Lee
Obstetrics. . . . . Darla Jones

NOTE: Hospital profiles are in alphabetical order by state, then city, then hospital within the city; Rankings are sorted by rate in descending order and exclude hospitals with less than 25 cases; (1) The number of cases is too small (n<25) for purposes of reliably predicting hospital performance; (2) Measure reflects the hospital's indication that its submission was based upon a sample of its relevant discharges; (3) Rate reflects fewer than the maximum possible quarters of data for the measure; (4) Inaccurate information submitted and suppressed for one or more quarters; (5) No data is available from the hospital for this measure; Please refer to the User's Guide for a full explanation of data

Outpatient Surgery. . . . . Dianne Scotten
Pulmonary Rehab/Respiratory Therapy . . . . Rick Poss

Measure	Cases	This Hospital	State Average	U.S. Average	Top Hospital
Heart Attack Care					
ACE Inhibitor or ARB for LVSD[1,3]	1	0%	78%	82%	100%
Aspirin at Arrival[1,3]	6	83%	96%	92%	100%
Aspirin at Discharge[1,3]	4	75%	85%	90%	100%
Beta Blocker at Arrival[1,3]	3	67%	81%	87%	100%
Beta Blocker at Discharge[1,3]	4	0%	80%	90%	100%
Fibrinolytic Medication Timing[3]	0	-	32%	31%	100%
PCI Within 90 Minutes of Arrival	0	-	73%	54%	95%
Smoking Cessation Advice[3]	0	-	87%	88%	100%
Heart Failure Care					
ACE Inhibitor or ARB for LVSD[1,3]	3	100%	83%	82%	100%
Discharge Instructions[1,3]	6	100%	47%	61%	93%
Evaluation of LVS Function[1,3]	13	46%	73%	83%	99%
Smoking Cessation Advice[1,3]	1	100%	74%	82%	100%
Pneumonia Care					
Appropriate Initial Antibiotic	34	82%	81%	83%	94%
Blood Culture Timing[1]	18	100%	93%	90%	100%
Influenza Vaccine[1]	7	100%	83%	70%	100%
Initial Antibiotic Timing	39	92%	87%	80%	93%
Oxygenation Assessment	42	100%	97%	99%	100%
Pneumococcal Vaccine	31	84%	79%	69%	94%
Smoking Cessation Advice[1]	6	83%	69%	80%	100%
Surgical Infection Prevention					
Prophylactic Antibiotic Given[3]	48	67%	86%	77%	95%
Prophylactic Antibiotic Selection[1]	17	94%	94%	90%	100%
Prophylactic Antibiotic Stopped[3]	48	90%	87%	72%	95%
Pregnancy Care					
Inpatient Neonatal Mortality	-	-	-	-	-
Third or Fourth Degree Laceration	-	-	-	3.63%	3.27%

Saint John's Lutheran Hospital

350 Louisiana Street
Libby, MT 59923
URL: www.sjlh.com
Ownership: Voluntary non-profit - Private
Emergency Services: Yes

Phone: 406-293-0100
Fax: 406-293-7931
Accredited: No
Licensed Beds: 15

Key Personnel:

CEO. . . . . Bill Patten
Chief Medical Staff. . . . . Lance Ercanbrack, MD
Emergency Room . . . . Mary Nelson
Emergency Room . . . . Jay Maloney, MD
Infection Control. . . . . Clarice Thompson
ICU . . . . Jackie Hare
Medical Surgical Nursing . . . . Clarice Thompson
Respiratory/Cardiopulmonary. . . . . Jackie Hare

Measure	Cases	This Hospital	State Average	U.S. Average	Top Hospital
Heart Attack Care					
ACE Inhibitor or ARB for LVSD[5]	-	-	78%	82%	100%
Aspirin at Arrival[5]	-	-	96%	92%	100%
Aspirin at Discharge[5]	-	-	85%	90%	100%
Beta Blocker at Arrival[5]	-	-	81%	87%	100%
Beta Blocker at Discharge[5]	-	-	80%	90%	100%
Fibrinolytic Medication Timing[5]	-	-	32%	31%	100%
PCI Within 90 Minutes of Arrival[5]	-	-	73%	54%	95%
Smoking Cessation Advice[5]	-	-	87%	88%	100%
Heart Failure Care					
ACE Inhibitor or ARB for LVSD[5]	-	-	83%	82%	100%
Discharge Instructions[5]	-	-	47%	61%	93%
Evaluation of LVS Function[5]	-	-	73%	83%	99%
Smoking Cessation Advice[5]	-	-	74%	82%	100%
Pneumonia Care					
Appropriate Initial Antibiotic[1,3]	17	88%	81%	83%	94%
Blood Culture Timing[1,3]	9	100%	93%	90%	100%
Influenza Vaccine[5]	-	-	83%	70%	100%
Initial Antibiotic Timing[1,3]	20	85%	87%	80%	93%
Oxygenation Assessment[1,3]	19	100%	97%	99%	100%
Pneumococcal Vaccine[1,3]	15	73%	79%	69%	94%
Smoking Cessation Advice[1,3]	8	12%	69%	80%	100%
Surgical Infection Prevention					
Prophylactic Antibiotic Given[5]	-	-	86%	77%	95%
Prophylactic Antibiotic Selection[5]	-	-	94%	90%	100%
Prophylactic Antibiotic Stopped[5]	-	-	87%	72%	95%
Pregnancy Care					
Inpatient Neonatal Mortality	-	-	-	-	-
Third or Fourth Degree Laceration	-	-	-	3.63%	3.27%

Livingston Memorial Hospital

504 S 13th Street
Livingston, MT 59047
Ownership: Voluntary non-profit - Private
Emergency Services: Yes

Phone: 406-222-3541
Fax: 406-222-5099
Accredited: No
Licensed Beds: 45

Key Personnel:

President/CEO. . . . . Richard Brown

Measure	Cases	This Hospital	State Average	U.S. Average	Top Hospital
Heart Attack Care					
ACE Inhibitor or ARB for LVSD[1,2]	2	50%	78%	82%	100%
Aspirin at Arrival[1,2]	7	100%	96%	92%	100%
Aspirin at Discharge[1,2]	4	100%	85%	90%	100%
Beta Blocker at Arrival[1,2]	7	100%	81%	87%	100%
Beta Blocker at Discharge[1,2]	5	80%	80%	90%	100%
Fibrinolytic Medication Timing[1,2]	9	67%	32%	31%	100%
PCI Within 90 Minutes of Arrival[2]	0	-	73%	54%	95%
Smoking Cessation Advice[2]	0	-	87%	88%	100%
Heart Failure Care					
ACE Inhibitor or ARB for LVSD[1,2]	5	100%	83%	82%	100%
Discharge Instructions[2]	27	63%	47%	61%	93%
Evaluation of LVS Function[2]	33	88%	73%	83%	99%
Smoking Cessation Advice[1,2]	1	0%	74%	82%	100%
Pneumonia Care					
Appropriate Initial Antibiotic[2]	50	78%	81%	83%	94%
Blood Culture Timing[2]	30	90%	93%	90%	100%
Influenza Vaccine[1,2]	8	100%	83%	70%	100%
Initial Antibiotic Timing[2]	57	89%	87%	80%	93%
Oxygenation Assessment[2]	67	100%	97%	99%	100%
Pneumococcal Vaccine[2]	47	94%	79%	69%	94%
Smoking Cessation Advice[1,2]	14	93%	69%	80%	100%
Surgical Infection Prevention					
Prophylactic Antibiotic Given[2]	74	81%	86%	77%	95%
Prophylactic Antibiotic Selection[1,2]	20	100%	94%	90%	100%
Prophylactic Antibiotic Stopped[2]	72	96%	87%	72%	95%
Pregnancy Care					
Inpatient Neonatal Mortality	-	-	-	-	-
Third or Fourth Degree Laceration	-	-	-	3.63%	3.27%

Holy Rosary Health Care

Alternate Name: Holy Rosary Hospital
2600 Wilson Street
Miles City, MT 59301

Ownership: Voluntary non-profit - Church
Emergency Services: Yes

Toll-Free: 800-843-3820
Phone: 406-233-2600
Fax: 406-233-2611
Accredited: Yes
Licensed Beds: 44

Key Personnel:

CEO. . . . . Greg Nielson

Measure	Cases	This Hospital	State Average	U.S. Average	Top Hospital
Heart Attack Care					
ACE Inhibitor or ARB for LVSD[1]	1	100%	78%	82%	100%
Aspirin at Arrival[1]	6	100%	96%	92%	100%
Aspirin at Discharge[1]	5	100%	85%	90%	100%
Beta Blocker at Arrival[1]	4	100%	81%	87%	100%
Beta Blocker at Discharge[1]	4	75%	80%	90%	100%
Fibrinolytic Medication Timing[1]	1	0%	32%	31%	100%
PCI Within 90 Minutes of Arrival	0	-	73%	54%	95%
Smoking Cessation Advice[1]	1	0%	87%	88%	100%
Heart Failure Care					
ACE Inhibitor or ARB for LVSD[1]	11	100%	83%	82%	100%
Discharge Instructions	34	82%	47%	61%	93%
Evaluation of LVS Function	50	64%	73%	83%	99%

NOTE: Hospital profiles are in alphabetical order by state, then city, then hospital within the city; Rankings are sorted by rate in descending order and exclude hospitals with less than 25 cases; (1) The number of cases is too small (n<25) for purposes of reliably predicting hospital performance; (2) Measure reflects the hospital's indication that its submission was based upon a sample of its relevant discharges; (3) Rate reflects fewer than the maximum possible quarters of data for the measure; (4) Inaccurate information submitted and suppressed for one or more quarters; (5) No data is available from the hospital for this measure; Please refer to the User's Guide for a full explanation of data

Measure	Cases	This Hospital	State Average	U.S. Average	Top Hospital
Smoking Cessation Advice[1]	5	60%	74%	82%	100%
Pneumonia Care					
Appropriate Initial Antibiotic	81	88%	81%	83%	94%
Blood Culture Timing	38	97%	93%	90%	100%
Influenza Vaccine[1]	11	100%	83%	70%	100%
Initial Antibiotic Timing	76	95%	87%	80%	93%
Oxygenation Assessment	95	100%	97%	99%	100%
Pneumococcal Vaccine	72	94%	79%	69%	94%
Smoking Cessation Advice[1]	11	82%	69%	80%	100%
Surgical Infection Prevention					
Prophylactic Antibiotic Given[2,3]	56	89%	86%	77%	95%
Prophylactic Antibiotic Selection[1,2]	23	96%	94%	90%	100%
Prophylactic Antibiotic Stopped[2,3]	56	89%	87%	72%	95%
Pregnancy Care					
Inpatient Neonatal Mortality	-	-	-	-	-
Third or Fourth Degree Laceration	-	-	-	3.63%	3.27%

Community Medical Center

Alternate Name: Missoula Communtiy Medical Center
2827 Fort Missoula Road — Phone: 406-728-4100
Missoula, MT 59804 — Fax: 406-327-4580
Ownership: Voluntary non-profit - Private — Accredited: Yes
Emergency Services: Yes — Licensed Beds: 125

Key Personnel:
CEO. . . . . Tom Moser
Chief of Medical Staff . . . . Frank Reed
Emergency Room . . . . Lisa Iakner

Measure	Cases	This Hospital	State Average	U.S. Average	Top Hospital
Heart Attack Care					
ACE Inhibitor or ARB for LVSD[1]	22	100%	78%	82%	100%
Aspirin at Arrival	49	100%	96%	92%	100%
Aspirin at Discharge	87	97%	85%	90%	100%
Beta Blocker at Arrival	45	98%	81%	87%	100%
Beta Blocker at Discharge	85	99%	80%	90%	100%
Fibrinolytic Medication Timing	0	-	32%	31%	100%
PCI Within 90 Minutes of Arrival[1]	4	75%	73%	54%	95%
Smoking Cessation Advice	37	92%	87%	88%	100%
Heart Failure Care					
ACE Inhibitor or ARB for LVSD[1]	20	90%	83%	82%	100%
Discharge Instructions	68	75%	47%	61%	93%
Evaluation of LVS Function	89	94%	73%	83%	99%
Smoking Cessation Advice[1]	13	100%	74%	82%	100%
Pneumonia Care					
Appropriate Initial Antibiotic	68	90%	81%	83%	94%
Blood Culture Timing	59	90%	93%	90%	100%
Influenza Vaccine[1]	11	82%	83%	70%	100%
Initial Antibiotic Timing	82	78%	87%	80%	93%
Oxygenation Assessment	98	100%	97%	99%	100%
Pneumococcal Vaccine	58	90%	79%	69%	94%
Smoking Cessation Advice	39	92%	69%	80%	100%
Surgical Infection Prevention					
Prophylactic Antibiotic Given[2]	621	93%	86%	77%	95%
Prophylactic Antibiotic Selection[2]	50	92%	94%	90%	100%
Prophylactic Antibiotic Stopped[2]	612	87%	87%	72%	95%
Pregnancy Care					
Inpatient Neonatal Mortality	-	-	-	-	-
Third or Fourth Degree Laceration	-	-	-	3.63%	3.27%

Saint Patrick Hosp and Health Sci Ctr

500 W Broadway — Phone: 406-543-7271
Missoula, MT 59802 — Fax: 406-329-5693
URL: www.saintpatrick.org
Ownership: Voluntary non-profit - Church — Accredited: No
Emergency Services: Yes — Licensed Beds: 213

Key Personnel:
President/CEO . . . . Jeff Fee
President Medical Staff . . . . Gary Willstein, MD
Chief Emergency Room . . . . Greg Kazemi, MD
Chief Surgery . . . . Matt Maxwell, MD
Chief Radiology . . . . Sarsfield Dougherty, MD
Supervisor Respiratory Therapy . . . . Randy Boehnke

Measure	Cases	This Hospital	State Average	U.S. Average	Top Hospital
Heart Attack Care					
ACE Inhibitor or ARB for LVSD	50	96%	78%	82%	100%
Aspirin at Arrival	125	99%	96%	92%	100%
Aspirin at Discharge	284	100%	85%	90%	100%
Beta Blocker at Arrival	111	99%	81%	87%	100%
Beta Blocker at Discharge	273	99%	80%	90%	100%
Fibrinolytic Medication Timing	0	-	32%	31%	100%
PCI Within 90 Minutes of Arrival[1]	10	90%	73%	54%	95%
Smoking Cessation Advice	85	100%	87%	88%	100%
Heart Failure Care					
ACE Inhibitor or ARB for LVSD	115	97%	83%	82%	100%
Discharge Instructions	189	69%	47%	61%	93%
Evaluation of LVS Function	220	100%	73%	83%	99%
Smoking Cessation Advice	35	100%	74%	82%	100%
Pneumonia Care					
Appropriate Initial Antibiotic	92	79%	81%	83%	94%
Blood Culture Timing	93	94%	93%	90%	100%
Influenza Vaccine[1]	24	96%	83%	70%	100%
Initial Antibiotic Timing	131	88%	87%	80%	93%
Oxygenation Assessment	159	100%	97%	99%	100%
Pneumococcal Vaccine	105	91%	79%	69%	94%
Smoking Cessation Advice	41	95%	69%	80%	100%
Surgical Infection Prevention					
Prophylactic Antibiotic Given[3]	402	93%	86%	77%	95%
Prophylactic Antibiotic Selection	152	98%	94%	90%	100%
Prophylactic Antibiotic Stopped[3]	391	92%	87%	72%	95%
Pregnancy Care					
Inpatient Neonatal Mortality	-	-	-	-	-
Third or Fourth Degree Laceration	-	-	-	3.63%	3.27%

Sheridan Memorial Hospital

440 West Laurel Avenue — Phone: 406-765-1420
Plentywood, MT 59254 — Fax: 406-765-1424
URL: www.sheridanmemorial.net
Ownership: Proprietary — Accredited: No
Emergency Services: Yes — Licensed Beds: 98

Key Personnel:
Administrator . . . . Ella Gutzke
Chief Medical Staff. . . . . Kirk Stoner, MD
Director Infection/Disease Control . . . . Debbie Somppi

Measure	Cases	This Hospital	State Average	U.S. Average	Top Hospital
Heart Attack Care					
ACE Inhibitor or ARB for LVSD[3]	0	-	78%	82%	100%
Aspirin at Arrival[1,3]	2	100%	96%	92%	100%
Aspirin at Discharge[1,3]	1	100%	85%	90%	100%
Beta Blocker at Arrival[1,3]	2	50%	81%	87%	100%
Beta Blocker at Discharge[3]	0	-	80%	90%	100%
Fibrinolytic Medication Timing[3]	0	-	32%	31%	100%
PCI Within 90 Minutes of Arrival	0	-	73%	54%	95%
Smoking Cessation Advice[3]	0	-	87%	88%	100%
Heart Failure Care					
ACE Inhibitor or ARB for LVSD[3]	0	-	83%	82%	100%
Discharge Instructions[1,3]	6	17%	47%	61%	93%
Evaluation of LVS Function[1,3]	10	50%	73%	83%	99%
Smoking Cessation Advice[1,3]	1	100%	74%	82%	100%
Pneumonia Care					
Appropriate Initial Antibiotic[1]	10	100%	81%	83%	94%
Blood Culture Timing[1]	2	100%	93%	90%	100%
Influenza Vaccine[1]	2	100%	83%	70%	100%
Initial Antibiotic Timing[1]	18	94%	87%	80%	93%
Oxygenation Assessment[1]	22	100%	97%	99%	100%
Pneumococcal Vaccine[1]	19	89%	79%	69%	94%
Smoking Cessation Advice	0	-	69%	80%	100%
Surgical Infection Prevention					
Prophylactic Antibiotic Given[5]	-	-	86%	77%	95%
Prophylactic Antibiotic Selection[5]	-	-	94%	90%	100%
Prophylactic Antibiotic Stopped[5]	-	-	87%	72%	95%
Pregnancy Care					
Inpatient Neonatal Mortality	-	-	-	-	-

NOTE: Hospital profiles are in alphabetical order by state, then city, then hospital within the city; Rankings are sorted by rate in descending order and exclude hospitals with less than 25 cases; (1) The number of cases is too small (n<25) for purposes of reliably predicting hospital performance; (2) Measure reflects the hospital's indication that its submission was based upon a sample of its relevant discharges; (3) Rate reflects fewer than the maximum possible quarters of data for the measure; (4) Inaccurate information submitted and suppressed for one or more quarters; (5) No data is available from the hospital for this measure; Please refer to the User's Guide for a full explanation of data

Third or Fourth Degree Laceration	-	-	-	3.63%	3.27%

Saint Joseph Hospital

PO Box 1010
Polson, MT 59860
Ownership: Voluntary non-profit - Church
Emergency Services: Yes
Phone: 406-883-5377
Fax: 406-883-8439
Accredited: Yes
Licensed Beds: 40

Key Personnel:
CEO. . . . . John Glueckert
Chief of Medical Staff. . . . . Karen Lund
Director of Cardiology/Cardiac Lab. . . . . Darleen Cooper
Director of Pulmonary/Respiratory Care. . . . . . . William Beckner

Measure	Cases	This Hospital	State Average	U.S. Average	Top Hospital
Heart Attack Care					
ACE Inhibitor or ARB for LVSD[5]	-	-	78%	82%	100%
Aspirin at Arrival[5]	-	-	96%	92%	100%
Aspirin at Discharge[5]	-	-	85%	90%	100%
Beta Blocker at Arrival[5]	-	-	81%	87%	100%
Beta Blocker at Discharge[5]	-	-	80%	90%	100%
Fibrinolytic Medication Timing[5]	-	-	32%	31%	100%
PCI Within 90 Minutes of Arrival[5]	-	-	73%	54%	95%
Smoking Cessation Advice[5]	-	-	87%	88%	100%
Heart Failure Care					
ACE Inhibitor or ARB for LVSD[1]	7	57%	83%	82%	100%
Discharge Instructions[1]	16	12%	47%	61%	93%
Evaluation of LVS Function[1]	22	73%	73%	83%	99%
Smoking Cessation Advice[1]	2	50%	74%	82%	100%
Pneumonia Care					
Appropriate Initial Antibiotic	32	75%	81%	83%	94%
Blood Culture Timing[1]	13	100%	93%	90%	100%
Influenza Vaccine[1]	3	33%	83%	70%	100%
Initial Antibiotic Timing	27	93%	87%	80%	93%
Oxygenation Assessment	33	100%	97%	99%	100%
Pneumococcal Vaccine[1]	22	64%	79%	69%	94%
Smoking Cessation Advice[1]	10	50%	69%	80%	100%
Surgical Infection Prevention					
Prophylactic Antibiotic Given	36	81%	86%	77%	95%
Prophylactic Antibiotic Selection[1]	9	100%	94%	90%	100%
Prophylactic Antibiotic Stopped	34	88%	87%	72%	95%
Pregnancy Care					
Inpatient Neonatal Mortality	-	-	-	-	-
Third or Fourth Degree Laceration	-	-	-	3.63%	3.27%

Northeast Montana Healthcare Poplar Hospital

Alternate Name: Poplar Community Hospital
Corner of H and Court Ave
Poplar, MT 59255
Ownership: Voluntary non-profit - Private
Emergency Services: Yes
Phone: 406-768-3452
Fax: 406-768-6160
Accredited: No
Licensed Beds: 22

Key Personnel:
CEO. . . . . Keg Morgaard, MD

Measure	Cases	This Hospital	State Average	U.S. Average	Top Hospital
Heart Attack Care					
ACE Inhibitor or ARB for LVSD[5]	-	-	78%	82%	100%
Aspirin at Arrival[5]	-	-	96%	92%	100%
Aspirin at Discharge[5]	-	-	85%	90%	100%
Beta Blocker at Arrival[5]	-	-	81%	87%	100%
Beta Blocker at Discharge[5]	-	-	80%	90%	100%
Fibrinolytic Medication Timing[5]	-	-	32%	31%	100%
PCI Within 90 Minutes of Arrival[5]	-	-	73%	54%	95%
Smoking Cessation Advice[5]	-	-	87%	88%	100%
Heart Failure Care					
ACE Inhibitor or ARB for LVSD[1]	3	67%	83%	82%	100%
Discharge Instructions[1]	12	8%	47%	61%	93%
Evaluation of LVS Function[1]	14	50%	73%	83%	99%
Smoking Cessation Advice[1]	2	50%	74%	82%	100%
Pneumonia Care					
Appropriate Initial Antibiotic[1]	21	76%	81%	83%	94%
Blood Culture Timing[1]	3	100%	93%	90%	100%
Influenza Vaccine[1]	7	43%	83%	70%	100%
Initial Antibiotic Timing	31	77%	87%	80%	93%
Oxygenation Assessment	32	100%	97%	99%	100%
Pneumococcal Vaccine[1]	9	67%	79%	69%	94%
Smoking Cessation Advice[1]	15	47%	69%	80%	100%
Surgical Infection Prevention					
Prophylactic Antibiotic Given[5]	-	-	86%	77%	95%
Prophylactic Antibiotic Selection[5]	-	-	94%	90%	100%
Prophylactic Antibiotic Stopped[5]	-	-	87%	72%	95%
Pregnancy Care					
Inpatient Neonatal Mortality	-	-	-	-	-
Third or Fourth Degree Laceration	-	-	-	3.63%	3.27%

Saint Luke Community Hospital

107 Sixth Avenue SW
Ronan, MT 59864
URL: www.stlukehealthnet.org
Ownership: Voluntary non-profit - Other
Emergency Services: Yes
Phone: 406-676-4441
Fax: 406-676-0835
Accredited: No
Licensed Beds: 15

Key Personnel:
CEO. . . . . Shane Robert
Chief Medical Staff. . . . . Steve Todd
Emergency Room . . . . Leah Amerson
OB/GYN Women's Health . . . . Daniel Bahnmiller, MD
Respiratory/Cardiopulmonary. . . . . Maggie Roddam

Measure	Cases	This Hospital	State Average	U.S. Average	Top Hospital
Heart Attack Care					
ACE Inhibitor or ARB for LVSD[5]	-	-	78%	82%	100%
Aspirin at Arrival[5]	-	-	96%	92%	100%
Aspirin at Discharge[5]	-	-	85%	90%	100%
Beta Blocker at Arrival[5]	-	-	81%	87%	100%
Beta Blocker at Discharge[5]	-	-	80%	90%	100%
Fibrinolytic Medication Timing[5]	-	-	32%	31%	100%
PCI Within 90 Minutes of Arrival[5]	-	-	73%	54%	95%
Smoking Cessation Advice[5]	-	-	87%	88%	100%
Heart Failure Care					
ACE Inhibitor or ARB for LVSD[1]	4	50%	83%	82%	100%
Discharge Instructions[1]	19	11%	47%	61%	93%
Evaluation of LVS Function	25	64%	73%	83%	99%
Smoking Cessation Advice[1]	6	17%	74%	82%	100%
Pneumonia Care					
Appropriate Initial Antibiotic	43	95%	81%	83%	94%
Blood Culture Timing	30	80%	93%	90%	100%
Influenza Vaccine[1]	7	100%	83%	70%	100%
Initial Antibiotic Timing	53	83%	87%	80%	93%
Oxygenation Assessment	61	100%	97%	99%	100%
Pneumococcal Vaccine	28	79%	79%	69%	94%
Smoking Cessation Advice[1]	22	50%	69%	80%	100%
Surgical Infection Prevention					
Prophylactic Antibiotic Given[5]	-	-	86%	77%	95%
Prophylactic Antibiotic Selection[5]	-	-	94%	90%	100%
Prophylactic Antibiotic Stopped[5]	-	-	87%	72%	95%
Pregnancy Care					
Inpatient Neonatal Mortality	-	-	-	-	-
Third or Fourth Degree Laceration	-	-	-	3.63%	3.27%

Roundup Memorial Hospital & Nursing Home

Alternate Name: Round Memorial Hospital
1202 3rd Street
PO Box 40
Roundup, MT 59072
E-mail: rmhclnh@midrivers.com
Ownership: Government - Local
Emergency Services: Yes
Phone: 406-323-2301
Fax: 406-323-1170
Accredited: No
Licensed Beds: 48

Key Personnel:
CEO. . . . . Lee Rhodes
Chief Medical Staff. . . . . Sunny Lageschulte
Emergency Room . . . . Dana Rutan
Emergency Room . . . . Brenda Dagley

Measure	Cases	This Hospital	State Average	U.S. Average	Top Hospital
Heart Attack Care					
ACE Inhibitor or ARB for LVSD[3]	0	-	78%	82%	100%

NOTE: Hospital profiles are in alphabetical order by state, then city, then hospital within the city; Rankings are sorted by rate in descending order and exclude hospitals with less than 25 cases; (1) The number of cases is too small (n<25) for purposes of reliably predicting hospital performance; (2) Measure reflects the hospital's indication that its submission was based upon a sample of its relevant discharges; (3) Rate reflects fewer than the maximum possible quarters of data for the measure; (4) Inaccurate information submitted and suppressed for one or more quarters; (5) No data is available from the hospital for this measure; Please refer to the User's Guide for a full explanation of data

Measure	Cases	This Hospital	State Average	U.S. Average	Top Hospital
Aspirin at Arrival[3]	0	-	96%	92%	100%
Aspirin at Discharge[3]	0	-	85%	90%	100%
Beta Blocker at Arrival[3]	0	-	81%	87%	100%
Beta Blocker at Discharge[3]	0	-	80%	90%	100%
Fibrinolytic Medication Timing[5]	-	-	32%	31%	100%
PCI Within 90 Minutes of Arrival[5]	-	-	73%	54%	95%
Smoking Cessation Advice[5]	-	-	87%	88%	100%
Heart Failure Care					
ACE Inhibitor or ARB for LVSD[1]	5	80%	83%	82%	100%
Discharge Instructions[1,3]	1	0%	47%	61%	93%
Evaluation of LVS Function	27	44%	73%	83%	99%
Smoking Cessation Advice[3]	0	-	74%	82%	100%
Pneumonia Care					
Appropriate Initial Antibiotic[1,3]	3	100%	81%	83%	94%
Blood Culture Timing[1,3]	1	100%	93%	90%	100%
Influenza Vaccine[5]	-	-	83%	70%	100%
Initial Antibiotic Timing	34	88%	87%	80%	93%
Oxygenation Assessment	38	100%	97%	99%	100%
Pneumococcal Vaccine[1]	23	9%	79%	69%	94%
Smoking Cessation Advice[1,3]	1	0%	69%	80%	100%
Surgical Infection Prevention					
Prophylactic Antibiotic Given[5]	-	-	86%	77%	95%
Prophylactic Antibiotic Selection[5]	-	-	94%	90%	100%
Prophylactic Antibiotic Stopped[5]	-	-	87%	72%	95%
Pregnancy Care					
Inpatient Neonatal Mortality	-	-	-	-	-
Third or Fourth Degree Laceration	-	-	-	3.63%	3.27%

Daniels Memorial Hospital & Nursing Home

105 5th Avenue E
Scobey, MT 59263
Phone: 406-487-2296
Fax: 406-487-2471
Ownership: Government - Local
Emergency Services: Yes
Accredited: No
Licensed Beds: 54

Key Personnel:

CEO. . . . . Davie Lloyd
Chief Medical Staff. . . . . William Escoffery, MD
Infection Control. . . . . Naomi Reed, RN

Measure	Cases	This Hospital	State Average	U.S. Average	Top Hospital
Heart Attack Care					
ACE Inhibitor or ARB for LVSD[5]	-	-	78%	82%	100%
Aspirin at Arrival[5]	-	-	96%	92%	100%
Aspirin at Discharge[5]	-	-	85%	90%	100%
Beta Blocker at Arrival[5]	-	-	81%	87%	100%
Beta Blocker at Discharge[5]	-	-	80%	90%	100%
Fibrinolytic Medication Timing[5]	-	-	32%	31%	100%
PCI Within 90 Minutes of Arrival[5]	-	-	73%	54%	95%
Smoking Cessation Advice[5]	-	-	87%	88%	100%
Heart Failure Care					
ACE Inhibitor or ARB for LVSD[3]	0	-	83%	82%	100%
Discharge Instructions[1,3]	1	0%	47%	61%	93%
Evaluation of LVS Function[1,3]	5	40%	73%	83%	99%
Smoking Cessation Advice[3]	0	-	74%	82%	100%
Pneumonia Care					
Appropriate Initial Antibiotic[1]	5	100%	81%	83%	94%
Blood Culture Timing[1]	4	100%	93%	90%	100%
Influenza Vaccine[1]	1	100%	83%	70%	100%
Initial Antibiotic Timing[1]	10	80%	87%	80%	93%
Oxygenation Assessment[1]	10	100%	97%	99%	100%
Pneumococcal Vaccine[1]	7	57%	79%	69%	94%
Smoking Cessation Advice	0	-	69%	80%	100%
Surgical Infection Prevention					
Prophylactic Antibiotic Given[5]	-	-	86%	77%	95%
Prophylactic Antibiotic Selection[5]	-	-	94%	90%	100%
Prophylactic Antibiotic Stopped[5]	-	-	87%	72%	95%
Pregnancy Care					
Inpatient Neonatal Mortality	-	-	-	-	-
Third or Fourth Degree Laceration	-	-	-	3.63%	3.27%

Marias Medical Center

640 Park Drive
PO Box 915
Shelby, MT 59474
Phone: 406-434-3200
Fax: 406-434-3213
URL: www.mmcmt.org
Ownership: Government - Local
Emergency Services: Yes
Accredited: No
Licensed Beds: 20

Key Personnel:

CEO. . . . . Mark Cross
Chief Medical Staff. . . . . Daniel Rausch, MD
Surgery Manager. . . . . Rod Keller, RN
Director Radiology . . . . Tom Carter
Respiratory Therapy. . . . . Randy Rideout

Measure	Cases	This Hospital	State Average	U.S. Average	Top Hospital
Heart Attack Care					
ACE Inhibitor or ARB for LVSD[3]	0	-	78%	82%	100%
Aspirin at Arrival[1,3]	2	100%	96%	92%	100%
Aspirin at Discharge[1,3]	1	100%	85%	90%	100%
Beta Blocker at Arrival[1,3]	2	100%	81%	87%	100%
Beta Blocker at Discharge[1,3]	2	100%	80%	90%	100%
Fibrinolytic Medication Timing[1,3]	1	0%	32%	31%	100%
PCI Within 90 Minutes of Arrival[5]	-	-	73%	54%	95%
Smoking Cessation Advice[3]	0	-	87%	88%	100%
Heart Failure Care					
ACE Inhibitor or ARB for LVSD[1]	1	0%	83%	82%	100%
Discharge Instructions[1]	6	50%	47%	61%	93%
Evaluation of LVS Function[1]	8	38%	73%	83%	99%
Smoking Cessation Advice[1]	1	0%	74%	82%	100%
Pneumonia Care					
Appropriate Initial Antibiotic[1]	20	80%	81%	83%	94%
Blood Culture Timing[1]	1	100%	93%	90%	100%
Influenza Vaccine[1]	7	100%	83%	70%	100%
Initial Antibiotic Timing[1]	24	96%	87%	80%	93%
Oxygenation Assessment	29	100%	97%	99%	100%
Pneumococcal Vaccine[1]	22	95%	79%	69%	94%
Smoking Cessation Advice[1]	7	57%	69%	80%	100%
Surgical Infection Prevention					
Prophylactic Antibiotic Given[5]	-	-	86%	77%	95%
Prophylactic Antibiotic Selection[5]	-	-	94%	90%	100%
Prophylactic Antibiotic Stopped[5]	-	-	87%	72%	95%
Pregnancy Care					
Inpatient Neonatal Mortality	-	-	-	-	-
Third or Fourth Degree Laceration	-	-	-	3.63%	3.27%

Sidney Health Center

Alternate Name: Community Memorial Hospital
216 14th Avenue SW
Sidney, MT 59270
Phone: 406-488-2100
Fax: 406-488-2115
URL: www.sidneyhealth.com
Ownership: Govt - Hospital District or Authority
Emergency Services: Yes
Accredited: No
Licensed Beds: 42

Key Personnel:

President/CEO. . . . . Don Rush
Chief Medical Staff. . . . . Edward Pierce, MD

Measure	Cases	This Hospital	State Average	U.S. Average	Top Hospital
Heart Attack Care					
ACE Inhibitor or ARB for LVSD[1]	1	0%	78%	82%	100%
Aspirin at Arrival[1]	5	80%	96%	92%	100%
Aspirin at Discharge[1]	4	50%	85%	90%	100%
Beta Blocker at Arrival[1]	5	80%	81%	87%	100%
Beta Blocker at Discharge[1]	4	50%	80%	90%	100%
Fibrinolytic Medication Timing[1]	2	0%	32%	31%	100%
PCI Within 90 Minutes of Arrival	0	-	73%	54%	95%
Smoking Cessation Advice	0	-	87%	88%	100%
Heart Failure Care					
ACE Inhibitor or ARB for LVSD[1]	5	40%	83%	82%	100%
Discharge Instructions	28	50%	47%	61%	93%
Evaluation of LVS Function	37	78%	73%	83%	99%
Smoking Cessation Advice[1]	7	100%	74%	82%	100%
Pneumonia Care					
Appropriate Initial Antibiotic[1]	13	69%	81%	83%	94%

NOTE: Hospital profiles are in alphabetical order by state, then city, then hospital within the city; Rankings are sorted by rate in descending order and exclude hospitals with less than 25 cases; (1) The number of cases is too small (n<25) for purposes of reliably predicting hospital performance; (2) Measure reflects the hospital's indication that its submission was based upon a sample of its relevant discharges; (3) Rate reflects fewer than the maximum possible quarters of data for the measure; (4) Inaccurate information submitted and suppressed for one or more quarters; (5) No data is available from the hospital for this measure; Please refer to the User's Guide for a full explanation of data

Measure	Cases	This Hospital	State Average	U.S. Average	Top Hospital
Blood Culture Timing[1]	7	86%	93%	90%	100%
Influenza Vaccine[1]	1	100%	83%	70%	100%
Initial Antibiotic Timing[1]	15	100%	87%	80%	93%
Oxygenation Assessment[1]	23	100%	97%	99%	100%
Pneumococcal Vaccine[1]	13	92%	79%	69%	94%
Smoking Cessation Advice[1]	3	67%	69%	80%	100%
Surgical Infection Prevention					
Prophylactic Antibiotic Given	53	96%	86%	77%	95%
Prophylactic Antibiotic Selection[1]	11	100%	94%	90%	100%
Prophylactic Antibiotic Stopped	53	81%	87%	72%	95%
Pregnancy Care					
Inpatient Neonatal Mortality	-	-	-	-	-
Third or Fourth Degree Laceration	-	-	-	3.63%	3.27%

Prairie Community Hospital

312 S Adams Avenue
Terry, MT 59349
Ownership: Voluntary non-profit - Other
Emergency Services: Yes
Phone: 406-635-5511
Fax: 406-635-5510
Accredited: No
Licensed Beds: 21

Key Personnel:
President/CEO. . . . . James Mantz

Measure	Cases	This Hospital	State Average	U.S. Average	Top Hospital
Heart Attack Care					
ACE Inhibitor or ARB for LVSD[5]	-	-	78%	82%	100%
Aspirin at Arrival[5]	-	-	96%	92%	100%
Aspirin at Discharge[5]	-	-	85%	90%	100%
Beta Blocker at Arrival[5]	-	-	81%	87%	100%
Beta Blocker at Discharge[5]	-	-	80%	90%	100%
Fibrinolytic Medication Timing[5]	-	-	32%	31%	100%
PCI Within 90 Minutes of Arrival[5]	-	-	73%	54%	95%
Smoking Cessation Advice[5]	-	-	87%	88%	100%
Heart Failure Care					
ACE Inhibitor or ARB for LVSD[5]	-	-	83%	82%	100%
Discharge Instructions[5]	-	-	47%	61%	93%
Evaluation of LVS Function[5]	-	-	73%	83%	99%
Smoking Cessation Advice[5]	-	-	74%	82%	100%
Pneumonia Care					
Appropriate Initial Antibiotic[5]	-	-	81%	83%	94%
Blood Culture Timing[5]	-	-	93%	90%	100%
Influenza Vaccine[5]	-	-	83%	70%	100%
Initial Antibiotic Timing[5]	-	-	87%	80%	93%
Oxygenation Assessment[5]	-	-	97%	99%	100%
Pneumococcal Vaccine[5]	-	-	79%	69%	94%
Smoking Cessation Advice[5]	-	-	69%	80%	100%
Surgical Infection Prevention					
Prophylactic Antibiotic Given[5]	-	-	86%	77%	95%
Prophylactic Antibiotic Selection[5]	-	-	94%	90%	100%
Prophylactic Antibiotic Stopped[5]	-	-	87%	72%	95%
Pregnancy Care					
Inpatient Neonatal Mortality	-	-	-	-	-
Third or Fourth Degree Laceration	-	-	-	3.63%	3.27%

Mountainview Medical Center

16 W Main Street
White Sulphur Springs, MT 59645
E-mail: info@mvmc.org
URL: www.mvmc.org
Ownership: Voluntary non-profit - Private
Emergency Services: Yes
Phone: 406-547-3321
Fax: 406-547-3589
Accredited: No
Licensed Beds: 6

Key Personnel:
CEO. . . . . Katharine Ann Campbell, CHE
Chief Medical Officer . . . . Marc Steinberg, MD

Measure	Cases	This Hospital	State Average	U.S. Average	Top Hospital
Heart Attack Care					
ACE Inhibitor or ARB for LVSD[5]	-	-	78%	82%	100%
Aspirin at Arrival[5]	-	-	96%	92%	100%
Aspirin at Discharge[5]	-	-	85%	90%	100%
Beta Blocker at Arrival[5]	-	-	81%	87%	100%
Beta Blocker at Discharge[5]	-	-	80%	90%	100%
Fibrinolytic Medication Timing[5]	-	-	32%	31%	100%
PCI Within 90 Minutes of Arrival[5]	-	-	73%	54%	95%
Smoking Cessation Advice[5]	-	-	87%	88%	100%
Heart Failure Care					
ACE Inhibitor or ARB for LVSD[3]	0	-	83%	82%	100%
Discharge Instructions[1,3]	1	100%	47%	61%	93%
Evaluation of LVS Function[1,3]	2	100%	73%	83%	99%
Smoking Cessation Advice[3]	0	-	74%	82%	100%
Pneumonia Care					
Appropriate Initial Antibiotic[1,3]	3	33%	81%	83%	94%
Blood Culture Timing[3]	0	-	93%	90%	100%
Influenza Vaccine[5]	-	-	83%	70%	100%
Initial Antibiotic Timing[1,3]	4	100%	87%	80%	93%
Oxygenation Assessment[1,3]	4	25%	97%	99%	100%
Pneumococcal Vaccine[1,3]	3	33%	79%	69%	94%
Smoking Cessation Advice[3]	0	-	69%	80%	100%
Surgical Infection Prevention					
Prophylactic Antibiotic Given[5]	-	-	86%	77%	95%
Prophylactic Antibiotic Selection[5]	-	-	94%	90%	100%
Prophylactic Antibiotic Stopped[5]	-	-	87%	72%	95%
Pregnancy Care					
Inpatient Neonatal Mortality	-	-	-	-	-
Third or Fourth Degree Laceration	-	-	-	3.63%	3.27%

North Valley Hospital

6575 Highway 93 South
Whitefish, MT 59937
Toll-Free: 888-815-5528
Phone: 406-863-3500
Fax: 406-862-2532

E-mail: nvhosp@nvhosp.org
URL: www.nvhosp.org
Ownership: Government - Federal
Accredited: No
Emergency Services: Yes

Key Personnel:
CEO. . . . . Craig Aasved
Chief Medical Staff. . . . . Randall Beach, MD
QI/RM/Infection Control . . . . Susan Fauntleroy
Medical/Surgical/Pediatric Nursing. . . . . Kathy Rea, RN
Maternity/Nursery. . . . . Cindy Walp, RNC
Respiratory Therapy/Home Oxygen. . . . . Erin Reed, RT

Measure	Cases	This Hospital	State Average	U.S. Average	Top Hospital
Heart Attack Care					
ACE Inhibitor or ARB for LVSD[3]	0	-	78%	82%	100%
Aspirin at Arrival[3]	0	-	96%	92%	100%
Aspirin at Discharge[3]	0	-	85%	90%	100%
Beta Blocker at Arrival[3]	0	-	81%	87%	100%
Beta Blocker at Discharge[3]	0	-	80%	90%	100%
Fibrinolytic Medication Timing[3]	0	-	32%	31%	100%
PCI Within 90 Minutes of Arrival[5]	-	-	73%	54%	95%
Smoking Cessation Advice[3]	0	-	87%	88%	100%
Heart Failure Care					
ACE Inhibitor or ARB for LVSD[1]	5	80%	83%	82%	100%
Discharge Instructions[1]	13	0%	47%	61%	93%
Evaluation of LVS Function[1]	15	100%	73%	83%	99%
Smoking Cessation Advice[1]	1	100%	74%	82%	100%
Pneumonia Care					
Appropriate Initial Antibiotic	43	72%	81%	83%	94%
Blood Culture Timing	31	90%	93%	90%	100%
Influenza Vaccine[1]	4	25%	83%	70%	100%
Initial Antibiotic Timing	51	94%	87%	80%	93%
Oxygenation Assessment	60	100%	97%	99%	100%
Pneumococcal Vaccine	40	88%	79%	69%	94%
Smoking Cessation Advice[1]	16	69%	69%	80%	100%
Surgical Infection Prevention					
Prophylactic Antibiotic Given	95	74%	86%	77%	95%
Prophylactic Antibiotic Selection[1]	12	83%	94%	90%	100%
Prophylactic Antibiotic Stopped	80	98%	87%	72%	95%
Pregnancy Care					
Inpatient Neonatal Mortality	-	-	-	-	-
Third or Fourth Degree Laceration	-	-	-	3.63%	3.27%

NOTE: Hospital profiles are in alphabetical order by state, then city, then hospital within the city; Rankings are sorted by rate in descending order and exclude hospitals with less than 25 cases; (1) The number of cases is too small (n<25) for purposes of reliably predicting hospital performance; (2) Measure reflects the hospital's indication that its submission was based upon a sample of its relevant discharges; (3) Rate reflects fewer than the maximum possible quarters of data for the measure; (4) Inaccurate information submitted and suppressed for one or more quarters; (5) No data is available from the hospital for this measure; Please refer to the User's Guide for a full explanation of data

Trinity Hospital

Alternate Name: Trinity Hospital
315 Knapp Street
Wolf Point, MT 59201
URL: www.nemhs.net
Ownership: Voluntary non-profit - Private
Emergency Services: Yes
Phone: 406-653-2100
Fax: 406-653-6592
Accredited: No
Licensed Beds: 20

Key Personnel:
CEO. . . . . Margaret Norgaard
Emergency Room . . . . Elaine Long, DON

Measure	Cases	This Hospital	State Average	U.S. Average	Top Hospital
Heart Attack Care					
ACE Inhibitor or ARB for LVSD[3]	0	-	78%	82%	100%
Aspirin at Arrival[1,3]	1	100%	96%	92%	100%
Aspirin at Discharge[3]	0	-	85%	90%	100%
Beta Blocker at Arrival[1,3]	1	0%	81%	87%	100%
Beta Blocker at Discharge[3]	0	-	80%	90%	100%
Fibrinolytic Medication Timing[3]	0	-	32%	31%	100%
PCI Within 90 Minutes of Arrival[5]	-	-	73%	54%	95%
Smoking Cessation Advice[3]	0	-	87%	88%	100%
Heart Failure Care					
ACE Inhibitor or ARB for LVSD[1]	4	100%	83%	82%	100%
Discharge Instructions	32	41%	47%	61%	93%
Evaluation of LVS Function	35	63%	73%	83%	99%
Smoking Cessation Advice[1]	4	75%	74%	82%	100%
Pneumonia Care					
Appropriate Initial Antibiotic[1]	20	85%	81%	83%	94%
Blood Culture Timing	0	-	93%	90%	100%
Influenza Vaccine[1]	7	86%	83%	70%	100%
Initial Antibiotic Timing	27	70%	87%	80%	93%
Oxygenation Assessment	31	100%	97%	99%	100%
Pneumococcal Vaccine[1]	18	100%	79%	69%	94%
Smoking Cessation Advice[1]	9	78%	69%	80%	100%
Surgical Infection Prevention					
Prophylactic Antibiotic Given[3]	0	-	86%	77%	95%
Prophylactic Antibiotic Selection	0	-	94%	90%	100%
Prophylactic Antibiotic Stopped[3]	0	-	87%	72%	95%
Pregnancy Care					
Inpatient Neonatal Mortality	-	-	-	-	-
Third or Fourth Degree Laceration	-	-	-	3.63%	3.27%

NOTE: Hospital profiles are in alphabetical order by state, then city, then hospital within the city; Rankings are sorted by rate in descending order and exclude hospitals with less than 25 cases; (1) The number of cases is too small (n<25) for purposes of reliably predicting hospital performance; (2) Measure reflects the hospital's indication that its submission was based upon a sample of its relevant discharges; (3) Rate reflects fewer than the maximum possible quarters of data for the measure; (4) Inaccurate information submitted and suppressed for one or more quarters; (5) No data is available from the hospital for this measure; Please refer to the User's Guide for a full explanation of data

Heart Attack Care

1. ACE Inhibitor or ARB for LVSD

Hospital Name	City	Rate	Cases
Carson-Tahoe Hospital	Carson City	96%	27
University Medical Center	Las Vegas	95%	39
MountainView Hospital	Las Vegas	90%	50
Renown Regional Medical Center	Reno	88%	84
Saint Mary's Regional Medical Center	Reno	87%	47
Sunrise Hospital & Medical Center	Las Vegas	86%	56
Saint Rose Dominican Hospital-Siena	Henderson	81%	36
Desert Springs Hospital	Las Vegas	72%	40
Valley Hospital Medical Center	Las Vegas	72%	57

2. Aspirin at Arrival

Hospital Name	City	Rate	Cases
Northeasetern Nevada Regional Hospital	Elko	100%	38
Saint Mary's Regional Medical Center	Reno	100%	210
Saint Rose Dominican Hospital-Siena	Henderson	100%	253
Saint Rose Dominican Hospital	Henderson	99%	165
Summerlin Hospital Medical Center	Las Vegas	99%	220
University Medical Center	Las Vegas	99%	206
MountainView Hospital	Las Vegas	98%	272
Southern Hills Hospital and Medical Center	Las Vegas	98%	53
Valley Hospital Medical Center	Las Vegas	98%	250
Renown Regional Medical Center	Reno	97%	173
Sunrise Hospital & Medical Center	Las Vegas	97%	271
Carson-Tahoe Hospital	Carson City	96%	143
North Vista Hospital	North Las Vegas	96%	89
Desert Springs Hospital	Las Vegas	95%	243
Northern Nevada Medical Center	Sparks	92%	38

3. Aspirin at Discharge

Hospital Name	City	Rate	Cases
MountainView Hospital	Las Vegas	98%	246
Renown Regional Medical Center	Reno	97%	362
Saint Mary's Regional Medical Center	Reno	97%	291
Saint Rose Dominican Hospital-Siena	Henderson	97%	261
University Medical Center	Las Vegas	97%	209
Sunrise Hospital & Medical Center	Las Vegas	96%	278
Saint Rose Dominican Hospital	Henderson	95%	119
Summerlin Hospital Medical Center	Las Vegas	95%	182
Carson-Tahoe Hospital	Carson City	92%	144
Valley Hospital Medical Center	Las Vegas	92%	293
Desert Springs Hospital	Las Vegas	90%	276
Southern Hills Hospital and Medical Center	Las Vegas	87%	31
North Vista Hospital	North Las Vegas	78%	36

4. Beta Blocker at Arrival

Hospital Name	City	Rate	Cases
Renown Regional Medical Center	Reno	99%	144
Saint Mary's Regional Medical Center	Reno	98%	186
Southern Hills Hospital and Medical Center	Las Vegas	98%	41
Carson-Tahoe Hospital	Carson City	96%	127
Saint Rose Dominican Hospital	Henderson	96%	133
University Medical Center	Las Vegas	96%	158
Northeasetern Nevada Regional Hospital	Elko	94%	31
Saint Rose Dominican Hospital-Siena	Henderson	94%	186
Summerlin Hospital Medical Center	Las Vegas	94%	177
MountainView Hospital	Las Vegas	92%	203
Valley Hospital Medical Center	Las Vegas	90%	189
North Vista Hospital	North Las Vegas	89%	73
Desert Springs Hospital	Las Vegas	87%	174
Sunrise Hospital & Medical Center	Las Vegas	86%	171
Northern Nevada Medical Center	Sparks	61%	38

5. Beta Blocker at Discharge

Hospital Name	City	Rate	Cases
Renown Regional Medical Center	Reno	99%	338
Saint Mary's Regional Medical Center	Reno	98%	307
Carson-Tahoe Hospital	Carson City	97%	150
MountainView Hospital	Las Vegas	96%	236
Saint Rose Dominican Hospital-Siena	Henderson	95%	241
Summerlin Hospital Medical Center	Las Vegas	95%	167
Saint Rose Dominican Hospital	Henderson	93%	124
Sunrise Hospital & Medical Center	Las Vegas	93%	295
University Medical Center	Las Vegas	93%	191
Southern Hills Hospital and Medical Center	Las Vegas	90%	29
Valley Hospital Medical Center	Las Vegas	89%	277
Desert Springs Hospital	Las Vegas	87%	259
North Vista Hospital	North Las Vegas	68%	34

8. Smoking Cessation Advice

Hospital Name	City	Rate	Cases
MountainView Hospital	Las Vegas	99%	97
Sunrise Hospital & Medical Center	Las Vegas	99%	153
Saint Rose Dominican Hospital	Henderson	96%	57
University Medical Center	Las Vegas	96%	97
Valley Hospital Medical Center	Las Vegas	95%	130
Saint Rose Dominican Hospital-Siena	Henderson	94%	103
Desert Springs Hospital	Las Vegas	93%	122
Saint Mary's Regional Medical Center	Reno	90%	118
Renown Regional Medical Center	Reno	85%	162
Summerlin Hospital Medical Center	Las Vegas	85%	66

Heart Failure Care

9. ACE Inhibitor or ARB for LVSD

Hospital Name	City	Rate	Cases
University Medical Center	Las Vegas	93%	180
Saint Mary's Regional Medical Center	Reno	90%	105
Carson-Tahoe Hospital	Carson City	88%	88
Renown Regional Medical Center	Reno	87%	157
MountainView Hospital	Las Vegas	83%	158
Summerlin Hospital Medical Center	Las Vegas	83%	78
Southern Hills Hospital and Medical Center	Las Vegas	80%	65
Saint Rose Dominican Hospital-Siena	Henderson	77%	115
Sunrise Hospital & Medical Center	Las Vegas	76%	334
Northern Nevada Medical Center	Sparks	75%	52
Valley Hospital Medical Center	Las Vegas	73%	154
Saint Rose Dominican Hospital	Henderson	71%	56
Desert Springs Hospital	Las Vegas	70%	83
North Vista Hospital	North Las Vegas	67%	99

10. Discharge Instructions

Hospital Name	City	Rate	Cases
Banner Churchill Community Hospital	Fallon	81%	36
University Medical Center	Las Vegas	75%	296
Summerlin Hospital Medical Center	Las Vegas	72%	187
Valley Hospital Medical Center	Las Vegas	72%	284
Saint Rose Dominican Hospital	Henderson	69%	162
Saint Rose Dominican Hospital-Siena	Henderson	65%	275
North Vista Hospital	North Las Vegas	63%	244
MountainView Hospital	Las Vegas	62%	402
Carson-Tahoe Hospital	Carson City	54%	50
Northeasetern Nevada Regional Hospital	Elko	49%	69
Renown South Meadows Medical Center	Reno	44%	45
Desert Springs Hospital	Las Vegas	41%	229
Southern Hills Hospital and Medical Center	Las Vegas	40%	147
Renown Regional Medical Center	Reno	37%	315
Sunrise Hospital & Medical Center	Las Vegas	36%	610
Northern Nevada Medical Center	Sparks	33%	93
Saint Mary's Regional Medical Center	Reno	31%	239

11. Evaluation of LVS Function

Hospital Name	City	Rate	Cases
Southern Hills Hospital and Medical Center	Las Vegas	99%	166
Saint Mary's Regional Medical Center	Reno	97%	282
Saint Rose Dominican Hospital-Siena	Henderson	97%	334
University Medical Center	Las Vegas	97%	326
Carson-Tahoe Hospital	Carson City	95%	245
MountainView Hospital	Las Vegas	95%	482
Renown Regional Medical Center	Reno	95%	354
Renown South Meadows Medical Center	Reno	95%	56
Summerlin Hospital Medical Center	Las Vegas	95%	243
Saint Rose Dominican Hospital	Henderson	93%	231
Sunrise Hospital & Medical Center	Las Vegas	92%	710
Valley Hospital Medical Center	Las Vegas	92%	338
Banner Churchill Community Hospital	Fallon	90%	39
Northern Nevada Medical Center	Sparks	88%	122
North Vista Hospital	North Las Vegas	87%	306
Desert Springs Hospital	Las Vegas	85%	291
Northeasetern Nevada Regional Hospital	Elko	82%	76

12. Smoking Cessation Advice

Hospital Name	City	Rate	Cases
North Vista Hospital	North Las Vegas	99%	105
Southern Hills Hospital and Medical Center	Las Vegas	97%	30
Saint Mary's Regional Medical Center	Reno	96%	50
Valley Hospital Medical Center	Las Vegas	96%	95
Desert Springs Hospital	Las Vegas	93%	54
Saint Rose Dominican Hospital-Siena	Henderson	90%	63
Saint Rose Dominican Hospital	Henderson	89%	61
Sunrise Hospital & Medical Center	Las Vegas	87%	213

NOTE: Hospital profiles are in alphabetical order by state, then city, then hospital within the city; Rankings are sorted by rate in descending order and exclude hospitals with less than 25 cases; (1) The number of cases is too small (n<25) for purposes of reliably predicting hospital performance; (2) Measure reflects the hospital's indication that its submission was based upon a sample of its relevant discharges; (3) Rate reflects fewer than the maximum possible quarters of data for the measure; (4) Inaccurate information submitted and suppressed for one or more quarters; (5) No data is available from the hospital for this measure; Please refer to the User's Guide for a full explanation of data

University Medical Center	Las Vegas	87%	142
MountainView Hospital	Las Vegas	85%	92
Summerlin Hospital Medical Center	Las Vegas	81%	32
Renown Regional Medical Center	Reno	77%	107
Northern Nevada Medical Center	Sparks	76%	34

Pneumonia Care

13. Appropriate Initial Antibiotic

Hospital Name	City	Rate	Cases
Northeasetern Nevada Regional Hospital	Elko	96%	72
Southern Hills Hospital and Medical Center	Las Vegas	94%	96
Valley Hospital Medical Center	Las Vegas	93%	96
MountainView Hospital	Las Vegas	92%	222
Renown South Meadows Medical Center	Reno	91%	68
Saint Mary's Regional Medical Center	Reno	91%	87
Desert Springs Hospital	Las Vegas	90%	100
Carson Valley Medical Center	Gardnerville	88%	34
North Vista Hospital	North Las Vegas	87%	172
Sunrise Hospital & Medical Center	Las Vegas	86%	403
Carson-Tahoe Hospital	Carson City	84%	49
Renown Regional Medical Center	Reno	82%	161
Summerlin Hospital Medical Center	Las Vegas	80%	124
Banner Churchill Community Hospital	Fallon	79%	89
Saint Rose Dominican Hospital	Henderson	79%	108
Saint Rose Dominican Hospital-Siena	Henderson	78%	122
University Medical Center	Las Vegas	78%	165
Northern Nevada Medical Center	Sparks	74%	76

14. Blood Culture Timing

Hospital Name	City	Rate	Cases
Renown South Meadows Medical Center	Reno	98%	52
Carson-Tahoe Hospital	Carson City	96%	55
MountainView Hospital	Las Vegas	94%	212
Southern Hills Hospital and Medical Center	Las Vegas	92%	99
Banner Churchill Community Hospital	Fallon	91%	55
North Vista Hospital	North Las Vegas	90%	151
Northern Nevada Medical Center	Sparks	86%	57
Saint Rose Dominican Hospital	Henderson	86%	71
Saint Rose Dominican Hospital-Siena	Henderson	86%	77
Renown Regional Medical Center	Reno	84%	127
Carson Valley Medical Center	Gardnerville	83%	29
Northeasetern Nevada Regional Hospital	Elko	83%	41
Sunrise Hospital & Medical Center	Las Vegas	79%	331
Saint Mary's Regional Medical Center	Reno	72%	101
Desert Springs Hospital	Las Vegas	68%	87
University Medical Center	Las Vegas	66%	76
Summerlin Hospital Medical Center	Las Vegas	63%	105
Valley Hospital Medical Center	Las Vegas	62%	104

15. Influenza Vaccine

Hospital Name	City	Rate	Cases
Summerlin Hospital Medical Center	Las Vegas	100%	28
Southern Hills Hospital and Medical Center	Las Vegas	57%	35
Saint Rose Dominican Hospital-Siena	Henderson	48%	27
MountainView Hospital	Las Vegas	46%	96
Sunrise Hospital & Medical Center	Las Vegas	36%	118
Desert Springs Hospital	Las Vegas	28%	25
North Vista Hospital	North Las Vegas	24%	41
University Medical Center	Las Vegas	12%	32

16. Initial Antibiotic Timing

Hospital Name	City	Rate	Cases
Northeasetern Nevada Regional Hospital	Elko	88%	78
Renown South Meadows Medical Center	Reno	87%	67
Banner Churchill Community Hospital	Fallon	84%	88
Northern Nevada Medical Center	Sparks	84%	81
South Lyon Medical Center	Yerington	84%	25
Carson Valley Medical Center	Gardnerville	82%	39
Renown Regional Medical Center	Reno	81%	204
Saint Mary's Regional Medical Center	Reno	80%	131
Saint Rose Dominican Hospital	Henderson	80%	131
Carson-Tahoe Hospital	Carson City	77%	315
Summerlin Hospital Medical Center	Las Vegas	70%	142
Southern Hills Hospital and Medical Center	Las Vegas	69%	112
North Vista Hospital	North Las Vegas	66%	209
Saint Rose Dominican Hospital-Siena	Henderson	66%	140
Sunrise Hospital & Medical Center	Las Vegas	65%	506
Valley Hospital Medical Center	Las Vegas	63%	138
Desert Springs Hospital	Las Vegas	54%	117
University Medical Center	Las Vegas	52%	206
MountainView Hospital	Las Vegas	51%	301

17. Oxygenation Assessment

Hospital Name	City	Rate	Cases
Banner Churchill Community Hospital	Fallon	100%	112
Carson Valley Medical Center	Gardnerville	100%	44
Carson-Tahoe Hospital	Carson City	100%	399
Desert Springs Hospital	Las Vegas	100%	167
Humboldt General Hospital	Winnemucca	100%	26
MountainView Hospital	Las Vegas	100%	398
North Vista Hospital	North Las Vegas	100%	252
Northeasetern Nevada Regional Hospital	Elko	100%	102
Northern Nevada Medical Center	Sparks	100%	96
Renown Regional Medical Center	Reno	100%	242
Renown South Meadows Medical Center	Reno	100%	86
Saint Mary's Regional Medical Center	Reno	100%	165
Saint Rose Dominican Hospital	Henderson	100%	169
Saint Rose Dominican Hospital-Siena	Henderson	100%	187
South Lyon Medical Center	Yerington	100%	28
Southern Hills Hospital and Medical Center	Las Vegas	100%	166
Summerlin Hospital Medical Center	Las Vegas	100%	194
Sunrise Hospital & Medical Center	Las Vegas	100%	655
University Medical Center	Las Vegas	100%	244
Valley Hospital Medical Center	Las Vegas	100%	164

18. Pneumococcal Vaccine

Hospital Name	City	Rate	Cases
Renown South Meadows Medical Center	Reno	86%	51
Carson Valley Medical Center	Gardnerville	79%	29
Renown Regional Medical Center	Reno	78%	120
MountainView Hospital	Las Vegas	75%	244
Saint Rose Dominican Hospital	Henderson	75%	97
Saint Rose Dominican Hospital-Siena	Henderson	75%	113
Summerlin Hospital Medical Center	Las Vegas	71%	109
Northeasetern Nevada Regional Hospital	Elko	69%	52
Banner Churchill Community Hospital	Fallon	68%	72
Saint Mary's Regional Medical Center	Reno	65%	101
Northern Nevada Medical Center	Sparks	60%	58
Southern Hills Hospital and Medical Center	Las Vegas	57%	91
Sunrise Hospital & Medical Center	Las Vegas	50%	333
Carson-Tahoe Hospital	Carson City	45%	283
Desert Springs Hospital	Las Vegas	43%	100
University Medical Center	Las Vegas	38%	64
Valley Hospital Medical Center	Las Vegas	26%	88
North Vista Hospital	North Las Vegas	18%	95

19. Smoking Cessation Advice

Hospital Name	City	Rate	Cases
Southern Hills Hospital and Medical Center	Las Vegas	98%	45
Valley Hospital Medical Center	Las Vegas	93%	46
North Vista Hospital	North Las Vegas	91%	100
Northern Nevada Medical Center	Sparks	88%	34
Saint Rose Dominican Hospital-Siena	Henderson	86%	49
Sunrise Hospital & Medical Center	Las Vegas	86%	208
University Medical Center	Las Vegas	86%	101
Saint Rose Dominican Hospital	Henderson	84%	45
Saint Mary's Regional Medical Center	Reno	81%	48
Northeasetern Nevada Regional Hospital	Elko	79%	28
Summerlin Hospital Medical Center	Las Vegas	79%	38
Renown Regional Medical Center	Reno	78%	76
Desert Springs Hospital	Las Vegas	74%	43
MountainView Hospital	Las Vegas	70%	105
Banner Churchill Community Hospital	Fallon	56%	32

Surgical Infection Prevention

20. Prophylactic Antibiotic Given

Hospital Name	City	Rate	Cases
Sierra Surgery & Imaging	Carson City	93%	94
Northern Nevada Medical Center	Sparks	92%	212
Saint Rose Dominican Hospital	Henderson	86%	140
Saint Mary's Regional Medical Center	Reno	85%	350
Renown South Meadows Medical Center	Reno	81%	70
Saint Rose Dominican Hospital-Siena	Henderson	78%	251
North Vista Hospital	North Las Vegas	77%	216
Valley Hospital Medical Center	Las Vegas	76%	401
Carson-Tahoe Hospital	Carson City	75%	77
Desert Springs Hospital	Las Vegas	74%	243
Renown Regional Medical Center	Reno	71%	494
MountainView Hospital	Las Vegas	70%	269
Banner Churchill Community Hospital	Fallon	67%	45
Summerlin Hospital Medical Center	Las Vegas	67%	304
Northeasetern Nevada Regional Hospital	Elko	60%	83
Sunrise Hospital & Medical Center	Las Vegas	59%	319

NOTE: Hospital profiles are in alphabetical order by state, then city, then hospital within the city; Rankings are sorted by rate in descending order and exclude hospitals with less than 25 cases; (1) The number of cases is too small (n<25) for purposes of reliably predicting hospital performance; (2) Measure reflects the hospital's indication that its submission was based upon a sample of its relevant discharges; (3) Rate reflects fewer than the maximum possible quarters of data for the measure; (4) Inaccurate information submitted and suppressed for one or more quarters; (5) No data is available from the hospital for this measure; Please refer to the User's Guide for a full explanation of data

Hospital Name	City	Rate	Cases
Southern Hills Hospital and Medical Center	Las Vegas	53%	164
University Medical Center	Las Vegas	37%	294

21. Prophylactic Antibiotic Selection

Hospital Name	City	Rate	Cases
Saint Mary's Regional Medical Center	Reno	98%	82
Northern Nevada Medical Center	Sparks	97%	39
North Vista Hospital	North Las Vegas	96%	46
Northeasetern Nevada Regional Hospital	Elko	96%	27
Southern Hills Hospital and Medical Center	Las Vegas	96%	98
Renown South Meadows Medical Center	Reno	94%	32
Saint Rose Dominican Hospital-Siena	Henderson	93%	90
Valley Hospital Medical Center	Las Vegas	93%	94
Desert Springs Hospital	Las Vegas	92%	61
MountainView Hospital	Las Vegas	91%	118
University Medical Center	Las Vegas	91%	57
Renown Regional Medical Center	Reno	90%	169
Saint Rose Dominican Hospital	Henderson	90%	51
Sunrise Hospital & Medical Center	Las Vegas	88%	162
Summerlin Hospital Medical Center	Las Vegas	87%	68

22. Prophylactic Antibiotic Stopped

Hospital Name	City	Rate	Cases
Carson-Tahoe Hospital	Carson City	83%	65
Sierra Surgery & Imaging	Carson City	80%	94
University Medical Center	Las Vegas	75%	271
Banner Churchill Community Hospital	Fallon	74%	42
Saint Mary's Regional Medical Center	Reno	72%	326
Sunrise Hospital & Medical Center	Las Vegas	71%	295
Summerlin Hospital Medical Center	Las Vegas	59%	286
MountainView Hospital	Las Vegas	57%	249
Renown Regional Medical Center	Reno	56%	481
Saint Rose Dominican Hospital	Henderson	45%	132
Saint Rose Dominican Hospital-Siena	Henderson	44%	229
Desert Springs Hospital	Las Vegas	42%	238
Valley Hospital Medical Center	Las Vegas	41%	380
Southern Hills Hospital and Medical Center	Las Vegas	39%	153
North Vista Hospital	North Las Vegas	36%	201
Renown South Meadows Medical Center	Reno	32%	68
Northeasetern Nevada Regional Hospital	Elko	26%	81
Northern Nevada Medical Center	Sparks	26%	208

Pregnancy Care

23. Inpatient Neonatal Mortality

Hospital Name	City	Rate	Cases
Saint Rose Dominican Hospital	Henderson	0.16%	3704
Renown Regional Medical Center	Reno	0.81%	992

24. Third or Fourth Degree Laceration

Hospital Name	City	Rate	Cases
Renown Regional Medical Center	Reno	3.79%	712
Saint Rose Dominican Hospital	Henderson	5.19%	2504

NOTE: Hospital profiles are in alphabetical order by state, then city, then hospital within the city; Rankings are sorted by rate in descending order and exclude hospitals with less than 25 cases; (1) The number of cases is too small (n<25) for purposes of reliably predicting hospital performance; (2) Measure reflects the hospital's indication that its submission was based upon a sample of its relevant discharges; (3) Rate reflects fewer than the maximum possible quarters of data for the measure; (4) Inaccurate information submitted and suppressed for one or more quarters; (5) No data is available from the hospital for this measure; Please refer to the User's Guide for a full explanation of data

Grover C Dils Medical Center

PO Box 1010
Caliente, NV 89008
URL: www.dilsmedicalcenter.org
Ownership: Govt - Hospital District or Authority
Emergency Services: Yes

Phone: 775-726-3171
Fax: 775-726-3797
Accredited: No
Licensed Beds: 20

Key Personnel:
CEO.................................. Shawn Wiscombe
Chief Medical Staff....................... R William Katschke Jr
Emergency Room .... Judy Johnson
Infection Control......................... Judy Johnson
Respiratory/Cardiopulmonary............... Merrillyn Budreau

Measure	Cases	This Hospital	State Average	U.S. Average	Top Hospital
Heart Attack Care					
ACE Inhibitor or ARB for LVSD[5]	-	-	78%	82%	100%
Aspirin at Arrival[5]	-	-	97%	92%	100%
Aspirin at Discharge[5]	-	-	86%	90%	100%
Beta Blocker at Arrival[5]	-	-	84%	87%	100%
Beta Blocker at Discharge[5]	-	-	84%	90%	100%
Fibrinolytic Medication Timing[5]	-	-	30%	31%	100%
PCI Within 90 Minutes of Arrival[5]	-	-	25%	54%	95%
Smoking Cessation Advice[5]	-	-	93%	88%	100%
Heart Failure Care					
ACE Inhibitor or ARB for LVSD[1,3]	1	100%	84%	82%	100%
Discharge Instructions[1,3]	1	0%	50%	61%	93%
Evaluation of LVS Function[1,3]	9	11%	83%	83%	99%
Smoking Cessation Advice[1,3]	1	0%	80%	82%	100%
Pneumonia Care					
Appropriate Initial Antibiotic[1,3]	4	100%	82%	83%	94%
Blood Culture Timing[3]	0	-	81%	90%	100%
Influenza Vaccine[5]	-	-	54%	70%	100%
Initial Antibiotic Timing[1,3]	12	58%	72%	80%	93%
Oxygenation Assessment[1,3]	13	100%	100%	99%	100%
Pneumococcal Vaccine[1,3]	7	0%	55%	69%	94%
Smoking Cessation Advice[1,3]	1	0%	75%	80%	100%
Surgical Infection Prevention					
Prophylactic Antibiotic Given[5]	-	-	72%	77%	95%
Prophylactic Antibiotic Selection[5]	-	-	93%	90%	100%
Prophylactic Antibiotic Stopped[5]	-	-	53%	72%	95%
Pregnancy Care					
Inpatient Neonatal Mortality	-	-	-	-	-
Third or Fourth Degree Laceration	-	-	-	3.63%	3.27%

Carson-Tahoe Hospital

1600 Medical Parkway
Carson City, NV 89703
E-mail: info@c-th.com
URL: www.carsontahoehospital.com
Ownership: Voluntary non-profit - Private
Emergency Services: Yes

Phone: 775-445-8000
Fax: 775-885-4447
Accredited: Yes
Licensed Beds: 128

Key Personnel:
Administrator/CEO....................... Steve Smith
Emergency Room .... Deena McKenzie
Director Infection/Disease Control .... Kim Neiman

Measure	Cases	This Hospital	State Average	U.S. Average	Top Hospital
Heart Attack Care					
ACE Inhibitor or ARB for LVSD	27	96%	78%	82%	100%
Aspirin at Arrival	143	96%	97%	92%	100%
Aspirin at Discharge	144	92%	86%	90%	100%
Beta Blocker at Arrival	127	96%	84%	87%	100%
Beta Blocker at Discharge	150	97%	84%	90%	100%
Fibrinolytic Medication Timing[3]	0	-	30%	31%	100%
PCI Within 90 Minutes of Arrival[1]	2	0%	25%	54%	95%
Smoking Cessation Advice[1,3]	12	100%	93%	88%	100%
Heart Failure Care					
ACE Inhibitor or ARB for LVSD	88	88%	84%	82%	100%
Discharge Instructions[3]	50	54%	50%	61%	93%
Evaluation of LVS Function	245	95%	83%	83%	99%
Smoking Cessation Advice[1,3]	10	90%	80%	82%	100%
Pneumonia Care					
Appropriate Initial Antibiotic[3]	49	84%	82%	83%	94%
Blood Culture Timing[3]	55	96%	81%	90%	100%
Influenza Vaccine[5]	-	-	54%	70%	100%
Initial Antibiotic Timing	315	77%	72%	80%	93%
Oxygenation Assessment	399	100%	100%	99%	100%
Pneumococcal Vaccine	283	45%	55%	69%	94%
Smoking Cessation Advice[1,3]	22	73%	75%	80%	100%
Surgical Infection Prevention					
Prophylactic Antibiotic Given[2,3]	77	75%	72%	77%	95%
Prophylactic Antibiotic Selection[5]	-	-	93%	90%	100%
Prophylactic Antibiotic Stopped[2,3]	65	83%	53%	72%	95%
Pregnancy Care					
Inpatient Neonatal Mortality	-	-	-	-	-
Third or Fourth Degree Laceration	-	-	-	3.63%	3.27%

Sierra Surgery & Imaging

1400 Medical Parkway
Carson City, NV 89703
Ownership: Proprietary
Emergency Services: No

Phone: 775-883-1700
Accredited: No

Measure	Cases	This Hospital	State Average	U.S. Average	Top Hospital
Heart Attack Care					
ACE Inhibitor or ARB for LVSD[5]	-	-	78%	82%	100%
Aspirin at Arrival[5]	-	-	97%	92%	100%
Aspirin at Discharge[5]	-	-	86%	90%	100%
Beta Blocker at Arrival[5]	-	-	84%	87%	100%
Beta Blocker at Discharge[5]	-	-	84%	90%	100%
Fibrinolytic Medication Timing[5]	-	-	30%	31%	100%
PCI Within 90 Minutes of Arrival[5]	-	-	25%	54%	95%
Smoking Cessation Advice[5]	-	-	93%	88%	100%
Heart Failure Care					
ACE Inhibitor or ARB for LVSD[5]	-	-	84%	82%	100%
Discharge Instructions[5]	-	-	50%	61%	93%
Evaluation of LVS Function[5]	-	-	83%	83%	99%
Smoking Cessation Advice[5]	-	-	80%	82%	100%
Pneumonia Care					
Appropriate Initial Antibiotic[5]	-	-	82%	83%	94%
Blood Culture Timing[5]	-	-	81%	90%	100%
Influenza Vaccine[5]	-	-	54%	70%	100%
Initial Antibiotic Timing[5]	-	-	72%	80%	93%
Oxygenation Assessment[5]	-	-	100%	99%	100%
Pneumococcal Vaccine[5]	-	-	55%	69%	94%
Smoking Cessation Advice[5]	-	-	75%	80%	100%
Surgical Infection Prevention					
Prophylactic Antibiotic Given[3]	94	93%	72%	77%	95%
Prophylactic Antibiotic Selection[5]	-	-	93%	90%	100%
Prophylactic Antibiotic Stopped[3]	94	80%	53%	72%	95%
Pregnancy Care					
Inpatient Neonatal Mortality	-	-	-	-	-
Third or Fourth Degree Laceration	-	-	-	3.63%	3.27%

Northeasetern Nevada Regional Hospital

2001 Errecart Boulevard
Elko, NV 89801
URL: www.nnrhospital.com
Ownership: Proprietary
Emergency Services: Yes

Phone: 775-738-5151
Fax: 775-748-2002
Accredited: Yes
Licensed Beds: 75

Key Personnel:
President/CEO.......................... Alex Poirier
Chief Medical Staff....................... Mitchell Miller, MD
Emergency Room .... Carol Laird
Emergency Room .... Robert Stefanko, MD
Infection Control......................... Lynn Gauthier
ICU .... Raquel Guerrero
Medical Surgical Nursing .... Raquel Guerrero
Respiratory/Cardiopulmonary............... Danny Warren

Measure	Cases	This Hospital	State Average	U.S. Average	Top Hospital
Heart Attack Care					
ACE Inhibitor or ARB for LVSD[1]	3	100%	78%	82%	100%
Aspirin at Arrival	38	100%	97%	92%	100%
Aspirin at Discharge[1]	13	85%	86%	90%	100%

NOTE: Hospital profiles are in alphabetical order by state, then city, then hospital within the city; Rankings are sorted by rate in descending order and exclude hospitals with less than 25 cases; (1) The number of cases is too small (n<25) for purposes of reliably predicting hospital performance; (2) Measure reflects the hospital's indication that its submission was based upon a sample of its relevant discharges; (3) Rate reflects fewer than the maximum possible quarters of data for the measure; (4) Inaccurate information submitted and suppressed for one or more quarters; (5) No data is available from the hospital for this measure; Please refer to the User's Guide for a full explanation of data

Beta Blocker at Arrival	31	94%	84%	87%	100%
Beta Blocker at Discharge[1]	11	100%	84%	90%	100%
Fibrinolytic Medication Timing[1]	15	47%	30%	31%	100%
PCI Within 90 Minutes of Arrival	0	-	25%	54%	95%
Smoking Cessation Advice[1]	5	40%	93%	88%	100%
Heart Failure Care					
ACE Inhibitor or ARB for LVSD[1]	20	100%	84%	82%	100%
Discharge Instructions	69	49%	50%	61%	93%
Evaluation of LVS Function	76	82%	83%	83%	99%
Smoking Cessation Advice[1]	21	67%	80%	82%	100%
Pneumonia Care					
Appropriate Initial Antibiotic	72	96%	82%	83%	94%
Blood Culture Timing	41	83%	81%	90%	100%
Influenza Vaccine[1]	12	75%	54%	70%	100%
Initial Antibiotic Timing	78	88%	72%	80%	93%
Oxygenation Assessment	102	100%	100%	99%	100%
Pneumococcal Vaccine	52	69%	55%	69%	94%
Smoking Cessation Advice	28	79%	75%	80%	100%
Surgical Infection Prevention					
Prophylactic Antibiotic Given[3]	83	60%	72%	77%	95%
Prophylactic Antibiotic Selection	27	96%	93%	90%	100%
Prophylactic Antibiotic Stopped[3]	81	26%	53%	72%	95%
Pregnancy Care					
Inpatient Neonatal Mortality	-	-	-	-	-
Third or Fourth Degree Laceration	-	-	-	3.63%	3.27%

Banner Churchill Community Hospital

801 East Williams Avenue
Fallon, NV 89406
Phone: 775-423-3151
Fax: 775-423-3793
Ownership: Voluntary non-profit - Private
Accredited: Yes
Emergency Services: Yes
Licensed Beds: 40

Key Personnel:

CEO. . . . . Charles Myers
Chief Medical Staff. . . . . Erick Herzog, MD
Emergency Room . . . . Brett Aikin, MD
Director Infection/Disease Control . . . . Arlene McDonnel, RN
Director Medical/Surgical Nursing . . . . Joan Andersen
OB/GYN Womens Health. . . . . Christopher Von Dippe
Director of Pulmonary/Respiratory Care. . . . . . . Al DeRose

Measure	Cases	This Hospital	State Average	U.S. Average	Top Hospital
Heart Attack Care					
ACE Inhibitor or ARB for LVSD[1]	2	50%	78%	82%	100%
Aspirin at Arrival[1]	10	80%	97%	92%	100%
Aspirin at Discharge[1]	5	80%	86%	90%	100%
Beta Blocker at Arrival[1]	12	75%	84%	87%	100%
Beta Blocker at Discharge[1]	8	100%	84%	90%	100%
Fibrinolytic Medication Timing[1]	3	33%	30%	31%	100%
PCI Within 90 Minutes of Arrival	0	-	25%	54%	95%
Smoking Cessation Advice[1]	2	100%	93%	88%	100%
Heart Failure Care					
ACE Inhibitor or ARB for LVSD[1]	12	83%	84%	82%	100%
Discharge Instructions	36	81%	50%	61%	93%
Evaluation of LVS Function	39	90%	83%	83%	99%
Smoking Cessation Advice[1]	6	83%	80%	82%	100%
Pneumonia Care					
Appropriate Initial Antibiotic	89	79%	82%	83%	94%
Blood Culture Timing	55	91%	81%	90%	100%
Influenza Vaccine[1]	19	84%	54%	70%	100%
Initial Antibiotic Timing	88	84%	72%	80%	93%
Oxygenation Assessment	112	100%	100%	99%	100%
Pneumococcal Vaccine	72	68%	55%	69%	94%
Smoking Cessation Advice	32	56%	75%	80%	100%
Surgical Infection Prevention					
Prophylactic Antibiotic Given	45	67%	72%	77%	95%
Prophylactic Antibiotic Selection[1]	12	100%	93%	90%	100%
Prophylactic Antibiotic Stopped	42	74%	53%	72%	95%
Pregnancy Care					
Inpatient Neonatal Mortality	-	-	-	-	-
Third or Fourth Degree Laceration	-	-	-	3.63%	3.27%

Carson Valley Medical Center

1107 Highway 395
Phone: 775-782-1500
Gardnerville, NV 89410
Ownership: Proprietary
Accredited: No
Emergency Services: Yes

Measure	Cases	This Hospital	State Average	U.S. Average	Top Hospital
Heart Attack Care					
ACE Inhibitor or ARB for LVSD[3]	0	-	78%	82%	100%
Aspirin at Arrival[1,3]	4	100%	97%	92%	100%
Aspirin at Discharge[1,3]	3	67%	86%	90%	100%
Beta Blocker at Arrival[1,3]	4	25%	84%	87%	100%
Beta Blocker at Discharge[1,3]	3	33%	84%	90%	100%
Fibrinolytic Medication Timing[3]	0	-	30%	31%	100%
PCI Within 90 Minutes of Arrival	0	-	25%	54%	95%
Smoking Cessation Advice[3]	0	-	93%	88%	100%
Heart Failure Care					
ACE Inhibitor or ARB for LVSD[1]	7	86%	84%	82%	100%
Discharge Instructions[1]	11	55%	50%	61%	93%
Evaluation of LVS Function[1]	11	64%	83%	83%	99%
Smoking Cessation Advice[1]	2	0%	80%	82%	100%
Pneumonia Care					
Appropriate Initial Antibiotic	34	88%	82%	83%	94%
Blood Culture Timing	29	83%	81%	90%	100%
Influenza Vaccine[1]	7	43%	54%	70%	100%
Initial Antibiotic Timing	39	82%	72%	80%	93%
Oxygenation Assessment	44	100%	100%	99%	100%
Pneumococcal Vaccine	29	79%	55%	69%	94%
Smoking Cessation Advice[1]	3	33%	75%	80%	100%
Surgical Infection Prevention					
Prophylactic Antibiotic Given[5]	-	-	72%	77%	95%
Prophylactic Antibiotic Selection[5]	-	-	93%	90%	100%
Prophylactic Antibiotic Stopped[5]	-	-	53%	72%	95%
Pregnancy Care					
Inpatient Neonatal Mortality	-	-	-	-	-
Third or Fourth Degree Laceration	-	-	-	3.63%	3.27%

Saint Rose Dominican Hospital

Alternate Name: Rose de Lima Campus
102 E Lake Mead Drive
Phone: 702-564-2622
Henderson, NV 89015
Fax: 702-616-4820
Ownership: Voluntary non-profit - Church
Accredited: Yes
Emergency Services: Yes
Licensed Beds: 143

Key Personnel:

Administrator/CEO. . . . . Rod A Davis
Chief Medical Staff. . . . . Matt McMahon, DO
Emergency Room . . . . Rick Henderson, MD
Director Infection/Disease Control . . . . Ann Jenkins
Manager CCU . . . . Linda Mayland, RN
OB/GYN Womens Health. . . . . Hesham A Sirsy, MD
Chief OB/GYN/Pediatrics . . . . Hesham A Sirsy, MD
Manager Respiratory Therapy . . . . Syd Rubecamp

Measure	Cases	This Hospital	State Average	U.S. Average	Top Hospital
Heart Attack Care					
ACE Inhibitor or ARB for LVSD[1]	16	88%	78%	82%	100%
Aspirin at Arrival	165	99%	97%	92%	100%
Aspirin at Discharge	119	95%	86%	90%	100%
Beta Blocker at Arrival	133	96%	84%	87%	100%
Beta Blocker at Discharge	124	93%	84%	90%	100%
Fibrinolytic Medication Timing[1]	9	67%	30%	31%	100%
PCI Within 90 Minutes of Arrival[1]	2	0%	25%	54%	95%
Smoking Cessation Advice	57	96%	93%	88%	100%
Heart Failure Care					
ACE Inhibitor or ARB for LVSD	56	71%	84%	82%	100%
Discharge Instructions	162	69%	50%	61%	93%
Evaluation of LVS Function	231	93%	83%	83%	99%
Smoking Cessation Advice	61	89%	80%	82%	100%
Pneumonia Care					
Appropriate Initial Antibiotic[2]	108	79%	82%	83%	94%
Blood Culture Timing[2]	71	86%	81%	90%	100%
Influenza Vaccine[4,5]	-	-	54%	70%	100%

NOTE: Hospital profiles are in alphabetical order by state, then city, then hospital within the city; Rankings are sorted by rate in descending order and exclude hospitals with less than 25 cases; (1) The number of cases is too small (n<25) for purposes of reliably predicting hospital performance; (2) Measure reflects the hospital's indication that its submission was based upon a sample of its relevant discharges; (3) Rate reflects fewer than the maximum possible quarters of data for the measure; (4) Inaccurate information submitted and suppressed for one or more quarters; (5) No data is available from the hospital for this measure; Please refer to the User's Guide for a full explanation of data

Initial Antibiotic Timing[2]	131	80%	72%	80%	93%
Oxygenation Assessment[2]	169	100%	100%	99%	100%
Pneumococcal Vaccine[2]	97	75%	55%	69%	94%
Smoking Cessation Advice[2]	45	84%	75%	80%	100%
Surgical Infection Prevention					
Prophylactic Antibiotic Given[2,3]	140	86%	72%	77%	95%
Prophylactic Antibiotic Selection[2]	51	90%	93%	90%	100%
Prophylactic Antibiotic Stopped[2,3]	132	45%	53%	72%	95%
Pregnancy Care					
Inpatient Neonatal Mortality	3,704	0.16%	-	-	-
Third or Fourth Degree Laceration	2,504	5.19%	-	3.63%	3.27%

Saint Rose Dominican Hospital-Siena

3001 Saint Rose Parkway
Henderson, NV 89052
Phone: 702-616-5000
Ownership: Voluntary non-profit - Church
Accredited: Yes
Emergency Services: Yes

Measure	Cases	This Hospital	State Average	U.S. Average	Top Hospital
Heart Attack Care					
ACE Inhibitor or ARB for LVSD	36	81%	78%	82%	100%
Aspirin at Arrival	253	100%	97%	92%	100%
Aspirin at Discharge	261	97%	86%	90%	100%
Beta Blocker at Arrival	186	94%	84%	87%	100%
Beta Blocker at Discharge	241	95%	84%	90%	100%
Fibrinolytic Medication Timing[1]	13	38%	30%	31%	100%
PCI Within 90 Minutes of Arrival[1]	3	100%	25%	54%	95%
Smoking Cessation Advice	103	94%	93%	88%	100%
Heart Failure Care					
ACE Inhibitor or ARB for LVSD	115	77%	84%	82%	100%
Discharge Instructions	275	65%	50%	61%	93%
Evaluation of LVS Function	334	97%	83%	83%	99%
Smoking Cessation Advice	63	90%	80%	82%	100%
Pneumonia Care					
Appropriate Initial Antibiotic[2]	122	78%	82%	83%	94%
Blood Culture Timing[2]	77	86%	81%	90%	100%
Influenza Vaccine	27	48%	54%	70%	100%
Initial Antibiotic Timing[2]	140	66%	72%	80%	93%
Oxygenation Assessment[2]	187	100%	100%	99%	100%
Pneumococcal Vaccine[2]	113	75%	55%	69%	94%
Smoking Cessation Advice[2]	49	86%	75%	80%	100%
Surgical Infection Prevention					
Prophylactic Antibiotic Given[2,3]	251	78%	72%	77%	95%
Prophylactic Antibiotic Selection[2]	90	93%	93%	90%	100%
Prophylactic Antibiotic Stopped[2,3]	229	44%	53%	72%	95%
Pregnancy Care					
Inpatient Neonatal Mortality	-	-	-	-	-
Third or Fourth Degree Laceration	-	-	-	3.63%	3.27%

Desert Springs Hospital

2075 East Flamingo Road
Las Vegas, NV 89119
Phone: 702-733-8800
Fax: 702-894-5654
URL: www.desertspringshospital.net/p12.html
Ownership: Proprietary
Accredited: Yes
Emergency Services: Yes
Licensed Beds: 286

Measure	Cases	This Hospital	State Average	U.S. Average	Top Hospital
Heart Attack Care					
ACE Inhibitor or ARB for LVSD[2]	40	72%	78%	82%	100%
Aspirin at Arrival[2]	243	95%	97%	92%	100%
Aspirin at Discharge[2]	276	90%	86%	90%	100%
Beta Blocker at Arrival[2]	174	87%	84%	87%	100%
Beta Blocker at Discharge[2]	259	87%	84%	90%	100%
Fibrinolytic Medication Timing[1,2]	12	67%	30%	31%	100%
PCI Within 90 Minutes of Arrival[1,2]	14	36%	25%	54%	95%
Smoking Cessation Advice[2]	122	93%	93%	88%	100%
Heart Failure Care					
ACE Inhibitor or ARB for LVSD[2]	83	70%	84%	82%	100%
Discharge Instructions[2]	229	41%	50%	61%	93%
Evaluation of LVS Function[2]	291	85%	83%	83%	99%
Smoking Cessation Advice[2]	54	93%	80%	82%	100%
Pneumonia Care					
Appropriate Initial Antibiotic[2]	100	90%	82%	83%	94%
Blood Culture Timing[2]	87	68%	81%	90%	100%
Influenza Vaccine[2]	25	28%	54%	70%	100%
Initial Antibiotic Timing[2]	117	54%	72%	80%	93%
Oxygenation Assessment[2]	167	100%	100%	99%	100%
Pneumococcal Vaccine[2]	100	43%	55%	69%	94%
Smoking Cessation Advice[2]	43	74%	75%	80%	100%
Surgical Infection Prevention					
Prophylactic Antibiotic Given[2]	243	74%	72%	77%	95%
Prophylactic Antibiotic Selection[2]	61	92%	93%	90%	100%
Prophylactic Antibiotic Stopped[2]	238	42%	53%	72%	95%
Pregnancy Care					
Inpatient Neonatal Mortality	-	-	-	-	-
Third or Fourth Degree Laceration	-	-	-	3.63%	3.27%

MountainView Hospital

3100 N Tenaya Way
Las Vegas, NV 89128
Phone: 792-255-5000
Fax: 702-255-5074
URL: www.mountainview-hospital.com
Ownership: Proprietary
Accredited: Yes
Emergency Services: Yes
Licensed Beds: 235
Key Personnel:
President/CEO. . . . . Mark J Howard

Measure	Cases	This Hospital	State Average	U.S. Average	Top Hospital
Heart Attack Care					
ACE Inhibitor or ARB for LVSD	50	90%	78%	82%	100%
Aspirin at Arrival	272	98%	97%	92%	100%
Aspirin at Discharge	246	98%	86%	90%	100%
Beta Blocker at Arrival	203	92%	84%	87%	100%
Beta Blocker at Discharge	236	96%	84%	90%	100%
Fibrinolytic Medication Timing[1]	13	23%	30%	31%	100%
PCI Within 90 Minutes of Arrival[1]	11	27%	25%	54%	95%
Smoking Cessation Advice	97	99%	93%	88%	100%
Heart Failure Care					
ACE Inhibitor or ARB for LVSD[2]	158	83%	84%	82%	100%
Discharge Instructions[2]	402	62%	50%	61%	93%
Evaluation of LVS Function[2]	482	95%	83%	83%	99%
Smoking Cessation Advice[2]	92	85%	80%	82%	100%
Pneumonia Care					
Appropriate Initial Antibiotic[2]	222	92%	82%	83%	94%
Blood Culture Timing[2]	212	94%	81%	90%	100%
Influenza Vaccine	96	46%	54%	70%	100%
Initial Antibiotic Timing[2]	301	51%	72%	80%	93%
Oxygenation Assessment[2]	398	100%	100%	99%	100%
Pneumococcal Vaccine[2]	244	75%	55%	69%	94%
Smoking Cessation Advice[2]	105	70%	75%	80%	100%
Surgical Infection Prevention					
Prophylactic Antibiotic Given[2,3]	269	70%	72%	77%	95%
Prophylactic Antibiotic Selection[2]	118	91%	93%	90%	100%
Prophylactic Antibiotic Stopped[2,3]	249	57%	53%	72%	95%
Pregnancy Care					
Inpatient Neonatal Mortality	-	-	-	-	-
Third or Fourth Degree Laceration	-	-	-	3.63%	3.27%

Southern Hills Hospital and Medical Center

9300 W Sunset Road
Las Vegas, NV 89148
Phone: 702-880-2100
Fax: 702-880-2961
URL: www.southernhillshospital.com
Ownership: Proprietary
Accredited: Yes
Emergency Services: Yes
Licensed Beds: 130
Key Personnel:
CEO. . . . . Steve Dixon

Measure	Cases	This Hospital	State Average	U.S. Average	Top Hospital
Heart Attack Care					
ACE Inhibitor or ARB for LVSD[1]	6	83%	78%	82%	100%
Aspirin at Arrival	53	98%	97%	92%	100%
Aspirin at Discharge	31	87%	86%	90%	100%
Beta Blocker at Arrival	41	98%	84%	87%	100%
Beta Blocker at Discharge	29	90%	84%	90%	100%
Fibrinolytic Medication Timing[1]	3	0%	30%	31%	100%

NOTE: Hospital profiles are in alphabetical order by state, then city, then hospital within the city; Rankings are sorted by rate in descending order and exclude hospitals with less than 25 cases; (1) The number of cases is too small (n<25) for purposes of reliably predicting hospital performance; (2) Measure reflects the hospital's indication that its submission was based upon a sample of its relevant discharges; (3) Rate reflects fewer than the maximum possible quarters of data for the measure; (4) Inaccurate information submitted and suppressed for one or more quarters; (5) No data is available from the hospital for this measure; Please refer to the User's Guide for a full explanation of data

PCI Within 90 Minutes of Arrival[1]	3	0%	25%	54%	95%
Smoking Cessation Advice[1]	9	100%	93%	88%	100%
Heart Failure Care					
ACE Inhibitor or ARB for LVSD	65	80%	84%	82%	100%
Discharge Instructions	147	40%	50%	61%	93%
Evaluation of LVS Function	166	99%	83%	83%	99%
Smoking Cessation Advice	30	97%	80%	82%	100%
Pneumonia Care					
Appropriate Initial Antibiotic	96	94%	82%	83%	94%
Blood Culture Timing	99	92%	81%	90%	100%
Influenza Vaccine	35	57%	54%	70%	100%
Initial Antibiotic Timing	112	69%	72%	80%	93%
Oxygenation Assessment	166	100%	100%	99%	100%
Pneumococcal Vaccine	91	57%	55%	69%	94%
Smoking Cessation Advice	45	98%	75%	80%	100%
Surgical Infection Prevention					
Prophylactic Antibiotic Given[2,3]	164	53%	72%	77%	95%
Prophylactic Antibiotic Selection[2]	98	96%	93%	90%	100%
Prophylactic Antibiotic Stopped[2,3]	153	39%	53%	72%	95%
Pregnancy Care					
Inpatient Neonatal Mortality	-	-	-	-	-
Third or Fourth Degree Laceration	-	-	-	3.63%	3.27%

Spring Valley Hospital

5400 South Rainbow Boulevard
Las Vegas, NM 89119
URL: www.springvalleyhospital.net
Ownership: Proprietary
Emergency Services: Yes

Phone: 702-853-3000
Fax: 702-853-3340
Accredited: Yes
Licensed Beds: 210

Key Personnel:

CEO. . . . . Karla Perez
Emergency Department . . . . Kevin Slaughter, DO
OB/GYN Department . . . . Steven Kramer, MD
Surgery Department. . . . . Randal Peoples, MD

Measure	Cases	This Hospital	State Average	U.S. Average	Top Hospital
Heart Attack Care					
ACE Inhibitor or ARB for LVSD[1]	13	77%	78%	82%	100%
Aspirin at Arrival	183	96%	97%	92%	100%
Aspirin at Discharge	80	91%	86%	90%	100%
Beta Blocker at Arrival	134	86%	84%	87%	100%
Beta Blocker at Discharge	80	81%	84%	90%	100%
Fibrinolytic Medication Timing[1]	17	65%	30%	31%	100%
PCI Within 90 Minutes of Arrival[1]	3	33%	25%	54%	95%
Smoking Cessation Advice	40	98%	93%	88%	100%
Heart Failure Care					
ACE Inhibitor or ARB for LVSD[2]	77	92%	84%	82%	100%
Discharge Instructions[2]	183	99%	50%	61%	93%
Evaluation of LVS Function[2]	234	98%	83%	83%	99%
Smoking Cessation Advice[2]	69	99%	80%	82%	100%
Pneumonia Care					
Appropriate Initial Antibiotic[2]	125	90%	82%	83%	94%
Blood Culture Timing[2]	70	80%	81%	90%	100%
Influenza Vaccine[1,2]	20	90%	54%	70%	100%
Initial Antibiotic Timing[2]	139	75%	72%	80%	93%
Oxygenation Assessment[2]	145	100%	100%	99%	100%
Pneumococcal Vaccine[2]	72	85%	55%	69%	94%
Smoking Cessation Advice[2]	48	96%	75%	80%	100%
Surgical Infection Prevention					
Prophylactic Antibiotic Given[2]	208	71%	72%	77%	95%
Prophylactic Antibiotic Selection[2]	50	88%	93%	90%	100%
Prophylactic Antibiotic Stopped[2]	200	54%	53%	72%	95%
Pregnancy Care					
Inpatient Neonatal Mortality	-	-	-	-	-
Third or Fourth Degree Laceration	-	-	-	3.63%	3.27%

Summerlin Hospital Medical Center

657 Town Center Drive
Las Vegas, NV 89144
URL: www.summerlinhospital.org
Ownership: Proprietary
Emergency Services: Yes

Phone: 702-233-7000
Fax: 702-233-7599
Accredited: Yes
Licensed Beds: 274

Key Personnel:

CEO/Managing Director. . . . . Tim Hingtgen
Director Cardiac Care Program . . . . Nancy Donahoe, MD
CNO. . . . . Ann Benson, RN

Measure	Cases	This Hospital	State Average	U.S. Average	Top Hospital
Heart Attack Care					
ACE Inhibitor or ARB for LVSD[1,2]	23	96%	78%	82%	100%
Aspirin at Arrival[2]	220	99%	97%	92%	100%
Aspirin at Discharge[2]	182	95%	86%	90%	100%
Beta Blocker at Arrival[2]	177	94%	84%	87%	100%
Beta Blocker at Discharge[2]	167	95%	84%	90%	100%
Fibrinolytic Medication Timing[1,2]	4	25%	30%	31%	100%
PCI Within 90 Minutes of Arrival[1,2]	5	20%	25%	54%	95%
Smoking Cessation Advice[2]	66	85%	93%	88%	100%
Heart Failure Care					
ACE Inhibitor or ARB for LVSD[2]	78	83%	84%	82%	100%
Discharge Instructions[2]	187	72%	50%	61%	93%
Evaluation of LVS Function[2]	243	95%	83%	83%	99%
Smoking Cessation Advice[2]	32	81%	80%	82%	100%
Pneumonia Care					
Appropriate Initial Antibiotic[2]	124	80%	82%	83%	94%
Blood Culture Timing[2]	105	63%	81%	90%	100%
Influenza Vaccine[2]	28	100%	54%	70%	100%
Initial Antibiotic Timing[2]	142	70%	72%	80%	93%
Oxygenation Assessment[2]	194	100%	100%	99%	100%
Pneumococcal Vaccine[2]	109	71%	55%	69%	94%
Smoking Cessation Advice[2]	38	79%	75%	80%	100%
Surgical Infection Prevention					
Prophylactic Antibiotic Given[2]	304	67%	72%	77%	95%
Prophylactic Antibiotic Selection[2]	68	87%	93%	90%	100%
Prophylactic Antibiotic Stopped[2]	286	59%	53%	72%	95%
Pregnancy Care					
Inpatient Neonatal Mortality	-	-	-	-	-
Third or Fourth Degree Laceration	-	-	-	3.63%	3.27%

Sunrise Hospital & Medical Center

Alternate Name: Sunrise Hospital & Medical Center
3186 S Maryland Parkway
Las Vegas, NV 89109
URL: www.sunrisehospital.com
Ownership: Proprietary
Emergency Services: Yes

Phone: 702-731-8000
Fax: 702-731-8668
Accredited: Yes
Licensed Beds: 701

Key Personnel:

President/CEO. . . . . Bryan Robinson
Chief Medical Staff. . . . . Edwin Kingsley, MD
Chair Emergency Room. . . . . Paul Fischer, MD
Cardiology . . . . John Adan
CNO. . . . . Dee Hicks
Chair OB/GYN . . . . David Kartzinel, MD
Director Surgical Services . . . . Candy Jensen
Pulmonary . . . . Joseph M Crawley

Measure	Cases	This Hospital	State Average	U.S. Average	Top Hospital
Heart Attack Care					
ACE Inhibitor or ARB for LVSD	56	86%	78%	82%	100%
Aspirin at Arrival	271	97%	97%	92%	100%
Aspirin at Discharge	278	96%	86%	90%	100%
Beta Blocker at Arrival	171	86%	84%	87%	100%
Beta Blocker at Discharge	295	93%	84%	90%	100%
Fibrinolytic Medication Timing[1]	4	0%	30%	31%	100%
PCI Within 90 Minutes of Arrival[1]	14	21%	25%	54%	95%
Smoking Cessation Advice	153	99%	93%	88%	100%
Heart Failure Care					
ACE Inhibitor or ARB for LVSD	334	76%	84%	82%	100%
Discharge Instructions	610	36%	50%	61%	93%
Evaluation of LVS Function	710	92%	83%	83%	99%

NOTE: Hospital profiles are in alphabetical order by state, then city, then hospital within the city; Rankings are sorted by rate in descending order and exclude hospitals with less than 25 cases; (1) The number of cases is too small (n<25) for purposes of reliably predicting hospital performance; (2) Measure reflects the hospital's indication that its submission was based upon a sample of its relevant discharges; (3) Rate reflects fewer than the maximum possible quarters of data for the measure; (4) Inaccurate information submitted and suppressed for one or more quarters; (5) No data is available from the hospital for this measure; Please refer to the User's Guide for a full explanation of data

Smoking Cessation Advice	213	87%	80%	82%	100%
Pneumonia Care					
Appropriate Initial Antibiotic	403	86%	82%	83%	94%
Blood Culture Timing	331	79%	81%	90%	100%
Influenza Vaccine	118	36%	54%	70%	100%
Initial Antibiotic Timing	506	65%	72%	80%	93%
Oxygenation Assessment	655	100%	100%	99%	100%
Pneumococcal Vaccine	333	50%	55%	69%	94%
Smoking Cessation Advice	208	86%	75%	80%	100%
Surgical Infection Prevention					
Prophylactic Antibiotic Given[2,3]	319	59%	72%	77%	95%
Prophylactic Antibiotic Selection[2]	162	88%	93%	90%	100%
Prophylactic Antibiotic Stopped[2,3]	295	71%	53%	72%	95%
Pregnancy Care					
Inpatient Neonatal Mortality	-	-	-	-	-
Third or Fourth Degree Laceration	-	-	-	3.63%	3.27%

University Medical Center

1800 W Charleston Blvd
Las Vegas, NV 89102
URL: www.umc-cares.org
Ownership: Government - Local
Emergency Services: Yes

Phone: 702-383-2000
Fax: 702-383-2067
Accredited: Yes
Licensed Beds: 542

Key Personnel:

Administrator/CEO . . . . William R Hale
Chief Medical Staff . . . . John Ellerton, MD
Cardiac Lab . . . . Joyce Perich
Catheterization Lab . . . . Joyce Perich
Emergency Room . . . . Connie Clemmons-Bworn
Emergency Room . . . . Scott Rolfe
Infection Control . . . . Barbara Quattelbaum
ICU . . . . Lindaara Williams
Medical Surgical Nursing . . . . Vicki Huber
OB/GYN Womens Health . . . . Lorainne Noonan
Respiratory . . . . Gerald Daine

Measure	Cases	This Hospital	State Average	U.S. Average	Top Hospital
Heart Attack Care					
ACE Inhibitor or ARB for LVSD[2]	39	95%	78%	82%	100%
Aspirin at Arrival[2]	206	99%	97%	92%	100%
Aspirin at Discharge[2]	209	97%	86%	90%	100%
Beta Blocker at Arrival[2]	158	96%	84%	87%	100%
Beta Blocker at Discharge[2]	191	93%	84%	90%	100%
Fibrinolytic Medication Timing[1,2]	4	25%	30%	31%	100%
PCI Within 90 Minutes of Arrival[1,2]	4	0%	25%	54%	95%
Smoking Cessation Advice[2]	97	96%	93%	88%	100%
Heart Failure Care					
ACE Inhibitor or ARB for LVSD[2]	180	93%	84%	82%	100%
Discharge Instructions[2]	296	75%	50%	61%	93%
Evaluation of LVS Function[2]	326	97%	83%	83%	99%
Smoking Cessation Advice[2]	142	87%	80%	82%	100%
Pneumonia Care					
Appropriate Initial Antibiotic[2]	165	78%	82%	83%	94%
Blood Culture Timing[2]	76	66%	81%	90%	100%
Influenza Vaccine[2]	32	12%	54%	70%	100%
Initial Antibiotic Timing[2]	206	52%	72%	80%	93%
Oxygenation Assessment[2]	244	100%	100%	99%	100%
Pneumococcal Vaccine[2]	64	38%	55%	69%	94%
Smoking Cessation Advice[2]	101	86%	75%	80%	100%
Surgical Infection Prevention					
Prophylactic Antibiotic Given[2,3]	294	37%	72%	77%	95%
Prophylactic Antibiotic Selection[2]	57	91%	93%	90%	100%
Prophylactic Antibiotic Stopped[2,3]	271	75%	53%	72%	95%
Pregnancy Care					
Inpatient Neonatal Mortality	-	-	-	-	-
Third or Fourth Degree Laceration	-	-	-	3.63%	3.27%

Valley Hospital Medical Center

620 Shadow Lane
Las Vegas, NV 89106
URL: www.valleyhealthsystem.org
Ownership: Proprietary
Emergency Services: Yes

Phone: 702-388-4000
Fax: 702-388-4618
Accredited: Yes
Licensed Beds: 409

Key Personnel:

CEO . . . . Gregory E Boyer
Chief Medical Staff . . . . Paul Heeren, MD
Cardiac Laboratory . . . . Diane Rybko
Catheterization Laboratory . . . . Diane Rybko, MD
Emergency Room . . . . Jeff Davidson, MD
Emergency Room . . . . Pam Turner, RN
OB/GYN Womens Health . . . . Midge Elkins, RN
Director Respiratory Therapy . . . . Dale Redfairn

Measure	Cases	This Hospital	State Average	U.S. Average	Top Hospital
Heart Attack Care					
ACE Inhibitor or ARB for LVSD[2]	57	72%	78%	82%	100%
Aspirin at Arrival[2]	250	98%	97%	92%	100%
Aspirin at Discharge[2]	293	92%	86%	90%	100%
Beta Blocker at Arrival[2]	189	90%	84%	87%	100%
Beta Blocker at Discharge[2]	277	89%	84%	90%	100%
Fibrinolytic Medication Timing[1,2]	24	33%	30%	31%	100%
PCI Within 90 Minutes of Arrival[1,2]	5	0%	25%	54%	95%
Smoking Cessation Advice[2]	130	95%	93%	88%	100%
Heart Failure Care					
ACE Inhibitor or ARB for LVSD[2]	154	73%	84%	82%	100%
Discharge Instructions[2]	284	72%	50%	61%	93%
Evaluation of LVS Function[2]	338	92%	83%	83%	99%
Smoking Cessation Advice[2]	95	96%	80%	82%	100%
Pneumonia Care					
Appropriate Initial Antibiotic[2]	96	93%	82%	83%	94%
Blood Culture Timing[2]	104	62%	81%	90%	100%
Influenza Vaccine[1,2]	23	30%	54%	70%	100%
Initial Antibiotic Timing[2]	138	63%	72%	80%	93%
Oxygenation Assessment[2]	164	100%	100%	99%	100%
Pneumococcal Vaccine[2]	88	26%	55%	69%	94%
Smoking Cessation Advice[2]	46	93%	75%	80%	100%
Surgical Infection Prevention					
Prophylactic Antibiotic Given[2]	401	76%	72%	77%	95%
Prophylactic Antibiotic Selection[2]	94	93%	93%	90%	100%
Prophylactic Antibiotic Stopped[2]	380	41%	53%	72%	95%
Pregnancy Care					
Inpatient Neonatal Mortality	-	-	-	-	-
Third or Fourth Degree Laceration	-	-	-	3.63%	3.27%

Mesa View Regional Hospital

1299 Bertha Howe Avenue
Mesquite, NV 89027
Ownership: Proprietary
Emergency Services: Yes

Phone: 702-346-8040
Accredited: No

Measure	Cases	This Hospital	State Average	U.S. Average	Top Hospital
Heart Attack Care					
ACE Inhibitor or ARB for LVSD[5]	-	-	78%	82%	100%
Aspirin at Arrival[5]	-	-	97%	92%	100%
Aspirin at Discharge[5]	-	-	86%	90%	100%
Beta Blocker at Arrival[5]	-	-	84%	87%	100%
Beta Blocker at Discharge[5]	-	-	84%	90%	100%
Fibrinolytic Medication Timing[5]	-	-	30%	31%	100%
PCI Within 90 Minutes of Arrival[5]	-	-	25%	54%	95%
Smoking Cessation Advice[5]	-	-	93%	88%	100%
Heart Failure Care					
ACE Inhibitor or ARB for LVSD[5]	-	-	84%	82%	100%
Discharge Instructions[5]	-	-	50%	61%	93%
Evaluation of LVS Function[5]	-	-	83%	83%	99%
Smoking Cessation Advice[5]	-	-	80%	82%	100%
Pneumonia Care					
Appropriate Initial Antibiotic[5]	-	-	82%	83%	94%
Blood Culture Timing[5]	-	-	81%	90%	100%
Influenza Vaccine[5]	-	-	54%	70%	100%

NOTE: Hospital profiles are in alphabetical order by state, then city, then hospital within the city; Rankings are sorted by rate in descending order and exclude hospitals with less than 25 cases; (1) The number of cases is too small (n<25) for purposes of reliably predicting hospital performance; (2) Measure reflects the hospital's indication that its submission was based upon a sample of its relevant discharges; (3) Rate reflects fewer than the maximum possible quarters of data for the measure; (4) Inaccurate information submitted and suppressed for one or more quarters; (5) No data is available from the hospital for this measure; Please refer to the User's Guide for a full explanation of data

Measure	Cases	This Hospital	State Average	U.S. Average	Top Hospital
Initial Antibiotic Timing[5]	-	-	72%	80%	93%
Oxygenation Assessment[5]	-	-	100%	99%	100%
Pneumococcal Vaccine[5]	-	-	55%	69%	94%
Smoking Cessation Advice[5]	-	-	75%	80%	100%
Surgical Infection Prevention					
Prophylactic Antibiotic Given[5]	-	-	72%	77%	95%
Prophylactic Antibiotic Selection[5]	-	-	93%	90%	100%
Prophylactic Antibiotic Stopped[5]	-	-	53%	72%	95%
Pregnancy Care					
Inpatient Neonatal Mortality	-	-	-	-	-
Third or Fourth Degree Laceration	-	-	-	3.63%	3.27%

North Vista Hospital

1409 East Lake Mead Boulevard — Phone: 702-649-7711
North Las Vegas, NV 89030 — Fax: 702-657-5605
URL: www.northvistahospital.com
Ownership: Proprietary — Accredited: Yes
Emergency Services: Yes — Licensed Beds: 198
Key Personnel:
CEO. . . . . Tony Marinello

Measure	Cases	This Hospital	State Average	U.S. Average	Top Hospital
Heart Attack Care					
ACE Inhibitor or ARB for LVSD[1]	8	75%	78%	82%	100%
Aspirin at Arrival	89	96%	97%	92%	100%
Aspirin at Discharge	36	78%	86%	90%	100%
Beta Blocker at Arrival	73	89%	84%	87%	100%
Beta Blocker at Discharge	34	68%	84%	90%	100%
Fibrinolytic Medication Timing[1]	21	19%	30%	31%	100%
PCI Within 90 Minutes of Arrival	0	-	25%	54%	95%
Smoking Cessation Advice[1]	10	90%	93%	88%	100%
Heart Failure Care					
ACE Inhibitor or ARB for LVSD	99	67%	84%	82%	100%
Discharge Instructions	244	63%	50%	61%	93%
Evaluation of LVS Function	306	87%	83%	83%	99%
Smoking Cessation Advice	105	99%	80%	82%	100%
Pneumonia Care					
Appropriate Initial Antibiotic	172	87%	82%	83%	94%
Blood Culture Timing	151	90%	81%	90%	100%
Influenza Vaccine	41	24%	54%	70%	100%
Initial Antibiotic Timing	209	66%	72%	80%	93%
Oxygenation Assessment	252	100%	100%	99%	100%
Pneumococcal Vaccine	95	18%	55%	69%	94%
Smoking Cessation Advice	100	91%	75%	80%	100%
Surgical Infection Prevention					
Prophylactic Antibiotic Given	216	77%	72%	77%	95%
Prophylactic Antibiotic Selection	46	96%	93%	90%	100%
Prophylactic Antibiotic Stopped	201	36%	53%	72%	95%
Pregnancy Care					
Inpatient Neonatal Mortality	-	-	-	-	-
Third or Fourth Degree Laceration	-	-	-	3.63%	3.27%

Renown Regional Medical Center

1155 Mill Street — Phone: 775-982-4100
Reno, NV 89502
Ownership: Voluntary non-profit - Other — Accredited: Yes
Emergency Services: Yes

Measure	Cases	This Hospital	State Average	U.S. Average	Top Hospital
Heart Attack Care					
ACE Inhibitor or ARB for LVSD	84	88%	78%	82%	100%
Aspirin at Arrival	173	97%	97%	92%	100%
Aspirin at Discharge	362	97%	86%	90%	100%
Beta Blocker at Arrival	144	99%	84%	87%	100%
Beta Blocker at Discharge	338	99%	84%	90%	100%
Fibrinolytic Medication Timing[1]	2	50%	30%	31%	100%
PCI Within 90 Minutes of Arrival[1]	15	53%	25%	54%	95%
Smoking Cessation Advice	162	85%	93%	88%	100%
Heart Failure Care					
ACE Inhibitor or ARB for LVSD	157	87%	84%	82%	100%
Discharge Instructions	315	37%	50%	61%	93%
Evaluation of LVS Function	354	95%	83%	83%	99%
Smoking Cessation Advice	107	77%	80%	82%	100%
Pneumonia Care					
Appropriate Initial Antibiotic	161	82%	82%	83%	94%
Blood Culture Timing	127	84%	81%	90%	100%
Influenza Vaccine[4,5]	-	-	54%	70%	100%
Initial Antibiotic Timing	204	81%	72%	80%	93%
Oxygenation Assessment	242	100%	100%	99%	100%
Pneumococcal Vaccine	120	78%	55%	69%	94%
Smoking Cessation Advice	76	78%	75%	80%	100%
Surgical Infection Prevention					
Prophylactic Antibiotic Given[3]	494	71%	72%	77%	95%
Prophylactic Antibiotic Selection	169	90%	93%	90%	100%
Prophylactic Antibiotic Stopped[3]	481	56%	53%	72%	95%
Pregnancy Care					
Inpatient Neonatal Mortality[2]	992	0.81%	-	-	-
Third or Fourth Degree Laceration[2]	712	3.79%	-	3.63%	3.27%

Renown South Meadows Medical Center

10101 Double R Blvd — Phone: 775-982-7000
Reno, NV 89521
Ownership: Voluntary non-profit - Private — Accredited: No
Emergency Services: Yes

Measure	Cases	This Hospital	State Average	U.S. Average	Top Hospital
Heart Attack Care					
ACE Inhibitor or ARB for LVSD[3]	0	-	78%	82%	100%
Aspirin at Arrival[1,3]	3	100%	97%	92%	100%
Aspirin at Discharge[1,3]	4	100%	86%	90%	100%
Beta Blocker at Arrival[1,3]	2	100%	84%	87%	100%
Beta Blocker at Discharge[1,3]	3	100%	84%	90%	100%
Fibrinolytic Medication Timing[1,3]	2	50%	30%	31%	100%
PCI Within 90 Minutes of Arrival	0	-	25%	54%	95%
Smoking Cessation Advice[1,3]	1	100%	93%	88%	100%
Heart Failure Care					
ACE Inhibitor or ARB for LVSD[1]	16	88%	84%	82%	100%
Discharge Instructions	45	44%	50%	61%	93%
Evaluation of LVS Function	56	95%	83%	83%	99%
Smoking Cessation Advice[1]	11	91%	80%	82%	100%
Pneumonia Care					
Appropriate Initial Antibiotic	68	91%	82%	83%	94%
Blood Culture Timing	52	98%	81%	90%	100%
Influenza Vaccine[1]	18	89%	54%	70%	100%
Initial Antibiotic Timing	67	87%	72%	80%	93%
Oxygenation Assessment	86	100%	100%	99%	100%
Pneumococcal Vaccine	51	86%	55%	69%	94%
Smoking Cessation Advice[1]	24	79%	75%	80%	100%
Surgical Infection Prevention					
Prophylactic Antibiotic Given	70	81%	72%	77%	95%
Prophylactic Antibiotic Selection	32	94%	93%	90%	100%
Prophylactic Antibiotic Stopped	68	32%	53%	72%	95%
Pregnancy Care					
Inpatient Neonatal Mortality	-	-	-	-	-
Third or Fourth Degree Laceration	-	-	-	3.63%	3.27%

Saint Mary's Regional Medical Center

235 West Sixth Street — Phone: 775-770-7100
Reno, NV 89503 — Fax: 775-770-3963
URL: www.saintmarysreno.com
Ownership: Voluntary non-profit - Private — Accredited: Yes
Emergency Services: No — Licensed Beds: 380
Key Personnel:
President/CEO. . . . . Jeff K Bills
Senior VP. . . . . Peter H Braunstein, MD
Manager Surgery . . . . Kit Landis, RN
Manager Emergency Room . . . . Ann Roberts, RN
Emergency Room . . . . Ann Roberts, RN
Coordinator Infection Control . . . . Cyndie Kern, RN
Director Maternal/Child Health Services. . . . . . . Terri Mishl, RN
Director Respiratory Care. . . . . Greg Ronaldson

Measure	Cases	This Hospital	State Average	U.S. Average	Top Hospital

NOTE: Hospital profiles are in alphabetical order by state, then city, then hospital within the city; Rankings are sorted by rate in descending order and exclude hospitals with less than 25 cases; (1) The number of cases is too small (n<25) for purposes of reliably predicting hospital performance; (2) Measure reflects the hospital's indication that its submission was based upon a sample of its relevant discharges; (3) Rate reflects fewer than the maximum possible quarters of data for the measure; (4) Inaccurate information submitted and suppressed for one or more quarters; (5) No data is available from the hospital for this measure; Please refer to the User's Guide for a full explanation of data

Heart Attack Care					
ACE Inhibitor or ARB for LVSD	47	87%	78%	82%	100%
Aspirin at Arrival	210	100%	97%	92%	100%
Aspirin at Discharge	291	97%	86%	90%	100%
Beta Blocker at Arrival	186	98%	84%	87%	100%
Beta Blocker at Discharge	307	98%	84%	90%	100%
Fibrinolytic Medication Timing[1]	1	0%	30%	31%	100%
PCI Within 90 Minutes of Arrival[1]	14	29%	25%	54%	95%
Smoking Cessation Advice	118	90%	93%	88%	100%
Heart Failure Care					
ACE Inhibitor or ARB for LVSD	105	90%	84%	82%	100%
Discharge Instructions	239	31%	50%	61%	93%
Evaluation of LVS Function	282	97%	83%	83%	99%
Smoking Cessation Advice	50	96%	80%	82%	100%
Pneumonia Care					
Appropriate Initial Antibiotic[2]	87	91%	82%	83%	94%
Blood Culture Timing[2]	101	72%	81%	90%	100%
Influenza Vaccine[1,2]	22	50%	54%	70%	100%
Initial Antibiotic Timing[2]	131	80%	72%	80%	93%
Oxygenation Assessment[2]	165	100%	100%	99%	100%
Pneumococcal Vaccine[2]	101	65%	55%	69%	94%
Smoking Cessation Advice[2]	48	81%	75%	80%	100%
Surgical Infection Prevention					
Prophylactic Antibiotic Given[2]	350	85%	72%	77%	95%
Prophylactic Antibiotic Selection[2]	82	98%	93%	90%	100%
Prophylactic Antibiotic Stopped[2]	326	72%	53%	72%	95%
Pregnancy Care					
Inpatient Neonatal Mortality	-	-	-	-	-
Third or Fourth Degree Laceration	-	-	-	3.63%	3.27%

Northern Nevada Medical Center

2375 E Prater Way
Sparks, NV 89434
Phone: 775-331-7000
Fax: 775-356-4901
URL: www.northernnvmed.com
Ownership: Proprietary
Accredited: Yes
Emergency Services: Yes
Licensed Beds: 100

Key Personnel:

CEO. . . . . Brandt Wright

Measure	Cases	This Hospital	State Average	U.S. Average	Top Hospital
Heart Attack Care					
ACE Inhibitor or ARB for LVSD[1]	3	67%	78%	82%	100%
Aspirin at Arrival	38	92%	97%	92%	100%
Aspirin at Discharge[1]	20	55%	86%	90%	100%
Beta Blocker at Arrival	38	61%	84%	87%	100%
Beta Blocker at Discharge[1]	21	52%	84%	90%	100%
Fibrinolytic Medication Timing[1]	1	0%	30%	31%	100%
PCI Within 90 Minutes of Arrival	0	-	25%	54%	95%
Smoking Cessation Advice[1]	5	100%	93%	88%	100%
Heart Failure Care					
ACE Inhibitor or ARB for LVSD	52	75%	84%	82%	100%
Discharge Instructions	93	33%	50%	61%	93%
Evaluation of LVS Function	122	88%	83%	83%	99%
Smoking Cessation Advice	34	76%	80%	82%	100%
Pneumonia Care					
Appropriate Initial Antibiotic	76	74%	82%	83%	94%
Blood Culture Timing	57	86%	81%	90%	100%
Influenza Vaccine[1]	12	67%	54%	70%	100%
Initial Antibiotic Timing	81	84%	72%	80%	93%
Oxygenation Assessment	96	100%	100%	99%	100%
Pneumococcal Vaccine	58	60%	55%	69%	94%
Smoking Cessation Advice	34	88%	75%	80%	100%
Surgical Infection Prevention					
Prophylactic Antibiotic Given	212	92%	72%	77%	95%
Prophylactic Antibiotic Selection	39	97%	93%	90%	100%
Prophylactic Antibiotic Stopped	208	26%	53%	72%	95%
Pregnancy Care					
Inpatient Neonatal Mortality	-	-	-	-	-
Third or Fourth Degree Laceration	-	-	-	3.63%	3.27%

Nye Regional Medical Center

825 S Main Street
Tonopah, NV 89049
Phone: 775-482-6233
Fax: 775-482-8272
URL: www.nyeregional.org
Ownership: Proprietary
Accredited: No
Emergency Services: Yes
Licensed Beds: 44

Key Personnel:

CEO. . . . . Rick Kilburn
Chief Medical Staff. . . . . Vincent Scoccia
Emergency Room . . . . Pat Steffens
Infection Control. . . . . Jessica Thompson
Respiratory . . . . Heather Zimmerman

Measure	Cases	This Hospital	State Average	U.S. Average	Top Hospital
Heart Attack Care					
ACE Inhibitor or ARB for LVSD[1,3]	1	0%	78%	82%	100%
Aspirin at Arrival[1,3]	1	100%	97%	92%	100%
Aspirin at Discharge[1,3]	1	100%	86%	90%	100%
Beta Blocker at Arrival[1,3]	1	100%	84%	87%	100%
Beta Blocker at Discharge[1,3]	1	100%	84%	90%	100%
Fibrinolytic Medication Timing[1,3]	1	0%	30%	31%	100%
PCI Within 90 Minutes of Arrival[5]	-	-	25%	54%	95%
Smoking Cessation Advice[1,3]	1	100%	93%	88%	100%
Heart Failure Care					
ACE Inhibitor or ARB for LVSD[3]	0	-	84%	82%	100%
Discharge Instructions[1,3]	24	17%	50%	61%	93%
Evaluation of LVS Function[1,3]	15	67%	83%	83%	99%
Smoking Cessation Advice[1,3]	8	88%	80%	82%	100%
Pneumonia Care					
Appropriate Initial Antibiotic[1,2]	23	22%	82%	83%	94%
Blood Culture Timing[1,2]	3	33%	81%	90%	100%
Influenza Vaccine[1]	2	50%	54%	70%	100%
Initial Antibiotic Timing[1,2]	23	70%	72%	80%	93%
Oxygenation Assessment[1,2]	24	100%	100%	99%	100%
Pneumococcal Vaccine[1,2]	13	31%	55%	69%	94%
Smoking Cessation Advice[1,2]	10	100%	75%	80%	100%
Surgical Infection Prevention					
Prophylactic Antibiotic Given[5]	-	-	72%	77%	95%
Prophylactic Antibiotic Selection[5]	-	-	93%	90%	100%
Prophylactic Antibiotic Stopped[5]	-	-	53%	72%	95%
Pregnancy Care					
Inpatient Neonatal Mortality	-	-	-	-	-
Third or Fourth Degree Laceration	-	-	-	3.63%	3.27%

Humboldt General Hospital

Alternate Name: Harmony Manor
118 E Haskell Street
Winnemucca, NV 89445
Phone: 775-623-5222
Fax: 775-623-5904
URL: www.hghospital.ws
Ownership: Govt - Hospital District or Authority
Accredited: No
Emergency Services: Yes
Licensed Beds: 22

Key Personnel:

President/CEO. . . . . James G Parrish
Chief Medical Staff. . . . . Richard Ingle
ER Unit Coordinator. . . . . Rita Clement, RN
Director Infection/Disease Control . . . . Robin Gillis, RN
Director Respiratory Therapy . . . . Arnie Prissing

Measure	Cases	This Hospital	State Average	U.S. Average	Top Hospital
Heart Attack Care					
ACE Inhibitor or ARB for LVSD[2,3]	0	-	78%	82%	100%
Aspirin at Arrival[1,2,3]	2	100%	97%	92%	100%
Aspirin at Discharge[1,2,3]	2	100%	86%	90%	100%
Beta Blocker at Arrival[1,2,3]	2	100%	84%	87%	100%
Beta Blocker at Discharge[1,2,3]	2	100%	84%	90%	100%
Fibrinolytic Medication Timing[2,3]	0	-	30%	31%	100%
PCI Within 90 Minutes of Arrival[5]	-	-	25%	54%	95%
Smoking Cessation Advice[2,3]	0	-	93%	88%	100%
Heart Failure Care					
ACE Inhibitor or ARB for LVSD[2,3]	0	-	84%	82%	100%
Discharge Instructions[1,2,3]	2	0%	50%	61%	93%
Evaluation of LVS Function[1,2,3]	2	50%	83%	83%	99%
Smoking Cessation Advice[1,2,3]	2	100%	80%	82%	100%

NOTE: Hospital profiles are in alphabetical order by state, then city, then hospital within the city; Rankings are sorted by rate in descending order and exclude hospitals with less than 25 cases; (1) The number of cases is too small (n<25) for purposes of reliably predicting hospital performance; (2) Measure reflects the hospital's indication that its submission was based upon a sample of its relevant discharges; (3) Rate reflects fewer than the maximum possible quarters of data for the measure; (4) Inaccurate information submitted and suppressed for one or more quarters; (5) No data is available from the hospital for this measure; Please refer to the User's Guide for a full explanation of data

Pneumonia Care					
Appropriate Initial Antibiotic[1,2]	20	75%	82%	83%	94%
Blood Culture Timing[1,2]	7	100%	81%	90%	100%
Influenza Vaccine[1,2]	2	50%	54%	70%	100%
Initial Antibiotic Timing[1,2]	22	77%	72%	80%	93%
Oxygenation Assessment[2]	26	100%	100%	99%	100%
Pneumococcal Vaccine[1,2]	17	65%	55%	69%	94%
Smoking Cessation Advice[1,2]	12	25%	75%	80%	100%
Surgical Infection Prevention					
Prophylactic Antibiotic Given[5]	-	-	72%	77%	95%
Prophylactic Antibiotic Selection[5]	-	-	93%	90%	100%
Prophylactic Antibiotic Stopped[5]	-	-	53%	72%	95%
Pregnancy Care					
Inpatient Neonatal Mortality	-	-	-	-	-
Third or Fourth Degree Laceration	-	-	-	3.63%	3.27%

South Lyon Medical Center

213 S Whitacre
Yerington, NV 89447
Ownership: Voluntary non-profit - Private
Emergency Services: Yes

Phone: 775-463-2301
Fax: 775-463-7864
Accredited: No
Licensed Beds: 63

Key Personnel:

CEO. . . . . John Hall
Chief Medical Staff. . . . . Charlie Hicks
Director Infection/Disease Control . . . . John Malek
Chief Radiology . . . . Rose Brown
Director Respiratory Therapy . . . . Ron Siler

Measure	Cases	This Hospital	State Average	U.S. Average	Top Hospital
Heart Attack Care					
ACE Inhibitor or ARB for LVSD[3]	0	-	78%	82%	100%
Aspirin at Arrival[1,3]	1	100%	97%	92%	100%
Aspirin at Discharge[1,3]	1	0%	86%	90%	100%
Beta Blocker at Arrival[1,3]	1	0%	84%	87%	100%
Beta Blocker at Discharge[1,3]	1	0%	84%	90%	100%
Fibrinolytic Medication Timing[5]	-	-	30%	31%	100%
PCI Within 90 Minutes of Arrival[5]	-	-	25%	54%	95%
Smoking Cessation Advice[5]	-	-	93%	88%	100%
Heart Failure Care					
ACE Inhibitor or ARB for LVSD[1]	1	100%	84%	82%	100%
Discharge Instructions[3]	0	-	50%	61%	93%
Evaluation of LVS Function[1]	13	46%	83%	83%	99%
Smoking Cessation Advice[3]	0	-	80%	82%	100%
Pneumonia Care					
Appropriate Initial Antibiotic[1,3]	3	67%	82%	83%	94%
Blood Culture Timing[1,3]	1	100%	81%	90%	100%
Influenza Vaccine[5]	-	-	54%	70%	100%
Initial Antibiotic Timing	25	84%	72%	80%	93%
Oxygenation Assessment	28	100%	100%	99%	100%
Pneumococcal Vaccine[1]	20	15%	55%	69%	94%
Smoking Cessation Advice[1,3]	1	100%	75%	80%	100%
Surgical Infection Prevention					
Prophylactic Antibiotic Given[5]	-	-	72%	77%	95%
Prophylactic Antibiotic Selection[5]	-	-	93%	90%	100%
Prophylactic Antibiotic Stopped[5]	-	-	53%	72%	95%
Pregnancy Care					
Inpatient Neonatal Mortality	-	-	-	-	-
Third or Fourth Degree Laceration	-	-	-	3.63%	3.27%

NOTE: Hospital profiles are in alphabetical order by state, then city, then hospital within the city; Rankings are sorted by rate in descending order and exclude hospitals with less than 25 cases; (1) The number of cases is too small (n<25) for purposes of reliably predicting hospital performance; (2) Measure reflects the hospital's indication that its submission was based upon a sample of its relevant discharges; (3) Rate reflects fewer than the maximum possible quarters of data for the measure; (4) Inaccurate information submitted and suppressed for one or more quarters; (5) No data is available from the hospital for this measure; Please refer to the User's Guide for a full explanation of data

Heart Attack Care

1. ACE Inhibitor or ARB for LVSD

Hospital Name	City	Rate	Cases
Saint Vincent Regional Medical Center	Santa Fe	100%	27
Lovelace Health Systems	Albuquerque	94%	53
Heart Hospital of New Mexico	Albuquerque	91%	192
Presbyterian Hospital	Albuquerque	72%	50
University of New Mexico Hospital	Albuquerque	71%	28
Mountain View Regional Medical Center	Las Cruces	65%	54
Memorial Medical Center	Las Cruces	58%	48

2. Aspirin at Arrival

Hospital Name	City	Rate	Cases
Heart Hospital of New Mexico	Albuquerque	99%	158
Lovelace Health Systems	Albuquerque	99%	201
Presbyterian Hospital	Albuquerque	99%	219
San Juan Regional Medical Center	Farmington	99%	85
Eastern New Mexico Medical Center	Roswell	98%	62
Carlsbad Medical Center	Carlsbad	97%	78
Saint Vincent Regional Medical Center	Santa Fe	97%	120
Spring Valley Hospital	Las Vegas	96%	183
University of New Mexico Hospital	Albuquerque	96%	135
Memorial Medical Center	Las Cruces	91%	70
Mountain View Regional Medical Center	Las Cruces	91%	85
Plains Regional Medical Center	Clovis	75%	28

3. Aspirin at Discharge

Hospital Name	City	Rate	Cases
Heart Hospital of New Mexico	Albuquerque	99%	644
Carlsbad Medical Center	Carlsbad	98%	60
Presbyterian Hospital	Albuquerque	98%	285
Lovelace Health Systems	Albuquerque	97%	250
Memorial Medical Center	Las Cruces	97%	137
University of New Mexico Hospital	Albuquerque	97%	146
Mountain View Regional Medical Center	Las Cruces	95%	145
Eastern New Mexico Medical Center	Roswell	94%	36
Saint Vincent Regional Medical Center	Santa Fe	93%	170
San Juan Regional Medical Center	Farmington	91%	45
Spring Valley Hospital	Las Vegas	91%	80
Plains Regional Medical Center	Clovis	43%	30

4. Beta Blocker at Arrival

Hospital Name	City	Rate	Cases
Heart Hospital of New Mexico	Albuquerque	99%	152
San Juan Regional Medical Center	Farmington	97%	70
Carlsbad Medical Center	Carlsbad	96%	70
University of New Mexico Hospital	Albuquerque	95%	128
Presbyterian Hospital	Albuquerque	94%	176
Saint Vincent Regional Medical Center	Santa Fe	94%	97
Lovelace Health Systems	Albuquerque	93%	182
Eastern New Mexico Medical Center	Roswell	89%	54
Spring Valley Hospital	Las Vegas	86%	134
Mountain View Regional Medical Center	Las Cruces	85%	62
Memorial Medical Center	Las Cruces	70%	63
Plains Regional Medical Center	Clovis	63%	27

5. Beta Blocker at Discharge

Hospital Name	City	Rate	Cases
Carlsbad Medical Center	Carlsbad	100%	61
Heart Hospital of New Mexico	Albuquerque	98%	646
Presbyterian Hospital	Albuquerque	97%	290
University of New Mexico Hospital	Albuquerque	97%	143
Saint Vincent Regional Medical Center	Santa Fe	96%	168
San Juan Regional Medical Center	Farmington	95%	44
Eastern New Mexico Medical Center	Roswell	93%	29
Lovelace Health Systems	Albuquerque	92%	250
Memorial Medical Center	Las Cruces	92%	167
Mountain View Regional Medical Center	Las Cruces	91%	159
Spring Valley Hospital	Las Vegas	81%	80
Plains Regional Medical Center	Clovis	42%	31

8. Smoking Cessation Advice

Hospital Name	City	Rate	Cases
Carlsbad Medical Center	Carlsbad	100%	26
Presbyterian Hospital	Albuquerque	98%	112
Spring Valley Hospital	Las Vegas	98%	40
Mountain View Regional Medical Center	Las Cruces	97%	63
University of New Mexico Hospital	Albuquerque	93%	69
Lovelace Health Systems	Albuquerque	90%	60
Saint Vincent Regional Medical Center	Santa Fe	90%	63
Heart Hospital of New Mexico	Albuquerque	86%	256
Memorial Medical Center	Las Cruces	79%	67

Heart Failure Care

9. ACE Inhibitor or ARB for LVSD

Hospital Name	City	Rate	Cases
San Juan Regional Medical Center	Farmington	97%	98
Carlsbad Medical Center	Carlsbad	93%	28
Lovelace Health Systems	Albuquerque	93%	122
Spring Valley Hospital	Las Vegas	92%	77
Saint Vincent Regional Medical Center	Santa Fe	91%	69
Eastern New Mexico Medical Center	Roswell	89%	47
University of New Mexico Hospital	Albuquerque	86%	96
Heart Hospital of New Mexico	Albuquerque	84%	154
Mountain View Regional Medical Center	Las Cruces	79%	73
Alta Vista Regional Hospital	Las Vegas	76%	25
Presbyterian Hospital	Albuquerque	76%	132
Memorial Medical Center	Las Cruces	73%	102
Gerald Champion Memorial Hospital	Alamogordo	71%	45
Plains Regional Medical Center	Clovis	66%	92

10. Discharge Instructions

Hospital Name	City	Rate	Cases
Spring Valley Hospital	Las Vegas	99%	183
Lovelace Health Systems	Albuquerque	89%	249
Carlsbad Medical Center	Carlsbad	77%	56
Espanola Hospital	Espanola	74%	50
Heart Hospital of New Mexico	Albuquerque	65%	254
Gerald Champion Memorial Hospital	Alamogordo	63%	153
Lea Regional Medical Center	Hobbs	59%	29
Plains Regional Medical Center	Clovis	58%	109
San Juan Regional Medical Center	Farmington	52%	165
Mountain View Regional Medical Center	Las Cruces	50%	141
Presbyterian Hospital	Albuquerque	48%	248
Eastern New Mexico Medical Center	Roswell	41%	155
Rehoboth McKinley Christian Health Care Svcs	Gallup	27%	66
Lovelace Westside Hospital	Albuquerque	22%	45
Holy Cross Hospital	Taos	18%	39
Gila Regional Medical Center	Silver City	16%	95
University of New Mexico Hospital	Albuquerque	15%	163
Loveless Medical Center-Downtown	Albuquerque	14%	36
Gallup Indian Medical Center	Gallup	11%	37
Memorial Medical Center	Las Cruces	10%	209
Roosevelt General Hospital	Portales	10%	48
Saint Vincent Regional Medical Center	Santa Fe	5%	152
Alta Vista Regional Hospital	Las Vegas	2%	63
Lincoln County Medical Center	Ruidoso	0%	37
Mimbres Memorial Hospital	Deming	0%	67

11. Evaluation of LVS Function

Hospital Name	City	Rate	Cases
Lovelace Health Systems	Albuquerque	99%	279
University of New Mexico Hospital	Albuquerque	99%	182
Gallup Indian Medical Center	Gallup	98%	40
Heart Hospital of New Mexico	Albuquerque	98%	277
Spring Valley Hospital	Las Vegas	98%	234
San Juan Regional Medical Center	Farmington	96%	198
Saint Vincent Regional Medical Center	Santa Fe	95%	169
Presbyterian Hospital	Albuquerque	94%	292
Carlsbad Medical Center	Carlsbad	93%	69
Lovelace Westside Hospital	Albuquerque	92%	51
Mountain View Regional Medical Center	Las Cruces	91%	163
Holy Cross Hospital	Taos	90%	49
Loveless Medical Center-Downtown	Albuquerque	89%	45
Lea Regional Medical Center	Hobbs	88%	49
Eastern New Mexico Medical Center	Roswell	86%	173
Presbyterian Kaseman Hospital	Albuquerque	84%	31
Memorial Medical Center	Las Cruces	81%	239
Alta Vista Regional Hospital	Las Vegas	77%	75
Plains Regional Medical Center	Clovis	75%	128
Espanola Hospital	Espanola	74%	54
Gerald Champion Memorial Hospital	Alamogordo	61%	179
Northern Navajo Medical Center	Shiprock	60%	42
Gila Regional Medical Center	Silver City	50%	117
Socorro General Hospital	Socorro	48%	31
Miners' Colfax Medical Center	Raton	47%	30
Rehoboth McKinley Christian Health Care Svcs	Gallup	40%	73
Mimbres Memorial Hospital	Deming	32%	80
Roosevelt General Hospital	Portales	25%	60
Lincoln County Medical Center	Ruidoso	5%	44

NOTE: Hospital profiles are in alphabetical order by state, then city, then hospital within the city; Rankings are sorted by rate in descending order and exclude hospitals with less than 25 cases; (1) The number of cases is too small (n<25) for purposes of reliably predicting hospital performance; (2) Measure reflects the hospital's indication that its submission was based upon a sample of its relevant discharges; (3) Rate reflects fewer than the maximum possible quarters of data for the measure; (4) Inaccurate information submitted and suppressed for one or more quarters; (5) No data is available from the hospital for this measure; Please refer to the User's Guide for a full explanation of data

12. Smoking Cessation Advice

Hospital Name	City	Rate	Cases
Spring Valley Hospital	Las Vegas	99%	69
Presbyterian Hospital	Albuquerque	93%	54
Eastern New Mexico Medical Center	Roswell	85%	33
Heart Hospital of New Mexico	Albuquerque	81%	31
University of New Mexico Hospital	Albuquerque	81%	58
Lovelace Health Systems	Albuquerque	68%	37
Gerald Champion Memorial Hospital	Alamogordo	67%	36
Memorial Medical Center	Las Cruces	59%	32
Plains Regional Medical Center	Clovis	34%	29

Pneumonia Care

13. Appropriate Initial Antibiotic

Hospital Name	City	Rate	Cases
Presbyterian Kaseman Hospital	Albuquerque	95%	42
Carlsbad Medical Center	Carlsbad	93%	100
Gila Regional Medical Center	Silver City	93%	103
Mimbres Memorial Hospital	Deming	93%	81
Presbyterian Hospital	Albuquerque	93%	55
Lea Regional Medical Center	Hobbs	90%	84
Spring Valley Hospital	Las Vegas	90%	125
Plains Regional Medical Center	Clovis	89%	101
Cibola General Hospital	Grants	88%	40
Lovelace Health Systems	Albuquerque	87%	252
Mountain View Regional Medical Center	Las Cruces	87%	127
San Juan Regional Medical Center	Farmington	87%	157
Gallup Indian Medical Center	Gallup	85%	97
Gerald Champion Memorial Hospital	Alamogordo	85%	96
Nor-Lea General Hospital	Lovington	85%	27
Holy Cross Hospital	Taos	84%	88
Saint Joseph's North East Heights Hospital	Albuquerque	84%	105
Los Alamos Medical Center	Los Alamos	83%	47
Saint Vincent Regional Medical Center	Santa Fe	83%	160
Memorial Medical Center	Las Cruces	82%	261
Lovelace Westside Hospital	Albuquerque	81%	108
Espanola Hospital	Espanola	80%	87
Loveless Medical Center-Downtown	Albuquerque	80%	121
Rehoboth McKinley Christian Health Care Svcs	Gallup	80%	108
University of New Mexico Hospital	Albuquerque	80%	121
Artesia General Hospital	Artesia	79%	48
Roosevelt General Hospital	Portales	79%	84
Socorro General Hospital	Socorro	79%	42
Alta Vista Regional Hospital	Las Vegas	77%	87
Doctor Dan C Trigg Memorial Hospital	Tucumcari	77%	26
Eastern New Mexico Medical Center	Roswell	76%	181
Lincoln County Medical Center	Ruidoso	74%	39

14. Blood Culture Timing

Hospital Name	City	Rate	Cases
Cibola General Hospital	Grants	100%	30
Plains Regional Medical Center	Clovis	98%	63
Eastern New Mexico Medical Center	Roswell	97%	127
Gila Regional Medical Center	Silver City	96%	74
Lovelace Health Systems	Albuquerque	96%	185
Mimbres Memorial Hospital	Deming	96%	26
Carlsbad Medical Center	Carlsbad	95%	107
Mountain View Regional Medical Center	Las Cruces	95%	126
Gallup Indian Medical Center	Gallup	93%	59
Loveless Medical Center-Downtown	Albuquerque	93%	110
Presbyterian Kaseman Hospital	Albuquerque	92%	66
Roosevelt General Hospital	Portales	92%	40
Lea Regional Medical Center	Hobbs	91%	75
Memorial Medical Center	Las Cruces	91%	193
Presbyterian Hospital	Albuquerque	90%	90
Lovelace Westside Hospital	Albuquerque	88%	68
Saint Joseph's North East Heights Hospital	Albuquerque	87%	71
San Juan Regional Medical Center	Farmington	87%	156
Espanola Hospital	Espanola	85%	62
Los Alamos Medical Center	Los Alamos	84%	32
Rehoboth McKinley Christian Health Care Svcs	Gallup	82%	80
University of New Mexico Hospital	Albuquerque	82%	115
Holy Cross Hospital	Taos	81%	91
Spring Valley Hospital	Las Vegas	80%	70
Alta Vista Regional Hospital	Las Vegas	79%	72
Gerald Champion Memorial Hospital	Alamogordo	74%	47
Saint Vincent Regional Medical Center	Santa Fe	73%	130

15. Influenza Vaccine

Hospital Name	City	Rate	Cases
Eastern New Mexico Medical Center	Roswell	94%	69
Carlsbad Medical Center	Carlsbad	88%	52
Mountain View Regional Medical Center	Las Cruces	81%	42
Lovelace Westside Hospital	Albuquerque	77%	26
Saint Joseph's North East Heights Hospital	Albuquerque	75%	28
San Juan Regional Medical Center	Farmington	66%	76
Plains Regional Medical Center	Clovis	60%	30
Memorial Medical Center	Las Cruces	57%	69
Presbyterian Hospital	Albuquerque	56%	25
University of New Mexico Hospital	Albuquerque	50%	26
Rehoboth McKinley Christian Health Care Svcs	Gallup	48%	33
Loveless Medical Center-Downtown	Albuquerque	46%	41
Gerald Champion Memorial Hospital	Alamogordo	45%	51

16. Initial Antibiotic Timing

Hospital Name	City	Rate	Cases
Espanola Hospital	Espanola	92%	100
Gila Regional Medical Center	Silver City	91%	141
Carlsbad Medical Center	Carlsbad	88%	137
Lincoln County Medical Center	Ruidoso	82%	40
Rehoboth McKinley Christian Health Care Svcs	Gallup	82%	125
San Juan Regional Medical Center	Farmington	82%	261
Holy Cross Hospital	Taos	81%	134
US Public Health Service Indian Hospital	Crownpoint	81%	43
Plains Regional Medical Center	Clovis	80%	138
Roosevelt General Hospital	Portales	80%	100
Los Alamos Medical Center	Los Alamos	79%	58
Northern Navajo Medical Center	Shiprock	78%	95
Sierra Vista Hospital	Truth or Conseq.	77%	39
ACL-IHS Hospital	San Fidel	76%	49
Miners' Colfax Medical Center	Raton	76%	49
Socorro General Hospital	Socorro	76%	41
Mimbres Memorial Hospital	Deming	75%	100
Presbyterian Kaseman Hospital	Albuquerque	75%	91
Saint Joseph's North East Heights Hospital	Albuquerque	75%	109
Spring Valley Hospital	Las Vegas	75%	139
Presbyterian Hospital	Albuquerque	74%	129
Saint Vincent Regional Medical Center	Santa Fe	74%	184
Alta Vista Regional Hospital	Las Vegas	73%	122
Gallup Indian Medical Center	Gallup	73%	112
Lea Regional Medical Center	Hobbs	73%	104
Doctor Dan C Trigg Memorial Hospital	Tucumcari	72%	36
Gerald Champion Memorial Hospital	Alamogordo	72%	162
Loveless Medical Center-Downtown	Albuquerque	71%	141
Lovelace Health Systems	Albuquerque	70%	284
Lovelace Westside Hospital	Albuquerque	70%	107
Mountain View Regional Medical Center	Las Cruces	70%	152
Eastern New Mexico Medical Center	Roswell	66%	271
Cibola General Hospital	Grants	61%	36
Nor-Lea General Hospital	Lovington	61%	31
Artesia General Hospital	Artesia	60%	52
Memorial Medical Center	Las Cruces	57%	337
University of New Mexico Hospital	Albuquerque	37%	161

17. Oxygenation Assessment

Hospital Name	City	Rate	Cases
Alta Vista Regional Hospital	Las Vegas	100%	136
Carlsbad Medical Center	Carlsbad	100%	168
Cibola General Hospital	Grants	100%	45
Doctor Dan C Trigg Memorial Hospital	Tucumcari	100%	40
Eastern New Mexico Medical Center	Roswell	100%	298
Espanola Hospital	Espanola	100%	111
Gerald Champion Memorial Hospital	Alamogordo	100%	197
Gila Regional Medical Center	Silver City	100%	144
Holy Cross Hospital	Taos	100%	163
Lea Regional Medical Center	Hobbs	100%	116
Lincoln County Medical Center	Ruidoso	100%	44
Los Alamos Medical Center	Los Alamos	100%	63
Lovelace Health Systems	Albuquerque	100%	349
Lovelace Westside Hospital	Albuquerque	100%	150
Loveless Medical Center-Downtown	Albuquerque	100%	193
Mimbres Memorial Hospital	Deming	100%	107
Miners' Colfax Medical Center	Raton	100%	57
Mountain View Regional Medical Center	Las Cruces	100%	193
Nor-Lea General Hospital	Lovington	100%	38
Presbyterian Hospital	Albuquerque	100%	158
Presbyterian Kaseman Hospital	Albuquerque	100%	112
Rehoboth McKinley Christian Health Care Svcs	Gallup	100%	161
Roosevelt General Hospital	Portales	100%	113
Saint Joseph's North East Heights Hospital	Albuquerque	100%	133
San Juan Regional Medical Center	Farmington	100%	317
Socorro General Hospital	Socorro	100%	46
Spring Valley Hospital	Las Vegas	100%	145
University of New Mexico Hospital	Albuquerque	100%	197
Gallup Indian Medical Center	Gallup	99%	136

NOTE: Hospital profiles are in alphabetical order by state, then city, then hospital within the city; Rankings are sorted by rate in descending order and exclude hospitals with less than 25 cases; (1) The number of cases is too small (n<25) for purposes of reliably predicting hospital performance; (2) Measure reflects the hospital's indication that its submission was based upon a sample of its relevant discharges; (3) Rate reflects fewer than the maximum possible quarters of data for the measure; (4) Inaccurate information submitted and suppressed for one or more quarters; (5) No data is available from the hospital for this measure; Please refer to the User's Guide for a full explanation of data

Plains Regional Medical Center	Clovis	99%	154
Saint Vincent Regional Medical Center	Santa Fe	99%	232
ACL-IHS Hospital	San Fidel	98%	50
Northern Navajo Medical Center	Shiprock	98%	120
Memorial Medical Center	Las Cruces	96%	369
Sierra Vista Hospital	Truth or Conseq.	96%	45
US Public Health Service Indian Hospital	Crownpoint	96%	57
Artesia General Hospital	Artesia	95%	60
Zuni Hospital	Zuni	94%	33

18. Pneumococcal Vaccine

Hospital Name	City	Rate	Cases
Lincoln County Medical Center	Ruidoso	93%	27
US Public Health Service Indian Hospital	Crownpoint	93%	41
Carlsbad Medical Center	Carlsbad	92%	100
ACL-IHS Hospital	San Fidel	90%	31
Mountain View Regional Medical Center	Las Cruces	89%	128
Eastern New Mexico Medical Center	Roswell	87%	175
Spring Valley Hospital	Las Vegas	85%	72
Gallup Indian Medical Center	Gallup	81%	67
Lea Regional Medical Center	Hobbs	78%	69
Lovelace Westside Hospital	Albuquerque	71%	78
Saint Joseph's North East Heights Hospital	Albuquerque	71%	92
Lovelace Health Systems	Albuquerque	68%	237
Espanola Hospital	Espanola	66%	70
Sierra Vista Hospital	Truth or Conseq.	66%	29
Miners' Colfax Medical Center	Raton	65%	37
Artesia General Hospital	Artesia	64%	36
San Juan Regional Medical Center	Farmington	62%	226
Socorro General Hospital	Socorro	59%	29
Alta Vista Regional Hospital	Las Vegas	53%	73
Saint Vincent Regional Medical Center	Santa Fe	51%	134
Loveless Medical Center-Downtown	Albuquerque	49%	127
Memorial Medical Center	Las Cruces	49%	219
Gila Regional Medical Center	Silver City	48%	90
Presbyterian Hospital	Albuquerque	48%	115
Gerald Champion Memorial Hospital	Alamogordo	46%	118
Plains Regional Medical Center	Clovis	45%	101
Holy Cross Hospital	Taos	44%	105
Cibola General Hospital	Grants	42%	26
Presbyterian Kaseman Hospital	Albuquerque	42%	89
Los Alamos Medical Center	Los Alamos	40%	35
Northern Navajo Medical Center	Shiprock	40%	84
Rehoboth McKinley Christian Health Care Svcs	Gallup	40%	91
University of New Mexico Hospital	Albuquerque	33%	73
Roosevelt General Hospital	Portales	14%	77
Doctor Dan C Trigg Memorial Hospital	Tucumcari	8%	26
Mimbres Memorial Hospital	Deming	8%	65

19. Smoking Cessation Advice

Hospital Name	City	Rate	Cases
Carlsbad Medical Center	Carlsbad	98%	43
Espanola Hospital	Espanola	96%	25
Spring Valley Hospital	Las Vegas	96%	48
Mountain View Regional Medical Center	Las Cruces	95%	38
Lea Regional Medical Center	Hobbs	85%	33
Eastern New Mexico Medical Center	Roswell	83%	75
Presbyterian Hospital	Albuquerque	82%	49
San Juan Regional Medical Center	Farmington	80%	45
Memorial Medical Center	Las Cruces	79%	66
Rehoboth McKinley Christian Health Care Svcs	Gallup	79%	29
Saint Joseph's North East Heights Hospital	Albuquerque	79%	34
Lovelace Health Systems	Albuquerque	77%	64
Loveless Medical Center-Downtown	Albuquerque	68%	50
Lovelace Westside Hospital	Albuquerque	65%	34
Alta Vista Regional Hospital	Las Vegas	62%	47
Saint Vincent Regional Medical Center	Santa Fe	57%	42
Gila Regional Medical Center	Silver City	48%	25
Plains Regional Medical Center	Clovis	44%	34
University of New Mexico Hospital	Albuquerque	38%	52
Gerald Champion Memorial Hospital	Alamogordo	37%	49
Mimbres Memorial Hospital	Deming	33%	30
Roosevelt General Hospital	Portales	22%	37

Surgical Infection Prevention

20. Prophylactic Antibiotic Given

Hospital Name	City	Rate	Cases
Carlsbad Medical Center	Carlsbad	97%	224
Presbyterian Kaseman Hospital	Albuquerque	96%	105
Heart Hospital of New Mexico	Albuquerque	95%	309
Presbyterian Hospital	Albuquerque	95%	436
Lea Regional Medical Center	Hobbs	94%	220
Lovelace Health Systems	Albuquerque	87%	164
Saint Joseph's North East Heights Hospital	Albuquerque	87%	30
Rehoboth McKinley Christian Health Care Svcs	Gallup	86%	63
Plains Regional Medical Center	Clovis	84%	321
University of New Mexico Hospital	Albuquerque	84%	390
Mountain View Regional Medical Center	Las Cruces	82%	536
San Juan Regional Medical Center	Farmington	82%	249
Loveless Medical Center-Downtown	Albuquerque	81%	36
Los Alamos Medical Center	Los Alamos	78%	79
Eastern New Mexico Medical Center	Roswell	77%	309
Espanola Hospital	Espanola	77%	44
Saint Vincent Regional Medical Center	Santa Fe	71%	732
Spring Valley Hospital	Las Vegas	71%	208
Memorial Medical Center	Las Cruces	69%	227
Gallup Indian Medical Center	Gallup	67%	33
Alta Vista Regional Hospital	Las Vegas	62%	52
Gerald Champion Memorial Hospital	Alamogordo	62%	143
Lincoln County Medical Center	Ruidoso	55%	49
Gila Regional Medical Center	Silver City	52%	223

21. Prophylactic Antibiotic Selection

Hospital Name	City	Rate	Cases
Carlsbad Medical Center	Carlsbad	100%	59
Heart Hospital of New Mexico	Albuquerque	100%	89
Lea Regional Medical Center	Hobbs	99%	73
Mountain View Regional Medical Center	Las Cruces	98%	124
Presbyterian Hospital	Albuquerque	98%	104
San Juan Regional Medical Center	Farmington	98%	64
University of New Mexico Hospital	Albuquerque	97%	67
Gerald Champion Memorial Hospital	Alamogordo	96%	76
Saint Joseph's North East Heights Hospital	Albuquerque	96%	28
Gila Regional Medical Center	Silver City	93%	71
Lovelace Health Systems	Albuquerque	93%	27
Memorial Medical Center	Las Cruces	93%	118
Saint Vincent Regional Medical Center	Santa Fe	92%	165
Eastern New Mexico Medical Center	Roswell	89%	74
Loveless Medical Center-Downtown	Albuquerque	89%	35
Spring Valley Hospital	Las Vegas	88%	50
Plains Regional Medical Center	Clovis	86%	72
Presbyterian Kaseman Hospital	Albuquerque	82%	28

22. Prophylactic Antibiotic Stopped

Hospital Name	City	Rate	Cases
Espanola Hospital	Espanola	95%	42
Heart Hospital of New Mexico	Albuquerque	91%	293
Eastern New Mexico Medical Center	Roswell	90%	301
Lea Regional Medical Center	Hobbs	88%	209
Carlsbad Medical Center	Carlsbad	85%	220
Mountain View Regional Medical Center	Las Cruces	85%	520
Lincoln County Medical Center	Ruidoso	81%	43
Loveless Medical Center-Downtown	Albuquerque	80%	35
Presbyterian Hospital	Albuquerque	80%	424
Presbyterian Kaseman Hospital	Albuquerque	80%	105
Rehoboth McKinley Christian Health Care Svcs	Gallup	80%	61
Gallup Indian Medical Center	Gallup	78%	32
Lovelace Health Systems	Albuquerque	78%	152
Plains Regional Medical Center	Clovis	78%	318
Alta Vista Regional Hospital	Las Vegas	76%	46
Saint Vincent Regional Medical Center	Santa Fe	74%	658
San Juan Regional Medical Center	Farmington	70%	241
University of New Mexico Hospital	Albuquerque	69%	383
Memorial Medical Center	Las Cruces	68%	223
Los Alamos Medical Center	Los Alamos	62%	79
Gerald Champion Memorial Hospital	Alamogordo	58%	137
Spring Valley Hospital	Las Vegas	54%	200
Saint Joseph's North East Heights Hospital	Albuquerque	52%	29
Gila Regional Medical Center	Silver City	44%	208

Pregnancy Care

23. Inpatient Neonatal Mortality

Hospital Name	City	Rate	Cases
Socorro General Hospital	Socorro	0.00%	222
Plains Regional Medical Center	Clovis	0.07%	1435
Lea Regional Medical Center	Hobbs	0.09%	1072
Espanola Hospital	Espanola	0.32%	310
Presbyterian Hospital	Albuquerque	0.40%	1005

24. Third or Fourth Degree Laceration

Hospital Name	City	Rate	Cases
Socorro General Hospital	Socorro	0.62%	161
Presbyterian Hospital	Albuquerque	1.74%	749

NOTE: Hospital profiles are in alphabetical order by state, then city, then hospital within the city; Rankings are sorted by rate in descending order and exclude hospitals with less than 25 cases; (1) The number of cases is too small (n<25) for purposes of reliably predicting hospital performance; (2) Measure reflects the hospital's indication that its submission was based upon a sample of its relevant discharges; (3) Rate reflects fewer than the maximum possible quarters of data for the measure; (4) Inaccurate information submitted and suppressed for one or more quarters; (5) No data is available from the hospital for this measure; Please refer to the User's Guide for a full explanation of data

Plains Regional Medical Center	Clovis	2.80%	1036
Lea Regional Medical Center	Hobbs	3.18%	785
Espanola Hospital	Espanola	3.29%	243

NOTE: Hospital profiles are in alphabetical order by state, then city, then hospital within the city; Rankings are sorted by rate in descending order and exclude hospitals with less than 25 cases; (1) The number of cases is too small (n<25) for purposes of reliably predicting hospital performance; (2) Measure reflects the hospital's indication that its submission was based upon a sample of its relevant discharges; (3) Rate reflects fewer than the maximum possible quarters of data for the measure; (4) Inaccurate information submitted and suppressed for one or more quarters; (5) No data is available from the hospital for this measure; Please refer to the User's Guide for a full explanation of data

Gerald Champion Memorial Hospital

2669 N Scenic Dr
Alamogordo, NM 88310
URL: www.gcrmc.org
Ownership: Voluntary non-profit - Other
Emergency Services: Yes
Phone: 505-439-6100
Fax: 505-443-7858
Accredited: No

Key Personnel:
CEO. . . . . Carl W Mantey

Measure	Cases	This Hospital	State Average	U.S. Average	Top Hospital
Heart Attack Care					
ACE Inhibitor or ARB for LVSD[1]	1	100%	71%	82%	100%
Aspirin at Arrival[1]	17	88%	87%	92%	100%
Aspirin at Discharge[1]	17	82%	87%	90%	100%
Beta Blocker at Arrival[1]	20	75%	76%	87%	100%
Beta Blocker at Discharge[1]	15	80%	83%	90%	100%
Fibrinolytic Medication Timing	0	-	21%	31%	100%
PCI Within 90 Minutes of Arrival	0	-	52%	54%	95%
Smoking Cessation Advice[1]	7	14%	78%	88%	100%
Heart Failure Care					
ACE Inhibitor or ARB for LVSD	45	71%	76%	82%	100%
Discharge Instructions	153	63%	27%	61%	93%
Evaluation of LVS Function	179	61%	66%	83%	99%
Smoking Cessation Advice	36	67%	51%	82%	100%
Pneumonia Care					
Appropriate Initial Antibiotic	96	85%	84%	83%	94%
Blood Culture Timing	47	74%	90%	90%	100%
Influenza Vaccine	51	45%	56%	70%	100%
Initial Antibiotic Timing	162	72%	73%	80%	93%
Oxygenation Assessment	197	100%	99%	99%	100%
Pneumococcal Vaccine	118	46%	56%	69%	94%
Smoking Cessation Advice	49	37%	58%	80%	100%
Surgical Infection Prevention					
Prophylactic Antibiotic Given[3]	143	62%	71%	77%	95%
Prophylactic Antibiotic Selection	76	96%	87%	90%	100%
Prophylactic Antibiotic Stopped[3]	137	58%	81%	72%	95%
Pregnancy Care					
Inpatient Neonatal Mortality	-	-	-	-	-
Third or Fourth Degree Laceration	-	-	-	3.63%	3.27%

Heart Hospital of New Mexico

504 Elm Street NE
Albuquerque, NM 87102
URL: www.hearthospitalnm.com
Ownership: Proprietary
Emergency Services: Yes
Phone: 505-724-2000
Fax: 505-246-9933
Accredited: Yes
Licensed Beds: 55

Key Personnel:
Interim CEO. . . . . Terry Odom
Interim CEO. . . . . Daune Scholer
Surgical Director. . . . . Richard Gerety, MD

Measure	Cases	This Hospital	State Average	U.S. Average	Top Hospital
Heart Attack Care					
ACE Inhibitor or ARB for LVSD	192	91%	71%	82%	100%
Aspirin at Arrival	158	99%	87%	92%	100%
Aspirin at Discharge	644	99%	87%	90%	100%
Beta Blocker at Arrival	152	99%	76%	87%	100%
Beta Blocker at Discharge	646	98%	83%	90%	100%
Fibrinolytic Medication Timing	0	-	21%	31%	100%
PCI Within 90 Minutes of Arrival[1]	13	77%	52%	54%	95%
Smoking Cessation Advice	256	86%	78%	88%	100%
Heart Failure Care					
ACE Inhibitor or ARB for LVSD	154	84%	76%	82%	100%
Discharge Instructions	254	65%	27%	61%	93%
Evaluation of LVS Function	277	98%	66%	83%	99%
Smoking Cessation Advice	31	81%	51%	82%	100%
Pneumonia Care					
Appropriate Initial Antibiotic[1]	6	83%	84%	83%	94%
Blood Culture Timing[1]	11	100%	90%	90%	100%
Influenza Vaccine[1]	5	20%	56%	70%	100%
Initial Antibiotic Timing[1]	16	69%	73%	80%	93%
Oxygenation Assessment[1]	18	100%	99%	99%	100%
Pneumococcal Vaccine[1]	18	61%	56%	69%	94%
Smoking Cessation Advice[1]	7	71%	58%	80%	100%
Surgical Infection Prevention					
Prophylactic Antibiotic Given[3]	309	95%	71%	77%	95%
Prophylactic Antibiotic Selection	89	100%	87%	90%	100%
Prophylactic Antibiotic Stopped[3]	293	91%	81%	72%	95%
Pregnancy Care					
Inpatient Neonatal Mortality	-	-	-	-	-
Third or Fourth Degree Laceration	-	-	-	3.63%	3.27%

Lovelace Health Systems

Alternate Name: Lovelace Medical Center
5400 Gibson Boulevard SE
Albuquerque, NM 87108
URL: www.lovelace.com
Ownership: Government - State
Emergency Services: Yes
Phone: 505-262-7000
Fax: 505-262-7729
Accredited: Yes
Licensed Beds: 225

Key Personnel:
Administrator/CEO. . . . . Martin Hickey, MD
Chief Medical Staff. . . . . Toby Merlin, MD
Chief Catheterization Laboratory . . . . Steve Ung, MD
Emergency Room . . . . John Martin, MD
Director Infection/Disease Control . . . . Janice Beene

Measure	Cases	This Hospital	State Average	U.S. Average	Top Hospital
Heart Attack Care					
ACE Inhibitor or ARB for LVSD	53	94%	71%	82%	100%
Aspirin at Arrival	201	99%	87%	92%	100%
Aspirin at Discharge	250	97%	87%	90%	100%
Beta Blocker at Arrival	182	93%	76%	87%	100%
Beta Blocker at Discharge	250	92%	83%	90%	100%
Fibrinolytic Medication Timing	0	-	21%	31%	100%
PCI Within 90 Minutes of Arrival[1]	11	73%	52%	54%	95%
Smoking Cessation Advice	60	90%	78%	88%	100%
Heart Failure Care					
ACE Inhibitor or ARB for LVSD	122	93%	76%	82%	100%
Discharge Instructions	249	89%	27%	61%	93%
Evaluation of LVS Function	279	99%	66%	83%	99%
Smoking Cessation Advice	37	68%	51%	82%	100%
Pneumonia Care					
Appropriate Initial Antibiotic[2]	252	87%	84%	83%	94%
Blood Culture Timing[2]	185	96%	90%	90%	100%
Influenza Vaccine[4,5]	-	-	56%	70%	100%
Initial Antibiotic Timing[2]	284	70%	73%	80%	93%
Oxygenation Assessment[2]	349	100%	99%	99%	100%
Pneumococcal Vaccine[2]	237	68%	56%	69%	94%
Smoking Cessation Advice[2]	64	77%	58%	80%	100%
Surgical Infection Prevention					
Prophylactic Antibiotic Given[2,3]	164	87%	71%	77%	95%
Prophylactic Antibiotic Selection[2]	27	93%	87%	90%	100%
Prophylactic Antibiotic Stopped[2,3]	152	78%	81%	72%	95%
Pregnancy Care					
Inpatient Neonatal Mortality	-	-	-	-	-
Third or Fourth Degree Laceration	-	-	-	3.63%	3.27%

Lovelace Westside Hospital

10501 Golf Course Road Nw
Albuquerque, NM 87114
Ownership: Voluntary non-profit - Church
Emergency Services: Yes
Phone: 505-727-7001
Accredited: Yes

Measure	Cases	This Hospital	State Average	U.S. Average	Top Hospital
Heart Attack Care					
ACE Inhibitor or ARB for LVSD[1,3]	1	100%	71%	82%	100%
Aspirin at Arrival[1,3]	4	75%	87%	92%	100%
Aspirin at Discharge[1,3]	4	75%	87%	90%	100%
Beta Blocker at Arrival[1,3]	6	67%	76%	87%	100%
Beta Blocker at Discharge[1,3]	4	100%	83%	90%	100%
Fibrinolytic Medication Timing[3]	0	-	21%	31%	100%
PCI Within 90 Minutes of Arrival[5]	-	-	52%	54%	95%
Smoking Cessation Advice[1,3]	1	100%	78%	88%	100%
Heart Failure Care					

NOTE: Hospital profiles are in alphabetical order by state, then city, then hospital within the city; Rankings are sorted by rate in descending order and exclude hospitals with less than 25 cases; (1) The number of cases is too small (n<25) for purposes of reliably predicting hospital performance; (2) Measure reflects the hospital's indication that its submission was based upon a sample of its relevant discharges; (3) Rate reflects fewer than the maximum possible quarters of data for the measure; (4) Inaccurate information submitted and suppressed for one or more quarters; (5) No data is available from the hospital for this measure; Please refer to the User's Guide for a full explanation of data

Measure	Cases	This Hospital	State Average	U.S. Average	Top Hospital
ACE Inhibitor or ARB for LVSD[1]	15	73%	76%	82%	100%
Discharge Instructions	45	22%	27%	61%	93%
Evaluation of LVS Function	51	92%	66%	83%	99%
Smoking Cessation Advice[1]	9	78%	51%	82%	100%
Pneumonia Care					
Appropriate Initial Antibiotic	108	81%	84%	83%	94%
Blood Culture Timing	68	88%	90%	90%	100%
Influenza Vaccine	26	77%	56%	70%	100%
Initial Antibiotic Timing	107	70%	73%	80%	93%
Oxygenation Assessment	150	100%	99%	99%	100%
Pneumococcal Vaccine	78	71%	56%	69%	94%
Smoking Cessation Advice	34	65%	58%	80%	100%
Surgical Infection Prevention					
Prophylactic Antibiotic Given[1,3]	14	100%	71%	77%	95%
Prophylactic Antibiotic Selection[1]	14	100%	87%	90%	100%
Prophylactic Antibiotic Stopped[1,3]	14	93%	81%	72%	95%
Pregnancy Care					
Inpatient Neonatal Mortality	-	-	-	-	-
Third or Fourth Degree Laceration	-	-	-	3.63%	3.27%

Loveless Medical Center-Downtown

601 Dr Martin Luther King Jr Ave NE | Phone: 505-727-8000
Albuquerque, NM 87102 | Fax: 505-727-8162
URL: www.lovelace.com
Ownership: Voluntary non-profit - Private | Accredited: Yes
Emergency Services: Yes | Licensed Beds: 254

Key Personnel:
President/CEO . . . . Michael O'Keefe
Chief Medical Staff . . . . William Mitchel
Emergency Room . . . . Erica Hamilton
Director of Respiratory . . . . Patrick Moya

Measure	Cases	This Hospital	State Average	U.S. Average	Top Hospital
Heart Attack Care					
ACE Inhibitor or ARB for LVSD[1]	3	100%	71%	82%	100%
Aspirin at Arrival[1]	6	100%	87%	92%	100%
Aspirin at Discharge[1]	9	89%	87%	90%	100%
Beta Blocker at Arrival[1]	8	50%	76%	87%	100%
Beta Blocker at Discharge[1]	9	78%	83%	90%	100%
Fibrinolytic Medication Timing	0	-	21%	31%	100%
PCI Within 90 Minutes of Arrival	0	-	52%	54%	95%
Smoking Cessation Advice[1]	1	100%	78%	88%	100%
Heart Failure Care					
ACE Inhibitor or ARB for LVSD[1]	13	85%	76%	82%	100%
Discharge Instructions	36	14%	27%	61%	93%
Evaluation of LVS Function	45	89%	66%	83%	99%
Smoking Cessation Advice[1]	8	25%	51%	82%	100%
Pneumonia Care					
Appropriate Initial Antibiotic	121	80%	84%	83%	94%
Blood Culture Timing	110	93%	90%	90%	100%
Influenza Vaccine	41	46%	56%	70%	100%
Initial Antibiotic Timing	141	71%	73%	80%	93%
Oxygenation Assessment	193	100%	99%	99%	100%
Pneumococcal Vaccine	127	49%	56%	69%	94%
Smoking Cessation Advice	50	68%	58%	80%	100%
Surgical Infection Prevention					
Prophylactic Antibiotic Given[3]	36	81%	71%	77%	95%
Prophylactic Antibiotic Selection	35	89%	87%	90%	100%
Prophylactic Antibiotic Stopped[3]	35	80%	81%	72%	95%
Pregnancy Care					
Inpatient Neonatal Mortality	-	-	-	-	-
Third or Fourth Degree Laceration	-	-	-	3.63%	3.27%

Presbyterian Hospital

1100 Centra Ave SE | Toll-Free: 800-672-8880
Albuquerque, NM 87106 | Phone: 505-841-1234
Fax: 505-841-1861

E-mail: info@phs.org
URL: www.phs.org
Ownership: Voluntary non-profit - Private | Accredited: Yes
Emergency Services: Yes | Licensed Beds: 453

Key Personnel:
Administrator/President . . . . James Hinton
Chief Medical Staff . . . . Lynn Bryant
Emergency Room . . . . George Molzen
Director Infection/Disease Control . . . . JoAnn Ferranti
CCU Spvg. Nurse . . . . Susan Finch
OB/GYN Womens Health . . . . Rebecca Shoden
Chief Radiology . . . . Ruth Lovvet
Director Pulmonary Services . . . . Donna Coon

Measure	Cases	This Hospital	State Average	U.S. Average	Top Hospital
Heart Attack Care					
ACE Inhibitor or ARB for LVSD[2]	50	72%	71%	82%	100%
Aspirin at Arrival[2]	219	99%	87%	92%	100%
Aspirin at Discharge[2]	285	98%	87%	90%	100%
Beta Blocker at Arrival[2]	176	94%	76%	87%	100%
Beta Blocker at Discharge[2]	290	97%	83%	90%	100%
Fibrinolytic Medication Timing[2]	0	-	21%	31%	100%
PCI Within 90 Minutes of Arrival[1,2]	19	84%	52%	54%	95%
Smoking Cessation Advice[2]	112	98%	78%	88%	100%
Heart Failure Care					
ACE Inhibitor or ARB for LVSD[2]	132	76%	76%	82%	100%
Discharge Instructions[2]	248	48%	27%	61%	93%
Evaluation of LVS Function[2]	292	94%	66%	83%	99%
Smoking Cessation Advice[2]	54	93%	51%	82%	100%
Pneumonia Care					
Appropriate Initial Antibiotic[2]	55	93%	84%	83%	94%
Blood Culture Timing[2]	90	90%	90%	90%	100%
Influenza Vaccine	25	56%	56%	70%	100%
Initial Antibiotic Timing[2]	129	74%	73%	80%	93%
Oxygenation Assessment[2]	158	100%	99%	99%	100%
Pneumococcal Vaccine[2]	115	48%	56%	69%	94%
Smoking Cessation Advice[2]	49	82%	58%	80%	100%
Surgical Infection Prevention					
Prophylactic Antibiotic Given[2]	436	95%	71%	77%	95%
Prophylactic Antibiotic Selection[2]	104	98%	87%	90%	100%
Prophylactic Antibiotic Stopped[2]	424	80%	81%	72%	95%
Pregnancy Care					
Inpatient Neonatal Mortality[2]	1,005	0.40%	-	-	-
Third or Fourth Degree Laceration[2]	749	1.74%	-	3.63%	3.27%

Presbyterian Kaseman Hospital

8300 Constitution Avenue NE | Phone: 505-291-2000
Albuquerque, NM 87110 | Fax: 505-291-2983
URL: www.phs.org
Ownership: Proprietary | Accredited: No
Emergency Services: Yes | Licensed Beds: 170

Key Personnel:
President/CEO . . . . Jim Hinton

Measure	Cases	This Hospital	State Average	U.S. Average	Top Hospital
Heart Attack Care					
ACE Inhibitor or ARB for LVSD[1,3]	1	0%	71%	82%	100%
Aspirin at Arrival[1,3]	6	100%	87%	92%	100%
Aspirin at Discharge[1,3]	5	100%	87%	90%	100%
Beta Blocker at Arrival[1,3]	6	50%	76%	87%	100%
Beta Blocker at Discharge[1,3]	4	100%	83%	90%	100%
Fibrinolytic Medication Timing[3]	0	-	21%	31%	100%
PCI Within 90 Minutes of Arrival	0	-	52%	54%	95%
Smoking Cessation Advice[3]	0	-	78%	88%	100%
Heart Failure Care					
ACE Inhibitor or ARB for LVSD[1]	10	90%	76%	82%	100%
Discharge Instructions[1]	22	5%	27%	61%	93%
Evaluation of LVS Function	31	84%	66%	83%	99%
Smoking Cessation Advice[1]	4	50%	51%	82%	100%
Pneumonia Care					
Appropriate Initial Antibiotic	42	95%	84%	83%	94%
Blood Culture Timing	66	92%	90%	90%	100%
Influenza Vaccine[1]	23	57%	56%	70%	100%
Initial Antibiotic Timing	91	75%	73%	80%	93%
Oxygenation Assessment	112	100%	99%	99%	100%
Pneumococcal Vaccine	89	42%	56%	69%	94%
Smoking Cessation Advice[1]	22	73%	58%	80%	100%

NOTE: Hospital profiles are in alphabetical order by state, then city, then hospital within the city; Rankings are sorted by rate in descending order and exclude hospitals with less than 25 cases; (1) The number of cases is too small (n<25) for purposes of reliably predicting hospital performance; (2) Measure reflects the hospital's indication that its submission was based upon a sample of its relevant discharges; (3) Rate reflects fewer than the maximum possible quarters of data for the measure; (4) Inaccurate information submitted and suppressed for one or more quarters; (5) No data is available from the hospital for this measure; Please refer to the User's Guide for a full explanation of data

Surgical Infection Prevention					
Prophylactic Antibiotic Given	105	96%	71%	77%	95%
Prophylactic Antibiotic Selection	28	82%	87%	90%	100%
Prophylactic Antibiotic Stopped	105	80%	81%	72%	95%
Pregnancy Care					
Inpatient Neonatal Mortality	-	-	-	-	-
Third or Fourth Degree Laceration	-	-	-	3.63%	3.27%

Saint Joseph's North East Heights Hospital

Alternate Name: Lovelace Women's Hospital
4701 Montgomery
Albuquerque, NM 87109
Phone: 505-727-8000
Fax: 505-727-7888
Ownership: Government - State
Accredited: Yes
Emergency Services: No
Licensed Beds: 112
Key Personnel:
Administrator . . . . Vincent Townsend

Measure	Cases	This Hospital	State Average	U.S. Average	Top Hospital
Heart Attack Care					
ACE Inhibitor or ARB for LVSD[1]	2	50%	71%	82%	100%
Aspirin at Arrival[1]	7	100%	87%	92%	100%
Aspirin at Discharge[1]	6	100%	87%	90%	100%
Beta Blocker at Arrival[1]	9	78%	76%	87%	100%
Beta Blocker at Discharge[1]	6	83%	83%	90%	100%
Fibrinolytic Medication Timing	0	-	21%	31%	100%
PCI Within 90 Minutes of Arrival	0	-	52%	54%	95%
Smoking Cessation Advice	0	-	78%	88%	100%
Heart Failure Care					
ACE Inhibitor or ARB for LVSD[1]	5	60%	76%	82%	100%
Discharge Instructions[1]	17	18%	27%	61%	93%
Evaluation of LVS Function[1]	23	96%	66%	83%	99%
Smoking Cessation Advice[1]	5	40%	51%	82%	100%
Pneumonia Care					
Appropriate Initial Antibiotic	105	84%	84%	83%	94%
Blood Culture Timing	71	87%	90%	90%	100%
Influenza Vaccine	28	75%	56%	70%	100%
Initial Antibiotic Timing	109	75%	73%	80%	93%
Oxygenation Assessment	133	100%	99%	99%	100%
Pneumococcal Vaccine	92	71%	56%	69%	94%
Smoking Cessation Advice	34	79%	58%	80%	100%
Surgical Infection Prevention					
Prophylactic Antibiotic Given[3]	30	87%	71%	77%	95%
Prophylactic Antibiotic Selection	28	96%	87%	90%	100%
Prophylactic Antibiotic Stopped[3]	29	52%	81%	72%	95%
Pregnancy Care					
Inpatient Neonatal Mortality[5]	0	0.00%	-	-	-
Third or Fourth Degree Laceration[5]	0	0.00%	-	3.63%	3.27%

University of New Mexico Hospital

2211 Lomas Boulevard NE
Albuquerque, NM 87106
Phone: 505-272-2111
Fax: 505-272-0940
E-mail: montiveros@salud.unm.edu
URL: hospitals.unm.edu/unmh
Ownership: Government - State
Accredited: Yes
Emergency Services: Yes
Licensed Beds: 333
Key Personnel:
CEO. . . . . Steve McKernan
Chief Medical Staff. . . . . RG Strickland, MD
Emergency Room . . . . Susan Harrison-Solt
Director Medical/Surgical Nursing Svcs . . . . Pam Demarest
OB/GYN Womens Health. . . . . Gloria Sarto, MD
Chief Radiology . . . . Fred Mettler, Jr, DM
Director Respiratory Therapy . . . . Bruce Riser

Measure	Cases	This Hospital	State Average	U.S. Average	Top Hospital
Heart Attack Care					
ACE Inhibitor or ARB for LVSD	28	71%	71%	82%	100%
Aspirin at Arrival	135	96%	87%	92%	100%
Aspirin at Discharge	146	97%	87%	90%	100%
Beta Blocker at Arrival	128	95%	76%	87%	100%
Beta Blocker at Discharge	143	97%	83%	90%	100%
Fibrinolytic Medication Timing	0	-	21%	31%	100%
PCI Within 90 Minutes of Arrival[1]	6	83%	52%	54%	95%
Smoking Cessation Advice	69	93%	78%	88%	100%
Heart Failure Care					
ACE Inhibitor or ARB for LVSD	96	86%	76%	82%	100%
Discharge Instructions	163	15%	27%	61%	93%
Evaluation of LVS Function	182	99%	66%	83%	99%
Smoking Cessation Advice	58	81%	51%	82%	100%
Pneumonia Care					
Appropriate Initial Antibiotic[2]	121	80%	84%	83%	94%
Blood Culture Timing[2]	115	82%	90%	90%	100%
Influenza Vaccine[2]	26	50%	56%	70%	100%
Initial Antibiotic Timing[2]	161	37%	73%	80%	93%
Oxygenation Assessment[2]	197	100%	99%	99%	100%
Pneumococcal Vaccine[2]	73	33%	56%	69%	94%
Smoking Cessation Advice[2]	52	38%	58%	80%	100%
Surgical Infection Prevention					
Prophylactic Antibiotic Given[2]	390	84%	71%	77%	95%
Prophylactic Antibiotic Selection[2]	67	97%	87%	90%	100%
Prophylactic Antibiotic Stopped[2]	383	69%	81%	72%	95%
Pregnancy Care					
Inpatient Neonatal Mortality	-	-	-	-	-
Third or Fourth Degree Laceration	-	-	-	3.63%	3.27%

Artesia General Hospital

702 N 13th Street
Artesia, NM 88210
Phone: 505-748-3333
Fax: 505-748-8377
Ownership: Voluntary non-profit - Private
Accredited: No
Emergency Services: Yes
Licensed Beds: 34
Key Personnel:
CEO. . . . . Claude Camp
Emergency Room . . . . Kelli Suto

Measure	Cases	This Hospital	State Average	U.S. Average	Top Hospital
Heart Attack Care					
ACE Inhibitor or ARB for LVSD[3]	0	-	71%	82%	100%
Aspirin at Arrival[1,3]	5	60%	87%	92%	100%
Aspirin at Discharge[1,3]	5	80%	87%	90%	100%
Beta Blocker at Arrival[1,3]	4	75%	76%	87%	100%
Beta Blocker at Discharge[1,3]	5	80%	83%	90%	100%
Fibrinolytic Medication Timing[3]	0	-	21%	31%	100%
PCI Within 90 Minutes of Arrival	0	-	52%	54%	95%
Smoking Cessation Advice[3]	0	-	78%	88%	100%
Heart Failure Care					
ACE Inhibitor or ARB for LVSD[1]	2	100%	76%	82%	100%
Discharge Instructions[1]	16	25%	27%	61%	93%
Evaluation of LVS Function[1]	18	17%	66%	83%	99%
Smoking Cessation Advice[1]	4	50%	51%	82%	100%
Pneumonia Care					
Appropriate Initial Antibiotic	48	79%	84%	83%	94%
Blood Culture Timing[1]	21	95%	90%	90%	100%
Influenza Vaccine[1]	11	82%	56%	70%	100%
Initial Antibiotic Timing	52	60%	73%	80%	93%
Oxygenation Assessment	60	95%	99%	99%	100%
Pneumococcal Vaccine	36	64%	56%	69%	94%
Smoking Cessation Advice[1]	19	32%	58%	80%	100%
Surgical Infection Prevention					
Prophylactic Antibiotic Given[1,3]	6	33%	71%	77%	95%
Prophylactic Antibiotic Selection[1]	4	75%	87%	90%	100%
Prophylactic Antibiotic Stopped[1,3]	6	83%	81%	72%	95%
Pregnancy Care					
Inpatient Neonatal Mortality	-	-	-	-	-
Third or Fourth Degree Laceration	-	-	-	3.63%	3.27%

Carlsbad Medical Center

2430 W Pierce Street
Carlsbad, NM 88220
Phone: 505-887-4100
Fax: 505-887-4256
URL: www.triadhospital.com
Ownership: Proprietary
Accredited: Yes
Emergency Services: Yes
Licensed Beds: 135
Key Personnel:
President/CEO. . . . . Fred Woody
Chief of Medical Staff . . . . Brad McGrath
Emergency Room . . . . Connie Willis

NOTE: Hospital profiles are in alphabetical order by state, then city, then hospital within the city; Rankings are sorted by rate in descending order and exclude hospitals with less than 25 cases; (1) The number of cases is too small (n<25) for purposes of reliably predicting hospital performance; (2) Measure reflects the hospital's indication that its submission was based upon a sample of its relevant discharges; (3) Rate reflects fewer than the maximum possible quarters of data for the measure; (4) Inaccurate information submitted and suppressed for one or more quarters; (5) No data is available from the hospital for this measure; Please refer to the User's Guide for a full explanation of data

Infection Control . . . . Marcia Westfall, RN
ICU . . . . Elizabeth Madison, RN
Medical/Surgical Nursing . . . . Carla Bradley
OB/GYN Womens Health . . . . Carla Welch, RN
Director Surgical Services . . . . Faith Johnston, RN
Respiratory/Cardiopulmonary . . . . Jeffery Molina

Measure	Cases	This Hospital	State Average	U.S. Average	Top Hospital
Heart Attack Care					
ACE Inhibitor or ARB for LVSD[1]	13	100%	71%	82%	100%
Aspirin at Arrival	78	97%	87%	92%	100%
Aspirin at Discharge	60	98%	87%	90%	100%
Beta Blocker at Arrival	70	96%	76%	87%	100%
Beta Blocker at Discharge	61	100%	83%	90%	100%
Fibrinolytic Medication Timing[1]	9	44%	21%	31%	100%
PCI Within 90 Minutes of Arrival[1]	1	0%	52%	54%	95%
Smoking Cessation Advice	26	100%	78%	88%	100%
Heart Failure Care					
ACE Inhibitor or ARB for LVSD	28	93%	76%	82%	100%
Discharge Instructions	56	77%	27%	61%	93%
Evaluation of LVS Function	69	93%	66%	83%	99%
Smoking Cessation Advice[1]	16	100%	51%	82%	100%
Pneumonia Care					
Appropriate Initial Antibiotic	100	93%	84%	83%	94%
Blood Culture Timing	107	95%	90%	90%	100%
Influenza Vaccine	52	88%	56%	70%	100%
Initial Antibiotic Timing	137	88%	73%	80%	93%
Oxygenation Assessment	168	100%	99%	99%	100%
Pneumococcal Vaccine	100	92%	56%	69%	94%
Smoking Cessation Advice	43	98%	58%	80%	100%
Surgical Infection Prevention					
Prophylactic Antibiotic Given	224	97%	71%	77%	95%
Prophylactic Antibiotic Selection	59	100%	87%	90%	100%
Prophylactic Antibiotic Stopped	220	85%	81%	72%	95%
Pregnancy Care					
Inpatient Neonatal Mortality	-	-	-	-	-
Third or Fourth Degree Laceration	-	-	-	3.63%	3.27%

Union County General Hospital

301 Harding Street
PO Box 489
Clayton, NM 88415
Phone: 505-374-2585
Fax: 505-374-8146
Ownership: Government - Local
Accredited: No
Emergency Services: Yes
Licensed Beds: 30

Key Personnel:
Chief Medical Staff . . . . Michael Jenkins
Director Infection/Disease Control . . . . Loretta Butler
Chief Radiology . . . . Gloria Rice
Director Respiratory Therapy . . . . Adelina Montoya

Measure	Cases	This Hospital	State Average	U.S. Average	Top Hospital
Heart Attack Care					
ACE Inhibitor or ARB for LVSD[3]	0	-	71%	82%	100%
Aspirin at Arrival[1,3]	1	100%	87%	92%	100%
Aspirin at Discharge[3]	0	-	87%	90%	100%
Beta Blocker at Arrival[1,3]	1	100%	76%	87%	100%
Beta Blocker at Discharge[3]	0	-	83%	90%	100%
Fibrinolytic Medication Timing[3]	0	-	21%	31%	100%
PCI Within 90 Minutes of Arrival	0	-	52%	54%	95%
Smoking Cessation Advice[3]	0	-	78%	88%	100%
Heart Failure Care					
ACE Inhibitor or ARB for LVSD[1,3]	2	50%	76%	82%	100%
Discharge Instructions[1,3]	5	20%	27%	61%	93%
Evaluation of LVS Function[1,3]	5	60%	66%	83%	99%
Smoking Cessation Advice[1,3]	1	0%	51%	82%	100%
Pneumonia Care					
Appropriate Initial Antibiotic[1,3]	10	60%	84%	83%	94%
Blood Culture Timing	0	-	90%	90%	100%
Influenza Vaccine[1]	6	67%	56%	70%	100%
Initial Antibiotic Timing[1,3]	17	82%	73%	80%	93%
Oxygenation Assessment[1,3]	19	100%	99%	99%	100%
Pneumococcal Vaccine[1,3]	15	80%	56%	69%	94%
Smoking Cessation Advice[1,3]	3	0%	58%	80%	100%
Surgical Infection Prevention					
Prophylactic Antibiotic Given[1,3]	8	75%	71%	77%	95%
Prophylactic Antibiotic Selection[1]	1	100%	87%	90%	100%
Prophylactic Antibiotic Stopped[1,3]	8	62%	81%	72%	95%
Pregnancy Care					
Inpatient Neonatal Mortality	-	-	-	-	-
Third or Fourth Degree Laceration	-	-	-	3.63%	3.27%

Plains Regional Medical Center

Alternate Name: Clovis High Plains Hospital
1600 W 21st Street
Clovis, NM 88102
URL: www.phs.org
Phone: 505-769-2141
Fax: 505-769-7526
Ownership: Voluntary non-profit - Private
Accredited: Yes
Emergency Services: Yes
Licensed Beds: 106

Key Personnel:
CEO . . . . Brian Betley
Chief Medical Staff . . . . Cynthia Smithnd
Emergency Room . . . . Cythia Smithnd
Director Infection/Disease Control . . . . Donna Chartien
Director Surgical Nursing . . . . Sheryll Plyler
OB/GYN Womens Health . . . . Richard Layman
Director Radiology . . . . Michael Luscombe
Respiratory Care . . . . Michael Luscombe

Measure	Cases	This Hospital	State Average	U.S. Average	Top Hospital
Heart Attack Care					
ACE Inhibitor or ARB for LVSD[1]	19	37%	71%	82%	100%
Aspirin at Arrival	28	75%	87%	92%	100%
Aspirin at Discharge	30	43%	87%	90%	100%
Beta Blocker at Arrival	27	63%	76%	87%	100%
Beta Blocker at Discharge	31	42%	83%	90%	100%
Fibrinolytic Medication Timing[1]	3	0%	21%	31%	100%
PCI Within 90 Minutes of Arrival	0	-	52%	54%	95%
Smoking Cessation Advice[1]	5	60%	78%	88%	100%
Heart Failure Care					
ACE Inhibitor or ARB for LVSD	92	66%	76%	82%	100%
Discharge Instructions	109	58%	27%	61%	93%
Evaluation of LVS Function	128	75%	66%	83%	99%
Smoking Cessation Advice	29	34%	51%	82%	100%
Pneumonia Care					
Appropriate Initial Antibiotic	101	89%	84%	83%	94%
Blood Culture Timing	63	98%	90%	90%	100%
Influenza Vaccine	30	60%	56%	70%	100%
Initial Antibiotic Timing	138	80%	73%	80%	93%
Oxygenation Assessment	154	99%	99%	99%	100%
Pneumococcal Vaccine	101	45%	56%	69%	94%
Smoking Cessation Advice	34	44%	58%	80%	100%
Surgical Infection Prevention					
Prophylactic Antibiotic Given	321	84%	71%	77%	95%
Prophylactic Antibiotic Selection	72	86%	87%	90%	100%
Prophylactic Antibiotic Stopped	318	78%	81%	72%	95%
Pregnancy Care					
Inpatient Neonatal Mortality	1,435	0.07%	-	-	-
Third or Fourth Degree Laceration	1,036	2.80%	-	3.63%	3.27%

US Public Health Service Indian Hospital

Alternate Name: Crownpoint PHS Indian Hospital
PO Box 358
Crownpoint, NM 87313
URL: www.ihs.gov
Phone: 928-729-8000
Fax: 928-729-8269
Ownership: Government - Federal
Accredited: No
Emergency Services: Yes
Licensed Beds: 39

Key Personnel:
CEO . . . . Anita Nuneta
Chief Medical Officer . . . . W Craig Vanderwagen, MD

Measure	Cases	This Hospital	State Average	U.S. Average	Top Hospital
Heart Attack Care					
ACE Inhibitor or ARB for LVSD[3]	0	-	71%	82%	100%
Aspirin at Arrival[3]	0	-	87%	92%	100%
Aspirin at Discharge[3]	0	-	87%	90%	100%

NOTE: Hospital profiles are in alphabetical order by state, then city, then hospital within the city; Rankings are sorted by rate in descending order and exclude hospitals with less than 25 cases; (1) The number of cases is too small (n<25) for purposes of reliably predicting hospital performance; (2) Measure reflects the hospital's indication that its submission was based upon a sample of its relevant discharges; (3) Rate reflects fewer than the maximum possible quarters of data for the measure; (4) Inaccurate information submitted and suppressed for one or more quarters; (5) No data is available from the hospital for this measure; Please refer to the User's Guide for a full explanation of data

Beta Blocker at Arrival[3]	0	-	76%	87%	100%
Beta Blocker at Discharge[3]	0	-	83%	90%	100%
Fibrinolytic Medication Timing[3]	0	-	21%	31%	100%
PCI Within 90 Minutes of Arrival	0	-	52%	54%	95%
Smoking Cessation Advice[3]	0	-	78%	88%	100%
Heart Failure Care					
ACE Inhibitor or ARB for LVSD[1,3]	2	50%	76%	82%	100%
Discharge Instructions[1,3]	5	0%	27%	61%	93%
Evaluation of LVS Function[1,3]	10	60%	66%	83%	99%
Smoking Cessation Advice[3]	0	-	51%	82%	100%
Pneumonia Care					
Appropriate Initial Antibiotic[1,3]	18	78%	84%	83%	94%
Blood Culture Timing[1,3]	12	100%	90%	90%	100%
Influenza Vaccine[5]	-	-	56%	70%	100%
Initial Antibiotic Timing	43	81%	73%	80%	93%
Oxygenation Assessment	57	96%	99%	99%	100%
Pneumococcal Vaccine	41	93%	56%	69%	94%
Smoking Cessation Advice[1,3]	1	0%	58%	80%	100%
Surgical Infection Prevention					
Prophylactic Antibiotic Given[5]	-	-	71%	77%	95%
Prophylactic Antibiotic Selection[5]	-	-	87%	90%	100%
Prophylactic Antibiotic Stopped[5]	-	-	81%	72%	95%
Pregnancy Care					
Inpatient Neonatal Mortality	-	-	-	-	-
Third or Fourth Degree Laceration	-	-	-	3.63%	3.27%

Mimbres Memorial Hospital

900 W Ash Street
Deming, NM 88030
Toll-Free: 888-464-6273
Phone: 505-546-2761
Fax: 505-543-6914

URL: www.mimbresmemorial.com
Ownership: Proprietary
Emergency Services: Yes
Accredited: No
Licensed Beds: 118

Key Personnel:
CEO. . . . . Derrick Uyu
Chief Medical Staff . . . . Joe Jone, MD
Emergency Room . . . . Joe Jone, MD
Director of Respiratory . . . . Sharon Holbrook

Measure	Cases	This Hospital	State Average	U.S. Average	Top Hospital
Heart Attack Care					
ACE Inhibitor or ARB for LVSD[1]	1	0%	71%	82%	100%
Aspirin at Arrival[1]	15	80%	87%	92%	100%
Aspirin at Discharge[1]	12	100%	87%	90%	100%
Beta Blocker at Arrival[1]	13	85%	76%	87%	100%
Beta Blocker at Discharge[1]	12	75%	83%	90%	100%
Fibrinolytic Medication Timing	0	-	21%	31%	100%
PCI Within 90 Minutes of Arrival	0	-	52%	54%	95%
Smoking Cessation Advice[1]	4	50%	78%	88%	100%
Heart Failure Care					
ACE Inhibitor or ARB for LVSD[1]	8	50%	76%	82%	100%
Discharge Instructions	67	0%	27%	61%	93%
Evaluation of LVS Function	80	32%	66%	83%	99%
Smoking Cessation Advice[1]	15	27%	51%	82%	100%
Pneumonia Care					
Appropriate Initial Antibiotic	81	93%	84%	83%	94%
Blood Culture Timing	26	96%	90%	90%	100%
Influenza Vaccine[4,5]	-	-	56%	70%	100%
Initial Antibiotic Timing	100	75%	73%	80%	93%
Oxygenation Assessment	107	100%	99%	99%	100%
Pneumococcal Vaccine	65	8%	56%	69%	94%
Smoking Cessation Advice	30	33%	58%	80%	100%
Surgical Infection Prevention					
Prophylactic Antibiotic Given[1,2,3]	18	39%	71%	77%	95%
Prophylactic Antibiotic Selection[1,2]	10	10%	87%	90%	100%
Prophylactic Antibiotic Stopped[1,2,3]	17	100%	81%	72%	95%
Pregnancy Care					
Inpatient Neonatal Mortality	-	-	-	-	-
Third or Fourth Degree Laceration	-	-	-	3.63%	3.27%

Espanola Hospital

1010 Spruce Street
Espanola, NM 87532
Phone: 505-753-7111
Fax: 505-753-1536
URL: www.phs.org
Ownership: Voluntary non-profit - Private
Emergency Services: Yes
Accredited: Yes
Licensed Beds: 180

Key Personnel:
Administrator . . . . Marcella Romera
Director Infection/Disease Control . . . . Susan Wagner, RN
Director Respiratory Therapy . . . . Mary Jo Metzger

Measure	Cases	This Hospital	State Average	U.S. Average	Top Hospital
Heart Attack Care					
ACE Inhibitor or ARB for LVSD	0	-	71%	82%	100%
Aspirin at Arrival[1]	5	100%	87%	92%	100%
Aspirin at Discharge[1]	1	100%	87%	90%	100%
Beta Blocker at Arrival[1]	5	60%	76%	87%	100%
Beta Blocker at Discharge[1]	1	100%	83%	90%	100%
Fibrinolytic Medication Timing	0	-	21%	31%	100%
PCI Within 90 Minutes of Arrival	0	-	52%	54%	95%
Smoking Cessation Advice	0	-	78%	88%	100%
Heart Failure Care					
ACE Inhibitor or ARB for LVSD[1]	17	82%	76%	82%	100%
Discharge Instructions	50	74%	27%	61%	93%
Evaluation of LVS Function	54	74%	66%	83%	99%
Smoking Cessation Advice[1]	8	100%	51%	82%	100%
Pneumonia Care					
Appropriate Initial Antibiotic	87	80%	84%	83%	94%
Blood Culture Timing	62	85%	90%	90%	100%
Influenza Vaccine[1]	21	76%	56%	70%	100%
Initial Antibiotic Timing	100	92%	73%	80%	93%
Oxygenation Assessment	111	100%	99%	99%	100%
Pneumococcal Vaccine	70	66%	56%	69%	94%
Smoking Cessation Advice	25	96%	58%	80%	100%
Surgical Infection Prevention					
Prophylactic Antibiotic Given[3]	44	77%	71%	77%	95%
Prophylactic Antibiotic Selection[1]	16	100%	87%	90%	100%
Prophylactic Antibiotic Stopped[3]	42	95%	81%	72%	95%
Pregnancy Care					
Inpatient Neonatal Mortality	310	0.32%	-	-	-
Third or Fourth Degree Laceration	243	3.29%	-	3.63%	3.27%

San Juan Regional Medical Center

801 W Maple Street
Farmington, NM 87401
Phone: 505-325-5011
Fax: 505-599-6249
URL: www.lifecowisehealth.com
Ownership: Government - Federal
Emergency Services: Yes
Accredited: Yes
Licensed Beds: 175

Key Personnel:
Administrator/CEO . . . . Steve Altmiller
ER Medical Director . . . . Dale Kester, MD
Emergency Room . . . . Mike Berve
Manager/Cardiopulmonary Special Services . . . Keith Johnson
Infection Control Professional. . . . . Penny Hill
Manager ICU/CCU. . . . . Kris Cuthair
Medical Staff Services . . . . Violet Kelley

Measure	Cases	This Hospital	State Average	U.S. Average	Top Hospital
Heart Attack Care					
ACE Inhibitor or ARB for LVSD[1]	14	100%	71%	82%	100%
Aspirin at Arrival	85	99%	87%	92%	100%
Aspirin at Discharge	45	91%	87%	90%	100%
Beta Blocker at Arrival	70	97%	76%	87%	100%
Beta Blocker at Discharge	44	95%	83%	90%	100%
Fibrinolytic Medication Timing[1]	15	53%	21%	31%	100%
PCI Within 90 Minutes of Arrival	0	-	52%	54%	95%
Smoking Cessation Advice[1]	11	82%	78%	88%	100%
Heart Failure Care					
ACE Inhibitor or ARB for LVSD	98	97%	76%	82%	100%
Discharge Instructions	165	52%	27%	61%	93%
Evaluation of LVS Function	198	96%	66%	83%	99%
Smoking Cessation Advice[1]	21	76%	51%	82%	100%
Pneumonia Care					

NOTE: Hospital profiles are in alphabetical order by state, then city, then hospital within the city; Rankings are sorted by rate in descending order and exclude hospitals with less than 25 cases; (1) The number of cases is too small (n<25) for purposes of reliably predicting hospital performance; (2) Measure reflects the hospital's indication that its submission was based upon a sample of its relevant discharges; (3) Rate reflects fewer than the maximum possible quarters of data for the measure; (4) Inaccurate information submitted and suppressed for one or more quarters; (5) No data is available from the hospital for this measure; Please refer to the User's Guide for a full explanation of data

Measure	Cases	This Hospital	State Average	U.S. Average	Top Hospital
Appropriate Initial Antibiotic	157	87%	84%	83%	94%
Blood Culture Timing	156	87%	90%	90%	100%
Influenza Vaccine	76	66%	56%	70%	100%
Initial Antibiotic Timing	261	82%	73%	80%	93%
Oxygenation Assessment	317	100%	99%	99%	100%
Pneumococcal Vaccine	226	62%	56%	69%	94%
Smoking Cessation Advice	45	80%	58%	80%	100%
Surgical Infection Prevention					
Prophylactic Antibiotic Given[2,3]	249	82%	71%	77%	95%
Prophylactic Antibiotic Selection[2]	64	98%	87%	90%	100%
Prophylactic Antibiotic Stopped[2,3]	241	70%	81%	72%	95%
Pregnancy Care					
Inpatient Neonatal Mortality	-	-	-	-	-
Third or Fourth Degree Laceration	-	-	-	3.63%	3.27%

Gallup Indian Medical Center

516 E Nizhoni Boulevard
Gallup, NM 87305
URL: www.ihs.gov/facilitiesservices
Ownership: Government - Federal
Emergency Services: Yes
Phone: 505-722-1000
Fax: 505-722-1386
Accredited: Yes
Licensed Beds: 99

Key Personnel:

President/CEO. . . . . Floyd Thompson
Chief Medical Staff. . . . . Jerome Alford, DDS
Emergency Room . . . . Kenneth Stewart
Emergency Room . . . . Carla Huber
Infection Control. . . . . Richard Nauman
ICU . . . . Karen Digman, RN
Medical/Surgical Nursing . . . . Pamela Atkins
Respiratory/Cardiopulmonary. . . . . Ernest Sandoval

Measure	Cases	This Hospital	State Average	U.S. Average	Top Hospital
Heart Attack Care					
ACE Inhibitor or ARB for LVSD[1,3]	1	0%	71%	82%	100%
Aspirin at Arrival[1,3]	2	100%	87%	92%	100%
Aspirin at Discharge[1,3]	1	100%	87%	90%	100%
Beta Blocker at Arrival[1,3]	1	100%	76%	87%	100%
Beta Blocker at Discharge[1,3]	1	100%	83%	90%	100%
Fibrinolytic Medication Timing[3]	0	-	21%	31%	100%
PCI Within 90 Minutes of Arrival	0	-	52%	54%	95%
Smoking Cessation Advice[3]	0	-	78%	88%	100%
Heart Failure Care					
ACE Inhibitor or ARB for LVSD[1]	22	82%	76%	82%	100%
Discharge Instructions	37	11%	27%	61%	93%
Evaluation of LVS Function	40	98%	66%	83%	99%
Smoking Cessation Advice[1]	1	0%	51%	82%	100%
Pneumonia Care					
Appropriate Initial Antibiotic[2]	97	85%	84%	83%	94%
Blood Culture Timing[2]	59	93%	90%	90%	100%
Influenza Vaccine[1]	21	71%	56%	70%	100%
Initial Antibiotic Timing[2]	112	73%	73%	80%	93%
Oxygenation Assessment[2]	136	99%	99%	99%	100%
Pneumococcal Vaccine[2]	67	81%	56%	69%	94%
Smoking Cessation Advice[1,2]	6	17%	58%	80%	100%
Surgical Infection Prevention					
Prophylactic Antibiotic Given	33	67%	71%	77%	95%
Prophylactic Antibiotic Selection[1]	8	88%	87%	90%	100%
Prophylactic Antibiotic Stopped	32	78%	81%	72%	95%
Pregnancy Care					
Inpatient Neonatal Mortality	-	-	-	-	-
Third or Fourth Degree Laceration	-	-	-	3.63%	3.27%

Rehoboth McKinley Christian Health Care Svcs

1901 Red Rock Drive
Gallup, NM 87301
URL: www.rmch.org
Ownership: Voluntary non-profit - Private
Emergency Services: Yes
Phone: 505-863-7000
Fax: 505-863-8920
Accredited: Yes
Licensed Beds: 109

Key Personnel:

President/CEO. . . . . David J Baltzer
Chief Medical Staff. . . . . Mary Poel
Emergency Room . . . . Alan Beamsley
Director Infection/Disease Control . . . . Jay Vink
Director Radiology . . . . John M Tafoya
Director Cardio-Pulmonary Services . . . . Randy Whitsitt

Measure	Cases	This Hospital	State Average	U.S. Average	Top Hospital
Heart Attack Care					
ACE Inhibitor or ARB for LVSD	0	-	71%	82%	100%
Aspirin at Arrival[1]	4	100%	87%	92%	100%
Aspirin at Discharge	0	-	87%	90%	100%
Beta Blocker at Arrival[1]	4	75%	76%	87%	100%
Beta Blocker at Discharge[1]	1	100%	83%	90%	100%
Fibrinolytic Medication Timing	0	-	21%	31%	100%
PCI Within 90 Minutes of Arrival	0	-	52%	54%	95%
Smoking Cessation Advice	0	-	78%	88%	100%
Heart Failure Care					
ACE Inhibitor or ARB for LVSD[1]	13	77%	76%	82%	100%
Discharge Instructions	66	27%	27%	61%	93%
Evaluation of LVS Function	73	40%	66%	83%	99%
Smoking Cessation Advice[1]	11	73%	51%	82%	100%
Pneumonia Care					
Appropriate Initial Antibiotic	108	80%	84%	83%	94%
Blood Culture Timing	80	82%	90%	90%	100%
Influenza Vaccine	33	48%	56%	70%	100%
Initial Antibiotic Timing	125	82%	73%	80%	93%
Oxygenation Assessment	161	100%	99%	99%	100%
Pneumococcal Vaccine	91	40%	56%	69%	94%
Smoking Cessation Advice	29	79%	58%	80%	100%
Surgical Infection Prevention					
Prophylactic Antibiotic Given	63	86%	71%	77%	95%
Prophylactic Antibiotic Selection[1]	18	89%	87%	90%	100%
Prophylactic Antibiotic Stopped	61	80%	81%	72%	95%
Pregnancy Care					
Inpatient Neonatal Mortality	-	-	-	-	-
Third or Fourth Degree Laceration	-	-	-	3.63%	3.27%

Cibola General Hospital

1016 E Rooseveltue
Grants, NM 87020
Ownership: Voluntary non-profit - Other
Emergency Services: Yes
Phone: 505-287-5300
Fax: 505-287-5309
Accredited: Yes
Licensed Beds: 25

Key Personnel:

President/CEO. . . . . Vincent Ashley
Chief Medical Staff. . . . . Janice Shipley, MD, CDS
Cardiac Lab . . . . Dennis Winter
Emergency Room . . . . Arnold Valdivia, MD
Director Medical/Surgical Nursing . . . . Dorcas Yates, RN
Respiratory Therapy. . . . . Dennis Winter

Measure	Cases	This Hospital	State Average	U.S. Average	Top Hospital
Heart Attack Care					
ACE Inhibitor or ARB for LVSD[3]	0	-	71%	82%	100%
Aspirin at Arrival[1,3]	3	100%	87%	92%	100%
Aspirin at Discharge[1,3]	3	100%	87%	90%	100%
Beta Blocker at Arrival[1,3]	3	67%	76%	87%	100%
Beta Blocker at Discharge[1,3]	3	100%	83%	90%	100%
Fibrinolytic Medication Timing[3]	0	-	21%	31%	100%
PCI Within 90 Minutes of Arrival	0	-	52%	54%	95%
Smoking Cessation Advice[1,3]	1	100%	78%	88%	100%
Heart Failure Care					
ACE Inhibitor or ARB for LVSD[1]	1	0%	76%	82%	100%
Discharge Instructions[1]	15	20%	27%	61%	93%
Evaluation of LVS Function[1]	17	24%	66%	83%	99%
Smoking Cessation Advice[1]	1	100%	51%	82%	100%
Pneumonia Care					
Appropriate Initial Antibiotic	40	88%	84%	83%	94%
Blood Culture Timing	30	100%	90%	90%	100%
Influenza Vaccine[1]	10	40%	56%	70%	100%
Initial Antibiotic Timing	36	61%	73%	80%	93%
Oxygenation Assessment	45	100%	99%	99%	100%
Pneumococcal Vaccine	26	42%	56%	69%	94%
Smoking Cessation Advice[1]	8	62%	58%	80%	100%
Surgical Infection Prevention					
Prophylactic Antibiotic Given[1,3]	20	50%	71%	77%	95%

NOTE: Hospital profiles are in alphabetical order by state, then city, then hospital within the city; Rankings are sorted by rate in descending order and exclude hospitals with less than 25 cases; (1) The number of cases is too small (n<25) for purposes of reliably predicting hospital performance; (2) Measure reflects the hospital's indication that its submission was based upon a sample of its relevant discharges; (3) Rate reflects fewer than the maximum possible quarters of data for the measure; (4) Inaccurate information submitted and suppressed for one or more quarters; (5) No data is available from the hospital for this measure; Please refer to the User's Guide for a full explanation of data

Prophylactic Antibiotic Selection[1]	6	83%	87%	90%	100%
Prophylactic Antibiotic Stopped[1,3]	19	100%	81%	72%	95%
Pregnancy Care					
Inpatient Neonatal Mortality	-	-	-	-	-
Third or Fourth Degree Laceration	-	-	-	3.63%	3.27%

Lea Regional Medical Center

Alternate Name: Columbia Lea Regional Medical Center
5419 N Lovington Highway
Hobbs, NM 88240
Phone: 505-492-5000
Fax: 505-492-5393
URL: www.learegionalmedical.com
Ownership: Proprietary
Accredited: Yes
Emergency Services: Yes
Licensed Beds: 250

Key Personnel:

CEO. . . . . Edmundo Castaneda
Chief Medical Staff. . . . . Andre Feria, MD
Emergency Room . . . . C Wilmes
Emergency Room . . . . Jamie Todd, RN
CNO. . . . . Wade Tyrrell
OB/GYN Womens Health. . . . . Anne Hale, MD
Chief Radiology . . . . Howard Nunn, MD
Director Respiratory Therapy . . . . Rubin Rossalo

Measure	Cases	This Hospital	State Average	U.S. Average	Top Hospital
Heart Attack Care					
ACE Inhibitor or ARB for LVSD	0	-	71%	82%	100%
Aspirin at Arrival[1]	11	100%	87%	92%	100%
Aspirin at Discharge[1]	6	100%	87%	90%	100%
Beta Blocker at Arrival[1]	11	82%	76%	87%	100%
Beta Blocker at Discharge[1]	6	100%	83%	90%	100%
Fibrinolytic Medication Timing[1]	1	0%	21%	31%	100%
PCI Within 90 Minutes of Arrival	0	-	52%	54%	95%
Smoking Cessation Advice[1]	5	80%	78%	88%	100%
Heart Failure Care					
ACE Inhibitor or ARB for LVSD[1]	13	92%	76%	82%	100%
Discharge Instructions	29	59%	27%	61%	93%
Evaluation of LVS Function	49	88%	66%	83%	99%
Smoking Cessation Advice[1]	13	92%	51%	82%	100%
Pneumonia Care					
Appropriate Initial Antibiotic	84	90%	84%	83%	94%
Blood Culture Timing	75	91%	90%	90%	100%
Influenza Vaccine[1]	21	48%	56%	70%	100%
Initial Antibiotic Timing	104	73%	73%	80%	93%
Oxygenation Assessment	116	100%	99%	99%	100%
Pneumococcal Vaccine	69	78%	56%	69%	94%
Smoking Cessation Advice	33	85%	58%	80%	100%
Surgical Infection Prevention					
Prophylactic Antibiotic Given	220	94%	71%	77%	95%
Prophylactic Antibiotic Selection	73	99%	87%	90%	100%
Prophylactic Antibiotic Stopped	209	88%	81%	72%	95%
Pregnancy Care					
Inpatient Neonatal Mortality	1,072	0.09%	-	-	-
Third or Fourth Degree Laceration	785	3.18%	-	3.63%	3.27%

Memorial Medical Center

2450 S Telshor Boulevard
Las Cruces, NM 88001
Phone: 505-522-8641
Fax: 505-556-5837
URL: www.mmclc.org
Ownership: Proprietary
Accredited: Yes
Emergency Services: Yes
Licensed Beds: 286

Key Personnel:

CEO. . . . . Paul Herzog
Chief Medical Officer . . . . Bruce D San Filippo, MD

Measure	Cases	This Hospital	State Average	U.S. Average	Top Hospital
Heart Attack Care					
ACE Inhibitor or ARB for LVSD	48	58%	71%	82%	100%
Aspirin at Arrival	70	91%	87%	92%	100%
Aspirin at Discharge	137	97%	87%	90%	100%
Beta Blocker at Arrival	63	70%	76%	87%	100%
Beta Blocker at Discharge	167	92%	83%	90%	100%
Fibrinolytic Medication Timing	0	-	21%	31%	100%
PCI Within 90 Minutes of Arrival[1]	7	43%	52%	54%	95%
Smoking Cessation Advice	67	79%	78%	88%	100%
Heart Failure Care					
ACE Inhibitor or ARB for LVSD	102	73%	76%	82%	100%
Discharge Instructions	209	10%	27%	61%	93%
Evaluation of LVS Function	239	81%	66%	83%	99%
Smoking Cessation Advice	32	59%	51%	82%	100%
Pneumonia Care					
Appropriate Initial Antibiotic	261	82%	84%	83%	94%
Blood Culture Timing	193	91%	90%	90%	100%
Influenza Vaccine	69	57%	56%	70%	100%
Initial Antibiotic Timing	337	57%	73%	80%	93%
Oxygenation Assessment	369	96%	99%	99%	100%
Pneumococcal Vaccine	219	49%	56%	69%	94%
Smoking Cessation Advice	66	79%	58%	80%	100%
Surgical Infection Prevention					
Prophylactic Antibiotic Given[2,3]	227	69%	71%	77%	95%
Prophylactic Antibiotic Selection[2]	118	93%	87%	90%	100%
Prophylactic Antibiotic Stopped[2,3]	223	68%	81%	72%	95%
Pregnancy Care					
Inpatient Neonatal Mortality	-	-	-	-	-
Third or Fourth Degree Laceration	-	-	-	3.63%	3.27%

Mountain View Regional Medical Center

4311 East Lohman Avenue
Las Cruces, NM 88001
Phone: 505-556-7600
Fax: 505-556-7619
URL: www.mountainviewregional.com
Ownership: Voluntary non-profit - Private
Accredited: Yes
Emergency Services: Yes
Licensed Beds: 168

Key Personnel:

CEO. . . . . Karen Springer
Chief Medical Staff. . . . . Laura Enn
Cardiac Lab . . . . Jose Tutierrev
Chief Pulmonary Care . . . . James Bately
Director Respiratory Care. . . . . Cirbuee Hibes

Measure	Cases	This Hospital	State Average	U.S. Average	Top Hospital
Heart Attack Care					
ACE Inhibitor or ARB for LVSD	54	65%	71%	82%	100%
Aspirin at Arrival	85	91%	87%	92%	100%
Aspirin at Discharge	145	95%	87%	90%	100%
Beta Blocker at Arrival	62	85%	76%	87%	100%
Beta Blocker at Discharge	159	91%	83%	90%	100%
Fibrinolytic Medication Timing	0	-	21%	31%	100%
PCI Within 90 Minutes of Arrival[1]	4	25%	52%	54%	95%
Smoking Cessation Advice	63	97%	78%	88%	100%
Heart Failure Care					
ACE Inhibitor or ARB for LVSD	73	79%	76%	82%	100%
Discharge Instructions	141	50%	27%	61%	93%
Evaluation of LVS Function	163	91%	66%	83%	99%
Smoking Cessation Advice[1]	22	91%	51%	82%	100%
Pneumonia Care					
Appropriate Initial Antibiotic	127	87%	84%	83%	94%
Blood Culture Timing	126	95%	90%	90%	100%
Influenza Vaccine	42	81%	56%	70%	100%
Initial Antibiotic Timing	152	70%	73%	80%	93%
Oxygenation Assessment	193	100%	99%	99%	100%
Pneumococcal Vaccine	128	89%	56%	69%	94%
Smoking Cessation Advice	38	95%	58%	80%	100%
Surgical Infection Prevention					
Prophylactic Antibiotic Given	536	82%	71%	77%	95%
Prophylactic Antibiotic Selection	124	98%	87%	90%	100%
Prophylactic Antibiotic Stopped	520	85%	81%	72%	95%
Pregnancy Care					
Inpatient Neonatal Mortality	-	-	-	-	-
Third or Fourth Degree Laceration	-	-	-	3.63%	3.27%

NOTE: Hospital profiles are in alphabetical order by state, then city, then hospital within the city; Rankings are sorted by rate in descending order and exclude hospitals with less than 25 cases; (1) The number of cases is too small (n<25) for purposes of reliably predicting hospital performance; (2) Measure reflects the hospital's indication that its submission was based upon a sample of its relevant discharges; (3) Rate reflects fewer than the maximum possible quarters of data for the measure; (4) Inaccurate information submitted and suppressed for one or more quarters; (5) No data is available from the hospital for this measure; Please refer to the User's Guide for a full explanation of data

Alta Vista Regional Hospital

104 Legion Drive
Las Vegas, NM 87701
URL: www.altavistaregioanlhospital.com
Phone: 505-426-3500
Fax: 505-426-3611

Ownership: Voluntary non-profit - Private
Accredited: Yes
Emergency Services: Yes
Licensed Beds: 54

Key Personnel:

CEO. . . . . Brian Gibbons
Director Cardiology . . . . Barbara Travis
Director Emergency Room. . . . . Bred Langdorg
Respiratory Care . . . . Rubie Mabs

Measure	Cases	This Hospital	State Average	U.S. Average	Top Hospital
Heart Attack Care					
ACE Inhibitor or ARB for LVSD[3]	0	-	71%	82%	100%
Aspirin at Arrival[1,3]	8	100%	87%	92%	100%
Aspirin at Discharge[1,3]	6	100%	87%	90%	100%
Beta Blocker at Arrival[1,3]	8	75%	76%	87%	100%
Beta Blocker at Discharge[1,3]	4	100%	83%	90%	100%
Fibrinolytic Medication Timing[3]	0	-	21%	31%	100%
PCI Within 90 Minutes of Arrival[5]	-	-	52%	54%	95%
Smoking Cessation Advice[1,3]	2	50%	78%	88%	100%
Heart Failure Care					
ACE Inhibitor or ARB for LVSD	25	76%	76%	82%	100%
Discharge Instructions	63	2%	27%	61%	93%
Evaluation of LVS Function	75	77%	66%	83%	99%
Smoking Cessation Advice[1]	19	37%	51%	82%	100%
Pneumonia Care					
Appropriate Initial Antibiotic	87	77%	84%	83%	94%
Blood Culture Timing	72	79%	90%	90%	100%
Influenza Vaccine[1]	21	33%	56%	70%	100%
Initial Antibiotic Timing	122	73%	73%	80%	93%
Oxygenation Assessment	136	100%	99%	99%	100%
Pneumococcal Vaccine	73	53%	56%	69%	94%
Smoking Cessation Advice	47	62%	58%	80%	100%
Surgical Infection Prevention					
Prophylactic Antibiotic Given[2,3]	52	62%	71%	77%	95%
Prophylactic Antibiotic Selection[1,2]	16	88%	87%	90%	100%
Prophylactic Antibiotic Stopped[2,3]	46	76%	81%	72%	95%
Pregnancy Care					
Inpatient Neonatal Mortality	-	-	-	-	-
Third or Fourth Degree Laceration	-	-	-	3.63%	3.27%

Los Alamos Medical Center

3917 West Road
Los Alamos, NM 87544
Phone: 505-662-4201
Fax: 505-661-9598

Ownership: Proprietary
Accredited: Yes
Emergency Services: Yes
Licensed Beds: 47

Key Personnel:

CEO. . . . . Gary Nichols
Chief of Medical Staff. Marylen Chanodi
Emergency Room . . . . Vallery Merl
Chief Radiology . . . . David Williams, MD
Director of Pulmonary/Respiratory Care. . . . . . . Joan Temple

Measure	Cases	This Hospital	State Average	U.S. Average	Top Hospital
Heart Attack Care					
ACE Inhibitor or ARB for LVSD[3]	0	-	71%	82%	100%
Aspirin at Arrival[1,3]	2	50%	87%	92%	100%
Aspirin at Discharge[1,3]	1	100%	87%	90%	100%
Beta Blocker at Arrival[1,3]	2	100%	76%	87%	100%
Beta Blocker at Discharge[1,3]	1	100%	83%	90%	100%
Fibrinolytic Medication Timing[3]	0	-	21%	31%	100%
PCI Within 90 Minutes of Arrival	0	-	52%	54%	95%
Smoking Cessation Advice[3]	0	-	78%	88%	100%
Heart Failure Care					
ACE Inhibitor or ARB for LVSD[1]	6	100%	76%	82%	100%
Discharge Instructions[1]	20	15%	27%	61%	93%
Evaluation of LVS Function[1]	22	64%	66%	83%	99%
Smoking Cessation Advice[1]	6	33%	51%	82%	100%
Pneumonia Care					
Appropriate Initial Antibiotic	47	83%	84%	83%	94%
Blood Culture Timing	32	84%	90%	90%	100%
Influenza Vaccine[4,5]	-	-	56%	70%	100%
Initial Antibiotic Timing	58	79%	73%	80%	93%
Oxygenation Assessment	63	100%	99%	99%	100%
Pneumococcal Vaccine	35	40%	56%	69%	94%
Smoking Cessation Advice[1]	7	43%	58%	80%	100%
Surgical Infection Prevention					
Prophylactic Antibiotic Given[3]	79	78%	71%	77%	95%
Prophylactic Antibiotic Selection[1]	24	96%	87%	90%	100%
Prophylactic Antibiotic Stopped[3]	79	62%	81%	72%	95%
Pregnancy Care					
Inpatient Neonatal Mortality	-	-	-	-	-
Third or Fourth Degree Laceration	-	-	-	3.63%	3.27%

Nor-Lea General Hospital

1600 N Main
Lovington, NM 88260
E-mail: carold@nlgh.org
URL: www.nlgh.org
Phone: 505-396-6611
Fax: 505-396-3729

Ownership: Govt - Hospital District or Authority
Accredited: No
Emergency Services: Yes
Licensed Beds: 28

Key Personnel:

Administrator/CEO. . . . . David Shaw
Chief Medical Staff. . . . . Ronald D Hopkins, DO
Emergency Room . . . . Ronald D Hopkins, DO
Director Infection/Disease Control . . . . Katie Sandovil
Coord. Medical & Surgical . . . . Brenda Shirley
Director Respiratory Therapy . . . . Dan Hamilton

Measure	Cases	This Hospital	State Average	U.S. Average	Top Hospital
Heart Attack Care					
ACE Inhibitor or ARB for LVSD[3]	0	-	71%	82%	100%
Aspirin at Arrival[1,3]	1	0%	87%	92%	100%
Aspirin at Discharge[1,3]	1	0%	87%	90%	100%
Beta Blocker at Arrival[1,3]	1	0%	76%	87%	100%
Beta Blocker at Discharge[1,3]	1	0%	83%	90%	100%
Fibrinolytic Medication Timing[3]	0	-	21%	31%	100%
PCI Within 90 Minutes of Arrival[5]	-	-	52%	54%	95%
Smoking Cessation Advice[3]	0	-	78%	88%	100%
Heart Failure Care					
ACE Inhibitor or ARB for LVSD[1,2,3]	4	75%	76%	82%	100%
Discharge Instructions[1,2,3]	13	8%	27%	61%	93%
Evaluation of LVS Function[1,2,3]	13	54%	66%	83%	99%
Smoking Cessation Advice[1,2,3]	2	0%	51%	82%	100%
Pneumonia Care					
Appropriate Initial Antibiotic[2,3]	27	85%	84%	83%	94%
Blood Culture Timing[1,2]	11	100%	90%	90%	100%
Influenza Vaccine[1,2]	13	0%	56%	70%	100%
Initial Antibiotic Timing[2,3]	31	61%	73%	80%	93%
Oxygenation Assessment[2,3]	38	100%	99%	99%	100%
Pneumococcal Vaccine[1,2,3]	20	55%	56%	69%	94%
Smoking Cessation Advice[1,2,3]	10	60%	58%	80%	100%
Surgical Infection Prevention					
Prophylactic Antibiotic Given[1,3]	5	20%	71%	77%	95%
Prophylactic Antibiotic Selection[5]	-	-	87%	90%	100%
Prophylactic Antibiotic Stopped[1,3]	4	100%	81%	72%	95%
Pregnancy Care					
Inpatient Neonatal Mortality	-	-	-	-	-
Third or Fourth Degree Laceration	-	-	-	3.63%	3.27%

Mescalero PHS Indian Hospital

PO Box 210
Mescalero, NM 88340
Phone: 505-464-4441

Ownership: Government - Federal
Accredited: Yes
Emergency Services: Yes

Measure	Cases	This Hospital	State Average	U.S. Average	Top Hospital
Heart Attack Care					
ACE Inhibitor or ARB for LVSD[5]	-	-	71%	82%	100%
Aspirin at Arrival[5]	-	-	87%	92%	100%
Aspirin at Discharge[5]	-	-	87%	90%	100%
Beta Blocker at Arrival[5]	-	-	76%	87%	100%
Beta Blocker at Discharge[5]	-	-	83%	90%	100%

NOTE: Hospital profiles are in alphabetical order by state, then city, then hospital within the city; Rankings are sorted by rate in descending order and exclude hospitals with less than 25 cases; (1) The number of cases is too small (n<25) for purposes of reliably predicting hospital performance; (2) Measure reflects the hospital's indication that its submission was based upon a sample of its relevant discharges; (3) Rate reflects fewer than the maximum possible quarters of data for the measure; (4) Inaccurate information submitted and suppressed for one or more quarters; (5) No data is available from the hospital for this measure; Please refer to the User's Guide for a full explanation of data

Measure	Cases	This Hospital	State Average	U.S. Average	Top Hospital
Fibrinolytic Medication Timing[5]	-	-	21%	31%	100%
PCI Within 90 Minutes of Arrival[5]	-	-	52%	54%	95%
Smoking Cessation Advice[5]	-	-	78%	88%	100%
Heart Failure Care					
ACE Inhibitor or ARB for LVSD[5]	-	-	76%	82%	100%
Discharge Instructions[5]	-	-	27%	61%	93%
Evaluation of LVS Function[5]	-	-	66%	83%	99%
Smoking Cessation Advice[5]	-	-	51%	82%	100%
Pneumonia Care					
Appropriate Initial Antibiotic[1,3]	2	100%	84%	83%	94%
Blood Culture Timing[3]	0	-	90%	90%	100%
Influenza Vaccine[5]	-	-	56%	70%	100%
Initial Antibiotic Timing[1,3]	1	0%	73%	80%	93%
Oxygenation Assessment[1,3]	2	100%	99%	99%	100%
Pneumococcal Vaccine[1,3]	1	0%	56%	69%	94%
Smoking Cessation Advice[3]	0	-	58%	80%	100%
Surgical Infection Prevention					
Prophylactic Antibiotic Given[5]	-	-	71%	77%	95%
Prophylactic Antibiotic Selection[5]	-	-	87%	90%	100%
Prophylactic Antibiotic Stopped[5]	-	-	81%	72%	95%
Pregnancy Care					
Inpatient Neonatal Mortality	-	-	-	-	-
Third or Fourth Degree Laceration	-	-	-	3.63%	3.27%

Roosevelt General Hospital

42121 Us Highway 70
Portales, NM 88130
Phone: 505-359-1800
Ownership: Voluntary non-profit - Other
Accredited: No
Emergency Services: Yes

Measure	Cases	This Hospital	State Average	U.S. Average	Top Hospital
Heart Attack Care					
ACE Inhibitor or ARB for LVSD[1,3]	1	100%	71%	82%	100%
Aspirin at Arrival[1,3]	2	50%	87%	92%	100%
Aspirin at Discharge[1,3]	3	67%	87%	90%	100%
Beta Blocker at Arrival[1,3]	2	50%	76%	87%	100%
Beta Blocker at Discharge[1,3]	3	0%	83%	90%	100%
Fibrinolytic Medication Timing[3]	0	-	21%	31%	100%
PCI Within 90 Minutes of Arrival	0	-	52%	54%	95%
Smoking Cessation Advice[1,3]	1	0%	78%	88%	100%
Heart Failure Care					
ACE Inhibitor or ARB for LVSD[1]	6	100%	76%	82%	100%
Discharge Instructions	48	10%	27%	61%	93%
Evaluation of LVS Function	60	25%	66%	83%	99%
Smoking Cessation Advice[1]	10	20%	51%	82%	100%
Pneumonia Care					
Appropriate Initial Antibiotic	84	79%	84%	83%	94%
Blood Culture Timing	40	92%	90%	90%	100%
Influenza Vaccine[1]	20	15%	56%	70%	100%
Initial Antibiotic Timing	100	80%	73%	80%	93%
Oxygenation Assessment	113	100%	99%	99%	100%
Pneumococcal Vaccine	77	14%	56%	69%	94%
Smoking Cessation Advice	37	22%	58%	80%	100%
Surgical Infection Prevention					
Prophylactic Antibiotic Given[1,3]	1	0%	71%	77%	95%
Prophylactic Antibiotic Selection	0	-	87%	90%	100%
Prophylactic Antibiotic Stopped[1,3]	1	100%	81%	72%	95%
Pregnancy Care					
Inpatient Neonatal Mortality	-	-	-	-	-
Third or Fourth Degree Laceration	-	-	-	3.63%	3.27%

Miners' Colfax Medical Center

200 Hospital Drive
Raton, NM 87740
Phone: 505-445-3661
Fax: 505-445-7875
URL: www.minershosp.com
Ownership: Government - State
Accredited: No
Emergency Services: Yes
Licensed Beds: 33

Key Personnel:

CEO. . . . . Donald Holl
Chief Medical Staff. . . . . Francis Visconte, MD
Emergency Room . . . . Valerie Ridolsi
Director of Pulmonary/Respiratory Care. . . . . . . Ken Ingram

Measure	Cases	This Hospital	State Average	U.S. Average	Top Hospital
Heart Attack Care					
ACE Inhibitor or ARB for LVSD	0	-	71%	82%	100%
Aspirin at Arrival[1]	8	100%	87%	92%	100%
Aspirin at Discharge[1]	7	86%	87%	90%	100%
Beta Blocker at Arrival[1]	6	83%	76%	87%	100%
Beta Blocker at Discharge[1]	8	62%	83%	90%	100%
Fibrinolytic Medication Timing[1,3]	2	50%	21%	31%	100%
PCI Within 90 Minutes of Arrival	0	-	52%	54%	95%
Smoking Cessation Advice[1,3]	1	100%	78%	88%	100%
Heart Failure Care					
ACE Inhibitor or ARB for LVSD[1]	4	75%	76%	82%	100%
Discharge Instructions[1,3]	18	6%	27%	61%	93%
Evaluation of LVS Function	30	47%	66%	83%	99%
Smoking Cessation Advice[1,3]	1	0%	51%	82%	100%
Pneumonia Care					
Appropriate Initial Antibiotic[1,3]	21	76%	84%	83%	94%
Blood Culture Timing[1]	20	100%	90%	90%	100%
Influenza Vaccine[1]	3	67%	56%	70%	100%
Initial Antibiotic Timing	49	76%	73%	80%	93%
Oxygenation Assessment	57	100%	99%	99%	100%
Pneumococcal Vaccine	37	65%	56%	69%	94%
Smoking Cessation Advice[1,3]	8	38%	58%	80%	100%
Surgical Infection Prevention					
Prophylactic Antibiotic Given[1,3]	9	22%	71%	77%	95%
Prophylactic Antibiotic Selection[1]	5	0%	87%	90%	100%
Prophylactic Antibiotic Stopped[1,3]	9	89%	81%	72%	95%
Pregnancy Care					
Inpatient Neonatal Mortality	-	-	-	-	-
Third or Fourth Degree Laceration	-	-	-	3.63%	3.27%

Eastern New Mexico Medical Center

405 W Country Club Road
Roswell, NM 88201
Phone: 505-622-8170
Fax: 505-624-8726
E-mail: enmmc@enmmc.com
URL: www.enmmc.com
Ownership: Proprietary
Accredited: Yes
Emergency Services: Yes
Licensed Beds: 162

Key Personnel:

CEO. . . . . Rich Robinson
Associate CEO. . . . . Brian Gibbons
Chief Medical Staff . . . . Madhu Sasidhar, MD
Catheterization Laboratory . . . . David Staleup
Emergency Room . . . . Jane Smith, RN
Director Infection/Disease Control . . . . Susan Esparsen
Chief ICU/ER. . . . . Jane Smith, RN
Director Medical Surgical Nursing . . . . Roman Jenks, RN
Director OB/GYN/Family Care Services. . . . . . . Alyce Cook, RN
Surgical Services Director . . . . Kay Haywood, RN
Director Radiology . . . . Terry Anderson
Director Respiratory Therapy . . . . Kevin Whitle

Measure	Cases	This Hospital	State Average	U.S. Average	Top Hospital
Heart Attack Care					
ACE Inhibitor or ARB for LVSD[1]	6	83%	71%	82%	100%
Aspirin at Arrival	62	98%	87%	92%	100%
Aspirin at Discharge	36	94%	87%	90%	100%
Beta Blocker at Arrival	54	89%	76%	87%	100%
Beta Blocker at Discharge	29	93%	83%	90%	100%
Fibrinolytic Medication Timing[1]	1	0%	21%	31%	100%
PCI Within 90 Minutes of Arrival	0	-	52%	54%	95%
Smoking Cessation Advice[1]	13	92%	78%	88%	100%
Heart Failure Care					
ACE Inhibitor or ARB for LVSD	47	89%	76%	82%	100%
Discharge Instructions	155	41%	27%	61%	93%
Evaluation of LVS Function	173	86%	66%	83%	99%
Smoking Cessation Advice	33	85%	51%	82%	100%
Pneumonia Care					
Appropriate Initial Antibiotic	181	76%	84%	83%	94%
Blood Culture Timing	127	97%	90%	90%	100%
Influenza Vaccine	69	94%	56%	70%	100%
Initial Antibiotic Timing	271	66%	73%	80%	93%

NOTE: Hospital profiles are in alphabetical order by state, then city, then hospital within the city; Rankings are sorted by rate in descending order and exclude hospitals with less than 25 cases; (1) The number of cases is too small (n<25) for purposes of reliably predicting hospital performance; (2) Measure reflects the hospital's indication that its submission was based upon a sample of its relevant discharges; (3) Rate reflects fewer than the maximum possible quarters of data for the measure; (4) Inaccurate information submitted and suppressed for one or more quarters; (5) No data is available from the hospital for this measure; Please refer to the User's Guide for a full explanation of data

Measure	Cases	This Hospital	State Average	U.S. Average	Top Hospital
Oxygenation Assessment	298	100%	99%	99%	100%
Pneumococcal Vaccine	175	87%	56%	69%	94%
Smoking Cessation Advice	75	83%	58%	80%	100%
Surgical Infection Prevention					
Prophylactic Antibiotic Given[2,3]	309	77%	71%	77%	95%
Prophylactic Antibiotic Selection[2]	74	89%	87%	90%	100%
Prophylactic Antibiotic Stopped[2,3]	301	90%	81%	72%	95%
Pregnancy Care					
Inpatient Neonatal Mortality	-	-	-	-	-
Third or Fourth Degree Laceration	-	-	-	3.63%	3.27%

Lincoln County Medical Center

211 Sudderth
Ruidoso, NM 88345
Ownership: Government - Local
Emergency Services: Yes

Phone: 505-257-8250
Fax: 505-630-4233
Accredited: No
Licensed Beds: 42

Key Personnel:
CEO. . . . . James Gibson

Measure	Cases	This Hospital	State Average	U.S. Average	Top Hospital
Heart Attack Care					
ACE Inhibitor or ARB for LVSD[3]	0	-	71%	82%	100%
Aspirin at Arrival[1,3]	5	100%	87%	92%	100%
Aspirin at Discharge[1,3]	5	80%	87%	90%	100%
Beta Blocker at Arrival[1,3]	4	50%	76%	87%	100%
Beta Blocker at Discharge[1,3]	5	80%	83%	90%	100%
Fibrinolytic Medication Timing[1,3]	4	0%	21%	31%	100%
PCI Within 90 Minutes of Arrival[5]	-	-	52%	54%	95%
Smoking Cessation Advice[3]	0	-	78%	88%	100%
Heart Failure Care					
ACE Inhibitor or ARB for LVSD	0	-	76%	82%	100%
Discharge Instructions	37	0%	27%	61%	93%
Evaluation of LVS Function	44	5%	66%	83%	99%
Smoking Cessation Advice[1]	8	38%	51%	82%	100%
Pneumonia Care					
Appropriate Initial Antibiotic	39	74%	84%	83%	94%
Blood Culture Timing[1]	20	100%	90%	90%	100%
Influenza Vaccine[1]	10	80%	56%	70%	100%
Initial Antibiotic Timing	40	82%	73%	80%	93%
Oxygenation Assessment	44	100%	99%	99%	100%
Pneumococcal Vaccine	27	93%	56%	69%	94%
Smoking Cessation Advice[1]	14	71%	58%	80%	100%
Surgical Infection Prevention					
Prophylactic Antibiotic Given[3]	49	55%	71%	77%	95%
Prophylactic Antibiotic Selection[1]	15	87%	87%	90%	100%
Prophylactic Antibiotic Stopped[3]	43	81%	81%	72%	95%
Pregnancy Care					
Inpatient Neonatal Mortality	-	-	-	-	-
Third or Fourth Degree Laceration	-	-	-	3.63%	3.27%

ACL-IHS Hospital

PO Box 130
San Fidel, NM 87049
URL: www.ihs.gov
Ownership: Government - Federal
Emergency Services: Yes

Phone: 505-552-5300
Fax: 505-552-5490
Accredited: Yes
Licensed Beds: 25

Key Personnel:
CEO. . . . . William Thorne Jr

Measure	Cases	This Hospital	State Average	U.S. Average	Top Hospital
Heart Attack Care					
ACE Inhibitor or ARB for LVSD[5]	-	-	71%	82%	100%
Aspirin at Arrival[5]	-	-	87%	92%	100%
Aspirin at Discharge[5]	-	-	87%	90%	100%
Beta Blocker at Arrival[5]	-	-	76%	87%	100%
Beta Blocker at Discharge[5]	-	-	83%	90%	100%
Fibrinolytic Medication Timing[5]	-	-	21%	31%	100%
PCI Within 90 Minutes of Arrival[5]	-	-	52%	54%	95%
Smoking Cessation Advice[5]	-	-	78%	88%	100%
Heart Failure Care					
ACE Inhibitor or ARB for LVSD[1,3]	2	50%	76%	82%	100%
Discharge Instructions[5]	-	-	27%	61%	93%
Evaluation of LVS Function[1,3]	3	100%	66%	83%	99%
Smoking Cessation Advice[5]	-	-	51%	82%	100%
Pneumonia Care					
Appropriate Initial Antibiotic[1,3]	3	100%	84%	83%	94%
Blood Culture Timing[1,3]	4	75%	90%	90%	100%
Influenza Vaccine[5]	-	-	56%	70%	100%
Initial Antibiotic Timing	49	76%	73%	80%	93%
Oxygenation Assessment	50	98%	99%	99%	100%
Pneumococcal Vaccine	31	90%	56%	69%	94%
Smoking Cessation Advice[3]	0	-	58%	80%	100%
Surgical Infection Prevention					
Prophylactic Antibiotic Given[5]	-	-	71%	77%	95%
Prophylactic Antibiotic Selection[5]	-	-	87%	90%	100%
Prophylactic Antibiotic Stopped[5]	-	-	81%	72%	95%
Pregnancy Care					
Inpatient Neonatal Mortality	-	-	-	-	-
Third or Fourth Degree Laceration	-	-	-	3.63%	3.27%

PHS Indian Hospital

1700 Cerrillos Road
Santa Fe, NM 87505

Toll-Free: 800-871-1562
Phone: 505-988-9821
Fax: 505-986-0751

URL: www.ihs.gov
Ownership: Government - Federal
Emergency Services: Yes

Accredited: Yes
Licensed Beds: 39

Key Personnel:
CEO. . . . . Richard Zethier

Measure	Cases	This Hospital	State Average	U.S. Average	Top Hospital
Heart Attack Care					
ACE Inhibitor or ARB for LVSD[3]	0	-	71%	82%	100%
Aspirin at Arrival[1,3]	2	0%	87%	92%	100%
Aspirin at Discharge[1,3]	1	0%	87%	90%	100%
Beta Blocker at Arrival[1,3]	2	0%	76%	87%	100%
Beta Blocker at Discharge[1,3]	1	0%	83%	90%	100%
Fibrinolytic Medication Timing[5]	-	-	21%	31%	100%
PCI Within 90 Minutes of Arrival[5]	-	-	52%	54%	95%
Smoking Cessation Advice[5]	-	-	78%	88%	100%
Heart Failure Care					
ACE Inhibitor or ARB for LVSD[3]	0	-	76%	82%	100%
Discharge Instructions[1,3]	2	0%	27%	61%	93%
Evaluation of LVS Function[1,3]	5	0%	66%	83%	99%
Smoking Cessation Advice[3]	0	-	51%	82%	100%
Pneumonia Care					
Appropriate Initial Antibiotic[5]	-	-	84%	83%	94%
Blood Culture Timing[5]	-	-	90%	90%	100%
Influenza Vaccine[5]	-	-	56%	70%	100%
Initial Antibiotic Timing[1,3]	6	83%	73%	80%	93%
Oxygenation Assessment[1,3]	18	100%	99%	99%	100%
Pneumococcal Vaccine[1,3]	12	92%	56%	69%	94%
Smoking Cessation Advice[5]	-	-	58%	80%	100%
Surgical Infection Prevention					
Prophylactic Antibiotic Given[5]	-	-	71%	77%	95%
Prophylactic Antibiotic Selection[5]	-	-	87%	90%	100%
Prophylactic Antibiotic Stopped[5]	-	-	81%	72%	95%
Pregnancy Care					
Inpatient Neonatal Mortality	-	-	-	-	-
Third or Fourth Degree Laceration	-	-	-	3.63%	3.27%

Saint Vincent Regional Medical Center

455 Saint Michael's Drive
Santa Fe, NM 87505
E-mail: ContactUs@stvin.org
URL: www.stvin.org
Ownership: Proprietary
Emergency Services: Yes

Phone: 505-983-3361
Fax: 505-989-6408

Accredited: Yes
Licensed Beds: 268

Key Personnel:
President/CEO. . . . . Alex Valdez, MD
Chief Medical Staff. . . . . Gary Frank, MD
OB/GYN Womens Health. . . . . Maria Rodriguez, MD

Measure	Cases	This Hospital	State Average	U.S. Average	Top Hospital

NOTE: Hospital profiles are in alphabetical order by state, then city, then hospital within the city; Rankings are sorted by rate in descending order and exclude hospitals with less than 25 cases; (1) The number of cases is too small (n<25) for purposes of reliably predicting hospital performance; (2) Measure reflects the hospital's indication that its submission was based upon a sample of its relevant discharges; (3) Rate reflects fewer than the maximum possible quarters of data for the measure; (4) Inaccurate information submitted and suppressed for one or more quarters; (5) No data is available from the hospital for this measure; Please refer to the User's Guide for a full explanation of data

Measure	Cases	This Hospital	State Average	U.S. Average	Top Hospital
Heart Attack Care					
ACE Inhibitor or ARB for LVSD	27	100%	71%	82%	100%
Aspirin at Arrival	120	97%	87%	92%	100%
Aspirin at Discharge	170	93%	87%	90%	100%
Beta Blocker at Arrival	97	94%	76%	87%	100%
Beta Blocker at Discharge	168	96%	83%	90%	100%
Fibrinolytic Medication Timing	0	-	21%	31%	100%
PCI Within 90 Minutes of Arrival[1]	7	29%	52%	54%	95%
Smoking Cessation Advice	63	90%	78%	88%	100%
Heart Failure Care					
ACE Inhibitor or ARB for LVSD	69	91%	76%	82%	100%
Discharge Instructions	152	5%	27%	61%	93%
Evaluation of LVS Function	169	95%	66%	83%	99%
Smoking Cessation Advice[1]	24	54%	51%	82%	100%
Pneumonia Care					
Appropriate Initial Antibiotic	160	83%	84%	83%	94%
Blood Culture Timing	130	73%	90%	90%	100%
Influenza Vaccine[4,5]	-	-	56%	70%	100%
Initial Antibiotic Timing	184	74%	73%	80%	93%
Oxygenation Assessment	232	99%	99%	99%	100%
Pneumococcal Vaccine	134	51%	56%	69%	94%
Smoking Cessation Advice	42	57%	58%	80%	100%
Surgical Infection Prevention					
Prophylactic Antibiotic Given	732	71%	71%	77%	95%
Prophylactic Antibiotic Selection	165	92%	87%	90%	100%
Prophylactic Antibiotic Stopped	658	74%	81%	72%	95%
Pregnancy Care					
Inpatient Neonatal Mortality	-	-	-	-	-
Third or Fourth Degree Laceration	-	-	-	3.63%	3.27%

Guadalupe County Hospital

535 Lake Drive
Santa Rosa, NM 88435
Ownership: Government - Local
Emergency Services: Yes
Phone: 505-472-3417
Fax: 505-472-4587
Accredited: No
Licensed Beds: 12

Key Personnel:

CEO. . . . . Christina Tampos
Chief Medical Staff. . . . . Mubarak Khawaja
Director Respiratory Therapy . . . . Anastacia Baka

Measure	Cases	This Hospital	State Average	U.S. Average	Top Hospital
Heart Attack Care					
ACE Inhibitor or ARB for LVSD[3]	0	-	71%	82%	100%
Aspirin at Arrival[1,3]	1	100%	87%	92%	100%
Aspirin at Discharge[1,3]	1	100%	87%	90%	100%
Beta Blocker at Arrival[3]	0	-	76%	87%	100%
Beta Blocker at Discharge[1,3]	1	100%	83%	90%	100%
Fibrinolytic Medication Timing[3]	0	-	21%	31%	100%
PCI Within 90 Minutes of Arrival	0	-	52%	54%	95%
Smoking Cessation Advice[1,3]	1	100%	78%	88%	100%
Heart Failure Care					
ACE Inhibitor or ARB for LVSD[1]	2	100%	76%	82%	100%
Discharge Instructions[1,3]	1	100%	27%	61%	93%
Evaluation of LVS Function[1]	10	90%	66%	83%	99%
Smoking Cessation Advice[3]	0	-	51%	82%	100%
Pneumonia Care					
Appropriate Initial Antibiotic[3]	0	-	84%	83%	94%
Blood Culture Timing[3]	0	-	90%	90%	100%
Influenza Vaccine[5]	-	-	56%	70%	100%
Initial Antibiotic Timing[1]	9	89%	73%	80%	93%
Oxygenation Assessment[1]	19	100%	99%	99%	100%
Pneumococcal Vaccine[1]	7	71%	56%	69%	94%
Smoking Cessation Advice[1,3]	1	100%	58%	80%	100%
Surgical Infection Prevention					
Prophylactic Antibiotic Given[5]	-	-	71%	77%	95%
Prophylactic Antibiotic Selection[5]	-	-	87%	90%	100%
Prophylactic Antibiotic Stopped[5]	-	-	81%	72%	95%
Pregnancy Care					
Inpatient Neonatal Mortality	-	-	-	-	-
Third or Fourth Degree Laceration	-	-	-	3.63%	3.27%

Northern Navajo Medical Center

Alternate Name: PHS Indian Hospital
PO Box 160
Shiprock, NM 87420
Ownership: Government - Federal
Emergency Services: Yes
Phone: 505-368-6001
Fax: 505-368-6260
Accredited: Yes
Licensed Beds: 75

Key Personnel:

CEO. . . . . Carla Baha-Al-Chesay
Chief of Medical Staff . . . . John Mohs
Emergency Room . . . . Elizabeth Israel
Emergency Room . . . . Steve Bowers
Director Infection/Disease Control . . . . Linda Schweigman, RN
Director Medical/Surgical Nursing . . . . Sandra Colins, RN
OB/GYN Womens Health. . . . . Phillip Weaver
Chief Radiology . . . . William Kauffman
Director Respiratory Therapy . . . . Marilyn Rodriquez-Bowma

Measure	Cases	This Hospital	State Average	U.S. Average	Top Hospital
Heart Attack Care					
ACE Inhibitor or ARB for LVSD[3]	0	-	71%	82%	100%
Aspirin at Arrival[1,3]	4	100%	87%	92%	100%
Aspirin at Discharge[1,3]	1	100%	87%	90%	100%
Beta Blocker at Arrival[1,3]	4	75%	76%	87%	100%
Beta Blocker at Discharge[1,3]	1	100%	83%	90%	100%
Fibrinolytic Medication Timing[3]	0	-	21%	31%	100%
PCI Within 90 Minutes of Arrival	0	-	52%	54%	95%
Smoking Cessation Advice[3]	0	-	78%	88%	100%
Heart Failure Care					
ACE Inhibitor or ARB for LVSD[1]	16	75%	76%	82%	100%
Discharge Instructions[1,3]	9	0%	27%	61%	93%
Evaluation of LVS Function	42	60%	66%	83%	99%
Smoking Cessation Advice[1,3]	2	0%	51%	82%	100%
Pneumonia Care					
Appropriate Initial Antibiotic[1,3]	19	95%	84%	83%	94%
Blood Culture Timing[1,3]	7	86%	90%	90%	100%
Influenza Vaccine[5]	-	-	56%	70%	100%
Initial Antibiotic Timing	95	78%	73%	80%	93%
Oxygenation Assessment	120	98%	99%	99%	100%
Pneumococcal Vaccine	84	40%	56%	69%	94%
Smoking Cessation Advice[1,3]	1	0%	58%	80%	100%
Surgical Infection Prevention					
Prophylactic Antibiotic Given[5]	-	-	71%	77%	95%
Prophylactic Antibiotic Selection[5]	-	-	87%	90%	100%
Prophylactic Antibiotic Stopped[5]	-	-	81%	72%	95%
Pregnancy Care					
Inpatient Neonatal Mortality	-	-	-	-	-
Third or Fourth Degree Laceration	-	-	-	3.63%	3.27%

Gila Regional Medical Center

1313 E 32nd Street
Silver City, NM 88061
Ownership: Govt - Hospital District or Authority
Emergency Services: No
Phone: 505-538-4000
Fax: 505-538-2824
Accredited: No
Licensed Beds: 68

Key Personnel:

CEO. . . . . Steven Daniel
Chief Medical Staff. . . . . Robert Wilcox, MD
Emergency Room . . . . Bill Neely, MD

Measure	Cases	This Hospital	State Average	U.S. Average	Top Hospital
Heart Attack Care					
ACE Inhibitor or ARB for LVSD	0	-	71%	82%	100%
Aspirin at Arrival[1]	9	100%	87%	92%	100%
Aspirin at Discharge[1]	6	83%	87%	90%	100%
Beta Blocker at Arrival[1]	9	100%	76%	87%	100%
Beta Blocker at Discharge[1]	6	100%	83%	90%	100%
Fibrinolytic Medication Timing[1]	11	45%	21%	31%	100%
PCI Within 90 Minutes of Arrival	0	-	52%	54%	95%
Smoking Cessation Advice[1]	1	100%	78%	88%	100%
Heart Failure Care					
ACE Inhibitor or ARB for LVSD[1]	20	70%	76%	82%	100%
Discharge Instructions	95	16%	27%	61%	93%
Evaluation of LVS Function	117	50%	66%	83%	99%
Smoking Cessation Advice[1]	11	27%	51%	82%	100%

NOTE: Hospital profiles are in alphabetical order by state, then city, then hospital within the city; Rankings are sorted by rate in descending order and exclude hospitals with less than 25 cases; (1) The number of cases is too small (n<25) for purposes of reliably predicting hospital performance; (2) Measure reflects the hospital's indication that its submission was based upon a sample of its relevant discharges; (3) Rate reflects fewer than the maximum possible quarters of data for the measure; (4) Inaccurate information submitted and suppressed for one or more quarters; (5) No data is available from the hospital for this measure; Please refer to the User's Guide for a full explanation of data

Pneumonia Care					
Appropriate Initial Antibiotic	103	93%	84%	83%	94%
Blood Culture Timing	74	96%	90%	90%	100%
Influenza Vaccine[1]	20	60%	56%	70%	100%
Initial Antibiotic Timing	141	91%	73%	80%	93%
Oxygenation Assessment	144	100%	99%	99%	100%
Pneumococcal Vaccine	90	48%	56%	69%	94%
Smoking Cessation Advice	25	48%	58%	80%	100%
Surgical Infection Prevention					
Prophylactic Antibiotic Given[3]	223	52%	71%	77%	95%
Prophylactic Antibiotic Selection	71	93%	87%	90%	100%
Prophylactic Antibiotic Stopped[3]	208	44%	81%	72%	95%
Pregnancy Care					
Inpatient Neonatal Mortality	-	-	-	-	-
Third or Fourth Degree Laceration	-	-	-	3.63%	3.27%

Socorro General Hospital

1202 Highway 60 W
PO Box 1009
Socorro, NM 87801
Phone: 505-835-1140
Fax: 505-835-8703
URL: www.phs.org
Ownership: Voluntary non-profit - Private
Accredited: Yes
Emergency Services: Yes

Measure	Cases	This Hospital	State Average	U.S. Average	Top Hospital
Heart Attack Care					
ACE Inhibitor or ARB for LVSD[3]	0	-	71%	82%	100%
Aspirin at Arrival[1,3]	1	100%	87%	92%	100%
Aspirin at Discharge[1,3]	1	100%	87%	90%	100%
Beta Blocker at Arrival[1,3]	1	100%	76%	87%	100%
Beta Blocker at Discharge[1,3]	1	100%	83%	90%	100%
Fibrinolytic Medication Timing[3]	0	-	21%	31%	100%
PCI Within 90 Minutes of Arrival[5]	-	-	52%	54%	95%
Smoking Cessation Advice[1,3]	1	100%	78%	88%	100%
Heart Failure Care					
ACE Inhibitor or ARB for LVSD[1]	11	64%	76%	82%	100%
Discharge Instructions[1]	19	26%	27%	61%	93%
Evaluation of LVS Function	31	48%	66%	83%	99%
Smoking Cessation Advice[1]	5	80%	51%	82%	100%
Pneumonia Care					
Appropriate Initial Antibiotic	42	79%	84%	83%	94%
Blood Culture Timing[1]	17	76%	90%	90%	100%
Influenza Vaccine[1]	12	83%	56%	70%	100%
Initial Antibiotic Timing	41	76%	73%	80%	93%
Oxygenation Assessment	46	100%	99%	99%	100%
Pneumococcal Vaccine	29	59%	56%	69%	94%
Smoking Cessation Advice[1]	18	72%	58%	80%	100%
Surgical Infection Prevention					
Prophylactic Antibiotic Given[1,3]	1	100%	71%	77%	95%
Prophylactic Antibiotic Selection[5]	-	-	87%	90%	100%
Prophylactic Antibiotic Stopped[1,3]	1	100%	81%	72%	95%
Pregnancy Care					
Inpatient Neonatal Mortality	222	0.00%	-	-	-
Third or Fourth Degree Laceration	161	0.62%	-	3.63%	3.27%

Sierra Vista Hospital

800 E 9th Avanue
Truth or Consequences, NM 87901
Phone: 505-894-2111
Fax: 505-894-7659
Ownership: Govt - Hospital District or Authority
Accredited: Yes
Emergency Services: Yes

Key Personnel:

Administrator/CEO. . . . . James J Cliborne, JR
Coordinator Emergency Room. . . . . Dolly Creller, RN
Infection Control. . . . . Mary Hubble, RN
Respiratory/Cardiopulmonary. . . . . Jamie Pruna, CRTT

Measure	Cases	This Hospital	State Average	U.S. Average	Top Hospital
Heart Attack Care					
ACE Inhibitor or ARB for LVSD[3]	0	-	71%	82%	100%
Aspirin at Arrival[3]	0	-	87%	92%	100%
Aspirin at Discharge[3]	0	-	87%	90%	100%
Beta Blocker at Arrival[3]	0	-	76%	87%	100%
Beta Blocker at Discharge[3]	0	-	83%	90%	100%
Fibrinolytic Medication Timing[3]	0	-	21%	31%	100%
PCI Within 90 Minutes of Arrival[5]	-	-	52%	54%	95%
Smoking Cessation Advice[3]	0	-	78%	88%	100%
Heart Failure Care					
ACE Inhibitor or ARB for LVSD	0	-	76%	82%	100%
Discharge Instructions[1]	16	6%	27%	61%	93%
Evaluation of LVS Function[1]	20	15%	66%	83%	99%
Smoking Cessation Advice[1]	3	0%	51%	82%	100%
Pneumonia Care					
Appropriate Initial Antibiotic[1]	23	74%	84%	83%	94%
Blood Culture Timing[1]	15	80%	90%	90%	100%
Influenza Vaccine[1]	5	40%	56%	70%	100%
Initial Antibiotic Timing	39	77%	73%	80%	93%
Oxygenation Assessment	45	96%	99%	99%	100%
Pneumococcal Vaccine	29	66%	56%	69%	94%
Smoking Cessation Advice[1]	13	31%	58%	80%	100%
Surgical Infection Prevention					
Prophylactic Antibiotic Given[5]	-	-	71%	77%	95%
Prophylactic Antibiotic Selection[5]	-	-	87%	90%	100%
Prophylactic Antibiotic Stopped[5]	-	-	81%	72%	95%
Pregnancy Care					
Inpatient Neonatal Mortality	-	-	-	-	-
Third or Fourth Degree Laceration	-	-	-	3.63%	3.27%

Holy Cross Hospital

1397 Weimer Road
PO Box DD
Taos, NM 87571
Toll-Free: 800-755-6236
Phone: 505-758-8883
Fax: 505-751-5719
E-mail: mcornum@taoshospital.org
URL: www.taoshospital.org
Ownership: Voluntary non-profit - Private
Accredited: No
Emergency Services: Yes
Licensed Beds: 49

Key Personnel:

CEO. . . . . Warren K Spellman
Emergency Room . . . . Lesa Fraker
Director Medical/Surgical Nursing . . . . Theresa Valerio
OB/GYN Womens Health. . . . . Sharon Mohling, MD
Director Respiratory Therapy . . . . Linda Hodapp

Measure	Cases	This Hospital	State Average	U.S. Average	Top Hospital
Heart Attack Care					
ACE Inhibitor or ARB for LVSD[1]	1	100%	71%	82%	100%
Aspirin at Arrival[1]	5	80%	87%	92%	100%
Aspirin at Discharge[1]	1	100%	87%	90%	100%
Beta Blocker at Arrival[1]	4	50%	76%	87%	100%
Beta Blocker at Discharge[1]	1	100%	83%	90%	100%
Fibrinolytic Medication Timing	0	-	21%	31%	100%
PCI Within 90 Minutes of Arrival	0	-	52%	54%	95%
Smoking Cessation Advice	0	-	78%	88%	100%
Heart Failure Care					
ACE Inhibitor or ARB for LVSD[1]	14	79%	76%	82%	100%
Discharge Instructions	39	18%	27%	61%	93%
Evaluation of LVS Function	49	90%	66%	83%	99%
Smoking Cessation Advice[1]	7	86%	51%	82%	100%
Pneumonia Care					
Appropriate Initial Antibiotic	88	84%	84%	83%	94%
Blood Culture Timing	91	81%	90%	90%	100%
Influenza Vaccine[4,5]	-	-	56%	70%	100%
Initial Antibiotic Timing	134	81%	73%	80%	93%
Oxygenation Assessment	163	100%	99%	99%	100%
Pneumococcal Vaccine	105	44%	56%	69%	94%
Smoking Cessation Advice[1]	19	95%	58%	80%	100%
Surgical Infection Prevention					
Prophylactic Antibiotic Given[1,3]	15	73%	71%	77%	95%
Prophylactic Antibiotic Selection[1]	15	100%	87%	90%	100%
Prophylactic Antibiotic Stopped[1,3]	14	100%	81%	72%	95%
Pregnancy Care					
Inpatient Neonatal Mortality	-	-	-	-	-
Third or Fourth Degree Laceration	-	-	-	3.63%	3.27%

NOTE: Hospital profiles are in alphabetical order by state, then city, then hospital within the city; Rankings are sorted by rate in descending order and exclude hospitals with less than 25 cases; (1) The number of cases is too small (n<25) for purposes of reliably predicting hospital performance; (2) Measure reflects the hospital's indication that its submission was based upon a sample of its relevant discharges; (3) Rate reflects fewer than the maximum possible quarters of data for the measure; (4) Inaccurate information submitted and suppressed for one or more quarters; (5) No data is available from the hospital for this measure; Please refer to the User's Guide for a full explanation of data

Doctor Dan C Trigg Memorial Hospital

301 E Miel de Luna
PO Box 608
Tucumcari, NM 88401
URL: www.phs.org
Ownership: Government - Federal
Emergency Services: No
Phone: 505-461-0141
Fax: 505-461-7272
Accredited: No
Licensed Beds: 25

Key Personnel:
CEO/President. . . . . Bo Beames
Chief Medical Staff. . . . . John Faith
Emergency Room Director. . . . . Debbie Stoner
Emergency Room . . . . Twila Loudder
Respiratory Care . . . . Vicki Kirby

Measure	Cases	This Hospital	State Average	U.S. Average	Top Hospital
Heart Attack Care					
ACE Inhibitor or ARB for LVSD[3]	0	-	71%	82%	100%
Aspirin at Arrival[1,3]	2	100%	87%	92%	100%
Aspirin at Discharge[1,3]	6	83%	87%	90%	100%
Beta Blocker at Arrival[1,3]	2	100%	76%	87%	100%
Beta Blocker at Discharge[1,3]	6	67%	83%	90%	100%
Fibrinolytic Medication Timing[1,3]	1	0%	21%	31%	100%
PCI Within 90 Minutes of Arrival	0	-	52%	54%	95%
Smoking Cessation Advice[1,3]	1	0%	78%	88%	100%
Heart Failure Care					
ACE Inhibitor or ARB for LVSD	0	-	76%	82%	100%
Discharge Instructions[1]	12	0%	27%	61%	93%
Evaluation of LVS Function[1]	17	0%	66%	83%	99%
Smoking Cessation Advice[1]	2	0%	51%	82%	100%
Pneumonia Care					
Appropriate Initial Antibiotic	26	77%	84%	83%	94%
Blood Culture Timing[1]	10	100%	90%	90%	100%
Influenza Vaccine[1]	9	0%	56%	70%	100%
Initial Antibiotic Timing	36	72%	73%	80%	93%
Oxygenation Assessment	40	100%	99%	99%	100%
Pneumococcal Vaccine	26	8%	56%	69%	94%
Smoking Cessation Advice[1]	6	33%	58%	80%	100%
Surgical Infection Prevention					
Prophylactic Antibiotic Given[5]	-	-	71%	77%	95%
Prophylactic Antibiotic Selection[5]	-	-	87%	90%	100%
Prophylactic Antibiotic Stopped[5]	-	-	81%	72%	95%
Pregnancy Care					
Inpatient Neonatal Mortality	-	-	-	-	-
Third or Fourth Degree Laceration	-	-	-	3.63%	3.27%

Zuni Hospital

Route 301 North B Street
Zuni, NM 87327
URL: www.ihs.gov
Ownership: Government - Federal
Emergency Services: Yes
Phone: 505-782-4431
Fax: 505-782-7405
Accredited: Yes
Licensed Beds: 45

Key Personnel:
Administrator . . . . Jean Othole
Chief Medical Staff. . . . . David Kessler
Director Infection/Disease Control . . . . Virginia Lasiloo
Chief Radiology . . . . Glorietta Laweka

Measure	Cases	This Hospital	State Average	U.S. Average	Top Hospital
Heart Attack Care					
ACE Inhibitor or ARB for LVSD[5]	-	-	71%	82%	100%
Aspirin at Arrival[5]	-	-	87%	92%	100%
Aspirin at Discharge[5]	-	-	87%	90%	100%
Beta Blocker at Arrival[5]	-	-	76%	87%	100%
Beta Blocker at Discharge[5]	-	-	83%	90%	100%
Fibrinolytic Medication Timing[5]	-	-	21%	31%	100%
PCI Within 90 Minutes of Arrival[5]	-	-	52%	54%	95%
Smoking Cessation Advice[5]	-	-	78%	88%	100%
Heart Failure Care					
ACE Inhibitor or ARB for LVSD[3]	0	-	76%	82%	100%
Discharge Instructions[1,3]	2	0%	27%	61%	93%
Evaluation of LVS Function[1,3]	2	50%	66%	83%	99%
Smoking Cessation Advice[3]	0	-	51%	82%	100%
Pneumonia Care					
Appropriate Initial Antibiotic[1,3]	2	100%	84%	83%	94%
Blood Culture Timing[1,3]	5	100%	90%	90%	100%
Influenza Vaccine[5]	-	-	56%	70%	100%
Initial Antibiotic Timing[1]	18	89%	73%	80%	93%
Oxygenation Assessment	33	94%	99%	99%	100%
Pneumococcal Vaccine[1]	22	5%	56%	69%	94%
Smoking Cessation Advice[3]	0	-	58%	80%	100%
Surgical Infection Prevention					
Prophylactic Antibiotic Given[5]	-	-	71%	77%	95%
Prophylactic Antibiotic Selection[5]	-	-	87%	90%	100%
Prophylactic Antibiotic Stopped[5]	-	-	81%	72%	95%
Pregnancy Care					
Inpatient Neonatal Mortality	-	-	-	-	-
Third or Fourth Degree Laceration	-	-	-	3.63%	3.27%

NOTE: Hospital profiles are in alphabetical order by state, then city, then hospital within the city; Rankings are sorted by rate in descending order and exclude hospitals with less than 25 cases; (1) The number of cases is too small (n<25) for purposes of reliably predicting hospital performance; (2) Measure reflects the hospital's indication that its submission was based upon a sample of its relevant discharges; (3) Rate reflects fewer than the maximum possible quarters of data for the measure; (4) Inaccurate information submitted and suppressed for one or more quarters; (5) No data is available from the hospital for this measure; Please refer to the User's Guide for a full explanation of data

Heart Attack Care

1. ACE Inhibitor or ARB for LVSD

Hospital Name	City	Rate	Cases
Providence Portland Medical Center	Portland	98%	106
Rogue Valley Medical Center	Medford	95%	58
Saint Charles Medical Center-Bend-Redmond	Bend	94%	48
Good Samaritan Regional Medical Center	Corvallis	90%	30
Providence Saint Vincent Medical Center	Portland	90%	136
Sacred Heart Medical Center	Eugene	89%	149
Oregon Health Sciences University	Portland	86%	28
Legacy Emanuel Hospital/Health Center	Portland	83%	35
Legacy Meridian Park Hospital	Tualatin	82%	34
Salem Hospital	Salem	73%	67
Legacy Good Samaritan Hospital	Portland	66%	76

2. Aspirin at Arrival

Hospital Name	City	Rate	Cases
Providence Milwaukie Hospital	Portland	100%	41
Good Samaritan Regional Medical Center	Corvallis	99%	96
Legacy Good Samaritan Hospital	Portland	99%	122
Oregon Health Sciences University	Portland	99%	73
Providence Saint Vincent Medical Center	Portland	99%	716
Rogue Valley Medical Center	Medford	99%	219
Salem Hospital	Salem	99%	343
Kaiser Sunnyside Medical Center	Clackamas	98%	137
Providence Medford Medical Center	Medford	98%	64
Providence Portland Medical Center	Portland	98%	389
Sacred Heart Medical Center	Eugene	98%	302
Saint Charles Medical Center-Bend-Redmond	Bend	98%	244
Legacy Emanuel Hospital/Health Center	Portland	97%	73
Legacy Mount Hood Medical Center	Gresham	97%	36
McKenzie-Willamette Medical Center	Springfield	97%	74
Mercy Medical Center	Roseburg	97%	76
Merle West Medical Center	Klamath Falls	96%	73
Portland Adventist Medical Center	Portland	96%	96
Tuality Community Hospital	Hillsboro	95%	131
Legacy Meridian Park Hospital	Tualatin	94%	108
Willamette Valley Medical Center	McMinnville	94%	36
Three Rivers Community Hospital/Health Center	Grants Pass	93%	83
Saint Charles Medical Center-Redmond	Redmond	92%	40
Willamette Falls Hospital	Oregon City	92%	52

3. Aspirin at Discharge

Hospital Name	City	Rate	Cases
Good Samaritan Regional Medical Center	Corvallis	100%	206
Kaiser Sunnyside Medical Center	Clackamas	100%	98
Providence Medford Medical Center	Medford	100%	45
Oregon Health Sciences University	Portland	99%	93
Providence Portland Medical Center	Portland	99%	545
Rogue Valley Medical Center	Medford	99%	421
Sacred Heart Medical Center	Eugene	99%	606
Legacy Emanuel Hospital/Health Center	Portland	98%	129
Legacy Good Samaritan Hospital	Portland	98%	272
Portland Adventist Medical Center	Portland	98%	88
Providence Saint Vincent Medical Center	Portland	98%	1008
Saint Charles Medical Center-Bend-Redmond	Bend	98%	339
Salem Hospital	Salem	98%	387
Merle West Medical Center	Klamath Falls	97%	65
Tuality Community Hospital	Hillsboro	94%	125
Legacy Meridian Park Hospital	Tualatin	92%	75
Providence Milwaukie Hospital	Portland	92%	25
McKenzie-Willamette Medical Center	Springfield	90%	39
Mercy Medical Center	Roseburg	90%	41
Three Rivers Community Hospital/Health Center	Grants Pass	88%	52
Saint Charles Medical Center-Redmond	Redmond	80%	25

4. Beta Blocker at Arrival

Hospital Name	City	Rate	Cases
Kaiser Sunnyside Medical Center	Clackamas	100%	132
Oregon Health Sciences University	Portland	98%	62
Providence Portland Medical Center	Portland	98%	336
Rogue Valley Medical Center	Medford	98%	162
Legacy Good Samaritan Hospital	Portland	97%	76
McKenzie-Willamette Medical Center	Springfield	97%	65
Providence Medford Medical Center	Medford	97%	60
Providence Milwaukie Hospital	Portland	97%	37
Salem Hospital	Salem	97%	296
Good Samaritan Regional Medical Center	Corvallis	96%	69
Providence Saint Vincent Medical Center	Portland	96%	648
Sacred Heart Medical Center	Eugene	96%	285
Mercy Medical Center	Roseburg	95%	81
Saint Charles Medical Center-Bend-Redmond	Bend	95%	195
Portland Adventist Medical Center	Portland	94%	50
Legacy Meridian Park Hospital	Tualatin	93%	75
Legacy Emanuel Hospital/Health Center	Portland	90%	42
Willamette Falls Hospital	Oregon City	90%	41
Merle West Medical Center	Klamath Falls	89%	57
Three Rivers Community Hospital/Health Center	Grants Pass	89%	72
Tuality Community Hospital	Hillsboro	85%	105
Saint Charles Medical Center-Redmond	Redmond	82%	34

5. Beta Blocker at Discharge

Hospital Name	City	Rate	Cases
Kaiser Sunnyside Medical Center	Clackamas	100%	112
Good Samaritan Regional Medical Center	Corvallis	99%	221
Legacy Emanuel Hospital/Health Center	Portland	99%	122
Oregon Health Sciences University	Portland	99%	93
Providence Portland Medical Center	Portland	99%	500
Sacred Heart Medical Center	Eugene	99%	665
Salem Hospital	Salem	99%	345
Portland Adventist Medical Center	Portland	98%	95
Rogue Valley Medical Center	Medford	97%	448
Legacy Meridian Park Hospital	Tualatin	96%	83
Providence Medford Medical Center	Medford	96%	52
Providence Milwaukie Hospital	Portland	96%	27
Providence Saint Vincent Medical Center	Portland	96%	923
Saint Charles Medical Center-Bend-Redmond	Bend	95%	293
Three Rivers Community Hospital/Health Center	Grants Pass	95%	43
Legacy Good Samaritan Hospital	Portland	94%	259
Mercy Medical Center	Roseburg	94%	48
Merle West Medical Center	Klamath Falls	92%	63
Tuality Community Hospital	Hillsboro	89%	130
McKenzie-Willamette Medical Center	Springfield	88%	42
Saint Charles Medical Center-Redmond	Redmond	85%	26

8. Smoking Cessation Advice

Hospital Name	City	Rate	Cases
Portland Adventist Medical Center	Portland	100%	32
Sacred Heart Medical Center	Eugene	99%	239
Saint Charles Medical Center-Bend-Redmond	Bend	98%	88
Providence Portland Medical Center	Portland	96%	154
Rogue Valley Medical Center	Medford	95%	142
Salem Hospital	Salem	95%	119
Good Samaritan Regional Medical Center	Corvallis	93%	86
Legacy Good Samaritan Hospital	Portland	91%	108
Legacy Emanuel Hospital/Health Center	Portland	89%	46
Providence Saint Vincent Medical Center	Portland	86%	297
Kaiser Sunnyside Medical Center	Clackamas	78%	32
Oregon Health Sciences University	Portland	77%	26
Tuality Community Hospital	Hillsboro	41%	37

Heart Failure Care

9. ACE Inhibitor or ARB for LVSD

Hospital Name	City	Rate	Cases
Oregon Health Sciences University	Portland	94%	108
Willamette Falls Hospital	Oregon City	94%	33
Portland Adventist Medical Center	Portland	93%	44
Providence Milwaukie Hospital	Portland	92%	37
Saint Charles Medical Center-Bend-Redmond	Bend	92%	84
Kaiser Sunnyside Medical Center	Clackamas	91%	85
Rogue Valley Medical Center	Medford	91%	221
Three Rivers Community Hospital/Health Center	Grants Pass	91%	65
Bay Area Hospital	Coos Bay	90%	80
Sacred Heart Medical Center	Eugene	90%	246
Merle West Medical Center	Klamath Falls	89%	46
Providence Portland Medical Center	Portland	89%	132
Good Samaritan Regional Medical Center	Corvallis	87%	63
Albany General Hospital	Albany	85%	40
Samaritan Lebanon Community Hospital	Lebanon	85%	26
Providence Saint Vincent Medical Center	Portland	80%	131
Willamette Valley Medical Center	McMinnville	79%	38
Legacy Emanuel Hospital/Health Center	Portland	77%	64
Mercy Medical Center	Roseburg	77%	61
Salem Hospital	Salem	77%	156
Legacy Meridian Park Hospital	Tualatin	75%	93
McKenzie-Willamette Medical Center	Springfield	74%	35
Providence Medford Medical Center	Medford	74%	39
Legacy Mount Hood Medical Center	Gresham	72%	36
Legacy Good Samaritan Hospital	Portland	66%	177
Tuality Community Hospital	Hillsboro	60%	47

NOTE: Hospital profiles are in alphabetical order by state, then city, then hospital within the city; Rankings are sorted by rate in descending order and exclude hospitals with less than 25 cases; (1) The number of cases is too small (n<25) for purposes of reliably predicting hospital performance; (2) Measure reflects the hospital's indication that its submission was based upon a sample of its relevant discharges; (3) Rate reflects fewer than the maximum possible quarters of data for the measure; (4) Inaccurate information submitted and suppressed for one or more quarters; (5) No data is available from the hospital for this measure; Please refer to the User's Guide for a full explanation of data

10. Discharge Instructions

Hospital Name	City	Rate	Cases
Mid-Columbia Medical Center	The Dalles	98%	50
Sacred Heart Medical Center	Eugene	93%	408
Willamette Valley Medical Center	McMinnville	85%	96
Tillamook County General Hospital	Tillamook	84%	38
Grande Ronde Hospital	La Grande	82%	45
Kaiser Sunnyside Medical Center	Clackamas	79%	246
McKenzie-Willamette Medical Center	Springfield	76%	91
Portland Adventist Medical Center	Portland	75%	133
Rogue Valley Medical Center	Medford	73%	402
Albany General Hospital	Albany	69%	97
Bay Area Hospital	Coos Bay	69%	106
Providence Portland Medical Center	Portland	61%	280
Salem Hospital	Salem	59%	303
Providence Saint Vincent Medical Center	Portland	57%	308
Good Samaritan Regional Medical Center	Corvallis	51%	123
Merle West Medical Center	Klamath Falls	51%	131
Saint Charles Medical Center-Bend-Redmond	Bend	49%	167
Samaritan Lebanon Community Hospital	Lebanon	46%	70
Columbia Memorial Hospital	Astoria	41%	44
Oregon Health Sciences University	Portland	41%	199
Saint Charles Medical Center-Redmond	Redmond	40%	40
Legacy Emanuel Hospital/Health Center	Portland	33%	107
Legacy Good Samaritan Hospital	Portland	30%	270
Legacy Meridian Park Hospital	Tualatin	30%	173
Holy Rosary Medical Center	Ontario	29%	51
Providence Milwaukie Hospital	Portland	27%	86
Tuality Community Hospital	Hillsboro	25%	134
Peace Harbor Hospital	Florence	24%	38
Samaritan North Lincoln Hospital	Lincoln City	24%	29
Samaritan Pacific Community Hospital	Newport	23%	39
Providence Newberg Hospital	Newberg	22%	41
Legacy Mount Hood Medical Center	Gresham	11%	84
Providence Medford Medical Center	Medford	10%	136
Providence Seaside Hospital	Seaside	10%	39
Three Rivers Community Hospital/Health Center	Grants Pass	6%	174
Mercy Medical Center	Roseburg	4%	215

11. Evaluation of LVS Function

Hospital Name	City	Rate	Cases
Willamette Valley Medical Center	McMinnville	100%	122
Sacred Heart Medical Center	Eugene	99%	476
Legacy Emanuel Hospital/Health Center	Portland	98%	126
Mid-Columbia Medical Center	The Dalles	98%	59
Oregon Health Sciences University	Portland	98%	216
Kaiser Sunnyside Medical Center	Clackamas	97%	274
Albany General Hospital	Albany	95%	123
Legacy Good Samaritan Hospital	Portland	95%	332
Portland Adventist Medical Center	Portland	95%	153
Salem Hospital	Salem	95%	388
McKenzie-Willamette Medical Center	Springfield	94%	131
Providence Portland Medical Center	Portland	94%	323
Rogue Valley Medical Center	Medford	94%	428
Grande Ronde Hospital	La Grande	93%	56
Legacy Meridian Park Hospital	Tualatin	93%	216
Legacy Mount Hood Medical Center	Gresham	93%	95
Providence Milwaukie Hospital	Portland	93%	105
Saint Charles Medical Center-Bend-Redmond	Bend	93%	178
Merle West Medical Center	Klamath Falls	92%	155
Providence Newberg Hospital	Newberg	91%	55
Peace Harbor Hospital	Florence	90%	39
Providence Saint Vincent Medical Center	Portland	90%	346
Saint Charles Medical Center-Redmond	Redmond	87%	45
Silverton Hospital	Silverton	87%	30
Willamette Falls Hospital	Oregon City	87%	118
Providence Medford Medical Center	Medford	85%	162
Good Samaritan Regional Medical Center	Corvallis	84%	149
Holy Rosary Medical Center	Ontario	82%	60
Three Rivers Community Hospital/Health Center	Grants Pass	82%	213
Tillamook County General Hospital	Tillamook	79%	38
Tuality Community Hospital	Hillsboro	78%	156
Samaritan Lebanon Community Hospital	Lebanon	77%	96
Bay Area Hospital	Coos Bay	76%	200
Samaritan Pacific Community Hospital	Newport	76%	37
Santiam Memorial Hospital	Stayton	76%	29
Mercy Medical Center	Roseburg	75%	240
Samaritan North Lincoln Hospital	Lincoln City	74%	43
Pioneer Memorial Hospital	Prineville	65%	34
Providence Seaside Hospital	Seaside	64%	45
Columbia Memorial Hospital	Astoria	47%	53

12. Smoking Cessation Advice

Hospital Name	City	Rate	Cases
Portland Adventist Medical Center	Portland	98%	45
Providence Portland Medical Center	Portland	98%	59
McKenzie-Willamette Medical Center	Springfield	96%	25
Willamette Valley Medical Center	McMinnville	96%	25
Sacred Heart Medical Center	Eugene	94%	79
Salem Hospital	Salem	92%	64
Saint Charles Medical Center-Bend-Redmond	Bend	87%	38
Rogue Valley Medical Center	Medford	85%	68
Kaiser Sunnyside Medical Center	Clackamas	80%	41
Legacy Emanuel Hospital/Health Center	Portland	79%	34
Providence Saint Vincent Medical Center	Portland	78%	41
Albany General Hospital	Albany	77%	26
Providence Milwaukie Hospital	Portland	73%	26
Mercy Medical Center	Roseburg	67%	27
Providence Medford Medical Center	Medford	65%	40
Legacy Good Samaritan Hospital	Portland	63%	62
Three Rivers Community Hospital/Health Center	Grants Pass	57%	35
Oregon Health Sciences University	Portland	49%	45

Pneumonia Care

13. Appropriate Initial Antibiotic

Hospital Name	City	Rate	Cases
Mountain View Hospital District	Madras	100%	28
Silverton Hospital	Silverton	94%	51
Sacred Heart Medical Center	Eugene	92%	295
Bay Area Hospital	Coos Bay	91%	93
Providence Hood River Memorial Hospital	Hood River	91%	43
Rogue Valley Medical Center	Medford	91%	188
Good Samaritan Regional Medical Center	Corvallis	90%	84
Legacy Mount Hood Medical Center	Gresham	90%	89
Merle West Medical Center	Klamath Falls	90%	139
Portland Adventist Medical Center	Portland	90%	164
Saint Charles Medical Center-Bend-Redmond	Bend	90%	136
Salem Hospital	Salem	90%	254
Tuality Community Hospital	Hillsboro	90%	128
Providence Saint Vincent Medical Center	Portland	89%	157
Mercy Medical Center	Roseburg	88%	139
Three Rivers Community Hospital/Health Center	Grants Pass	88%	232
Willamette Valley Medical Center	McMinnville	88%	132
Legacy Good Samaritan Hospital	Portland	87%	78
McKenzie-Willamette Medical Center	Springfield	87%	150
Providence Portland Medical Center	Portland	86%	125
Samaritan Lebanon Community Hospital	Lebanon	86%	95
Albany General Hospital	Albany	84%	142
Legacy Emanuel Hospital/Health Center	Portland	84%	69
Pioneer Memorial Hospital	Prineville	84%	25
Columbia Memorial Hospital	Astoria	83%	99
Good Shepherd Health Care System	Hermiston	83%	42
Providence Medford Medical Center	Medford	83%	107
Providence Seaside Hospital	Seaside	83%	41
Willamette Falls Hospital	Oregon City	83%	92
Ashland Community Hospital	Ashland	82%	33
Peace Harbor Hospital	Florence	82%	34
Tillamook County General Hospital	Tillamook	82%	50
Saint Charles Medical Center-Redmond	Redmond	81%	53
Samaritan Pacific Community Hospital	Newport	80%	49
Kaiser Sunnyside Medical Center	Clackamas	79%	90
Legacy Meridian Park Hospital	Tualatin	79%	89
Mid-Columbia Medical Center	The Dalles	79%	70
Southern Coos Hospital & Health Center	Bandon	79%	34
Cottage Grove Community Hospital	Cottage Grove	77%	44
Grande Ronde Hospital	La Grande	76%	89
Providence Milwaukie Hospital	Portland	76%	98
Santiam Memorial Hospital	Stayton	76%	42
Providence Newberg Hospital	Newberg	74%	50
Oregon Health Sciences University	Portland	72%	68
Samaritan North Lincoln Hospital	Lincoln City	72%	39
Holy Rosary Medical Center	Ontario	67%	83

14. Blood Culture Timing

Hospital Name	City	Rate	Cases
Three Rivers Community Hospital/Health Center	Grants Pass	98%	80
Legacy Mount Hood Medical Center	Gresham	97%	61
Portland Adventist Medical Center	Portland	97%	167
Willamette Valley Medical Center	McMinnville	97%	147
Legacy Good Samaritan Hospital	Portland	96%	67
Legacy Meridian Park Hospital	Tualatin	96%	72
Mid-Columbia Medical Center	The Dalles	96%	71
Rogue Valley Medical Center	Medford	96%	176
Oregon Health Sciences University	Portland	95%	84

NOTE: Hospital profiles are in alphabetical order by state, then city, then hospital within the city; Rankings are sorted by rate in descending order and exclude hospitals with less than 25 cases; (1) The number of cases is too small (n<25) for purposes of reliably predicting hospital performance; (2) Measure reflects the hospital's indication that its submission was based upon a sample of its relevant discharges; (3) Rate reflects fewer than the maximum possible quarters of data for the measure; (4) Inaccurate information submitted and suppressed for one or more quarters; (5) No data is available from the hospital for this measure; Please refer to the User's Guide for a full explanation of data

Hospital Name	City	Rate	Cases
Providence Portland Medical Center	Portland	94%	123
Sacred Heart Medical Center	Eugene	94%	345
Tuality Community Hospital	Hillsboro	94%	112
Willamette Falls Hospital	Oregon City	93%	56
Albany General Hospital	Albany	92%	118
Kaiser Sunnyside Medical Center	Clackamas	92%	86
McKenzie-Willamette Medical Center	Springfield	92%	142
Providence Newberg Hospital	Newberg	92%	36
Samaritan Lebanon Community Hospital	Lebanon	92%	61
Salem Hospital	Salem	91%	245
Silverton Hospital	Silverton	91%	34
Good Samaritan Regional Medical Center	Corvallis	90%	67
Providence Saint Vincent Medical Center	Portland	90%	147
Mercy Medical Center	Roseburg	88%	82
Merle West Medical Center	Klamath Falls	88%	105
Peace Harbor Hospital	Florence	88%	26
Bay Area Hospital	Coos Bay	86%	111
Legacy Emanuel Hospital/Health Center	Portland	86%	65
Providence Milwaukie Hospital	Portland	86%	79
Tillamook County General Hospital	Tillamook	86%	28
Saint Charles Medical Center-Bend-Redmond	Bend	85%	124
Providence Medford Medical Center	Medford	82%	68
Grande Ronde Hospital	La Grande	80%	41
Saint Charles Medical Center-Redmond	Redmond	80%	45
Holy Rosary Medical Center	Ontario	77%	30

15. Influenza Vaccine

Hospital Name	City	Rate	Cases
McKenzie-Willamette Medical Center	Springfield	97%	30
Willamette Valley Medical Center	McMinnville	96%	45
Salem Hospital	Salem	95%	78
Portland Adventist Medical Center	Portland	93%	42
Providence Portland Medical Center	Portland	92%	25
Albany General Hospital	Albany	90%	39
Grande Ronde Hospital	La Grande	89%	28
Sacred Heart Medical Center	Eugene	83%	112
Providence Milwaukie Hospital	Portland	74%	27
Rogue Valley Medical Center	Medford	69%	62
Bay Area Hospital	Coos Bay	67%	33
Merle West Medical Center	Klamath Falls	66%	35
Tuality Community Hospital	Hillsboro	62%	39
Providence Saint Vincent Medical Center	Portland	57%	28
Three Rivers Community Hospital/Health Center	Grants Pass	49%	59
Legacy Mount Hood Medical Center	Gresham	41%	27
Saint Charles Medical Center-Bend-Redmond	Bend	20%	41
Mercy Medical Center	Roseburg	8%	37

16. Initial Antibiotic Timing

Hospital Name	City	Rate	Cases
Tillamook County General Hospital	Tillamook	93%	45
Samaritan Lebanon Community Hospital	Lebanon	92%	118
Good Samaritan Regional Medical Center	Corvallis	91%	127
Legacy Meridian Park Hospital	Tualatin	91%	172
Silverton Hospital	Silverton	91%	53
Albany General Hospital	Albany	90%	176
Providence Hood River Memorial Hospital	Hood River	90%	48
Willamette Falls Hospital	Oregon City	90%	104
Bay Area Hospital	Coos Bay	89%	173
Mid-Columbia Medical Center	The Dalles	89%	83
Legacy Mount Hood Medical Center	Gresham	86%	140
Samaritan Pacific Community Hospital	Newport	86%	42
Columbia Memorial Hospital	Astoria	85%	100
McKenzie-Willamette Medical Center	Springfield	85%	206
Pioneer Memorial Hospital	Prineville	85%	34
Southern Coos Hospital & Health Center	Bandon	85%	39
Three Rivers Community Hospital/Health Center	Grants Pass	85%	275
Mountain View Hospital District	Madras	84%	37
Providence Milwaukie Hospital	Portland	84%	129
Tuality Community Hospital	Hillsboro	84%	172
Merle West Medical Center	Klamath Falls	83%	167
Ashland Community Hospital	Ashland	82%	34
Peace Harbor Hospital	Florence	82%	38
Providence Newberg Hospital	Newberg	82%	62
Portland Adventist Medical Center	Portland	81%	236
Sacred Heart Medical Center	Eugene	81%	526
Mercy Medical Center	Roseburg	80%	132
Providence Seaside Hospital	Seaside	80%	45
Providence Portland Medical Center	Portland	78%	179
Providence Saint Vincent Medical Center	Portland	78%	185
Saint Charles Medical Center-Redmond	Redmond	78%	69
Salem Hospital	Salem	78%	371
Willamette Valley Medical Center	McMinnville	78%	180
Samaritan North Lincoln Hospital	Lincoln City	77%	48
Grande Ronde Hospital	La Grande	76%	103
Holy Rosary Medical Center	Ontario	76%	84
Rogue Valley Medical Center	Medford	76%	259
Saint Charles Medical Center-Bend-Redmond	Bend	76%	184
Kaiser Sunnyside Medical Center	Clackamas	71%	122
Legacy Good Samaritan Hospital	Portland	71%	134
Good Shepherd Health Care System	Hermiston	70%	37
Providence Medford Medical Center	Medford	70%	132
Legacy Emanuel Hospital/Health Center	Portland	68%	102
Oregon Health Sciences University	Portland	64%	135
Santiam Memorial Hospital	Stayton	63%	43
Cottage Grove Community Hospital	Cottage Grove	61%	49

17. Oxygenation Assessment

Hospital Name	City	Rate	Cases
Albany General Hospital	Albany	100%	210
Ashland Community Hospital	Ashland	100%	48
Bay Area Hospital	Coos Bay	100%	211
Columbia Memorial Hospital	Astoria	100%	116
Coquille Valley Hospital	Coquille	100%	28
Cottage Grove Community Hospital	Cottage Grove	100%	60
Good Samaritan Regional Medical Center	Corvallis	100%	163
Kaiser Sunnyside Medical Center	Clackamas	100%	150
Legacy Good Samaritan Hospital	Portland	100%	152
Legacy Meridian Park Hospital	Tualatin	100%	186
Legacy Mount Hood Medical Center	Gresham	100%	159
McKenzie-Willamette Medical Center	Springfield	100%	249
Mercy Medical Center	Roseburg	100%	182
Merle West Medical Center	Klamath Falls	100%	199
Mid-Columbia Medical Center	The Dalles	100%	103
Mountain View Hospital District	Madras	100%	42
Oregon Health Sciences University	Portland	100%	167
Peace Harbor Hospital	Florence	100%	51
Pioneer Memorial Hospital	Prineville	100%	40
Portland Adventist Medical Center	Portland	100%	304
Providence Hood River Memorial Hospital	Hood River	100%	61
Providence Medford Medical Center	Medford	100%	166
Providence Milwaukie Hospital	Portland	100%	156
Providence Newberg Hospital	Newberg	100%	78
Providence Portland Medical Center	Portland	100%	215
Providence Saint Vincent Medical Center	Portland	100%	230
Providence Seaside Hospital	Seaside	100%	56
Rogue Valley Medical Center	Medford	100%	325
Sacred Heart Medical Center	Eugene	100%	624
Saint Charles Medical Center-Bend-Redmond	Bend	100%	226
Saint Charles Medical Center-Redmond	Redmond	100%	81
Salem Hospital	Salem	100%	478
Samaritan Lebanon Community Hospital	Lebanon	100%	139
Samaritan North Lincoln Hospital	Lincoln City	100%	59
Samaritan Pacific Community Hospital	Newport	100%	58
Santiam Memorial Hospital	Stayton	100%	61
Silverton Hospital	Silverton	100%	67
Southern Coos Hospital & Health Center	Bandon	100%	45
Three Rivers Community Hospital/Health Center	Grants Pass	100%	323
Tillamook County General Hospital	Tillamook	100%	59
Tuality Community Hospital	Hillsboro	100%	209
Willamette Falls Hospital	Oregon City	100%	129
Willamette Valley Medical Center	McMinnville	100%	224
Grande Ronde Hospital	La Grande	99%	128
Holy Rosary Medical Center	Ontario	99%	106
Legacy Emanuel Hospital/Health Center	Portland	99%	110
Good Shepherd Health Care System	Hermiston	96%	45

18. Pneumococcal Vaccine

Hospital Name	City	Rate	Cases
Peace Harbor Hospital	Florence	91%	35
Providence Seaside Hospital	Seaside	91%	33
Providence Hood River Memorial Hospital	Hood River	90%	49
Cottage Grove Community Hospital	Cottage Grove	88%	43
Willamette Valley Medical Center	McMinnville	88%	155
Salem Hospital	Salem	87%	303
Kaiser Sunnyside Medical Center	Clackamas	85%	88
Albany General Hospital	Albany	84%	136
Portland Adventist Medical Center	Portland	84%	204
McKenzie-Willamette Medical Center	Springfield	83%	149
Mid-Columbia Medical Center	The Dalles	82%	65
Providence Saint Vincent Medical Center	Portland	82%	164
Merle West Medical Center	Klamath Falls	80%	125
Tillamook County General Hospital	Tillamook	80%	35
Ashland Community Hospital	Ashland	77%	31
Providence Portland Medical Center	Portland	77%	123
Sacred Heart Medical Center	Eugene	76%	388
Willamette Falls Hospital	Oregon City	75%	79
Providence Milwaukie Hospital	Portland	74%	99
Samaritan Lebanon Community Hospital	Lebanon	70%	105

NOTE: Hospital profiles are in alphabetical order by state, then city, then hospital within the city; Rankings are sorted by rate in descending order and exclude hospitals with less than 25 cases; (1) The number of cases is too small (n<25) for purposes of reliably predicting hospital performance; (2) Measure reflects the hospital's indication that its submission was based upon a sample of its relevant discharges; (3) Rate reflects fewer than the maximum possible quarters of data for the measure; (4) Inaccurate information submitted and suppressed for one or more quarters; (5) No data is available from the hospital for this measure; Please refer to the User's Guide for a full explanation of data

Bay Area Hospital	Coos Bay	69%	144
Grande Ronde Hospital	La Grande	68%	87
Silverton Hospital	Silverton	68%	44
Oregon Health Sciences University	Portland	67%	51
Rogue Valley Medical Center	Medford	67%	230
Columbia Memorial Hospital	Astoria	66%	65
Good Samaritan Regional Medical Center	Corvallis	63%	123
Legacy Emanuel Hospital/Health Center	Portland	56%	50
Legacy Good Samaritan Hospital	Portland	56%	95
Three Rivers Community Hospital/Health Center	Grants Pass	56%	229
Legacy Meridian Park Hospital	Tualatin	53%	133
Samaritan Pacific Community Hospital	Newport	52%	31
Tuality Community Hospital	Hillsboro	52%	156
Santiam Memorial Hospital	Stayton	47%	36
Good Shepherd Health Care System	Hermiston	45%	31
Providence Medford Medical Center	Medford	45%	115
Legacy Mount Hood Medical Center	Gresham	44%	86
Samaritan North Lincoln Hospital	Lincoln City	44%	41
Providence Newberg Hospital	Newberg	37%	49
Mercy Medical Center	Roseburg	35%	108
Holy Rosary Medical Center	Ontario	34%	79
Southern Coos Hospital & Health Center	Bandon	31%	32
Saint Charles Medical Center-Bend-Redmond	Bend	24%	137
Saint Charles Medical Center-Redmond	Redmond	20%	50

19. Smoking Cessation Advice

Hospital Name	City	Rate	Cases
Providence Portland Medical Center	Portland	98%	56
Sacred Heart Medical Center	Eugene	97%	215
Willamette Valley Medical Center	McMinnville	96%	55
Rogue Valley Medical Center	Medford	94%	77
Samaritan Lebanon Community Hospital	Lebanon	94%	36
McKenzie-Willamette Medical Center	Springfield	92%	78
Salem Hospital	Salem	88%	112
Portland Adventist Medical Center	Portland	83%	76
Kaiser Sunnyside Medical Center	Clackamas	82%	34
Providence Medford Medical Center	Medford	80%	50
Providence Milwaukie Hospital	Portland	79%	43
Mercy Medical Center	Roseburg	75%	48
Bay Area Hospital	Coos Bay	74%	46
Legacy Good Samaritan Hospital	Portland	72%	54
Providence Saint Vincent Medical Center	Portland	72%	47
Legacy Emanuel Hospital/Health Center	Portland	70%	47
Albany General Hospital	Albany	69%	55
Legacy Meridian Park Hospital	Tualatin	68%	25
Good Samaritan Regional Medical Center	Corvallis	66%	35
Legacy Mount Hood Medical Center	Gresham	66%	47
Three Rivers Community Hospital/Health Center	Grants Pass	65%	84
Oregon Health Sciences University	Portland	63%	62
Merle West Medical Center	Klamath Falls	62%	56
Saint Charles Medical Center-Bend-Redmond	Bend	62%	45
Tuality Community Hospital	Hillsboro	50%	48

Surgical Infection Prevention

20. Prophylactic Antibiotic Given

Hospital Name	City	Rate	Cases
Providence Hood River Memorial Hospital	Hood River	96%	125
Willamette Valley Medical Center	McMinnville	96%	230
Mid-Columbia Medical Center	The Dalles	93%	163
Providence Newberg Hospital	Newberg	93%	99
Pioneer Memorial Hospital	Prineville	92%	37
Providence Saint Vincent Medical Center	Portland	92%	263
Albany General Hospital	Albany	89%	266
Saint Charles Medical Center-Redmond	Redmond	88%	204
Columbia Memorial Hospital	Astoria	87%	70
Portland Adventist Medical Center	Portland	84%	158
Providence Portland Medical Center	Portland	84%	222
Sacred Heart Medical Center	Eugene	83%	148
Samaritan Lebanon Community Hospital	Lebanon	83%	88
Rogue Valley Medical Center	Medford	82%	590
Salem Hospital	Salem	82%	1171
Merle West Medical Center	Klamath Falls	80%	97
Samaritan Pacific Community Hospital	Newport	80%	54
Kaiser Sunnyside Medical Center	Clackamas	79%	47
Legacy Mount Hood Medical Center	Gresham	79%	73
Saint Charles Medical Center-Bend-Redmond	Bend	79%	1197
Good Samaritan Regional Medical Center	Corvallis	78%	1049
Silverton Hospital	Silverton	78%	110
Legacy Meridian Park Hospital	Tualatin	77%	98
Ashland Community Hospital	Ashland	76%	181
Three Rivers Community Hospital/Health Center	Grants Pass	75%	231
Oregon Health Sciences University	Portland	74%	373
Bay Area Hospital	Coos Bay	72%	299
Good Shepherd Health Care System	Hermiston	72%	58
McKenzie-Willamette Medical Center	Springfield	72%	196
Providence Milwaukie Hospital	Portland	69%	113
Tuality Community Hospital	Hillsboro	69%	288
Mercy Medical Center	Roseburg	68%	240
Legacy Emanuel Hospital/Health Center	Portland	67%	124
Providence Medford Medical Center	Medford	65%	108
Samaritan North Lincoln Hospital	Lincoln City	59%	64
Tillamook County General Hospital	Tillamook	57%	75
Legacy Good Samaritan Hospital	Portland	51%	138
Holy Rosary Medical Center	Ontario	50%	133
Willamette Falls Hospital	Oregon City	40%	45

21. Prophylactic Antibiotic Selection

Hospital Name	City	Rate	Cases
Ashland Community Hospital	Ashland	100%	59
Mid-Columbia Medical Center	The Dalles	100%	58
Providence Hood River Memorial Hospital	Hood River	100%	44
Providence Saint Vincent Medical Center	Portland	99%	94
Rogue Valley Medical Center	Medford	99%	78
Albany General Hospital	Albany	98%	56
Legacy Meridian Park Hospital	Tualatin	98%	50
Saint Charles Medical Center-Bend-Redmond	Bend	98%	308
Legacy Good Samaritan Hospital	Portland	97%	71
Three Rivers Community Hospital/Health Center	Grants Pass	97%	35
Kaiser Sunnyside Medical Center	Clackamas	96%	48
Willamette Valley Medical Center	McMinnville	96%	51
Legacy Emanuel Hospital/Health Center	Portland	95%	58
Legacy Mount Hood Medical Center	Gresham	95%	40
Providence Milwaukie Hospital	Portland	95%	39
Providence Newberg Hospital	Newberg	95%	37
Providence Portland Medical Center	Portland	95%	79
Oregon Health Sciences University	Portland	93%	83
Sacred Heart Medical Center	Eugene	93%	150
Willamette Falls Hospital	Oregon City	93%	43
Bay Area Hospital	Coos Bay	91%	98
McKenzie-Willamette Medical Center	Springfield	91%	74
Saint Charles Medical Center-Redmond	Redmond	91%	45
Tuality Community Hospital	Hillsboro	91%	110
Portland Adventist Medical Center	Portland	90%	52
Good Samaritan Regional Medical Center	Corvallis	89%	182
Providence Medford Medical Center	Medford	85%	27
Silverton Hospital	Silverton	72%	29
Mercy Medical Center	Roseburg	70%	60
Holy Rosary Medical Center	Ontario	63%	43
Merle West Medical Center	Klamath Falls	62%	97
Salem Hospital	Salem	62%	277

22. Prophylactic Antibiotic Stopped

Hospital Name	City	Rate	Cases
Willamette Falls Hospital	Oregon City	98%	40
Albany General Hospital	Albany	93%	263
Samaritan Lebanon Community Hospital	Lebanon	92%	85
Legacy Good Samaritan Hospital	Portland	90%	128
Providence Newberg Hospital	Newberg	89%	96
Salem Hospital	Salem	89%	1109
McKenzie-Willamette Medical Center	Springfield	87%	192
Willamette Valley Medical Center	McMinnville	86%	222
Columbia Memorial Hospital	Astoria	85%	65
Rogue Valley Medical Center	Medford	84%	574
Providence Saint Vincent Medical Center	Portland	83%	259
Samaritan Pacific Community Hospital	Newport	82%	51
Mid-Columbia Medical Center	The Dalles	81%	164
Silverton Hospital	Silverton	81%	101
Oregon Health Sciences University	Portland	80%	373
Good Samaritan Regional Medical Center	Corvallis	79%	1034
Providence Medford Medical Center	Medford	78%	108
Legacy Emanuel Hospital/Health Center	Portland	77%	114
Legacy Meridian Park Hospital	Tualatin	74%	92
Providence Hood River Memorial Hospital	Hood River	74%	125
Pioneer Memorial Hospital	Prineville	73%	37
Three Rivers Community Hospital/Health Center	Grants Pass	72%	214
Sacred Heart Medical Center	Eugene	70%	142
Portland Adventist Medical Center	Portland	68%	153
Saint Charles Medical Center-Bend-Redmond	Bend	68%	1149
Kaiser Sunnyside Medical Center	Clackamas	64%	47
Bay Area Hospital	Coos Bay	59%	275
Saint Charles Medical Center-Redmond	Redmond	56%	194
Providence Milwaukie Hospital	Portland	55%	105
Providence Portland Medical Center	Portland	55%	215
Mercy Medical Center	Roseburg	49%	231
Tuality Community Hospital	Hillsboro	49%	284
Legacy Mount Hood Medical Center	Gresham	44%	70
Merle West Medical Center	Klamath Falls	41%	95

NOTE: Hospital profiles are in alphabetical order by state, then city, then hospital within the city; Rankings are sorted by rate in descending order and exclude hospitals with less than 25 cases; (1) The number of cases is too small (n<25) for purposes of reliably predicting hospital performance; (2) Measure reflects the hospital's indication that its submission was based upon a sample of its relevant discharges; (3) Rate reflects fewer than the maximum possible quarters of data for the measure; (4) Inaccurate information submitted and suppressed for one or more quarters; (5) No data is available from the hospital for this measure; Please refer to the User's Guide for a full explanation of data

Samaritan North Lincoln Hospital	Lincoln City	35%	60
Holy Rosary Medical Center	Ontario	34%	131
Tillamook County General Hospital	Tillamook	34%	77
Good Shepherd Health Care System	Hermiston	32%	53
Ashland Community Hospital	Ashland	29%	175

Pregnancy Care

23. Inpatient Neonatal Mortality

Hospital Name	City	Rate	Cases
McKenzie-Willamette Medical Center	Springfield	0.00%	799
Saint Charles Medical Center-Redmond	Redmond	0.00%	255
Willamette Falls Hospital	Oregon City	0.09%	1125
Saint Charles Medical Center-Bend-Redmond	Bend	0.10%	1998
Bay Area Hospital	Coos Bay	0.15%	649
Holy Rosary Medical Center	Ontario	0.15%	663
Mercy Medical Center	Roseburg	0.19%	1042
Merle West Medical Center	Klamath Falls	0.23%	870
Albany General Hospital	Albany	0.28%	715
Ashland Community Hospital	Ashland	0.32%	312

24. Third or Fourth Degree Laceration

Hospital Name	City	Rate	Cases
Holy Rosary Medical Center	Ontario	1.04%	479
Ashland Community Hospital	Ashland	1.25%	240
Albany General Hospital	Albany	1.76%	510
Saint Charles Medical Center-Bend-Redmond	Bend	2.02%	1487
Bay Area Hospital	Coos Bay	2.39%	460
Mercy Medical Center	Roseburg	3.31%	756
McKenzie-Willamette Medical Center	Springfield	3.42%	555
Saint Charles Medical Center-Redmond	Redmond	3.55%	197
Willamette Falls Hospital	Oregon City	4.05%	839
Merle West Medical Center	Klamath Falls	5.25%	591

NOTE: Hospital profiles are in alphabetical order by state, then city, then hospital within the city; Rankings are sorted by rate in descending order and exclude hospitals with less than 25 cases; (1) The number of cases is too small (n<25) for purposes of reliably predicting hospital performance; (2) Measure reflects the hospital's indication that its submission was based upon a sample of its relevant discharges; (3) Rate reflects fewer than the maximum possible quarters of data for the measure; (4) Inaccurate information submitted and suppressed for one or more quarters; (5) No data is available from the hospital for this measure; Please refer to the User's Guide for a full explanation of data

Albany General Hospital

1046 SW Sixth Avenue
Albany, OR 97321
Ownership: Voluntary non-profit - Private
Emergency Services: Yes

Phone: 541-812-4000
Fax: 541-812-4610
Accredited: Yes
Licensed Beds: 106

Key Personnel:

President . . . . David Triebes
Chief Medical Staff . . . . Thomas Rafalski, MD
Director Infection/Disease Control . . . . Kim Forrester, RN
Director Medical/Surgical Nursing . . . . Sharon Smith, RN
OB/GYN Womens Health . . . . Rodney Wren, MD
Chief Radiology . . . . W Purnell, Jr, DM
Director Respiratory Therapy . . . . Steve Kalb

Measure	Cases	This Hospital	State Average	U.S. Average	Top Hospital
Heart Attack Care					
ACE Inhibitor or ARB for LVSD[1]	8	88%	88%	82%	100%
Aspirin at Arrival[1]	24	88%	93%	92%	100%
Aspirin at Discharge[1]	15	100%	93%	90%	100%
Beta Blocker at Arrival[1]	20	90%	92%	87%	100%
Beta Blocker at Discharge[1]	20	100%	95%	90%	100%
Fibrinolytic Medication Timing	0	-	29%	31%	100%
PCI Within 90 Minutes of Arrival	0	-	63%	54%	95%
Smoking Cessation Advice[1]	3	100%	77%	88%	100%
Heart Failure Care					
ACE Inhibitor or ARB for LVSD	40	85%	84%	82%	100%
Discharge Instructions	97	69%	46%	61%	93%
Evaluation of LVS Function	123	95%	82%	83%	99%
Smoking Cessation Advice	26	77%	70%	82%	100%
Pneumonia Care					
Appropriate Initial Antibiotic	142	84%	84%	83%	94%
Blood Culture Timing	118	92%	90%	90%	100%
Influenza Vaccine	39	90%	64%	70%	100%
Initial Antibiotic Timing	176	90%	81%	80%	93%
Oxygenation Assessment	210	100%	100%	99%	100%
Pneumococcal Vaccine	136	84%	63%	69%	94%
Smoking Cessation Advice	55	69%	70%	80%	100%
Surgical Infection Prevention					
Prophylactic Antibiotic Given[2]	266	89%	71%	77%	95%
Prophylactic Antibiotic Selection[2]	56	98%	89%	90%	100%
Prophylactic Antibiotic Stopped[2]	263	93%	65%	72%	95%
Pregnancy Care					
Inpatient Neonatal Mortality	715	0.28%	-	-	-
Third or Fourth Degree Laceration	510	1.76%	3.10%	3.63%	3.27%

Ashland Community Hospital

280 Maple Street
PO Box 98
Ashland, OR 97520
E-mail: bhamlett@ashlandhospital.org
URL: www.ashlandhospital.org
Ownership: Government - Local
Emergency Services: Yes

Phone: 541-482-2441
Fax: 541-488-7417
Accredited: Yes
Licensed Beds: 49

Key Personnel:

President . . . . Linda Jackson
CEO . . . . Mark Marchetti
Chief Medical Staff . . . . Thomas Marguilies, MD
Emergency Room . . . . Carl Griesser, MD
Director Infection/Disease Control . . . . Erin Coke
CCU Spvg. Nurse . . . . Cindy Lilley, RN
OB/GYN Womens Health . . . . Miriam Soriano, MD
Chief Radiology . . . . Donald Ryan, MD
Director Respiratory Therapy . . . . John Clark

Measure	Cases	This Hospital	State Average	U.S. Average	Top Hospital
Heart Attack Care					
ACE Inhibitor or ARB for LVSD[1]	1	100%	88%	82%	100%
Aspirin at Arrival[1]	7	57%	93%	92%	100%
Aspirin at Discharge[1]	7	86%	93%	90%	100%
Beta Blocker at Arrival[1]	6	83%	92%	87%	100%
Beta Blocker at Discharge[1]	7	86%	95%	90%	100%
Fibrinolytic Medication Timing	0	-	29%	31%	100%
PCI Within 90 Minutes of Arrival	0	-	63%	54%	95%
Smoking Cessation Advice[1]	1	100%	77%	88%	100%
Heart Failure Care					
ACE Inhibitor or ARB for LVSD[1]	6	67%	84%	82%	100%
Discharge Instructions[1]	22	77%	46%	61%	93%
Evaluation of LVS Function[1]	24	79%	82%	83%	99%
Smoking Cessation Advice[1]	3	67%	70%	82%	100%
Pneumonia Care					
Appropriate Initial Antibiotic	33	82%	84%	83%	94%
Blood Culture Timing[1]	23	87%	90%	90%	100%
Influenza Vaccine[1]	9	78%	64%	70%	100%
Initial Antibiotic Timing	34	82%	81%	80%	93%
Oxygenation Assessment	48	100%	100%	99%	100%
Pneumococcal Vaccine	31	77%	63%	69%	94%
Smoking Cessation Advice[1]	10	60%	70%	80%	100%
Surgical Infection Prevention					
Prophylactic Antibiotic Given[3]	181	76%	71%	77%	95%
Prophylactic Antibiotic Selection	59	100%	89%	90%	100%
Prophylactic Antibiotic Stopped[3]	175	29%	65%	72%	95%
Pregnancy Care					
Inpatient Neonatal Mortality	312	0.32%	-	-	-
Third or Fourth Degree Laceration	240	1.25%	3.10%	3.63%	3.27%

Columbia Memorial Hospital

2111 Exchange Street
Astoria, OR 97103
Ownership: Proprietary
Emergency Services: Yes

Phone: 503-325-4321

Accredited: No

Measure	Cases	This Hospital	State Average	U.S. Average	Top Hospital
Heart Attack Care					
ACE Inhibitor or ARB for LVSD[1]	1	100%	88%	82%	100%
Aspirin at Arrival[1]	17	100%	93%	92%	100%
Aspirin at Discharge[1]	5	80%	93%	90%	100%
Beta Blocker at Arrival[1]	12	92%	92%	87%	100%
Beta Blocker at Discharge[1]	6	100%	95%	90%	100%
Fibrinolytic Medication Timing[1]	2	50%	29%	31%	100%
PCI Within 90 Minutes of Arrival	0	-	63%	54%	95%
Smoking Cessation Advice[1]	1	100%	77%	88%	100%
Heart Failure Care					
ACE Inhibitor or ARB for LVSD[1]	14	79%	84%	82%	100%
Discharge Instructions	44	41%	46%	61%	93%
Evaluation of LVS Function	53	47%	82%	83%	99%
Smoking Cessation Advice[1]	10	50%	70%	82%	100%
Pneumonia Care					
Appropriate Initial Antibiotic	99	83%	84%	83%	94%
Blood Culture Timing[1]	21	90%	90%	90%	100%
Influenza Vaccine[1]	16	69%	64%	70%	100%
Initial Antibiotic Timing	100	85%	81%	80%	93%
Oxygenation Assessment	116	100%	100%	99%	100%
Pneumococcal Vaccine	65	66%	63%	69%	94%
Smoking Cessation Advice[1]	19	58%	70%	80%	100%
Surgical Infection Prevention					
Prophylactic Antibiotic Given	70	87%	71%	77%	95%
Prophylactic Antibiotic Selection[1]	13	100%	89%	90%	100%
Prophylactic Antibiotic Stopped	65	85%	65%	72%	95%
Pregnancy Care					
Inpatient Neonatal Mortality	-	-	-	-	-
Third or Fourth Degree Laceration	-	-	3.10%	3.63%	3.27%

Saint Elizabeth Health Services

3325 Pocahontas Road
Baker City, OR 97814
Ownership: Voluntary non-profit - Church
Emergency Services: Yes

Phone: 541-523-6461
Fax: 541-523-8151
Accredited: Yes
Licensed Beds: 36

Key Personnel:

President/CEO . . . . George Winn
Chief Medical Staff . . . . Neal Jacobson
Emergency Room . . . . Deana Chesiak
ICU . . . . Dave Mc Closkey

Measure	Cases	This Hospital	State Average	U.S. Average	Top Hospital
Heart Attack Care					

NOTE: Hospital profiles are in alphabetical order by state, then city, then hospital within the city; Rankings are sorted by rate in descending order and exclude hospitals with less than 25 cases; (1) The number of cases is too small (n<25) for purposes of reliably predicting hospital performance; (2) Measure reflects the hospital's indication that its submission was based upon a sample of its relevant discharges; (3) Rate reflects fewer than the maximum possible quarters of data for the measure; (4) Inaccurate information submitted and suppressed for one or more quarters; (5) No data is available from the hospital for this measure; Please refer to the User's Guide for a full explanation of data

Measure	Cases	This Hospital	State Average	U.S. Average	Top Hospital
ACE Inhibitor or ARB for LVSD[5]	-	-	88%	82%	100%
Aspirin at Arrival[5]	-	-	93%	92%	100%
Aspirin at Discharge[5]	-	-	93%	90%	100%
Beta Blocker at Arrival[5]	-	-	92%	87%	100%
Beta Blocker at Discharge[5]	-	-	95%	90%	100%
Fibrinolytic Medication Timing[5]	-	-	29%	31%	100%
PCI Within 90 Minutes of Arrival[5]	-	-	63%	54%	95%
Smoking Cessation Advice[5]	-	-	77%	88%	100%
Heart Failure Care					
ACE Inhibitor or ARB for LVSD[5]	-	-	84%	82%	100%
Discharge Instructions[5]	-	-	46%	61%	93%
Evaluation of LVS Function[5]	-	-	82%	83%	99%
Smoking Cessation Advice[5]	-	-	70%	82%	100%
Pneumonia Care					
Appropriate Initial Antibiotic[5]	-	-	84%	83%	94%
Blood Culture Timing[5]	-	-	90%	90%	100%
Influenza Vaccine[5]	-	-	64%	70%	100%
Initial Antibiotic Timing[5]	-	-	81%	80%	93%
Oxygenation Assessment[5]	-	-	100%	99%	100%
Pneumococcal Vaccine[5]	-	-	63%	69%	94%
Smoking Cessation Advice[5]	-	-	70%	80%	100%
Surgical Infection Prevention					
Prophylactic Antibiotic Given[5]	-	-	71%	77%	95%
Prophylactic Antibiotic Selection[5]	-	-	89%	90%	100%
Prophylactic Antibiotic Stopped[5]	-	-	65%	72%	95%
Pregnancy Care					
Inpatient Neonatal Mortality	-	-	-	-	-
Third or Fourth Degree Laceration	-	-	3.10%	3.63%	3.27%

Southern Coos Hospital & Health Center

900 11th Street — Phone: 541-347-2426
Bandon, OR 97411 — Fax: 541-347-3923
Ownership: Voluntary non-profit - Other — Accredited: No
Emergency Services: Yes — Licensed Beds: 21

Key Personnel:
President/CEO . . . . James A Wathen

Measure	Cases	This Hospital	State Average	U.S. Average	Top Hospital
Heart Attack Care					
ACE Inhibitor or ARB for LVSD[3]	0	-	88%	82%	100%
Aspirin at Arrival[1,3]	1	100%	93%	92%	100%
Aspirin at Discharge[3]	0	-	93%	90%	100%
Beta Blocker at Arrival[1,3]	1	100%	92%	87%	100%
Beta Blocker at Discharge[3]	0	-	95%	90%	100%
Fibrinolytic Medication Timing[1,3]	1	0%	29%	31%	100%
PCI Within 90 Minutes of Arrival	0	-	63%	54%	95%
Smoking Cessation Advice[3]	0	-	77%	88%	100%
Heart Failure Care					
ACE Inhibitor or ARB for LVSD[5]	-	-	84%	82%	100%
Discharge Instructions[5]	-	-	46%	61%	93%
Evaluation of LVS Function[5]	-	-	82%	83%	99%
Smoking Cessation Advice[5]	-	-	70%	82%	100%
Pneumonia Care					
Appropriate Initial Antibiotic	34	79%	84%	83%	94%
Blood Culture Timing[1]	9	100%	90%	90%	100%
Influenza Vaccine[1]	7	29%	64%	70%	100%
Initial Antibiotic Timing	39	85%	81%	80%	93%
Oxygenation Assessment	45	100%	100%	99%	100%
Pneumococcal Vaccine	32	31%	63%	69%	94%
Smoking Cessation Advice[1]	10	90%	70%	80%	100%
Surgical Infection Prevention					
Prophylactic Antibiotic Given[1]	20	50%	71%	77%	95%
Prophylactic Antibiotic Selection[1]	2	50%	89%	90%	100%
Prophylactic Antibiotic Stopped[1]	20	30%	65%	72%	95%
Pregnancy Care					
Inpatient Neonatal Mortality	-	-	-	-	-
Third or Fourth Degree Laceration	-	-	3.10%	3.63%	3.27%

Saint Charles Medical Center-Bend-Redmond

2500 NE Neff Road — Phone: 541-382-4321
Bend, OR 97701 — Fax: 541-388-7791
E-mail: scmc@scmc.org
URL: www.scmc.org
Ownership: Voluntary non-profit - Private — Accredited: Yes
Emergency Services: Yes — Licensed Beds: 220

Key Personnel:
Administrator/CEO . . . . James T Lussier
Medical Staff President . . . . Gary Buchholz
Leader/Manager Emergency Room . . . . Marty Betsch
Infection Control . . . . Merlene Morris
ICU Supervising Nurse . . . . Dorothy Barrow, RN
Leader/Manager ICCU . . . . Dorothy Barrows
Leader/Manager Medical/Surgical Nursing . . . . . Karon Hack
Director Radiology . . . . Doug Clevenger
Leader/Manager Respiratory . . . . Dorothy Barrows

Measure	Cases	This Hospital	State Average	U.S. Average	Top Hospital
Heart Attack Care					
ACE Inhibitor or ARB for LVSD	48	94%	88%	82%	100%
Aspirin at Arrival	244	98%	93%	92%	100%
Aspirin at Discharge	339	98%	93%	90%	100%
Beta Blocker at Arrival	195	95%	92%	87%	100%
Beta Blocker at Discharge	293	95%	95%	90%	100%
Fibrinolytic Medication Timing	0	-	29%	31%	100%
PCI Within 90 Minutes of Arrival[1]	15	73%	63%	54%	95%
Smoking Cessation Advice	88	98%	77%	88%	100%
Heart Failure Care					
ACE Inhibitor or ARB for LVSD	84	92%	84%	82%	100%
Discharge Instructions	167	49%	46%	61%	93%
Evaluation of LVS Function	178	93%	82%	83%	99%
Smoking Cessation Advice	38	87%	70%	82%	100%
Pneumonia Care					
Appropriate Initial Antibiotic	136	90%	84%	83%	94%
Blood Culture Timing	124	85%	90%	90%	100%
Influenza Vaccine	41	20%	64%	70%	100%
Initial Antibiotic Timing	184	76%	81%	80%	93%
Oxygenation Assessment	226	100%	100%	99%	100%
Pneumococcal Vaccine	137	24%	63%	69%	94%
Smoking Cessation Advice	45	62%	70%	80%	100%
Surgical Infection Prevention					
Prophylactic Antibiotic Given[2]	1,197	79%	71%	77%	95%
Prophylactic Antibiotic Selection[2]	308	98%	89%	90%	100%
Prophylactic Antibiotic Stopped[2]	1,149	68%	65%	72%	95%
Pregnancy Care					
Inpatient Neonatal Mortality	1,998	0.10%	-	-	-
Third or Fourth Degree Laceration	1,487	2.02%	3.10%	3.63%	3.27%

Kaiser Sunnyside Medical Center

10180 SE Sunnyside Road — Toll-Free: 800-813-2000
Clackamas, OR 97015 — Phone: 503-652-2880
Fax: 503-571-2671
Ownership: Voluntary non-profit - Other — Accredited: Yes
Emergency Services: Yes — Licensed Beds: 196

Key Personnel:
Administrator . . . . Kathleen Wegener
Chief Medical Staff . . . . Tom Harburg, MD
Emergency Room . . . . Jeremy Ota, MD
Director Infection/Disease Control . . . . Joseph Kane, MD
CCU Spvg. Nurse . . . . Brenda Cusick
Director Medical/Surgical Nursing . . . . Jane Gilronen
OB/GYN Womens Health . . . . Robert House, MD
Chief Radiology . . . . Brian Markey, MD
Director Respiratory Therapy . . . . Joe Dwan

Measure	Cases	This Hospital	State Average	U.S. Average	Top Hospital
Heart Attack Care					
ACE Inhibitor or ARB for LVSD[1]	18	83%	88%	82%	100%
Aspirin at Arrival	137	98%	93%	92%	100%
Aspirin at Discharge	98	100%	93%	90%	100%
Beta Blocker at Arrival	132	100%	92%	87%	100%
Beta Blocker at Discharge	112	100%	95%	90%	100%

NOTE: Hospital profiles are in alphabetical order by state, then city, then hospital within the city; Rankings are sorted by rate in descending order and exclude hospitals with less than 25 cases; (1) The number of cases is too small (n<25) for purposes of reliably predicting hospital performance; (2) Measure reflects the hospital's indication that its submission was based upon a sample of its relevant discharges; (3) Rate reflects fewer than the maximum possible quarters of data for the measure; (4) Inaccurate information submitted and suppressed for one or more quarters; (5) No data is available from the hospital for this measure; Please refer to the User's Guide for a full explanation of data

Measure	Cases	This Hospital	State Average	U.S. Average	Top Hospital
Fibrinolytic Medication Timing[1]	2	0%	29%	31%	100%
PCI Within 90 Minutes of Arrival	0	-	63%	54%	95%
Smoking Cessation Advice	32	78%	77%	88%	100%
Heart Failure Care					
ACE Inhibitor or ARB for LVSD	85	91%	84%	82%	100%
Discharge Instructions	246	79%	46%	61%	93%
Evaluation of LVS Function	274	97%	82%	83%	99%
Smoking Cessation Advice	41	80%	70%	82%	100%
Pneumonia Care					
Appropriate Initial Antibiotic	90	79%	84%	83%	94%
Blood Culture Timing	86	92%	90%	90%	100%
Influenza Vaccine[1]	24	58%	64%	70%	100%
Initial Antibiotic Timing	122	71%	81%	80%	93%
Oxygenation Assessment	150	100%	100%	99%	100%
Pneumococcal Vaccine	88	85%	63%	69%	94%
Smoking Cessation Advice	34	82%	70%	80%	100%
Surgical Infection Prevention					
Prophylactic Antibiotic Given[3]	47	79%	71%	77%	95%
Prophylactic Antibiotic Selection	48	96%	89%	90%	100%
Prophylactic Antibiotic Stopped[3]	47	64%	65%	72%	95%
Pregnancy Care					
Inpatient Neonatal Mortality	-	-	-	-	-
Third or Fourth Degree Laceration	-	-	3.10%	3.63%	3.27%

Bay Area Hospital

1775 Thompson Road
Coos Bay, OR 97420
Phone: 541-269-8111
Fax: 541-267-7057
E-mail: cacace@bayareahospital.org
Ownership: Govt - Hospital District or Authority
Accredited: Yes
Emergency Services: Yes
Licensed Beds: 172

Key Personnel:

CEO. . . . . Dan Smith
Chief Medical Staff. . . . . Shaun Hobson, MD
Emergency Room . . . . Bridget Berlin
Emergency Room . . . . Clyde Hill
Surgical Services. . . . . Lori Krenos
Respiratory Care . . . . Glen Lyon

Measure	Cases	This Hospital	State Average	U.S. Average	Top Hospital
Heart Attack Care					
ACE Inhibitor or ARB for LVSD	0	-	88%	82%	100%
Aspirin at Arrival[1]	16	94%	93%	92%	100%
Aspirin at Discharge[1]	2	100%	93%	90%	100%
Beta Blocker at Arrival[1]	16	88%	92%	87%	100%
Beta Blocker at Discharge[1]	2	100%	95%	90%	100%
Fibrinolytic Medication Timing[1,3]	6	17%	29%	31%	100%
PCI Within 90 Minutes of Arrival	0	-	63%	54%	95%
Smoking Cessation Advice[3]	0	-	77%	88%	100%
Heart Failure Care					
ACE Inhibitor or ARB for LVSD	80	90%	84%	82%	100%
Discharge Instructions[3]	106	69%	46%	61%	93%
Evaluation of LVS Function	200	76%	82%	83%	99%
Smoking Cessation Advice[1,3]	18	78%	70%	82%	100%
Pneumonia Care					
Appropriate Initial Antibiotic[3]	93	91%	84%	83%	94%
Blood Culture Timing	111	86%	90%	90%	100%
Influenza Vaccine	33	67%	64%	70%	100%
Initial Antibiotic Timing	173	89%	81%	80%	93%
Oxygenation Assessment	211	100%	100%	99%	100%
Pneumococcal Vaccine	144	69%	63%	69%	94%
Smoking Cessation Advice[3]	46	74%	70%	80%	100%
Surgical Infection Prevention					
Prophylactic Antibiotic Given[3]	299	72%	71%	77%	95%
Prophylactic Antibiotic Selection	98	91%	89%	90%	100%
Prophylactic Antibiotic Stopped[3]	275	59%	65%	72%	95%
Pregnancy Care					
Inpatient Neonatal Mortality	649	0.15%	-	-	-
Third or Fourth Degree Laceration	460	2.39%	3.10%	3.63%	3.27%

Coquille Valley Hospital

940 East Fifth Street
Coquille, OR 97423
Phone: 541-396-3101
Fax: 541-396-5760
URL: www.cvhospital.org
Ownership: Voluntary non-profit - Private
Accredited: No
Emergency Services: Yes
Licensed Beds: 25

Key Personnel:

President/CEO. . . . . Dennis Zielinski
Chief Medical Staff. . . . . James J Sinnott
Emergency Room . . . . James Sinnott
Infection Control. . . . . Renee Marineau
Respiratory/Cardiopulmonary. . . . . Rosemary Carter

Measure	Cases	This Hospital	State Average	U.S. Average	Top Hospital
Heart Attack Care					
ACE Inhibitor or ARB for LVSD[1,3]	1	100%	88%	82%	100%
Aspirin at Arrival[1,3]	8	75%	93%	92%	100%
Aspirin at Discharge[1,3]	6	83%	93%	90%	100%
Beta Blocker at Arrival[1,3]	8	75%	92%	87%	100%
Beta Blocker at Discharge[1,3]	6	83%	95%	90%	100%
Fibrinolytic Medication Timing[1,3]	2	50%	29%	31%	100%
PCI Within 90 Minutes of Arrival	0	-	63%	54%	95%
Smoking Cessation Advice[1,3]	2	50%	77%	88%	100%
Heart Failure Care					
ACE Inhibitor or ARB for LVSD[1,3]	1	100%	84%	82%	100%
Discharge Instructions[1,3]	14	0%	46%	61%	93%
Evaluation of LVS Function[1,3]	16	12%	82%	83%	99%
Smoking Cessation Advice[1,3]	3	33%	70%	82%	100%
Pneumonia Care					
Appropriate Initial Antibiotic[1,3]	21	57%	84%	83%	94%
Blood Culture Timing[1]	7	71%	90%	90%	100%
Influenza Vaccine[1]	5	0%	64%	70%	100%
Initial Antibiotic Timing[1,3]	24	75%	81%	80%	93%
Oxygenation Assessment[3]	28	100%	100%	99%	100%
Pneumococcal Vaccine[1,3]	16	0%	63%	69%	94%
Smoking Cessation Advice[1,3]	12	33%	70%	80%	100%
Surgical Infection Prevention					
Prophylactic Antibiotic Given[1,3]	3	0%	71%	77%	95%
Prophylactic Antibiotic Selection[1]	1	100%	89%	90%	100%
Prophylactic Antibiotic Stopped[1,3]	1	0%	65%	72%	95%
Pregnancy Care					
Inpatient Neonatal Mortality	-	-	-	-	-
Third or Fourth Degree Laceration	-	-	3.10%	3.63%	3.27%

Good Samaritan Regional Medical Center

3600 NW Samaritan Drive
Corvallis, OR 97330
Phone: 541-757-5111
Fax: 541-768-6400
Ownership: Voluntary non-profit - Private
Accredited: Yes
Emergency Services: Yes
Licensed Beds: 188

Key Personnel:

President/CEO. . . . . Larry A Mullins
Chief of Medical Staff. . . . . Steven Athay
Head of Emergency Room. . . . . Chriss Boos
Medical/Surgical Nursing . . . . Jim Beecroft
OB/GYN Womens Health. . . . . Debbie Heim
Respiratory/Cardiopulmonary. . . . . Bob Vanderford

Measure	Cases	This Hospital	State Average	U.S. Average	Top Hospital
Heart Attack Care					
ACE Inhibitor or ARB for LVSD	30	90%	88%	82%	100%
Aspirin at Arrival	96	99%	93%	92%	100%
Aspirin at Discharge	206	100%	93%	90%	100%
Beta Blocker at Arrival	69	96%	92%	87%	100%
Beta Blocker at Discharge	221	99%	95%	90%	100%
Fibrinolytic Medication Timing	0	-	29%	31%	100%
PCI Within 90 Minutes of Arrival[1]	8	88%	63%	54%	95%
Smoking Cessation Advice	86	93%	77%	88%	100%
Heart Failure Care					
ACE Inhibitor or ARB for LVSD	63	87%	84%	82%	100%
Discharge Instructions	123	51%	46%	61%	93%
Evaluation of LVS Function	149	84%	82%	83%	99%
Smoking Cessation Advice[1]	21	90%	70%	82%	100%
Pneumonia Care					

NOTE: Hospital profiles are in alphabetical order by state, then city, then hospital within the city; Rankings are sorted by rate in descending order and exclude hospitals with less than 25 cases; (1) The number of cases is too small (n<25) for purposes of reliably predicting hospital performance; (2) Measure reflects the hospital's indication that its submission was based upon a sample of its relevant discharges; (3) Rate reflects fewer than the maximum possible quarters of data for the measure; (4) Inaccurate information submitted and suppressed for one or more quarters; (5) No data is available from the hospital for this measure; Please refer to the User's Guide for a full explanation of data

Appropriate Initial Antibiotic	84	90%	84%	83%	94%
Blood Culture Timing	67	90%	90%	90%	100%
Influenza Vaccine[1]	24	75%	64%	70%	100%
Initial Antibiotic Timing	127	91%	81%	80%	93%
Oxygenation Assessment	163	100%	100%	99%	100%
Pneumococcal Vaccine	123	63%	63%	69%	94%
Smoking Cessation Advice	35	66%	70%	80%	100%
Surgical Infection Prevention					
Prophylactic Antibiotic Given[2]	1,049	78%	71%	77%	95%
Prophylactic Antibiotic Selection[2]	182	89%	89%	90%	100%
Prophylactic Antibiotic Stopped[2]	1,034	79%	65%	72%	95%
Pregnancy Care					
Inpatient Neonatal Mortality	-	-	-	-	-
Third or Fourth Degree Laceration	-	-	3.10%	3.63%	3.27%

Cottage Grove Community Hospital

Alternate Name: Cottage Grove Hospital
1340 Birch Avenue — Phone: 541-942-0511
Cottage Grove, OR 97424 — Fax: 541-942-0353
Ownership: Voluntary non-profit - Other — Accredited: No
Emergency Services: Yes — Licensed Beds: 11

Key Personnel:

Administrator . . . . Patria Tulley

Measure	Cases	This Hospital	State Average	U.S. Average	Top Hospital
Heart Attack Care					
ACE Inhibitor or ARB for LVSD[5]	-	-	88%	82%	100%
Aspirin at Arrival[5]	-	-	93%	92%	100%
Aspirin at Discharge[5]	-	-	93%	90%	100%
Beta Blocker at Arrival[5]	-	-	92%	87%	100%
Beta Blocker at Discharge[5]	-	-	95%	90%	100%
Fibrinolytic Medication Timing[5]	-	-	29%	31%	100%
PCI Within 90 Minutes of Arrival[5]	-	-	63%	54%	95%
Smoking Cessation Advice[5]	-	-	77%	88%	100%
Heart Failure Care					
ACE Inhibitor or ARB for LVSD[5]	-	-	84%	82%	100%
Discharge Instructions[5]	-	-	46%	61%	93%
Evaluation of LVS Function[5]	-	-	82%	83%	99%
Smoking Cessation Advice[5]	-	-	70%	82%	100%
Pneumonia Care					
Appropriate Initial Antibiotic	44	77%	84%	83%	94%
Blood Culture Timing[1]	18	100%	90%	90%	100%
Influenza Vaccine[1]	17	94%	64%	70%	100%
Initial Antibiotic Timing	49	61%	81%	80%	93%
Oxygenation Assessment	60	100%	100%	99%	100%
Pneumococcal Vaccine	43	88%	63%	69%	94%
Smoking Cessation Advice[1]	11	73%	70%	80%	100%
Surgical Infection Prevention					
Prophylactic Antibiotic Given[5]	-	-	71%	77%	95%
Prophylactic Antibiotic Selection[5]	-	-	89%	90%	100%
Prophylactic Antibiotic Stopped[5]	-	-	65%	72%	95%
Pregnancy Care					
Inpatient Neonatal Mortality	-	-	-	-	-
Third or Fourth Degree Laceration	-	-	3.10%	3.63%	3.27%

West Valley Hospital

525 Se Washington Street — Phone: 503-623-8301
Dallas, OR 97338
Ownership: Govt - Hospital District or Authority — Accredited: No
Emergency Services: Yes

Measure	Cases	This Hospital	State Average	U.S. Average	Top Hospital
Heart Attack Care					
ACE Inhibitor or ARB for LVSD[5]	-	-	88%	82%	100%
Aspirin at Arrival[5]	-	-	93%	92%	100%
Aspirin at Discharge[5]	-	-	93%	90%	100%
Beta Blocker at Arrival[5]	-	-	92%	87%	100%
Beta Blocker at Discharge[5]	-	-	95%	90%	100%
Fibrinolytic Medication Timing[5]	-	-	29%	31%	100%
PCI Within 90 Minutes of Arrival[5]	-	-	63%	54%	95%
Smoking Cessation Advice[5]	-	-	77%	88%	100%
Heart Failure Care					
ACE Inhibitor or ARB for LVSD[5]	-	-	84%	82%	100%
Discharge Instructions[5]	-	-	46%	61%	93%
Evaluation of LVS Function[5]	-	-	82%	83%	99%
Smoking Cessation Advice[5]	-	-	70%	82%	100%
Pneumonia Care					
Appropriate Initial Antibiotic[5]	-	-	84%	83%	94%
Blood Culture Timing[5]	-	-	90%	90%	100%
Influenza Vaccine[5]	-	-	64%	70%	100%
Initial Antibiotic Timing[5]	-	-	81%	80%	93%
Oxygenation Assessment[5]	-	-	100%	99%	100%
Pneumococcal Vaccine[5]	-	-	63%	69%	94%
Smoking Cessation Advice[5]	-	-	70%	80%	100%
Surgical Infection Prevention					
Prophylactic Antibiotic Given[5]	-	-	71%	77%	95%
Prophylactic Antibiotic Selection[5]	-	-	89%	90%	100%
Prophylactic Antibiotic Stopped[5]	-	-	65%	72%	95%
Pregnancy Care					
Inpatient Neonatal Mortality	-	-	-	-	-
Third or Fourth Degree Laceration	-	-	3.10%	3.63%	3.27%

Sacred Heart Medical Center

1255 Hilyard Street — Phone: 541-686-7300
Eugene, OR 97401 — Fax: 541-686-7005
URL: www.peacehealth.org
Ownership: Voluntary non-profit - Church — Accredited: Yes
Emergency Services: Yes — Licensed Beds: 432

Key Personnel:

CEO. . . . . Allen Yordy
Chief Medical Staff. . . . . Phyllis Brown, MD
Cardiac Lab . . . . Chris Berry
Catheterization Lab . . . . Carol Doyle
Emergency Room . . . . Tim Herrman, RN
Infection Control. . . . . Susan Kline
ICU . . . . Joy Cresci
Intensive/Coronary Care . . . . Angela Christensen
Medical/Surgical Nursing . . . . Linda Rankin
OB/GYN Womens Health. . . . . Mary Duke, RN
Respiratory/Cardiopulmonary. . . . . Janet Sale

Measure	Cases	This Hospital	State Average	U.S. Average	Top Hospital
Heart Attack Care					
ACE Inhibitor or ARB for LVSD	149	89%	88%	82%	100%
Aspirin at Arrival	302	98%	93%	92%	100%
Aspirin at Discharge	606	99%	93%	90%	100%
Beta Blocker at Arrival	285	96%	92%	87%	100%
Beta Blocker at Discharge	665	99%	95%	90%	100%
Fibrinolytic Medication Timing	0	-	29%	31%	100%
PCI Within 90 Minutes of Arrival[1]	21	71%	63%	54%	95%
Smoking Cessation Advice	239	99%	77%	88%	100%
Heart Failure Care					
ACE Inhibitor or ARB for LVSD	246	90%	84%	82%	100%
Discharge Instructions	408	93%	46%	61%	93%
Evaluation of LVS Function	476	99%	82%	83%	99%
Smoking Cessation Advice	79	94%	70%	82%	100%
Pneumonia Care					
Appropriate Initial Antibiotic	295	92%	84%	83%	94%
Blood Culture Timing	345	94%	90%	90%	100%
Influenza Vaccine	112	83%	64%	70%	100%
Initial Antibiotic Timing	526	81%	81%	80%	93%
Oxygenation Assessment	624	100%	100%	99%	100%
Pneumococcal Vaccine	388	76%	63%	69%	94%
Smoking Cessation Advice	215	97%	70%	80%	100%
Surgical Infection Prevention					
Prophylactic Antibiotic Given[2,3]	148	83%	71%	77%	95%
Prophylactic Antibiotic Selection[2]	150	93%	89%	90%	100%
Prophylactic Antibiotic Stopped[2,3]	142	70%	65%	72%	95%
Pregnancy Care					
Inpatient Neonatal Mortality	-	-	-	-	-
Third or Fourth Degree Laceration	-	-	3.10%	3.63%	3.27%

NOTE: Hospital profiles are in alphabetical order by state, then city, then hospital within the city; Rankings are sorted by rate in descending order and exclude hospitals with less than 25 cases; (1) The number of cases is too small (n<25) for purposes of reliably predicting hospital performance; (2) Measure reflects the hospital's indication that its submission was based upon a sample of its relevant discharges; (3) Rate reflects fewer than the maximum possible quarters of data for the measure; (4) Inaccurate information submitted and suppressed for one or more quarters; (5) No data is available from the hospital for this measure; Please refer to the User's Guide for a full explanation of data

Peace Harbor Hospital

400 9th Street
Florence, OR 97439
Ownership: Voluntary non-profit - Church
Emergency Services: Yes

Phone: 541-997-8412
Fax: 541-997-9155
Accredited: Yes
Licensed Beds: 21

Key Personnel:
CEO/President . . . . James Barnhart
Chief Medical Staff . . . . Ronald Shearer
Emergency Room . . . . Mathew Valentine
Emergency Room . . . . Jim Wiley, RN
Director Infection/Disease Control . . . . Leslie Weaver
Chief Radiology . . . . Ann Henry
Director Respiratory Therapy . . . . Mike Hill

Measure	Cases	This Hospital	State Average	U.S. Average	Top Hospital
Heart Attack Care					
ACE Inhibitor or ARB for LVSD[1]	1	100%	88%	82%	100%
Aspirin at Arrival[1]	5	80%	93%	92%	100%
Aspirin at Discharge[1]	3	100%	93%	90%	100%
Beta Blocker at Arrival[1]	7	71%	92%	87%	100%
Beta Blocker at Discharge[1]	6	100%	95%	90%	100%
Fibrinolytic Medication Timing	0	-	29%	31%	100%
PCI Within 90 Minutes of Arrival	0	-	63%	54%	95%
Smoking Cessation Advice[1]	1	0%	77%	88%	100%
Heart Failure Care					
ACE Inhibitor or ARB for LVSD[1]	12	92%	84%	82%	100%
Discharge Instructions	38	24%	46%	61%	93%
Evaluation of LVS Function	39	90%	82%	83%	99%
Smoking Cessation Advice[1]	5	80%	70%	82%	100%
Pneumonia Care					
Appropriate Initial Antibiotic	34	82%	84%	83%	94%
Blood Culture Timing	26	88%	90%	90%	100%
Influenza Vaccine[1]	3	100%	64%	70%	100%
Initial Antibiotic Timing	38	82%	81%	80%	93%
Oxygenation Assessment	51	100%	100%	99%	100%
Pneumococcal Vaccine	35	91%	63%	69%	94%
Smoking Cessation Advice[1]	11	82%	70%	80%	100%
Surgical Infection Prevention					
Prophylactic Antibiotic Given[1,3]	18	78%	71%	77%	95%
Prophylactic Antibiotic Selection[1]	17	100%	89%	90%	100%
Prophylactic Antibiotic Stopped[1,3]	16	81%	65%	72%	95%
Pregnancy Care					
Inpatient Neonatal Mortality	-	-	-	-	-
Third or Fourth Degree Laceration	-	-	3.10%	3.63%	3.27%

Three Rivers Community Hospital/Health Center

500 SW Ramsey
Grants Pass, OR 97527
E-mail: pmckeen@asante.org
URL: www.asante.org
Ownership: Voluntary non-profit - Other
Emergency Services: Yes

Phone: 541-472-7000
Fax: 541-472-7381
Accredited: Yes
Licensed Beds: 150

Key Personnel:
President/CEO . . . . Roy Vinyard
Chief Medical Staff . . . . Kelley Burnett
Director Infection/Disease Control . . . . Sheri Thomson, RN
CCU Spvg. Nurse . . . . Sherri Dague, RN
Director Medical/Surgical Nursing . . . . Marylin Watkins, RN
OB/GYN Womens Health . . . . T Collins, MD
Manager Radiology . . . . Rod Graham
Director Respiratory Therapy . . . . Chris Sorensen

Measure	Cases	This Hospital	State Average	U.S. Average	Top Hospital
Heart Attack Care					
ACE Inhibitor or ARB for LVSD[1]	11	91%	88%	82%	100%
Aspirin at Arrival	83	93%	93%	92%	100%
Aspirin at Discharge	52	88%	93%	90%	100%
Beta Blocker at Arrival	72	89%	92%	87%	100%
Beta Blocker at Discharge	43	95%	95%	90%	100%
Fibrinolytic Medication Timing	0	-	29%	31%	100%
PCI Within 90 Minutes of Arrival	0	-	63%	54%	95%
Smoking Cessation Advice[1]	9	56%	77%	88%	100%
Heart Failure Care					
ACE Inhibitor or ARB for LVSD	65	91%	84%	82%	100%
Discharge Instructions	174	6%	46%	61%	93%
Evaluation of LVS Function	213	82%	82%	83%	99%
Smoking Cessation Advice	35	57%	70%	82%	100%
Pneumonia Care					
Appropriate Initial Antibiotic	232	88%	84%	83%	94%
Blood Culture Timing	80	98%	90%	90%	100%
Influenza Vaccine	59	49%	64%	70%	100%
Initial Antibiotic Timing	275	85%	81%	80%	93%
Oxygenation Assessment	323	100%	100%	99%	100%
Pneumococcal Vaccine	229	56%	63%	69%	94%
Smoking Cessation Advice	84	65%	70%	80%	100%
Surgical Infection Prevention					
Prophylactic Antibiotic Given[2,3]	231	75%	71%	77%	95%
Prophylactic Antibiotic Selection[2]	35	97%	89%	90%	100%
Prophylactic Antibiotic Stopped[2,3]	214	72%	65%	72%	95%
Pregnancy Care					
Inpatient Neonatal Mortality	-	-	-	-	-
Third or Fourth Degree Laceration	-	-	3.10%	3.63%	3.27%

Legacy Mount Hood Medical Center

Alternate Name: Mount Hood Medical Center
24800 SE Stark
Gresham, OR 97030
Ownership: Voluntary non-profit - Private
Emergency Services: Yes

Phone: 503-413-2500
Fax: 503-415-5954
Accredited: Yes
Licensed Beds: 115

Key Personnel:
President/CEO . . . . Bob Pallari
Chief Medical Staff . . . . Kelly Carter
Emergency Room . . . . Joel Brenner
Director Infection/Disease Control . . . . Kelly Eagan
CCU Spvg. Nurse . . . . Shannon Muse
Director Medical/Surgical Nursing . . . . Lani Gaskill
Director Respiratory Therapy . . . . Jan White

Measure	Cases	This Hospital	State Average	U.S. Average	Top Hospital
Heart Attack Care					
ACE Inhibitor or ARB for LVSD[1,2]	7	71%	88%	82%	100%
Aspirin at Arrival[2]	36	97%	93%	92%	100%
Aspirin at Discharge[1,2]	16	88%	93%	90%	100%
Beta Blocker at Arrival[1,2]	20	100%	92%	87%	100%
Beta Blocker at Discharge[1,2]	18	83%	95%	90%	100%
Fibrinolytic Medication Timing[1,2]	3	33%	29%	31%	100%
PCI Within 90 Minutes of Arrival[2]	0	-	63%	54%	95%
Smoking Cessation Advice[1,2]	5	40%	77%	88%	100%
Heart Failure Care					
ACE Inhibitor or ARB for LVSD[2]	36	72%	84%	82%	100%
Discharge Instructions[2]	84	11%	46%	61%	93%
Evaluation of LVS Function[2]	95	93%	82%	83%	99%
Smoking Cessation Advice[1,2]	16	50%	70%	82%	100%
Pneumonia Care					
Appropriate Initial Antibiotic[2]	89	90%	84%	83%	94%
Blood Culture Timing[2]	61	97%	90%	90%	100%
Influenza Vaccine	27	41%	64%	70%	100%
Initial Antibiotic Timing[2]	140	86%	81%	80%	93%
Oxygenation Assessment[2]	159	100%	100%	99%	100%
Pneumococcal Vaccine[2]	86	44%	63%	69%	94%
Smoking Cessation Advice[2]	47	66%	70%	80%	100%
Surgical Infection Prevention					
Prophylactic Antibiotic Given[2,3]	73	79%	71%	77%	95%
Prophylactic Antibiotic Selection[2]	40	95%	89%	90%	100%
Prophylactic Antibiotic Stopped[2,3]	70	44%	65%	72%	95%
Pregnancy Care					
Inpatient Neonatal Mortality	-	-	-	-	-
Third or Fourth Degree Laceration	-	-	3.10%	3.63%	3.27%

Pioneer Memorial Hospital

Alternate Name: Morrow County Health District

NOTE: Hospital profiles are in alphabetical order by state, then city, then hospital within the city; Rankings are sorted by rate in descending order and exclude hospitals with less than 25 cases; (1) The number of cases is too small (n<25) for purposes of reliably predicting hospital performance; (2) Measure reflects the hospital's indication that its submission was based upon a sample of its relevant discharges; (3) Rate reflects fewer than the maximum possible quarters of data for the measure; (4) Inaccurate information submitted and suppressed for one or more quarters; (5) No data is available from the hospital for this measure; Please refer to the User's Guide for a full explanation of data

564 E Pioneer Drive
PO Box 9
Heppner, OR 97836
Phone: 541-676-9133
Fax: 541-676-2900
Ownership: Govt - Hospital District or Authority
Accredited: No
Emergency Services: No
Licensed Beds: 12

Key Personnel:

Administrator . . . . Victor Vander Does
Chief Medical Staff. . . . . Kenneth F Wenberg, MD
Emergency Room . . . . Kenneth F Wenberg, MD
Director Infection/Disease Control . . . . Jay Straley
ICU . . . . Molly Rhea, RN
Director Respiratory Therapy . . . . Pennie Miller

Measure	Cases	This Hospital	State Average	U.S. Average	Top Hospital
Heart Attack Care					
ACE Inhibitor or ARB for LVSD[5]	-	-	88%	82%	100%
Aspirin at Arrival[5]	-	-	93%	92%	100%
Aspirin at Discharge[5]	-	-	93%	90%	100%
Beta Blocker at Arrival[5]	-	-	92%	87%	100%
Beta Blocker at Discharge[5]	-	-	95%	90%	100%
Fibrinolytic Medication Timing[5]	-	-	29%	31%	100%
PCI Within 90 Minutes of Arrival[5]	-	-	63%	54%	95%
Smoking Cessation Advice[5]	-	-	77%	88%	100%
Heart Failure Care					
ACE Inhibitor or ARB for LVSD[5]	-	-	84%	82%	100%
Discharge Instructions[5]	-	-	46%	61%	93%
Evaluation of LVS Function[5]	-	-	82%	83%	99%
Smoking Cessation Advice[5]	-	-	70%	82%	100%
Pneumonia Care					
Appropriate Initial Antibiotic[5]	-	-	84%	83%	94%
Blood Culture Timing[5]	-	-	90%	90%	100%
Influenza Vaccine[5]	-	-	64%	70%	100%
Initial Antibiotic Timing[5]	-	-	81%	80%	93%
Oxygenation Assessment[5]	-	-	100%	99%	100%
Pneumococcal Vaccine[5]	-	-	63%	69%	94%
Smoking Cessation Advice[5]	-	-	70%	80%	100%
Surgical Infection Prevention					
Prophylactic Antibiotic Given[5]	-	-	71%	77%	95%
Prophylactic Antibiotic Selection[5]	-	-	89%	90%	100%
Prophylactic Antibiotic Stopped[5]	-	-	65%	72%	95%
Pregnancy Care					
Inpatient Neonatal Mortality	-	-	-	-	-
Third or Fourth Degree Laceration	-	-	3.10%	3.63%	3.27%

Good Shepherd Health Care System

Alternate Name: Good Shepherd Community Hospital
610 NW 11th Street
Hermiston, OR 97838
Phone: 541-667-3400
Fax: 541-667-3414
URL: www.gshealth.org
Ownership: Govt - Hospital District or Authority
Accredited: No
Emergency Services: Yes
Licensed Beds: 49

Key Personnel:

CEO. . . . . Dennis Eurke
Chief Medical Staff. . . . . Dr. Richard Flaiz
Chief Medical Staff. . . . . Winn Gregory
Emergency Room . . . . Ken Franz

Measure	Cases	This Hospital	State Average	U.S. Average	Top Hospital
Heart Attack Care					
ACE Inhibitor or ARB for LVSD[1,3]	1	100%	88%	82%	100%
Aspirin at Arrival[1,3]	3	100%	93%	92%	100%
Aspirin at Discharge[1,3]	2	100%	93%	90%	100%
Beta Blocker at Arrival[1,3]	2	100%	92%	87%	100%
Beta Blocker at Discharge[1,3]	1	100%	95%	90%	100%
Fibrinolytic Medication Timing[3]	0	-	29%	31%	100%
PCI Within 90 Minutes of Arrival[5]	-	-	63%	54%	95%
Smoking Cessation Advice[1,3]	1	0%	77%	88%	100%
Heart Failure Care					
ACE Inhibitor or ARB for LVSD[1,3]	8	100%	84%	82%	100%
Discharge Instructions[1,3]	20	85%	46%	61%	93%
Evaluation of LVS Function[1,3]	24	75%	82%	83%	99%
Smoking Cessation Advice[1,3]	3	67%	70%	82%	100%
Pneumonia Care					
Appropriate Initial Antibiotic[2,3]	42	83%	84%	83%	94%
Blood Culture Timing[1,2]	20	90%	90%	90%	100%
Influenza Vaccine[1]	3	67%	64%	70%	100%
Initial Antibiotic Timing[2,3]	37	70%	81%	80%	93%
Oxygenation Assessment[2,3]	45	96%	100%	99%	100%
Pneumococcal Vaccine[2,3]	31	45%	63%	69%	94%
Smoking Cessation Advice[1,2,3]	12	50%	70%	80%	100%
Surgical Infection Prevention					
Prophylactic Antibiotic Given[3]	58	72%	71%	77%	95%
Prophylactic Antibiotic Selection[1]	24	88%	89%	90%	100%
Prophylactic Antibiotic Stopped[3]	53	32%	65%	72%	95%
Pregnancy Care					
Inpatient Neonatal Mortality	-	-	-	-	-
Third or Fourth Degree Laceration	-	-	3.10%	3.63%	3.27%

Tuality Community Hospital

335 SE Eighth Ave
Hillsboro, OR 97123
Phone: 503-681-1111
Fax: 503-681-1695
URL: www.tuality.com
Ownership: Voluntary non-profit - Private
Accredited: Yes
Emergency Services: Yes
Licensed Beds: 167

Key Personnel:

President/CEO. . . . . Dick Stenson
Chief Medical Staff. . . . . Nicholas G Ortonekis, MD
Chief Catheterization Laboratory . . . . Vincent Reyes, MD
Director Emergency Services. . . . . Tom Hoffman, MD
Director Medical/Surgical Nursing . . . . Chris Chandler
OB/GYN Womens Health. . . . . Susan Nestrutt
Director Surgical Services . . . . Susan Terry
Director Radiology . . . . Dave Foster
Respiratory Therapy Manager . . . . Pat McClone

Measure	Cases	This Hospital	State Average	U.S. Average	Top Hospital
Heart Attack Care					
ACE Inhibitor or ARB for LVSD[1]	10	20%	88%	82%	100%
Aspirin at Arrival	131	95%	93%	92%	100%
Aspirin at Discharge	125	94%	93%	90%	100%
Beta Blocker at Arrival	105	85%	92%	87%	100%
Beta Blocker at Discharge	130	89%	95%	90%	100%
Fibrinolytic Medication Timing[1]	1	0%	29%	31%	100%
PCI Within 90 Minutes of Arrival[1]	5	40%	63%	54%	95%
Smoking Cessation Advice	37	41%	77%	88%	100%
Heart Failure Care					
ACE Inhibitor or ARB for LVSD	47	60%	84%	82%	100%
Discharge Instructions	134	25%	46%	61%	93%
Evaluation of LVS Function	156	78%	82%	83%	99%
Smoking Cessation Advice[1]	22	41%	70%	82%	100%
Pneumonia Care					
Appropriate Initial Antibiotic	128	90%	84%	83%	94%
Blood Culture Timing	112	94%	90%	90%	100%
Influenza Vaccine	39	62%	64%	70%	100%
Initial Antibiotic Timing	172	84%	81%	80%	93%
Oxygenation Assessment	209	100%	100%	99%	100%
Pneumococcal Vaccine	156	52%	63%	69%	94%
Smoking Cessation Advice	48	50%	70%	80%	100%
Surgical Infection Prevention					
Prophylactic Antibiotic Given[2,3]	288	69%	71%	77%	95%
Prophylactic Antibiotic Selection[2]	110	91%	89%	90%	100%
Prophylactic Antibiotic Stopped[2,3]	284	49%	65%	72%	95%
Pregnancy Care					
Inpatient Neonatal Mortality	-	-	-	-	-
Third or Fourth Degree Laceration	-	-	3.10%	3.63%	3.27%

Providence Hood River Memorial Hospital

Alternate Name: Hood River Memorial Hospital
13th & May Streets
Hood River, OR 97031
Phone: 541-386-3911
Fax: 541-387-6462
Ownership: Voluntary non-profit - Other
Accredited: No
Emergency Services: Yes
Licensed Beds: 32

Key Personnel:

CEO. . . . . Larry Beth
Emergency Room . . . . Thomas Wilhelm

NOTE: Hospital profiles are in alphabetical order by state, then city, then hospital within the city; Rankings are sorted by rate in descending order and exclude hospitals with less than 25 cases; (1) The number of cases is too small (n<25) for purposes of reliably predicting hospital performance; (2) Measure reflects the hospital's indication that its submission was based upon a sample of its relevant discharges; (3) Rate reflects fewer than the maximum possible quarters of data for the measure; (4) Inaccurate information submitted and suppressed for one or more quarters; (5) No data is available from the hospital for this measure; Please refer to the User's Guide for a full explanation of data

Measure	Cases	This Hospital	State Average	U.S. Average	Top Hospital
Heart Attack Care					
ACE Inhibitor or ARB for LVSD[1]	3	100%	88%	82%	100%
Aspirin at Arrival[1]	16	100%	93%	92%	100%
Aspirin at Discharge[1]	9	100%	93%	90%	100%
Beta Blocker at Arrival[1]	14	100%	92%	87%	100%
Beta Blocker at Discharge[1]	9	100%	95%	90%	100%
Fibrinolytic Medication Timing[1]	2	0%	29%	31%	100%
PCI Within 90 Minutes of Arrival	0	-	63%	54%	95%
Smoking Cessation Advice[1]	2	0%	77%	88%	100%
Heart Failure Care					
ACE Inhibitor or ARB for LVSD[1]	9	100%	84%	82%	100%
Discharge Instructions[1]	20	10%	46%	61%	93%
Evaluation of LVS Function[1]	23	74%	82%	83%	99%
Smoking Cessation Advice[1]	2	50%	70%	82%	100%
Pneumonia Care					
Appropriate Initial Antibiotic	43	91%	84%	83%	94%
Blood Culture Timing[1]	11	91%	90%	90%	100%
Influenza Vaccine[1]	7	86%	64%	70%	100%
Initial Antibiotic Timing	48	90%	81%	80%	93%
Oxygenation Assessment	61	100%	100%	99%	100%
Pneumococcal Vaccine	49	90%	63%	69%	94%
Smoking Cessation Advice[1]	4	25%	70%	80%	100%
Surgical Infection Prevention					
Prophylactic Antibiotic Given[3]	125	96%	71%	77%	95%
Prophylactic Antibiotic Selection	44	100%	89%	90%	100%
Prophylactic Antibiotic Stopped[3]	125	74%	65%	72%	95%
Pregnancy Care					
Inpatient Neonatal Mortality	-	-	-	-	-
Third or Fourth Degree Laceration	-	-	3.10%	3.63%	3.27%

Blue Mountain Hospital District

170 Ford Road Phone: 541-575-1311
John Day, OR 97845
Ownership: Govt - Hospital District or Authority Accredited: No
Emergency Services: Yes

Measure	Cases	This Hospital	State Average	U.S. Average	Top Hospital
Heart Attack Care					
ACE Inhibitor or ARB for LVSD[1,3]	1	100%	88%	82%	100%
Aspirin at Arrival[1,3]	4	100%	93%	92%	100%
Aspirin at Discharge[1,3]	2	100%	93%	90%	100%
Beta Blocker at Arrival[1,3]	4	75%	92%	87%	100%
Beta Blocker at Discharge[1,3]	2	100%	95%	90%	100%
Fibrinolytic Medication Timing[1,3]	1	0%	29%	31%	100%
PCI Within 90 Minutes of Arrival[5]	-	-	63%	54%	95%
Smoking Cessation Advice[3]	0	-	77%	88%	100%
Heart Failure Care					
ACE Inhibitor or ARB for LVSD[1,3]	1	0%	84%	82%	100%
Discharge Instructions[1,3]	7	14%	46%	61%	93%
Evaluation of LVS Function[1,3]	9	22%	82%	83%	99%
Smoking Cessation Advice[1,3]	1	0%	70%	82%	100%
Pneumonia Care					
Appropriate Initial Antibiotic[1,2]	15	93%	84%	83%	94%
Blood Culture Timing[1,2]	11	91%	90%	90%	100%
Influenza Vaccine[1]	2	100%	64%	70%	100%
Initial Antibiotic Timing[1,2]	11	82%	81%	80%	93%
Oxygenation Assessment[1,2]	18	100%	100%	99%	100%
Pneumococcal Vaccine[1,2]	12	67%	63%	69%	94%
Smoking Cessation Advice[1,2]	3	0%	70%	80%	100%
Surgical Infection Prevention					
Prophylactic Antibiotic Given[5]	-	-	71%	77%	95%
Prophylactic Antibiotic Selection[5]	-	-	89%	90%	100%
Prophylactic Antibiotic Stopped[5]	-	-	65%	72%	95%
Pregnancy Care					
Inpatient Neonatal Mortality	-	-	-	-	-
Third or Fourth Degree Laceration	-	-	3.10%	3.63%	3.27%

Merle West Medical Center

2865 Daggett Avenue Phone: 541-882-6311
Klamath Falls, OR 97601 Fax: 541-885-6725
URL: www.mwmc.org
Ownership: Voluntary non-profit - Private Accredited: Yes
Emergency Services: Yes Licensed Beds: 176

Key Personnel:

President/CEO . . . . Paul R Stewart
Chief Medical Staff . . . . Kathy Bakke, MD
Catheterization Lab . . . . Paul Mee
Emergency Room . . . . Gretchen Garza
Emergency Room . . . . Bryan Stuart, MD
Infection Control . . . . Laurie Gerskey, RN
ICU . . . . Cindy Neubauer, RN
Intensive/Coronary Care . . . . Don Hundley
Medical/Surgical Nursing . . . . Michael Hughes, RN
Respiratory/Cardiopulmonary . . . . Ki Rabbe

Measure	Cases	This Hospital	State Average	U.S. Average	Top Hospital
Heart Attack Care					
ACE Inhibitor or ARB for LVSD[1]	11	64%	88%	82%	100%
Aspirin at Arrival	73	96%	93%	92%	100%
Aspirin at Discharge	65	97%	93%	90%	100%
Beta Blocker at Arrival	57	89%	92%	87%	100%
Beta Blocker at Discharge	63	92%	95%	90%	100%
Fibrinolytic Medication Timing[1]	1	0%	29%	31%	100%
PCI Within 90 Minutes of Arrival[1]	9	44%	63%	54%	95%
Smoking Cessation Advice[1]	18	89%	77%	88%	100%
Heart Failure Care					
ACE Inhibitor or ARB for LVSD	46	89%	84%	82%	100%
Discharge Instructions	131	51%	46%	61%	93%
Evaluation of LVS Function	155	92%	82%	83%	99%
Smoking Cessation Advice[1]	22	73%	70%	82%	100%
Pneumonia Care					
Appropriate Initial Antibiotic	139	90%	84%	83%	94%
Blood Culture Timing	105	88%	90%	90%	100%
Influenza Vaccine	35	66%	64%	70%	100%
Initial Antibiotic Timing	167	83%	81%	80%	93%
Oxygenation Assessment	199	100%	100%	99%	100%
Pneumococcal Vaccine	125	80%	63%	69%	94%
Smoking Cessation Advice	56	62%	70%	80%	100%
Surgical Infection Prevention					
Prophylactic Antibiotic Given[3]	97	80%	71%	77%	95%
Prophylactic Antibiotic Selection	97	62%	89%	90%	100%
Prophylactic Antibiotic Stopped[3]	95	41%	65%	72%	95%
Pregnancy Care					
Inpatient Neonatal Mortality	870	0.23%	-	-	-
Third or Fourth Degree Laceration	591	5.25%	3.10%	3.63%	3.27%

Grande Ronde Hospital

900 Sunset Drive Phone: 541-963-8421
PO Box 3290 Fax: 541-963-1485
La Grande, OR 97850
E-mail: wkr0@grh.org
URL: www.grh.org
Ownership: Voluntary non-profit - Private Accredited: No
Emergency Services: Yes Licensed Beds: 49

Key Personnel:

President/CEO . . . . James A Mattes
Medical Staff President . . . . Stephen Bump, MD
Manager Emergency Room . . . . Debi Akers, RN
Director Emergency Room . . . . Ken Chasteem, MD
Manager Infection/Disease Control . . . . Vicki Hill-Brown, RN
Medical Surgical Nursing . . . . Robin Mitchell, RN
Manager Radiology . . . . Troy Juniper
Manager Respiratory Therapy . . . . Norman Kerr

Measure	Cases	This Hospital	State Average	U.S. Average	Top Hospital
Heart Attack Care					
ACE Inhibitor or ARB for LVSD[1]	2	50%	88%	82%	100%
Aspirin at Arrival[1]	19	100%	93%	92%	100%
Aspirin at Discharge[1]	10	80%	93%	90%	100%
Beta Blocker at Arrival[1]	17	100%	92%	87%	100%

NOTE: Hospital profiles are in alphabetical order by state, then city, then hospital within the city; Rankings are sorted by rate in descending order and exclude hospitals with less than 25 cases; (1) The number of cases is too small (n<25) for purposes of reliably predicting hospital performance; (2) Measure reflects the hospital's indication that its submission was based upon a sample of its relevant discharges; (3) Rate reflects fewer than the maximum possible quarters of data for the measure; (4) Inaccurate information submitted and suppressed for one or more quarters; (5) No data is available from the hospital for this measure; Please refer to the User's Guide for a full explanation of data

Measure	Cases	This Hospital	State Average	U.S. Average	Top Hospital
Beta Blocker at Discharge[1]	11	100%	95%	90%	100%
Fibrinolytic Medication Timing[1]	4	0%	29%	31%	100%
PCI Within 90 Minutes of Arrival	0	-	63%	54%	95%
Smoking Cessation Advice[1]	1	100%	77%	88%	100%
Heart Failure Care					
ACE Inhibitor or ARB for LVSD[1]	15	87%	84%	82%	100%
Discharge Instructions	45	82%	46%	61%	93%
Evaluation of LVS Function	56	93%	82%	83%	99%
Smoking Cessation Advice[1]	5	60%	70%	82%	100%
Pneumonia Care					
Appropriate Initial Antibiotic	89	76%	84%	83%	94%
Blood Culture Timing	41	80%	90%	90%	100%
Influenza Vaccine	28	89%	64%	70%	100%
Initial Antibiotic Timing	103	76%	81%	80%	93%
Oxygenation Assessment	128	99%	100%	99%	100%
Pneumococcal Vaccine	87	68%	63%	69%	94%
Smoking Cessation Advice[1]	12	42%	70%	80%	100%
Surgical Infection Prevention					
Prophylactic Antibiotic Given[5]	-	-	71%	77%	95%
Prophylactic Antibiotic Selection[5]	-	-	89%	90%	100%
Prophylactic Antibiotic Stopped[5]	-	-	65%	72%	95%
Pregnancy Care					
Inpatient Neonatal Mortality	-	-	-	-	-
Third or Fourth Degree Laceration	-	-	3.10%	3.63%	3.27%

Lake District Hospital

700 South J Street Phone: 541-947-2114
Lakeview, OR 97630
Ownership: Govt - Hospital District or Authority Accredited: No
Emergency Services: Yes

Measure	Cases	This Hospital	State Average	U.S. Average	Top Hospital
Heart Attack Care					
ACE Inhibitor or ARB for LVSD[5]	-	-	88%	82%	100%
Aspirin at Arrival[3]	0	-	93%	92%	100%
Aspirin at Discharge[3]	0	-	93%	90%	100%
Beta Blocker at Arrival[3]	0	-	92%	87%	100%
Beta Blocker at Discharge[3]	0	-	95%	90%	100%
Fibrinolytic Medication Timing[3]	0	-	29%	31%	100%
PCI Within 90 Minutes of Arrival[5]	-	-	63%	54%	95%
Smoking Cessation Advice[3]	0	-	77%	88%	100%
Heart Failure Care					
ACE Inhibitor or ARB for LVSD[5]	-	-	84%	82%	100%
Discharge Instructions[1,3]	5	20%	46%	61%	93%
Evaluation of LVS Function[5]	-	-	82%	83%	99%
Smoking Cessation Advice[3]	0	-	70%	82%	100%
Pneumonia Care					
Appropriate Initial Antibiotic[3]	0	-	84%	83%	94%
Blood Culture Timing[3]	0	-	90%	90%	100%
Influenza Vaccine[5]	-	-	64%	70%	100%
Initial Antibiotic Timing[5]	-	-	81%	80%	93%
Oxygenation Assessment[1,3]	1	100%	100%	99%	100%
Pneumococcal Vaccine[3]	0	-	63%	69%	94%
Smoking Cessation Advice[3]	0	-	70%	80%	100%
Surgical Infection Prevention					
Prophylactic Antibiotic Given[5]	-	-	71%	77%	95%
Prophylactic Antibiotic Selection[5]	-	-	89%	90%	100%
Prophylactic Antibiotic Stopped[5]	-	-	65%	72%	95%
Pregnancy Care					
Inpatient Neonatal Mortality	-	-	-	-	-
Third or Fourth Degree Laceration	-	-	3.10%	3.63%	3.27%

Samaritan Lebanon Community Hospital

525 N Santiam Highway Phone: 541-258-2101
Lebanon, OR 97355 Fax: 541-768-5124
URL: www.samhealth.org
Ownership: Voluntary non-profit - Church Accredited: No
Emergency Services: Yes Licensed Beds: 49
Key Personnel:
CEO. . . . . Becky A Pape
Cardiac Services Program Manager . . . . Randy Cox

Measure	Cases	This Hospital	State Average	U.S. Average	Top Hospital
Heart Attack Care					
ACE Inhibitor or ARB for LVSD[1]	2	50%	88%	82%	100%
Aspirin at Arrival[1]	23	96%	93%	92%	100%
Aspirin at Discharge[1]	15	93%	93%	90%	100%
Beta Blocker at Arrival[1]	23	83%	92%	87%	100%
Beta Blocker at Discharge[1]	19	95%	95%	90%	100%
Fibrinolytic Medication Timing	0	-	29%	31%	100%
PCI Within 90 Minutes of Arrival	0	-	63%	54%	95%
Smoking Cessation Advice[1]	2	100%	77%	88%	100%
Heart Failure Care					
ACE Inhibitor or ARB for LVSD	26	85%	84%	82%	100%
Discharge Instructions	70	46%	46%	61%	93%
Evaluation of LVS Function	96	77%	82%	83%	99%
Smoking Cessation Advice[1]	17	100%	70%	82%	100%
Pneumonia Care					
Appropriate Initial Antibiotic	95	86%	84%	83%	94%
Blood Culture Timing	61	92%	90%	90%	100%
Influenza Vaccine[1]	23	74%	64%	70%	100%
Initial Antibiotic Timing	118	92%	81%	80%	93%
Oxygenation Assessment	139	100%	100%	99%	100%
Pneumococcal Vaccine	105	70%	63%	69%	94%
Smoking Cessation Advice	36	94%	70%	80%	100%
Surgical Infection Prevention					
Prophylactic Antibiotic Given[2]	88	83%	71%	77%	95%
Prophylactic Antibiotic Selection[1,2]	17	100%	89%	90%	100%
Prophylactic Antibiotic Stopped[2]	85	92%	65%	72%	95%
Pregnancy Care					
Inpatient Neonatal Mortality	-	-	-	-	-
Third or Fourth Degree Laceration	-	-	3.10%	3.63%	3.27%

Samaritan North Lincoln Hospital

PO Box 767 Phone: 541-994-3661
Lincoln City, OR 97367 Fax: 541-996-7386
Ownership: Voluntary non-profit - Private Accredited: Yes
Emergency Services: Yes Licensed Beds: 37
Key Personnel:
Administrator/CEO. . . . . Jack Flaig
Chief Medical Staff. . . . . David Rosencrentz
Director Infection/Disease Control . . . . Leah Baker-Fones, RN
CCU Spvg. Nurse . . . . Willa Espinoza, RN
Director Medical/Surgical Nursing . . . . Judy Mori
Director Respiratory Therapy. . . . . Tim Lindsey

Measure	Cases	This Hospital	State Average	U.S. Average	Top Hospital
Heart Attack Care					
ACE Inhibitor or ARB for LVSD[1]	2	100%	88%	82%	100%
Aspirin at Arrival[1]	10	100%	93%	92%	100%
Aspirin at Discharge[1]	10	80%	93%	90%	100%
Beta Blocker at Arrival[1]	5	80%	92%	87%	100%
Beta Blocker at Discharge[1]	6	83%	95%	90%	100%
Fibrinolytic Medication Timing	0	-	29%	31%	100%
PCI Within 90 Minutes of Arrival	0	-	63%	54%	95%
Smoking Cessation Advice[1]	1	100%	77%	88%	100%
Heart Failure Care					
ACE Inhibitor or ARB for LVSD[1]	11	82%	84%	82%	100%
Discharge Instructions	29	24%	46%	61%	93%
Evaluation of LVS Function	43	74%	82%	83%	99%
Smoking Cessation Advice[1]	10	40%	70%	82%	100%
Pneumonia Care					
Appropriate Initial Antibiotic	39	72%	84%	83%	94%
Blood Culture Timing[1]	22	91%	90%	90%	100%
Influenza Vaccine[1]	9	44%	64%	70%	100%
Initial Antibiotic Timing	48	77%	81%	80%	93%
Oxygenation Assessment	59	100%	100%	99%	100%
Pneumococcal Vaccine	41	44%	63%	69%	94%
Smoking Cessation Advice[1]	23	43%	70%	80%	100%
Surgical Infection Prevention					
Prophylactic Antibiotic Given	64	59%	71%	77%	95%
Prophylactic Antibiotic Selection[1]	9	44%	89%	90%	100%
Prophylactic Antibiotic Stopped	60	35%	65%	72%	95%
Pregnancy Care					

NOTE: Hospital profiles are in alphabetical order by state, then city, then hospital within the city; Rankings are sorted by rate in descending order and exclude hospitals with less than 25 cases; (1) The number of cases is too small (n<25) for purposes of reliably predicting hospital performance; (2) Measure reflects the hospital's indication that its submission was based upon a sample of its relevant discharges; (3) Rate reflects fewer than the maximum possible quarters of data for the measure; (4) Inaccurate information submitted and suppressed for one or more quarters; (5) No data is available from the hospital for this measure; Please refer to the User's Guide for a full explanation of data

Inpatient Neonatal Mortality	-	-	-	-	-
Third or Fourth Degree Laceration	-	-	3.10%	3.63%	3.27%

Mountain View Hospital District

470 NE A Street
Madras, OR 97741
Ownership: Voluntary non-profit - Other
Emergency Services: Yes
Phone: 541-475-3882
Fax: 541-475-4804
Accredited: No
Licensed Beds: 106

Key Personnel:

Administrator . . . . Susan McGough
Chief Medical Staff . . . . Carlos Kemper, MD
Emergency Room . . . . Leland Beamer, MD
Director Infection/Disease Control . . . . Cathy Luther, RN
Director Radiology . . . . Greg Kemper
Director Respiratory Therapy . . . . Charles Hayes

Measure	Cases	This Hospital	State Average	U.S. Average	Top Hospital
Heart Attack Care					
ACE Inhibitor or ARB for LVSD[3]	0	-	88%	82%	100%
Aspirin at Arrival[1,3]	3	67%	93%	92%	100%
Aspirin at Discharge[1,3]	3	100%	93%	90%	100%
Beta Blocker at Arrival[1,3]	3	67%	92%	87%	100%
Beta Blocker at Discharge[1,3]	3	67%	95%	90%	100%
Fibrinolytic Medication Timing[3]	0	-	29%	31%	100%
PCI Within 90 Minutes of Arrival[5]	-	-	63%	54%	95%
Smoking Cessation Advice[3]	0	-	77%	88%	100%
Heart Failure Care					
ACE Inhibitor or ARB for LVSD[1,3]	2	100%	84%	82%	100%
Discharge Instructions[1,3]	16	25%	46%	61%	93%
Evaluation of LVS Function[1,3]	20	30%	82%	83%	99%
Smoking Cessation Advice[1,3]	8	62%	70%	82%	100%
Pneumonia Care					
Appropriate Initial Antibiotic	28	100%	84%	83%	94%
Blood Culture Timing[1]	20	95%	90%	90%	100%
Influenza Vaccine[1]	5	80%	64%	70%	100%
Initial Antibiotic Timing	37	84%	81%	80%	93%
Oxygenation Assessment	42	100%	100%	99%	100%
Pneumococcal Vaccine[1]	23	87%	63%	69%	94%
Smoking Cessation Advice[1]	12	75%	70%	80%	100%
Surgical Infection Prevention					
Prophylactic Antibiotic Given[1]	22	45%	71%	77%	95%
Prophylactic Antibiotic Selection[1]	9	89%	89%	90%	100%
Prophylactic Antibiotic Stopped[1]	22	82%	65%	72%	95%
Pregnancy Care					
Inpatient Neonatal Mortality	-	-	-	-	-
Third or Fourth Degree Laceration	-	-	3.10%	3.63%	3.27%

Willamette Valley Medical Center

Alternate Name: McMinnville Community Hospital
2700 Three Mile Lane
McMinnville, OR 97128
Ownership: Voluntary non-profit - Private
Emergency Services: Yes
Phone: 503-472-6131
Fax: 503-472-8691
Accredited: Yes
Licensed Beds: 80

Key Personnel:

CEO . . . . Rosemary Davis
Chief Medical Staff . . . . John Topping
Emergency Room . . . . John Sandberg, MD
Director Medical/Surgical Nursing . . . . Alice Cooper
Chief Radiology . . . . Steven H Edelman, MD
Director Respiratory Therapy . . . . Will Lutsock

Measure	Cases	This Hospital	State Average	U.S. Average	Top Hospital
Heart Attack Care					
ACE Inhibitor or ARB for LVSD[1]	4	100%	88%	82%	100%
Aspirin at Arrival	36	94%	93%	92%	100%
Aspirin at Discharge[1]	21	100%	93%	90%	100%
Beta Blocker at Arrival[1]	23	96%	92%	87%	100%
Beta Blocker at Discharge[1]	21	90%	95%	90%	100%
Fibrinolytic Medication Timing[1]	3	0%	29%	31%	100%
PCI Within 90 Minutes of Arrival	0	-	63%	54%	95%
Smoking Cessation Advice[1]	7	100%	77%	88%	100%
Heart Failure Care					
ACE Inhibitor or ARB for LVSD	38	79%	84%	82%	100%
Discharge Instructions	96	85%	46%	61%	93%
Evaluation of LVS Function	122	100%	82%	83%	99%
Smoking Cessation Advice	25	96%	70%	82%	100%
Pneumonia Care					
Appropriate Initial Antibiotic	132	88%	84%	83%	94%
Blood Culture Timing	147	97%	90%	90%	100%
Influenza Vaccine	45	96%	64%	70%	100%
Initial Antibiotic Timing	180	78%	81%	80%	93%
Oxygenation Assessment	224	100%	100%	99%	100%
Pneumococcal Vaccine	155	88%	63%	69%	94%
Smoking Cessation Advice	55	96%	70%	80%	100%
Surgical Infection Prevention					
Prophylactic Antibiotic Given	230	96%	71%	77%	95%
Prophylactic Antibiotic Selection	51	96%	89%	90%	100%
Prophylactic Antibiotic Stopped	222	86%	65%	72%	95%
Pregnancy Care					
Inpatient Neonatal Mortality	-	-	-	-	-
Third or Fourth Degree Laceration	-	-	3.10%	3.63%	3.27%

Providence Medford Medical Center

Alternate Name: Providence Hospital
1111 Crater Lake Avenue
Medford, OR 97504
Ownership: Voluntary non-profit - Church
Emergency Services: Yes
Phone: 541-732-5000
Fax: 541-732-5872
Accredited: Yes
Licensed Beds: 168

Key Personnel:

President/CEO . . . . Charles T Wright
Chief Medical Staff . . . . Erich Weber, MD
Emergency Room . . . . Gordon Everett
Infection Control . . . . Carleen Lawence
Respiratory Therapy . . . . Becky Rauschenberger

Measure	Cases	This Hospital	State Average	U.S. Average	Top Hospital
Heart Attack Care					
ACE Inhibitor or ARB for LVSD[1]	11	91%	88%	82%	100%
Aspirin at Arrival	64	98%	93%	92%	100%
Aspirin at Discharge	45	100%	93%	90%	100%
Beta Blocker at Arrival	60	97%	92%	87%	100%
Beta Blocker at Discharge	52	96%	95%	90%	100%
Fibrinolytic Medication Timing	0	-	29%	31%	100%
PCI Within 90 Minutes of Arrival	0	-	63%	54%	95%
Smoking Cessation Advice[1]	11	82%	77%	88%	100%
Heart Failure Care					
ACE Inhibitor or ARB for LVSD[2]	39	74%	84%	82%	100%
Discharge Instructions[2]	136	10%	46%	61%	93%
Evaluation of LVS Function[2]	162	85%	82%	83%	99%
Smoking Cessation Advice[2]	40	65%	70%	82%	100%
Pneumonia Care					
Appropriate Initial Antibiotic[2]	107	83%	84%	83%	94%
Blood Culture Timing[2]	68	82%	90%	90%	100%
Influenza Vaccine[1,2]	24	83%	64%	70%	100%
Initial Antibiotic Timing[2]	132	70%	81%	80%	93%
Oxygenation Assessment[2]	166	100%	100%	99%	100%
Pneumococcal Vaccine[2]	115	45%	63%	69%	94%
Smoking Cessation Advice[2]	50	80%	70%	80%	100%
Surgical Infection Prevention					
Prophylactic Antibiotic Given[2,3]	108	65%	71%	77%	95%
Prophylactic Antibiotic Selection[2]	27	85%	89%	90%	100%
Prophylactic Antibiotic Stopped[2,3]	108	78%	65%	72%	95%
Pregnancy Care					
Inpatient Neonatal Mortality	-	-	-	-	-
Third or Fourth Degree Laceration	-	-	3.10%	3.63%	3.27%

Rogue Valley Medical Center

2825 E Barnett Road
Medford, OR 97504
URL: www.asante.org
Ownership: Voluntary non-profit - Other
Emergency Services: Yes
Phone: 541-789-7000
Fax: 541-789-5870
Accredited: Yes
Licensed Beds: 305

Key Personnel:

CEO . . . . Roy Vineyard
Emergency Room . . . . Ken Rhee

NOTE: Hospital profiles are in alphabetical order by state, then city, then hospital within the city; Rankings are sorted by rate in descending order and exclude hospitals with less than 25 cases; (1) The number of cases is too small (n<25) for purposes of reliably predicting hospital performance; (2) Measure reflects the hospital's indication that its submission was based upon a sample of its relevant discharges; (3) Rate reflects fewer than the maximum possible quarters of data for the measure; (4) Inaccurate information submitted and suppressed for one or more quarters; (5) No data is available from the hospital for this measure; Please refer to the User's Guide for a full explanation of data

Director Radiology . . . . Bob James
Manager Respiratory Therapy . . . . Dan Coons

Measure	Cases	This Hospital	State Average	U.S. Average	Top Hospital
Heart Attack Care					
ACE Inhibitor or ARB for LVSD	58	95%	88%	82%	100%
Aspirin at Arrival	219	99%	93%	92%	100%
Aspirin at Discharge	421	99%	93%	90%	100%
Beta Blocker at Arrival	162	98%	92%	87%	100%
Beta Blocker at Discharge	448	97%	95%	90%	100%
Fibrinolytic Medication Timing	0	-	29%	31%	100%
PCI Within 90 Minutes of Arrival[1]	19	53%	63%	54%	95%
Smoking Cessation Advice	142	95%	77%	88%	100%
Heart Failure Care					
ACE Inhibitor or ARB for LVSD	221	91%	84%	82%	100%
Discharge Instructions	402	73%	46%	61%	93%
Evaluation of LVS Function	428	94%	82%	83%	99%
Smoking Cessation Advice	68	85%	70%	82%	100%
Pneumonia Care					
Appropriate Initial Antibiotic	188	91%	84%	83%	94%
Blood Culture Timing	176	96%	90%	90%	100%
Influenza Vaccine	62	69%	64%	70%	100%
Initial Antibiotic Timing	259	76%	81%	80%	93%
Oxygenation Assessment	325	100%	100%	99%	100%
Pneumococcal Vaccine	230	67%	63%	69%	94%
Smoking Cessation Advice	77	94%	70%	80%	100%
Surgical Infection Prevention					
Prophylactic Antibiotic Given[2,3]	590	82%	71%	77%	95%
Prophylactic Antibiotic Selection[2]	78	99%	89%	90%	100%
Prophylactic Antibiotic Stopped[2,3]	574	84%	65%	72%	95%
Pregnancy Care					
Inpatient Neonatal Mortality	-	-	-	-	-
Third or Fourth Degree Laceration	-	-	3.10%	3.63%	3.27%

Providence Milwaukie Hospital

10150 SE 32nd Avenue
Portland, OR 97222
URL: www.providence.org
Ownership: Voluntary non-profit - Church
Emergency Services: Yes
Phone: 503-513-8300
Fax: 503-513-8463
Accredited: Yes
Licensed Beds: 77

Key Personnel:

Chief of Medical Staff . . . . Sindy Talbot
Head of Emergency Room . . . . Fred Underwood
Head of Respiratory Care . . . . Marry Kirschbaum

Measure	Cases	This Hospital	State Average	U.S. Average	Top Hospital
Heart Attack Care					
ACE Inhibitor or ARB for LVSD[1]	5	100%	88%	82%	100%
Aspirin at Arrival	41	100%	93%	92%	100%
Aspirin at Discharge	25	92%	93%	90%	100%
Beta Blocker at Arrival	37	97%	92%	87%	100%
Beta Blocker at Discharge	27	96%	95%	90%	100%
Fibrinolytic Medication Timing	0	-	29%	31%	100%
PCI Within 90 Minutes of Arrival	0	-	63%	54%	95%
Smoking Cessation Advice[1]	4	75%	77%	88%	100%
Heart Failure Care					
ACE Inhibitor or ARB for LVSD[2]	37	92%	84%	82%	100%
Discharge Instructions[2]	86	27%	46%	61%	93%
Evaluation of LVS Function[2]	105	93%	82%	83%	99%
Smoking Cessation Advice[2]	26	73%	70%	82%	100%
Pneumonia Care					
Appropriate Initial Antibiotic[2]	98	76%	84%	83%	94%
Blood Culture Timing[2]	79	86%	90%	90%	100%
Influenza Vaccine[2]	27	74%	64%	70%	100%
Initial Antibiotic Timing[2]	129	84%	81%	80%	93%
Oxygenation Assessment[2]	156	100%	100%	99%	100%
Pneumococcal Vaccine[2]	99	74%	63%	69%	94%
Smoking Cessation Advice[2]	43	79%	70%	80%	100%
Surgical Infection Prevention					
Prophylactic Antibiotic Given[2,3]	113	69%	71%	77%	95%
Prophylactic Antibiotic Selection[2]	39	95%	89%	90%	100%
Prophylactic Antibiotic Stopped[2,3]	105	55%	65%	72%	95%
Pregnancy Care					
Inpatient Neonatal Mortality	-	-	-	-	-
Third or Fourth Degree Laceration	-	-	3.10%	3.63%	3.27%

Providence Newberg Hospital

Alternate Name: Newberg Community Hospital
501 Villa Road
Newberg, OR 97132
Ownership: Voluntary non-profit - Church
Emergency Services: Yes
Phone: 503-537-1555
Fax: 503-537-1815
Accredited: Yes
Licensed Beds: 35

Key Personnel:

President/CEO . . . . Mark W Meinert
Chief Medical Staff . . . . Steve Townsend, MD
Emergency Room . . . . John Van Eaton, MD
Director Medical/Surgical Nursing . . . . Kathleen Macken

Measure	Cases	This Hospital	State Average	U.S. Average	Top Hospital
Heart Attack Care					
ACE Inhibitor or ARB for LVSD[1]	1	100%	88%	82%	100%
Aspirin at Arrival[1]	15	100%	93%	92%	100%
Aspirin at Discharge[1]	9	100%	93%	90%	100%
Beta Blocker at Arrival[1]	15	93%	92%	87%	100%
Beta Blocker at Discharge[1]	11	100%	95%	90%	100%
Fibrinolytic Medication Timing[1]	2	50%	29%	31%	100%
PCI Within 90 Minutes of Arrival	0	-	63%	54%	95%
Smoking Cessation Advice	0	-	77%	88%	100%
Heart Failure Care					
ACE Inhibitor or ARB for LVSD[1,2]	14	57%	84%	82%	100%
Discharge Instructions[2]	41	22%	46%	61%	93%
Evaluation of LVS Function[2]	55	91%	82%	83%	99%
Smoking Cessation Advice[1,2]	8	25%	70%	82%	100%
Pneumonia Care					
Appropriate Initial Antibiotic[2]	50	74%	84%	83%	94%
Blood Culture Timing[2]	36	92%	90%	90%	100%
Influenza Vaccine[1,2]	7	57%	64%	70%	100%
Initial Antibiotic Timing[2]	62	82%	81%	80%	93%
Oxygenation Assessment[2]	78	100%	100%	99%	100%
Pneumococcal Vaccine[2]	49	37%	63%	69%	94%
Smoking Cessation Advice[1,2]	13	62%	70%	80%	100%
Surgical Infection Prevention					
Prophylactic Antibiotic Given[2,3]	99	93%	71%	77%	95%
Prophylactic Antibiotic Selection[2]	37	95%	89%	90%	100%
Prophylactic Antibiotic Stopped[2,3]	96	89%	65%	72%	95%
Pregnancy Care					
Inpatient Neonatal Mortality	-	-	-	-	-
Third or Fourth Degree Laceration	-	-	3.10%	3.63%	3.27%

Samaritan Pacific Community Hospital

930 SW Abbey Street
Newport, OR 97365
Toll-Free: 800-863-5241
Phone: 541-265-2244
Fax: 541-574-4664
URL: www.samhealth.org
Ownership: Voluntary non-profit - Private
Emergency Services: Yes
Accredited: Yes
Licensed Beds: 48

Key Personnel:

CEO . . . . David C Bigelow

Measure	Cases	This Hospital	State Average	U.S. Average	Top Hospital
Heart Attack Care					
ACE Inhibitor or ARB for LVSD[1]	2	100%	88%	82%	100%
Aspirin at Arrival[1]	15	80%	93%	92%	100%
Aspirin at Discharge[1]	13	77%	93%	90%	100%
Beta Blocker at Arrival[1]	11	100%	92%	87%	100%
Beta Blocker at Discharge[1]	11	100%	95%	90%	100%
Fibrinolytic Medication Timing	0	-	29%	31%	100%
PCI Within 90 Minutes of Arrival	0	-	63%	54%	95%
Smoking Cessation Advice[1]	3	33%	77%	88%	100%
Heart Failure Care					
ACE Inhibitor or ARB for LVSD[1]	9	78%	84%	82%	100%
Discharge Instructions	39	23%	46%	61%	93%
Evaluation of LVS Function	37	76%	82%	83%	99%
Smoking Cessation Advice[1]	10	70%	70%	82%	100%

NOTE: Hospital profiles are in alphabetical order by state, then city, then hospital within the city; Rankings are sorted by rate in descending order and exclude hospitals with less than 25 cases; (1) The number of cases is too small (n<25) for purposes of reliably predicting hospital performance; (2) Measure reflects the hospital's indication that its submission was based upon a sample of its relevant discharges; (3) Rate reflects fewer than the maximum possible quarters of data for the measure; (4) Inaccurate information submitted and suppressed for one or more quarters; (5) No data is available from the hospital for this measure; Please refer to the User's Guide for a full explanation of data

Pneumonia Care					
Appropriate Initial Antibiotic	49	80%	84%	83%	94%
Blood Culture Timing[1]	23	83%	90%	90%	100%
Influenza Vaccine[1]	9	33%	64%	70%	100%
Initial Antibiotic Timing	42	86%	81%	80%	93%
Oxygenation Assessment	58	100%	100%	99%	100%
Pneumococcal Vaccine	31	52%	63%	69%	94%
Smoking Cessation Advice[1]	16	81%	70%	80%	100%
Surgical Infection Prevention					
Prophylactic Antibiotic Given	54	80%	71%	77%	95%
Prophylactic Antibiotic Selection[1]	10	100%	89%	90%	100%
Prophylactic Antibiotic Stopped	51	82%	65%	72%	95%
Pregnancy Care					
Inpatient Neonatal Mortality	-	-	-	-	-
Third or Fourth Degree Laceration	-	-	3.10%	3.63%	3.27%

Holy Rosary Medical Center

351 SW Ninth Street
Ontario, OR 97914
Phone: 541-881-7000
Fax: 541-881-7184
URL: www.holyrosary-ontario.org
Ownership: Voluntary non-profit - Private
Accredited: Yes
Emergency Services: Yes
Licensed Beds: 92

Key Personnel:

Administrator . . . . Bruce Jensen
Patient Care Manager Medical/Surgery . . . . Linda Hoffman
OB/GYN Womens Health. . . . . Kathy Rice
Surgery Director. . . . . Carol Wininger
Director Maternal/Child Services . . . . Kathy Rice
Director Respiratory/Cardiopulmonary . . . . John Mayberry

Measure	Cases	This Hospital	State Average	U.S. Average	Top Hospital
Heart Attack Care					
ACE Inhibitor or ARB for LVSD[1]	5	80%	88%	82%	100%
Aspirin at Arrival[1]	14	100%	93%	92%	100%
Aspirin at Discharge[1]	10	70%	93%	90%	100%
Beta Blocker at Arrival[1]	12	92%	92%	87%	100%
Beta Blocker at Discharge[1]	10	100%	95%	90%	100%
Fibrinolytic Medication Timing	0	-	29%	31%	100%
PCI Within 90 Minutes of Arrival	0	-	63%	54%	95%
Smoking Cessation Advice[1]	1	100%	77%	88%	100%
Heart Failure Care					
ACE Inhibitor or ARB for LVSD[1]	14	71%	84%	82%	100%
Discharge Instructions	51	29%	46%	61%	93%
Evaluation of LVS Function	60	82%	82%	83%	99%
Smoking Cessation Advice[1]	9	100%	70%	82%	100%
Pneumonia Care					
Appropriate Initial Antibiotic	83	67%	84%	83%	94%
Blood Culture Timing	30	77%	90%	90%	100%
Influenza Vaccine[1]	16	31%	64%	70%	100%
Initial Antibiotic Timing	84	76%	81%	80%	93%
Oxygenation Assessment	106	99%	100%	99%	100%
Pneumococcal Vaccine	79	34%	63%	69%	94%
Smoking Cessation Advice[1]	19	74%	70%	80%	100%
Surgical Infection Prevention					
Prophylactic Antibiotic Given[3]	133	50%	71%	77%	95%
Prophylactic Antibiotic Selection	43	63%	89%	90%	100%
Prophylactic Antibiotic Stopped[3]	131	34%	65%	72%	95%
Pregnancy Care					
Inpatient Neonatal Mortality	663	0.15%	-	-	-
Third or Fourth Degree Laceration	479	1.04%	3.10%	3.63%	3.27%

Willamette Falls Hospital

1500 Division Street
Oregon City, OR 97045
Phone: 503-656-1631
Fax: 503-557-2101
E-mail: wfh@wfhonline.org
URL: www.willamettefallshospital.org
Ownership: Voluntary non-profit - Private
Accredited: Yes
Emergency Services: Yes
Licensed Beds: 143

Key Personnel:

CEO. . . . . Russ Reinhard

Measure	Cases	This Hospital	State Average	U.S. Average	Top Hospital
Heart Attack Care					
ACE Inhibitor or ARB for LVSD[1]	3	100%	88%	82%	100%
Aspirin at Arrival	52	92%	93%	92%	100%
Aspirin at Discharge[1]	18	100%	93%	90%	100%
Beta Blocker at Arrival	41	90%	92%	87%	100%
Beta Blocker at Discharge[1]	22	82%	95%	90%	100%
Fibrinolytic Medication Timing[3]	0	-	29%	31%	100%
PCI Within 90 Minutes of Arrival	0	-	63%	54%	95%
Smoking Cessation Advice[1]	5	60%	77%	88%	100%
Heart Failure Care					
ACE Inhibitor or ARB for LVSD	33	94%	84%	82%	100%
Discharge Instructions[1,3]	16	75%	46%	61%	93%
Evaluation of LVS Function	118	87%	82%	83%	99%
Smoking Cessation Advice[1,3]	2	50%	70%	82%	100%
Pneumonia Care					
Appropriate Initial Antibiotic	92	83%	84%	83%	94%
Blood Culture Timing	56	93%	90%	90%	100%
Influenza Vaccine[5]	-	-	64%	70%	100%
Initial Antibiotic Timing	104	90%	81%	80%	93%
Oxygenation Assessment	129	100%	100%	99%	100%
Pneumococcal Vaccine	79	75%	63%	69%	94%
Smoking Cessation Advice[1,3]	7	71%	70%	80%	100%
Surgical Infection Prevention					
Prophylactic Antibiotic Given[2,3]	45	40%	71%	77%	95%
Prophylactic Antibiotic Selection[2]	43	93%	89%	90%	100%
Prophylactic Antibiotic Stopped[2,3]	40	98%	65%	72%	95%
Pregnancy Care					
Inpatient Neonatal Mortality	1,125	0.09%	-	-	-
Third or Fourth Degree Laceration	839	4.05%	3.10%	3.63%	3.27%

Legacy Emanuel Hospital/Health Center

2801 N Gantenbein Avenue
Portland, OR 97227
Phone: 503-413-2200
Fax: 503-415-5777
URL: www.legacyhealth.org
Ownership: Govt - Hospital District or Authority
Accredited: Yes
Emergency Services: Yes
Licensed Beds: 554

Key Personnel:

President/CEO. . . . . Lee Domanico

Measure	Cases	This Hospital	State Average	U.S. Average	Top Hospital
Heart Attack Care					
ACE Inhibitor or ARB for LVSD[2]	35	83%	88%	82%	100%
Aspirin at Arrival[2]	73	97%	93%	92%	100%
Aspirin at Discharge[2]	129	98%	93%	90%	100%
Beta Blocker at Arrival[2]	42	90%	92%	87%	100%
Beta Blocker at Discharge[2]	122	99%	95%	90%	100%
Fibrinolytic Medication Timing[1,2]	1	100%	29%	31%	100%
PCI Within 90 Minutes of Arrival[1,2]	4	75%	63%	54%	95%
Smoking Cessation Advice[2]	46	89%	77%	88%	100%
Heart Failure Care					
ACE Inhibitor or ARB for LVSD[2]	64	77%	84%	82%	100%
Discharge Instructions[2]	107	33%	46%	61%	93%
Evaluation of LVS Function[2]	126	98%	82%	83%	99%
Smoking Cessation Advice[2]	34	79%	70%	82%	100%
Pneumonia Care					
Appropriate Initial Antibiotic[2]	69	84%	84%	83%	94%
Blood Culture Timing[2]	65	86%	90%	90%	100%
Influenza Vaccine[1]	20	45%	64%	70%	100%
Initial Antibiotic Timing[2]	102	68%	81%	80%	93%
Oxygenation Assessment[2]	110	99%	100%	99%	100%
Pneumococcal Vaccine[2]	50	56%	63%	69%	94%
Smoking Cessation Advice[2]	47	70%	70%	80%	100%
Surgical Infection Prevention					
Prophylactic Antibiotic Given[2,3]	124	67%	71%	77%	95%
Prophylactic Antibiotic Selection[2]	58	95%	89%	90%	100%
Prophylactic Antibiotic Stopped[2,3]	114	77%	65%	72%	95%
Pregnancy Care					
Inpatient Neonatal Mortality	-	-	-	-	-
Third or Fourth Degree Laceration	-	-	3.10%	3.63%	3.27%

Legacy Good Samaritan Hospital

Alternate Name: Legacy Portland Hospitals

NOTE: Hospital profiles are in alphabetical order by state, then city, then hospital within the city; Rankings are sorted by rate in descending order and exclude hospitals with less than 25 cases; (1) The number of cases is too small (n<25) for purposes of reliably predicting hospital performance; (2) Measure reflects the hospital's indication that its submission was based upon a sample of its relevant discharges; (3) Rate reflects fewer than the maximum possible quarters of data for the measure; (4) Inaccurate information submitted and suppressed for one or more quarters; (5) No data is available from the hospital for this measure; Please refer to the User's Guide for a full explanation of data

1015 NW 22nd Avenue
Portland, OR 97210
Phone: 503-413-7711
Fax: 503-413-6347
Ownership: Voluntary non-profit - Church
Accredited: Yes
Emergency Services: Yes
Licensed Beds: 539

Key Personnel:

President/CEO . . . . Robert Pallari
Chief Medical Staff . . . . Keith Marton, MD
Cardiac Lab . . . . Margaret Allee
Catheterization Lab . . . . Margaret Allee
Emergency Room . . . . Ginny Posey
Manager Infection Control . . . . Julia Marcotte
ICU . . . . Cindy Lilley
Intensive/Coronary Care . . . . Sue Lilley
Medical/Surgical Nursing . . . . Vicky Kraushar
OB/GYN Womens Health . . . . Cheryl Purvis
Respiratory/Cardiopulmonary . . . . Margaret Allee

Measure	Cases	This Hospital	State Average	U.S. Average	Top Hospital
Heart Attack Care					
ACE Inhibitor or ARB for LVSD[2]	76	66%	88%	82%	100%
Aspirin at Arrival[2]	122	99%	93%	92%	100%
Aspirin at Discharge[2]	272	98%	93%	90%	100%
Beta Blocker at Arrival[2]	76	97%	92%	87%	100%
Beta Blocker at Discharge[2]	259	94%	95%	90%	100%
Fibrinolytic Medication Timing[2]	0	-	29%	31%	100%
PCI Within 90 Minutes of Arrival[1,2]	11	27%	63%	54%	95%
Smoking Cessation Advice[2]	108	91%	77%	88%	100%
Heart Failure Care					
ACE Inhibitor or ARB for LVSD[2]	177	66%	84%	82%	100%
Discharge Instructions[2]	270	30%	46%	61%	93%
Evaluation of LVS Function[2]	332	95%	82%	83%	99%
Smoking Cessation Advice[2]	62	63%	70%	82%	100%
Pneumonia Care					
Appropriate Initial Antibiotic[2]	78	87%	84%	83%	94%
Blood Culture Timing[2]	67	96%	90%	90%	100%
Influenza Vaccine[1]	20	60%	64%	70%	100%
Initial Antibiotic Timing[2]	134	71%	81%	80%	93%
Oxygenation Assessment[2]	152	100%	100%	99%	100%
Pneumococcal Vaccine[2]	95	56%	63%	69%	94%
Smoking Cessation Advice[2]	54	72%	70%	80%	100%
Surgical Infection Prevention					
Prophylactic Antibiotic Given[2,3]	138	51%	71%	77%	95%
Prophylactic Antibiotic Selection[2]	71	97%	89%	90%	100%
Prophylactic Antibiotic Stopped[2,3]	128	90%	65%	72%	95%
Pregnancy Care					
Inpatient Neonatal Mortality	-	-	-	-	-
Third or Fourth Degree Laceration	-	-	3.10%	3.63%	3.27%

Oregon Health Sciences University

3181 SW Sam Jackson Park Road
Portland, OR 97201
Phone: 503-494-8311
Fax: 503-494-6469
URL: www.ohsu.edu
Ownership: Voluntary non-profit - Other
Accredited: Yes
Emergency Services: Yes
Licensed Beds: 509

Key Personnel:

President . . . . Joseph Robertson, Jr, MD, MBA
Chief Catheterization Laboratory . . . . Leonard Christie, MD
Emergency Room . . . . Jerris Hedges, MD
Director Infection/Disease Control . . . . Paul Lewis, MD
Director Medical/Surgical Nursing . . . . Bonnie Driggers, RN
OB/GYN Womens Health . . . . E Paul Kirk, MD
Chief Radiology . . . . Fred Keller, MD
Director Respiratory Therapy . . . . Gene Ellis

Measure	Cases	This Hospital	State Average	U.S. Average	Top Hospital
Heart Attack Care					
ACE Inhibitor or ARB for LVSD	28	86%	88%	82%	100%
Aspirin at Arrival	73	99%	93%	92%	100%
Aspirin at Discharge	93	99%	93%	90%	100%
Beta Blocker at Arrival	62	98%	92%	87%	100%
Beta Blocker at Discharge	93	99%	95%	90%	100%
Fibrinolytic Medication Timing	0	-	29%	31%	100%
PCI Within 90 Minutes of Arrival[1]	1	100%	63%	54%	95%
Smoking Cessation Advice	26	77%	77%	88%	100%
Heart Failure Care					
ACE Inhibitor or ARB for LVSD	108	94%	84%	82%	100%
Discharge Instructions	199	41%	46%	61%	93%
Evaluation of LVS Function	216	98%	82%	83%	99%
Smoking Cessation Advice	45	49%	70%	82%	100%
Pneumonia Care					
Appropriate Initial Antibiotic[2]	68	72%	84%	83%	94%
Blood Culture Timing[2]	84	95%	90%	90%	100%
Influenza Vaccine[1,2]	23	26%	64%	70%	100%
Initial Antibiotic Timing[2]	135	64%	81%	80%	93%
Oxygenation Assessment[2]	167	100%	100%	99%	100%
Pneumococcal Vaccine[2]	51	67%	63%	69%	94%
Smoking Cessation Advice[2]	62	63%	70%	80%	100%
Surgical Infection Prevention					
Prophylactic Antibiotic Given[2,3]	373	74%	71%	77%	95%
Prophylactic Antibiotic Selection[2]	83	93%	89%	90%	100%
Prophylactic Antibiotic Stopped[2,3]	373	80%	65%	72%	95%
Pregnancy Care					
Inpatient Neonatal Mortality	-	-	-	-	-
Third or Fourth Degree Laceration	-	-	3.10%	3.63%	3.27%

Portland Adventist Medical Center

10123 SE Market Street
Portland, OR 97216
Phone: 503-257-2500
Fax: 503-251-6318
URL: www.adventisthealth.com
Ownership: Voluntary non-profit - Church
Accredited: Yes
Emergency Services: Yes
Licensed Beds: 302

Key Personnel:

CEO . . . . Deryl L Jones
Chief Medical Staff . . . . Curtis R Nevness, MD
Director of Cardiology/Cardiac Lab . . . . Larry Popplewell
Emergency Room Director . . . . Joyce Goitein
Director Medical/Surgical Nursing . . . . Gloria Santos
OB/GYN Womens Health . . . . Alan M Fisher, MD
Chief Radiology . . . . Lucien Burke, MD

Measure	Cases	This Hospital	State Average	U.S. Average	Top Hospital
Heart Attack Care					
ACE Inhibitor or ARB for LVSD[1]	15	87%	88%	82%	100%
Aspirin at Arrival	96	96%	93%	92%	100%
Aspirin at Discharge	88	98%	93%	90%	100%
Beta Blocker at Arrival	50	94%	92%	87%	100%
Beta Blocker at Discharge	95	98%	95%	90%	100%
Fibrinolytic Medication Timing	0	-	29%	31%	100%
PCI Within 90 Minutes of Arrival[1]	10	50%	63%	54%	95%
Smoking Cessation Advice	32	100%	77%	88%	100%
Heart Failure Care					
ACE Inhibitor or ARB for LVSD	44	93%	84%	82%	100%
Discharge Instructions	133	75%	46%	61%	93%
Evaluation of LVS Function	153	95%	82%	83%	99%
Smoking Cessation Advice	45	98%	70%	82%	100%
Pneumonia Care					
Appropriate Initial Antibiotic	164	90%	84%	83%	94%
Blood Culture Timing	167	97%	90%	90%	100%
Influenza Vaccine	42	93%	64%	70%	100%
Initial Antibiotic Timing	236	81%	81%	80%	93%
Oxygenation Assessment	304	100%	100%	99%	100%
Pneumococcal Vaccine	204	84%	63%	69%	94%
Smoking Cessation Advice	76	83%	70%	80%	100%
Surgical Infection Prevention					
Prophylactic Antibiotic Given[2,3]	158	84%	71%	77%	95%
Prophylactic Antibiotic Selection[2]	52	90%	89%	90%	100%
Prophylactic Antibiotic Stopped[2,3]	153	68%	65%	72%	95%
Pregnancy Care					
Inpatient Neonatal Mortality	-	-	-	-	-
Third or Fourth Degree Laceration	-	-	3.10%	3.63%	3.27%

Providence Portland Medical Center

Alternate Name: Providence Medical Center

NOTE: Hospital profiles are in alphabetical order by state, then city, then hospital within the city; Rankings are sorted by rate in descending order and exclude hospitals with less than 25 cases; (1) The number of cases is too small (n<25) for purposes of reliably predicting hospital performance; (2) Measure reflects the hospital's indication that its submission was based upon a sample of its relevant discharges; (3) Rate reflects fewer than the maximum possible quarters of data for the measure; (4) Inaccurate information submitted and suppressed for one or more quarters; (5) No data is available from the hospital for this measure; Please refer to the User's Guide for a full explanation of data

4805 NE Glisan Street
Portland, OR 97213
URL: www.providence.org/oregon
Ownership: Voluntary non-profit - Church
Emergency Services: Yes

Phone: 503-215-1111
Fax: 503-215-0431
Accredited: Yes
Licensed Beds: 483

Key Personnel:

Administrator . . . . Lisa Vance
Executive Director . . . . Kelly Buechler
Emergency Room . . . . Jene Williamson
Director Infection/Disease Control . . . . Joanne Jackson
President Medical Staff . . . . E Charles Douville, MD

Measure	Cases	This Hospital	State Average	U.S. Average	Top Hospital
Heart Attack Care					
ACE Inhibitor or ARB for LVSD	106	98%	88%	82%	100%
Aspirin at Arrival	389	98%	93%	92%	100%
Aspirin at Discharge	545	99%	93%	90%	100%
Beta Blocker at Arrival	336	98%	92%	87%	100%
Beta Blocker at Discharge	500	99%	95%	90%	100%
Fibrinolytic Medication Timing[1]	2	0%	29%	31%	100%
PCI Within 90 Minutes of Arrival[1]	23	70%	63%	54%	95%
Smoking Cessation Advice	154	96%	77%	88%	100%
Heart Failure Care					
ACE Inhibitor or ARB for LVSD[2]	132	89%	84%	82%	100%
Discharge Instructions[2]	280	61%	46%	61%	93%
Evaluation of LVS Function[2]	323	94%	82%	83%	99%
Smoking Cessation Advice[2]	59	98%	70%	82%	100%
Pneumonia Care					
Appropriate Initial Antibiotic[2]	125	86%	84%	83%	94%
Blood Culture Timing[2]	123	94%	90%	90%	100%
Influenza Vaccine[2]	25	92%	64%	70%	100%
Initial Antibiotic Timing[2]	179	78%	81%	80%	93%
Oxygenation Assessment[2]	215	100%	100%	99%	100%
Pneumococcal Vaccine[2]	123	77%	63%	69%	94%
Smoking Cessation Advice[2]	56	98%	70%	80%	100%
Surgical Infection Prevention					
Prophylactic Antibiotic Given[2,3]	222	84%	71%	77%	95%
Prophylactic Antibiotic Selection[2]	79	95%	89%	90%	100%
Prophylactic Antibiotic Stopped[2,3]	215	55%	65%	72%	95%
Pregnancy Care					
Inpatient Neonatal Mortality	-	-	-	-	-
Third or Fourth Degree Laceration	-	-	3.10%	3.63%	3.27%

Providence Saint Vincent Medical Center

Alternate Name: Saint Vincent Hospital and Medical Center
9205 SW Barnes Road
Portland, OR 97225
URL: www.providence.org
Ownership: Voluntary non-profit - Church
Emergency Services: Yes

Phone: 503-216-1234
Fax: 503-216-4659
Accredited: Yes
Licensed Beds: 451

Key Personnel:

President . . . . Frederick Waller, MD
Chief Medical Staff . . . . Kenneth Melvin, MD
Emergency Room . . . . Daniel Craig, MD
Director Infection/Disease Control . . . . Woodruff English, MD
CCU Spvg. Nurse . . . . Joyce Rountree, RN
OB/GYN Womens Health. . . . . Larry Veltman, MD
Director Respiratory Therapy . . . . Keith Hyde

Measure	Cases	This Hospital	State Average	U.S. Average	Top Hospital
Heart Attack Care					
ACE Inhibitor or ARB for LVSD	136	90%	88%	82%	100%
Aspirin at Arrival	716	99%	93%	92%	100%
Aspirin at Discharge	1,008	98%	93%	90%	100%
Beta Blocker at Arrival	648	96%	92%	87%	100%
Beta Blocker at Discharge	923	96%	95%	90%	100%
Fibrinolytic Medication Timing[1]	1	100%	29%	31%	100%
PCI Within 90 Minutes of Arrival[1]	23	78%	63%	54%	95%
Smoking Cessation Advice	297	86%	77%	88%	100%
Heart Failure Care					
ACE Inhibitor or ARB for LVSD[2]	131	80%	84%	82%	100%
Discharge Instructions[2]	308	57%	46%	61%	93%
Evaluation of LVS Function[2]	346	90%	82%	83%	99%
Smoking Cessation Advice[2]	41	78%	70%	82%	100%
Pneumonia Care					
Appropriate Initial Antibiotic[2]	157	89%	84%	83%	94%
Blood Culture Timing[2]	147	90%	90%	90%	100%
Influenza Vaccine[2]	28	57%	64%	70%	100%
Initial Antibiotic Timing[2]	185	78%	81%	80%	93%
Oxygenation Assessment[2]	230	100%	100%	99%	100%
Pneumococcal Vaccine[2]	164	82%	63%	69%	94%
Smoking Cessation Advice[2]	47	72%	70%	80%	100%
Surgical Infection Prevention					
Prophylactic Antibiotic Given[2,3]	263	92%	71%	77%	95%
Prophylactic Antibiotic Selection[2]	94	99%	89%	90%	100%
Prophylactic Antibiotic Stopped[2,3]	259	83%	65%	72%	95%
Pregnancy Care					
Inpatient Neonatal Mortality	-	-	-	-	-
Third or Fourth Degree Laceration	-	-	3.10%	3.63%	3.27%

Pioneer Memorial Hospital

1201 NE Elm Street
Prineville, OR 97754
URL: www.pmhprineville.org
Ownership: Voluntary non-profit - Private
Emergency Services: Yes

Phone: 541-447-6254
Fax: 541-447-6705
Accredited: No
Licensed Beds: 35

Key Personnel:

CEO. . . . . Don Wee

Measure	Cases	This Hospital	State Average	U.S. Average	Top Hospital
Heart Attack Care					
ACE Inhibitor or ARB for LVSD	0	-	88%	82%	100%
Aspirin at Arrival[1]	4	50%	93%	92%	100%
Aspirin at Discharge[1]	2	100%	93%	90%	100%
Beta Blocker at Arrival[1]	1	100%	92%	87%	100%
Beta Blocker at Discharge[1]	1	100%	95%	90%	100%
Fibrinolytic Medication Timing	0	-	29%	31%	100%
PCI Within 90 Minutes of Arrival	0	-	63%	54%	95%
Smoking Cessation Advice	0	-	77%	88%	100%
Heart Failure Care					
ACE Inhibitor or ARB for LVSD[1]	5	100%	84%	82%	100%
Discharge Instructions[5]	-	-	46%	61%	93%
Evaluation of LVS Function	34	65%	82%	83%	99%
Smoking Cessation Advice[1]	3	33%	70%	82%	100%
Pneumonia Care					
Appropriate Initial Antibiotic	25	84%	84%	83%	94%
Blood Culture Timing[1]	23	96%	90%	90%	100%
Influenza Vaccine[5]	-	-	64%	70%	100%
Initial Antibiotic Timing	34	85%	81%	80%	93%
Oxygenation Assessment	40	100%	100%	99%	100%
Pneumococcal Vaccine[1]	20	45%	63%	69%	94%
Smoking Cessation Advice[1]	9	22%	70%	80%	100%
Surgical Infection Prevention					
Prophylactic Antibiotic Given	37	92%	71%	77%	95%
Prophylactic Antibiotic Selection[1]	9	89%	89%	90%	100%
Prophylactic Antibiotic Stopped	37	73%	65%	72%	95%
Pregnancy Care					
Inpatient Neonatal Mortality	-	-	-	-	-
Third or Fourth Degree Laceration	-	-	3.10%	3.63%	3.27%

Saint Charles Medical Center-Redmond

1253 N Canal Boulevard
Redmond, OR 97756
URL: www.scmc.org
Ownership: Voluntary non-profit - Private
Emergency Services: Yes

Phone: 541-548-8131
Fax: 541-388-7791
Accredited: Yes
Licensed Beds: 48

Key Personnel:

Administrator . . . . Jim R Hobbs

Measure	Cases	This Hospital	State Average	U.S. Average	Top Hospital
Heart Attack Care					
ACE Inhibitor or ARB for LVSD[1]	6	100%	88%	82%	100%
Aspirin at Arrival	40	92%	93%	92%	100%
Aspirin at Discharge	25	80%	93%	90%	100%
Beta Blocker at Arrival	34	82%	92%	87%	100%

NOTE: Hospital profiles are in alphabetical order by state, then city, then hospital within the city; Rankings are sorted by rate in descending order and exclude hospitals with less than 25 cases; (1) The number of cases is too small (n<25) for purposes of reliably predicting hospital performance; (2) Measure reflects the hospital's indication that its submission was based upon a sample of its relevant discharges; (3) Rate reflects fewer than the maximum possible quarters of data for the measure; (4) Inaccurate information submitted and suppressed for one or more quarters; (5) No data is available from the hospital for this measure; Please refer to the User's Guide for a full explanation of data

Beta Blocker at Discharge	26	85%	95%	90%	100%
Fibrinolytic Medication Timing	0	-	29%	31%	100%
PCI Within 90 Minutes of Arrival	0	-	63%	54%	95%
Smoking Cessation Advice[1]	1	0%	77%	88%	100%
Heart Failure Care					
ACE Inhibitor or ARB for LVSD[1]	16	88%	84%	82%	100%
Discharge Instructions	40	40%	46%	61%	93%
Evaluation of LVS Function	45	87%	82%	83%	99%
Smoking Cessation Advice[1]	8	88%	70%	82%	100%
Pneumonia Care					
Appropriate Initial Antibiotic	53	81%	84%	83%	94%
Blood Culture Timing	45	80%	90%	90%	100%
Influenza Vaccine[1]	13	15%	64%	70%	100%
Initial Antibiotic Timing	69	78%	81%	80%	93%
Oxygenation Assessment	81	100%	100%	99%	100%
Pneumococcal Vaccine	50	20%	63%	69%	94%
Smoking Cessation Advice[1]	19	68%	70%	80%	100%
Surgical Infection Prevention					
Prophylactic Antibiotic Given[2]	204	88%	71%	77%	95%
Prophylactic Antibiotic Selection[2]	45	91%	89%	90%	100%
Prophylactic Antibiotic Stopped[2]	194	56%	65%	72%	95%
Pregnancy Care					
Inpatient Neonatal Mortality	255	0.00%	-	-	-
Third or Fourth Degree Laceration	197	3.55%	3.10%	3.63%	3.27%

Mercy Medical Center

2700 Stewart Parkway
Roseburg, OR 97470
URL: www.mercyrose.org
Ownership: Govt - Hospital District or Authority
Emergency Services: Yes

Phone: 541-673-0611
Fax: 541-677-4830
Accredited: Yes
Licensed Beds: 153

Key Personnel:

President/CEO . . . . Victor J Fresolone, FACHE
Chief Medical Staff . . . . Timothy McCarter, MD
Cardiac Coordinator . . . . Connie Kinman
Director Emergency Room . . . . Ann Fuller
Medical Director Emergency Department . . . . . . Ronald Ennick, MD
Infection Control Coordinator . . . . Sharon Standiford
Director Intensive Coronary . . . . Cheryl Palmer
Director Surgical Services . . . . Laurie Hayes
Director Radiology . . . . Ed Cox
Director Respiratory/Cardiopulmonary . . . . Richard Cleveland

Measure	Cases	This Hospital	State Average	U.S. Average	Top Hospital
Heart Attack Care					
ACE Inhibitor or ARB for LVSD[1]	9	100%	88%	82%	100%
Aspirin at Arrival	76	97%	93%	92%	100%
Aspirin at Discharge	41	90%	93%	90%	100%
Beta Blocker at Arrival	81	95%	92%	87%	100%
Beta Blocker at Discharge	48	94%	95%	90%	100%
Fibrinolytic Medication Timing[1]	19	63%	29%	31%	100%
PCI Within 90 Minutes of Arrival	0	-	63%	54%	95%
Smoking Cessation Advice[1]	14	100%	77%	88%	100%
Heart Failure Care					
ACE Inhibitor or ARB for LVSD	61	77%	84%	82%	100%
Discharge Instructions	215	4%	46%	61%	93%
Evaluation of LVS Function	240	75%	82%	83%	99%
Smoking Cessation Advice	27	67%	70%	82%	100%
Pneumonia Care					
Appropriate Initial Antibiotic	139	88%	84%	83%	94%
Blood Culture Timing	82	88%	90%	90%	100%
Influenza Vaccine	37	8%	64%	70%	100%
Initial Antibiotic Timing	132	80%	81%	80%	93%
Oxygenation Assessment	182	100%	100%	99%	100%
Pneumococcal Vaccine	108	35%	63%	69%	94%
Smoking Cessation Advice	48	75%	70%	80%	100%
Surgical Infection Prevention					
Prophylactic Antibiotic Given	240	68%	71%	77%	95%
Prophylactic Antibiotic Selection	60	70%	89%	90%	100%
Prophylactic Antibiotic Stopped	231	49%	65%	72%	95%
Pregnancy Care					
Inpatient Neonatal Mortality	1,042	0.19%	-	-	-
Third or Fourth Degree Laceration	756	3.31%	3.10%	3.63%	3.27%

Salem Hospital

665 Winter Street SE
Salem, OR 97301
Ownership: Voluntary non-profit - Other
Emergency Services: Yes

Phone: 503-561-5200
Fax: 503-561-4734
Accredited: Yes
Licensed Beds: 454

Key Personnel:

Administrator/CEO . . . . Dennis Noonan
Chief Medical Staff . . . . George Miller
Emergency Room . . . . Susie Mendoza
Director Infection/Disease Control . . . . Pat Mason, RN
CCU Spvg. Nurse . . . . Cindy Armstrong

Measure	Cases	This Hospital	State Average	U.S. Average	Top Hospital
Heart Attack Care					
ACE Inhibitor or ARB for LVSD	67	73%	88%	82%	100%
Aspirin at Arrival	343	99%	93%	92%	100%
Aspirin at Discharge	387	98%	93%	90%	100%
Beta Blocker at Arrival	296	97%	92%	87%	100%
Beta Blocker at Discharge	345	99%	95%	90%	100%
Fibrinolytic Medication Timing[1]	7	57%	29%	31%	100%
PCI Within 90 Minutes of Arrival[1]	15	73%	63%	54%	95%
Smoking Cessation Advice	119	95%	77%	88%	100%
Heart Failure Care					
ACE Inhibitor or ARB for LVSD[2]	156	77%	84%	82%	100%
Discharge Instructions[2]	303	59%	46%	61%	93%
Evaluation of LVS Function[2]	388	95%	82%	83%	99%
Smoking Cessation Advice[2]	64	92%	70%	82%	100%
Pneumonia Care					
Appropriate Initial Antibiotic	254	90%	84%	83%	94%
Blood Culture Timing	245	91%	90%	90%	100%
Influenza Vaccine	78	95%	64%	70%	100%
Initial Antibiotic Timing	371	78%	81%	80%	93%
Oxygenation Assessment	478	100%	100%	99%	100%
Pneumococcal Vaccine	303	87%	63%	69%	94%
Smoking Cessation Advice	112	88%	70%	80%	100%
Surgical Infection Prevention					
Prophylactic Antibiotic Given[2]	1,171	82%	71%	77%	95%
Prophylactic Antibiotic Selection[2]	277	62%	89%	90%	100%
Prophylactic Antibiotic Stopped[2]	1,109	89%	65%	72%	95%
Pregnancy Care					
Inpatient Neonatal Mortality	-	-	-	-	-
Third or Fourth Degree Laceration	-	-	3.10%	3.63%	3.27%

Providence Seaside Hospital

725 S Wahanna Road
Seaside, OR 97138
URL: www.providence.org/northcoast
Ownership: Voluntary non-profit - Church
Emergency Services: Yes

Phone: 503-717-7000
Fax: 503-717-7505
Accredited: Yes
Licensed Beds: 56

Key Personnel:

Administrator . . . . William P Sexton
Emergency Room . . . . Jim Sisk, MD

Measure	Cases	This Hospital	State Average	U.S. Average	Top Hospital
Heart Attack Care					
ACE Inhibitor or ARB for LVSD[1]	2	100%	88%	82%	100%
Aspirin at Arrival[1]	17	100%	93%	92%	100%
Aspirin at Discharge[1]	9	89%	93%	90%	100%
Beta Blocker at Arrival[1]	18	89%	92%	87%	100%
Beta Blocker at Discharge[1]	10	100%	95%	90%	100%
Fibrinolytic Medication Timing	0	-	29%	31%	100%
PCI Within 90 Minutes of Arrival	0	-	63%	54%	95%
Smoking Cessation Advice[1]	2	50%	77%	88%	100%
Heart Failure Care					
ACE Inhibitor or ARB for LVSD[1]	8	88%	84%	82%	100%
Discharge Instructions	39	10%	46%	61%	93%
Evaluation of LVS Function	45	64%	82%	83%	99%
Smoking Cessation Advice[1]	9	78%	70%	82%	100%
Pneumonia Care					
Appropriate Initial Antibiotic	41	83%	84%	83%	94%
Blood Culture Timing[1]	20	75%	90%	90%	100%
Influenza Vaccine[1]	14	79%	64%	70%	100%

NOTE: Hospital profiles are in alphabetical order by state, then city, then hospital within the city; Rankings are sorted by rate in descending order and exclude hospitals with less than 25 cases; (1) The number of cases is too small (n<25) for purposes of reliably predicting hospital performance; (2) Measure reflects the hospital's indication that its submission was based upon a sample of its relevant discharges; (3) Rate reflects fewer than the maximum possible quarters of data for the measure; (4) Inaccurate information submitted and suppressed for one or more quarters; (5) No data is available from the hospital for this measure; Please refer to the User's Guide for a full explanation of data

Initial Antibiotic Timing	45	80%	81%	80%	93%
Oxygenation Assessment	56	100%	100%	99%	100%
Pneumococcal Vaccine	33	91%	63%	69%	94%
Smoking Cessation Advice[1]	8	75%	70%	80%	100%
Surgical Infection Prevention					
Prophylactic Antibiotic Given[1,2,3]	8	38%	71%	77%	95%
Prophylactic Antibiotic Selection[1,2]	1	100%	89%	90%	100%
Prophylactic Antibiotic Stopped[1,2,3]	8	75%	65%	72%	95%
Pregnancy Care					
Inpatient Neonatal Mortality	-	-	-	-	-
Third or Fourth Degree Laceration	-	-	3.10%	3.63%	3.27%

Silverton Hospital

342 Fairview Street
Silverton, OR 97381

Toll-Free: 888-873-1500
Phone: 503-873-1500
Fax: 503-873-1534

URL: www.silvertonhospital.org
Ownership: Voluntary non-profit - Private
Emergency Services: Yes

Accredited: Yes
Licensed Beds: 48

Key Personnel:
Administrator . . . . William E Winter
Chief Medical Staff. . . . . Michael Grady, MD
Catheterization Lab . . . . Renee Angstrom
Manager ER. . . . . Lisa Jeffers, RN
Emergency Room . . . . Frank Lord
ICU Supervising Nurse. Maureen Murphy, RN
Coronary Care Unit Supervising Nurse . . . . Maureen Murphy, RN
OB/GYN/Women's Health . . . . Konnette Donaldson, RN
Director Respiratory Therapy . . . . Renee Angstrom

Measure	Cases	This Hospital	State Average	U.S. Average	Top Hospital
Heart Attack Care					
ACE Inhibitor or ARB for LVSD[1]	4	75%	88%	82%	100%
Aspirin at Arrival[1]	23	83%	93%	92%	100%
Aspirin at Discharge[1]	14	100%	93%	90%	100%
Beta Blocker at Arrival[1]	14	93%	92%	87%	100%
Beta Blocker at Discharge[1]	11	82%	95%	90%	100%
Fibrinolytic Medication Timing	0	-	29%	31%	100%
PCI Within 90 Minutes of Arrival	0	-	63%	54%	95%
Smoking Cessation Advice[1]	1	100%	77%	88%	100%
Heart Failure Care					
ACE Inhibitor or ARB for LVSD[1,3]	8	100%	84%	82%	100%
Discharge Instructions[1,3]	24	75%	46%	61%	93%
Evaluation of LVS Function[3]	30	87%	82%	83%	99%
Smoking Cessation Advice[1,3]	2	100%	70%	82%	100%
Pneumonia Care					
Appropriate Initial Antibiotic	51	94%	84%	83%	94%
Blood Culture Timing	34	91%	90%	90%	100%
Influenza Vaccine[1]	11	73%	64%	70%	100%
Initial Antibiotic Timing	53	91%	81%	80%	93%
Oxygenation Assessment	67	100%	100%	99%	100%
Pneumococcal Vaccine	44	68%	63%	69%	94%
Smoking Cessation Advice[1]	11	45%	70%	80%	100%
Surgical Infection Prevention					
Prophylactic Antibiotic Given	110	78%	71%	77%	95%
Prophylactic Antibiotic Selection	29	72%	89%	90%	100%
Prophylactic Antibiotic Stopped	101	81%	65%	72%	95%
Pregnancy Care					
Inpatient Neonatal Mortality	-	-	-	-	-
Third or Fourth Degree Laceration	-	-	3.10%	3.63%	3.27%

McKenzie-Willamette Medical Center

1460 G Street
Springfield, OR 97477
E-mail: royorr@mckweb.com
URL: www.mckweb.com
Ownership: Voluntary non-profit - Private
Emergency Services: Yes

Phone: 541-726-4400
Fax: 541-726-4540

Accredited: Yes
Licensed Beds: 114

Key Personnel:
CEO. . . . . Roy J Orr
Chief Medical Staff. . . . . Larry Vinis, MD
Emergency Room . . . . Alex Morley, MD
Medical/Surgical Nursing Director . . . . Gail Ragsdale, RN
OB/GYN/Womens Health. . . . . Zena Monji, MD
Chief Radiology . . . . Robert Gunderman, MD
Respiratory Therapy Director . . . . Warren Logan

Measure	Cases	This Hospital	State Average	U.S. Average	Top Hospital
Heart Attack Care					
ACE Inhibitor or ARB for LVSD[1]	8	100%	88%	82%	100%
Aspirin at Arrival	74	97%	93%	92%	100%
Aspirin at Discharge	39	90%	93%	90%	100%
Beta Blocker at Arrival	65	97%	92%	87%	100%
Beta Blocker at Discharge	42	88%	95%	90%	100%
Fibrinolytic Medication Timing	0	-	29%	31%	100%
PCI Within 90 Minutes of Arrival	0	-	63%	54%	95%
Smoking Cessation Advice[1]	7	100%	77%	88%	100%
Heart Failure Care					
ACE Inhibitor or ARB for LVSD	35	74%	84%	82%	100%
Discharge Instructions	91	76%	46%	61%	93%
Evaluation of LVS Function	131	94%	82%	83%	99%
Smoking Cessation Advice	25	96%	70%	82%	100%
Pneumonia Care					
Appropriate Initial Antibiotic	150	87%	84%	83%	94%
Blood Culture Timing	142	92%	90%	90%	100%
Influenza Vaccine	30	97%	64%	70%	100%
Initial Antibiotic Timing	206	85%	81%	80%	93%
Oxygenation Assessment	249	100%	100%	99%	100%
Pneumococcal Vaccine	149	83%	63%	69%	94%
Smoking Cessation Advice	78	92%	70%	80%	100%
Surgical Infection Prevention					
Prophylactic Antibiotic Given	196	72%	71%	77%	95%
Prophylactic Antibiotic Selection	74	91%	89%	90%	100%
Prophylactic Antibiotic Stopped	192	87%	65%	72%	95%
Pregnancy Care					
Inpatient Neonatal Mortality	799	0.00%	-	-	-
Third or Fourth Degree Laceration	555	3.42%	3.10%	3.63%	3.27%

Santiam Memorial Hospital

1401 N 10th Avenue
Stayton, OR 97383
URL: www.santiamhospital.com
Ownership: Voluntary non-profit - Other
Emergency Services: Yes

Phone: 503-769-2175
Fax: 503-769-5877

Accredited: Yes
Licensed Beds: 40

Key Personnel:
President/CEO. . . . . Tery Fletchall
Chief of Medical Staff . . . . Thomas Vanveen
Emergency Room . . . . Jenie Baldwin
Director of Pulmonary/Respiratory Care. . . . . . . Joe Zeanella

Measure	Cases	This Hospital	State Average	U.S. Average	Top Hospital
Heart Attack Care					
ACE Inhibitor or ARB for LVSD	0	-	88%	82%	100%
Aspirin at Arrival[1]	6	67%	93%	92%	100%
Aspirin at Discharge[1]	5	60%	93%	90%	100%
Beta Blocker at Arrival[1]	4	100%	92%	87%	100%
Beta Blocker at Discharge[1]	3	100%	95%	90%	100%
Fibrinolytic Medication Timing	0	-	29%	31%	100%
PCI Within 90 Minutes of Arrival	0	-	63%	54%	95%
Smoking Cessation Advice[1]	1	100%	77%	88%	100%
Heart Failure Care					
ACE Inhibitor or ARB for LVSD[1]	3	100%	84%	82%	100%
Discharge Instructions[1]	24	67%	46%	61%	93%
Evaluation of LVS Function	29	76%	82%	83%	99%
Smoking Cessation Advice[1]	2	50%	70%	82%	100%
Pneumonia Care					
Appropriate Initial Antibiotic	42	76%	84%	83%	94%
Blood Culture Timing[1]	18	72%	90%	90%	100%
Influenza Vaccine[1]	9	78%	64%	70%	100%
Initial Antibiotic Timing	43	63%	81%	80%	93%
Oxygenation Assessment	61	100%	100%	99%	100%
Pneumococcal Vaccine	36	47%	63%	69%	94%
Smoking Cessation Advice[1]	12	100%	70%	80%	100%
Surgical Infection Prevention					
Prophylactic Antibiotic Given[1,3]	2	0%	71%	77%	95%

NOTE: Hospital profiles are in alphabetical order by state, then city, then hospital within the city; Rankings are sorted by rate in descending order and exclude hospitals with less than 25 cases; (1) The number of cases is too small (n<25) for purposes of reliably predicting hospital performance; (2) Measure reflects the hospital's indication that its submission was based upon a sample of its relevant discharges; (3) Rate reflects fewer than the maximum possible quarters of data for the measure; (4) Inaccurate information submitted and suppressed for one or more quarters; (5) No data is available from the hospital for this measure; Please refer to the User's Guide for a full explanation of data

Prophylactic Antibiotic Selection[1]	2	50%	89%	90%	100%
Prophylactic Antibiotic Stopped[1,3]	2	0%	65%	72%	95%
Pregnancy Care					
Inpatient Neonatal Mortality	-	-	-	-	-
Third or Fourth Degree Laceration	-	-	3.10%	3.63%	3.27%

Mid-Columbia Medical Center

1700 E 19th Street
The Dalles, OR 97058
URL: www.mcmc.net
Ownership: Voluntary non-profit - Other
Emergency Services: Yes
Phone: 541-296-7273
Fax: 541-296-7600
Accredited: Yes
Licensed Beds: 49

Key Personnel:

Administrator . . . . Mark Scott
Chief Medical Staff . . . . Changes Annually
Emergency Room . . . . John Jacobson, MD
Director Infection/Disease Control . . . . Catherine Sessions
CCU Spvg. Nurse . . . . Shelley Reynolds-Wacker
Director Respiratory Therapy . . . . Joyce Powell Morin

Measure	Cases	This Hospital	State Average	U.S. Average	Top Hospital
Heart Attack Care					
ACE Inhibitor or ARB for LVSD[1]	1	100%	88%	82%	100%
Aspirin at Arrival[1]	18	100%	93%	92%	100%
Aspirin at Discharge[1]	6	100%	93%	90%	100%
Beta Blocker at Arrival[1]	16	94%	92%	87%	100%
Beta Blocker at Discharge[1]	8	100%	95%	90%	100%
Fibrinolytic Medication Timing[1]	4	50%	29%	31%	100%
PCI Within 90 Minutes of Arrival	0	-	63%	54%	95%
Smoking Cessation Advice[1]	2	100%	77%	88%	100%
Heart Failure Care					
ACE Inhibitor or ARB for LVSD[1]	15	93%	84%	82%	100%
Discharge Instructions	50	98%	46%	61%	93%
Evaluation of LVS Function	59	98%	82%	83%	99%
Smoking Cessation Advice[1]	17	100%	70%	82%	100%
Pneumonia Care					
Appropriate Initial Antibiotic	70	79%	84%	83%	94%
Blood Culture Timing	71	96%	90%	90%	100%
Influenza Vaccine[1]	19	58%	64%	70%	100%
Initial Antibiotic Timing	83	89%	81%	80%	93%
Oxygenation Assessment	103	100%	100%	99%	100%
Pneumococcal Vaccine	65	82%	63%	69%	94%
Smoking Cessation Advice[1]	22	100%	70%	80%	100%
Surgical Infection Prevention					
Prophylactic Antibiotic Given[2]	163	93%	71%	77%	95%
Prophylactic Antibiotic Selection[2]	58	100%	89%	90%	100%
Prophylactic Antibiotic Stopped[2]	164	81%	65%	72%	95%
Pregnancy Care					
Inpatient Neonatal Mortality	-	-	-	-	-
Third or Fourth Degree Laceration	-	-	3.10%	3.63%	3.27%

Tillamook County General Hospital

1000 3rd Street
Tillamook, OR 97141
E-mail: morrispa@ah.org
URL: www.tcgh.com
Ownership: Voluntary non-profit - Church
Emergency Services: Yes
Phone: 503-842-4444
Fax: 503-842-3062
Accredited: Yes
Licensed Beds: 49

Key Personnel:

President . . . . Wendell Hesselgine
President . . . . June Johnson
Chief Medical Staff . . . . Matt Turney
Emergency Room . . . . Larry Hamelton, RN
Director Infection/Disease Control . . . . Pat Valenti
Director Medical/Surgical Nursing . . . . Velda Handler
OB/GYN Womens Health . . . . Fred Roesener, MD
Chief Radiology . . . . Gordon Johnson, MD

Measure	Cases	This Hospital	State Average	U.S. Average	Top Hospital
Heart Attack Care					
ACE Inhibitor or ARB for LVSD[1]	1	100%	88%	82%	100%
Aspirin at Arrival[1]	14	100%	93%	92%	100%
Aspirin at Discharge[1]	9	100%	93%	90%	100%
Beta Blocker at Arrival[1]	13	100%	92%	87%	100%
Beta Blocker at Discharge[1]	10	100%	95%	90%	100%
Fibrinolytic Medication Timing[1]	4	0%	29%	31%	100%
PCI Within 90 Minutes of Arrival	0	-	63%	54%	95%
Smoking Cessation Advice[1]	3	100%	77%	88%	100%
Heart Failure Care					
ACE Inhibitor or ARB for LVSD[1]	5	100%	84%	82%	100%
Discharge Instructions	38	84%	46%	61%	93%
Evaluation of LVS Function	38	79%	82%	83%	99%
Smoking Cessation Advice[1]	10	90%	70%	82%	100%
Pneumonia Care					
Appropriate Initial Antibiotic	50	82%	84%	83%	94%
Blood Culture Timing	28	86%	90%	90%	100%
Influenza Vaccine[1]	12	83%	64%	70%	100%
Initial Antibiotic Timing	45	93%	81%	80%	93%
Oxygenation Assessment	59	100%	100%	99%	100%
Pneumococcal Vaccine	35	80%	63%	69%	94%
Smoking Cessation Advice[1]	12	100%	70%	80%	100%
Surgical Infection Prevention					
Prophylactic Antibiotic Given[3]	75	57%	71%	77%	95%
Prophylactic Antibiotic Selection[1]	19	89%	89%	90%	100%
Prophylactic Antibiotic Stopped[3]	77	34%	65%	72%	95%
Pregnancy Care					
Inpatient Neonatal Mortality	-	-	-	-	-
Third or Fourth Degree Laceration	-	-	3.10%	3.63%	3.27%

Legacy Meridian Park Hospital

Alternate Name: Meridian Park Hospital
19300 SW 65th Street
Tualatin, OR 97062
URL: www.legacyhealth.org
Ownership: Voluntary non-profit - Private
Emergency Services: Yes
Phone: 503-692-1212
Fax: 503-691-0919
Accredited: Yes
Licensed Beds: 150

Key Personnel:

Administrator . . . . Allyson Anderson
Chief Medical Staff . . . . John Braddock, MD
Emergency Room . . . . M Scott Miller, MD
Infection Control . . . . Mary Shanks, RN
ICU . . . . Sue Ellison, RN
Medical Surgical Nursing . . . . Joyce Perry, RN
OB/GYN Womens Health . . . . Lusanne Wisecaver, RN
Respiratory Therapy . . . . Janise White

Measure	Cases	This Hospital	State Average	U.S. Average	Top Hospital
Heart Attack Care					
ACE Inhibitor or ARB for LVSD[2]	34	82%	88%	82%	100%
Aspirin at Arrival[2]	108	94%	93%	92%	100%
Aspirin at Discharge[2]	75	92%	93%	90%	100%
Beta Blocker at Arrival[2]	75	93%	92%	87%	100%
Beta Blocker at Discharge[2]	83	96%	95%	90%	100%
Fibrinolytic Medication Timing[1,2]	3	33%	29%	31%	100%
PCI Within 90 Minutes of Arrival[1,2]	3	33%	63%	54%	95%
Smoking Cessation Advice[1,2]	18	94%	77%	88%	100%
Heart Failure Care					
ACE Inhibitor or ARB for LVSD[2]	93	75%	84%	82%	100%
Discharge Instructions[2]	173	30%	46%	61%	93%
Evaluation of LVS Function[2]	216	93%	82%	83%	99%
Smoking Cessation Advice[1,2]	11	82%	70%	82%	100%
Pneumonia Care					
Appropriate Initial Antibiotic[2]	89	79%	84%	83%	94%
Blood Culture Timing[2]	72	96%	90%	90%	100%
Influenza Vaccine[1]	22	36%	64%	70%	100%
Initial Antibiotic Timing[2]	172	91%	81%	80%	93%
Oxygenation Assessment[2]	186	100%	100%	99%	100%
Pneumococcal Vaccine[2]	133	53%	63%	69%	94%
Smoking Cessation Advice[2]	25	68%	70%	80%	100%
Surgical Infection Prevention					
Prophylactic Antibiotic Given[2,3]	98	77%	71%	77%	95%
Prophylactic Antibiotic Selection[2]	50	98%	89%	90%	100%
Prophylactic Antibiotic Stopped[2,3]	92	74%	65%	72%	95%
Pregnancy Care					
Inpatient Neonatal Mortality	-	-	-	-	-
Third or Fourth Degree Laceration	-	-	3.10%	3.63%	3.27%

NOTE: Hospital profiles are in alphabetical order by state, then city, then hospital within the city; Rankings are sorted by rate in descending order and exclude hospitals with less than 25 cases; (1) The number of cases is too small (n<25) for purposes of reliably predicting hospital performance; (2) Measure reflects the hospital's indication that its submission was based upon a sample of its relevant discharges; (3) Rate reflects fewer than the maximum possible quarters of data for the measure; (4) Inaccurate information submitted and suppressed for one or more quarters; (5) No data is available from the hospital for this measure; Please refer to the User's Guide for a full explanation of data

Heart Attack Care

1. ACE Inhibitor or ARB for LVSD

Hospital Name	City	Rate	Cases
Dixie Regional Medical Center	Saint George	100%	32
McKay-Dee Hospital Center	Ogden	96%	25
University Health Care/Univ of Utah Hosp	Salt Lake City	90%	42
Utah Valley Regional Medical Center	Provo	89%	37
LDS Hospital	Salt Lake City	80%	70
Saint Mark's Hospital	Salt Lake City	79%	28

2. Aspirin at Arrival

Hospital Name	City	Rate	Cases
Jordan Valley Hospital	West Jordan	100%	25
Lakeview Hospital	Bountiful	100%	66
McKay-Dee Hospital Center	Ogden	99%	177
Ogden Regional Medical Center	Ogden	99%	81
Dixie Regional Medical Center	Saint George	98%	170
Pioneer Valley Hospital	West Valley City	98%	89
Saint Mark's Hospital	Salt Lake City	98%	132
Utah Valley Regional Medical Center	Provo	98%	157
LDS Hospital	Salt Lake City	96%	178
University Health Care/Univ of Utah Hosp	Salt Lake City	96%	85
Mountain View Hospital	Payson	95%	39
Davis Hospital and Medical Center	Layton	93%	107
Cottonwood Hospital	Murray	92%	127
Timpanogos Regional Hospital	Orem	88%	26

3. Aspirin at Discharge

Hospital Name	City	Rate	Cases
Lakeview Hospital	Bountiful	100%	60
Dixie Regional Medical Center	Saint George	99%	216
LDS Hospital	Salt Lake City	99%	393
Pioneer Valley Hospital	West Valley City	99%	113
Saint Mark's Hospital	Salt Lake City	98%	174
University Health Care/Univ of Utah Hosp	Salt Lake City	98%	165
Utah Valley Regional Medical Center	Provo	98%	334
Davis Hospital and Medical Center	Layton	97%	100
McKay-Dee Hospital Center	Ogden	97%	248
Ogden Regional Medical Center	Ogden	97%	105
Mountain View Hospital	Payson	95%	39
Cottonwood Hospital	Murray	93%	106
Timpanogos Regional Hospital	Orem	92%	26
Salt Lake Regional Medical Center	Salt Lake City	90%	52

4. Beta Blocker at Arrival

Hospital Name	City	Rate	Cases
Dixie Regional Medical Center	Saint George	96%	145
Lakeview Hospital	Bountiful	95%	55
Saint Mark's Hospital	Salt Lake City	95%	106
University Health Care/Univ of Utah Hosp	Salt Lake City	95%	78
Ogden Regional Medical Center	Ogden	94%	62
Utah Valley Regional Medical Center	Provo	94%	135
Cottonwood Hospital	Murray	93%	104
LDS Hospital	Salt Lake City	93%	148
Pioneer Valley Hospital	West Valley City	91%	66
Davis Hospital and Medical Center	Layton	89%	93
McKay-Dee Hospital Center	Ogden	88%	144
Mountain View Hospital	Payson	85%	26
Timpanogos Regional Hospital	Orem	85%	27

5. Beta Blocker at Discharge

Hospital Name	City	Rate	Cases
Dixie Regional Medical Center	Saint George	100%	244
Lakeview Hospital	Bountiful	100%	56
Ogden Regional Medical Center	Ogden	98%	104
Davis Hospital and Medical Center	Layton	97%	98
Utah Valley Regional Medical Center	Provo	96%	305
McKay-Dee Hospital Center	Ogden	95%	229
Cottonwood Hospital	Murray	94%	117
LDS Hospital	Salt Lake City	93%	387
University Health Care/Univ of Utah Hosp	Salt Lake City	92%	172
Pioneer Valley Hospital	West Valley City	91%	101
Timpanogos Regional Hospital	Orem	90%	31
Mountain View Hospital	Payson	89%	35
Saint Mark's Hospital	Salt Lake City	86%	169
Salt Lake Regional Medical Center	Salt Lake City	73%	44

8. Smoking Cessation Advice

Hospital Name	City	Rate	Cases
Utah Valley Regional Medical Center	Provo	100%	82
LDS Hospital	Salt Lake City	99%	95
Dixie Regional Medical Center	Saint George	98%	57
McKay-Dee Hospital Center	Ogden	97%	68
Pioneer Valley Hospital	West Valley City	95%	55
University Health Care/Univ of Utah Hosp	Salt Lake City	95%	74
Cottonwood Hospital	Murray	94%	31
Davis Hospital and Medical Center	Layton	93%	29
Ogden Regional Medical Center	Ogden	92%	38
Saint Mark's Hospital	Salt Lake City	86%	49

Heart Failure Care

9. ACE Inhibitor or ARB for LVSD

Hospital Name	City	Rate	Cases
Dixie Regional Medical Center	Saint George	100%	79
McKay-Dee Hospital Center	Ogden	93%	116
Davis Hospital and Medical Center	Layton	90%	29
Pioneer Valley Hospital	West Valley City	90%	31
Ogden Regional Medical Center	Ogden	89%	38
University Health Care/Univ of Utah Hosp	Salt Lake City	88%	121
Saint Mark's Hospital	Salt Lake City	85%	100
Utah Valley Regional Medical Center	Provo	80%	82
LDS Hospital	Salt Lake City	78%	190
Cottonwood Hospital	Murray	77%	30
Salt Lake Regional Medical Center	Salt Lake City	75%	32

10. Discharge Instructions

Hospital Name	City	Rate	Cases
Dixie Regional Medical Center	Saint George	93%	147
LDS Hospital	Salt Lake City	89%	337
Logan Regional Hospital	Logan	89%	38
American Fork Hospital	American Fork	88%	65
Cottonwood Hospital	Murray	88%	91
Utah Valley Regional Medical Center	Provo	86%	187
McKay-Dee Hospital Center	Ogden	83%	221
Alta View Hospital	Sandy	69%	45
Timpanogos Regional Hospital	Orem	61%	36
Jordan Valley Hospital	West Jordan	57%	67
University Health Care/Univ of Utah Hosp	Salt Lake City	57%	153
Saint Mark's Hospital	Salt Lake City	56%	186
Lakeview Hospital	Bountiful	55%	38
Ogden Regional Medical Center	Ogden	54%	78
Davis Hospital and Medical Center	Layton	53%	72
Mountain View Hospital	Payson	53%	45
Salt Lake Regional Medical Center	Salt Lake City	35%	66
Pioneer Valley Hospital	West Valley City	29%	78
Mountain West Medical Center	Tooele	18%	28

11. Evaluation of LVS Function

Hospital Name	City	Rate	Cases
LDS Hospital	Salt Lake City	100%	369
Dixie Regional Medical Center	Saint George	99%	187
McKay-Dee Hospital Center	Ogden	98%	256
Mountain View Hospital	Payson	98%	57
University Health Care/Univ of Utah Hosp	Salt Lake City	98%	183
Utah Valley Regional Medical Center	Provo	98%	236
Saint Mark's Hospital	Salt Lake City	96%	222
Alta View Hospital	Sandy	95%	65
American Fork Hospital	American Fork	94%	87
Lakeview Hospital	Bountiful	94%	52
Pioneer Valley Hospital	West Valley City	94%	88
Cottonwood Hospital	Murray	92%	105
Ogden Regional Medical Center	Ogden	92%	109
Timpanogos Regional Hospital	Orem	91%	46
Davis Hospital and Medical Center	Layton	89%	89
Jordan Valley Hospital	West Jordan	87%	79
Mountain West Medical Center	Tooele	87%	39
Salt Lake Regional Medical Center	Salt Lake City	87%	86
Logan Regional Hospital	Logan	85%	47
Castleview Hospital	Price	67%	33
Central Valley Medical Center	Nephi	64%	25

12. Smoking Cessation Advice

Hospital Name	City	Rate	Cases
McKay-Dee Hospital Center	Ogden	96%	27
Utah Valley Regional Medical Center	Provo	93%	29
Saint Mark's Hospital	Salt Lake City	89%	36
LDS Hospital	Salt Lake City	86%	58
University Health Care/Univ of Utah Hosp	Salt Lake City	53%	34

NOTE: Hospital profiles are in alphabetical order by state, then city, then hospital within the city; Rankings are sorted by rate in descending order and exclude hospitals with less than 25 cases; (1) The number of cases is too small (n<25) for purposes of reliably predicting hospital performance; (2) Measure reflects the hospital's indication that its submission was based upon a sample of its relevant discharges; (3) Rate reflects fewer than the maximum possible quarters of data for the measure; (4) Inaccurate information submitted and suppressed for one or more quarters; (5) No data is available from the hospital for this measure; Please refer to the User's Guide for a full explanation of data

Pneumonia Care

13. Appropriate Initial Antibiotic

Hospital Name	City	Rate	Cases
Beaver Valley Hospital	Beaver	96%	53
Garfield Memorial Hospital & Clinics	Panguitch	94%	34
Saint Mark's Hospital	Salt Lake City	93%	269
McKay-Dee Hospital Center	Ogden	92%	292
Davis Hospital and Medical Center	Layton	90%	125
Utah Valley Regional Medical Center	Provo	90%	149
Jordan Valley Hospital	West Jordan	89%	151
Ogden Regional Medical Center	Ogden	89%	129
Bear River Valley Hospital	Tremonton	88%	26
Mountain West Medical Center	Tooele	86%	43
LDS Hospital	Salt Lake City	85%	169
Salt Lake Regional Medical Center	Salt Lake City	85%	68
Valley View Medical Center	Cedar City	85%	79
Alta View Hospital	Sandy	84%	110
Ashley Valley Medical Center	Vernal	84%	45
Cottonwood Hospital	Murray	84%	257
Heber Valley Medical Center	Heber City	84%	37
Lakeview Hospital	Bountiful	84%	115
Dixie Regional Medical Center	Saint George	83%	202
Mountain View Hospital	Payson	83%	72
Sanpete Valley Hospital	Mount Pleasant	82%	44
American Fork Hospital	American Fork	81%	112
Central Valley Medical Center	Nephi	81%	27
Pioneer Valley Hospital	West Valley City	81%	183
University Health Care/Univ of Utah Hosp	Salt Lake City	81%	52
Sevier Valley Hospital	Richfield	80%	61
Gunnison Valley Hospital	Gunnison	78%	40
Logan Regional Hospital	Logan	78%	83
Castleview Hospital	Price	72%	101
Kane County Hospital	Kanab	72%	47
Timpanogos Regional Hospital	Orem	71%	63

14. Blood Culture Timing

Hospital Name	City	Rate	Cases
Castleview Hospital	Price	99%	88
Saint Mark's Hospital	Salt Lake City	97%	261
Alta View Hospital	Sandy	96%	100
Jordan Valley Hospital	West Jordan	95%	112
Mountain View Hospital	Payson	95%	60
American Fork Hospital	American Fork	94%	65
Cottonwood Hospital	Murray	94%	163
University Health Care/Univ of Utah Hosp	Salt Lake City	94%	72
Pioneer Valley Hospital	West Valley City	93%	135
Lakeview Hospital	Bountiful	91%	100
Mountain West Medical Center	Tooele	91%	32
Dixie Regional Medical Center	Saint George	89%	178
LDS Hospital	Salt Lake City	89%	132
Davis Hospital and Medical Center	Layton	87%	79
Timpanogos Regional Hospital	Orem	87%	53
Utah Valley Regional Medical Center	Provo	87%	119
Logan Regional Hospital	Logan	85%	62
McKay-Dee Hospital Center	Ogden	84%	231
Ogden Regional Medical Center	Ogden	84%	75
Valley View Medical Center	Cedar City	81%	42
Salt Lake Regional Medical Center	Salt Lake City	61%	54

15. Influenza Vaccine

Hospital Name	City	Rate	Cases
Jordan Valley Hospital	West Jordan	100%	35
Pioneer Valley Hospital	West Valley City	98%	44
Dixie Regional Medical Center	Saint George	90%	83
Ogden Regional Medical Center	Ogden	90%	40
Mountain View Hospital	Payson	88%	33
Logan Regional Hospital	Logan	86%	28
Cottonwood Hospital	Murray	84%	67
McKay-Dee Hospital Center	Ogden	82%	62
Lakeview Hospital	Bountiful	81%	36
Saint Mark's Hospital	Salt Lake City	78%	94
Utah Valley Regional Medical Center	Provo	75%	51
Davis Hospital and Medical Center	Layton	74%	35
Castleview Hospital	Price	73%	33
LDS Hospital	Salt Lake City	65%	60

16. Initial Antibiotic Timing

Hospital Name	City	Rate	Cases
Garfield Memorial Hospital & Clinics	Panguitch	100%	34
Beaver Valley Hospital	Beaver	98%	54
Ashley Valley Medical Center	Vernal	93%	54
Castleview Hospital	Price	90%	123
Logan Regional Hospital	Logan	90%	116
McKay-Dee Hospital Center	Ogden	90%	323
Ogden Regional Medical Center	Ogden	90%	145
American Fork Hospital	American Fork	89%	126
Valley View Medical Center	Cedar City	86%	83
Alta View Hospital	Sandy	85%	160
Central Valley Medical Center	Nephi	85%	34
Heber Valley Medical Center	Heber City	85%	34
Jordan Valley Hospital	West Jordan	84%	177
Gunnison Valley Hospital	Gunnison	83%	36
Dixie Regional Medical Center	Saint George	82%	288
Davis Hospital and Medical Center	Layton	81%	134
Kane County Hospital	Kanab	81%	47
Lakeview Hospital	Bountiful	81%	134
Uintah Basin Medical Center	Roosevelt	81%	26
Mountain View Hospital	Payson	80%	99
LDS Hospital	Salt Lake City	79%	225
Pioneer Valley Hospital	West Valley City	79%	202
Timpanogos Regional Hospital	Orem	79%	82
Saint Mark's Hospital	Salt Lake City	78%	361
Sevier Valley Hospital	Richfield	78%	68
Utah Valley Regional Medical Center	Provo	78%	211
Salt Lake Regional Medical Center	Salt Lake City	77%	78
Mountain West Medical Center	Tooele	76%	55
Sanpete Valley Hospital	Mount Pleasant	74%	47
Cottonwood Hospital	Murray	73%	329
University Health Care/Univ of Utah Hosp	Salt Lake City	55%	103

17. Oxygenation Assessment

Hospital Name	City	Rate	Cases
Alta View Hospital	Sandy	100%	194
American Fork Hospital	American Fork	100%	156
Ashley Valley Medical Center	Vernal	100%	56
Bear River Valley Hospital	Tremonton	100%	28
Beaver Valley Hospital	Beaver	100%	70
Brigham City Community Hospital	Brigham City	100%	31
Castleview Hospital	Price	100%	151
Central Valley Medical Center	Nephi	100%	42
Davis Hospital and Medical Center	Layton	100%	178
Delta Community Medical Center	Delta	100%	26
Dixie Regional Medical Center	Saint George	100%	364
Garfield Memorial Hospital & Clinics	Panguitch	100%	40
Gunnison Valley Hospital	Gunnison	100%	47
Jordan Valley Hospital	West Jordan	100%	211
Kane County Hospital	Kanab	100%	53
LDS Hospital	Salt Lake City	100%	314
Lakeview Hospital	Bountiful	100%	184
Logan Regional Hospital	Logan	100%	159
McKay-Dee Hospital Center	Ogden	100%	444
Mountain View Hospital	Payson	100%	124
Mountain West Medical Center	Tooele	100%	63
Ogden Regional Medical Center	Ogden	100%	174
Pioneer Valley Hospital	West Valley City	100%	226
Saint Mark's Hospital	Salt Lake City	100%	472
Salt Lake Regional Medical Center	Salt Lake City	100%	93
Sanpete Valley Hospital	Mount Pleasant	100%	49
Sevier Valley Hospital	Richfield	100%	79
Timpanogos Regional Hospital	Orem	100%	111
Uintah Basin Medical Center	Roosevelt	100%	33
University Health Care/Univ of Utah Hosp	Salt Lake City	100%	208
Utah Valley Regional Medical Center	Provo	100%	272
Valley View Medical Center	Cedar City	100%	111
Cottonwood Hospital	Murray	99%	382
Heber Valley Medical Center	Heber City	98%	42

18. Pneumococcal Vaccine

Hospital Name	City	Rate	Cases
Ashley Valley Medical Center	Vernal	100%	31
Jordan Valley Hospital	West Jordan	97%	98
Valley View Medical Center	Cedar City	90%	58
Logan Regional Hospital	Logan	87%	109
Ogden Regional Medical Center	Ogden	86%	119
Mountain View Hospital	Payson	85%	79
Pioneer Valley Hospital	West Valley City	84%	128
Salt Lake Regional Medical Center	Salt Lake City	84%	44
American Fork Hospital	American Fork	83%	92
Alta View Hospital	Sandy	82%	119
Timpanogos Regional Hospital	Orem	80%	56
Cottonwood Hospital	Murray	79%	212
Utah Valley Regional Medical Center	Provo	78%	155
Dixie Regional Medical Center	Saint George	77%	269
Gunnison Valley Hospital	Gunnison	77%	26
Lakeview Hospital	Bountiful	73%	127
Saint Mark's Hospital	Salt Lake City	73%	311

NOTE: Hospital profiles are in alphabetical order by state, then city, then hospital within the city; Rankings are sorted by rate in descending order and exclude hospitals with less than 25 cases; (1) The number of cases is too small (n<25) for purposes of reliably predicting hospital performance; (2) Measure reflects the hospital's indication that its submission was based upon a sample of its relevant discharges; (3) Rate reflects fewer than the maximum possible quarters of data for the measure; (4) Inaccurate information submitted and suppressed for one or more quarters; (5) No data is available from the hospital for this measure; Please refer to the User's Guide for a full explanation of data

Hospital Name	City	Rate	Cases
McKay-Dee Hospital Center	Ogden	71%	268
Castleview Hospital	Price	70%	87
Davis Hospital and Medical Center	Layton	68%	107
University Health Care/Univ of Utah Hosp	Salt Lake City	66%	74
Garfield Memorial Hospital & Clinics	Panguitch	58%	26
LDS Hospital	Salt Lake City	58%	170
Sanpete Valley Hospital	Mount Pleasant	58%	33
Beaver Valley Hospital	Beaver	57%	54
Sevier Valley Hospital	Richfield	52%	42
Mountain West Medical Center	Tooele	51%	37
Kane County Hospital	Kanab	8%	36

19. Smoking Cessation Advice

Hospital Name	City	Rate	Cases
Jordan Valley Hospital	West Jordan	100%	49
Dixie Regional Medical Center	Saint George	94%	50
Castleview Hospital	Price	92%	37
Alta View Hospital	Sandy	91%	33
Pioneer Valley Hospital	West Valley City	88%	59
McKay-Dee Hospital Center	Ogden	86%	101
Cottonwood Hospital	Murray	85%	74
Ogden Regional Medical Center	Ogden	85%	39
Davis Hospital and Medical Center	Layton	79%	34
LDS Hospital	Salt Lake City	76%	70
Saint Mark's Hospital	Salt Lake City	68%	85
Salt Lake Regional Medical Center	Salt Lake City	62%	29
Utah Valley Regional Medical Center	Provo	57%	35
University Health Care/Univ of Utah Hosp	Salt Lake City	39%	46

Surgical Infection Prevention

20. Prophylactic Antibiotic Given

Hospital Name	City	Rate	Cases
Alta View Hospital	Sandy	95%	261
Mountain View Hospital	Payson	94%	138
Dixie Regional Medical Center	Saint George	93%	518
American Fork Hospital	American Fork	92%	219
Lakeview Hospital	Bountiful	91%	218
Saint Mark's Hospital	Salt Lake City	91%	290
Central Valley Medical Center	Nephi	90%	50
McKay-Dee Hospital Center	Ogden	88%	508
The Orthopedic Specialty Hospital	Murray	87%	194
Castleview Hospital	Price	85%	129
Timpanogos Regional Hospital	Orem	85%	152
Davis Hospital and Medical Center	Layton	84%	476
LDS Hospital	Salt Lake City	84%	549
Sevier Valley Hospital	Richfield	83%	29
Cottonwood Hospital	Murray	81%	260
Logan Regional Hospital	Logan	79%	242
University Health Care/Univ of Utah Hosp	Salt Lake City	79%	385
Utah Valley Regional Medical Center	Provo	79%	534
Ashley Valley Medical Center	Vernal	78%	32
Salt Lake Regional Medical Center	Salt Lake City	78%	211
Valley View Medical Center	Cedar City	78%	228
Pioneer Valley Hospital	West Valley City	71%	190
Jordan Valley Hospital	West Jordan	70%	341
Ogden Regional Medical Center	Ogden	64%	199
Brigham City Community Hospital	Brigham City	40%	70
Heber Valley Medical Center	Heber City	38%	76
Uintah Basin Medical Center	Roosevelt	36%	36
Mountain West Medical Center	Tooele	32%	75
Cache Valley Speciality Hospital	North Logan	16%	64

21. Prophylactic Antibiotic Selection

Hospital Name	City	Rate	Cases
Alta View Hospital	Sandy	100%	81
Castleview Hospital	Price	100%	57
Salt Lake Regional Medical Center	Salt Lake City	100%	52
Lakeview Hospital	Bountiful	99%	134
The Orthopedic Specialty Hospital	Murray	99%	71
Jordan Valley Hospital	West Jordan	98%	92
Pioneer Valley Hospital	West Valley City	98%	54
American Fork Hospital	American Fork	97%	60
Logan Regional Hospital	Logan	97%	69
Timpanogos Regional Hospital	Orem	97%	65
University Health Care/Univ of Utah Hosp	Salt Lake City	96%	83
Dixie Regional Medical Center	Saint George	95%	172
Saint Mark's Hospital	Salt Lake City	95%	134
Utah Valley Regional Medical Center	Provo	95%	169
Davis Hospital and Medical Center	Layton	94%	111
Ogden Regional Medical Center	Ogden	93%	94
Cottonwood Hospital	Murray	92%	78
LDS Hospital	Salt Lake City	92%	196
McKay-Dee Hospital Center	Ogden	92%	173
Valley View Medical Center	Cedar City	92%	50
Cache Valley Speciality Hospital	North Logan	91%	64
Mountain View Hospital	Payson	89%	61
Brigham City Community Hospital	Brigham City	80%	25

22. Prophylactic Antibiotic Stopped

Hospital Name	City	Rate	Cases
Brigham City Community Hospital	Brigham City	100%	68
Central Valley Medical Center	Nephi	96%	48
Mountain View Hospital	Payson	89%	133
Timpanogos Regional Hospital	Orem	88%	146
University Health Care/Univ of Utah Hosp	Salt Lake City	85%	382
Castleview Hospital	Price	84%	121
Dixie Regional Medical Center	Saint George	83%	496
Salt Lake Regional Medical Center	Salt Lake City	83%	193
Saint Mark's Hospital	Salt Lake City	81%	283
Alta View Hospital	Sandy	77%	260
American Fork Hospital	American Fork	77%	216
Davis Hospital and Medical Center	Layton	77%	463
Utah Valley Regional Medical Center	Provo	77%	520
Ogden Regional Medical Center	Ogden	72%	198
Pioneer Valley Hospital	West Valley City	72%	179
Heber Valley Medical Center	Heber City	71%	77
Logan Regional Hospital	Logan	70%	235
McKay-Dee Hospital Center	Ogden	69%	498
LDS Hospital	Salt Lake City	67%	548
Jordan Valley Hospital	West Jordan	63%	329
Cottonwood Hospital	Murray	62%	254
Sevier Valley Hospital	Richfield	56%	27
Uintah Basin Medical Center	Roosevelt	56%	34
Ashley Valley Medical Center	Vernal	38%	32
The Orthopedic Specialty Hospital	Murray	34%	194
Valley View Medical Center	Cedar City	30%	224
Lakeview Hospital	Bountiful	24%	215
Mountain West Medical Center	Tooele	21%	62
Cache Valley Speciality Hospital	North Logan	17%	64

Pregnancy Care

23. Inpatient Neonatal Mortality

Hospital Name	City	Rate	Cases
American Fork Hospital	American Fork	0.00%	2845
Cottonwood Hospital	Murray	0.00%	3852
Davis Hospital and Medical Center	Layton	0.00%	753
Logan Regional Hospital	Logan	0.00%	2645
Pioneer Valley Hospital	West Valley City	0.00%	287
Salt Lake Regional Medical Center	Salt Lake City	0.00%	814
Jordan Valley Hospital	West Jordan	0.07%	1502
Alta View Hospital	Sandy	0.09%	2234
Timpanogos Regional Hospital	Orem	0.11%	1852
Ogden Regional Medical Center	Ogden	0.12%	2431
McKay-Dee Hospital Center	Ogden	0.20%	3920
Dixie Regional Medical Center	Saint George	0.21%	2875
Ashley Valley Medical Center	Vernal	0.28%	352
Brigham City Community Hospital	Brigham City	0.28%	358
Utah Valley Regional Medical Center	Provo	0.34%	5901
Valley View Medical Center	Cedar City	0.34%	885
Sevier Valley Hospital	Richfield	0.38%	265
LDS Hospital	Salt Lake City	0.55%	4215
University Health Care/Univ of Utah Hosp	Salt Lake City	1.03%	679

24. Third or Fourth Degree Laceration

Hospital Name	City	Rate	Cases
Ogden Regional Medical Center	Ogden	0.79%	1768
Brigham City Community Hospital	Brigham City	1.46%	274
Pioneer Valley Hospital	West Valley City	1.86%	215
Timpanogos Regional Hospital	Orem	2.11%	1471
Davis Hospital and Medical Center	Layton	2.14%	562
McKay-Dee Hospital Center	Ogden	2.14%	2849
Salt Lake Regional Medical Center	Salt Lake City	2.20%	682
Valley View Medical Center	Cedar City	2.51%	718
Logan Regional Hospital	Logan	2.89%	2147
Jordan Valley Hospital	West Jordan	3.05%	1213
American Fork Hospital	American Fork	3.09%	2397
LDS Hospital	Salt Lake City	3.34%	3169
Utah Valley Regional Medical Center	Provo	3.39%	4579
Dixie Regional Medical Center	Saint George	3.40%	2296
Cottonwood Hospital	Murray	3.51%	2992
Alta View Hospital	Sandy	3.65%	1780
Ashley Valley Medical Center	Vernal	3.80%	263
University Health Care/Univ of Utah Hosp	Salt Lake City	3.87%	2349
Sevier Valley Hospital	Richfield	4.35%	207

NOTE: Hospital profiles are in alphabetical order by state, then city, then hospital within the city; Rankings are sorted by rate in descending order and exclude hospitals with less than 25 cases; (1) The number of cases is too small (n<25) for purposes of reliably predicting hospital performance; (2) Measure reflects the hospital's indication that its submission was based upon a sample of its relevant discharges; (3) Rate reflects fewer than the maximum possible quarters of data for the measure; (4) Inaccurate information submitted and suppressed for one or more quarters; (5) No data is available from the hospital for this measure; Please refer to the User's Guide for a full explanation of data

American Fork Hospital

170 North 1100 East
American Fork, UT 84003
URL: www.ihc.com/facility/facilityresults.jsp
Ownership: Voluntary non-profit - Other
Emergency Services: Yes
Phone: 801-855-3300
Fax: 801-855-3586
Accredited: Yes
Licensed Beds: 117

Key Personnel:
President/CEO . . . . William H Nelson
Administrator . . . . Michael R Olson

Measure	Cases	This Hospital	State Average	U.S. Average	Top Hospital
Heart Attack Care					
ACE Inhibitor or ARB for LVSD[3]	0	-	83%	82%	100%
Aspirin at Arrival[1,3]	3	100%	91%	92%	100%
Aspirin at Discharge[1,3]	1	100%	81%	90%	100%
Beta Blocker at Arrival[1,3]	3	67%	71%	87%	100%
Beta Blocker at Discharge[1,3]	2	50%	70%	90%	100%
Fibrinolytic Medication Timing[3]	0	-	15%	31%	100%
PCI Within 90 Minutes of Arrival	0	-	58%	54%	95%
Smoking Cessation Advice[3]	0	-	94%	88%	100%
Heart Failure Care					
ACE Inhibitor or ARB for LVSD[1]	12	67%	81%	82%	100%
Discharge Instructions	65	88%	51%	61%	93%
Evaluation of LVS Function	87	94%	75%	83%	99%
Smoking Cessation Advice[1]	7	86%	78%	82%	100%
Pneumonia Care					
Appropriate Initial Antibiotic	112	81%	84%	83%	94%
Blood Culture Timing	65	94%	89%	90%	100%
Influenza Vaccine[1]	19	84%	73%	70%	100%
Initial Antibiotic Timing	126	89%	80%	80%	93%
Oxygenation Assessment	156	100%	100%	99%	100%
Pneumococcal Vaccine	92	83%	68%	69%	94%
Smoking Cessation Advice[1]	21	48%	64%	80%	100%
Surgical Infection Prevention					
Prophylactic Antibiotic Given[2]	219	92%	70%	77%	95%
Prophylactic Antibiotic Selection[2]	60	97%	92%	90%	100%
Prophylactic Antibiotic Stopped[2]	216	77%	69%	72%	95%
Pregnancy Care					
Inpatient Neonatal Mortality	2,845	0.00%	-	-	-
Third or Fourth Degree Laceration[2]	2,397	3.09%	2.98%	3.63%	3.27%

Beaver Valley Hospital

1109 North 100 West
Beaver, UT 84713
Ownership: Government - Local
Emergency Services: Yes
Phone: 435-438-2531
Fax: 435-438-7138
Accredited: No
Licensed Beds: 57

Key Personnel:
Administrator . . . . Craig Val Davidson

Measure	Cases	This Hospital	State Average	U.S. Average	Top Hospital
Heart Attack Care					
ACE Inhibitor or ARB for LVSD[1,3]	1	0%	83%	82%	100%
Aspirin at Arrival[1,3]	2	100%	91%	92%	100%
Aspirin at Discharge[1,3]	2	50%	81%	90%	100%
Beta Blocker at Arrival[1,3]	3	33%	71%	87%	100%
Beta Blocker at Discharge[1,3]	3	33%	70%	90%	100%
Fibrinolytic Medication Timing[3]	0	-	15%	31%	100%
PCI Within 90 Minutes of Arrival[5]	-	-	58%	54%	95%
Smoking Cessation Advice[3]	0	-	94%	88%	100%
Heart Failure Care					
ACE Inhibitor or ARB for LVSD	0	-	81%	82%	100%
Discharge Instructions[1]	15	13%	51%	61%	93%
Evaluation of LVS Function[1]	20	15%	75%	83%	99%
Smoking Cessation Advice[1]	3	33%	78%	82%	100%
Pneumonia Care					
Appropriate Initial Antibiotic	53	96%	84%	83%	94%
Blood Culture Timing[1]	5	100%	89%	90%	100%
Influenza Vaccine[1]	15	27%	73%	70%	100%
Initial Antibiotic Timing	54	98%	80%	80%	93%
Oxygenation Assessment	70	100%	100%	99%	100%
Pneumococcal Vaccine	54	57%	68%	69%	94%
Smoking Cessation Advice[1]	7	14%	64%	80%	100%
Surgical Infection Prevention					
Prophylactic Antibiotic Given[1,3]	1	0%	70%	77%	95%
Prophylactic Antibiotic Selection	0	-	92%	90%	100%
Prophylactic Antibiotic Stopped[1,3]	1	100%	69%	72%	95%
Pregnancy Care					
Inpatient Neonatal Mortality	-	-	-	-	-
Third or Fourth Degree Laceration	-	-	2.98%	3.63%	3.27%

Lakeview Hospital

630 E Medical Drive
Bountiful, UT 84010
Ownership: Proprietary
Emergency Services: Yes
Phone: 801-292-6231
Fax: 801-299-2198
Accredited: Yes
Licensed Beds: 128

Key Personnel:
CEO . . . . Craig Preston
Chief Medical Staff . . . . Mark Boschert
Chief Catheterization Laboratory . . . . John Angel
Emergency Room . . . . Mark Flammer, MD
Director Infection/Disease Control . . . . Pam Clark
CCU Spvg. Nurse . . . . Jolene Casper
Director Medical/Surgical Nursing . . . . Jeonelle Wright
OB/GYN Womens Health . . . . David Lewis
Chief Radiology . . . . Richard Hartvigson, MD
Director Respiratory Therapy . . . . Jerry Lake

Measure	Cases	This Hospital	State Average	U.S. Average	Top Hospital
Heart Attack Care					
ACE Inhibitor or ARB for LVSD[1]	7	100%	83%	82%	100%
Aspirin at Arrival	66	100%	91%	92%	100%
Aspirin at Discharge	60	100%	81%	90%	100%
Beta Blocker at Arrival	55	95%	71%	87%	100%
Beta Blocker at Discharge	56	100%	70%	90%	100%
Fibrinolytic Medication Timing[1]	2	0%	15%	31%	100%
PCI Within 90 Minutes of Arrival[1]	7	100%	58%	54%	95%
Smoking Cessation Advice[1]	7	100%	94%	88%	100%
Heart Failure Care					
ACE Inhibitor or ARB for LVSD[1]	16	88%	81%	82%	100%
Discharge Instructions	38	55%	51%	61%	93%
Evaluation of LVS Function	52	94%	75%	83%	99%
Smoking Cessation Advice	0	-	78%	82%	100%
Pneumonia Care					
Appropriate Initial Antibiotic	115	84%	84%	83%	94%
Blood Culture Timing	100	91%	89%	90%	100%
Influenza Vaccine	36	81%	73%	70%	100%
Initial Antibiotic Timing	134	81%	80%	80%	93%
Oxygenation Assessment	184	100%	100%	99%	100%
Pneumococcal Vaccine	127	73%	68%	69%	94%
Smoking Cessation Advice[1]	21	62%	64%	80%	100%
Surgical Infection Prevention					
Prophylactic Antibiotic Given[2,3]	218	91%	70%	77%	95%
Prophylactic Antibiotic Selection[2]	134	99%	92%	90%	100%
Prophylactic Antibiotic Stopped[2,3]	215	24%	69%	72%	95%
Pregnancy Care					
Inpatient Neonatal Mortality	-	-	-	-	-
Third or Fourth Degree Laceration	-	-	2.98%	3.63%	3.27%

Brigham City Community Hospital

950 S Medical Drive
Brigham City, UT 84302
Toll-Free: 800-439-4162
Phone: 435-734-9471
Fax: 435-723-5085
URL: www.brighamcityhospital.com
Ownership: Proprietary
Emergency Services: Yes
Accredited: Yes
Licensed Beds: 49

Key Personnel:
CEO . . . . Steven B Bateman
Chief Medical Staff . . . . Michael Sumko, DO
Emergency Room . . . . Corey Johnson, MD
Infection Control . . . . Kelli Cox, RN
ICU . . . . Susan Thompson, RN
Medical Surgical Nursing . . . . Chris Midget, RN
OB/GYN Womens Health . . . . Kari Griffin, RN

NOTE: Hospital profiles are in alphabetical order by state, then city, then hospital within the city; Rankings are sorted by rate in descending order and exclude hospitals with less than 25 cases; (1) The number of cases is too small (n<25) for purposes of reliably predicting hospital performance; (2) Measure reflects the hospital's indication that its submission was based upon a sample of its relevant discharges; (3) Rate reflects fewer than the maximum possible quarters of data for the measure; (4) Inaccurate information submitted and suppressed for one or more quarters; (5) No data is available from the hospital for this measure; Please refer to the User's Guide for a full explanation of data

Measure	Cases	This Hospital	State Average	U.S. Average	Top Hospital
Heart Attack Care					
ACE Inhibitor or ARB for LVSD[3]	0	-	83%	82%	100%
Aspirin at Arrival[3]	0	-	91%	92%	100%
Aspirin at Discharge[3]	0	-	81%	90%	100%
Beta Blocker at Arrival[3]	0	-	71%	87%	100%
Beta Blocker at Discharge[3]	0	-	70%	90%	100%
Fibrinolytic Medication Timing[3]	0	-	15%	31%	100%
PCI Within 90 Minutes of Arrival	0	-	58%	54%	95%
Smoking Cessation Advice[3]	0	-	94%	88%	100%
Heart Failure Care					
ACE Inhibitor or ARB for LVSD[1]	1	100%	81%	82%	100%
Discharge Instructions[1]	4	0%	51%	61%	93%
Evaluation of LVS Function[1]	8	75%	75%	83%	99%
Smoking Cessation Advice[1]	1	100%	78%	82%	100%
Pneumonia Care					
Appropriate Initial Antibiotic[1]	23	83%	84%	83%	94%
Blood Culture Timing[1]	5	80%	89%	90%	100%
Influenza Vaccine[1]	8	88%	73%	70%	100%
Initial Antibiotic Timing[1]	23	91%	80%	80%	93%
Oxygenation Assessment	31	100%	100%	99%	100%
Pneumococcal Vaccine[1]	21	90%	68%	69%	94%
Smoking Cessation Advice[1]	5	60%	64%	80%	100%
Surgical Infection Prevention					
Prophylactic Antibiotic Given[2,3]	70	40%	70%	77%	95%
Prophylactic Antibiotic Selection[2]	25	80%	92%	90%	100%
Prophylactic Antibiotic Stopped[2,3]	68	100%	69%	72%	95%
Pregnancy Care					
Inpatient Neonatal Mortality	358	0.28%	-	-	-
Third or Fourth Degree Laceration	274	1.46%	2.98%	3.63%	3.27%

Valley View Medical Center

595 S 75 E Street
Cedar City, UT 84720
E-mail: vvjfeike@ihc.com
Ownership: Voluntary non-profit - Private
Emergency Services: Yes

Phone: 435-868-5000
Fax: 435-868-5814
Accredited: Yes
Licensed Beds: 48

Key Personnel:

Administrator . . . . Craig Smedley
Chief Medical Staff. . . . . E Alfaro, MD
Emergency Room . . . . G Kim Rowland, MD
Director Infection/Disease Control . . . . Cyndi Wallace, RN
CCU Spvg. Nurse . . . . Kathy Caldwell, RN
Director Medical/Surgical Nursing . . . . Kathy Caldwell, RN
OB/GYN Womens Health. . . . . Ralph Oler, MD
Chief Radiology . . . . S Douglas Phillips, MD
Director Respiratory Therapy . . . . Robert Spangler

Measure	Cases	This Hospital	State Average	U.S. Average	Top Hospital
Heart Attack Care					
ACE Inhibitor or ARB for LVSD	0	-	83%	82%	100%
Aspirin at Arrival[1]	4	75%	91%	92%	100%
Aspirin at Discharge[1]	1	100%	81%	90%	100%
Beta Blocker at Arrival[1]	4	50%	71%	87%	100%
Beta Blocker at Discharge[1]	2	50%	70%	90%	100%
Fibrinolytic Medication Timing	0	-	15%	31%	100%
PCI Within 90 Minutes of Arrival	0	-	58%	54%	95%
Smoking Cessation Advice[1]	1	100%	94%	88%	100%
Heart Failure Care					
ACE Inhibitor or ARB for LVSD[1]	9	78%	81%	82%	100%
Discharge Instructions[1]	20	65%	51%	61%	93%
Evaluation of LVS Function[1]	23	96%	75%	83%	99%
Smoking Cessation Advice[1]	7	57%	78%	82%	100%
Pneumonia Care					
Appropriate Initial Antibiotic	79	85%	84%	83%	94%
Blood Culture Timing	42	81%	89%	90%	100%
Influenza Vaccine[1]	16	100%	73%	70%	100%
Initial Antibiotic Timing	83	86%	80%	80%	93%
Oxygenation Assessment	111	100%	100%	99%	100%
Pneumococcal Vaccine	58	90%	68%	69%	94%
Smoking Cessation Advice[1]	20	70%	64%	80%	100%
Surgical Infection Prevention					
Prophylactic Antibiotic Given[2]	228	78%	70%	77%	95%
Prophylactic Antibiotic Selection[2]	50	92%	92%	90%	100%
Prophylactic Antibiotic Stopped[2]	224	30%	69%	72%	95%
Pregnancy Care					
Inpatient Neonatal Mortality	885	0.34%	-	-	-
Third or Fourth Degree Laceration[2]	718	2.51%	2.98%	3.63%	3.27%

Delta Community Medical Center

126 S White Sage Avenue
Delta, UT 84624
URL: www.ihc.com/delta
Ownership: Voluntary non-profit - Private
Emergency Services: Yes

Phone: 435-864-5591
Fax: 435-864-4186
Accredited: No
Licensed Beds: 20

Key Personnel:

CEO. . . . . James Beckstrand
Chief Medical Staff. . . . . Steven W Shamo

Measure	Cases	This Hospital	State Average	U.S. Average	Top Hospital
Heart Attack Care					
ACE Inhibitor or ARB for LVSD[3]	0	-	83%	82%	100%
Aspirin at Arrival[1,3]	2	0%	91%	92%	100%
Aspirin at Discharge[1,3]	1	0%	81%	90%	100%
Beta Blocker at Arrival[1,3]	2	50%	71%	87%	100%
Beta Blocker at Discharge[1,3]	1	0%	70%	90%	100%
Fibrinolytic Medication Timing[3]	0	-	15%	31%	100%
PCI Within 90 Minutes of Arrival[5]	-	-	58%	54%	95%
Smoking Cessation Advice[3]	0	-	94%	88%	100%
Heart Failure Care					
ACE Inhibitor or ARB for LVSD	0	-	81%	82%	100%
Discharge Instructions[1]	7	86%	51%	61%	93%
Evaluation of LVS Function[1]	9	67%	75%	83%	99%
Smoking Cessation Advice	0	-	78%	82%	100%
Pneumonia Care					
Appropriate Initial Antibiotic[1]	21	81%	84%	83%	94%
Blood Culture Timing[1]	5	80%	89%	90%	100%
Influenza Vaccine[1]	5	80%	73%	70%	100%
Initial Antibiotic Timing[1]	23	87%	80%	80%	93%
Oxygenation Assessment	26	100%	100%	99%	100%
Pneumococcal Vaccine[1]	17	65%	68%	69%	94%
Smoking Cessation Advice[1]	3	0%	64%	80%	100%
Surgical Infection Prevention					
Prophylactic Antibiotic Given[3]	0	-	70%	77%	95%
Prophylactic Antibiotic Selection	0	-	92%	90%	100%
Prophylactic Antibiotic Stopped[3]	0	-	69%	72%	95%
Pregnancy Care					
Inpatient Neonatal Mortality	-	-	-	-	-
Third or Fourth Degree Laceration	-	-	2.98%	3.63%	3.27%

Fillmore Community Medical Center

674 S Highway 99
Fillmore, UT 84631
URL: www.ihc.com
Ownership: Voluntary non-profit - Private
Emergency Services: Yes

Phone: 435-743-5591
Fax: 435-743-6312
Accredited: No
Licensed Beds: 20

Key Personnel:

Administrator/CEO . . . . James Beckstrand
Emergency Room . . . . Paul Blad
Chief Radiology . . . . Shelli Richardson

Measure	Cases	This Hospital	State Average	U.S. Average	Top Hospital
Heart Attack Care					
ACE Inhibitor or ARB for LVSD[3]	0	-	83%	82%	100%
Aspirin at Arrival[1,3]	1	100%	91%	92%	100%
Aspirin at Discharge[3]	0	-	81%	90%	100%
Beta Blocker at Arrival[1,3]	1	100%	71%	87%	100%
Beta Blocker at Discharge[3]	0	-	70%	90%	100%
Fibrinolytic Medication Timing[3]	0	-	15%	31%	100%
PCI Within 90 Minutes of Arrival	0	-	58%	54%	95%
Smoking Cessation Advice[3]	0	-	94%	88%	100%
Heart Failure Care					
ACE Inhibitor or ARB for LVSD[5]	-	-	81%	82%	100%

NOTE: Hospital profiles are in alphabetical order by state, then city, then hospital within the city; Rankings are sorted by rate in descending order and exclude hospitals with less than 25 cases; (1) The number of cases is too small (n<25) for purposes of reliably predicting hospital performance; (2) Measure reflects the hospital's indication that its submission was based upon a sample of its relevant discharges; (3) Rate reflects fewer than the maximum possible quarters of data for the measure; (4) Inaccurate information submitted and suppressed for one or more quarters; (5) No data is available from the hospital for this measure; Please refer to the User's Guide for a full explanation of data

Discharge Instructions[5]	-	-	51%	61%	93%
Evaluation of LVS Function[5]	-	-	75%	83%	99%
Smoking Cessation Advice[5]	-	-	78%	82%	100%
Pneumonia Care					
Appropriate Initial Antibiotic[1,3]	11	73%	84%	83%	94%
Blood Culture Timing[1,3]	1	0%	89%	90%	100%
Influenza Vaccine[1]	1	100%	73%	70%	100%
Initial Antibiotic Timing[1,3]	12	67%	80%	80%	93%
Oxygenation Assessment[1,3]	15	100%	100%	99%	100%
Pneumococcal Vaccine[1,3]	10	80%	68%	69%	94%
Smoking Cessation Advice[1,3]	2	50%	64%	80%	100%
Surgical Infection Prevention					
Prophylactic Antibiotic Given[3]	0	-	70%	77%	95%
Prophylactic Antibiotic Selection	0	-	92%	90%	100%
Prophylactic Antibiotic Stopped[3]	0	-	69%	72%	95%
Pregnancy Care					
Inpatient Neonatal Mortality	-	-	-	-	-
Third or Fourth Degree Laceration	-	-	2.98%	3.63%	3.27%

Gunnison Valley Hospital

64 E 100 N
PO Box 759
Gunnison, UT 84634
E-mail: greg.rosenvall@utahtelehealth.net
Phone: 435-528-7246
Fax: 435-528-2190
Ownership: Voluntary non-profit - Other
Emergency Services: Yes
Accredited: No
Licensed Beds: 21

Key Personnel:
Administrator/CEO....................... Greg Rosenvall
Chief/Medical Staff....................... Richard Anderson, MD
Emergency Room .... Brenda Batholomew
Infection Control......................... Brenda Bartholomew
Director Respiratory Therapy............... Kay C Caldwell

Measure	Cases	This Hospital	State Average	U.S. Average	Top Hospital
Heart Attack Care					
ACE Inhibitor or ARB for LVSD[5]	-	-	83%	82%	100%
Aspirin at Arrival[5]	-	-	91%	92%	100%
Aspirin at Discharge[5]	-	-	81%	90%	100%
Beta Blocker at Arrival[5]	-	-	71%	87%	100%
Beta Blocker at Discharge[5]	-	-	70%	90%	100%
Fibrinolytic Medication Timing[5]	-	-	15%	31%	100%
PCI Within 90 Minutes of Arrival[5]	-	-	58%	54%	95%
Smoking Cessation Advice[5]	-	-	94%	88%	100%
Heart Failure Care					
ACE Inhibitor or ARB for LVSD	0	-	81%	82%	100%
Discharge Instructions[1]	11	27%	51%	61%	93%
Evaluation of LVS Function[1]	16	44%	75%	83%	99%
Smoking Cessation Advice[1]	2	100%	78%	82%	100%
Pneumonia Care					
Appropriate Initial Antibiotic	40	78%	84%	83%	94%
Blood Culture Timing[1]	5	100%	89%	90%	100%
Influenza Vaccine[1]	4	50%	73%	70%	100%
Initial Antibiotic Timing	36	83%	80%	80%	93%
Oxygenation Assessment	47	100%	100%	99%	100%
Pneumococcal Vaccine	26	77%	68%	69%	94%
Smoking Cessation Advice[1]	7	57%	64%	80%	100%
Surgical Infection Prevention					
Prophylactic Antibiotic Given[3]	0	-	70%	77%	95%
Prophylactic Antibiotic Selection	0	-	92%	90%	100%
Prophylactic Antibiotic Stopped[3]	0	-	69%	72%	95%
Pregnancy Care					
Inpatient Neonatal Mortality	-	-	-	-	-
Third or Fourth Degree Laceration	-	-	2.98%	3.63%	3.27%

Heber Valley Medical Center

Alternate Name: Wasatch County Hospital
1485 South Highway 40
Heber City, UT 84032
URL: www.ihc.com
Phone: 435-654-2500
Fax: 435-654-2576
Ownership: Voluntary non-profit - Private
Emergency Services: Yes
Accredited: No
Licensed Beds: 25

Key Personnel:
Administrator.......................... Ezra Segura
President/CEO.......................... Randall Prebet
Chief Medical Staff....................... George Pitts, MD
Emergency Room .... Dorothy Sullivan
Infection Control......................... Michele Ludlow
OB/GYN Women's Health .... Kathy Coleman

Measure	Cases	This Hospital	State Average	U.S. Average	Top Hospital
Heart Attack Care					
ACE Inhibitor or ARB for LVSD[3]	0	-	83%	82%	100%
Aspirin at Arrival[1,3]	1	100%	91%	92%	100%
Aspirin at Discharge[1,3]	1	0%	81%	90%	100%
Beta Blocker at Arrival[1,3]	1	0%	71%	87%	100%
Beta Blocker at Discharge[1,3]	1	0%	70%	90%	100%
Fibrinolytic Medication Timing[3]	0	-	15%	31%	100%
PCI Within 90 Minutes of Arrival[5]	-	-	58%	54%	95%
Smoking Cessation Advice[3]	0	-	94%	88%	100%
Heart Failure Care					
ACE Inhibitor or ARB for LVSD[3]	0	-	81%	82%	100%
Discharge Instructions[1,3]	5	40%	51%	61%	93%
Evaluation of LVS Function[1,3]	8	38%	75%	83%	99%
Smoking Cessation Advice[1,3]	1	0%	78%	82%	100%
Pneumonia Care					
Appropriate Initial Antibiotic	37	84%	84%	83%	94%
Blood Culture Timing[1]	8	100%	89%	90%	100%
Influenza Vaccine[1]	11	73%	73%	70%	100%
Initial Antibiotic Timing	34	85%	80%	80%	93%
Oxygenation Assessment	42	98%	100%	99%	100%
Pneumococcal Vaccine[1]	20	65%	68%	69%	94%
Smoking Cessation Advice[1]	7	29%	64%	80%	100%
Surgical Infection Prevention					
Prophylactic Antibiotic Given[2]	76	38%	70%	77%	95%
Prophylactic Antibiotic Selection[1,2]	18	89%	92%	90%	100%
Prophylactic Antibiotic Stopped[2]	77	71%	69%	72%	95%
Pregnancy Care					
Inpatient Neonatal Mortality	-	-	-	-	-
Third or Fourth Degree Laceration	-	-	2.98%	3.63%	3.27%

Kane County Hospital

355 N Main Street
Kanab, UT 84741
Phone: 435-644-5811
Fax: 435-644-4140
Ownership: Govt - Hospital District or Authority
Emergency Services: Yes
Accredited: No
Licensed Beds: 38

Key Personnel:
Administrator .... Tom Mitchell
Chief Medical Staff....................... Avnish P Pandyah, MD
Emergency Room .... K Mortenson, MD

Measure	Cases	This Hospital	State Average	U.S. Average	Top Hospital
Heart Attack Care					
ACE Inhibitor or ARB for LVSD[3]	0	-	83%	82%	100%
Aspirin at Arrival[1,3]	1	100%	91%	92%	100%
Aspirin at Discharge[1,3]	1	0%	81%	90%	100%
Beta Blocker at Arrival[1,3]	1	100%	71%	87%	100%
Beta Blocker at Discharge[1,3]	1	100%	70%	90%	100%
Fibrinolytic Medication Timing[3]	0	-	15%	31%	100%
PCI Within 90 Minutes of Arrival	0	-	58%	54%	95%
Smoking Cessation Advice[3]	0	-	94%	88%	100%
Heart Failure Care					
ACE Inhibitor or ARB for LVSD	0	-	81%	82%	100%
Discharge Instructions[1]	10	0%	51%	61%	93%
Evaluation of LVS Function[1]	12	0%	75%	83%	99%
Smoking Cessation Advice	0	-	78%	82%	100%
Pneumonia Care					
Appropriate Initial Antibiotic	47	72%	84%	83%	94%
Blood Culture Timing[1]	2	100%	89%	90%	100%
Influenza Vaccine[1]	9	0%	73%	70%	100%
Initial Antibiotic Timing	47	81%	80%	80%	93%
Oxygenation Assessment	53	100%	100%	99%	100%
Pneumococcal Vaccine	36	8%	68%	69%	94%
Smoking Cessation Advice[1]	7	0%	64%	80%	100%
Surgical Infection Prevention					
Prophylactic Antibiotic Given[1]	5	40%	70%	77%	95%

NOTE: Hospital profiles are in alphabetical order by state, then city, then hospital within the city; Rankings are sorted by rate in descending order and exclude hospitals with less than 25 cases; (1) The number of cases is too small (n<25) for purposes of reliably predicting hospital performance; (2) Measure reflects the hospital's indication that its submission was based upon a sample of its relevant discharges; (3) Rate reflects fewer than the maximum possible quarters of data for the measure; (4) Inaccurate information submitted and suppressed for one or more quarters; (5) No data is available from the hospital for this measure; Please refer to the User's Guide for a full explanation of data

Measure	Cases	This Hospital	State Average	U.S. Average	Top Hospital
Prophylactic Antibiotic Selection[1]	2	100%	92%	90%	100%
Prophylactic Antibiotic Stopped[1]	5	100%	69%	72%	95%
Pregnancy Care					
Inpatient Neonatal Mortality	-	-	-	-	-
Third or Fourth Degree Laceration	-	-	2.98%	3.63%	3.27%

Davis Hospital and Medical Center

Alternate Name: Humana Hospital Davis North
1600 W Antelope Drive
Layton, UT 84041
Ownership: Proprietary
Emergency Services: Yes

Phone: 801-807-1000
Fax: 801-774-7045
Accredited: Yes
Licensed Beds: 126

Key Personnel:
Administrator/President . . . . Bruce A Baldwin
Chief Medical Staff . . . . Stephen Tucker, MD
Chief Catheterization Laboratory . . . . Stephanie Olsen
Emergency Room . . . . Bart Nilson
Director Infection/Disease Control . . . . Cindy Johnston
Director Medical/Surgical Nursing . . . . Debbie Thurman
OB/GYN Womens Health . . . . Joseph Bell, DO
Director Respiratory Therapy . . . . Sara Worrall

Measure	Cases	This Hospital	State Average	U.S. Average	Top Hospital
Heart Attack Care					
ACE Inhibitor or ARB for LVSD[1]	17	94%	83%	82%	100%
Aspirin at Arrival	107	93%	91%	92%	100%
Aspirin at Discharge	100	97%	81%	90%	100%
Beta Blocker at Arrival	93	89%	71%	87%	100%
Beta Blocker at Discharge	98	97%	70%	90%	100%
Fibrinolytic Medication Timing	0	-	15%	31%	100%
PCI Within 90 Minutes of Arrival[1]	8	75%	58%	54%	95%
Smoking Cessation Advice	29	93%	94%	88%	100%
Heart Failure Care					
ACE Inhibitor or ARB for LVSD	29	90%	81%	82%	100%
Discharge Instructions	72	53%	51%	61%	93%
Evaluation of LVS Function	89	89%	75%	83%	99%
Smoking Cessation Advice[1]	16	94%	78%	82%	100%
Pneumonia Care					
Appropriate Initial Antibiotic	125	90%	84%	83%	94%
Blood Culture Timing	79	87%	89%	90%	100%
Influenza Vaccine	35	74%	73%	70%	100%
Initial Antibiotic Timing	134	81%	80%	80%	93%
Oxygenation Assessment	178	100%	100%	99%	100%
Pneumococcal Vaccine	107	68%	68%	69%	94%
Smoking Cessation Advice	34	79%	64%	80%	100%
Surgical Infection Prevention					
Prophylactic Antibiotic Given	476	84%	70%	77%	95%
Prophylactic Antibiotic Selection	111	94%	92%	90%	100%
Prophylactic Antibiotic Stopped	463	77%	69%	72%	95%
Pregnancy Care					
Inpatient Neonatal Mortality[2]	753	0.00%	-	-	-
Third or Fourth Degree Laceration[2]	562	2.14%	2.98%	3.63%	3.27%

Logan Regional Hospital

500 East 1400 North
Logan, UT 84341
URL: www.intermountainhealthcare.org
Ownership: Voluntary non-profit - Private
Emergency Services: Yes

Phone: 435-716-1000
Fax: 435-716-5409
Accredited: Yes
Licensed Beds: 148

Key Personnel:
Administrator . . . . Richard J Smith
Chief Medical Staff . . . . Bryan Larsen
Chief Catheterization Laboratory . . . . Jana Huffman
Emergency Room . . . . James Davis
Director Infection/Disease Control . . . . Debbi Moore
CCU Spvg. Nurse . . . . Sharlene Moe
Director Medical/Surgical Nursing . . . . Sharlene Moe
OB/GYN Womens Health . . . . F Neal Mortenson, MD
Director Respiratory Therapy . . . . Don Huffman

Measure	Cases	This Hospital	State Average	U.S. Average	Top Hospital
Heart Attack Care					
ACE Inhibitor or ARB for LVSD	0	-	83%	82%	100%
Aspirin at Arrival[1]	14	100%	91%	92%	100%
Aspirin at Discharge[1]	5	100%	81%	90%	100%
Beta Blocker at Arrival[1]	11	100%	71%	87%	100%
Beta Blocker at Discharge[1]	4	100%	70%	90%	100%
Fibrinolytic Medication Timing	0	-	15%	31%	100%
PCI Within 90 Minutes of Arrival	0	-	58%	54%	95%
Smoking Cessation Advice	0	-	94%	88%	100%
Heart Failure Care					
ACE Inhibitor or ARB for LVSD[1]	6	67%	81%	82%	100%
Discharge Instructions	38	89%	51%	61%	93%
Evaluation of LVS Function	47	85%	75%	83%	99%
Smoking Cessation Advice[1]	7	100%	78%	82%	100%
Pneumonia Care					
Appropriate Initial Antibiotic	83	78%	84%	83%	94%
Blood Culture Timing	62	85%	89%	90%	100%
Influenza Vaccine	28	86%	73%	70%	100%
Initial Antibiotic Timing	116	90%	80%	80%	93%
Oxygenation Assessment	159	100%	100%	99%	100%
Pneumococcal Vaccine	109	87%	68%	69%	94%
Smoking Cessation Advice[1]	9	67%	64%	80%	100%
Surgical Infection Prevention					
Prophylactic Antibiotic Given[2]	242	79%	70%	77%	95%
Prophylactic Antibiotic Selection[2]	69	97%	92%	90%	100%
Prophylactic Antibiotic Stopped[2]	235	70%	69%	72%	95%
Pregnancy Care					
Inpatient Neonatal Mortality	2,645	0.00%	-	-	-
Third or Fourth Degree Laceration[2]	2,147	2.89%	2.98%	3.63%	3.27%

Sanpete Valley Hospital

1100 S Medical Drive
Mount Pleasant, UT 84647
URL: www.ihc.com
Ownership: Voluntary non-profit - Private
Emergency Services: Yes

Phone: 435-462-2441
Fax: 435-462-2609
Accredited: No
Licensed Beds: 20

Key Personnel:
Chief Medical Staff . . . . Robert Amstrong, MD
Infection Control . . . . Suana Olsen, RN
Medical Surgical Nursing . . . . Warren Benincosa, RN
OB/GYN/Women's Health . . . . Suzy Zahler, RN
Respiratory/Cardiopulmonary . . . . Kerry Durfey

Measure	Cases	This Hospital	State Average	U.S. Average	Top Hospital
Heart Attack Care					
ACE Inhibitor or ARB for LVSD[3]	0	-	83%	82%	100%
Aspirin at Arrival[3]	0	-	91%	92%	100%
Aspirin at Discharge[3]	0	-	81%	90%	100%
Beta Blocker at Arrival[1,3]	1	0%	71%	87%	100%
Beta Blocker at Discharge[1,3]	1	0%	70%	90%	100%
Fibrinolytic Medication Timing[3]	0	-	15%	31%	100%
PCI Within 90 Minutes of Arrival	0	-	58%	54%	95%
Smoking Cessation Advice[3]	0	-	94%	88%	100%
Heart Failure Care					
ACE Inhibitor or ARB for LVSD[3]	0	-	81%	82%	100%
Discharge Instructions[1,3]	3	33%	51%	61%	93%
Evaluation of LVS Function[1,3]	3	0%	75%	83%	99%
Smoking Cessation Advice[3]	0	-	78%	82%	100%
Pneumonia Care					
Appropriate Initial Antibiotic	44	82%	84%	83%	94%
Blood Culture Timing[1]	8	88%	89%	90%	100%
Influenza Vaccine[1]	11	82%	73%	70%	100%
Initial Antibiotic Timing	47	74%	80%	80%	93%
Oxygenation Assessment	49	100%	100%	99%	100%
Pneumococcal Vaccine	33	58%	68%	69%	94%
Smoking Cessation Advice[1]	7	14%	64%	80%	100%
Surgical Infection Prevention					
Prophylactic Antibiotic Given[1]	9	33%	70%	77%	95%
Prophylactic Antibiotic Selection[1]	3	100%	92%	90%	100%
Prophylactic Antibiotic Stopped[1]	9	44%	69%	72%	95%
Pregnancy Care					
Inpatient Neonatal Mortality	-	-	-	-	-
Third or Fourth Degree Laceration	-	-	2.98%	3.63%	3.27%

NOTE: Hospital profiles are in alphabetical order by state, then city, then hospital within the city; Rankings are sorted by rate in descending order and exclude hospitals with less than 25 cases; (1) The number of cases is too small (n<25) for purposes of reliably predicting hospital performance; (2) Measure reflects the hospital's indication that its submission was based upon a sample of its relevant discharges; (3) Rate reflects fewer than the maximum possible quarters of data for the measure; (4) Inaccurate information submitted and suppressed for one or more quarters; (5) No data is available from the hospital for this measure; Please refer to the User's Guide for a full explanation of data

Cottonwood Hospital

5770 South 300 East
Murray, UT 84107
Phone: 801-314-5300
Ownership: Voluntary non-profit - Private
Accredited: Yes
Emergency Services: Yes

Measure	Cases	This Hospital	State Average	U.S. Average	Top Hospital
Heart Attack Care					
ACE Inhibitor or ARB for LVSD[1]	13	77%	83%	82%	100%
Aspirin at Arrival	127	92%	91%	92%	100%
Aspirin at Discharge	106	93%	81%	90%	100%
Beta Blocker at Arrival	104	93%	71%	87%	100%
Beta Blocker at Discharge	117	94%	70%	90%	100%
Fibrinolytic Medication Timing	0	-	15%	31%	100%
PCI Within 90 Minutes of Arrival[1]	7	43%	58%	54%	95%
Smoking Cessation Advice	31	94%	94%	88%	100%
Heart Failure Care					
ACE Inhibitor or ARB for LVSD	30	77%	81%	82%	100%
Discharge Instructions	91	88%	51%	61%	93%
Evaluation of LVS Function	105	92%	75%	83%	99%
Smoking Cessation Advice[1]	20	85%	78%	82%	100%
Pneumonia Care					
Appropriate Initial Antibiotic	257	84%	84%	83%	94%
Blood Culture Timing	163	94%	89%	90%	100%
Influenza Vaccine	67	84%	73%	70%	100%
Initial Antibiotic Timing	329	73%	80%	80%	93%
Oxygenation Assessment	382	99%	100%	99%	100%
Pneumococcal Vaccine	212	79%	68%	69%	94%
Smoking Cessation Advice	74	85%	64%	80%	100%
Surgical Infection Prevention					
Prophylactic Antibiotic Given[2]	260	81%	70%	77%	95%
Prophylactic Antibiotic Selection[2]	78	92%	92%	90%	100%
Prophylactic Antibiotic Stopped[2]	254	62%	69%	72%	95%
Pregnancy Care					
Inpatient Neonatal Mortality	3,852	0.00%	-	-	-
Third or Fourth Degree Laceration[2]	2,992	3.51%	2.98%	3.63%	3.27%

The Orthopedic Specialty Hospital

5848 South 300 East
Murray, UT 84107
Phone: 801-314-4100
Ownership: Voluntary non-profit - Private
Accredited: Yes
Emergency Services: No

Measure	Cases	This Hospital	State Average	U.S. Average	Top Hospital
Heart Attack Care					
ACE Inhibitor or ARB for LVSD[5]	-	-	83%	82%	100%
Aspirin at Arrival[5]	-	-	91%	92%	100%
Aspirin at Discharge[5]	-	-	81%	90%	100%
Beta Blocker at Arrival[5]	-	-	71%	87%	100%
Beta Blocker at Discharge[5]	-	-	70%	90%	100%
Fibrinolytic Medication Timing[5]	-	-	15%	31%	100%
PCI Within 90 Minutes of Arrival[5]	-	-	58%	54%	95%
Smoking Cessation Advice[5]	-	-	94%	88%	100%
Heart Failure Care					
ACE Inhibitor or ARB for LVSD[5]	-	-	81%	82%	100%
Discharge Instructions[5]	-	-	51%	61%	93%
Evaluation of LVS Function[5]	-	-	75%	83%	99%
Smoking Cessation Advice[5]	-	-	78%	82%	100%
Pneumonia Care					
Appropriate Initial Antibiotic[5]	-	-	84%	83%	94%
Blood Culture Timing[5]	-	-	89%	90%	100%
Influenza Vaccine[5]	-	-	73%	70%	100%
Initial Antibiotic Timing[5]	-	-	80%	80%	93%
Oxygenation Assessment[5]	-	-	100%	99%	100%
Pneumococcal Vaccine[5]	-	-	68%	69%	94%
Smoking Cessation Advice[5]	-	-	64%	80%	100%
Surgical Infection Prevention					
Prophylactic Antibiotic Given[2]	194	87%	70%	77%	95%
Prophylactic Antibiotic Selection[2]	71	99%	92%	90%	100%
Prophylactic Antibiotic Stopped[2]	194	34%	69%	72%	95%
Pregnancy Care					
Inpatient Neonatal Mortality	-	-	-	-	-
Third or Fourth Degree Laceration	-	-	2.98%	3.63%	3.27%

Central Valley Medical Center

48 W 5100 N
Nephi, UT 84648
Phone: 435-623-3000
Fax: 435-623-3290
E-mail: banks@outreach.med.utah.edu
Ownership: Voluntary non-profit - Private
Accredited: No
Emergency Services: Yes
Licensed Beds: 19

Key Personnel:

CEO. . . . . Mark Stoddard
Chief of Medical Staff. . . . . Mark Oveson, MD
Emergency Room . . . . Grant Rasmussen, MD
Ob/Gyn/Womens Health . . . . Rachelle Benson, RN
Respiratory/Cardiopulmonary. . . . . Mike Cannell

Measure	Cases	This Hospital	State Average	U.S. Average	Top Hospital
Heart Attack Care					
ACE Inhibitor or ARB for LVSD[5]	-	-	83%	82%	100%
Aspirin at Arrival[5]	-	-	91%	92%	100%
Aspirin at Discharge[5]	-	-	81%	90%	100%
Beta Blocker at Arrival[5]	-	-	71%	87%	100%
Beta Blocker at Discharge[5]	-	-	70%	90%	100%
Fibrinolytic Medication Timing[5]	-	-	15%	31%	100%
PCI Within 90 Minutes of Arrival[5]	-	-	58%	54%	95%
Smoking Cessation Advice[5]	-	-	94%	88%	100%
Heart Failure Care					
ACE Inhibitor or ARB for LVSD[1]	3	100%	81%	82%	100%
Discharge Instructions[1]	18	11%	51%	61%	93%
Evaluation of LVS Function	25	64%	75%	83%	99%
Smoking Cessation Advice[1]	1	100%	78%	82%	100%
Pneumonia Care					
Appropriate Initial Antibiotic	27	81%	84%	83%	94%
Blood Culture Timing[1]	4	100%	89%	90%	100%
Influenza Vaccine[1]	12	8%	73%	70%	100%
Initial Antibiotic Timing	34	85%	80%	80%	93%
Oxygenation Assessment	42	100%	100%	99%	100%
Pneumococcal Vaccine[1]	22	18%	68%	69%	94%
Smoking Cessation Advice[1]	5	60%	64%	80%	100%
Surgical Infection Prevention					
Prophylactic Antibiotic Given	50	90%	70%	77%	95%
Prophylactic Antibiotic Selection[1]	17	100%	92%	90%	100%
Prophylactic Antibiotic Stopped	48	96%	69%	72%	95%
Pregnancy Care					
Inpatient Neonatal Mortality	-	-	-	-	-
Third or Fourth Degree Laceration	-	-	2.98%	3.63%	3.27%

Cache Valley Speciality Hospital

2380 North 400 East
North Logan, UT 84341
Phone: 435-713-9700
Ownership: Voluntary non-profit - Private
Accredited: Yes
Emergency Services: No

Measure	Cases	This Hospital	State Average	U.S. Average	Top Hospital
Heart Attack Care					
ACE Inhibitor or ARB for LVSD[5]	-	-	83%	82%	100%
Aspirin at Arrival[5]	-	-	91%	92%	100%
Aspirin at Discharge[5]	-	-	81%	90%	100%
Beta Blocker at Arrival[5]	-	-	71%	87%	100%
Beta Blocker at Discharge[5]	-	-	70%	90%	100%
Fibrinolytic Medication Timing[5]	-	-	15%	31%	100%
PCI Within 90 Minutes of Arrival[5]	-	-	58%	54%	95%
Smoking Cessation Advice[5]	-	-	94%	88%	100%
Heart Failure Care					
ACE Inhibitor or ARB for LVSD[2,3]	0	-	81%	82%	100%
Discharge Instructions[1,2,3]	2	0%	51%	61%	93%
Evaluation of LVS Function[1,2,3]	2	50%	75%	83%	99%
Smoking Cessation Advice[2,3]	0	-	78%	82%	100%
Pneumonia Care					
Appropriate Initial Antibiotic[1,2,3]	1	100%	84%	83%	94%
Blood Culture Timing[2,3]	0	-	89%	90%	100%
Influenza Vaccine[5]	-	-	73%	70%	100%

NOTE: Hospital profiles are in alphabetical order by state, then city, then hospital within the city; Rankings are sorted by rate in descending order and exclude hospitals with less than 25 cases; (1) The number of cases is too small (n<25) for purposes of reliably predicting hospital performance; (2) Measure reflects the hospital's indication that its submission was based upon a sample of its relevant discharges; (3) Rate reflects fewer than the maximum possible quarters of data for the measure; (4) Inaccurate information submitted and suppressed for one or more quarters; (5) No data is available from the hospital for this measure; Please refer to the User's Guide for a full explanation of data

Measure	Cases	This Hospital	State Average	U.S. Average	Top Hospital
Initial Antibiotic Timing[1,2,3]	1	0%	80%	80%	93%
Oxygenation Assessment[1,2,3]	1	100%	100%	99%	100%
Pneumococcal Vaccine[1,2,3]	1	0%	68%	69%	94%
Smoking Cessation Advice[2,3]	0	-	64%	80%	100%
Surgical Infection Prevention					
Prophylactic Antibiotic Given[2,3]	64	16%	70%	77%	95%
Prophylactic Antibiotic Selection[2]	64	91%	92%	90%	100%
Prophylactic Antibiotic Stopped[2,3]	64	17%	69%	72%	95%
Pregnancy Care					
Inpatient Neonatal Mortality	-	-	-	-	-
Third or Fourth Degree Laceration	-	-	2.98%	3.63%	3.27%

McKay-Dee Hospital Center

4401 Harrison Boulevard
Ogden, UT 84403

Toll-Free: 800-308-1907
Phone: 801-627-2800
Fax: 801-387-7755

URL: www.ihc.com/mckay-dee
Ownership: Voluntary non-profit - Other
Emergency Services: Yes
Accredited: Yes
Licensed Beds: 335

Key Personnel:
CEO/President. . . . . Tim Pehrson
Chief Medical Staff. . . . . Richard Arbogast, MD
Director of Cardiology/Cardiac Lab. . . . . Ruth Brockman
President Medical Staff . . . . Steven Cain, MD
OB/Gyn/Women's Health. . . . . Sherry Monson

Measure	Cases	This Hospital	State Average	U.S. Average	Top Hospital
Heart Attack Care					
ACE Inhibitor or ARB for LVSD	25	96%	83%	82%	100%
Aspirin at Arrival	177	99%	91%	92%	100%
Aspirin at Discharge	248	97%	81%	90%	100%
Beta Blocker at Arrival	144	88%	71%	87%	100%
Beta Blocker at Discharge	229	95%	70%	90%	100%
Fibrinolytic Medication Timing	0	-	15%	31%	100%
PCI Within 90 Minutes of Arrival[1]	8	75%	58%	54%	95%
Smoking Cessation Advice	68	97%	94%	88%	100%
Heart Failure Care					
ACE Inhibitor or ARB for LVSD	116	93%	81%	82%	100%
Discharge Instructions	221	83%	51%	61%	93%
Evaluation of LVS Function	256	98%	75%	83%	99%
Smoking Cessation Advice	27	96%	78%	82%	100%
Pneumonia Care					
Appropriate Initial Antibiotic	292	92%	84%	83%	94%
Blood Culture Timing	231	84%	89%	90%	100%
Influenza Vaccine	62	82%	73%	70%	100%
Initial Antibiotic Timing	323	90%	80%	80%	93%
Oxygenation Assessment	444	100%	100%	99%	100%
Pneumococcal Vaccine	268	71%	68%	69%	94%
Smoking Cessation Advice	101	86%	64%	80%	100%
Surgical Infection Prevention					
Prophylactic Antibiotic Given[2]	508	88%	70%	77%	95%
Prophylactic Antibiotic Selection[2]	173	92%	92%	90%	100%
Prophylactic Antibiotic Stopped[2]	498	69%	69%	72%	95%
Pregnancy Care					
Inpatient Neonatal Mortality	3,920	0.20%	-	-	-
Third or Fourth Degree Laceration[2]	2,849	2.14%	2.98%	3.63%	3.27%

Ogden Regional Medical Center

Alternate Name: Saint Benedict's Hospital
5475 S 500 E
Ogden, UT 84405
Ownership: Proprietary
Emergency Services: Yes

Phone: 801-479-2111
Fax: 801-479-2091
Accredited: Yes
Licensed Beds: 227

Key Personnel:
CEO. . . . . Steven B Bateman
Chief Medical Staff. . . . . Douglas K Anderson, MD
Emergency Room . . . . William Sheffield, MD
Infection Control. . . . . Jeanette Smyth
Medical/Surgical Nursing . . . . Linda Baxter
OB/GYN Womens Health. . . . . Shirley Garcia, MD
Respiratory Therapy. . . . . Kurt Park

Measure	Cases	This Hospital	State Average	U.S. Average	Top Hospital
Heart Attack Care					
ACE Inhibitor or ARB for LVSD[1]	10	100%	83%	82%	100%
Aspirin at Arrival	81	99%	91%	92%	100%
Aspirin at Discharge	105	97%	81%	90%	100%
Beta Blocker at Arrival	62	94%	71%	87%	100%
Beta Blocker at Discharge	104	98%	70%	90%	100%
Fibrinolytic Medication Timing[1]	1	0%	15%	31%	100%
PCI Within 90 Minutes of Arrival[1]	8	25%	58%	54%	95%
Smoking Cessation Advice	38	92%	94%	88%	100%
Heart Failure Care					
ACE Inhibitor or ARB for LVSD	38	89%	81%	82%	100%
Discharge Instructions	78	54%	51%	61%	93%
Evaluation of LVS Function	109	92%	75%	83%	99%
Smoking Cessation Advice[1]	13	100%	78%	82%	100%
Pneumonia Care					
Appropriate Initial Antibiotic	129	89%	84%	83%	94%
Blood Culture Timing	75	84%	89%	90%	100%
Influenza Vaccine	40	90%	73%	70%	100%
Initial Antibiotic Timing	145	90%	80%	80%	93%
Oxygenation Assessment	174	100%	100%	99%	100%
Pneumococcal Vaccine	119	86%	68%	69%	94%
Smoking Cessation Advice	39	85%	64%	80%	100%
Surgical Infection Prevention					
Prophylactic Antibiotic Given[2,3]	199	64%	70%	77%	95%
Prophylactic Antibiotic Selection[2]	94	93%	92%	90%	100%
Prophylactic Antibiotic Stopped[2,3]	198	72%	69%	72%	95%
Pregnancy Care					
Inpatient Neonatal Mortality	2,431	0.12%	-	-	-
Third or Fourth Degree Laceration	1,768	0.79%	2.98%	3.63%	3.27%

Orem Community Hospital

331 North 400 West
Orem, UT 84057
URL: www.ihc.com/och
Ownership: Voluntary non-profit - Private
Emergency Services: Yes

Phone: 801-224-4080
Fax: 801-226-7831
Accredited: Yes
Licensed Beds: 20

Key Personnel:
Administrator/CEO . . . . Chris Coons
Chief Medical Staff. . . . . Clark Bishop, MD
Emergency Room . . . . Keith Hooker
Director Infection/Disease Control . . . . Steve Freestone, MD
CCU Spvg. Nurse . . . . Cynthia Capel
OB/GYN Womens Health. . . . . Jay Baxter, MD
Chief Radiology . . . . Gary Watts, MD
Director Respiratory Therapy . . . . Karl Ludwig

Measure	Cases	This Hospital	State Average	U.S. Average	Top Hospital
Heart Attack Care					
ACE Inhibitor or ARB for LVSD[5]	-	-	83%	82%	100%
Aspirin at Arrival[5]	-	-	91%	92%	100%
Aspirin at Discharge[5]	-	-	81%	90%	100%
Beta Blocker at Arrival[5]	-	-	71%	87%	100%
Beta Blocker at Discharge[5]	-	-	70%	90%	100%
Fibrinolytic Medication Timing[5]	-	-	15%	31%	100%
PCI Within 90 Minutes of Arrival[5]	-	-	58%	54%	95%
Smoking Cessation Advice[5]	-	-	94%	88%	100%
Heart Failure Care					
ACE Inhibitor or ARB for LVSD[5]	-	-	81%	82%	100%
Discharge Instructions[5]	-	-	51%	61%	93%
Evaluation of LVS Function[5]	-	-	75%	83%	99%
Smoking Cessation Advice[5]	-	-	78%	82%	100%
Pneumonia Care					
Appropriate Initial Antibiotic[5]	-	-	84%	83%	94%
Blood Culture Timing[5]	-	-	89%	90%	100%
Influenza Vaccine[5]	-	-	73%	70%	100%
Initial Antibiotic Timing[5]	-	-	80%	80%	93%
Oxygenation Assessment[5]	-	-	100%	99%	100%
Pneumococcal Vaccine[5]	-	-	68%	69%	94%
Smoking Cessation Advice[5]	-	-	64%	80%	100%
Surgical Infection Prevention					
Prophylactic Antibiotic Given[1,2]	18	100%	70%	77%	95%

NOTE: Hospital profiles are in alphabetical order by state, then city, then hospital within the city; Rankings are sorted by rate in descending order and exclude hospitals with less than 25 cases; (1) The number of cases is too small (n<25) for purposes of reliably predicting hospital performance; (2) Measure reflects the hospital's indication that its submission was based upon a sample of its relevant discharges; (3) Rate reflects fewer than the maximum possible quarters of data for the measure; (4) Inaccurate information submitted and suppressed for one or more quarters; (5) No data is available from the hospital for this measure; Please refer to the User's Guide for a full explanation of data

Measure	Cases	This Hospital	State Average	U.S. Average	Top Hospital
Prophylactic Antibiotic Selection[1,2]	3	100%	92%	90%	100%
Prophylactic Antibiotic Stopped[1,2]	18	100%	69%	72%	95%
Pregnancy Care					
Inpatient Neonatal Mortality	-	-	-	-	-
Third or Fourth Degree Laceration	-	-	2.98%	3.63%	3.27%

Timpanogos Regional Hospital

750 West 800 North
Orem, UT 84057
URL: www.timpanogosregionalhopsital.com
Ownership: Proprietary
Emergency Services: Yes
Phone: 801-714-6000
Fax: 801-714-6597
Accredited: Yes
Licensed Beds: 51

Key Personnel:

CEO. . . . . Keith D Tintle

Measure	Cases	This Hospital	State Average	U.S. Average	Top Hospital
Heart Attack Care					
ACE Inhibitor or ARB for LVSD[1]	8	50%	83%	82%	100%
Aspirin at Arrival	26	88%	91%	92%	100%
Aspirin at Discharge	26	92%	81%	90%	100%
Beta Blocker at Arrival	27	85%	71%	87%	100%
Beta Blocker at Discharge	31	90%	70%	90%	100%
Fibrinolytic Medication Timing	0	-	15%	31%	100%
PCI Within 90 Minutes of Arrival	0	-	58%	54%	95%
Smoking Cessation Advice[1]	5	80%	94%	88%	100%
Heart Failure Care					
ACE Inhibitor or ARB for LVSD[1]	20	75%	81%	82%	100%
Discharge Instructions	36	61%	51%	61%	93%
Evaluation of LVS Function	46	91%	75%	83%	99%
Smoking Cessation Advice[1]	2	100%	78%	82%	100%
Pneumonia Care					
Appropriate Initial Antibiotic	63	71%	84%	83%	94%
Blood Culture Timing	53	87%	89%	90%	100%
Influenza Vaccine[1]	17	82%	73%	70%	100%
Initial Antibiotic Timing	82	79%	80%	80%	93%
Oxygenation Assessment	111	100%	100%	99%	100%
Pneumococcal Vaccine	56	80%	68%	69%	94%
Smoking Cessation Advice[1]	15	80%	64%	80%	100%
Surgical Infection Prevention					
Prophylactic Antibiotic Given[2,3]	152	85%	70%	77%	95%
Prophylactic Antibiotic Selection[2]	65	97%	92%	90%	100%
Prophylactic Antibiotic Stopped[2,3]	146	88%	69%	72%	95%
Pregnancy Care					
Inpatient Neonatal Mortality	1,852	0.11%	-	-	-
Third or Fourth Degree Laceration	1,471	2.11%	2.98%	3.63%	3.27%

Garfield Memorial Hospital & Clinics

200N Fourth E
Panguitch, UT 84759
URL: www.intermountainhealthcare.org
Ownership: Voluntary non-profit - Other
Emergency Services: Yes
Phone: 435-676-8811
Fax: 435-676-2679
Accredited: No
Licensed Beds: 44

Key Personnel:

Administrator . . . . Alberto Vasquez
Medical Staff President . . . . Shaun Shurtliff, DO

Measure	Cases	This Hospital	State Average	U.S. Average	Top Hospital
Heart Attack Care					
ACE Inhibitor or ARB for LVSD[3]	0	-	83%	82%	100%
Aspirin at Arrival[3]	0	-	91%	92%	100%
Aspirin at Discharge[3]	0	-	81%	90%	100%
Beta Blocker at Arrival[3]	0	-	71%	87%	100%
Beta Blocker at Discharge[3]	0	-	70%	90%	100%
Fibrinolytic Medication Timing[3]	0	-	15%	31%	100%
PCI Within 90 Minutes of Arrival	0	-	58%	54%	95%
Smoking Cessation Advice[3]	0	-	94%	88%	100%
Heart Failure Care					
ACE Inhibitor or ARB for LVSD[1]	1	0%	81%	82%	100%
Discharge Instructions[1]	8	25%	51%	61%	93%
Evaluation of LVS Function[1]	12	42%	75%	83%	99%
Smoking Cessation Advice[1]	1	100%	78%	82%	100%
Pneumonia Care					
Appropriate Initial Antibiotic	34	94%	84%	83%	94%
Blood Culture Timing[1]	2	100%	89%	90%	100%
Influenza Vaccine[1]	4	50%	73%	70%	100%
Initial Antibiotic Timing	34	100%	80%	80%	93%
Oxygenation Assessment	40	100%	100%	99%	100%
Pneumococcal Vaccine	26	58%	68%	69%	94%
Smoking Cessation Advice[1]	9	78%	64%	80%	100%
Surgical Infection Prevention					
Prophylactic Antibiotic Given[3]	0	-	70%	77%	95%
Prophylactic Antibiotic Selection	0	-	92%	90%	100%
Prophylactic Antibiotic Stopped[3]	0	-	69%	72%	95%
Pregnancy Care					
Inpatient Neonatal Mortality	-	-	-	-	-
Third or Fourth Degree Laceration	-	-	2.98%	3.63%	3.27%

Mountain View Hospital

Alternate Name: Mountain View Hospital
1000 E 100 N
Payson, UT 84651
E-mail: kevin.johnson@columbia.net
Ownership: Proprietary
Emergency Services: Yes
Phone: 801-465-7100
Fax: 801-465-7170
Accredited: Yes
Licensed Beds: 136

Key Personnel:

CEO. . . . . Kevin Johnson
Emergency Room . . . . Cimby Ford
OB/GYN/Women's Health . . . . Marguerite Smith, RN
Respiratory/Cardiopulmonary. . . . . Ric Johnson

Measure	Cases	This Hospital	State Average	U.S. Average	Top Hospital
Heart Attack Care					
ACE Inhibitor or ARB for LVSD[1]	4	100%	83%	82%	100%
Aspirin at Arrival	39	95%	91%	92%	100%
Aspirin at Discharge	39	95%	81%	90%	100%
Beta Blocker at Arrival	26	85%	71%	87%	100%
Beta Blocker at Discharge	35	89%	70%	90%	100%
Fibrinolytic Medication Timing	0	-	15%	31%	100%
PCI Within 90 Minutes of Arrival[1]	4	50%	58%	54%	95%
Smoking Cessation Advice[1]	6	100%	94%	88%	100%
Heart Failure Care					
ACE Inhibitor or ARB for LVSD[1]	13	92%	81%	82%	100%
Discharge Instructions	45	53%	51%	61%	93%
Evaluation of LVS Function	57	98%	75%	83%	99%
Smoking Cessation Advice[1]	6	100%	78%	82%	100%
Pneumonia Care					
Appropriate Initial Antibiotic	72	83%	84%	83%	94%
Blood Culture Timing	60	95%	89%	90%	100%
Influenza Vaccine	33	88%	73%	70%	100%
Initial Antibiotic Timing	99	80%	80%	80%	93%
Oxygenation Assessment	124	100%	100%	99%	100%
Pneumococcal Vaccine	79	85%	68%	69%	94%
Smoking Cessation Advice[1]	20	100%	64%	80%	100%
Surgical Infection Prevention					
Prophylactic Antibiotic Given[2,3]	138	94%	70%	77%	95%
Prophylactic Antibiotic Selection[2]	61	89%	92%	90%	100%
Prophylactic Antibiotic Stopped[2,3]	133	89%	69%	72%	95%
Pregnancy Care					
Inpatient Neonatal Mortality	-	-	-	-	-
Third or Fourth Degree Laceration	-	-	2.98%	3.63%	3.27%

Castleview Hospital

Alternate Name: Columbia Castleview Hospital
300 North Hospital Drive
Price, UT 84501
URL: www.castleviewhospital.net
Ownership: Proprietary
Emergency Services: Yes
Phone: 435-637-4800
Fax: 435-637-9513
Accredited: Yes
Licensed Beds: 88

Key Personnel:

Administrator . . . . Allen Penry
CEO. . . . . Jeff Manley
Chief Medical Staff. . . . . Kurt King, MD
Emergency Room . . . . Terry Watkins
Director Infection/Disease Control . . . . Pam Konakis

NOTE: Hospital profiles are in alphabetical order by state, then city, then hospital within the city; Rankings are sorted by rate in descending order and exclude hospitals with less than 25 cases; (1) The number of cases is too small (n<25) for purposes of reliably predicting hospital performance; (2) Measure reflects the hospital's indication that its submission was based upon a sample of its relevant discharges; (3) Rate reflects fewer than the maximum possible quarters of data for the measure; (4) Inaccurate information submitted and suppressed for one or more quarters; (5) No data is available from the hospital for this measure; Please refer to the User's Guide for a full explanation of data

Measure	Cases	This Hospital	State Average	U.S. Average	Top Hospital
Heart Attack Care					
ACE Inhibitor or ARB for LVSD	0	-	83%	82%	100%
Aspirin at Arrival[1]	1	100%	91%	92%	100%
Aspirin at Discharge[1]	1	100%	81%	90%	100%
Beta Blocker at Arrival[1]	2	100%	71%	87%	100%
Beta Blocker at Discharge[1]	1	100%	70%	90%	100%
Fibrinolytic Medication Timing	0	-	15%	31%	100%
PCI Within 90 Minutes of Arrival	0	-	58%	54%	95%
Smoking Cessation Advice	0	-	94%	88%	100%
Heart Failure Care					
ACE Inhibitor or ARB for LVSD[1]	5	100%	81%	82%	100%
Discharge Instructions[1]	19	58%	51%	61%	93%
Evaluation of LVS Function	33	67%	75%	83%	99%
Smoking Cessation Advice[1]	7	71%	78%	82%	100%
Pneumonia Care					
Appropriate Initial Antibiotic	101	72%	84%	83%	94%
Blood Culture Timing	88	99%	89%	90%	100%
Influenza Vaccine	33	73%	73%	70%	100%
Initial Antibiotic Timing	123	90%	80%	80%	93%
Oxygenation Assessment	151	100%	100%	99%	100%
Pneumococcal Vaccine	87	70%	68%	69%	94%
Smoking Cessation Advice	37	92%	64%	80%	100%
Surgical Infection Prevention					
Prophylactic Antibiotic Given[2,3]	129	85%	70%	77%	95%
Prophylactic Antibiotic Selection[2]	57	100%	92%	90%	100%
Prophylactic Antibiotic Stopped[2,3]	121	84%	69%	72%	95%
Pregnancy Care					
Inpatient Neonatal Mortality	-	-	-	-	-
Third or Fourth Degree Laceration	-	-	2.98%	3.63%	3.27%

Utah Valley Regional Medical Center

1034 North 500 West
Provo, UT 84604
Phone: 801-373-7850
Fax: 801-357-7590
Ownership: Voluntary non-profit - Private
Accredited: Yes
Emergency Services: Yes
Licensed Beds: 409

Key Personnel:

Administrator . . . . Mary Nann Young
Chief Medical Staff. . . . . Clark Bishop, MD
Director Infection/Disease Control . . . . Joan Golden
CCU Spvg. Nurse . . . . Kim Henrickson
Director Medical/Surgical Nursing . . . . Nan Nicponski
Director Respiratory Therapy . . . . Ed Trammell

Measure	Cases	This Hospital	State Average	U.S. Average	Top Hospital
Heart Attack Care					
ACE Inhibitor or ARB for LVSD	37	89%	83%	82%	100%
Aspirin at Arrival	157	98%	91%	92%	100%
Aspirin at Discharge	334	98%	81%	90%	100%
Beta Blocker at Arrival	135	94%	71%	87%	100%
Beta Blocker at Discharge	305	96%	70%	90%	100%
Fibrinolytic Medication Timing	0	-	15%	31%	100%
PCI Within 90 Minutes of Arrival[1]	10	70%	58%	54%	95%
Smoking Cessation Advice	82	100%	94%	88%	100%
Heart Failure Care					
ACE Inhibitor or ARB for LVSD	82	80%	81%	82%	100%
Discharge Instructions	187	86%	51%	61%	93%
Evaluation of LVS Function	236	98%	75%	83%	99%
Smoking Cessation Advice	29	93%	78%	82%	100%
Pneumonia Care					
Appropriate Initial Antibiotic	149	90%	84%	83%	94%
Blood Culture Timing	119	87%	89%	90%	100%
Influenza Vaccine	51	75%	73%	70%	100%
Initial Antibiotic Timing	211	78%	80%	80%	93%
Oxygenation Assessment	272	100%	100%	99%	100%
Pneumococcal Vaccine	155	78%	68%	69%	94%
Smoking Cessation Advice	35	57%	64%	80%	100%
Surgical Infection Prevention					
Prophylactic Antibiotic Given[2]	534	79%	70%	77%	95%
Prophylactic Antibiotic Selection[2]	169	95%	92%	90%	100%
Prophylactic Antibiotic Stopped[2]	520	77%	69%	72%	95%

Measure	Cases	This Hospital	State Average	U.S. Average	Top Hospital
Pregnancy Care					
Inpatient Neonatal Mortality	5,901	0.34%	-	-	-
Third or Fourth Degree Laceration[2]	4,579	3.39%	2.98%	3.63%	3.27%

Sevier Valley Hospital

1100 N Main Street
Richfield, UT 84701
Phone: 435-896-8271
Fax: 435-896-9449
URL: www.intermountainhealthcare.org
Ownership: Voluntary non-profit - Private
Accredited: Yes
Emergency Services: Yes
Licensed Beds: 42

Key Personnel:

Administrator . . . . Gary Beck
Medical Staff President . . . . David Pope, MD

Measure	Cases	This Hospital	State Average	U.S. Average	Top Hospital
Heart Attack Care					
ACE Inhibitor or ARB for LVSD[3]	0	-	83%	82%	100%
Aspirin at Arrival[1,3]	1	100%	91%	92%	100%
Aspirin at Discharge[3]	0	-	81%	90%	100%
Beta Blocker at Arrival[1,3]	1	0%	71%	87%	100%
Beta Blocker at Discharge[3]	0	-	70%	90%	100%
Fibrinolytic Medication Timing[3]	0	-	15%	31%	100%
PCI Within 90 Minutes of Arrival[5]	-	-	58%	54%	95%
Smoking Cessation Advice[3]	0	-	94%	88%	100%
Heart Failure Care					
ACE Inhibitor or ARB for LVSD[1]	2	50%	81%	82%	100%
Discharge Instructions[1]	20	30%	51%	61%	93%
Evaluation of LVS Function[1]	23	43%	75%	83%	99%
Smoking Cessation Advice[1]	2	50%	78%	82%	100%
Pneumonia Care					
Appropriate Initial Antibiotic	61	80%	84%	83%	94%
Blood Culture Timing[1]	17	100%	89%	90%	100%
Influenza Vaccine[1]	9	89%	73%	70%	100%
Initial Antibiotic Timing	68	78%	80%	80%	93%
Oxygenation Assessment	79	100%	100%	99%	100%
Pneumococcal Vaccine	42	52%	68%	69%	94%
Smoking Cessation Advice[1]	17	47%	64%	80%	100%
Surgical Infection Prevention					
Prophylactic Antibiotic Given	29	83%	70%	77%	95%
Prophylactic Antibiotic Selection[1]	6	83%	92%	90%	100%
Prophylactic Antibiotic Stopped	27	56%	69%	72%	95%
Pregnancy Care					
Inpatient Neonatal Mortality	265	0.38%	-	-	-
Third or Fourth Degree Laceration	207	4.35%	2.98%	3.63%	3.27%

Uintah Basin Medical Center

Alternate Name: Duchense County Hospital
250 W 300 N (75-2)
Roosevelt, UT 84066
Phone: 435-722-6163
Fax: 435-722-9291
Ownership: Voluntary non-profit - Private
Accredited: No
Emergency Services: Yes
Licensed Beds: 42

Key Personnel:

Administrator . . . . Bradley D LeBaron
Chief Medical Staff. . . . . Dr. Glenn Robertson
Director Infection/Disease Control . . . . Louise lorg
Director Medical/Surgical Nursing . . . . Carol Allred, RN
OB/GYN Womens Health. . . . . Keith Evans
Chief Radiology . . . . Wayne Stewart, MD
Director Respiratory Therapy . . . . Jim Richardson

Measure	Cases	This Hospital	State Average	U.S. Average	Top Hospital
Heart Attack Care					
ACE Inhibitor or ARB for LVSD[1]	1	100%	83%	82%	100%
Aspirin at Arrival[1]	4	50%	91%	92%	100%
Aspirin at Discharge[1]	4	50%	81%	90%	100%
Beta Blocker at Arrival[1]	4	75%	71%	87%	100%
Beta Blocker at Discharge[1]	4	75%	70%	90%	100%
Fibrinolytic Medication Timing	0	-	15%	31%	100%
PCI Within 90 Minutes of Arrival	0	-	58%	54%	95%
Smoking Cessation Advice	0	-	94%	88%	100%
Heart Failure Care					
ACE Inhibitor or ARB for LVSD[1]	4	100%	81%	82%	100%

NOTE: Hospital profiles are in alphabetical order by state, then city, then hospital within the city; Rankings are sorted by rate in descending order and exclude hospitals with less than 25 cases; (1) The number of cases is too small (n<25) for purposes of reliably predicting hospital performance; (2) Measure reflects the hospital's indication that its submission was based upon a sample of its relevant discharges; (3) Rate reflects fewer than the maximum possible quarters of data for the measure; (4) Inaccurate information submitted and suppressed for one or more quarters; (5) No data is available from the hospital for this measure; Please refer to the User's Guide for a full explanation of data

Measure	Cases	This Hospital	State Average	U.S. Average	Top Hospital
Discharge Instructions[1]	16	0%	51%	61%	93%
Evaluation of LVS Function[1]	21	67%	75%	83%	99%
Smoking Cessation Advice[1]	4	0%	78%	82%	100%
Pneumonia Care					
Appropriate Initial Antibiotic[1,2]	21	86%	84%	83%	94%
Blood Culture Timing[1,2]	11	82%	89%	90%	100%
Influenza Vaccine[1,2]	3	33%	73%	70%	100%
Initial Antibiotic Timing[2]	26	81%	80%	80%	93%
Oxygenation Assessment[2]	33	100%	100%	99%	100%
Pneumococcal Vaccine[1,2]	17	12%	68%	69%	94%
Smoking Cessation Advice[1,2]	7	43%	64%	80%	100%
Surgical Infection Prevention					
Prophylactic Antibiotic Given[2]	36	36%	70%	77%	95%
Prophylactic Antibiotic Selection[1,2]	14	100%	92%	90%	100%
Prophylactic Antibiotic Stopped[2]	34	56%	69%	72%	95%
Pregnancy Care					
Inpatient Neonatal Mortality	-	-	-	-	-
Third or Fourth Degree Laceration	-	-	2.98%	3.63%	3.27%

Dixie Regional Medical Center

1380 East Medical Center Drive
Saint George, UT 84790
Phone: 435-688-4000
Ownership: Voluntary non-profit - Private
Accredited: Yes
Emergency Services: No

Measure	Cases	This Hospital	State Average	U.S. Average	Top Hospital
Heart Attack Care					
ACE Inhibitor or ARB for LVSD	32	100%	83%	82%	100%
Aspirin at Arrival	170	98%	91%	92%	100%
Aspirin at Discharge	216	99%	81%	90%	100%
Beta Blocker at Arrival	145	96%	71%	87%	100%
Beta Blocker at Discharge	244	100%	70%	90%	100%
Fibrinolytic Medication Timing	0	-	15%	31%	100%
PCI Within 90 Minutes of Arrival[1]	12	58%	58%	54%	95%
Smoking Cessation Advice	57	98%	94%	88%	100%
Heart Failure Care					
ACE Inhibitor or ARB for LVSD	79	100%	81%	82%	100%
Discharge Instructions	147	93%	51%	61%	93%
Evaluation of LVS Function	187	99%	75%	83%	99%
Smoking Cessation Advice[1]	22	100%	78%	82%	100%
Pneumonia Care					
Appropriate Initial Antibiotic	202	83%	84%	83%	94%
Blood Culture Timing	178	89%	89%	90%	100%
Influenza Vaccine	83	90%	73%	70%	100%
Initial Antibiotic Timing	288	82%	80%	80%	93%
Oxygenation Assessment	364	100%	100%	99%	100%
Pneumococcal Vaccine	269	77%	68%	69%	94%
Smoking Cessation Advice	50	94%	64%	80%	100%
Surgical Infection Prevention					
Prophylactic Antibiotic Given[2]	518	93%	70%	77%	95%
Prophylactic Antibiotic Selection[2]	172	95%	92%	90%	100%
Prophylactic Antibiotic Stopped[2]	496	83%	69%	72%	95%
Pregnancy Care					
Inpatient Neonatal Mortality	2,875	0.21%	-	-	-
Third or Fourth Degree Laceration[2]	2,296	3.40%	2.98%	3.63%	3.27%

LDS Hospital

8th Avenue & C Street
Salt Lake City, UT 84143
Phone: 801-408-1100
Fax: 801-408-1663
URL: www.intermountainhealthcare.org
Ownership: Voluntary non-profit - Private
Accredited: Yes
Emergency Services: Yes
Licensed Beds: 520

Key Personnel:
President/CEO. . . . . Scott Anderson
OB/GYN Womens Health. . . . . Gary Johnson, MD
Director Respiratory Therapy . . . . Loren Greenway

Measure	Cases	This Hospital	State Average	U.S. Average	Top Hospital
Heart Attack Care					
ACE Inhibitor or ARB for LVSD	70	80%	83%	82%	100%
Aspirin at Arrival	178	96%	91%	92%	100%
Aspirin at Discharge	393	99%	81%	90%	100%
Beta Blocker at Arrival	148	93%	71%	87%	100%
Beta Blocker at Discharge	387	93%	70%	90%	100%
Fibrinolytic Medication Timing	0	-	15%	31%	100%
PCI Within 90 Minutes of Arrival[1]	18	72%	58%	54%	95%
Smoking Cessation Advice	95	99%	94%	88%	100%
Heart Failure Care					
ACE Inhibitor or ARB for LVSD	190	78%	81%	82%	100%
Discharge Instructions	337	89%	51%	61%	93%
Evaluation of LVS Function	369	100%	75%	83%	99%
Smoking Cessation Advice	58	86%	78%	82%	100%
Pneumonia Care					
Appropriate Initial Antibiotic	169	85%	84%	83%	94%
Blood Culture Timing	132	89%	89%	90%	100%
Influenza Vaccine	60	65%	73%	70%	100%
Initial Antibiotic Timing	225	79%	80%	80%	93%
Oxygenation Assessment	314	100%	100%	99%	100%
Pneumococcal Vaccine	170	58%	68%	69%	94%
Smoking Cessation Advice	70	76%	64%	80%	100%
Surgical Infection Prevention					
Prophylactic Antibiotic Given[2]	549	84%	70%	77%	95%
Prophylactic Antibiotic Selection[2]	196	92%	92%	90%	100%
Prophylactic Antibiotic Stopped[2]	548	67%	69%	72%	95%
Pregnancy Care					
Inpatient Neonatal Mortality	4,215	0.55%	-	-	-
Third or Fourth Degree Laceration[2]	3,169	3.34%	2.98%	3.63%	3.27%

Saint Mark's Hospital

1200 East 3900 South
Salt Lake City, UT 84124
Phone: 801-268-7111
Fax: 801-270-3353
URL: www.stmarkshospital.com
Ownership: Proprietary
Accredited: Yes
Emergency Services: Yes
Licensed Beds: 317

Key Personnel:
CEO. . . . . John Hanshaw
Catheterization Lab . . . . Tom Pachelli
Emergency Room . . . . Glenda Hochstetler
Infection Control. . . . . Lorie Gilette
ICU . . . . CJ Cooper
Intensive Coronary. . . . . CJ Cooper
Director Medical/Surgical Nursing . . . . Janelle Smothers
OB/GYN/Women's Health . . . . Sandy Osmond
Director Respiratory Therapy . . . . Jack Fried

Measure	Cases	This Hospital	State Average	U.S. Average	Top Hospital
Heart Attack Care					
ACE Inhibitor or ARB for LVSD	28	79%	83%	82%	100%
Aspirin at Arrival	132	98%	91%	92%	100%
Aspirin at Discharge	174	98%	81%	90%	100%
Beta Blocker at Arrival	106	95%	71%	87%	100%
Beta Blocker at Discharge	169	86%	70%	90%	100%
Fibrinolytic Medication Timing[1]	1	0%	15%	31%	100%
PCI Within 90 Minutes of Arrival[1]	16	56%	58%	54%	95%
Smoking Cessation Advice	49	86%	94%	88%	100%
Heart Failure Care					
ACE Inhibitor or ARB for LVSD	100	85%	81%	82%	100%
Discharge Instructions	186	56%	51%	61%	93%
Evaluation of LVS Function	222	96%	75%	83%	99%
Smoking Cessation Advice	36	89%	78%	82%	100%
Pneumonia Care					
Appropriate Initial Antibiotic[2]	269	93%	84%	83%	94%
Blood Culture Timing[2]	261	97%	89%	90%	100%
Influenza Vaccine	94	78%	73%	70%	100%
Initial Antibiotic Timing[2]	361	78%	80%	80%	93%
Oxygenation Assessment[2]	472	100%	100%	99%	100%
Pneumococcal Vaccine[2]	311	73%	68%	69%	94%
Smoking Cessation Advice[2]	85	68%	64%	80%	100%
Surgical Infection Prevention					
Prophylactic Antibiotic Given[2,3]	290	91%	70%	77%	95%
Prophylactic Antibiotic Selection[2]	134	95%	92%	90%	100%
Prophylactic Antibiotic Stopped[2,3]	283	81%	69%	72%	95%
Pregnancy Care					

NOTE: Hospital profiles are in alphabetical order by state, then city, then hospital within the city; Rankings are sorted by rate in descending order and exclude hospitals with less than 25 cases; (1) The number of cases is too small (n<25) for purposes of reliably predicting hospital performance; (2) Measure reflects the hospital's indication that its submission was based upon a sample of its relevant discharges; (3) Rate reflects fewer than the maximum possible quarters of data for the measure; (4) Inaccurate information submitted and suppressed for one or more quarters; (5) No data is available from the hospital for this measure; Please refer to the User's Guide for a full explanation of data

Inpatient Neonatal Mortality	-	-	-	-	-
Third or Fourth Degree Laceration	-	-	2.98%	3.63%	3.27%

Salt Lake Regional Medical Center

Alternate Name: Holy Cross Hospital
1050 East South Temple
Salt Lake City, UT 84102
Phone: 801-350-4111
Fax: 801-350-4323
E-mail: info@iasishealthcare.com
URL: www.saltlakeregional.com
Ownership: Proprietary
Accredited: Yes
Emergency Services: Yes
Licensed Beds: 200

Key Personnel:

CEO. . . . . Brian E Dunn
Chief Medical Staff. . . . . Kevin McKuster, MD
Director Cardiac Lab . . . . Sarah Evans
Director Catheterization Lab. . . . . Sarah Evans
Emergency Room . . . . Guy Thompson
Infection Control Coordinator . . . . Chris Martin
ICU . . . . Guy Thompson, CNO
Intensive Coronary Care . . . . Guy Thompson, CNO
Director Medical Surgical Nursing . . . . T'Ann Ularich
Director OB/GYN/Women's Health. . . . . Chris Monson
Director Respiratory/Cardiopulmonary . . . . Sarah Evans

Measure	Cases	This Hospital	State Average	U.S. Average	Top Hospital
Heart Attack Care					
ACE Inhibitor or ARB for LVSD[1]	7	71%	83%	82%	100%
Aspirin at Arrival[1]	20	75%	91%	92%	100%
Aspirin at Discharge	52	90%	81%	90%	100%
Beta Blocker at Arrival[1]	16	69%	71%	87%	100%
Beta Blocker at Discharge	44	73%	70%	90%	100%
Fibrinolytic Medication Timing	0	-	15%	31%	100%
PCI Within 90 Minutes of Arrival[1]	2	100%	58%	54%	95%
Smoking Cessation Advice[1]	20	75%	94%	88%	100%
Heart Failure Care					
ACE Inhibitor or ARB for LVSD	32	75%	81%	82%	100%
Discharge Instructions	66	35%	51%	61%	93%
Evaluation of LVS Function	86	87%	75%	83%	99%
Smoking Cessation Advice[1]	18	44%	78%	82%	100%
Pneumonia Care					
Appropriate Initial Antibiotic	68	85%	84%	83%	94%
Blood Culture Timing	54	61%	89%	90%	100%
Influenza Vaccine[1]	19	89%	73%	70%	100%
Initial Antibiotic Timing	78	77%	80%	80%	93%
Oxygenation Assessment	93	100%	100%	99%	100%
Pneumococcal Vaccine	44	84%	68%	69%	94%
Smoking Cessation Advice	29	62%	64%	80%	100%
Surgical Infection Prevention					
Prophylactic Antibiotic Given	211	78%	70%	77%	95%
Prophylactic Antibiotic Selection	52	100%	92%	90%	100%
Prophylactic Antibiotic Stopped	193	83%	69%	72%	95%
Pregnancy Care					
Inpatient Neonatal Mortality[2]	814	0.00%	-	-	-
Third or Fourth Degree Laceration[2]	682	2.20%	2.98%	3.63%	3.27%

University Health Care/Univ of Utah Hosp

50 North Medical Drive
Salt Lake City, UT 84132
Phone: 801-581-2121
Ownership: Government - State
Accredited: Yes
Emergency Services: Yes

Measure	Cases	This Hospital	State Average	U.S. Average	Top Hospital
Heart Attack Care					
ACE Inhibitor or ARB for LVSD	42	90%	83%	82%	100%
Aspirin at Arrival	85	96%	91%	92%	100%
Aspirin at Discharge	165	98%	81%	90%	100%
Beta Blocker at Arrival	78	95%	71%	87%	100%
Beta Blocker at Discharge	172	92%	70%	90%	100%
Fibrinolytic Medication Timing[1]	1	0%	15%	31%	100%
PCI Within 90 Minutes of Arrival[1]	9	22%	58%	54%	95%
Smoking Cessation Advice	74	95%	94%	88%	100%
Heart Failure Care					
ACE Inhibitor or ARB for LVSD	121	88%	81%	82%	100%
Discharge Instructions	153	57%	51%	61%	93%
Evaluation of LVS Function	183	98%	75%	83%	99%
Smoking Cessation Advice	34	53%	78%	82%	100%
Pneumonia Care					
Appropriate Initial Antibiotic[2]	52	81%	84%	83%	94%
Blood Culture Timing[2]	72	94%	89%	90%	100%
Influenza Vaccine[1,2]	18	50%	73%	70%	100%
Initial Antibiotic Timing[2]	103	55%	80%	80%	93%
Oxygenation Assessment[2]	208	100%	100%	99%	100%
Pneumococcal Vaccine[2]	74	66%	68%	69%	94%
Smoking Cessation Advice[2]	46	39%	64%	80%	100%
Surgical Infection Prevention					
Prophylactic Antibiotic Given[2,3]	385	79%	70%	77%	95%
Prophylactic Antibiotic Selection[2]	83	96%	92%	90%	100%
Prophylactic Antibiotic Stopped[2,3]	382	85%	69%	72%	95%
Pregnancy Care					
Inpatient Neonatal Mortality[2]	679	1.03%	-	-	-
Third or Fourth Degree Laceration	2,349	3.87%	2.98%	3.63%	3.27%

Alta View Hospital

9660 S 1300 E
Sandy, UT 84094
Phone: 801-501-2600
Fax: 801-501-2043
URL: www.intermountainhealthcare.org
Ownership: Voluntary non-profit - Private
Accredited: Yes
Emergency Services: Yes
Licensed Beds: 72

Key Personnel:

Administrator/CEO. . . . . Tim Brinker

Measure	Cases	This Hospital	State Average	U.S. Average	Top Hospital
Heart Attack Care					
ACE Inhibitor or ARB for LVSD	0	-	83%	82%	100%
Aspirin at Arrival[1]	7	100%	91%	92%	100%
Aspirin at Discharge[1]	5	40%	81%	90%	100%
Beta Blocker at Arrival[1]	8	75%	71%	87%	100%
Beta Blocker at Discharge[1]	6	67%	70%	90%	100%
Fibrinolytic Medication Timing	0	-	15%	31%	100%
PCI Within 90 Minutes of Arrival	0	-	58%	54%	95%
Smoking Cessation Advice	0	-	94%	88%	100%
Heart Failure Care					
ACE Inhibitor or ARB for LVSD[1]	18	83%	81%	82%	100%
Discharge Instructions	45	69%	51%	61%	93%
Evaluation of LVS Function	65	95%	75%	83%	99%
Smoking Cessation Advice[1]	3	67%	78%	82%	100%
Pneumonia Care					
Appropriate Initial Antibiotic	110	84%	84%	83%	94%
Blood Culture Timing	100	96%	89%	90%	100%
Influenza Vaccine[4,5]	-	-	73%	70%	100%
Initial Antibiotic Timing	160	85%	80%	80%	93%
Oxygenation Assessment	194	100%	100%	99%	100%
Pneumococcal Vaccine	119	82%	68%	69%	94%
Smoking Cessation Advice	33	91%	64%	80%	100%
Surgical Infection Prevention					
Prophylactic Antibiotic Given[2]	261	95%	70%	77%	95%
Prophylactic Antibiotic Selection[2]	81	100%	92%	90%	100%
Prophylactic Antibiotic Stopped[2]	260	77%	69%	72%	95%
Pregnancy Care					
Inpatient Neonatal Mortality	2,234	0.09%	-	-	-
Third or Fourth Degree Laceration[2]	1,780	3.65%	2.98%	3.63%	3.27%

Mountain West Medical Center

Alternate Name: Tooele Valley Regional Medical Center
2055 North Main
Tooele, UT 84074
Phone: 435-843-2794
Fax: 435-843-3753
URL: www.mountainwestmc.com
Ownership: Proprietary
Accredited: Yes
Emergency Services: Yes
Licensed Beds: 38

Key Personnel:

CEO. . . . . Charles A Davis

Measure	Cases	This Hospital	State Average	U.S. Average	Top Hospital

NOTE: Hospital profiles are in alphabetical order by state, then city, then hospital within the city; Rankings are sorted by rate in descending order and exclude hospitals with less than 25 cases; (1) The number of cases is too small (n<25) for purposes of reliably predicting hospital performance; (2) Measure reflects the hospital's indication that its submission was based upon a sample of its relevant discharges; (3) Rate reflects fewer than the maximum possible quarters of data for the measure; (4) Inaccurate information submitted and suppressed for one or more quarters; (5) No data is available from the hospital for this measure; Please refer to the User's Guide for a full explanation of data

Measure	Cases	This Hospital	State Average	U.S. Average	Top Hospital
Heart Attack Care					
ACE Inhibitor or ARB for LVSD	0	-	83%	82%	100%
Aspirin at Arrival[1]	4	100%	91%	92%	100%
Aspirin at Discharge[1]	4	100%	81%	90%	100%
Beta Blocker at Arrival[1]	2	100%	71%	87%	100%
Beta Blocker at Discharge[1]	4	75%	70%	90%	100%
Fibrinolytic Medication Timing	0	-	15%	31%	100%
PCI Within 90 Minutes of Arrival	0	-	58%	54%	95%
Smoking Cessation Advice	0	-	94%	88%	100%
Heart Failure Care					
ACE Inhibitor or ARB for LVSD[1]	12	67%	81%	82%	100%
Discharge Instructions	28	18%	51%	61%	93%
Evaluation of LVS Function	39	87%	75%	83%	99%
Smoking Cessation Advice[1]	10	60%	78%	82%	100%
Pneumonia Care					
Appropriate Initial Antibiotic	43	86%	84%	83%	94%
Blood Culture Timing	32	91%	89%	90%	100%
Influenza Vaccine[1]	8	62%	73%	70%	100%
Initial Antibiotic Timing	55	76%	80%	80%	93%
Oxygenation Assessment	63	100%	100%	99%	100%
Pneumococcal Vaccine	37	51%	68%	69%	94%
Smoking Cessation Advice[1]	13	77%	64%	80%	100%
Surgical Infection Prevention					
Prophylactic Antibiotic Given[2,3]	75	32%	70%	77%	95%
Prophylactic Antibiotic Selection[1,2]	23	43%	92%	90%	100%
Prophylactic Antibiotic Stopped[2,3]	62	21%	69%	72%	95%
Pregnancy Care					
Inpatient Neonatal Mortality	-	-	-	-	-
Third or Fourth Degree Laceration	-	-	2.98%	3.63%	3.27%

Bear River Valley Hospital

440 W 600 N
Tremonton, UT 84337
Phone: 435-257-7441
Fax: 435-257-4386
Ownership: Voluntary non-profit - Private
Accredited: No
Emergency Services: Yes
Licensed Beds: 20

Key Personnel:

Administrator . . . . Robert Jex
Emergency Room . . . . Rod Merrell, MD
Director Infection/Disease Control . . . . Rhonda Merryweather
Director Medical/Surgical Nursing . . . . Rhonda Merryweather

Measure	Cases	This Hospital	State Average	U.S. Average	Top Hospital
Heart Attack Care					
ACE Inhibitor or ARB for LVSD[3]	0	-	83%	82%	100%
Aspirin at Arrival[3]	0	-	91%	92%	100%
Aspirin at Discharge[3]	0	-	81%	90%	100%
Beta Blocker at Arrival[1,3]	1	0%	71%	87%	100%
Beta Blocker at Discharge[1,3]	1	0%	70%	90%	100%
Fibrinolytic Medication Timing[3]	0	-	15%	31%	100%
PCI Within 90 Minutes of Arrival[5]	-	-	58%	54%	95%
Smoking Cessation Advice[3]	0	-	94%	88%	100%
Heart Failure Care					
ACE Inhibitor or ARB for LVSD[3]	0	-	81%	82%	100%
Discharge Instructions[1,3]	10	80%	51%	61%	93%
Evaluation of LVS Function[1,3]	9	89%	75%	83%	99%
Smoking Cessation Advice[3]	0	-	78%	82%	100%
Pneumonia Care					
Appropriate Initial Antibiotic	26	88%	84%	83%	94%
Blood Culture Timing[1]	2	100%	89%	90%	100%
Influenza Vaccine[1]	4	75%	73%	70%	100%
Initial Antibiotic Timing[1]	22	86%	80%	80%	93%
Oxygenation Assessment	28	100%	100%	99%	100%
Pneumococcal Vaccine[1]	18	72%	68%	69%	94%
Smoking Cessation Advice[1]	6	83%	64%	80%	100%
Surgical Infection Prevention					
Prophylactic Antibiotic Given[1]	19	47%	70%	77%	95%
Prophylactic Antibiotic Selection[1]	4	50%	92%	90%	100%
Prophylactic Antibiotic Stopped[1]	19	84%	69%	72%	95%
Pregnancy Care					
Inpatient Neonatal Mortality	-	-	-	-	-
Third or Fourth Degree Laceration	-	-	2.98%	3.63%	3.27%

Ashley Valley Medical Center

151 West 200 North
Vernal, UT 84078
Toll-Free: 866-725-2862
Phone: 435-789-3342
Fax: 435-789-1314
URL: www.avmc-hospital.com
Ownership: Proprietary
Accredited: Yes
Emergency Services: Yes
Licensed Beds: 39

Key Personnel:

Administrator/CEO . . . . Si Hutt
Chief Medical Staff . . . . Jon Hughes, MD
Emergency Room . . . . Norman Nielson, MD
Director Infection/Disease Control . . . . Beth Christensen
CCU Spvg. Nurse . . . . Susie Tenderholt
Chief Radiology . . . . David Perry, MD

Measure	Cases	This Hospital	State Average	U.S. Average	Top Hospital
Heart Attack Care					
ACE Inhibitor or ARB for LVSD[3]	0	-	83%	82%	100%
Aspirin at Arrival[1,3]	1	100%	91%	92%	100%
Aspirin at Discharge[1,3]	1	100%	81%	90%	100%
Beta Blocker at Arrival[1,3]	1	0%	71%	87%	100%
Beta Blocker at Discharge[1,3]	1	0%	70%	90%	100%
Fibrinolytic Medication Timing[3]	0	-	15%	31%	100%
PCI Within 90 Minutes of Arrival	0	-	58%	54%	95%
Smoking Cessation Advice[3]	0	-	94%	88%	100%
Heart Failure Care					
ACE Inhibitor or ARB for LVSD[1]	4	100%	81%	82%	100%
Discharge Instructions[1]	14	86%	51%	61%	93%
Evaluation of LVS Function[1]	18	100%	75%	83%	99%
Smoking Cessation Advice[1]	6	100%	78%	82%	100%
Pneumonia Care					
Appropriate Initial Antibiotic	45	84%	84%	83%	94%
Blood Culture Timing[1]	23	100%	89%	90%	100%
Influenza Vaccine[1]	6	100%	73%	70%	100%
Initial Antibiotic Timing	54	93%	80%	80%	93%
Oxygenation Assessment	56	100%	100%	99%	100%
Pneumococcal Vaccine	31	100%	68%	69%	94%
Smoking Cessation Advice[1]	21	100%	64%	80%	100%
Surgical Infection Prevention					
Prophylactic Antibiotic Given[2,3]	32	78%	70%	77%	95%
Prophylactic Antibiotic Selection[1,2]	9	100%	92%	90%	100%
Prophylactic Antibiotic Stopped[2,3]	32	38%	69%	72%	95%
Pregnancy Care					
Inpatient Neonatal Mortality	352	0.28%	-	-	-
Third or Fourth Degree Laceration	263	3.80%	2.98%	3.63%	3.27%

Jordan Valley Hospital

3580 West 9000 South
West Jordan, UT 84088
Phone: 801-561-8888
Fax: 801-569-8723
E-mail: info@iasishealthcare.com
URL: www.jordanvalleyhospital.com
Ownership: Proprietary
Accredited: Yes
Emergency Services: Yes
Licensed Beds: 92

Key Personnel:

CEO . . . . Bryanie Swilley
Chief Medical Staff . . . . R Bart Johansen, MD
Emergency Room . . . . Jon Butterfield, RN
ICU . . . . Julia Nokes, RN
Medical/Surgical Nursing . . . . Julia Nokes
OB/GYN Womens Health . . . . Lynette Tulka, RN
Director Radiology . . . . Doug Madsen
Director Respiratory/Cardiopulmonary . . . . Mike Jimenez

Measure	Cases	This Hospital	State Average	U.S. Average	Top Hospital
Heart Attack Care					
ACE Inhibitor or ARB for LVSD[1]	3	100%	83%	82%	100%
Aspirin at Arrival	25	100%	91%	92%	100%
Aspirin at Discharge[1]	18	89%	81%	90%	100%
Beta Blocker at Arrival[1]	23	91%	71%	87%	100%
Beta Blocker at Discharge[1]	15	87%	70%	90%	100%
Fibrinolytic Medication Timing[1]	3	67%	15%	31%	100%
PCI Within 90 Minutes of Arrival[1]	6	33%	58%	54%	95%
Smoking Cessation Advice[1]	6	100%	94%	88%	100%

NOTE: Hospital profiles are in alphabetical order by state, then city, then hospital within the city; Rankings are sorted by rate in descending order and exclude hospitals with less than 25 cases; (1) The number of cases is too small (n<25) for purposes of reliably predicting hospital performance; (2) Measure reflects the hospital's indication that its submission was based upon a sample of its relevant discharges; (3) Rate reflects fewer than the maximum possible quarters of data for the measure; (4) Inaccurate information submitted and suppressed for one or more quarters; (5) No data is available from the hospital for this measure; Please refer to the User's Guide for a full explanation of data

Heart Failure Care					
ACE Inhibitor or ARB for LVSD[1]	15	87%	81%	82%	100%
Discharge Instructions	67	57%	51%	61%	93%
Evaluation of LVS Function	79	87%	75%	83%	99%
Smoking Cessation Advice[1]	14	100%	78%	82%	100%
Pneumonia Care					
Appropriate Initial Antibiotic	151	89%	84%	83%	94%
Blood Culture Timing	112	95%	89%	90%	100%
Influenza Vaccine	35	100%	73%	70%	100%
Initial Antibiotic Timing	177	84%	80%	80%	93%
Oxygenation Assessment	211	100%	100%	99%	100%
Pneumococcal Vaccine	98	97%	68%	69%	94%
Smoking Cessation Advice	49	100%	64%	80%	100%
Surgical Infection Prevention					
Prophylactic Antibiotic Given	341	70%	70%	77%	95%
Prophylactic Antibiotic Selection	92	98%	92%	90%	100%
Prophylactic Antibiotic Stopped	329	63%	69%	72%	95%
Pregnancy Care					
Inpatient Neonatal Mortality[2]	1,502	0.07%	-	-	-
Third or Fourth Degree Laceration[2]	1,213	3.05%	2.98%	3.63%	3.27%

Pioneer Valley Hospital

3460 South Pioneer Parkway
West Valley City, UT 84120
Ownership: Proprietary
Emergency Services: Yes

Phone: 801-964-3100

Accredited: Yes

Measure	Cases	This Hospital	State Average	U.S. Average	Top Hospital
Heart Attack Care					
ACE Inhibitor or ARB for LVSD[1]	17	76%	83%	82%	100%
Aspirin at Arrival	89	98%	91%	92%	100%
Aspirin at Discharge	113	99%	81%	90%	100%
Beta Blocker at Arrival	66	91%	71%	87%	100%
Beta Blocker at Discharge	101	91%	70%	90%	100%
Fibrinolytic Medication Timing[1]	8	25%	15%	31%	100%
PCI Within 90 Minutes of Arrival[1]	16	38%	58%	54%	95%
Smoking Cessation Advice	55	95%	94%	88%	100%
Heart Failure Care					
ACE Inhibitor or ARB for LVSD	31	90%	81%	82%	100%
Discharge Instructions	78	29%	51%	61%	93%
Evaluation of LVS Function	88	94%	75%	83%	99%
Smoking Cessation Advice[1]	23	87%	78%	82%	100%
Pneumonia Care					
Appropriate Initial Antibiotic	183	81%	84%	83%	94%
Blood Culture Timing	135	93%	89%	90%	100%
Influenza Vaccine	44	98%	73%	70%	100%
Initial Antibiotic Timing	202	79%	80%	80%	93%
Oxygenation Assessment	226	100%	100%	99%	100%
Pneumococcal Vaccine	128	84%	68%	69%	94%
Smoking Cessation Advice	59	88%	64%	80%	100%
Surgical Infection Prevention					
Prophylactic Antibiotic Given	190	71%	70%	77%	95%
Prophylactic Antibiotic Selection	54	98%	92%	90%	100%
Prophylactic Antibiotic Stopped	179	72%	69%	72%	95%
Pregnancy Care					
Inpatient Neonatal Mortality[2]	287	0.00%	-	-	-
Third or Fourth Degree Laceration[2]	215	1.86%	2.98%	3.63%	3.27%

NOTE: Hospital profiles are in alphabetical order by state, then city, then hospital within the city; Rankings are sorted by rate in descending order and exclude hospitals with less than 25 cases; (1) The number of cases is too small (n<25) for purposes of reliably predicting hospital performance; (2) Measure reflects the hospital's indication that its submission was based upon a sample of its relevant discharges; (3) Rate reflects fewer than the maximum possible quarters of data for the measure; (4) Inaccurate information submitted and suppressed for one or more quarters; (5) No data is available from the hospital for this measure; Please refer to the User's Guide for a full explanation of data

Heart Attack Care

1. ACE Inhibitor or ARB for LVSD

Hospital Name	City	Rate	Cases
Evergreen Hospital Medical Center	Kirkland	98%	46
Yakima Regional Medical & Cardiac Center	Yakima	98%	56
Sacred Heart Medical Center	Spokane	97%	97
Saint Joseph Hospital	Bellingham	95%	59
Saint Francis Hospital	Federal Way	94%	31
Northwest Hospital and Medical Center	Seattle	93%	29
Good Samaritan Hospital & Rehab Center	Puyallup	91%	33
Harrison Medical Center	Bremerton	91%	47
Deaconess Medical Center	Spokane	89%	70
Virginia Mason Medical Center	Seattle	88%	48
Saint Joseph Medical Center	Tacoma	86%	100
Tacoma General Hospital	Tacoma	85%	71
Valley Medical Center	Renton	85%	40
Kadlec Medical Center	Richland	84%	55
Central Washington Hospital	Wenatchee	82%	33
Skagit Valley Hospital	Mount Vernon	81%	26
Providence Saint Peter Hospital	Olympia	80%	103
Southwest Washington Medical Center	Vancouver	80%	85
Overlake Hospital Medical Center	Bellevue	78%	77
Swedish Medical Center/Providence	Seattle	78%	36
Providence Everett Medical Center	Everett	76%	62
Swedish Medical Center	Seattle	76%	42
Auburn Regional Medical Center	Auburn	62%	55

2. Aspirin at Arrival

Hospital Name	City	Rate	Cases
Central Washington Hospital	Wenatchee	100%	100
Harborview Medical Center	Seattle	100%	98
Legacy Salmon Creek Hospital	Vancouver	100%	39
Sacred Heart Medical Center	Spokane	100%	193
Saint John Medical Center	Longview	100%	115
Saint Joseph Hospital	Bellingham	100%	283
Skagit Valley Hospital	Mount Vernon	100%	88
Southwest Washington Medical Center	Vancouver	100%	415
University of Washington Medical Center	Seattle	100%	51
Deaconess Medical Center	Spokane	99%	105
Evergreen Hospital Medical Center	Kirkland	99%	205
Good Samaritan Hospital & Rehab Center	Puyallup	99%	225
Highline Community Hospital	Burien	99%	85
Holy Family Hospital	Spokane	99%	97
Providence Everett Medical Center	Everett	99%	406
Saint Joseph Medical Center	Tacoma	99%	296
Providence Centralia Hospital	Centralia	98%	43
Saint Clare Hospital	Lakewood	98%	47
Saint Francis Hospital	Federal Way	98%	145
Swedish Medical Center	Seattle	98%	152
Swedish Medical Center/Providence	Seattle	98%	99
Virginia Mason Medical Center	Seattle	98%	139
Group Health Eastside Hospital	Redmond	97%	31
Providence Saint Peter Hospital	Olympia	97%	377
Valley Medical Center	Renton	97%	261
Yakima Regional Medical & Cardiac Center	Yakima	97%	95
Yakima Valley Memorial Hospital	Yakima	97%	161
Tacoma General Hospital	Tacoma	96%	210
Harrison Medical Center	Bremerton	95%	239
Northwest Hospital and Medical Center	Seattle	95%	114
Overlake Hospital Medical Center	Bellevue	94%	213
Auburn Regional Medical Center	Auburn	93%	142
Saint Mary Medical Center	Walla Walla	93%	28
Stevens Hospital	Edmonds	93%	115
Olympic Medical Center	Port Angeles	91%	35
Capital Medical Center	Olympia	90%	29
Kadlec Medical Center	Richland	90%	115
Kennewick General Hospital	Kennewick	82%	33
Grays Harbor Community Hospital-West Campus	Aberdeen	78%	50

3. Aspirin at Discharge

Hospital Name	City	Rate	Cases
Deaconess Medical Center	Spokane	100%	270
Harborview Medical Center	Seattle	100%	63
Sacred Heart Medical Center	Spokane	100%	530
Saint Clare Hospital	Lakewood	100%	26
Saint Francis Hospital	Federal Way	100%	109
Yakima Valley Memorial Hospital	Yakima	100%	128
Central Washington Hospital	Wenatchee	99%	161
Holy Family Hospital	Spokane	99%	73
Northwest Hospital and Medical Center	Seattle	99%	101
Stevens Hospital	Edmonds	99%	88
Swedish Medical Center/Providence	Seattle	99%	168
Tacoma General Hospital	Tacoma	99%	251
University of Washington Medical Center	Seattle	99%	82
Virginia Mason Medical Center	Seattle	99%	244
Yakima Regional Medical & Cardiac Center	Yakima	99%	180
Harrison Medical Center	Bremerton	98%	288
Overlake Hospital Medical Center	Bellevue	98%	253
Providence Everett Medical Center	Everett	98%	453
Saint Joseph Hospital	Bellingham	98%	306
Auburn Regional Medical Center	Auburn	97%	118
Evergreen Hospital Medical Center	Kirkland	97%	191
Providence Saint Peter Hospital	Olympia	97%	570
Saint John Medical Center	Longview	97%	64
Saint Joseph Medical Center	Tacoma	97%	363
Southwest Washington Medical Center	Vancouver	97%	456
Valley Medical Center	Renton	97%	209
Kadlec Medical Center	Richland	96%	298
Skagit Valley Hospital	Mount Vernon	96%	91
Swedish Medical Center	Seattle	96%	196
Capital Medical Center	Olympia	95%	42
Highline Community Hospital	Burien	94%	79
Providence Centralia Hospital	Centralia	94%	33
Good Samaritan Hospital & Rehab Center	Puyallup	91%	188
Legacy Salmon Creek Hospital	Vancouver	90%	29

4. Beta Blocker at Arrival

Hospital Name	City	Rate	Cases
Harborview Medical Center	Seattle	100%	61
Saint Mary Medical Center	Walla Walla	100%	27
Virginia Mason Medical Center	Seattle	100%	125
Good Samaritan Hospital & Rehab Center	Puyallup	99%	206
Highline Community Hospital	Burien	99%	70
Holy Family Hospital	Spokane	99%	86
Sacred Heart Medical Center	Spokane	99%	168
Saint John Medical Center	Longview	99%	90
Providence Everett Medical Center	Everett	98%	394
Saint Joseph Hospital	Bellingham	98%	237
Southwest Washington Medical Center	Vancouver	98%	369
Tacoma General Hospital	Tacoma	98%	163
Yakima Valley Memorial Hospital	Yakima	98%	121
Stevens Hospital	Edmonds	97%	63
Swedish Medical Center/Providence	Seattle	97%	88
Deaconess Medical Center	Spokane	96%	92
Harrison Medical Center	Bremerton	96%	209
Northwest Hospital and Medical Center	Seattle	96%	89
Olympic Medical Center	Port Angeles	96%	27
Saint Joseph Medical Center	Tacoma	96%	157
Skagit Valley Hospital	Mount Vernon	96%	79
Valley Medical Center	Renton	96%	223
Yakima Regional Medical & Cardiac Center	Yakima	96%	71
Auburn Regional Medical Center	Auburn	95%	147
Saint Francis Hospital	Federal Way	95%	61
University of Washington Medical Center	Seattle	95%	42
Evergreen Hospital Medical Center	Kirkland	94%	136
Providence Saint Peter Hospital	Olympia	93%	338
Swedish Medical Center	Seattle	92%	145
Central Washington Hospital	Wenatchee	90%	88
Capital Medical Center	Olympia	88%	25
Grays Harbor Community Hospital-West Campus	Aberdeen	86%	43
Overlake Hospital Medical Center	Bellevue	86%	149
Providence Centralia Hospital	Centralia	85%	34
Kadlec Medical Center	Richland	82%	106
Kennewick General Hospital	Kennewick	73%	33

5. Beta Blocker at Discharge

Hospital Name	City	Rate	Cases
Harborview Medical Center	Seattle	100%	80
Northwest Hospital and Medical Center	Seattle	100%	114
Saint Clare Hospital	Lakewood	100%	28
Saint Francis Hospital	Federal Way	100%	111
Deaconess Medical Center	Spokane	99%	297
Providence Everett Medical Center	Everett	99%	450
Sacred Heart Medical Center	Spokane	99%	527
Saint John Medical Center	Longview	99%	69
Saint Joseph Hospital	Bellingham	99%	318
Saint Joseph Medical Center	Tacoma	99%	360
University of Washington Medical Center	Seattle	99%	105
Yakima Regional Medical & Cardiac Center	Yakima	99%	177
Yakima Valley Memorial Hospital	Yakima	99%	130
Evergreen Hospital Medical Center	Kirkland	98%	181
Harrison Medical Center	Bremerton	98%	304
Skagit Valley Hospital	Mount Vernon	98%	113
Southwest Washington Medical Center	Vancouver	98%	489
Virginia Mason Medical Center	Seattle	98%	240
Overlake Hospital Medical Center	Bellevue	97%	265

NOTE: Hospital profiles are in alphabetical order by state, then city, then hospital within the city; Rankings are sorted by rate in descending order and exclude hospitals with less than 25 cases; (1) The number of cases is too small (n<25) for purposes of reliably predicting hospital performance; (2) Measure reflects the hospital's indication that its submission was based upon a sample of its relevant discharges; (3) Rate reflects fewer than the maximum possible quarters of data for the measure; (4) Inaccurate information submitted and suppressed for one or more quarters; (5) No data is available from the hospital for this measure; Please refer to the User's Guide for a full explanation of data

Providence Centralia Hospital	Centralia	97%	32
Stevens Hospital	Edmonds	97%	73
Holy Family Hospital	Spokane	96%	72
Tacoma General Hospital	Tacoma	96%	279
Valley Medical Center	Renton	96%	200
Central Washington Hospital	Wenatchee	95%	172
Good Samaritan Hospital & Rehab Center	Puyallup	95%	190
Swedish Medical Center	Seattle	94%	216
Swedish Medical Center/Providence	Seattle	93%	176
Capital Medical Center	Olympia	92%	39
Highline Community Hospital	Burien	92%	78
Kadlec Medical Center	Richland	92%	275
Providence Saint Peter Hospital	Olympia	90%	540
Auburn Regional Medical Center	Auburn	89%	119
Kennewick General Hospital	Kennewick	77%	26

6. Fibrinolytic Medication Timing

Hospital Name	City	Rate	Cases
Auburn Regional Medical Center	Auburn	52%	27

7. PCI Within 90 Minutes of Arrival

Hospital Name	City	Rate	Cases
Providence Everett Medical Center	Everett	70%	30

8. Smoking Cessation Advice

Hospital Name	City	Rate	Cases
Deaconess Medical Center	Spokane	100%	107
Highline Community Hospital	Burien	100%	30
Sacred Heart Medical Center	Spokane	100%	196
University of Washington Medical Center	Seattle	100%	36
Yakima Regional Medical & Cardiac Center	Yakima	100%	89
Yakima Valley Memorial Hospital	Yakima	100%	47
Virginia Mason Medical Center	Seattle	98%	47
Holy Family Hospital	Spokane	97%	29
Northwest Hospital and Medical Center	Seattle	97%	32
Good Samaritan Hospital & Rehab Center	Puyallup	96%	68
Saint Joseph Medical Center	Tacoma	94%	135
Skagit Valley Hospital	Mount Vernon	94%	31
Stevens Hospital	Edmonds	94%	33
Providence Everett Medical Center	Everett	93%	142
Saint Francis Hospital	Federal Way	93%	28
Tacoma General Hospital	Tacoma	93%	113
Central Washington Hospital	Wenatchee	92%	62
Overlake Hospital Medical Center	Bellevue	92%	59
Harborview Medical Center	Seattle	91%	54
Saint Joseph Hospital	Bellingham	90%	82
Southwest Washington Medical Center	Vancouver	90%	173
Harrison Medical Center	Bremerton	86%	85
Evergreen Hospital Medical Center	Kirkland	82%	56
Auburn Regional Medical Center	Auburn	81%	42
Providence Saint Peter Hospital	Olympia	81%	213
Swedish Medical Center/Providence	Seattle	80%	49
Swedish Medical Center	Seattle	79%	53

Heart Failure Care

9. ACE Inhibitor or ARB for LVSD

Hospital Name	City	Rate	Cases
Sacred Heart Medical Center	Spokane	98%	245
University of Washington Medical Center	Seattle	97%	231
Saint Clare Hospital	Lakewood	96%	77
Providence Everett Medical Center	Everett	95%	115
Saint Francis Hospital	Federal Way	95%	57
Saint Joseph Hospital	Bellingham	95%	174
Yakima Regional Medical & Cardiac Center	Yakima	93%	67
Providence Centralia Hospital	Centralia	92%	50
Providence Saint Peter Hospital	Olympia	92%	161
Deaconess Medical Center	Spokane	91%	128
Toppenish Community Hospital	Toppenish	91%	34
Grays Harbor Community Hospital-West Campus	Aberdeen	90%	41
Harborview Medical Center	Seattle	90%	113
Mason General Hospital	Shelton	90%	29
Southwest Washington Medical Center	Vancouver	90%	185
Evergreen Hospital Medical Center	Kirkland	89%	80
Group Health Eastside Hospital	Redmond	89%	54
Olympic Medical Center	Port Angeles	89%	62
Central Washington Hospital	Wenatchee	88%	72
Tacoma General Hospital	Tacoma	88%	161
Valley Medical Center	Renton	88%	113
Harrison Medical Center	Bremerton	86%	151
Northwest Hospital and Medical Center	Seattle	86%	85
Good Samaritan Hospital & Rehab Center	Puyallup	85%	82
Swedish Medical Center/Providence	Seattle	85%	124
Saint Joseph Medical Center	Tacoma	83%	223
Saint John Medical Center	Longview	82%	93
Holy Family Hospital	Spokane	81%	53
Swedish Medical Center	Seattle	81%	150
Stevens Hospital	Edmonds	79%	47
Overlake Hospital Medical Center	Bellevue	77%	134
Virginia Mason Medical Center	Seattle	77%	123
Auburn Regional Medical Center	Auburn	76%	79
Yakima Valley Memorial Hospital	Yakima	76%	84
Highline Community Hospital	Burien	74%	57
Skagit Valley Hospital	Mount Vernon	72%	54
Kennewick General Hospital	Kennewick	69%	35
Kadlec Medical Center	Richland	67%	67
Legacy Salmon Creek Hospital	Vancouver	66%	62
Saint Mary Medical Center	Walla Walla	60%	25

10. Discharge Instructions

Hospital Name	City	Rate	Cases
Mount Carmel Hospital	Colville	97%	34
Sacred Heart Medical Center	Spokane	96%	414
Valley General Hospital	Monroe	90%	39
Deaconess Medical Center	Spokane	85%	217
Olympic Medical Center	Port Angeles	84%	128
Providence Centralia Hospital	Centralia	80%	133
Toppenish Community Hospital	Toppenish	79%	81
Yakima Regional Medical & Cardiac Center	Yakima	78%	170
Saint John Medical Center	Longview	76%	172
Saint Joseph Hospital	Bellingham	71%	268
Valley Medical Center	Renton	71%	55
Northwest Hospital and Medical Center	Seattle	69%	158
Lourdes Medical Center	Pasco	67%	30
Holy Family Hospital	Spokane	66%	129
Evergreen Hospital Medical Center	Kirkland	63%	175
Kennewick General Hospital	Kennewick	62%	92
Mason General Hospital	Shelton	62%	45
Saint Clare Hospital	Lakewood	60%	203
Central Washington Hospital	Wenatchee	59%	157
Harborview Medical Center	Seattle	59%	176
Virginia Mason Medical Center	Seattle	59%	288
Southwest Washington Medical Center	Vancouver	58%	481
Tacoma General Hospital	Tacoma	58%	351
Tri-State Memorial Hospital	Clarkston	58%	26
Auburn Regional Medical Center	Auburn	56%	124
Skagit Valley Hospital	Mount Vernon	54%	127
Harrison Medical Center	Bremerton	53%	300
Saint Mary Medical Center	Walla Walla	53%	68
Providence Everett Medical Center	Everett	51%	255
University of Washington Medical Center	Seattle	51%	333
Highline Community Hospital	Burien	48%	157
Island Hospital	Anacortes	47%	38
Group Health Eastside Hospital	Redmond	46%	35
Cascade Valley Hosp/N Snohomish Co Sys	Arlington	44%	43
Walla Walla General Hospital	Walla Walla	43%	30
Saint Joseph Medical Center	Tacoma	42%	471
Kadlec Medical Center	Richland	41%	32
Providence Saint Peter Hospital	Olympia	41%	355
Whidbey General Hospital	Coupeville	41%	27
Stevens Hospital	Edmonds	40%	112
Saint Francis Hospital	Federal Way	39%	145
Valley Hospital & Medical Center	Spokane	36%	56
Yakima Valley Memorial Hospital	Yakima	36%	220
Good Samaritan Hospital & Rehab Center	Puyallup	35%	211
Samaritan Healthcare	Moses Lake	35%	51
Grays Harbor Community Hospital-West Campus	Aberdeen	32%	192
Legacy Salmon Creek Hospital	Vancouver	31%	147
Swedish Medical Center/Providence	Seattle	27%	222
Jefferson General Hospital	Port Townsend	25%	36
Swedish Medical Center	Seattle	22%	361
Capital Medical Center	Olympia	19%	42
Sunnyside Community Hospital	Sunnyside	19%	27
Overlake Hospital Medical Center	Bellevue	16%	269

11. Evaluation of LVS Function

Hospital Name	City	Rate	Cases
Group Health Eastside Hospital	Redmond	99%	149
Sacred Heart Medical Center	Spokane	99%	457
Saint Francis Hospital	Federal Way	99%	194
Saint Joseph Hospital	Bellingham	99%	337
University of Washington Medical Center	Seattle	99%	352
Harborview Medical Center	Seattle	98%	199
Olympic Medical Center	Port Angeles	98%	172
Saint Clare Hospital	Lakewood	98%	263
Valley General Hospital	Monroe	98%	49

NOTE: Hospital profiles are in alphabetical order by state, then city, then hospital within the city; Rankings are sorted by rate in descending order and exclude hospitals with less than 25 cases; (1) The number of cases is too small (n<25) for purposes of reliably predicting hospital performance; (2) Measure reflects the hospital's indication that its submission was based upon a sample of its relevant discharges; (3) Rate reflects fewer than the maximum possible quarters of data for the measure; (4) Inaccurate information submitted and suppressed for one or more quarters; (5) No data is available from the hospital for this measure; Please refer to the User's Guide for a full explanation of data

Hospital Name	City	Rate	Cases
Overlake Hospital Medical Center	Bellevue	97%	344
Virginia Mason Medical Center	Seattle	97%	375
Skagit Valley Hospital	Mount Vernon	96%	172
Walla Walla General Hospital	Walla Walla	96%	47
Evergreen Hospital Medical Center	Kirkland	95%	223
Saint Mary Medical Center	Walla Walla	95%	98
Tacoma General Hospital	Tacoma	95%	454
Deaconess Medical Center	Spokane	94%	252
Saint Joseph Medical Center	Tacoma	94%	559
Swedish Medical Center/Providence	Seattle	94%	271
Mount Carmel Hospital	Colville	93%	41
Providence Centralia Hospital	Centralia	92%	157
Harrison Medical Center	Bremerton	91%	439
Saint John Medical Center	Longview	91%	209
Swedish Medical Center	Seattle	91%	453
United General Hospital	Sedro Woolley	91%	34
Yakima Regional Medical & Cardiac Center	Yakima	91%	192
Central Washington Hospital	Wenatchee	90%	185
Good Samaritan Hospital & Rehab Center	Puyallup	90%	292
Kittitas Valley Community Hospital	Ellensburg	90%	31
Southwest Washington Medical Center	Vancouver	90%	551
Kadlec Medical Center	Richland	89%	161
Northwest Hospital and Medical Center	Seattle	89%	218
Providence Everett Medical Center	Everett	89%	331
Stevens Hospital	Edmonds	89%	137
Legacy Salmon Creek Hospital	Vancouver	88%	185
Highline Community Hospital	Burien	87%	186
Providence Saint Peter Hospital	Olympia	87%	431
Holy Family Hospital	Spokane	86%	165
Yakima Valley Memorial Hospital	Yakima	86%	261
Capital Medical Center	Olympia	84%	68
Island Hospital	Anacortes	84%	44
Valley Medical Center	Renton	84%	303
Jefferson General Hospital	Port Townsend	83%	46
Kennewick General Hospital	Kennewick	83%	118
Valley Hospital & Medical Center	Spokane	83%	86
Toppenish Community Hospital	Toppenish	82%	87
Enumclaw Regional Hospital	Enumclaw	81%	26
Cascade Valley Hosp/N Snohomish Co Sys	Arlington	75%	61
Mason General Hospital	Shelton	74%	68
Lourdes Medical Center	Pasco	73%	37
Grays Harbor Community Hospital-West Campus	Aberdeen	72%	224
Auburn Regional Medical Center	Auburn	70%	156
Sunnyside Community Hospital	Sunnyside	70%	27
Whidbey General Hospital	Coupeville	70%	37
Samaritan Healthcare	Moses Lake	63%	73
Tri-State Memorial Hospital	Clarkston	52%	56

12. Smoking Cessation Advice

Hospital Name	City	Rate	Cases
Sacred Heart Medical Center	Spokane	100%	70
University of Washington Medical Center	Seattle	100%	63
Deaconess Medical Center	Spokane	97%	62
Yakima Valley Memorial Hospital	Yakima	96%	28
Saint John Medical Center	Longview	94%	50
Providence Everett Medical Center	Everett	93%	46
Northwest Hospital and Medical Center	Seattle	92%	26
Saint Joseph Hospital	Bellingham	92%	49
Yakima Regional Medical & Cardiac Center	Yakima	92%	40
Central Washington Hospital	Wenatchee	91%	35
Saint Francis Hospital	Federal Way	91%	34
Highline Community Hospital	Burien	90%	41
Tacoma General Hospital	Tacoma	90%	103
Saint Clare Hospital	Lakewood	86%	56
Auburn Regional Medical Center	Auburn	85%	33
Providence Centralia Hospital	Centralia	80%	25
Legacy Salmon Creek Hospital	Vancouver	78%	41
Providence Saint Peter Hospital	Olympia	78%	79
Good Samaritan Hospital & Rehab Center	Puyallup	75%	40
Harborview Medical Center	Seattle	74%	102
Grays Harbor Community Hospital-West Campus	Aberdeen	72%	43
Saint Joseph Medical Center	Tacoma	72%	95
Harrison Medical Center	Bremerton	67%	60
Southwest Washington Medical Center	Vancouver	64%	97
Swedish Medical Center/Providence	Seattle	54%	63
Swedish Medical Center	Seattle	48%	61

Pneumonia Care

13. Appropriate Initial Antibiotic

Hospital Name	City	Rate	Cases
Saint Francis Hospital	Federal Way	96%	110
Virginia Mason Medical Center	Seattle	96%	177
Saint Joseph Medical Center	Tacoma	95%	205
Saint Clare Hospital	Lakewood	94%	197
United General Hospital	Sedro Woolley	94%	107
Yakima Valley Memorial Hospital	Yakima	94%	187
Kittitas Valley Community Hospital	Ellensburg	93%	29
Saint Joseph's Hospital	Chewelah	92%	59
Skagit Valley Hospital	Mount Vernon	92%	108
Legacy Salmon Creek Hospital	Vancouver	91%	88
Yakima Regional Medical & Cardiac Center	Yakima	90%	87
Capital Medical Center	Olympia	89%	53
Central Washington Hospital	Wenatchee	89%	99
Olympic Medical Center	Port Angeles	89%	150
Saint Joseph Hospital	Bellingham	89%	172
Walla Walla General Hospital	Walla Walla	89%	47
Providence Centralia Hospital	Centralia	88%	154
Deaconess Medical Center	Spokane	87%	91
Holy Family Hospital	Spokane	87%	280
Tacoma General Hospital	Tacoma	87%	249
Evergreen Hospital Medical Center	Kirkland	86%	146
Saint Mary Medical Center	Walla Walla	86%	79
University of Washington Medical Center	Seattle	86%	83
Enumclaw Regional Hospital	Enumclaw	85%	26
Swedish Medical Center/Providence	Seattle	84%	88
Harborview Medical Center	Seattle	83%	121
Highline Community Hospital	Burien	83%	177
Jefferson General Hospital	Port Townsend	83%	48
Stevens Hospital	Edmonds	83%	186
Overlake Hospital Medical Center	Bellevue	82%	130
Sacred Heart Medical Center	Spokane	82%	219
Saint John Medical Center	Longview	82%	140
Sunnyside Community Hospital	Sunnyside	82%	33
Island Hospital	Anacortes	81%	63
Harrison Medical Center	Bremerton	80%	246
Mount Carmel Hospital	Colville	80%	82
Valley Hospital & Medical Center	Spokane	80%	82
Auburn Regional Medical Center	Auburn	79%	159
Swedish Medical Center	Seattle	79%	261
Samaritan Healthcare	Moses Lake	78%	54
Providence Everett Medical Center	Everett	77%	104
Good Samaritan Hospital & Rehab Center	Puyallup	76%	147
Kadlec Medical Center	Richland	76%	25
Providence Saint Peter Hospital	Olympia	76%	242
Kennewick General Hospital	Kennewick	75%	76
Grays Harbor Community Hospital-West Campus	Aberdeen	74%	189
Lourdes Medical Center	Pasco	74%	54
Valley General Hospital	Monroe	74%	54
Northwest Hospital and Medical Center	Seattle	72%	119
Whidbey General Hospital	Coupeville	70%	82
Toppenish Community Hospital	Toppenish	51%	59
Cascade Valley Hosp/N Snohomish Co Sys	Arlington	50%	58
Southwest Washington Medical Center	Vancouver	39%	119

14. Blood Culture Timing

Hospital Name	City	Rate	Cases
Mount Carmel Hospital	Colville	98%	63
Overlake Hospital Medical Center	Bellevue	98%	142
Capital Medical Center	Olympia	97%	35
Saint Joseph Hospital	Bellingham	97%	180
Saint Joseph's Hospital	Chewelah	97%	29
Samaritan Healthcare	Moses Lake	97%	38
University of Washington Medical Center	Seattle	97%	97
United General Hospital	Sedro Woolley	96%	50
Valley Hospital & Medical Center	Spokane	96%	73
Walla Walla General Hospital	Walla Walla	96%	47
Yakima Valley Memorial Hospital	Yakima	96%	70
Grays Harbor Community Hospital-West Campus	Aberdeen	95%	116
Holy Family Hospital	Spokane	95%	240
Evergreen Hospital Medical Center	Kirkland	94%	166
Tacoma General Hospital	Tacoma	94%	214
Group Health Eastside Hospital	Redmond	93%	27
Harrison Medical Center	Bremerton	93%	251
Kadlec Medical Center	Richland	93%	30
Olympic Medical Center	Port Angeles	93%	155
Saint John Medical Center	Longview	93%	125
Saint Joseph Medical Center	Tacoma	93%	257
Stevens Hospital	Edmonds	93%	170
Swedish Medical Center/Providence	Seattle	93%	74
Highline Community Hospital	Burien	92%	188
Jefferson General Hospital	Port Townsend	92%	36
Kennewick General Hospital	Kennewick	92%	86
Legacy Salmon Creek Hospital	Vancouver	92%	65
Providence Everett Medical Center	Everett	92%	95
Saint Mary Medical Center	Walla Walla	92%	77
Toppenish Community Hospital	Toppenish	92%	50
Northwest Hospital and Medical Center	Seattle	91%	125

NOTE: Hospital profiles are in alphabetical order by state, then city, then hospital within the city; Rankings are sorted by rate in descending order and exclude hospitals with less than 25 cases; (1) The number of cases is too small (n<25) for purposes of reliably predicting hospital performance; (2) Measure reflects the hospital's indication that its submission was based upon a sample of its relevant discharges; (3) Rate reflects fewer than the maximum possible quarters of data for the measure; (4) Inaccurate information submitted and suppressed for one or more quarters; (5) No data is available from the hospital for this measure; Please refer to the User's Guide for a full explanation of data

Providence Saint Peter Hospital	Olympia	91%	225
Sacred Heart Medical Center	Spokane	91%	267
Saint Francis Hospital	Federal Way	90%	121
Valley Medical Center	Renton	90%	30
Whidbey General Hospital	Coupeville	90%	49
Central Washington Hospital	Wenatchee	89%	116
Deaconess Medical Center	Spokane	89%	76
Good Samaritan Hospital & Rehab Center	Puyallup	89%	120
Saint Clare Hospital	Lakewood	89%	191
Southwest Washington Medical Center	Vancouver	89%	103
Tri-State Memorial Hospital	Clarkston	89%	36
Island Hospital	Anacortes	88%	64
Mason General Hospital	Shelton	88%	40
Swedish Medical Center	Seattle	88%	249
Cascade Valley Hosp/N Snohomish Co Sys	Arlington	87%	54
Lourdes Medical Center	Pasco	87%	38
Valley General Hospital	Monroe	87%	53
Virginia Mason Medical Center	Seattle	87%	202
Auburn Regional Medical Center	Auburn	86%	97
Yakima Regional Medical & Cardiac Center	Yakima	82%	88
Skagit Valley Hospital	Mount Vernon	81%	121
Harborview Medical Center	Seattle	80%	119
Providence Centralia Hospital	Centralia	78%	109

15. Influenza Vaccine

Hospital Name	City	Rate	Cases
Saint John Medical Center	Longview	100%	62
Evergreen Hospital Medical Center	Kirkland	89%	44
Holy Family Hospital	Spokane	88%	64
Sacred Heart Medical Center	Spokane	84%	61
Saint Joseph Hospital	Bellingham	82%	61
Highline Community Hospital	Burien	79%	53
Central Washington Hospital	Wenatchee	77%	35
Virginia Mason Medical Center	Seattle	74%	78
Deaconess Medical Center	Spokane	71%	31
Stevens Hospital	Edmonds	70%	37
Good Samaritan Hospital & Rehab Center	Puyallup	68%	28
Skagit Valley Hospital	Mount Vernon	68%	34
Saint Joseph Medical Center	Tacoma	67%	64
Olympic Medical Center	Port Angeles	65%	60
Southwest Washington Medical Center	Vancouver	65%	31
Swedish Medical Center	Seattle	63%	92
Saint Francis Hospital	Federal Way	61%	28
Saint Clare Hospital	Lakewood	54%	56
Yakima Valley Memorial Hospital	Yakima	54%	48
Auburn Regional Medical Center	Auburn	53%	32
Providence Saint Peter Hospital	Olympia	48%	52
Grays Harbor Community Hospital-West Campus	Aberdeen	38%	45
University of Washington Medical Center	Seattle	33%	30
Providence Everett Medical Center	Everett	29%	31
Overlake Hospital Medical Center	Bellevue	19%	53

16. Initial Antibiotic Timing

Hospital Name	City	Rate	Cases
Saint Joseph's Hospital	Chewelah	91%	86
Kennewick General Hospital	Kennewick	90%	119
Central Washington Hospital	Wenatchee	88%	172
Highline Community Hospital	Burien	88%	269
Kittitas Valley Community Hospital	Ellensburg	88%	32
Mason General Hospital	Shelton	88%	83
Mount Carmel Hospital	Colville	88%	95
Jefferson General Hospital	Port Townsend	87%	63
Saint Mary Medical Center	Walla Walla	86%	98
Cascade Valley Hosp/N Snohomish Co Sys	Arlington	85%	72
Saint John Medical Center	Longview	85%	335
Walla Walla General Hospital	Walla Walla	85%	52
Yakima Valley Memorial Hospital	Yakima	85%	275
Legacy Salmon Creek Hospital	Vancouver	84%	142
Saint Francis Hospital	Federal Way	84%	153
Saint Joseph Medical Center	Tacoma	84%	320
Yakima Regional Medical & Cardiac Center	Yakima	84%	117
Saint Clare Hospital	Lakewood	83%	254
Tacoma General Hospital	Tacoma	83%	311
Auburn Regional Medical Center	Auburn	82%	163
Providence Saint Peter Hospital	Olympia	82%	311
Skagit Valley Hospital	Mount Vernon	82%	147
United General Hospital	Sedro Woolley	82%	92
Group Health Eastside Hospital	Redmond	81%	125
Saint Joseph Hospital	Bellingham	81%	318
Virginia Mason Medical Center	Seattle	81%	235
Whidbey General Hospital	Coupeville	81%	83
Grays Harbor Community Hospital-West Campus	Aberdeen	80%	231
Providence Centralia Hospital	Centralia	80%	180
Olympic Medical Center	Port Angeles	79%	225
Holy Family Hospital	Spokane	78%	310
Kadlec Medical Center	Richland	78%	156
Stevens Hospital	Edmonds	78%	245
Swedish Medical Center	Seattle	78%	399
Overlake Hospital Medical Center	Bellevue	76%	197
Swedish Medical Center/Providence	Seattle	76%	114
Toppenish Community Hospital	Toppenish	76%	63
Valley General Hospital	Monroe	76%	79
Evergreen Hospital Medical Center	Kirkland	75%	207
Lourdes Medical Center	Pasco	75%	55
Pullman Memorial Hospital	Pullman	75%	32
Sacred Heart Medical Center	Spokane	75%	391
Tri-State Memorial Hospital	Clarkston	75%	36
Island Hospital	Anacortes	74%	84
Samaritan Healthcare	Moses Lake	74%	85
Capital Medical Center	Olympia	73%	52
Deaconess Medical Center	Spokane	73%	146
Good Samaritan Hospital & Rehab Center	Puyallup	73%	176
Northwest Hospital and Medical Center	Seattle	73%	145
Southwest Washington Medical Center	Vancouver	73%	156
Sunnyside Community Hospital	Sunnyside	72%	36
Harrison Medical Center	Bremerton	70%	371
Harborview Medical Center	Seattle	68%	177
Valley Hospital & Medical Center	Spokane	68%	110
Enumclaw Regional Hospital	Enumclaw	67%	33
Valley Medical Center	Renton	61%	239
Providence Everett Medical Center	Everett	57%	152
University of Washington Medical Center	Seattle	47%	173

17. Oxygenation Assessment

Hospital Name	City	Rate	Cases
Auburn Regional Medical Center	Auburn	100%	201
Capital Medical Center	Olympia	100%	67
Cascade Valley Hosp/N Snohomish Co Sys	Arlington	100%	93
Central Washington Hospital	Wenatchee	100%	206
Deaconess Medical Center	Spokane	100%	186
Enumclaw Regional Hospital	Enumclaw	100%	42
Evergreen Hospital Medical Center	Kirkland	100%	254
Grays Harbor Community Hospital-West Campus	Aberdeen	100%	254
Group Health Eastside Hospital	Redmond	100%	177
Harborview Medical Center	Seattle	100%	214
Harrison Medical Center	Bremerton	100%	448
Highline Community Hospital	Burien	100%	318
Holy Family Hospital	Spokane	100%	393
Island Hospital	Anacortes	100%	114
Jefferson General Hospital	Port Townsend	100%	77
Kadlec Medical Center	Richland	100%	211
Kennewick General Hospital	Kennewick	100%	157
Kittitas Valley Community Hospital	Ellensburg	100%	36
Legacy Salmon Creek Hospital	Vancouver	100%	161
Mason General Hospital	Shelton	100%	99
Mount Carmel Hospital	Colville	100%	112
Northwest Hospital and Medical Center	Seattle	100%	188
Olympic Medical Center	Port Angeles	100%	269
Overlake Hospital Medical Center	Bellevue	100%	245
Providence Centralia Hospital	Centralia	100%	226
Providence Everett Medical Center	Everett	100%	189
Pullman Memorial Hospital	Pullman	100%	42
Sacred Heart Medical Center	Spokane	100%	476
Saint Clare Hospital	Lakewood	100%	327
Saint Francis Hospital	Federal Way	100%	181
Saint John Medical Center	Longview	100%	428
Saint Joseph Hospital	Bellingham	100%	372
Saint Joseph Medical Center	Tacoma	100%	392
Saint Joseph's Hospital	Chewelah	100%	100
Saint Mary Medical Center	Walla Walla	100%	129
Samaritan Healthcare	Moses Lake	100%	103
Skagit Valley Hospital	Mount Vernon	100%	195
Southwest Washington Medical Center	Vancouver	100%	204
Stevens Hospital	Edmonds	100%	272
Sunnyside Community Hospital	Sunnyside	100%	37
Swedish Medical Center	Seattle	100%	506
Swedish Medical Center/Providence	Seattle	100%	142
Tacoma General Hospital	Tacoma	100%	405
Toppenish Community Hospital	Toppenish	100%	94
Tri-State Memorial Hospital	Clarkston	100%	63
United General Hospital	Sedro Woolley	100%	113
University of Washington Medical Center	Seattle	100%	200
Valley General Hospital	Monroe	100%	83
Valley Hospital & Medical Center	Spokane	100%	152
Valley Medical Center	Renton	100%	284
Virginia Mason Medical Center	Seattle	100%	352
Walla Walla General Hospital	Walla Walla	100%	70
Whidbey General Hospital	Coupeville	100%	101

NOTE: Hospital profiles are in alphabetical order by state, then city, then hospital within the city; Rankings are sorted by rate in descending order and exclude hospitals with less than 25 cases; (1) The number of cases is too small (n<25) for purposes of reliably predicting hospital performance; (2) Measure reflects the hospital's indication that its submission was based upon a sample of its relevant discharges; (3) Rate reflects fewer than the maximum possible quarters of data for the measure; (4) Inaccurate information submitted and suppressed for one or more quarters; (5) No data is available from the hospital for this measure; Please refer to the User's Guide for a full explanation of data

Hospital Name	City	Rate	Cases
Yakima Regional Medical & Cardiac Center	Yakima	100%	144
Yakima Valley Memorial Hospital	Yakima	100%	333
Good Samaritan Hospital & Rehab Center	Puyallup	99%	229
Lourdes Medical Center	Pasco	99%	83
Providence Saint Peter Hospital	Olympia	99%	401

18. Pneumococcal Vaccine

Hospital Name	City	Rate	Cases
Mount Carmel Hospital	Colville	99%	80
Island Hospital	Anacortes	96%	85
United General Hospital	Sedro Woolley	96%	79
Group Health Eastside Hospital	Redmond	92%	163
Northwest Hospital and Medical Center	Seattle	92%	125
Saint Joseph Hospital	Bellingham	89%	267
Evergreen Hospital Medical Center	Kirkland	88%	146
Kennewick General Hospital	Kennewick	88%	109
Kadlec Medical Center	Richland	86%	123
Saint Joseph's Hospital	Chewelah	86%	57
Highline Community Hospital	Burien	85%	199
Providence Centralia Hospital	Centralia	85%	145
Central Washington Hospital	Wenatchee	84%	154
Holy Family Hospital	Spokane	83%	252
Mason General Hospital	Shelton	83%	58
Saint Francis Hospital	Federal Way	82%	105
Valley General Hospital	Monroe	82%	49
Skagit Valley Hospital	Mount Vernon	81%	135
Sacred Heart Medical Center	Spokane	80%	285
Harrison Medical Center	Bremerton	79%	325
Saint Clare Hospital	Lakewood	79%	205
Saint Mary Medical Center	Walla Walla	78%	77
Providence Everett Medical Center	Everett	77%	125
Saint Joseph Medical Center	Tacoma	74%	209
Toppenish Community Hospital	Toppenish	74%	46
Stevens Hospital	Edmonds	73%	174
Yakima Regional Medical & Cardiac Center	Yakima	73%	79
Swedish Medical Center	Seattle	71%	329
Tri-State Memorial Hospital	Clarkston	71%	49
Yakima Valley Memorial Hospital	Yakima	71%	221
Olympic Medical Center	Port Angeles	69%	199
Walla Walla General Hospital	Walla Walla	67%	48
Southwest Washington Medical Center	Vancouver	66%	145
Capital Medical Center	Olympia	65%	43
Jefferson General Hospital	Port Townsend	62%	50
Providence Saint Peter Hospital	Olympia	62%	261
Saint John Medical Center	Longview	62%	227
Auburn Regional Medical Center	Auburn	61%	111
Valley Hospital & Medical Center	Spokane	61%	98
Virginia Mason Medical Center	Seattle	61%	266
Deaconess Medical Center	Spokane	60%	125
Swedish Medical Center/Providence	Seattle	60%	90
Legacy Salmon Creek Hospital	Vancouver	59%	112
Enumclaw Regional Hospital	Enumclaw	58%	26
Valley Medical Center	Renton	57%	169
Cascade Valley Hosp/N Snohomish Co Sys	Arlington	49%	65
Harborview Medical Center	Seattle	46%	68
Good Samaritan Hospital & Rehab Center	Puyallup	45%	140
Grays Harbor Community Hospital-West Campus	Aberdeen	44%	153
Lourdes Medical Center	Pasco	44%	54
Whidbey General Hospital	Coupeville	44%	79
Samaritan Healthcare	Moses Lake	41%	61
University of Washington Medical Center	Seattle	38%	87
Pullman Memorial Hospital	Pullman	34%	32
Tacoma General Hospital	Tacoma	27%	224
Overlake Hospital Medical Center	Bellevue	23%	175

19. Smoking Cessation Advice

Hospital Name	City	Rate	Cases
Sacred Heart Medical Center	Spokane	100%	112
University of Washington Medical Center	Seattle	100%	51
Saint John Medical Center	Longview	98%	102
Virginia Mason Medical Center	Seattle	98%	61
Yakima Regional Medical & Cardiac Center	Yakima	98%	56
Highline Community Hospital	Burien	97%	74
Saint Joseph Hospital	Bellingham	97%	73
Valley Hospital & Medical Center	Spokane	97%	33
Yakima Valley Memorial Hospital	Yakima	97%	78
Kennewick General Hospital	Kennewick	96%	25
Saint Joseph's Hospital	Chewelah	93%	27
Central Washington Hospital	Wenatchee	92%	50
Holy Family Hospital	Spokane	92%	95
Providence Everett Medical Center	Everett	92%	60
Skagit Valley Hospital	Mount Vernon	92%	38
Deaconess Medical Center	Spokane	88%	58
Swedish Medical Center/Providence	Seattle	87%	45
Saint Francis Hospital	Federal Way	86%	44
Swedish Medical Center	Seattle	86%	116
Cascade Valley Hosp/N Snohomish Co Sys	Arlington	85%	34
Tacoma General Hospital	Tacoma	85%	116
Providence Centralia Hospital	Centralia	84%	49
Saint Clare Hospital	Lakewood	83%	94
Saint Joseph Medical Center	Tacoma	82%	112
Evergreen Hospital Medical Center	Kirkland	81%	43
Legacy Salmon Creek Hospital	Vancouver	81%	36
Olympic Medical Center	Port Angeles	79%	52
Northwest Hospital and Medical Center	Seattle	78%	41
Southwest Washington Medical Center	Vancouver	77%	52
Stevens Hospital	Edmonds	72%	57
Saint Mary Medical Center	Walla Walla	71%	34
Overlake Hospital Medical Center	Bellevue	70%	40
Harborview Medical Center	Seattle	66%	119
Grays Harbor Community Hospital-West Campus	Aberdeen	64%	72
Good Samaritan Hospital & Rehab Center	Puyallup	61%	44
Auburn Regional Medical Center	Auburn	57%	44
Harrison Medical Center	Bremerton	56%	114
Providence Saint Peter Hospital	Olympia	52%	118

Surgical Infection Prevention

20. Prophylactic Antibiotic Given

Hospital Name	City	Rate	Cases
Wenatchee Valley Hospital	Wenatchee	100%	66
Yakima Valley Memorial Hospital	Yakima	99%	819
Saint Joseph Hospital	Bellingham	97%	804
Toppenish Community Hospital	Toppenish	97%	31
Kittitas Valley Community Hospital	Ellensburg	94%	65
Saint Clare Hospital	Lakewood	94%	314
Yakima Regional Medical & Cardiac Center	Yakima	94%	282
Capital Medical Center	Olympia	93%	91
Highline Community Hospital	Burien	93%	293
Saint Mary Medical Center	Walla Walla	91%	341
Deaconess Medical Center	Spokane	90%	351
Group Health Eastside Hospital	Redmond	90%	199
Providence Everett Medical Center	Everett	90%	225
Sacred Heart Medical Center	Spokane	90%	239
Saint Joseph Medical Center	Tacoma	90%	1348
Jefferson General Hospital	Port Townsend	89%	152
Southwest Washington Medical Center	Vancouver	89%	243
Valley Hospital & Medical Center	Spokane	89%	227
Auburn Regional Medical Center	Auburn	88%	388
Mount Carmel Hospital	Colville	88%	25
Holy Family Hospital	Spokane	87%	151
Walla Walla General Hospital	Walla Walla	87%	110
Central Washington Hospital	Wenatchee	86%	285
Harrison Medical Center	Bremerton	86%	792
Providence Saint Peter Hospital	Olympia	86%	310
Saint Francis Hospital	Federal Way	86%	251
Whidbey General Hospital	Coupeville	84%	62
Evergreen Hospital Medical Center	Kirkland	83%	128
Valley General Hospital	Monroe	83%	75
University of Washington Medical Center	Seattle	81%	343
Olympic Medical Center	Port Angeles	80%	319
Saint John Medical Center	Longview	80%	152
Kennewick General Hospital	Kennewick	79%	162
Skagit Valley Hospital	Mount Vernon	79%	355
Stevens Hospital	Edmonds	79%	490
Swedish Medical Center	Seattle	79%	270
Tacoma General Hospital	Tacoma	78%	539
Grays Harbor Community Hospital-West Campus	Aberdeen	77%	146
Harborview Medical Center	Seattle	76%	133
Northwest Hospital and Medical Center	Seattle	76%	363
Swedish Medical Center/Providence	Seattle	73%	149
Kadlec Medical Center	Richland	70%	60
Virginia Mason Medical Center	Seattle	70%	524
Island Hospital	Anacortes	69%	35
Legacy Salmon Creek Hospital	Vancouver	67%	93
Providence Centralia Hospital	Centralia	67%	203
Valley Medical Center	Renton	67%	64
Samaritan Healthcare	Moses Lake	64%	213
Overlake Hospital Medical Center	Bellevue	63%	220
Cascade Valley Hosp/N Snohomish Co Sys	Arlington	56%	63
Good Samaritan Hospital & Rehab Center	Puyallup	55%	247

21. Prophylactic Antibiotic Selection

Hospital Name	City	Rate	Cases
Swedish Medical Center/Providence	Seattle	100%	60
Walla Walla General Hospital	Walla Walla	100%	41
Highline Community Hospital	Burien	99%	99
Central Washington Hospital	Wenatchee	98%	104

NOTE: Hospital profiles are in alphabetical order by state, then city, then hospital within the city; Rankings are sorted by rate in descending order and exclude hospitals with less than 25 cases; (1) The number of cases is too small (n<25) for purposes of reliably predicting hospital performance; (2) Measure reflects the hospital's indication that its submission was based upon a sample of its relevant discharges; (3) Rate reflects fewer than the maximum possible quarters of data for the measure; (4) Inaccurate information submitted and suppressed for one or more quarters; (5) No data is available from the hospital for this measure; Please refer to the User's Guide for a full explanation of data

Hospital Name	City	Rate	Cases
Saint Joseph Hospital	Bellingham	98%	261
Samaritan Healthcare	Moses Lake	98%	47
Swedish Medical Center	Seattle	98%	93
Yakima Regional Medical & Cardiac Center	Yakima	98%	50
Saint Mary Medical Center	Walla Walla	97%	64
Southwest Washington Medical Center	Vancouver	97%	77
Valley Hospital & Medical Center	Spokane	97%	66
Yakima Valley Memorial Hospital	Yakima	97%	192
Auburn Regional Medical Center	Auburn	96%	98
Capital Medical Center	Olympia	96%	93
Deaconess Medical Center	Spokane	96%	103
Good Samaritan Hospital & Rehab Center	Puyallup	96%	90
Providence Centralia Hospital	Centralia	96%	72
Sacred Heart Medical Center	Spokane	96%	84
Saint Clare Hospital	Lakewood	96%	46
Saint Francis Hospital	Federal Way	96%	56
Saint Joseph Medical Center	Tacoma	96%	252
Evergreen Hospital Medical Center	Kirkland	95%	39
Providence Everett Medical Center	Everett	95%	82
Tacoma General Hospital	Tacoma	95%	157
Holy Family Hospital	Spokane	94%	47
Virginia Mason Medical Center	Seattle	94%	134
Grays Harbor Community Hospital-West Campus	Aberdeen	92%	53
Island Hospital	Anacortes	92%	36
Kennewick General Hospital	Kennewick	92%	59
Providence Saint Peter Hospital	Olympia	92%	132
University of Washington Medical Center	Seattle	92%	74
Legacy Salmon Creek Hospital	Vancouver	91%	46
Valley Medical Center	Renton	91%	66
Cascade Valley Hosp/N Snohomish Co Sys	Arlington	90%	30
Saint John Medical Center	Longview	88%	155
Stevens Hospital	Edmonds	88%	111
Overlake Hospital Medical Center	Bellevue	85%	79
Harborview Medical Center	Seattle	83%	36
Northwest Hospital and Medical Center	Seattle	83%	60
Skagit Valley Hospital	Mount Vernon	83%	54
Olympic Medical Center	Port Angeles	81%	70
Valley General Hospital	Monroe	81%	31
Jefferson General Hospital	Port Townsend	76%	46
Harrison Medical Center	Bremerton	74%	297

22. Prophylactic Antibiotic Stopped

Hospital Name	City	Rate	Cases
Wenatchee Valley Hospital	Wenatchee	100%	66
Highline Community Hospital	Burien	94%	283
Saint Joseph Hospital	Bellingham	93%	782
Olympic Medical Center	Port Angeles	91%	306
Saint Clare Hospital	Lakewood	91%	303
Virginia Mason Medical Center	Seattle	91%	496
Sacred Heart Medical Center	Spokane	90%	233
Valley Hospital & Medical Center	Spokane	88%	222
Good Samaritan Hospital & Rehab Center	Puyallup	87%	222
Skagit Valley Hospital	Mount Vernon	86%	341
Island Hospital	Anacortes	85%	33
Kittitas Valley Community Hospital	Ellensburg	85%	62
Providence Centralia Hospital	Centralia	85%	184
Saint Mary Medical Center	Walla Walla	84%	329
Valley Medical Center	Renton	84%	64
Yakima Valley Memorial Hospital	Yakima	84%	806
Group Health Eastside Hospital	Redmond	83%	192
Holy Family Hospital	Spokane	82%	145
Providence Everett Medical Center	Everett	82%	214
Auburn Regional Medical Center	Auburn	81%	388
Toppenish Community Hospital	Toppenish	81%	31
Valley General Hospital	Monroe	81%	73
Whidbey General Hospital	Coupeville	81%	59
Overlake Hospital Medical Center	Bellevue	80%	210
Saint John Medical Center	Longview	80%	146
Evergreen Hospital Medical Center	Kirkland	79%	123
Walla Walla General Hospital	Walla Walla	79%	109
Harborview Medical Center	Seattle	78%	131
Central Washington Hospital	Wenatchee	77%	282
Saint Francis Hospital	Federal Way	77%	248
Southwest Washington Medical Center	Vancouver	77%	232
Grays Harbor Community Hospital-West Campus	Aberdeen	75%	138
Saint Joseph Medical Center	Tacoma	75%	1295
Kadlec Medical Center	Richland	74%	57
Stevens Hospital	Edmonds	73%	478
Tacoma General Hospital	Tacoma	70%	514
Swedish Medical Center/Providence	Seattle	69%	145
Cascade Valley Hosp/N Snohomish Co Sys	Arlington	68%	60
Deaconess Medical Center	Spokane	68%	345
Mount Carmel Hospital	Colville	68%	25
Capital Medical Center	Olympia	67%	90
Harrison Medical Center	Bremerton	65%	761
Jefferson General Hospital	Port Townsend	65%	151
Providence Saint Peter Hospital	Olympia	60%	305
Yakima Regional Medical & Cardiac Center	Yakima	59%	280
Northwest Hospital and Medical Center	Seattle	56%	349
University of Washington Medical Center	Seattle	56%	331
Swedish Medical Center	Seattle	52%	263
Samaritan Healthcare	Moses Lake	48%	207
Kennewick General Hospital	Kennewick	47%	152
Legacy Salmon Creek Hospital	Vancouver	47%	86

Pregnancy Care

23. Inpatient Neonatal Mortality

Hospital Name	City	Rate	Cases
Highline Community Hospital	Burien	0.00%	1252
Holy Family Hospital	Spokane	0.00%	1150
Northwest Hospital and Medical Center	Seattle	0.00%	999
Saint Mary Medical Center	Walla Walla	0.00%	635
Overlake Hospital Medical Center	Bellevue	0.02%	4155
Saint Joseph Medical Center	Tacoma	0.02%	5174
Southwest Washington Medical Center	Vancouver	0.02%	4044
Stevens Hospital	Edmonds	0.08%	1208
Providence Everett Medical Center	Everett	0.13%	1516
Valley Medical Center	Renton	0.14%	3571
Walla Walla General Hospital	Walla Walla	0.31%	323
Valley General Hospital	Monroe	0.50%	401
Tacoma General Hospital	Tacoma	0.72%	3316

24. Third or Fourth Degree Laceration

Hospital Name	City	Rate	Cases
Valley General Hospital	Monroe	1.76%	284
Highline Community Hospital	Burien	1.90%	843
Holy Family Hospital	Spokane	2.63%	876
Saint Mary Medical Center	Walla Walla	2.84%	457
Walla Walla General Hospital	Walla Walla	3.00%	233
Saint Joseph Medical Center	Tacoma	3.07%	3741
Providence Everett Medical Center	Everett	3.16%	1013
Tacoma General Hospital	Tacoma	3.79%	2113
Southwest Washington Medical Center	Vancouver	4.13%	2909
Valley Medical Center	Renton	4.19%	2243
Stevens Hospital	Edmonds	4.50%	866
Overlake Hospital Medical Center	Bellevue	5.66%	2703
Northwest Hospital and Medical Center	Seattle	6.75%	696

NOTE: Hospital profiles are in alphabetical order by state, then city, then hospital within the city; Rankings are sorted by rate in descending order and exclude hospitals with less than 25 cases; (1) The number of cases is too small (n<25) for purposes of reliably predicting hospital performance; (2) Measure reflects the hospital's indication that its submission was based upon a sample of its relevant discharges; (3) Rate reflects fewer than the maximum possible quarters of data for the measure; (4) Inaccurate information submitted and suppressed for one or more quarters; (5) No data is available from the hospital for this measure; Please refer to the User's Guide for a full explanation of data

Grays Harbor Community Hospital-West Campus

915 Anderson Drive
Aberdeen, WA 98520
Phone: 360-537-8330
Fax: 360-537-5039
URL: www.ghchwa.org
Ownership: Voluntary non-profit - Other
Accredited: Yes
Emergency Services: Yes
Licensed Beds: 200

Key Personnel:

President/CEO . . . . John Mitchell
Chief Medical Staff . . . . Timothy Troeh, MD
Emergency Room . . . . Murray Rice, MD
Director Infection/Disease Control . . . . Lin Boulay, RN
CCU Spvg. Nurse . . . . Mary Lynn Kluver
Director Medical/Surgical Nursing . . . . Ruth Fischer, RN
Chief Radiology . . . . Michael Cagan, MD
Director Cardio-Pulmonary Services . . . . Dan Lightfoot

Measure	Cases	This Hospital	State Average	U.S. Average	Top Hospital
Heart Attack Care					
ACE Inhibitor or ARB for LVSD[1]	2	100%	84%	82%	100%
Aspirin at Arrival	50	78%	95%	92%	100%
Aspirin at Discharge[1]	22	82%	95%	90%	100%
Beta Blocker at Arrival	43	86%	91%	87%	100%
Beta Blocker at Discharge[1]	24	83%	95%	90%	100%
Fibrinolytic Medication Timing[1]	9	22%	28%	31%	100%
PCI Within 90 Minutes of Arrival	0	-	60%	54%	95%
Smoking Cessation Advice[1]	9	67%	85%	88%	100%
Heart Failure Care					
ACE Inhibitor or ARB for LVSD	41	90%	85%	82%	100%
Discharge Instructions	192	32%	53%	61%	93%
Evaluation of LVS Function	224	72%	85%	83%	99%
Smoking Cessation Advice	43	72%	75%	82%	100%
Pneumonia Care					
Appropriate Initial Antibiotic	189	74%	82%	83%	94%
Blood Culture Timing	116	95%	91%	90%	100%
Influenza Vaccine	45	38%	60%	70%	100%
Initial Antibiotic Timing	231	80%	77%	80%	93%
Oxygenation Assessment	254	100%	100%	99%	100%
Pneumococcal Vaccine	153	44%	68%	69%	94%
Smoking Cessation Advice	72	64%	79%	80%	100%
Surgical Infection Prevention					
Prophylactic Antibiotic Given[3]	146	77%	82%	77%	95%
Prophylactic Antibiotic Selection	53	92%	91%	90%	100%
Prophylactic Antibiotic Stopped[3]	138	75%	75%	72%	95%
Pregnancy Care					
Inpatient Neonatal Mortality	-	-	-	-	-
Third or Fourth Degree Laceration	-	-	3.98%	3.63%	3.27%

Island Hospital

1211 24th Street
Anacortes, WA 98221
Phone: 360-299-1325
Fax: 360-299-1384
E-mail: kitm@island-health.org
URL: www.islandhealth.org
Ownership: Govt - Hospital District or Authority
Accredited: Yes
Emergency Services: Yes
Licensed Beds: 44

Key Personnel:

CEO/President . . . . Vincent C Oliver
Chief Medical Staff . . . . Judy Tempelton
Director of Cardiology/Cardiac Lab . . . . Richard E Gubner
Emergency Room . . . . Vicky Nostrant
Emergency Room . . . . R Apter, MD
Director Infection/Disease Control . . . . Gary Preston
CCU Spvg. Nurse . . . . Lois Pate
Director Medical/Surgical Nursing . . . . Bojan Kuure, RN
OB/GYN Womens Health . . . . R Prins, MD
Director Respiratory Therapy . . . . Bruce Cox

Measure	Cases	This Hospital	State Average	U.S. Average	Top Hospital
Heart Attack Care					
ACE Inhibitor or ARB for LVSD[1]	4	100%	84%	82%	100%
Aspirin at Arrival[1]	19	84%	95%	92%	100%
Aspirin at Discharge[1]	13	100%	95%	90%	100%
Beta Blocker at Arrival[1]	16	88%	91%	87%	100%
Beta Blocker at Discharge[1]	17	100%	95%	90%	100%
Fibrinolytic Medication Timing	0	-	28%	31%	100%
PCI Within 90 Minutes of Arrival	0	-	60%	54%	95%
Smoking Cessation Advice[1]	1	0%	85%	88%	100%
Heart Failure Care					
ACE Inhibitor or ARB for LVSD[1]	12	75%	85%	82%	100%
Discharge Instructions	38	47%	53%	61%	93%
Evaluation of LVS Function	44	84%	85%	83%	99%
Smoking Cessation Advice[1]	4	100%	75%	82%	100%
Pneumonia Care					
Appropriate Initial Antibiotic	63	81%	82%	83%	94%
Blood Culture Timing	64	88%	91%	90%	100%
Influenza Vaccine[1]	23	83%	60%	70%	100%
Initial Antibiotic Timing	84	74%	77%	80%	93%
Oxygenation Assessment	114	100%	100%	99%	100%
Pneumococcal Vaccine	85	96%	68%	69%	94%
Smoking Cessation Advice[1]	21	100%	79%	80%	100%
Surgical Infection Prevention					
Prophylactic Antibiotic Given[3]	35	69%	82%	77%	95%
Prophylactic Antibiotic Selection	36	92%	91%	90%	100%
Prophylactic Antibiotic Stopped[3]	33	85%	75%	72%	95%
Pregnancy Care					
Inpatient Neonatal Mortality	-	-	-	-	-
Third or Fourth Degree Laceration	-	-	3.98%	3.63%	3.27%

Cascade Valley Hosp/N Snohomish Co Sys

330 S Stillaguamish Avenue
Arlington, WA 98223
Phone: 360-435-2133
Fax: 360-435-0513
Ownership: Govt - Hospital District or Authority
Accredited: Yes
Emergency Services: Yes
Licensed Beds: 48

Key Personnel:

Administrator . . . . Patti Brache
Chief Medical Staff . . . . Roff Hartling
Emergency Room . . . . Gerald Hook
Respiratory . . . . Emmanuel Yruma

Measure	Cases	This Hospital	State Average	U.S. Average	Top Hospital
Heart Attack Care					
ACE Inhibitor or ARB for LVSD[1]	2	50%	84%	82%	100%
Aspirin at Arrival[1]	19	89%	95%	92%	100%
Aspirin at Discharge[1]	16	100%	95%	90%	100%
Beta Blocker at Arrival[1]	13	85%	91%	87%	100%
Beta Blocker at Discharge[1]	17	88%	95%	90%	100%
Fibrinolytic Medication Timing	0	-	28%	31%	100%
PCI Within 90 Minutes of Arrival	0	-	60%	54%	95%
Smoking Cessation Advice[1]	4	75%	85%	88%	100%
Heart Failure Care					
ACE Inhibitor or ARB for LVSD[1]	12	67%	85%	82%	100%
Discharge Instructions	43	44%	53%	61%	93%
Evaluation of LVS Function	61	75%	85%	83%	99%
Smoking Cessation Advice[1]	11	36%	75%	82%	100%
Pneumonia Care					
Appropriate Initial Antibiotic	58	50%	82%	83%	94%
Blood Culture Timing	54	87%	91%	90%	100%
Influenza Vaccine[1]	14	14%	60%	70%	100%
Initial Antibiotic Timing	72	85%	77%	80%	93%
Oxygenation Assessment	93	100%	100%	99%	100%
Pneumococcal Vaccine	65	49%	68%	69%	94%
Smoking Cessation Advice	34	85%	79%	80%	100%
Surgical Infection Prevention					
Prophylactic Antibiotic Given[3]	63	56%	82%	77%	95%
Prophylactic Antibiotic Selection	30	90%	91%	90%	100%
Prophylactic Antibiotic Stopped[3]	60	68%	75%	72%	95%
Pregnancy Care					
Inpatient Neonatal Mortality	-	-	-	-	-
Third or Fourth Degree Laceration	-	-	3.98%	3.63%	3.27%

Auburn Regional Medical Center

Alternate Name: Auburn General Hospital

NOTE: Hospital profiles are in alphabetical order by state, then city, then hospital within the city; Rankings are sorted by rate in descending order and exclude hospitals with less than 25 cases; (1) The number of cases is too small (n<25) for purposes of reliably predicting hospital performance; (2) Measure reflects the hospital's indication that its submission was based upon a sample of its relevant discharges; (3) Rate reflects fewer than the maximum possible quarters of data for the measure; (4) Inaccurate information submitted and suppressed for one or more quarters; (5) No data is available from the hospital for this measure; Please refer to the User's Guide for a full explanation of data

Plaza One, 202 N Division Street
Auburn, WA 98001
URL: www.armcuhs.com/p1.html
Ownership: Proprietary
Emergency Services: Yes
Phone: 253-833-7711
Fax: 253-939-2376
Accredited: Yes
Licensed Beds: 149

Key Personnel:
CEO . . . . Leonard Freehof
Emergency Room . . . . Vicki Seaman
Infection Control . . . . Beth Scott
Medical Surgical Nursing . . . . Debbie Gibbons
Respiratory/Cardiopulmonary . . . . Andre House

Measure	Cases	This Hospital	State Average	U.S. Average	Top Hospital
Heart Attack Care					
ACE Inhibitor or ARB for LVSD	55	62%	84%	82%	100%
Aspirin at Arrival	142	93%	95%	92%	100%
Aspirin at Discharge	118	97%	95%	90%	100%
Beta Blocker at Arrival	147	95%	91%	87%	100%
Beta Blocker at Discharge	119	89%	95%	90%	100%
Fibrinolytic Medication Timing	27	52%	28%	31%	100%
PCI Within 90 Minutes of Arrival[1]	10	20%	60%	54%	95%
Smoking Cessation Advice	42	81%	85%	88%	100%
Heart Failure Care					
ACE Inhibitor or ARB for LVSD	79	76%	85%	82%	100%
Discharge Instructions	124	56%	53%	61%	93%
Evaluation of LVS Function	156	70%	85%	83%	99%
Smoking Cessation Advice	33	85%	75%	82%	100%
Pneumonia Care					
Appropriate Initial Antibiotic	159	79%	82%	83%	94%
Blood Culture Timing	97	86%	91%	90%	100%
Influenza Vaccine	32	53%	60%	70%	100%
Initial Antibiotic Timing	163	82%	77%	80%	93%
Oxygenation Assessment	201	100%	100%	99%	100%
Pneumococcal Vaccine	111	61%	68%	69%	94%
Smoking Cessation Advice	44	57%	79%	80%	100%
Surgical Infection Prevention					
Prophylactic Antibiotic Given	388	88%	82%	77%	95%
Prophylactic Antibiotic Selection	98	96%	91%	90%	100%
Prophylactic Antibiotic Stopped	388	81%	75%	72%	95%
Pregnancy Care					
Inpatient Neonatal Mortality	-	-	-	-	-
Third or Fourth Degree Laceration	-	-	3.98%	3.63%	3.27%

Overlake Hospital Medical Center

1035 116th Avenue NE
Bellevue, WA 98004
URL: www.overlakehospital.org
Ownership: Voluntary non-profit - Other
Emergency Services: Yes
Phone: 425-688-5000
Fax: 425-688-5959
Accredited: Yes
Licensed Beds: 337

Key Personnel:
President/CEO . . . . Kenneth Graham
Chief Medical Staff . . . . Walter Smith, MD
Chairperson of Cardiology . . . . Peter Kures, MD
Catheterization Lab . . . . Randy Schwartz, MD
Infection Control . . . . Peter Hashisaki, MD
Director Woman/Child Services . . . . Julie Wehmeyer, MD
Director Surgical Services . . . . Mahin Wright
Director Respiratory Therapy . . . . Terry Smith

Measure	Cases	This Hospital	State Average	U.S. Average	Top Hospital
Heart Attack Care					
ACE Inhibitor or ARB for LVSD	77	78%	84%	82%	100%
Aspirin at Arrival	213	94%	95%	92%	100%
Aspirin at Discharge	253	98%	95%	90%	100%
Beta Blocker at Arrival	149	86%	91%	87%	100%
Beta Blocker at Discharge	265	97%	95%	90%	100%
Fibrinolytic Medication Timing[1]	2	0%	28%	31%	100%
PCI Within 90 Minutes of Arrival[1]	13	46%	60%	54%	95%
Smoking Cessation Advice	59	92%	85%	88%	100%
Heart Failure Care					
ACE Inhibitor or ARB for LVSD	134	77%	85%	82%	100%
Discharge Instructions	269	16%	53%	61%	93%
Evaluation of LVS Function	344	97%	85%	83%	99%
Smoking Cessation Advice[1]	22	68%	75%	82%	100%
Pneumonia Care					
Appropriate Initial Antibiotic	130	82%	82%	83%	94%
Blood Culture Timing	142	98%	91%	90%	100%
Influenza Vaccine	53	19%	60%	70%	100%
Initial Antibiotic Timing	197	76%	77%	80%	93%
Oxygenation Assessment	245	100%	100%	99%	100%
Pneumococcal Vaccine	175	23%	68%	69%	94%
Smoking Cessation Advice	40	70%	79%	80%	100%
Surgical Infection Prevention					
Prophylactic Antibiotic Given[2,3]	220	63%	82%	77%	95%
Prophylactic Antibiotic Selection[2]	79	85%	91%	90%	100%
Prophylactic Antibiotic Stopped[2,3]	210	80%	75%	72%	95%
Pregnancy Care					
Inpatient Neonatal Mortality	4,155	0.02%	-	-	-
Third or Fourth Degree Laceration	2,703	5.66%	3.98%	3.63%	3.27%

Saint Joseph Hospital

2901 Squalicum Parkway
Bellingham, WA 98225
Ownership: Voluntary non-profit - Other
Emergency Services: Yes
Phone: 360-734-5400
Fax: 360-738-6393
Accredited: Yes
Licensed Beds: 253

Key Personnel:
Administrator/CEO . . . . Nancy Bitting
Chief Medical Staff . . . . Ian Thompson, MD
Director Emergency Room . . . . Pat Wentworth
Emergency Room . . . . Greg Brown, MD

Measure	Cases	This Hospital	State Average	U.S. Average	Top Hospital
Heart Attack Care					
ACE Inhibitor or ARB for LVSD	59	95%	84%	82%	100%
Aspirin at Arrival	283	100%	95%	92%	100%
Aspirin at Discharge	306	98%	95%	90%	100%
Beta Blocker at Arrival	237	98%	91%	87%	100%
Beta Blocker at Discharge	318	99%	95%	90%	100%
Fibrinolytic Medication Timing[1]	1	100%	28%	31%	100%
PCI Within 90 Minutes of Arrival[1]	14	71%	60%	54%	95%
Smoking Cessation Advice	82	90%	85%	88%	100%
Heart Failure Care					
ACE Inhibitor or ARB for LVSD	174	95%	85%	82%	100%
Discharge Instructions	268	71%	53%	61%	93%
Evaluation of LVS Function	337	99%	85%	83%	99%
Smoking Cessation Advice	49	92%	75%	82%	100%
Pneumonia Care					
Appropriate Initial Antibiotic	172	89%	82%	83%	94%
Blood Culture Timing	180	97%	91%	90%	100%
Influenza Vaccine	61	82%	60%	70%	100%
Initial Antibiotic Timing	318	81%	77%	80%	93%
Oxygenation Assessment	372	100%	100%	99%	100%
Pneumococcal Vaccine	267	89%	68%	69%	94%
Smoking Cessation Advice	73	97%	79%	80%	100%
Surgical Infection Prevention					
Prophylactic Antibiotic Given[3]	804	97%	82%	77%	95%
Prophylactic Antibiotic Selection	261	98%	91%	90%	100%
Prophylactic Antibiotic Stopped[3]	782	93%	75%	72%	95%
Pregnancy Care					
Inpatient Neonatal Mortality	-	-	-	-	-
Third or Fourth Degree Laceration	-	-	3.98%	3.63%	3.27%

Harrison Medical Center

2520 Cherry Avenue
Bremerton, WA 98310
E-mail: ljull@hmh.westsound.net
URL: www.harrisonhospital.org
Ownership: Voluntary non-profit - Private
Emergency Services: Yes
Phone: 360-377-3911
Fax: 360-792-6515
Accredited: Yes
Licensed Beds: 297

Key Personnel:
President/CEO . . . . Scott Bosch
Chief Medical Staff . . . . Mark Abrams
Director Medical/Surgical Nursing . . . . Doris Babcock, RN
OB/GYN Womens Health . . . . Glen Christen, MD
Chief Radiology . . . . David Matsenbaugh, MD
Director Respiratory Therapy . . . . Eric Anderson

NOTE: Hospital profiles are in alphabetical order by state, then city, then hospital within the city; Rankings are sorted by rate in descending order and exclude hospitals with less than 25 cases; (1) The number of cases is too small (n<25) for purposes of reliably predicting hospital performance; (2) Measure reflects the hospital's indication that its submission was based upon a sample of its relevant discharges; (3) Rate reflects fewer than the maximum possible quarters of data for the measure; (4) Inaccurate information submitted and suppressed for one or more quarters; (5) No data is available from the hospital for this measure; Please refer to the User's Guide for a full explanation of data

Measure	Cases	This Hospital	State Average	U.S. Average	Top Hospital
Heart Attack Care					
ACE Inhibitor or ARB for LVSD	47	91%	84%	82%	100%
Aspirin at Arrival	239	95%	95%	92%	100%
Aspirin at Discharge	288	98%	95%	90%	100%
Beta Blocker at Arrival	209	96%	91%	87%	100%
Beta Blocker at Discharge	304	98%	95%	90%	100%
Fibrinolytic Medication Timing	0	-	28%	31%	100%
PCI Within 90 Minutes of Arrival[1]	12	58%	60%	54%	95%
Smoking Cessation Advice	85	86%	85%	88%	100%
Heart Failure Care					
ACE Inhibitor or ARB for LVSD	151	86%	85%	82%	100%
Discharge Instructions	300	53%	53%	61%	93%
Evaluation of LVS Function	439	91%	85%	83%	99%
Smoking Cessation Advice	60	67%	75%	82%	100%
Pneumonia Care					
Appropriate Initial Antibiotic	246	80%	82%	83%	94%
Blood Culture Timing	251	93%	91%	90%	100%
Influenza Vaccine[4,5]	-	-	60%	70%	100%
Initial Antibiotic Timing	371	70%	77%	80%	93%
Oxygenation Assessment	448	100%	100%	99%	100%
Pneumococcal Vaccine	325	79%	68%	69%	94%
Smoking Cessation Advice	114	56%	79%	80%	100%
Surgical Infection Prevention					
Prophylactic Antibiotic Given[3]	792	86%	82%	77%	95%
Prophylactic Antibiotic Selection	297	74%	91%	90%	100%
Prophylactic Antibiotic Stopped[3]	761	65%	75%	72%	95%
Pregnancy Care					
Inpatient Neonatal Mortality	-	-	-	-	-
Third or Fourth Degree Laceration	-	-	3.98%	3.63%	3.27%

Highline Community Hospital

16251 Sylvester Road SW
Burien, WA 98166
Phone: 206-244-9970
Fax: 206-246-5385
URL: www.hchnet.org
Ownership: Voluntary non-profit - Other
Accredited: Yes
Emergency Services: Yes
Licensed Beds: 296

Key Personnel:

President/CEO . . . . Paul Tucker
Chief Medical Staff . . . . Ismat Rajabali
Emergency Room . . . . Shirley Merkle
Director Infection/Disease Control . . . . Bevelrly Haggan
CCU Spvg. Nurse . . . . Laura McHenry, RN
Director Medical/Surgical Nursing . . . . Candace Smith
Director Respiratory Therapy . . . . John Lovelace

Measure	Cases	This Hospital	State Average	U.S. Average	Top Hospital
Heart Attack Care					
ACE Inhibitor or ARB for LVSD[1]	10	80%	84%	82%	100%
Aspirin at Arrival	85	99%	95%	92%	100%
Aspirin at Discharge	79	94%	95%	90%	100%
Beta Blocker at Arrival	70	99%	91%	87%	100%
Beta Blocker at Discharge	78	92%	95%	90%	100%
Fibrinolytic Medication Timing	0	-	28%	31%	100%
PCI Within 90 Minutes of Arrival[1]	4	100%	60%	54%	95%
Smoking Cessation Advice	30	100%	85%	88%	100%
Heart Failure Care					
ACE Inhibitor or ARB for LVSD	57	74%	85%	82%	100%
Discharge Instructions	157	48%	53%	61%	93%
Evaluation of LVS Function	186	87%	85%	83%	99%
Smoking Cessation Advice	41	90%	75%	82%	100%
Pneumonia Care					
Appropriate Initial Antibiotic	177	83%	82%	83%	94%
Blood Culture Timing	188	92%	91%	90%	100%
Influenza Vaccine	53	79%	60%	70%	100%
Initial Antibiotic Timing	269	88%	77%	80%	93%
Oxygenation Assessment	318	100%	100%	99%	100%
Pneumococcal Vaccine	199	85%	68%	69%	94%
Smoking Cessation Advice	74	97%	79%	80%	100%
Surgical Infection Prevention					
Prophylactic Antibiotic Given[3]	293	93%	82%	77%	95%
Prophylactic Antibiotic Selection	99	99%	91%	90%	100%
Prophylactic Antibiotic Stopped[3]	283	94%	75%	72%	95%
Pregnancy Care					
Inpatient Neonatal Mortality	1,252	0.00%	-	-	-
Third or Fourth Degree Laceration	843	1.90%	3.98%	3.63%	3.27%

Providence Centralia Hospital

914 S Scheuber Road
Centralia, WA 98531
Toll-Free: 866-321-4790
Phone: 360-736-2803
Fax: 360-330-8576
E-mail: chris.thomas@providence.org
URL: www.providence.org/swsa
Ownership: Voluntary non-profit - Church
Accredited: Yes
Emergency Services: Yes
Licensed Beds: 191

Key Personnel:

President & CEO . . . . Scott Bondn
Chief of Medical Staff . . . . Greg Carter
Chair/Department of Anesthesia/Surgery . . . . . . John McCord, DPM
Manager Emergency Room . . . . John Viglo, RN
Medical Director Emergency Department . . . . . . Doug Hayden
Infection Control . . . . Barbara Wagner
Manager Intensive Coronary Care . . . . Iva Fulmer, RN
Respiratory/Cardiopulmonary . . . . Kumar Arulampalaam

Measure	Cases	This Hospital	State Average	U.S. Average	Top Hospital
Heart Attack Care					
ACE Inhibitor or ARB for LVSD[1]	5	80%	84%	82%	100%
Aspirin at Arrival	43	98%	95%	92%	100%
Aspirin at Discharge	33	94%	95%	90%	100%
Beta Blocker at Arrival	34	85%	91%	87%	100%
Beta Blocker at Discharge	32	97%	95%	90%	100%
Fibrinolytic Medication Timing	0	-	28%	31%	100%
PCI Within 90 Minutes of Arrival	0	-	60%	54%	95%
Smoking Cessation Advice[1]	6	100%	85%	88%	100%
Heart Failure Care					
ACE Inhibitor or ARB for LVSD	50	92%	85%	82%	100%
Discharge Instructions	133	80%	53%	61%	93%
Evaluation of LVS Function	157	92%	85%	83%	99%
Smoking Cessation Advice	25	80%	75%	82%	100%
Pneumonia Care					
Appropriate Initial Antibiotic	154	88%	82%	83%	94%
Blood Culture Timing	109	78%	91%	90%	100%
Influenza Vaccine[1]	24	67%	60%	70%	100%
Initial Antibiotic Timing	180	80%	77%	80%	93%
Oxygenation Assessment	226	100%	100%	99%	100%
Pneumococcal Vaccine	145	85%	68%	69%	94%
Smoking Cessation Advice	49	84%	79%	80%	100%
Surgical Infection Prevention					
Prophylactic Antibiotic Given[2,3]	203	67%	82%	77%	95%
Prophylactic Antibiotic Selection[2]	72	96%	91%	90%	100%
Prophylactic Antibiotic Stopped[2,3]	184	85%	75%	72%	95%
Pregnancy Care					
Inpatient Neonatal Mortality	-	-	-	-	-
Third or Fourth Degree Laceration	-	-	3.98%	3.63%	3.27%

Lake Chelan Community Hospital

503 E Highland Avenue
PO Box 908
Chelan, WA 98816
Phone: 509-682-3300
Fax: 509-682-6116
E-mail: info@lakechelancommunityhospital.com
URL: www.lakechelancommunityhospital.com
Ownership: Govt - Hospital District or Authority
Accredited: No
Emergency Services: Yes
Licensed Beds: 34

Key Personnel:

Administrator . . . . Larry Peterson
Chief Medical Staff . . . . Bill Cagoe
Emergency Room . . . . Nan Bolomney
Director Infection/Disease Control . . . . Lee Tinsley, RN
Director Medical/Surgical Nursing . . . . Teresa Smith, RN

Measure	Cases	This Hospital	State Average	U.S. Average	Top Hospital
Heart Attack Care					
ACE Inhibitor or ARB for LVSD[3]	0	-	84%	82%	100%
Aspirin at Arrival[3]	0	-	95%	92%	100%

NOTE: Hospital profiles are in alphabetical order by state, then city, then hospital within the city; Rankings are sorted by rate in descending order and exclude hospitals with less than 25 cases; (1) The number of cases is too small (n<25) for purposes of reliably predicting hospital performance; (2) Measure reflects the hospital's indication that its submission was based upon a sample of its relevant discharges; (3) Rate reflects fewer than the maximum possible quarters of data for the measure; (4) Inaccurate information submitted and suppressed for one or more quarters; (5) No data is available from the hospital for this measure; Please refer to the User's Guide for a full explanation of data

Aspirin at Discharge[3]	0	-	95%	90%	100%
Beta Blocker at Arrival[3]	0	-	91%	87%	100%
Beta Blocker at Discharge[3]	0	-	95%	90%	100%
Fibrinolytic Medication Timing[1,3]	1	0%	28%	31%	100%
PCI Within 90 Minutes of Arrival	0	-	60%	54%	95%
Smoking Cessation Advice[3]	0	-	85%	88%	100%
Heart Failure Care					
ACE Inhibitor or ARB for LVSD[3]	0	-	85%	82%	100%
Discharge Instructions[1,3]	1	100%	53%	61%	93%
Evaluation of LVS Function[1,3]	2	0%	85%	83%	99%
Smoking Cessation Advice[3]	0	-	75%	82%	100%
Pneumonia Care					
Appropriate Initial Antibiotic[1,3]	3	67%	82%	83%	94%
Blood Culture Timing[1,3]	1	100%	91%	90%	100%
Influenza Vaccine[1]	1	0%	60%	70%	100%
Initial Antibiotic Timing[1,3]	3	100%	77%	80%	93%
Oxygenation Assessment[1,3]	3	100%	100%	99%	100%
Pneumococcal Vaccine[1,3]	2	0%	68%	69%	94%
Smoking Cessation Advice[3]	0	-	79%	80%	100%
Surgical Infection Prevention					
Prophylactic Antibiotic Given[5]	-	-	82%	77%	95%
Prophylactic Antibiotic Selection[5]	-	-	91%	90%	100%
Prophylactic Antibiotic Stopped[5]	-	-	75%	72%	95%
Pregnancy Care					
Inpatient Neonatal Mortality	-	-	-	-	-
Third or Fourth Degree Laceration	-	-	3.98%	3.63%	3.27%

Saint Joseph's Hospital

500 East Webster
PO Box 197
Chewelah, WA 99109
Phone: 509-935-8211
Fax: 509-935-5257
URL: www.sjhospital.org
Ownership: Voluntary non-profit - Church
Accredited: No
Emergency Services: Yes
Licensed Beds: 65

Key Personnel:

Administrator/CEO . . . . Gary V Peck
Chief Medical Staff . . . . Dr Tom Boone
Director Infection/Disease Control . . . . Becky Miner
Director Respiratory Therapy . . . . Harry Lewis

Measure	Cases	This Hospital	State Average	U.S. Average	Top Hospital
Heart Attack Care					
ACE Inhibitor or ARB for LVSD	0	-	84%	82%	100%
Aspirin at Arrival[1]	5	100%	95%	92%	100%
Aspirin at Discharge[1]	7	86%	95%	90%	100%
Beta Blocker at Arrival[1]	6	67%	91%	87%	100%
Beta Blocker at Discharge[1]	5	60%	95%	90%	100%
Fibrinolytic Medication Timing	0	-	28%	31%	100%
PCI Within 90 Minutes of Arrival	0	-	60%	54%	95%
Smoking Cessation Advice	0	-	85%	88%	100%
Heart Failure Care					
ACE Inhibitor or ARB for LVSD[1]	4	75%	85%	82%	100%
Discharge Instructions[1]	21	90%	53%	61%	93%
Evaluation of LVS Function[1]	23	91%	85%	83%	99%
Smoking Cessation Advice[1]	1	100%	75%	82%	100%
Pneumonia Care					
Appropriate Initial Antibiotic	59	92%	82%	83%	94%
Blood Culture Timing	29	97%	91%	90%	100%
Influenza Vaccine[1]	10	100%	60%	70%	100%
Initial Antibiotic Timing	86	91%	77%	80%	93%
Oxygenation Assessment	100	100%	100%	99%	100%
Pneumococcal Vaccine	57	86%	68%	69%	94%
Smoking Cessation Advice	27	93%	79%	80%	100%
Surgical Infection Prevention					
Prophylactic Antibiotic Given[1,3]	2	50%	82%	77%	95%
Prophylactic Antibiotic Selection[1]	1	100%	91%	90%	100%
Prophylactic Antibiotic Stopped[1,3]	2	50%	75%	72%	95%
Pregnancy Care					
Inpatient Neonatal Mortality	-	-	-	-	-
Third or Fourth Degree Laceration	-	-	3.98%	3.63%	3.27%

Tri-State Memorial Hospital

1221 Highland
Clarkston, WA 99403
Phone: 509-758-5511
Fax: 509-758-3566
E-mail: triadmin@clarkston.com
URL: www.tri-statehospital.com
Ownership: Government - Local
Accredited: Yes
Emergency Services: Yes
Licensed Beds: 62

Key Personnel:

Administrator/CEO . . . . Joseph K Lillard
Chief Medical Staff . . . . Morgan Wilson, MD
Director Infection/Disease Control . . . . Tenna Pennick-Sutton
ICU Supervising Nurse . . . . Kalene Gatz, RN
Director Medical/Surgical Nursing . . . . Kathy Cleghorn, RN
Director Respiratory Therapy . . . . Ken Miller

Measure	Cases	This Hospital	State Average	U.S. Average	Top Hospital
Heart Attack Care					
ACE Inhibitor or ARB for LVSD[1]	2	0%	84%	82%	100%
Aspirin at Arrival[1]	11	82%	95%	92%	100%
Aspirin at Discharge[1]	6	67%	95%	90%	100%
Beta Blocker at Arrival[1]	12	67%	91%	87%	100%
Beta Blocker at Discharge[1]	5	80%	95%	90%	100%
Fibrinolytic Medication Timing[3]	0	-	28%	31%	100%
PCI Within 90 Minutes of Arrival	0	-	60%	54%	95%
Smoking Cessation Advice[3]	0	-	85%	88%	100%
Heart Failure Care					
ACE Inhibitor or ARB for LVSD[1]	9	78%	85%	82%	100%
Discharge Instructions[3]	26	58%	53%	61%	93%
Evaluation of LVS Function	56	52%	85%	83%	99%
Smoking Cessation Advice[1,3]	7	57%	75%	82%	100%
Pneumonia Care					
Appropriate Initial Antibiotic[1,3]	4	100%	82%	83%	94%
Blood Culture Timing	36	89%	91%	90%	100%
Influenza Vaccine[5]	-	-	60%	70%	100%
Initial Antibiotic Timing	36	75%	77%	80%	93%
Oxygenation Assessment	63	100%	100%	99%	100%
Pneumococcal Vaccine	49	71%	68%	69%	94%
Smoking Cessation Advice[1,3]	9	33%	79%	80%	100%
Surgical Infection Prevention					
Prophylactic Antibiotic Given[5]	-	-	82%	77%	95%
Prophylactic Antibiotic Selection[5]	-	-	91%	90%	100%
Prophylactic Antibiotic Stopped[5]	-	-	75%	72%	95%
Pregnancy Care					
Inpatient Neonatal Mortality	-	-	-	-	-
Third or Fourth Degree Laceration	-	-	3.98%	3.63%	3.27%

Mount Carmel Hospital

982 East Columbia
Colville, WA 99114
Phone: 509-684-2561
Fax: 509-685-2492
URL: www.mtcarmelhospital.org
Ownership: Voluntary non-profit - Church
Accredited: Yes
Emergency Services: No
Licensed Beds: 55

Key Personnel:

President . . . . Gordon Mc Lean
Chief of Medical Staff . . . . Dr. Kathleen Schuerman, DO
Emergency Room . . . . Lisa Barber
Infection Control . . . . Ellen Imsland
Respiratory/Cardiopulmonary . . . . Terri Gordon

Measure	Cases	This Hospital	State Average	U.S. Average	Top Hospital
Heart Attack Care					
ACE Inhibitor or ARB for LVSD[1]	1	100%	84%	82%	100%
Aspirin at Arrival[1]	7	100%	95%	92%	100%
Aspirin at Discharge[1]	8	100%	95%	90%	100%
Beta Blocker at Arrival[1]	10	100%	91%	87%	100%
Beta Blocker at Discharge[1]	8	100%	95%	90%	100%
Fibrinolytic Medication Timing[1]	1	0%	28%	31%	100%
PCI Within 90 Minutes of Arrival	0	-	60%	54%	95%
Smoking Cessation Advice	0	-	85%	88%	100%
Heart Failure Care					
ACE Inhibitor or ARB for LVSD[1]	14	100%	85%	82%	100%
Discharge Instructions	34	97%	53%	61%	93%
Evaluation of LVS Function	41	93%	85%	83%	99%

NOTE: Hospital profiles are in alphabetical order by state, then city, then hospital within the city; Rankings are sorted by rate in descending order and exclude hospitals with less than 25 cases; (1) The number of cases is too small (n<25) for purposes of reliably predicting hospital performance; (2) Measure reflects the hospital's indication that its submission was based upon a sample of its relevant discharges; (3) Rate reflects fewer than the maximum possible quarters of data for the measure; (4) Inaccurate information submitted and suppressed for one or more quarters; (5) No data is available from the hospital for this measure; Please refer to the User's Guide for a full explanation of data

Smoking Cessation Advice[1]	5	100%	75%	82%	100%
Pneumonia Care					
Appropriate Initial Antibiotic	82	80%	82%	83%	94%
Blood Culture Timing	63	98%	91%	90%	100%
Influenza Vaccine[1]	18	100%	60%	70%	100%
Initial Antibiotic Timing	95	88%	77%	80%	93%
Oxygenation Assessment	112	100%	100%	99%	100%
Pneumococcal Vaccine	80	99%	68%	69%	94%
Smoking Cessation Advice[1]	23	91%	79%	80%	100%
Surgical Infection Prevention					
Prophylactic Antibiotic Given[3]	25	88%	82%	77%	95%
Prophylactic Antibiotic Selection[1]	9	100%	91%	90%	100%
Prophylactic Antibiotic Stopped[3]	25	68%	75%	72%	95%
Pregnancy Care					
Inpatient Neonatal Mortality	-	-	-	-	-
Third or Fourth Degree Laceration	-	-	3.98%	3.63%	3.27%

Whidbey General Hospital

101 N Main
PO Box 400
Coupeville, WA 98239
E-mail: rhines@whidbeygen.com
URL: www.whidbeygen.org
Toll-Free: 888-903-2345
Phone: 360-678-5151
Fax: 360-678-0945
Ownership: Govt - Hospital District or Authority
Accredited: No
Emergency Services: Yes
Licensed Beds: 51

Key Personnel:

President/CEO.......................... Scott Rhine
Chief of Medical Staff..................... D Terry Lee
Head Emergency Room................... John Bidding
Director Respiratory Care.................. Dave Virakle

Measure	Cases	This Hospital	State Average	U.S. Average	Top Hospital
Heart Attack Care					
ACE Inhibitor or ARB for LVSD[1]	2	100%	84%	82%	100%
Aspirin at Arrival[1]	22	95%	95%	92%	100%
Aspirin at Discharge[1]	9	100%	95%	90%	100%
Beta Blocker at Arrival[1]	18	89%	91%	87%	100%
Beta Blocker at Discharge[1]	10	100%	95%	90%	100%
Fibrinolytic Medication Timing[1]	1	100%	28%	31%	100%
PCI Within 90 Minutes of Arrival	0	-	60%	54%	95%
Smoking Cessation Advice[1]	2	0%	85%	88%	100%
Heart Failure Care					
ACE Inhibitor or ARB for LVSD[1]	13	77%	85%	82%	100%
Discharge Instructions	27	41%	53%	61%	93%
Evaluation of LVS Function	37	70%	85%	83%	99%
Smoking Cessation Advice[1]	3	33%	75%	82%	100%
Pneumonia Care					
Appropriate Initial Antibiotic	82	70%	82%	83%	94%
Blood Culture Timing	49	90%	91%	90%	100%
Influenza Vaccine[1]	19	58%	60%	70%	100%
Initial Antibiotic Timing	83	81%	77%	80%	93%
Oxygenation Assessment	101	100%	100%	99%	100%
Pneumococcal Vaccine	79	44%	68%	69%	94%
Smoking Cessation Advice[1]	9	67%	79%	80%	100%
Surgical Infection Prevention					
Prophylactic Antibiotic Given[3]	62	84%	82%	77%	95%
Prophylactic Antibiotic Selection[1]	20	90%	91%	90%	100%
Prophylactic Antibiotic Stopped[3]	59	81%	75%	72%	95%
Pregnancy Care					
Inpatient Neonatal Mortality	-	-	-	-	-
Third or Fourth Degree Laceration	-	-	3.98%	3.63%	3.27%

Lincoln Hospital

10 Nichols Street
Davenport, WA 99122
E-mail: tmsrtin@fanrc.org
URL: www.lincolnhospital.org
Phone: 509-725-7101
Fax: 509-725-2112
Ownership: Govt - Hospital District or Authority
Accredited: No
Emergency Services: Yes
Licensed Beds: 88

Key Personnel:

Administrator .... Thomas J Martin
Chief Medical Staff....................... Rolf Parke, DO
Emergency Room .... Cheryl Nelson, RN
Infection Control......................... Cindy McCall

Measure	Cases	This Hospital	State Average	U.S. Average	Top Hospital
Heart Attack Care					
ACE Inhibitor or ARB for LVSD[5]	-	-	84%	82%	100%
Aspirin at Arrival[5]	-	-	95%	92%	100%
Aspirin at Discharge[5]	-	-	95%	90%	100%
Beta Blocker at Arrival[5]	-	-	91%	87%	100%
Beta Blocker at Discharge[5]	-	-	95%	90%	100%
Fibrinolytic Medication Timing[5]	-	-	28%	31%	100%
PCI Within 90 Minutes of Arrival[5]	-	-	60%	54%	95%
Smoking Cessation Advice[5]	-	-	85%	88%	100%
Heart Failure Care					
ACE Inhibitor or ARB for LVSD[1,3]	2	100%	85%	82%	100%
Discharge Instructions[1,3]	1	100%	53%	61%	93%
Evaluation of LVS Function[1,3]	2	100%	85%	83%	99%
Smoking Cessation Advice[1,3]	2	50%	75%	82%	100%
Pneumonia Care					
Appropriate Initial Antibiotic[1,3]	6	100%	82%	83%	94%
Blood Culture Timing[3]	0	-	91%	90%	100%
Influenza Vaccine[5]	-	-	60%	70%	100%
Initial Antibiotic Timing[1,3]	6	50%	77%	80%	93%
Oxygenation Assessment[1,3]	7	100%	100%	99%	100%
Pneumococcal Vaccine[1,3]	4	50%	68%	69%	94%
Smoking Cessation Advice[1,3]	1	100%	79%	80%	100%
Surgical Infection Prevention					
Prophylactic Antibiotic Given[1,3]	7	100%	82%	77%	95%
Prophylactic Antibiotic Selection[5]	-	-	91%	90%	100%
Prophylactic Antibiotic Stopped[1,3]	7	100%	75%	72%	95%
Pregnancy Care					
Inpatient Neonatal Mortality	-	-	-	-	-
Third or Fourth Degree Laceration	-	-	3.98%	3.63%	3.27%

Deer Park Health Center & Hospital

1015 East D Street
Deer Park, WA 99006
Phone: 509-276-3504
Ownership: Voluntary non-profit - Church
Accredited: No
Emergency Services: Yes

Measure	Cases	This Hospital	State Average	U.S. Average	Top Hospital
Heart Attack Care					
ACE Inhibitor or ARB for LVSD[5]	-	-	84%	82%	100%
Aspirin at Arrival[5]	-	-	95%	92%	100%
Aspirin at Discharge[5]	-	-	95%	90%	100%
Beta Blocker at Arrival[5]	-	-	91%	87%	100%
Beta Blocker at Discharge[5]	-	-	95%	90%	100%
Fibrinolytic Medication Timing[5]	-	-	28%	31%	100%
PCI Within 90 Minutes of Arrival[5]	-	-	60%	54%	95%
Smoking Cessation Advice[5]	-	-	85%	88%	100%
Heart Failure Care					
ACE Inhibitor or ARB for LVSD[3]	0	-	85%	82%	100%
Discharge Instructions[1,3]	1	0%	53%	61%	93%
Evaluation of LVS Function[1,3]	1	100%	85%	83%	99%
Smoking Cessation Advice[3]	0	-	75%	82%	100%
Pneumonia Care					
Appropriate Initial Antibiotic[1,3]	2	100%	82%	83%	94%
Blood Culture Timing[3]	0	-	91%	90%	100%
Influenza Vaccine[5]	-	-	60%	70%	100%
Initial Antibiotic Timing[1,3]	1	0%	77%	80%	93%
Oxygenation Assessment[1,3]	2	100%	100%	99%	100%
Pneumococcal Vaccine[1,3]	2	100%	68%	69%	94%
Smoking Cessation Advice[3]	0	-	79%	80%	100%
Surgical Infection Prevention					
Prophylactic Antibiotic Given[5]	-	-	82%	77%	95%
Prophylactic Antibiotic Selection[5]	-	-	91%	90%	100%
Prophylactic Antibiotic Stopped[5]	-	-	75%	72%	95%
Pregnancy Care					
Inpatient Neonatal Mortality	-	-	-	-	-
Third or Fourth Degree Laceration	-	-	3.98%	3.63%	3.27%

NOTE: Hospital profiles are in alphabetical order by state, then city, then hospital within the city; Rankings are sorted by rate in descending order and exclude hospitals with less than 25 cases; (1) The number of cases is too small (n<25) for purposes of reliably predicting hospital performance; (2) Measure reflects the hospital's indication that its submission was based upon a sample of its relevant discharges; (3) Rate reflects fewer than the maximum possible quarters of data for the measure; (4) Inaccurate information submitted and suppressed for one or more quarters; (5) No data is available from the hospital for this measure; Please refer to the User's Guide for a full explanation of data

Stevens Hospital

21601 76th Avenue W
Edmonds, WA 98026
URL: www.stevenshealthcare.org
Ownership: Govt - Hospital District or Authority
Emergency Services: Yes

Phone: 425-640-4000
Fax: 425-640-4010
Accredited: Yes
Licensed Beds: 217

Key Personnel:

CEO . . . . John M Todd, MD
Chief Medical Staff . . . . Gary Dines, MD
Director Medical/Surgical Nursing . . . . Janet Hanna
OB/GYN Womens Health . . . . Debra Sciscoe, MD
Director Respiratory Therapy . . . . Cathy Mohns

Measure	Cases	This Hospital	State Average	U.S. Average	Top Hospital
Heart Attack Care					
ACE Inhibitor or ARB for LVSD[1]	22	95%	84%	82%	100%
Aspirin at Arrival	115	93%	95%	92%	100%
Aspirin at Discharge	88	99%	95%	90%	100%
Beta Blocker at Arrival	63	97%	91%	87%	100%
Beta Blocker at Discharge	73	97%	95%	90%	100%
Fibrinolytic Medication Timing	0	-	28%	31%	100%
PCI Within 90 Minutes of Arrival[1]	5	20%	60%	54%	95%
Smoking Cessation Advice	33	94%	85%	88%	100%
Heart Failure Care					
ACE Inhibitor or ARB for LVSD	47	79%	85%	82%	100%
Discharge Instructions	112	40%	53%	61%	93%
Evaluation of LVS Function	137	89%	85%	83%	99%
Smoking Cessation Advice[1]	23	70%	75%	82%	100%
Pneumonia Care					
Appropriate Initial Antibiotic	186	83%	82%	83%	94%
Blood Culture Timing	170	93%	91%	90%	100%
Influenza Vaccine	37	70%	60%	70%	100%
Initial Antibiotic Timing	245	78%	77%	80%	93%
Oxygenation Assessment	272	100%	100%	99%	100%
Pneumococcal Vaccine	174	73%	68%	69%	94%
Smoking Cessation Advice	57	72%	79%	80%	100%
Surgical Infection Prevention					
Prophylactic Antibiotic Given	490	79%	82%	77%	95%
Prophylactic Antibiotic Selection	111	88%	91%	90%	100%
Prophylactic Antibiotic Stopped	478	73%	75%	72%	95%
Pregnancy Care					
Inpatient Neonatal Mortality	1,208	0.08%	-	-	-
Third or Fourth Degree Laceration	866	4.50%	3.98%	3.63%	3.27%

Kittitas Valley Community Hospital

603 S Chestnut Street
Ellensburg, WA 98926
Ownership: Govt - Hospital District or Authority
Emergency Services: Yes

Phone: 509-962-7301
Fax: 509-925-8485
Accredited: No
Licensed Beds: 50

Key Personnel:

CEO . . . . Eric Jensen
Chief Medical Staff . . . . Richard Johnson
Emergency Room . . . . Jack Horsley
Chief CCU . . . . Vicki Machorro
Chief Radiology . . . . Sharon Davis
Director Respiratory Therapy . . . . Jim Allen

Measure	Cases	This Hospital	State Average	U.S. Average	Top Hospital
Heart Attack Care					
ACE Inhibitor or ARB for LVSD[1]	2	100%	84%	82%	100%
Aspirin at Arrival[1]	7	100%	95%	92%	100%
Aspirin at Discharge[1]	8	100%	95%	90%	100%
Beta Blocker at Arrival[1]	5	100%	91%	87%	100%
Beta Blocker at Discharge[1]	5	100%	95%	90%	100%
Fibrinolytic Medication Timing	0	-	28%	31%	100%
PCI Within 90 Minutes of Arrival	0	-	60%	54%	95%
Smoking Cessation Advice	0	-	85%	88%	100%
Heart Failure Care					
ACE Inhibitor or ARB for LVSD[1]	4	100%	85%	82%	100%
Discharge Instructions[1]	24	67%	53%	61%	93%
Evaluation of LVS Function	31	90%	85%	83%	99%
Smoking Cessation Advice[1]	3	100%	75%	82%	100%
Pneumonia Care					
Appropriate Initial Antibiotic	29	93%	82%	83%	94%
Blood Culture Timing[1]	21	95%	91%	90%	100%
Influenza Vaccine[1]	6	83%	60%	70%	100%
Initial Antibiotic Timing	32	88%	77%	80%	93%
Oxygenation Assessment	36	100%	100%	99%	100%
Pneumococcal Vaccine[1]	23	65%	68%	69%	94%
Smoking Cessation Advice[1]	8	88%	79%	80%	100%
Surgical Infection Prevention					
Prophylactic Antibiotic Given	65	94%	82%	77%	95%
Prophylactic Antibiotic Selection[1]	12	100%	91%	90%	100%
Prophylactic Antibiotic Stopped	62	85%	75%	72%	95%
Pregnancy Care					
Inpatient Neonatal Mortality	-	-	-	-	-
Third or Fourth Degree Laceration	-	-	3.98%	3.63%	3.27%

Enumclaw Regional Hospital

1450 Battersby Avenue
Enumclaw, WA 98022
URL: www.enumclawhospital.org
Ownership: Voluntary non-profit - Private
Emergency Services: No

Phone: 360-825-2505
Fax: 360-802-3274
Accredited: No
Licensed Beds: 38

Key Personnel:

Administrator . . . . Dennis Popp
Manager Emergency Department . . . . Richard Dickson
Medical/Surgical Nurse Manager . . . . Michelle Wylie
Manager Surgery . . . . Debbie Sutphin
Manager Radiology . . . . Richard Rosser

Measure	Cases	This Hospital	State Average	U.S. Average	Top Hospital
Heart Attack Care					
ACE Inhibitor or ARB for LVSD[1,3]	2	50%	84%	82%	100%
Aspirin at Arrival[1,3]	4	100%	95%	92%	100%
Aspirin at Discharge[1,3]	3	100%	95%	90%	100%
Beta Blocker at Arrival[1,3]	4	75%	91%	87%	100%
Beta Blocker at Discharge[1,3]	3	100%	95%	90%	100%
Fibrinolytic Medication Timing[3]	0	-	28%	31%	100%
PCI Within 90 Minutes of Arrival[5]	-	-	60%	54%	95%
Smoking Cessation Advice[3]	0	-	85%	88%	100%
Heart Failure Care					
ACE Inhibitor or ARB for LVSD[1]	4	75%	85%	82%	100%
Discharge Instructions[1]	19	21%	53%	61%	93%
Evaluation of LVS Function	26	81%	85%	83%	99%
Smoking Cessation Advice[1]	3	67%	75%	82%	100%
Pneumonia Care					
Appropriate Initial Antibiotic[2]	26	85%	82%	83%	94%
Blood Culture Timing[1,2]	14	79%	91%	90%	100%
Influenza Vaccine[1]	6	50%	60%	70%	100%
Initial Antibiotic Timing[2]	33	67%	77%	80%	93%
Oxygenation Assessment[2]	42	100%	100%	99%	100%
Pneumococcal Vaccine[2]	26	58%	68%	69%	94%
Smoking Cessation Advice[1,2]	8	62%	79%	80%	100%
Surgical Infection Prevention					
Prophylactic Antibiotic Given[5]	-	-	82%	77%	95%
Prophylactic Antibiotic Selection[5]	-	-	91%	90%	100%
Prophylactic Antibiotic Stopped[5]	-	-	75%	72%	95%
Pregnancy Care					
Inpatient Neonatal Mortality	-	-	-	-	-
Third or Fourth Degree Laceration	-	-	3.98%	3.63%	3.27%

Providence Everett Medical Center

1321 Colby Avenue
Everett, WA 98206
URL: www.providence.org
Ownership: Voluntary non-profit - Church
Emergency Services: Yes

Phone: 425-261-2000
Fax: 425-261-4051
Accredited: Yes
Licensed Beds: 362

Key Personnel:

CEO . . . . Gail C Larson

Measure	Cases	This Hospital	State Average	U.S. Average	Top Hospital
Heart Attack Care					
ACE Inhibitor or ARB for LVSD	62	76%	84%	82%	100%
Aspirin at Arrival	406	99%	95%	92%	100%

NOTE: Hospital profiles are in alphabetical order by state, then city, then hospital within the city; Rankings are sorted by rate in descending order and exclude hospitals with less than 25 cases; (1) The number of cases is too small (n<25) for purposes of reliably predicting hospital performance; (2) Measure reflects the hospital's indication that its submission was based upon a sample of its relevant discharges; (3) Rate reflects fewer than the maximum possible quarters of data for the measure; (4) Inaccurate information submitted and suppressed for one or more quarters; (5) No data is available from the hospital for this measure; Please refer to the User's Guide for a full explanation of data

Aspirin at Discharge	453	98%	95%	90%	100%
Beta Blocker at Arrival	394	98%	91%	87%	100%
Beta Blocker at Discharge	450	99%	95%	90%	100%
Fibrinolytic Medication Timing	0	-	28%	31%	100%
PCI Within 90 Minutes of Arrival	30	70%	60%	54%	95%
Smoking Cessation Advice	142	93%	85%	88%	100%
Heart Failure Care					
ACE Inhibitor or ARB for LVSD	115	95%	85%	82%	100%
Discharge Instructions	255	51%	53%	61%	93%
Evaluation of LVS Function	331	89%	85%	83%	99%
Smoking Cessation Advice	46	93%	75%	82%	100%
Pneumonia Care					
Appropriate Initial Antibiotic[2]	104	77%	82%	83%	94%
Blood Culture Timing[2]	95	92%	91%	90%	100%
Influenza Vaccine[2]	31	29%	60%	70%	100%
Initial Antibiotic Timing[2]	152	57%	77%	80%	93%
Oxygenation Assessment[2]	189	100%	100%	99%	100%
Pneumococcal Vaccine[2]	125	77%	68%	69%	94%
Smoking Cessation Advice[2]	60	92%	79%	80%	100%
Surgical Infection Prevention					
Prophylactic Antibiotic Given[2,3]	225	90%	82%	77%	95%
Prophylactic Antibiotic Selection[2]	82	95%	91%	90%	100%
Prophylactic Antibiotic Stopped[2,3]	214	82%	75%	72%	95%
Pregnancy Care					
Inpatient Neonatal Mortality[2]	1,516	0.13%	-	-	-
Third or Fourth Degree Laceration[2]	1,013	3.16%	3.98%	3.63%	3.27%

Saint Francis Hospital

Alternate Name: Saint Francis Community Hospital
34515 9th Avenue S
Federal Way, WA 98003
Phone: 253-838-9700
Fax: 253-952-7988
URL: www.fhshealth.org
Ownership: Voluntary non-profit - Church
Accredited: Yes
Emergency Services: Yes
Licensed Beds: 110

Key Personnel:

CEO. . . . . Joe Wilczek
Chief Medical Staff. . . . . Frank Senecal, MD
Emergency Room . . . . Bif Fink
CCU Spvg. Nurse . . . . Susan Merian-Tresch
Director Respiratory Therapy . . . . Paul Thackara

Measure	Cases	This Hospital	State Average	U.S. Average	Top Hospital
Heart Attack Care					
ACE Inhibitor or ARB for LVSD	31	94%	84%	82%	100%
Aspirin at Arrival	145	98%	95%	92%	100%
Aspirin at Discharge	109	100%	95%	90%	100%
Beta Blocker at Arrival	61	95%	91%	87%	100%
Beta Blocker at Discharge	111	100%	95%	90%	100%
Fibrinolytic Medication Timing	0	-	28%	31%	100%
PCI Within 90 Minutes of Arrival[1]	10	90%	60%	54%	95%
Smoking Cessation Advice	28	93%	85%	88%	100%
Heart Failure Care					
ACE Inhibitor or ARB for LVSD	57	95%	85%	82%	100%
Discharge Instructions	145	39%	53%	61%	93%
Evaluation of LVS Function	194	99%	85%	83%	99%
Smoking Cessation Advice	34	91%	75%	82%	100%
Pneumonia Care					
Appropriate Initial Antibiotic	110	96%	82%	83%	94%
Blood Culture Timing	121	90%	91%	90%	100%
Influenza Vaccine	28	61%	60%	70%	100%
Initial Antibiotic Timing	153	84%	77%	80%	93%
Oxygenation Assessment	181	100%	100%	99%	100%
Pneumococcal Vaccine	105	82%	68%	69%	94%
Smoking Cessation Advice	44	86%	79%	80%	100%
Surgical Infection Prevention					
Prophylactic Antibiotic Given[3]	251	86%	82%	77%	95%
Prophylactic Antibiotic Selection	56	96%	91%	90%	100%
Prophylactic Antibiotic Stopped[3]	248	77%	75%	72%	95%
Pregnancy Care					
Inpatient Neonatal Mortality	-	-	-	-	-
Third or Fourth Degree Laceration	-	-	3.98%	3.63%	3.27%

Coulee Community Hospital

411 Fortuyn Road
Grand Coulee, WA 99133
Phone: 509-633-1753
Fax: 509-633-0295
Ownership: Govt - Hospital District or Authority
Accredited: No
Emergency Services: Yes
Licensed Beds: 48

Key Personnel:

CEO. . . . . Jerry Lane
Chief Medical Staff. . . . . Andrew Castrodale

Measure	Cases	This Hospital	State Average	U.S. Average	Top Hospital
Heart Attack Care					
ACE Inhibitor or ARB for LVSD[5]	-	-	84%	82%	100%
Aspirin at Arrival[5]	-	-	95%	92%	100%
Aspirin at Discharge[5]	-	-	95%	90%	100%
Beta Blocker at Arrival[5]	-	-	91%	87%	100%
Beta Blocker at Discharge[5]	-	-	95%	90%	100%
Fibrinolytic Medication Timing[5]	-	-	28%	31%	100%
PCI Within 90 Minutes of Arrival[5]	-	-	60%	54%	95%
Smoking Cessation Advice[5]	-	-	85%	88%	100%
Heart Failure Care					
ACE Inhibitor or ARB for LVSD[5]	-	-	85%	82%	100%
Discharge Instructions[5]	-	-	53%	61%	93%
Evaluation of LVS Function[5]	-	-	85%	83%	99%
Smoking Cessation Advice[5]	-	-	75%	82%	100%
Pneumonia Care					
Appropriate Initial Antibiotic[5]	-	-	82%	83%	94%
Blood Culture Timing[5]	-	-	91%	90%	100%
Influenza Vaccine[5]	-	-	60%	70%	100%
Initial Antibiotic Timing[5]	-	-	77%	80%	93%
Oxygenation Assessment[5]	-	-	100%	99%	100%
Pneumococcal Vaccine[5]	-	-	68%	69%	94%
Smoking Cessation Advice[5]	-	-	79%	80%	100%
Surgical Infection Prevention					
Prophylactic Antibiotic Given[5]	-	-	82%	77%	95%
Prophylactic Antibiotic Selection[5]	-	-	91%	90%	100%
Prophylactic Antibiotic Stopped[5]	-	-	75%	72%	95%
Pregnancy Care					
Inpatient Neonatal Mortality	-	-	-	-	-
Third or Fourth Degree Laceration	-	-	3.98%	3.63%	3.27%

Ocean Beach Hospital

174 1st Avenue N
Ilwaco, WA 98624
Phone: 360-642-3181
Fax: 360-642-8070
Ownership: Govt - Hospital District or Authority
Accredited: No
Emergency Services: No
Licensed Beds: 25

Key Personnel:

President/CEO. . . . . James Robertson Jr
Chief Medical Staff. . . . . Michael Sthay, MD

Measure	Cases	This Hospital	State Average	U.S. Average	Top Hospital
Heart Attack Care					
ACE Inhibitor or ARB for LVSD[5]	-	-	84%	82%	100%
Aspirin at Arrival[5]	-	-	95%	92%	100%
Aspirin at Discharge[5]	-	-	95%	90%	100%
Beta Blocker at Arrival[5]	-	-	91%	87%	100%
Beta Blocker at Discharge[5]	-	-	95%	90%	100%
Fibrinolytic Medication Timing[5]	-	-	28%	31%	100%
PCI Within 90 Minutes of Arrival[5]	-	-	60%	54%	95%
Smoking Cessation Advice[5]	-	-	85%	88%	100%
Heart Failure Care					
ACE Inhibitor or ARB for LVSD[1,3]	1	100%	85%	82%	100%
Discharge Instructions[1,3]	3	67%	53%	61%	93%
Evaluation of LVS Function[1,3]	3	100%	85%	83%	99%
Smoking Cessation Advice[3]	0	-	75%	82%	100%
Pneumonia Care					
Appropriate Initial Antibiotic[5]	-	-	82%	83%	94%
Blood Culture Timing[5]	-	-	91%	90%	100%
Influenza Vaccine[5]	-	-	60%	70%	100%
Initial Antibiotic Timing[5]	-	-	77%	80%	93%
Oxygenation Assessment[5]	-	-	100%	99%	100%
Pneumococcal Vaccine[5]	-	-	68%	69%	94%
Smoking Cessation Advice[5]	-	-	79%	80%	100%

NOTE: Hospital profiles are in alphabetical order by state, then city, then hospital within the city; Rankings are sorted by rate in descending order and exclude hospitals with less than 25 cases; (1) The number of cases is too small (n<25) for purposes of reliably predicting hospital performance; (2) Measure reflects the hospital's indication that its submission was based upon a sample of its relevant discharges; (3) Rate reflects fewer than the maximum possible quarters of data for the measure; (4) Inaccurate information submitted and suppressed for one or more quarters; (5) No data is available from the hospital for this measure; Please refer to the User's Guide for a full explanation of data

Surgical Infection Prevention					
Prophylactic Antibiotic Given[5]	-	-	82%	77%	95%
Prophylactic Antibiotic Selection[5]	-	-	91%	90%	100%
Prophylactic Antibiotic Stopped[5]	-	-	75%	72%	95%
Pregnancy Care					
Inpatient Neonatal Mortality	-	-	-	-	-
Third or Fourth Degree Laceration	-	-	3.98%	3.63%	3.27%

Kennewick General Hospital

900 South Auburn Street Phone: 509-586-6111
Kennewick, WA 99336
Ownership: Govt - Hospital District or Authority Accredited: Yes
Emergency Services: No

Measure	Cases	This Hospital	State Average	U.S. Average	Top Hospital
Heart Attack Care					
ACE Inhibitor or ARB for LVSD[1]	9	89%	84%	82%	100%
Aspirin at Arrival	33	82%	95%	92%	100%
Aspirin at Discharge[1]	23	70%	95%	90%	100%
Beta Blocker at Arrival	33	73%	91%	87%	100%
Beta Blocker at Discharge	26	77%	95%	90%	100%
Fibrinolytic Medication Timing	0	-	28%	31%	100%
PCI Within 90 Minutes of Arrival	0	-	60%	54%	95%
Smoking Cessation Advice[1]	4	100%	85%	88%	100%
Heart Failure Care					
ACE Inhibitor or ARB for LVSD	35	69%	85%	82%	100%
Discharge Instructions	92	62%	53%	61%	93%
Evaluation of LVS Function	118	83%	85%	83%	99%
Smoking Cessation Advice[1]	22	91%	75%	82%	100%
Pneumonia Care					
Appropriate Initial Antibiotic	76	75%	82%	83%	94%
Blood Culture Timing	86	92%	91%	90%	100%
Influenza Vaccine[4,5]	-	-	60%	70%	100%
Initial Antibiotic Timing	119	90%	77%	80%	93%
Oxygenation Assessment	157	100%	100%	99%	100%
Pneumococcal Vaccine	109	88%	68%	69%	94%
Smoking Cessation Advice	25	96%	79%	80%	100%
Surgical Infection Prevention					
Prophylactic Antibiotic Given[3]	162	79%	82%	77%	95%
Prophylactic Antibiotic Selection	59	92%	91%	90%	100%
Prophylactic Antibiotic Stopped[3]	152	47%	75%	72%	95%
Pregnancy Care					
Inpatient Neonatal Mortality	-	-	-	-	-
Third or Fourth Degree Laceration	-	-	3.98%	3.63%	3.27%

Evergreen Hospital Medical Center

Alternate Name: Evergreen Community Healthcare
12040 NE 128th Street Phone: 425-899-1000
Kirkland, WA 98034 Fax: 425-899-2759
E-mail: info@evergreenhealthcare.org
URL: www.evergreenhealthcare.org
Ownership: Govt - Hospital District or Authority Accredited: Yes
Emergency Services: Yes Licensed Beds: 244
Key Personnel:
CEO. . . . . Steven E Brown, FACHE

Measure	Cases	This Hospital	State Average	U.S. Average	Top Hospital
Heart Attack Care					
ACE Inhibitor or ARB for LVSD	46	98%	84%	82%	100%
Aspirin at Arrival	205	99%	95%	92%	100%
Aspirin at Discharge	191	97%	95%	90%	100%
Beta Blocker at Arrival	136	94%	91%	87%	100%
Beta Blocker at Discharge	181	98%	95%	90%	100%
Fibrinolytic Medication Timing	0	-	28%	31%	100%
PCI Within 90 Minutes of Arrival[1]	15	47%	60%	54%	95%
Smoking Cessation Advice	56	82%	85%	88%	100%
Heart Failure Care					
ACE Inhibitor or ARB for LVSD	80	89%	85%	82%	100%
Discharge Instructions	175	63%	53%	61%	93%
Evaluation of LVS Function	223	95%	85%	83%	99%
Smoking Cessation Advice[1]	19	74%	75%	82%	100%
Pneumonia Care					
Appropriate Initial Antibiotic[2]	146	86%	82%	83%	94%
Blood Culture Timing[2]	166	94%	91%	90%	100%
Influenza Vaccine	44	89%	60%	70%	100%
Initial Antibiotic Timing[2]	207	75%	77%	80%	93%
Oxygenation Assessment[2]	254	100%	100%	99%	100%
Pneumococcal Vaccine[2]	146	88%	68%	69%	94%
Smoking Cessation Advice[2]	43	81%	79%	80%	100%
Surgical Infection Prevention					
Prophylactic Antibiotic Given[3]	128	83%	82%	77%	95%
Prophylactic Antibiotic Selection	39	95%	91%	90%	100%
Prophylactic Antibiotic Stopped[3]	123	79%	75%	72%	95%
Pregnancy Care					
Inpatient Neonatal Mortality	-	-	-	-	-
Third or Fourth Degree Laceration	-	-	3.98%	3.63%	3.27%

Providence St Peter Chemical Dependency Ctr

4800 College Street SE Toll-Free: 800-332-0465
Lacey, WA 98503 Phone: 360-456-7575
Fax: 360-493-5088
E-mail: recovery@providence.org
URL: www.providence.org/susa/services
Ownership: Voluntary non-profit - Church Accredited: Yes
Emergency Services: No Licensed Beds: 50
Key Personnel:
CEO. . . . . Mike Kerlin
Chief Medical Staff. . . . . George Chappell

Measure	Cases	This Hospital	State Average	U.S. Average	Top Hospital
Heart Attack Care					
ACE Inhibitor or ARB for LVSD[5]	-	-	84%	82%	100%
Aspirin at Arrival[5]	-	-	95%	92%	100%
Aspirin at Discharge[5]	-	-	95%	90%	100%
Beta Blocker at Arrival[5]	-	-	91%	87%	100%
Beta Blocker at Discharge[5]	-	-	95%	90%	100%
Fibrinolytic Medication Timing[5]	-	-	28%	31%	100%
PCI Within 90 Minutes of Arrival[5]	-	-	60%	54%	95%
Smoking Cessation Advice[5]	-	-	85%	88%	100%
Heart Failure Care					
ACE Inhibitor or ARB for LVSD[5]	-	-	85%	82%	100%
Discharge Instructions[5]	-	-	53%	61%	93%
Evaluation of LVS Function[5]	-	-	85%	83%	99%
Smoking Cessation Advice[5]	-	-	75%	82%	100%
Pneumonia Care					
Appropriate Initial Antibiotic[5]	-	-	82%	83%	94%
Blood Culture Timing[5]	-	-	91%	90%	100%
Influenza Vaccine[5]	-	-	60%	70%	100%
Initial Antibiotic Timing[5]	-	-	77%	80%	93%
Oxygenation Assessment[5]	-	-	100%	99%	100%
Pneumococcal Vaccine[5]	-	-	68%	69%	94%
Smoking Cessation Advice[5]	-	-	79%	80%	100%
Surgical Infection Prevention					
Prophylactic Antibiotic Given[5]	-	-	82%	77%	95%
Prophylactic Antibiotic Selection[5]	-	-	91%	90%	100%
Prophylactic Antibiotic Stopped[5]	-	-	75%	72%	95%
Pregnancy Care					
Inpatient Neonatal Mortality	-	-	-	-	-
Third or Fourth Degree Laceration	-	-	3.98%	3.63%	3.27%

Saint Clare Hospital

11315 Bridgeport Way SW Phone: 253-588-1711
Lakewood, WA 98499 Fax: 253-512-2708
URL: www.fhshealth.org
Ownership: Voluntary non-profit - Church Accredited: Yes
Emergency Services: Yes Licensed Beds: 106
Key Personnel:
President/CEO. . . . . Joseph W Wilczek

Measure	Cases	This Hospital	State Average	U.S. Average	Top Hospital
Heart Attack Care					
ACE Inhibitor or ARB for LVSD[1]	7	100%	84%	82%	100%
Aspirin at Arrival	47	98%	95%	92%	100%
Aspirin at Discharge	26	100%	95%	90%	100%

NOTE: Hospital profiles are in alphabetical order by state, then city, then hospital within the city; Rankings are sorted by rate in descending order and exclude hospitals with less than 25 cases; (1) The number of cases is too small (n<25) for purposes of reliably predicting hospital performance; (2) Measure reflects the hospital's indication that its submission was based upon a sample of its relevant discharges; (3) Rate reflects fewer than the maximum possible quarters of data for the measure; (4) Inaccurate information submitted and suppressed for one or more quarters; (5) No data is available from the hospital for this measure; Please refer to the User's Guide for a full explanation of data

Measure	Cases	This Hospital	State Average	U.S. Average	Top Hospital
Beta Blocker at Arrival[1]	21	95%	91%	87%	100%
Beta Blocker at Discharge	28	100%	95%	90%	100%
Fibrinolytic Medication Timing[1]	1	0%	28%	31%	100%
PCI Within 90 Minutes of Arrival	0	-	60%	54%	95%
Smoking Cessation Advice[1]	3	100%	85%	88%	100%
Heart Failure Care					
ACE Inhibitor or ARB for LVSD	77	96%	85%	82%	100%
Discharge Instructions	203	60%	53%	61%	93%
Evaluation of LVS Function	263	98%	85%	83%	99%
Smoking Cessation Advice	56	86%	75%	82%	100%
Pneumonia Care					
Appropriate Initial Antibiotic	197	94%	82%	83%	94%
Blood Culture Timing	191	89%	91%	90%	100%
Influenza Vaccine	56	54%	60%	70%	100%
Initial Antibiotic Timing	254	83%	77%	80%	93%
Oxygenation Assessment	327	100%	100%	99%	100%
Pneumococcal Vaccine	205	79%	68%	69%	94%
Smoking Cessation Advice	94	83%	79%	80%	100%
Surgical Infection Prevention					
Prophylactic Antibiotic Given[3]	314	94%	82%	77%	95%
Prophylactic Antibiotic Selection	46	96%	91%	90%	100%
Prophylactic Antibiotic Stopped[3]	303	91%	75%	72%	95%
Pregnancy Care					
Inpatient Neonatal Mortality	-	-	-	-	-
Third or Fourth Degree Laceration	-	-	3.98%	3.63%	3.27%

Hospice Care Center Hospital

1035 11th Avenue
Longview, WA 98632
Ownership: Proprietary
Emergency Services: No

Phone: 360-425-8510
Accredited: No

Measure	Cases	This Hospital	State Average	U.S. Average	Top Hospital
Heart Attack Care					
ACE Inhibitor or ARB for LVSD[5]	-	-	84%	82%	100%
Aspirin at Arrival[5]	-	-	95%	92%	100%
Aspirin at Discharge[5]	-	-	95%	90%	100%
Beta Blocker at Arrival[5]	-	-	91%	87%	100%
Beta Blocker at Discharge[5]	-	-	95%	90%	100%
Fibrinolytic Medication Timing[5]	-	-	28%	31%	100%
PCI Within 90 Minutes of Arrival[5]	-	-	60%	54%	95%
Smoking Cessation Advice[5]	-	-	85%	88%	100%
Heart Failure Care					
ACE Inhibitor or ARB for LVSD[5]	-	-	85%	82%	100%
Discharge Instructions[5]	-	-	53%	61%	93%
Evaluation of LVS Function[5]	-	-	85%	83%	99%
Smoking Cessation Advice[5]	-	-	75%	82%	100%
Pneumonia Care					
Appropriate Initial Antibiotic[5]	-	-	82%	83%	94%
Blood Culture Timing[5]	-	-	91%	90%	100%
Influenza Vaccine[5]	-	-	60%	70%	100%
Initial Antibiotic Timing[5]	-	-	77%	80%	93%
Oxygenation Assessment[5]	-	-	100%	99%	100%
Pneumococcal Vaccine[5]	-	-	68%	69%	94%
Smoking Cessation Advice[5]	-	-	79%	80%	100%
Surgical Infection Prevention					
Prophylactic Antibiotic Given[5]	-	-	82%	77%	95%
Prophylactic Antibiotic Selection[5]	-	-	91%	90%	100%
Prophylactic Antibiotic Stopped[5]	-	-	75%	72%	95%
Pregnancy Care					
Inpatient Neonatal Mortality	-	-	-	-	-
Third or Fourth Degree Laceration	-	-	3.98%	3.63%	3.27%

Saint John Medical Center

Alternate Name: Saint John's Hospital

1615 Delaware Street
PO Box 3002
Longview, WA 98632
URL: www.peacehealth.org
Ownership: Voluntary non-profit - Church
Emergency Services: Yes

Toll-Free: 800-438-7562
Phone: 360-414-2000
Fax: 360-414-7550
Accredited: Yes
Licensed Beds: 368

Key Personnel:
Regional CEO . . . . Medrice M Coluccio
Regional COO . . . . Jim Meskew
Chief Staff . . . . Steven X Cabrales, MD

Measure	Cases	This Hospital	State Average	U.S. Average	Top Hospital
Heart Attack Care					
ACE Inhibitor or ARB for LVSD[1]	22	82%	84%	82%	100%
Aspirin at Arrival	115	100%	95%	92%	100%
Aspirin at Discharge	64	97%	95%	90%	100%
Beta Blocker at Arrival	90	99%	91%	87%	100%
Beta Blocker at Discharge	69	99%	95%	90%	100%
Fibrinolytic Medication Timing[1]	11	18%	28%	31%	100%
PCI Within 90 Minutes of Arrival	0	-	60%	54%	95%
Smoking Cessation Advice[1]	13	100%	85%	88%	100%
Heart Failure Care					
ACE Inhibitor or ARB for LVSD	93	82%	85%	82%	100%
Discharge Instructions	172	76%	53%	61%	93%
Evaluation of LVS Function	209	91%	85%	83%	99%
Smoking Cessation Advice	50	94%	75%	82%	100%
Pneumonia Care					
Appropriate Initial Antibiotic	140	82%	82%	83%	94%
Blood Culture Timing	125	93%	91%	90%	100%
Influenza Vaccine	62	100%	60%	70%	100%
Initial Antibiotic Timing	335	85%	77%	80%	93%
Oxygenation Assessment	428	100%	100%	99%	100%
Pneumococcal Vaccine	227	62%	68%	69%	94%
Smoking Cessation Advice	102	98%	79%	80%	100%
Surgical Infection Prevention					
Prophylactic Antibiotic Given[3]	152	80%	82%	77%	95%
Prophylactic Antibiotic Selection	155	88%	91%	90%	100%
Prophylactic Antibiotic Stopped[3]	146	80%	75%	72%	95%
Pregnancy Care					
Inpatient Neonatal Mortality	-	-	-	-	-
Third or Fourth Degree Laceration	-	-	3.98%	3.63%	3.27%

Mark Reed Hospital

322 S Birch Street
McCleary, WA 98557
Ownership: Govt - Hospital District or Authority
Emergency Services: No

Phone: 360-495-3244
Fax: 360-495-4566
Accredited: No
Licensed Beds: 24

Key Personnel:
CEO. . . . . Georgett Hiles
Chief Medical Staff. . . . . Edward Macke, MD
Director Emergency Room. . . . . Robert Billings, MD

Measure	Cases	This Hospital	State Average	U.S. Average	Top Hospital
Heart Attack Care					
ACE Inhibitor or ARB for LVSD[5]	-	-	84%	82%	100%
Aspirin at Arrival[5]	-	-	95%	92%	100%
Aspirin at Discharge[5]	-	-	95%	90%	100%
Beta Blocker at Arrival[5]	-	-	91%	87%	100%
Beta Blocker at Discharge[5]	-	-	95%	90%	100%
Fibrinolytic Medication Timing[5]	-	-	28%	31%	100%
PCI Within 90 Minutes of Arrival[5]	-	-	60%	54%	95%
Smoking Cessation Advice[5]	-	-	85%	88%	100%
Heart Failure Care					
ACE Inhibitor or ARB for LVSD[5]	-	-	85%	82%	100%
Discharge Instructions[5]	-	-	53%	61%	93%
Evaluation of LVS Function[5]	-	-	85%	83%	99%
Smoking Cessation Advice[5]	-	-	75%	82%	100%
Pneumonia Care					
Appropriate Initial Antibiotic[1]	12	92%	82%	83%	94%
Blood Culture Timing[1]	4	100%	91%	90%	100%
Influenza Vaccine[1]	4	100%	60%	70%	100%
Initial Antibiotic Timing[1]	11	91%	77%	80%	93%
Oxygenation Assessment[1]	12	100%	100%	99%	100%

NOTE: Hospital profiles are in alphabetical order by state, then city, then hospital within the city; Rankings are sorted by rate in descending order and exclude hospitals with less than 25 cases; (1) The number of cases is too small (n<25) for purposes of reliably predicting hospital performance; (2) Measure reflects the hospital's indication that its submission was based upon a sample of its relevant discharges; (3) Rate reflects fewer than the maximum possible quarters of data for the measure; (4) Inaccurate information submitted and suppressed for one or more quarters; (5) No data is available from the hospital for this measure; Please refer to the User's Guide for a full explanation of data

Measure	Cases	This Hospital	State Average	U.S. Average	Top Hospital
Pneumococcal Vaccine[1]	6	100%	68%	69%	94%
Smoking Cessation Advice[1]	4	75%	79%	80%	100%
Surgical Infection Prevention					
Prophylactic Antibiotic Given[5]	-	-	82%	77%	95%
Prophylactic Antibiotic Selection[5]	-	-	91%	90%	100%
Prophylactic Antibiotic Stopped[5]	-	-	75%	72%	95%
Pregnancy Care					
Inpatient Neonatal Mortality	-	-	-	-	-
Third or Fourth Degree Laceration	-	-	3.98%	3.63%	3.27%

Valley General Hospital

14701 179th SE
PO Box 646
Monroe, WA 98272
URL: www.valleygeneral.com
Phone: 360-794-7497
Fax: 360-794-1486
Ownership: Govt - Hospital District or Authority
Accredited: Yes
Emergency Services: Yes
Licensed Beds: 72

Key Personnel:

Administrator/CEO . . . . Mark Judy
Chief Medical Staff. . . . . Bill Thor, MD
Director Medical Emergency Department. . . . . . Eric M Fields, DO
Infection Control. . . . . Gary Preston, MD
Director Medical/Surgical Nursing . . . . Brenda Rogers
Surgical Services . . . . Jeanne Bennetts, RN
Respiratory . . . . Brenda Rogers, RN

Measure	Cases	This Hospital	State Average	U.S. Average	Top Hospital
Heart Attack Care					
ACE Inhibitor or ARB for LVSD[1]	2	100%	84%	82%	100%
Aspirin at Arrival[1]	7	100%	95%	92%	100%
Aspirin at Discharge[1]	5	100%	95%	90%	100%
Beta Blocker at Arrival[1]	6	100%	91%	87%	100%
Beta Blocker at Discharge[1]	7	100%	95%	90%	100%
Fibrinolytic Medication Timing	0	-	28%	31%	100%
PCI Within 90 Minutes of Arrival	0	-	60%	54%	95%
Smoking Cessation Advice[1]	1	100%	85%	88%	100%
Heart Failure Care					
ACE Inhibitor or ARB for LVSD[1]	13	100%	85%	82%	100%
Discharge Instructions	39	90%	53%	61%	93%
Evaluation of LVS Function	49	98%	85%	83%	99%
Smoking Cessation Advice[1]	12	83%	75%	82%	100%
Pneumonia Care					
Appropriate Initial Antibiotic	54	74%	82%	83%	94%
Blood Culture Timing	53	87%	91%	90%	100%
Influenza Vaccine[4,5]	-	-	60%	70%	100%
Initial Antibiotic Timing	79	76%	77%	80%	93%
Oxygenation Assessment	83	100%	100%	99%	100%
Pneumococcal Vaccine	49	82%	68%	69%	94%
Smoking Cessation Advice[1]	17	76%	79%	80%	100%
Surgical Infection Prevention					
Prophylactic Antibiotic Given[3]	75	83%	82%	77%	95%
Prophylactic Antibiotic Selection	31	81%	91%	90%	100%
Prophylactic Antibiotic Stopped[3]	73	81%	75%	72%	95%
Pregnancy Care					
Inpatient Neonatal Mortality	401	0.50%	-	-	-
Third or Fourth Degree Laceration	284	1.76%	3.98%	3.63%	3.27%

Samaritan Healthcare

Alternate Name: Samaritan Hospital
801 E Wheeler Road
Moses Lake, WA 98837
URL: www.samaritanhealthcare.com
Phone: 509-765-5606
Fax: 509-764-6507
Ownership: Govt - Hospital District or Authority
Accredited: No
Emergency Services: Yes
Licensed Beds: 50

Key Personnel:

President/CEO. . . . . John White
Chief Medical Staff. . . . . Ed Hoover
Emergency Room . . . . Steve Rusnock
Infection Control. . . . . Pat Harrington
CCU Spvg. Nurse . . . . Maureen King
Director Medical/Surgical Nursing . . . . Michael Owen
Surgical Services . . . . Emily Webster
Chief Radiology . . . . Steve Schindler
Director Respiratory Therapy . . . . Margie Stansbury

Measure	Cases	This Hospital	State Average	U.S. Average	Top Hospital
Heart Attack Care					
ACE Inhibitor or ARB for LVSD[1]	1	100%	84%	82%	100%
Aspirin at Arrival[1]	24	79%	95%	92%	100%
Aspirin at Discharge[1]	14	100%	95%	90%	100%
Beta Blocker at Arrival[1]	18	89%	91%	87%	100%
Beta Blocker at Discharge[1]	12	92%	95%	90%	100%
Fibrinolytic Medication Timing	0	-	28%	31%	100%
PCI Within 90 Minutes of Arrival	0	-	60%	54%	95%
Smoking Cessation Advice[1]	2	100%	85%	88%	100%
Heart Failure Care					
ACE Inhibitor or ARB for LVSD[1]	12	83%	85%	82%	100%
Discharge Instructions	51	35%	53%	61%	93%
Evaluation of LVS Function	73	63%	85%	83%	99%
Smoking Cessation Advice[1]	8	50%	75%	82%	100%
Pneumonia Care					
Appropriate Initial Antibiotic	54	78%	82%	83%	94%
Blood Culture Timing	38	97%	91%	90%	100%
Influenza Vaccine[1]	17	18%	60%	70%	100%
Initial Antibiotic Timing	85	74%	77%	80%	93%
Oxygenation Assessment	103	100%	100%	99%	100%
Pneumococcal Vaccine	61	41%	68%	69%	94%
Smoking Cessation Advice[1]	16	94%	79%	80%	100%
Surgical Infection Prevention					
Prophylactic Antibiotic Given	213	64%	82%	77%	95%
Prophylactic Antibiotic Selection	47	98%	91%	90%	100%
Prophylactic Antibiotic Stopped	207	48%	75%	72%	95%
Pregnancy Care					
Inpatient Neonatal Mortality	-	-	-	-	-
Third or Fourth Degree Laceration	-	-	3.98%	3.63%	3.27%

Skagit Valley Hospital

1415 E Kincaid
PO Box 1376
Mount Vernon, WA 98273
E-mail: kranten@skagitvalleyhospital.org
URL: www.skagitvalleyhospital.org
Phone: 360-424-4111
Fax: 360-428-2416
Ownership: Govt - Hospital District or Authority
Accredited: Yes
Emergency Services: Yes
Licensed Beds: 115

Key Personnel:

President . . . . Stan Olson
CEO. . . . . Gregg Davidson, FACHE

Measure	Cases	This Hospital	State Average	U.S. Average	Top Hospital
Heart Attack Care					
ACE Inhibitor or ARB for LVSD	26	81%	84%	82%	100%
Aspirin at Arrival	88	100%	95%	92%	100%
Aspirin at Discharge	91	96%	95%	90%	100%
Beta Blocker at Arrival	79	96%	91%	87%	100%
Beta Blocker at Discharge	113	98%	95%	90%	100%
Fibrinolytic Medication Timing	0	-	28%	31%	100%
PCI Within 90 Minutes of Arrival[1]	5	80%	60%	54%	95%
Smoking Cessation Advice	31	94%	85%	88%	100%
Heart Failure Care					
ACE Inhibitor or ARB for LVSD	54	72%	85%	82%	100%
Discharge Instructions	127	54%	53%	61%	93%
Evaluation of LVS Function	172	96%	85%	83%	99%
Smoking Cessation Advice[1]	22	68%	75%	82%	100%
Pneumonia Care					
Appropriate Initial Antibiotic[2]	108	92%	82%	83%	94%
Blood Culture Timing[2]	121	81%	91%	90%	100%
Influenza Vaccine	34	68%	60%	70%	100%
Initial Antibiotic Timing[2]	147	82%	77%	80%	93%
Oxygenation Assessment[2]	195	100%	100%	99%	100%
Pneumococcal Vaccine[2]	135	81%	68%	69%	94%
Smoking Cessation Advice[2]	38	92%	79%	80%	100%
Surgical Infection Prevention					
Prophylactic Antibiotic Given[2,3]	355	79%	82%	77%	95%
Prophylactic Antibiotic Selection[2]	54	83%	91%	90%	100%
Prophylactic Antibiotic Stopped[2,3]	341	86%	75%	72%	95%

NOTE: Hospital profiles are in alphabetical order by state, then city, then hospital within the city; Rankings are sorted by rate in descending order and exclude hospitals with less than 25 cases; (1) The number of cases is too small (n<25) for purposes of reliably predicting hospital performance; (2) Measure reflects the hospital's indication that its submission was based upon a sample of its relevant discharges; (3) Rate reflects fewer than the maximum possible quarters of data for the measure; (4) Inaccurate information submitted and suppressed for one or more quarters; (5) No data is available from the hospital for this measure; Please refer to the User's Guide for a full explanation of data

Pregnancy Care					
Inpatient Neonatal Mortality	-	-	-	-	-
Third or Fourth Degree Laceration	-	-	3.98%	3.63%	3.27%

Capital Medical Center

Alternate Name: Columbia Capital Medical Center
3900 Capitol Mall Drive SW
Olympia, WA 98502
Toll-Free: 888-633-5101
Phone: 360-754-5858
Fax: 360-956-2574

URL: www.capitalmedical.com
Ownership: Proprietary
Emergency Services: Yes
Accredited: Yes
Licensed Beds: 119

Key Personnel:
Administrator/CEO . . . . Joseph Sharp
Chief Medical Staff. . . . . Marnee Obendorf
Emergency Room . . . . Cynthia Wolfe, MD
Director Infection/Disease Control . . . . Ira Rice, RN
CCU Spvg. Nurse . . . . Dona Kravis
Director Medical/Surgical Nursing . . . . Rhonda Osgood
Director Respiratory Therapy . . . . Wanda Shirreff

Measure	Cases	This Hospital	State Average	U.S. Average	Top Hospital
Heart Attack Care					
ACE Inhibitor or ARB for LVSD[1]	12	92%	84%	82%	100%
Aspirin at Arrival	29	90%	95%	92%	100%
Aspirin at Discharge	42	95%	95%	90%	100%
Beta Blocker at Arrival	25	88%	91%	87%	100%
Beta Blocker at Discharge	39	92%	95%	90%	100%
Fibrinolytic Medication Timing	0	-	28%	31%	100%
PCI Within 90 Minutes of Arrival[1]	4	0%	60%	54%	95%
Smoking Cessation Advice[1]	17	82%	85%	88%	100%
Heart Failure Care					
ACE Inhibitor or ARB for LVSD[1]	19	79%	85%	82%	100%
Discharge Instructions	42	19%	53%	61%	93%
Evaluation of LVS Function	68	84%	85%	83%	99%
Smoking Cessation Advice[1]	4	75%	75%	82%	100%
Pneumonia Care					
Appropriate Initial Antibiotic	53	89%	82%	83%	94%
Blood Culture Timing	35	97%	91%	90%	100%
Influenza Vaccine[1]	16	56%	60%	70%	100%
Initial Antibiotic Timing	52	73%	77%	80%	93%
Oxygenation Assessment	67	100%	100%	99%	100%
Pneumococcal Vaccine	43	65%	68%	69%	94%
Smoking Cessation Advice[1]	13	31%	79%	80%	100%
Surgical Infection Prevention					
Prophylactic Antibiotic Given[2,3]	91	93%	82%	77%	95%
Prophylactic Antibiotic Selection[2]	93	96%	91%	90%	100%
Prophylactic Antibiotic Stopped[2,3]	90	67%	75%	72%	95%
Pregnancy Care					
Inpatient Neonatal Mortality	-	-	-	-	-
Third or Fourth Degree Laceration	-	-	3.98%	3.63%	3.27%

Providence Saint Peter Hospital

413 Lilly Road NE
Olympia, WA 98506
Toll-Free: 888-492-9480
Phone: 360-491-9480
Fax: 360-493-7268

URL: www.providence.org/swsa
Ownership: Voluntary non-profit - Church
Emergency Services: Yes
Accredited: Yes
Licensed Beds: 390

Key Personnel:
President/CEO . . . . Scott Bond
Chief Medical Staff. . . . . Mike Matiock, MD
Cardiac Lab . . . . Kurt Miller
Catheterization Lab . . . . Kurt Miller
Emergency Room . . . . Brad Massey
Infection Control. . . . . Lou Hilken
ICU . . . . Cheryl Hartsook
Intensive/Coronary Care . . . . Cheryl Hartsook
Medical/Surgical Nursing . . . . Linda Foss
OB/GYN Womens Health. . . . . Connie Bololes
Respiratory/Cardiopulmonary. . . . . Kim Chase

Measure	Cases	This Hospital	State Average	U.S. Average	Top Hospital
Heart Attack Care					
ACE Inhibitor or ARB for LVSD	103	80%	84%	82%	100%
Aspirin at Arrival	377	97%	95%	92%	100%
Aspirin at Discharge	570	97%	95%	90%	100%
Beta Blocker at Arrival	338	93%	91%	87%	100%
Beta Blocker at Discharge	540	90%	95%	90%	100%
Fibrinolytic Medication Timing	0	-	28%	31%	100%
PCI Within 90 Minutes of Arrival[1]	22	50%	60%	54%	95%
Smoking Cessation Advice	213	81%	85%	88%	100%
Heart Failure Care					
ACE Inhibitor or ARB for LVSD	161	92%	85%	82%	100%
Discharge Instructions	355	41%	53%	61%	93%
Evaluation of LVS Function	431	87%	85%	83%	99%
Smoking Cessation Advice	79	78%	75%	82%	100%
Pneumonia Care					
Appropriate Initial Antibiotic	242	76%	82%	83%	94%
Blood Culture Timing	225	91%	91%	90%	100%
Influenza Vaccine	52	48%	60%	70%	100%
Initial Antibiotic Timing	311	82%	77%	80%	93%
Oxygenation Assessment	401	99%	100%	99%	100%
Pneumococcal Vaccine	261	62%	68%	69%	94%
Smoking Cessation Advice	118	52%	79%	80%	100%
Surgical Infection Prevention					
Prophylactic Antibiotic Given[2,3]	310	86%	82%	77%	95%
Prophylactic Antibiotic Selection[2]	132	92%	91%	90%	100%
Prophylactic Antibiotic Stopped[2,3]	305	60%	75%	72%	95%
Pregnancy Care					
Inpatient Neonatal Mortality	-	-	-	-	-
Third or Fourth Degree Laceration	-	-	3.98%	3.63%	3.27%

Othello Community Hospital

315 N 14th Street
Othello, WA 99344
Phone: 509-488-2636
Fax: 509-488-3857
Ownership: Govt - Hospital District or Authority
Emergency Services: No
Accredited: No
Licensed Beds: 49

Key Personnel:
Administrator . . . . Jay Coats
Chief Medical Staff. . . . . Fay Coats
Director Infection/Disease Control . . . . Mary McCourtie
Director Respiratory Therapy . . . . Greg Hanoff

Measure	Cases	This Hospital	State Average	U.S. Average	Top Hospital
Heart Attack Care					
ACE Inhibitor or ARB for LVSD[3]	0	-	84%	82%	100%
Aspirin at Arrival[1,3]	1	100%	95%	92%	100%
Aspirin at Discharge[3]	0	-	95%	90%	100%
Beta Blocker at Arrival[1,3]	1	0%	91%	87%	100%
Beta Blocker at Discharge[3]	0	-	95%	90%	100%
Fibrinolytic Medication Timing[3]	0	-	28%	31%	100%
PCI Within 90 Minutes of Arrival[5]	-	-	60%	54%	95%
Smoking Cessation Advice[3]	0	-	85%	88%	100%
Heart Failure Care					
ACE Inhibitor or ARB for LVSD[1]	8	100%	85%	82%	100%
Discharge Instructions[1]	19	79%	53%	61%	93%
Evaluation of LVS Function[1]	20	80%	85%	83%	99%
Smoking Cessation Advice[1]	7	71%	75%	82%	100%
Pneumonia Care					
Appropriate Initial Antibiotic[5]	-	-	82%	83%	94%
Blood Culture Timing[1]	4	100%	91%	90%	100%
Influenza Vaccine[1]	3	67%	60%	70%	100%
Initial Antibiotic Timing[1]	11	64%	77%	80%	93%
Oxygenation Assessment[1]	16	100%	100%	99%	100%
Pneumococcal Vaccine[1]	11	100%	68%	69%	94%
Smoking Cessation Advice	0	-	79%	80%	100%
Surgical Infection Prevention					
Prophylactic Antibiotic Given[5]	-	-	82%	77%	95%
Prophylactic Antibiotic Selection[5]	-	-	91%	90%	100%
Prophylactic Antibiotic Stopped[5]	-	-	75%	72%	95%
Pregnancy Care					
Inpatient Neonatal Mortality	-	-	-	-	-
Third or Fourth Degree Laceration	-	-	3.98%	3.63%	3.27%

NOTE: Hospital profiles are in alphabetical order by state, then city, then hospital within the city; Rankings are sorted by rate in descending order and exclude hospitals with less than 25 cases; (1) The number of cases is too small (n<25) for purposes of reliably predicting hospital performance; (2) Measure reflects the hospital's indication that its submission was based upon a sample of its relevant discharges; (3) Rate reflects fewer than the maximum possible quarters of data for the measure; (4) Inaccurate information submitted and suppressed for one or more quarters; (5) No data is available from the hospital for this measure; Please refer to the User's Guide for a full explanation of data

Lourdes Medical Center

Alternate Name: Our Lady of Lourdes Health Center
520 North 4th Avenue
PO Box 2568
Pasco, WA 99301
E-mail: ollhc@ibm.net
URL: www.lourdesonline.org
Toll-Free: 800-383-7515
Phone: 509-547-7704
Fax: 509-546-2291
Ownership: Voluntary non-profit - Church
Emergency Services: Yes
Accredited: Yes
Licensed Beds: 132

Key Personnel:

President/CEO . . . . John Serle
Chief Medical Officer . . . . Laurie T Zimmerman, MD
Chief Medical Staff . . . . Richard Shallman, MD
Director Emergency Room . . . . Barbara Edwards
Supervisor Infection Control . . . . Joanne Dixon
Director Medical/Surgical Nursing . . . . Dee Hazel
Director OB/GYN/Women's Health . . . . Sara Barron
Director Radiology . . . . Dari Ellsworth
Respiratory/Cardiopulmonary . . . . Mark Rogers

Measure	Cases	This Hospital	State Average	U.S. Average	Top Hospital
Heart Attack Care					
ACE Inhibitor or ARB for LVSD[1]	5	60%	84%	82%	100%
Aspirin at Arrival[1]	12	75%	95%	92%	100%
Aspirin at Discharge[1]	7	71%	95%	90%	100%
Beta Blocker at Arrival[1]	8	75%	91%	87%	100%
Beta Blocker at Discharge[1]	9	78%	95%	90%	100%
Fibrinolytic Medication Timing	0	-	28%	31%	100%
PCI Within 90 Minutes of Arrival	0	-	60%	54%	95%
Smoking Cessation Advice[1]	3	67%	85%	88%	100%
Heart Failure Care					
ACE Inhibitor or ARB for LVSD[1]	7	57%	85%	82%	100%
Discharge Instructions	30	67%	53%	61%	93%
Evaluation of LVS Function	37	73%	85%	83%	99%
Smoking Cessation Advice[1]	7	29%	75%	82%	100%
Pneumonia Care					
Appropriate Initial Antibiotic	54	74%	82%	83%	94%
Blood Culture Timing	38	87%	91%	90%	100%
Influenza Vaccine[1]	12	0%	60%	70%	100%
Initial Antibiotic Timing	55	75%	77%	80%	93%
Oxygenation Assessment	83	99%	100%	99%	100%
Pneumococcal Vaccine	54	44%	68%	69%	94%
Smoking Cessation Advice[1]	15	73%	79%	80%	100%
Surgical Infection Prevention					
Prophylactic Antibiotic Given[5]	-	-	82%	77%	95%
Prophylactic Antibiotic Selection[5]	-	-	91%	90%	100%
Prophylactic Antibiotic Stopped[5]	-	-	75%	72%	95%
Pregnancy Care					
Inpatient Neonatal Mortality	-	-	-	-	-
Third or Fourth Degree Laceration	-	-	3.98%	3.63%	3.27%

Olympic Medical Center

Alternate Name: Olympic Memorial Hospital
939 Caroline Street
Port Angeles, WA 98362
URL: www.olympicmedical.org
Phone: 360-417-7000
Fax: 360-417-7307
Ownership: Govt - Hospital District or Authority
Emergency Services: Yes
Accredited: Yes
Licensed Beds: 126

Key Personnel:

CEO . . . . Mike Glenn

Measure	Cases	This Hospital	State Average	U.S. Average	Top Hospital
Heart Attack Care					
ACE Inhibitor or ARB for LVSD[1]	7	100%	84%	82%	100%
Aspirin at Arrival	35	91%	95%	92%	100%
Aspirin at Discharge[1]	20	85%	95%	90%	100%
Beta Blocker at Arrival	27	96%	91%	87%	100%
Beta Blocker at Discharge[1]	19	95%	95%	90%	100%
Fibrinolytic Medication Timing[1]	5	60%	28%	31%	100%
PCI Within 90 Minutes of Arrival	0	-	60%	54%	95%
Smoking Cessation Advice[1]	5	60%	85%	88%	100%
Heart Failure Care					
ACE Inhibitor or ARB for LVSD	62	89%	85%	82%	100%
Discharge Instructions	128	84%	53%	61%	93%
Evaluation of LVS Function	172	98%	85%	83%	99%
Smoking Cessation Advice[1]	15	67%	75%	82%	100%
Pneumonia Care					
Appropriate Initial Antibiotic	150	89%	82%	83%	94%
Blood Culture Timing	155	93%	91%	90%	100%
Influenza Vaccine	60	65%	60%	70%	100%
Initial Antibiotic Timing	225	79%	77%	80%	93%
Oxygenation Assessment	269	100%	100%	99%	100%
Pneumococcal Vaccine	199	69%	68%	69%	94%
Smoking Cessation Advice	52	79%	79%	80%	100%
Surgical Infection Prevention					
Prophylactic Antibiotic Given	319	80%	82%	77%	95%
Prophylactic Antibiotic Selection	70	81%	91%	90%	100%
Prophylactic Antibiotic Stopped	306	91%	75%	72%	95%
Pregnancy Care					
Inpatient Neonatal Mortality	-	-	-	-	-
Third or Fourth Degree Laceration	-	-	3.98%	3.63%	3.27%

Jefferson General Hospital

834 Sheridan Avenue
Port Townsend, WA 98368
URL: www.jgh.org
Toll-Free: 800-244-8917
Phone: 360-385-2200
Fax: 360-385-1548
Ownership: Govt - Hospital District or Authority
Emergency Services: Yes
Accredited: No
Licensed Beds: 43

Key Personnel:

CEO . . . . Victor Dirksen
Chief of Medical Staff . . . . Grace Lawson
Emergency Room . . . . Jim Decianne
Director Infection/Disease Control . . . . Joanne Clyde
Director Respiratory Therapy . . . . Hank Brakebush

Measure	Cases	This Hospital	State Average	U.S. Average	Top Hospital
Heart Attack Care					
ACE Inhibitor or ARB for LVSD	0	-	84%	82%	100%
Aspirin at Arrival[1]	6	83%	95%	92%	100%
Aspirin at Discharge[1]	4	75%	95%	90%	100%
Beta Blocker at Arrival[1]	5	100%	91%	87%	100%
Beta Blocker at Discharge[1]	3	100%	95%	90%	100%
Fibrinolytic Medication Timing	0	-	28%	31%	100%
PCI Within 90 Minutes of Arrival	0	-	60%	54%	95%
Smoking Cessation Advice	0	-	85%	88%	100%
Heart Failure Care					
ACE Inhibitor or ARB for LVSD[1]	16	81%	85%	82%	100%
Discharge Instructions	36	25%	53%	61%	93%
Evaluation of LVS Function	46	83%	85%	83%	99%
Smoking Cessation Advice[1]	10	40%	75%	82%	100%
Pneumonia Care					
Appropriate Initial Antibiotic	48	83%	82%	83%	94%
Blood Culture Timing	36	92%	91%	90%	100%
Influenza Vaccine[1]	12	58%	60%	70%	100%
Initial Antibiotic Timing	63	87%	77%	80%	93%
Oxygenation Assessment	77	100%	100%	99%	100%
Pneumococcal Vaccine	50	62%	68%	69%	94%
Smoking Cessation Advice[1]	10	70%	79%	80%	100%
Surgical Infection Prevention					
Prophylactic Antibiotic Given	152	89%	82%	77%	95%
Prophylactic Antibiotic Selection	46	76%	91%	90%	100%
Prophylactic Antibiotic Stopped	151	65%	75%	72%	95%
Pregnancy Care					
Inpatient Neonatal Mortality	-	-	-	-	-
Third or Fourth Degree Laceration	-	-	3.98%	3.63%	3.27%

Prosser Memorial Hospital

723 Memorial Street
Prosser, WA 99350
E-mail: administration@pphdwa.org
URL: www.prosserhospital.com
Phone: 509-786-2222
Fax: 509-786-6683
Ownership: Govt - Hospital District or Authority
Emergency Services: Yes
Accredited: No

Key Personnel:

Administrator/CEO . . . . Jim Tavary

NOTE: Hospital profiles are in alphabetical order by state, then city, then hospital within the city; Rankings are sorted by rate in descending order and exclude hospitals with less than 25 cases; (1) The number of cases is too small (n<25) for purposes of reliably predicting hospital performance; (2) Measure reflects the hospital's indication that its submission was based upon a sample of its relevant discharges; (3) Rate reflects fewer than the maximum possible quarters of data for the measure; (4) Inaccurate information submitted and suppressed for one or more quarters; (5) No data is available from the hospital for this measure; Please refer to the User's Guide for a full explanation of data

Chief Medical Staff. . . . . Ben Sonnichsen
Emergency Room . . . . Kathy Horsager
Director Infection/Disease Control . . . . Susan Flory
Medical/Surgical Nursing . . . . Susan McCoy
Director Respiratory Therapy . . . . Thomas Anderson

Measure	Cases	This Hospital	State Average	U.S. Average	Top Hospital
Heart Attack Care					
ACE Inhibitor or ARB for LVSD[5]	-	-	84%	82%	100%
Aspirin at Arrival[5]	-	-	95%	92%	100%
Aspirin at Discharge[5]	-	-	95%	90%	100%
Beta Blocker at Arrival[5]	-	-	91%	87%	100%
Beta Blocker at Discharge[5]	-	-	95%	90%	100%
Fibrinolytic Medication Timing[5]	-	-	28%	31%	100%
PCI Within 90 Minutes of Arrival[5]	-	-	60%	54%	95%
Smoking Cessation Advice[5]	-	-	85%	88%	100%
Heart Failure Care					
ACE Inhibitor or ARB for LVSD[1,3]	1	100%	85%	82%	100%
Discharge Instructions[1,3]	7	0%	53%	61%	93%
Evaluation of LVS Function[1,3]	11	18%	85%	83%	99%
Smoking Cessation Advice[1,3]	4	0%	75%	82%	100%
Pneumonia Care					
Appropriate Initial Antibiotic[1,3]	15	73%	82%	83%	94%
Blood Culture Timing[1]	9	89%	91%	90%	100%
Influenza Vaccine[1]	5	40%	60%	70%	100%
Initial Antibiotic Timing[1,3]	13	69%	77%	80%	93%
Oxygenation Assessment[1,3]	15	100%	100%	99%	100%
Pneumococcal Vaccine[1,3]	12	58%	68%	69%	94%
Smoking Cessation Advice[1,3]	2	0%	79%	80%	100%
Surgical Infection Prevention					
Prophylactic Antibiotic Given[1,3]	19	58%	82%	77%	95%
Prophylactic Antibiotic Selection[1]	8	88%	91%	90%	100%
Prophylactic Antibiotic Stopped[1,3]	18	83%	75%	72%	95%
Pregnancy Care					
Inpatient Neonatal Mortality	-	-	-	-	-
Third or Fourth Degree Laceration	-	-	3.98%	3.63%	3.27%

Pullman Memorial Hospital

1125 NE Washington Avenue
Pullman, WA 99163
Phone: 509-332-2541
Fax: 509-332-6767
E-mail: sadams@complete.bbs.com
URL: www.pullmanhospital.org
Ownership: Govt - Hospital District or Authority
Accredited: No
Emergency Services: Yes
Licensed Beds: 42

Key Personnel:

Administrator . . . . Scott Adams
Chief Medical Staff. . . . . Gordon Teel
Emergency Room . . . . Richard Caggiano
Infection Control. . . . . Karen Cannon
Medical Surgical Nursing . . . . Dennise Stannard
OB/GYN/Women's Health . . . . Jeannie Eylar
Respiratory/Cardiopulmonary. . . . . Steve Dunning

Measure	Cases	This Hospital	State Average	U.S. Average	Top Hospital
Heart Attack Care					
ACE Inhibitor or ARB for LVSD[1]	1	100%	84%	82%	100%
Aspirin at Arrival[1]	4	100%	95%	92%	100%
Aspirin at Discharge[1]	4	100%	95%	90%	100%
Beta Blocker at Arrival[1]	4	75%	91%	87%	100%
Beta Blocker at Discharge[1]	4	100%	95%	90%	100%
Fibrinolytic Medication Timing[1,3]	2	0%	28%	31%	100%
PCI Within 90 Minutes of Arrival	0	-	60%	54%	95%
Smoking Cessation Advice[3]	0	-	85%	88%	100%
Heart Failure Care					
ACE Inhibitor or ARB for LVSD[1,3]	1	100%	85%	82%	100%
Discharge Instructions[1,3]	5	20%	53%	61%	93%
Evaluation of LVS Function[1,3]	9	33%	85%	83%	99%
Smoking Cessation Advice[1,3]	1	0%	75%	82%	100%
Pneumonia Care					
Appropriate Initial Antibiotic[1,3]	7	43%	82%	83%	94%
Blood Culture Timing[1]	22	77%	91%	90%	100%
Influenza Vaccine[5]	-	-	60%	70%	100%
Initial Antibiotic Timing	32	75%	77%	80%	93%
Oxygenation Assessment	42	100%	100%	99%	100%
Pneumococcal Vaccine	32	34%	68%	69%	94%
Smoking Cessation Advice[1,3]	3	0%	79%	80%	100%
Surgical Infection Prevention					
Prophylactic Antibiotic Given[5]	-	-	82%	77%	95%
Prophylactic Antibiotic Selection[5]	-	-	91%	90%	100%
Prophylactic Antibiotic Stopped[5]	-	-	75%	72%	95%
Pregnancy Care					
Inpatient Neonatal Mortality	-	-	-	-	-
Third or Fourth Degree Laceration	-	-	3.98%	3.63%	3.27%

Good Samaritan Hospital & Rehab Center

407 14th Ave Se
Phone: 253-848-6661
Puyallup, WA 98371
Ownership: Voluntary non-profit - Private
Accredited: Yes
Emergency Services: Yes

Measure	Cases	This Hospital	State Average	U.S. Average	Top Hospital
Heart Attack Care					
ACE Inhibitor or ARB for LVSD	33	91%	84%	82%	100%
Aspirin at Arrival	225	99%	95%	92%	100%
Aspirin at Discharge	188	91%	95%	90%	100%
Beta Blocker at Arrival	206	99%	91%	87%	100%
Beta Blocker at Discharge	190	95%	95%	90%	100%
Fibrinolytic Medication Timing	0	-	28%	31%	100%
PCI Within 90 Minutes of Arrival[1]	15	33%	60%	54%	95%
Smoking Cessation Advice	68	96%	85%	88%	100%
Heart Failure Care					
ACE Inhibitor or ARB for LVSD	82	85%	85%	82%	100%
Discharge Instructions	211	35%	53%	61%	93%
Evaluation of LVS Function	292	90%	85%	83%	99%
Smoking Cessation Advice	40	75%	75%	82%	100%
Pneumonia Care					
Appropriate Initial Antibiotic	147	76%	82%	83%	94%
Blood Culture Timing	120	89%	91%	90%	100%
Influenza Vaccine	28	68%	60%	70%	100%
Initial Antibiotic Timing	176	73%	77%	80%	93%
Oxygenation Assessment	229	99%	100%	99%	100%
Pneumococcal Vaccine	140	45%	68%	69%	94%
Smoking Cessation Advice	44	61%	79%	80%	100%
Surgical Infection Prevention					
Prophylactic Antibiotic Given[3]	247	55%	82%	77%	95%
Prophylactic Antibiotic Selection	90	96%	91%	90%	100%
Prophylactic Antibiotic Stopped[3]	222	87%	75%	72%	95%
Pregnancy Care					
Inpatient Neonatal Mortality	-	-	-	-	-
Third or Fourth Degree Laceration	-	-	3.98%	3.63%	3.27%

Group Health Eastside Hospital

2700 152nd Avenue NE
Redmond, WA 98052
Toll-Free: 800-231-6935
Phone: 425-883-5151
Fax: 425-883-5638
URL: www.ghc.org
Ownership: Voluntary non-profit - Other
Accredited: Yes
Emergency Services: Yes
Licensed Beds: 125

Key Personnel:

President/CEO. . . . . Cheryl M Scott
Administrator . . . . Susan Kropelnicki

Measure	Cases	This Hospital	State Average	U.S. Average	Top Hospital
Heart Attack Care					
ACE Inhibitor or ARB for LVSD[1]	8	100%	84%	82%	100%
Aspirin at Arrival	31	97%	95%	92%	100%
Aspirin at Discharge[1]	17	100%	95%	90%	100%
Beta Blocker at Arrival[1]	22	100%	91%	87%	100%
Beta Blocker at Discharge[1]	23	100%	95%	90%	100%
Fibrinolytic Medication Timing[3]	0	-	28%	31%	100%
PCI Within 90 Minutes of Arrival	0	-	60%	54%	95%
Smoking Cessation Advice[3]	0	-	85%	88%	100%
Heart Failure Care					
ACE Inhibitor or ARB for LVSD	54	89%	85%	82%	100%

NOTE: Hospital profiles are in alphabetical order by state, then city, then hospital within the city; Rankings are sorted by rate in descending order and exclude hospitals with less than 25 cases; (1) The number of cases is too small (n<25) for purposes of reliably predicting hospital performance; (2) Measure reflects the hospital's indication that its submission was based upon a sample of its relevant discharges; (3) Rate reflects fewer than the maximum possible quarters of data for the measure; (4) Inaccurate information submitted and suppressed for one or more quarters; (5) No data is available from the hospital for this measure; Please refer to the User's Guide for a full explanation of data

Discharge Instructions[3]	35	46%	53%	61%	93%
Evaluation of LVS Function	149	99%	85%	83%	99%
Smoking Cessation Advice[1,3]	2	100%	75%	82%	100%
Pneumonia Care					
Appropriate Initial Antibiotic[1,3]	20	90%	82%	83%	94%
Blood Culture Timing[3]	27	93%	91%	90%	100%
Influenza Vaccine[5]	-	-	60%	70%	100%
Initial Antibiotic Timing	125	81%	77%	80%	93%
Oxygenation Assessment	177	100%	100%	99%	100%
Pneumococcal Vaccine	163	92%	68%	69%	94%
Smoking Cessation Advice[1,3]	5	80%	79%	80%	100%
Surgical Infection Prevention					
Prophylactic Antibiotic Given[3]	199	90%	82%	77%	95%
Prophylactic Antibiotic Selection[5]	-	-	91%	90%	100%
Prophylactic Antibiotic Stopped[3]	192	83%	75%	72%	95%
Pregnancy Care					
Inpatient Neonatal Mortality	-	-	-	-	-
Third or Fourth Degree Laceration	-	-	3.98%	3.63%	3.27%

Valley Medical Center

400 S 43rd Street
PO Box 50010
Renton, WA 98055
Phone: 425-228-3450
Fax: 425-656-4202
URL: www.valleymed.org
Ownership: Govt - Hospital District or Authority
Accredited: Yes
Emergency Services: Yes
Licensed Beds: 303

Key Personnel:

CEO . . . . Richard D Roodman
Chief Medical Officer . . . . Tori McFall, MD
Manager Emergency Services . . . . Kayett Asuquo, RN
Director Respiratory Therapy . . . . Maryann Albenisius

Measure	Cases	This Hospital	State Average	U.S. Average	Top Hospital
Heart Attack Care					
ACE Inhibitor or ARB for LVSD	40	85%	84%	82%	100%
Aspirin at Arrival	261	97%	95%	92%	100%
Aspirin at Discharge	209	97%	95%	90%	100%
Beta Blocker at Arrival	223	96%	91%	87%	100%
Beta Blocker at Discharge	200	96%	95%	90%	100%
Fibrinolytic Medication Timing[3]	0	-	28%	31%	100%
PCI Within 90 Minutes of Arrival[1]	17	88%	60%	54%	95%
Smoking Cessation Advice[1,3]	20	85%	85%	88%	100%
Heart Failure Care					
ACE Inhibitor or ARB for LVSD	113	88%	85%	82%	100%
Discharge Instructions[3]	55	71%	53%	61%	93%
Evaluation of LVS Function	303	84%	85%	83%	99%
Smoking Cessation Advice[1,3]	9	67%	75%	82%	100%
Pneumonia Care					
Appropriate Initial Antibiotic[1,3]	20	90%	82%	83%	94%
Blood Culture Timing[3]	30	90%	91%	90%	100%
Influenza Vaccine[5]	-	-	60%	70%	100%
Initial Antibiotic Timing	239	61%	77%	80%	93%
Oxygenation Assessment	284	100%	100%	99%	100%
Pneumococcal Vaccine	169	57%	68%	69%	94%
Smoking Cessation Advice[1,3]	8	88%	79%	80%	100%
Surgical Infection Prevention					
Prophylactic Antibiotic Given[2,3]	64	67%	82%	77%	95%
Prophylactic Antibiotic Selection[2]	66	91%	91%	90%	100%
Prophylactic Antibiotic Stopped[2,3]	64	84%	75%	72%	95%
Pregnancy Care					
Inpatient Neonatal Mortality	3,571	0.14%	-	-	-
Third or Fourth Degree Laceration	2,243	4.19%	3.98%	3.63%	3.27%

Kadlec Medical Center

888 Swift Boulevard
Richland, WA 99352
Toll-Free: 800-765-1140
Phone: 509-946-4611
Fax: 509-942-2634
URL: www.kodlemed.org
Ownership: Voluntary non-profit - Other
Accredited: Yes
Emergency Services: Yes
Licensed Beds: 153

Key Personnel:

President/CEO . . . . Julie Meek
Chief of Medical Staff . . . . Thomas Radl
Director of Cardiology/Cardiac Lab. . . . . Brent O'Brian
Emergency Room Director . . . . Greg Brown
Respiratory Care Manager . . . . Angela Ohohdro

Measure	Cases	This Hospital	State Average	U.S. Average	Top Hospital
Heart Attack Care					
ACE Inhibitor or ARB for LVSD	55	84%	84%	82%	100%
Aspirin at Arrival	115	90%	95%	92%	100%
Aspirin at Discharge	298	96%	95%	90%	100%
Beta Blocker at Arrival	106	82%	91%	87%	100%
Beta Blocker at Discharge	275	92%	95%	90%	100%
Fibrinolytic Medication Timing[3]	0	-	28%	31%	100%
PCI Within 90 Minutes of Arrival[1]	15	80%	60%	54%	95%
Smoking Cessation Advice[1,3]	19	63%	85%	88%	100%
Heart Failure Care					
ACE Inhibitor or ARB for LVSD	67	67%	85%	82%	100%
Discharge Instructions[3]	32	41%	53%	61%	93%
Evaluation of LVS Function	161	89%	85%	83%	99%
Smoking Cessation Advice[1,3]	4	75%	75%	82%	100%
Pneumonia Care					
Appropriate Initial Antibiotic[3]	25	76%	82%	83%	94%
Blood Culture Timing[3]	30	93%	91%	90%	100%
Influenza Vaccine[4,5]	-	-	60%	70%	100%
Initial Antibiotic Timing	156	78%	77%	80%	93%
Oxygenation Assessment	211	100%	100%	99%	100%
Pneumococcal Vaccine	123	86%	68%	69%	94%
Smoking Cessation Advice[1,3]	4	100%	79%	80%	100%
Surgical Infection Prevention					
Prophylactic Antibiotic Given[3]	60	70%	82%	77%	95%
Prophylactic Antibiotic Selection[5]	-	-	91%	90%	100%
Prophylactic Antibiotic Stopped[3]	57	74%	75%	72%	95%
Pregnancy Care					
Inpatient Neonatal Mortality	-	-	-	-	-
Third or Fourth Degree Laceration	-	-	3.98%	3.63%	3.27%

Harborview Medical Center

325 9th Avenue
Seattle, WA 98104
Phone: 206-731-3036
Fax: 206-731-8551
URL: www.harborview.org
Ownership: Government - Local
Accredited: Yes
Emergency Services: Yes
Licensed Beds: 411

Key Personnel:

CEO/Executive Director . . . . David Jaffe
Chief Medical Staff . . . . Scott Barnnan
Emergency Room . . . . Michael Copass, MD
Director Infection/Disease Control . . . . Walter Stamm, MD
CCU Supervising Nurse . . . . Pattyra Calver
OB/GYN Womens Health. . . . . Kirk Shy, MD
Chief Radiology . . . . Lee Talner, MD
Director Respiratory Therapy . . . . David Pierson, MD

Measure	Cases	This Hospital	State Average	U.S. Average	Top Hospital
Heart Attack Care					
ACE Inhibitor or ARB for LVSD[1]	24	96%	84%	82%	100%
Aspirin at Arrival	98	100%	95%	92%	100%
Aspirin at Discharge	63	100%	95%	90%	100%
Beta Blocker at Arrival	61	100%	91%	87%	100%
Beta Blocker at Discharge	80	100%	95%	90%	100%
Fibrinolytic Medication Timing	0	-	28%	31%	100%
PCI Within 90 Minutes of Arrival[1]	9	67%	60%	54%	95%
Smoking Cessation Advice	54	91%	85%	88%	100%
Heart Failure Care					
ACE Inhibitor or ARB for LVSD[2]	113	90%	85%	82%	100%
Discharge Instructions[2]	176	59%	53%	61%	93%
Evaluation of LVS Function[2]	199	98%	85%	83%	99%
Smoking Cessation Advice[2]	102	74%	75%	82%	100%
Pneumonia Care					
Appropriate Initial Antibiotic[2]	121	83%	82%	83%	94%
Blood Culture Timing[2]	119	80%	91%	90%	100%
Influenza Vaccine[1,2]	24	21%	60%	70%	100%
Initial Antibiotic Timing[2]	177	68%	77%	80%	93%
Oxygenation Assessment[2]	214	100%	100%	99%	100%

NOTE: Hospital profiles are in alphabetical order by state, then city, then hospital within the city; Rankings are sorted by rate in descending order and exclude hospitals with less than 25 cases; (1) The number of cases is too small (n<25) for purposes of reliably predicting hospital performance; (2) Measure reflects the hospital's indication that its submission was based upon a sample of its relevant discharges; (3) Rate reflects fewer than the maximum possible quarters of data for the measure; (4) Inaccurate information submitted and suppressed for one or more quarters; (5) No data is available from the hospital for this measure; Please refer to the User's Guide for a full explanation of data

Measure	Cases	This Hospital	State Average	U.S. Average	Top Hospital
Pneumococcal Vaccine[2]	68	46%	68%	69%	94%
Smoking Cessation Advice[2]	119	66%	79%	80%	100%
Surgical Infection Prevention					
Prophylactic Antibiotic Given[2]	133	76%	82%	77%	95%
Prophylactic Antibiotic Selection[2]	36	83%	91%	90%	100%
Prophylactic Antibiotic Stopped[2]	131	78%	75%	72%	95%
Pregnancy Care					
Inpatient Neonatal Mortality	-	-	-	-	-
Third or Fourth Degree Laceration	-	-	3.98%	3.63%	3.27%

Northwest Hospital and Medical Center

1550 N 115th Street
Seattle, WA 98133
URL: www.nwhospital.org
Ownership: Voluntary non-profit - Other
Emergency Services: Yes

Phone: 206-364-0500
Fax: 206-368-1990
Accredited: Yes
Licensed Beds: 345

Key Personnel:

CEO. . . . . Will Sthenider
OB/GYN Womens Health. . . . . Barry Lawson, MD
Chief Radiology . . . . Thaddeus Paprocki, MD
Manager Respiratory Therapy . . . . Steve Crogan

Measure	Cases	This Hospital	State Average	U.S. Average	Top Hospital
Heart Attack Care					
ACE Inhibitor or ARB for LVSD	29	93%	84%	82%	100%
Aspirin at Arrival	114	95%	95%	92%	100%
Aspirin at Discharge	101	99%	95%	90%	100%
Beta Blocker at Arrival	89	96%	91%	87%	100%
Beta Blocker at Discharge	114	100%	95%	90%	100%
Fibrinolytic Medication Timing	0	-	28%	31%	100%
PCI Within 90 Minutes of Arrival[1]	10	50%	60%	54%	95%
Smoking Cessation Advice	32	97%	85%	88%	100%
Heart Failure Care					
ACE Inhibitor or ARB for LVSD	85	86%	85%	82%	100%
Discharge Instructions	158	69%	53%	61%	93%
Evaluation of LVS Function	218	89%	85%	83%	99%
Smoking Cessation Advice	26	92%	75%	82%	100%
Pneumonia Care					
Appropriate Initial Antibiotic	119	72%	82%	83%	94%
Blood Culture Timing	125	91%	91%	90%	100%
Influenza Vaccine[4,5]	-	-	60%	70%	100%
Initial Antibiotic Timing	145	73%	77%	80%	93%
Oxygenation Assessment	188	100%	100%	99%	100%
Pneumococcal Vaccine	125	92%	68%	69%	94%
Smoking Cessation Advice	41	78%	79%	80%	100%
Surgical Infection Prevention					
Prophylactic Antibiotic Given[3]	363	76%	82%	77%	95%
Prophylactic Antibiotic Selection	60	83%	91%	90%	100%
Prophylactic Antibiotic Stopped[3]	349	56%	75%	72%	95%
Pregnancy Care					
Inpatient Neonatal Mortality	999	0.00%	-	-	-
Third or Fourth Degree Laceration	696	6.75%	3.98%	3.63%	3.27%

Schick-Shadel Hospital

12101 Ambaum Boulevard SW
Seattle, WA 98146

Toll-Free: 800-272-8464
Phone: 206-244-8100
Fax: 206-431-9142

E-mail: contact-us@schick-shadel.com
URL: www.schick-shadel.com
Ownership: Proprietary
Emergency Services: No

Accredited: No
Licensed Beds: 63

Key Personnel:

CEO. . . . . James P Graham

Measure	Cases	This Hospital	State Average	U.S. Average	Top Hospital
Heart Attack Care					
ACE Inhibitor or ARB for LVSD[5]	-	-	84%	82%	100%
Aspirin at Arrival[5]	-	-	95%	92%	100%
Aspirin at Discharge[5]	-	-	95%	90%	100%
Beta Blocker at Arrival[5]	-	-	91%	87%	100%
Beta Blocker at Discharge[5]	-	-	95%	90%	100%
Fibrinolytic Medication Timing[5]	-	-	28%	31%	100%
PCI Within 90 Minutes of Arrival[5]	-	-	60%	54%	95%
Smoking Cessation Advice[5]	-	-	85%	88%	100%
Heart Failure Care					
ACE Inhibitor or ARB for LVSD[5]	-	-	85%	82%	100%
Discharge Instructions[5]	-	-	53%	61%	93%
Evaluation of LVS Function[5]	-	-	85%	83%	99%
Smoking Cessation Advice[5]	-	-	75%	82%	100%
Pneumonia Care					
Appropriate Initial Antibiotic[5]	-	-	82%	83%	94%
Blood Culture Timing[5]	-	-	91%	90%	100%
Influenza Vaccine[5]	-	-	60%	70%	100%
Initial Antibiotic Timing[5]	-	-	77%	80%	93%
Oxygenation Assessment[5]	-	-	100%	99%	100%
Pneumococcal Vaccine[5]	-	-	68%	69%	94%
Smoking Cessation Advice[5]	-	-	79%	80%	100%
Surgical Infection Prevention					
Prophylactic Antibiotic Given[5]	-	-	82%	77%	95%
Prophylactic Antibiotic Selection[5]	-	-	91%	90%	100%
Prophylactic Antibiotic Stopped[5]	-	-	75%	72%	95%
Pregnancy Care					
Inpatient Neonatal Mortality	-	-	-	-	-
Third or Fourth Degree Laceration	-	-	3.98%	3.63%	3.27%

Swedish Medical Center

First Hill Campus
747 Broadway
Seattle, WA 98122
URL: www.swedish.org
Ownership: Voluntary non-profit - Other
Emergency Services: Yes

Toll-Free: 800-833-6385
Phone: 206-386-6000
Fax: 206-386-6138
Accredited: Yes
Licensed Beds: 697

Key Personnel:

CEO. . . . . Rodney F Hochman, MD
Chief Medical Officer . . . . Nancy J Auer, MD
Emergency Room . . . . Ron Dobson, MD
Director Infection/Disease Control . . . . Will Shelton
OB/GYN Womens Health. . . . . David Luthy, MD
Chief Radiology . . . . Timothy Larson, MD
Director Respiratory Therapy . . . . Cal Cederblom

Measure	Cases	This Hospital	State Average	U.S. Average	Top Hospital
Heart Attack Care					
ACE Inhibitor or ARB for LVSD	42	76%	84%	82%	100%
Aspirin at Arrival	152	98%	95%	92%	100%
Aspirin at Discharge	196	96%	95%	90%	100%
Beta Blocker at Arrival	145	92%	91%	87%	100%
Beta Blocker at Discharge	216	94%	95%	90%	100%
Fibrinolytic Medication Timing	0	-	28%	31%	100%
PCI Within 90 Minutes of Arrival[1]	2	0%	60%	54%	95%
Smoking Cessation Advice	53	79%	85%	88%	100%
Heart Failure Care					
ACE Inhibitor or ARB for LVSD	150	81%	85%	82%	100%
Discharge Instructions	361	22%	53%	61%	93%
Evaluation of LVS Function	453	91%	85%	83%	99%
Smoking Cessation Advice	61	48%	75%	82%	100%
Pneumonia Care					
Appropriate Initial Antibiotic	261	79%	82%	83%	94%
Blood Culture Timing	249	88%	91%	90%	100%
Influenza Vaccine	92	63%	60%	70%	100%
Initial Antibiotic Timing	399	78%	77%	80%	93%
Oxygenation Assessment	506	100%	100%	99%	100%
Pneumococcal Vaccine	329	71%	68%	69%	94%
Smoking Cessation Advice	116	86%	79%	80%	100%
Surgical Infection Prevention					
Prophylactic Antibiotic Given[2,3]	270	79%	82%	77%	95%
Prophylactic Antibiotic Selection[2]	93	98%	91%	90%	100%
Prophylactic Antibiotic Stopped[2,3]	263	52%	75%	72%	95%
Pregnancy Care					
Inpatient Neonatal Mortality	-	-	-	-	-
Third or Fourth Degree Laceration	-	-	3.98%	3.63%	3.27%

NOTE: Hospital profiles are in alphabetical order by state, then city, then hospital within the city; Rankings are sorted by rate in descending order and exclude hospitals with less than 25 cases; (1) The number of cases is too small (n<25) for purposes of reliably predicting hospital performance; (2) Measure reflects the hospital's indication that its submission was based upon a sample of its relevant discharges; (3) Rate reflects fewer than the maximum possible quarters of data for the measure; (4) Inaccurate information submitted and suppressed for one or more quarters; (5) No data is available from the hospital for this measure; Please refer to the User's Guide for a full explanation of data

Swedish Medical Center/Providence

500 17th Avenue Phone: 206-320-2000
Seattle, WA 98122
Ownership: Voluntary non-profit - Church Accredited: Yes
Emergency Services: Yes

Measure	Cases	This Hospital	State Average	U.S. Average	Top Hospital
Heart Attack Care					
ACE Inhibitor or ARB for LVSD	36	78%	84%	82%	100%
Aspirin at Arrival	99	98%	95%	92%	100%
Aspirin at Discharge	168	99%	95%	90%	100%
Beta Blocker at Arrival	88	97%	91%	87%	100%
Beta Blocker at Discharge	176	93%	95%	90%	100%
Fibrinolytic Medication Timing	0	-	28%	31%	100%
PCI Within 90 Minutes of Arrival[1]	7	43%	60%	54%	95%
Smoking Cessation Advice	49	80%	85%	88%	100%
Heart Failure Care					
ACE Inhibitor or ARB for LVSD	124	85%	85%	82%	100%
Discharge Instructions	222	27%	53%	61%	93%
Evaluation of LVS Function	271	94%	85%	83%	99%
Smoking Cessation Advice	63	54%	75%	82%	100%
Pneumonia Care					
Appropriate Initial Antibiotic	88	84%	82%	83%	94%
Blood Culture Timing	74	93%	91%	90%	100%
Influenza Vaccine[1]	23	61%	60%	70%	100%
Initial Antibiotic Timing	114	76%	77%	80%	93%
Oxygenation Assessment	142	100%	100%	99%	100%
Pneumococcal Vaccine	90	60%	68%	69%	94%
Smoking Cessation Advice	45	87%	79%	80%	100%
Surgical Infection Prevention					
Prophylactic Antibiotic Given[2,3]	149	73%	82%	77%	95%
Prophylactic Antibiotic Selection[2]	60	100%	91%	90%	100%
Prophylactic Antibiotic Stopped[2,3]	145	69%	75%	72%	95%
Pregnancy Care					
Inpatient Neonatal Mortality	-	-	-	-	-
Third or Fourth Degree Laceration	-	-	3.98%	3.63%	3.27%

University of Washington Medical Center

1959 NE Pacific Toll-Free: 800-489-3887
Seattle, WA 98195 Phone: 206-598-3300
Fax: 206-598-4610
URL: www.washington.edu/medical/UWMC
Ownership: Government - State Accredited: Yes
Emergency Services: Yes Licensed Beds: 450

Key Personnel:

CEO. . . . . Kathleen Sellick
Chief Medical Staff. . . . . Ed Walker
Director Cardiac Laboratory . . . . Larry Dean, MD
Catheterization Laboratory. . . . . Larry Dean, MD
Intensive Coronary. . . . . Susan Grant
OB/GYN Womens Health. . . . . Stephanie Uhrich
Respiratory/Cardiopulmonary. . . . . Sal Ramirez

Measure	Cases	This Hospital	State Average	U.S. Average	Top Hospital
Heart Attack Care					
ACE Inhibitor or ARB for LVSD[1]	22	91%	84%	82%	100%
Aspirin at Arrival	51	100%	95%	92%	100%
Aspirin at Discharge	82	99%	95%	90%	100%
Beta Blocker at Arrival	42	95%	91%	87%	100%
Beta Blocker at Discharge	105	99%	95%	90%	100%
Fibrinolytic Medication Timing	0	-	28%	31%	100%
PCI Within 90 Minutes of Arrival[1]	4	50%	60%	54%	95%
Smoking Cessation Advice	36	100%	85%	88%	100%
Heart Failure Care					
ACE Inhibitor or ARB for LVSD	231	97%	85%	82%	100%
Discharge Instructions	333	51%	53%	61%	93%
Evaluation of LVS Function	352	99%	85%	83%	99%
Smoking Cessation Advice	63	100%	75%	82%	100%
Pneumonia Care					
Appropriate Initial Antibiotic	83	86%	82%	83%	94%
Blood Culture Timing	97	97%	91%	90%	100%
Influenza Vaccine	30	33%	60%	70%	100%
Initial Antibiotic Timing	173	47%	77%	80%	93%
Oxygenation Assessment	200	100%	100%	99%	100%
Pneumococcal Vaccine	87	38%	68%	69%	94%
Smoking Cessation Advice	51	100%	79%	80%	100%
Surgical Infection Prevention					
Prophylactic Antibiotic Given[2,3]	343	81%	82%	77%	95%
Prophylactic Antibiotic Selection[2]	74	92%	91%	90%	100%
Prophylactic Antibiotic Stopped[2,3]	331	56%	75%	72%	95%
Pregnancy Care					
Inpatient Neonatal Mortality	-	-	-	-	-
Third or Fourth Degree Laceration	-	-	3.98%	3.63%	3.27%

Virginia Mason Medical Center

1100 Ninth Avenue Phone: 206-223-6600
Seattle, WA 98101 Fax: 206-223-6976
URL: www.vmmc.org
Ownership: Voluntary non-profit - Private Accredited: Yes
Emergency Services: Yes Licensed Beds: 336

Key Personnel:

CEO. . . . . Gary Kaplan
Chief Medical Staff. . . . . Daniel Paull
Director of Cardiology/Cardiac Lab. . . . . Christopher Fellows
Emergency Room . . . . Chris Moore
Emergency Room . . . . Michael Glenn
Director Medical/Surgical Nursing . . . . Patti Crome
OB/GYN Womens Health. . . . . Michael Klotz, MD
Director of Pulmonary/Respiratory Care. . . . . . . Michael Weinstein

Measure	Cases	This Hospital	State Average	U.S. Average	Top Hospital
Heart Attack Care					
ACE Inhibitor or ARB for LVSD	48	88%	84%	82%	100%
Aspirin at Arrival	139	98%	95%	92%	100%
Aspirin at Discharge	244	99%	95%	90%	100%
Beta Blocker at Arrival	125	100%	91%	87%	100%
Beta Blocker at Discharge	240	98%	95%	90%	100%
Fibrinolytic Medication Timing	0	-	28%	31%	100%
PCI Within 90 Minutes of Arrival[1]	8	50%	60%	54%	95%
Smoking Cessation Advice	47	98%	85%	88%	100%
Heart Failure Care					
ACE Inhibitor or ARB for LVSD	123	77%	85%	82%	100%
Discharge Instructions	288	59%	53%	61%	93%
Evaluation of LVS Function	375	97%	85%	83%	99%
Smoking Cessation Advice[1]	15	100%	75%	82%	100%
Pneumonia Care					
Appropriate Initial Antibiotic[2]	177	96%	82%	83%	94%
Blood Culture Timing[2]	202	87%	91%	90%	100%
Influenza Vaccine	78	74%	60%	70%	100%
Initial Antibiotic Timing[2]	235	81%	77%	80%	93%
Oxygenation Assessment[2]	352	100%	100%	99%	100%
Pneumococcal Vaccine[2]	266	61%	68%	69%	94%
Smoking Cessation Advice[2]	61	98%	79%	80%	100%
Surgical Infection Prevention					
Prophylactic Antibiotic Given[2]	524	70%	82%	77%	95%
Prophylactic Antibiotic Selection[2]	134	94%	91%	90%	100%
Prophylactic Antibiotic Stopped[2]	496	91%	75%	72%	95%
Pregnancy Care					
Inpatient Neonatal Mortality	-	-	-	-	-
Third or Fourth Degree Laceration	-	-	3.98%	3.63%	3.27%

United General Hospital

2000 Hospital Drive Phone: 360-856-6021
Sedro Woolley, WA 98284
Ownership: Govt - Hospital District or Authority Accredited: Yes
Emergency Services: Yes

Measure	Cases	This Hospital	State Average	U.S. Average	Top Hospital
Heart Attack Care					
ACE Inhibitor or ARB for LVSD[1]	1	100%	84%	82%	100%
Aspirin at Arrival[1]	6	100%	95%	92%	100%
Aspirin at Discharge[1]	5	100%	95%	90%	100%
Beta Blocker at Arrival[1]	3	100%	91%	87%	100%
Beta Blocker at Discharge[1]	3	100%	95%	90%	100%
Fibrinolytic Medication Timing	0	-	28%	31%	100%

NOTE: Hospital profiles are in alphabetical order by state, then city, then hospital within the city; Rankings are sorted by rate in descending order and exclude hospitals with less than 25 cases; (1) The number of cases is too small (n<25) for purposes of reliably predicting hospital performance; (2) Measure reflects the hospital's indication that its submission was based upon a sample of its relevant discharges; (3) Rate reflects fewer than the maximum possible quarters of data for the measure; (4) Inaccurate information submitted and suppressed for one or more quarters; (5) No data is available from the hospital for this measure; Please refer to the User's Guide for a full explanation of data

Measure	Cases	This Hospital	State Average	U.S. Average	Top Hospital
PCI Within 90 Minutes of Arrival	0	-	60%	54%	95%
Smoking Cessation Advice	0	-	85%	88%	100%
Heart Failure Care					
ACE Inhibitor or ARB for LVSD[1]	14	100%	85%	82%	100%
Discharge Instructions[1]	24	88%	53%	61%	93%
Evaluation of LVS Function	34	91%	85%	83%	99%
Smoking Cessation Advice[1]	3	100%	75%	82%	100%
Pneumonia Care					
Appropriate Initial Antibiotic	107	94%	82%	83%	94%
Blood Culture Timing	50	96%	91%	90%	100%
Influenza Vaccine[1]	16	62%	60%	70%	100%
Initial Antibiotic Timing	92	82%	77%	80%	93%
Oxygenation Assessment	113	100%	100%	99%	100%
Pneumococcal Vaccine	79	96%	68%	69%	94%
Smoking Cessation Advice[1]	24	100%	79%	80%	100%
Surgical Infection Prevention					
Prophylactic Antibiotic Given[1,3]	1	100%	82%	77%	95%
Prophylactic Antibiotic Selection[1]	1	0%	91%	90%	100%
Prophylactic Antibiotic Stopped[1,3]	1	0%	75%	72%	95%
Pregnancy Care					
Inpatient Neonatal Mortality	-	-	-	-	-
Third or Fourth Degree Laceration	-	-	3.98%	3.63%	3.27%

Mason General Hospital

901 Mt View Drive
Building 1
Shelton, WA 98584
URL: www.masongeneral.com
Phone: 360-426-1611
Fax: 360-427-3603
Ownership: Govt - Hospital District or Authority
Accredited: No
Emergency Services: Yes
Licensed Beds: 68

Key Personnel:
CEO. . . . . Bob Appel

Measure	Cases	This Hospital	State Average	U.S. Average	Top Hospital
Heart Attack Care					
ACE Inhibitor or ARB for LVSD[1]	3	67%	84%	82%	100%
Aspirin at Arrival[1]	18	100%	95%	92%	100%
Aspirin at Discharge[1]	7	86%	95%	90%	100%
Beta Blocker at Arrival[1]	18	83%	91%	87%	100%
Beta Blocker at Discharge[1]	7	71%	95%	90%	100%
Fibrinolytic Medication Timing[3]	0	-	28%	31%	100%
PCI Within 90 Minutes of Arrival	0	-	60%	54%	95%
Smoking Cessation Advice[3]	0	-	85%	88%	100%
Heart Failure Care					
ACE Inhibitor or ARB for LVSD	29	90%	85%	82%	100%
Discharge Instructions[3]	45	62%	53%	61%	93%
Evaluation of LVS Function	68	74%	85%	83%	99%
Smoking Cessation Advice[1,3]	19	89%	75%	82%	100%
Pneumonia Care					
Appropriate Initial Antibiotic[1,3]	12	58%	82%	83%	94%
Blood Culture Timing	40	88%	91%	90%	100%
Influenza Vaccine[5]	-	-	60%	70%	100%
Initial Antibiotic Timing	83	88%	77%	80%	93%
Oxygenation Assessment	99	100%	100%	99%	100%
Pneumococcal Vaccine	58	83%	68%	69%	94%
Smoking Cessation Advice[1,3]	16	94%	79%	80%	100%
Surgical Infection Prevention					
Prophylactic Antibiotic Given[5]	-	-	82%	77%	95%
Prophylactic Antibiotic Selection[5]	-	-	91%	90%	100%
Prophylactic Antibiotic Stopped[5]	-	-	75%	72%	95%
Pregnancy Care					
Inpatient Neonatal Mortality	-	-	-	-	-
Third or Fourth Degree Laceration	-	-	3.98%	3.63%	3.27%

Snoqualmie Valley Hospital

9575 Ethan Wade Way Se
Snoqualmie, WA 98065
Phone: 425-831-2300
Ownership: Govt - Hospital District or Authority
Accredited: No
Emergency Services: Yes

Measure	Cases	This Hospital	State Average	U.S. Average	Top Hospital
Heart Attack Care					
ACE Inhibitor or ARB for LVSD[5]	-	-	84%	82%	100%
Aspirin at Arrival[5]	-	-	95%	92%	100%
Aspirin at Discharge[5]	-	-	95%	90%	100%
Beta Blocker at Arrival[5]	-	-	91%	87%	100%
Beta Blocker at Discharge[5]	-	-	95%	90%	100%
Fibrinolytic Medication Timing[5]	-	-	28%	31%	100%
PCI Within 90 Minutes of Arrival[5]	-	-	60%	54%	95%
Smoking Cessation Advice[5]	-	-	85%	88%	100%
Heart Failure Care					
ACE Inhibitor or ARB for LVSD[1]	1	100%	85%	82%	100%
Discharge Instructions[1]	5	0%	53%	61%	93%
Evaluation of LVS Function[1]	8	62%	85%	83%	99%
Smoking Cessation Advice	0	-	75%	82%	100%
Pneumonia Care					
Appropriate Initial Antibiotic[1]	9	67%	82%	83%	94%
Blood Culture Timing[1]	4	75%	91%	90%	100%
Influenza Vaccine[1]	2	50%	60%	70%	100%
Initial Antibiotic Timing[1]	10	70%	77%	80%	93%
Oxygenation Assessment[1]	12	100%	100%	99%	100%
Pneumococcal Vaccine[1]	6	50%	68%	69%	94%
Smoking Cessation Advice[1]	1	100%	79%	80%	100%
Surgical Infection Prevention					
Prophylactic Antibiotic Given[5]	-	-	82%	77%	95%
Prophylactic Antibiotic Selection[5]	-	-	91%	90%	100%
Prophylactic Antibiotic Stopped[5]	-	-	75%	72%	95%
Pregnancy Care					
Inpatient Neonatal Mortality	-	-	-	-	-
Third or Fourth Degree Laceration	-	-	3.98%	3.63%	3.27%

Deaconess Medical Center

800 W Fifth Avenue
Spokane, WA 99204
E-mail: Deaconess@empirehealth.org
URL: deaconessmedicalcenter.org
Phone: 509-458-5800
Fax: 509-473-7684
Ownership: Voluntary non-profit - Private
Accredited: Yes
Emergency Services: Yes
Licensed Beds: 388

Key Personnel:
President/CEO. . . . . Thomas White
Chief Medical Staff. . . . . Angie O'Brien
Manager Catheterization Laboratory . . . . Kim Davis
Emergency Room . . . . Pat Yost
Director Medical/Surgical Nursing . . . . Peggy Currie
Manager Respiratory Therapy . . . . Darrel Moss

Measure	Cases	This Hospital	State Average	U.S. Average	Top Hospital
Heart Attack Care					
ACE Inhibitor or ARB for LVSD	70	89%	84%	82%	100%
Aspirin at Arrival	105	99%	95%	92%	100%
Aspirin at Discharge	270	100%	95%	90%	100%
Beta Blocker at Arrival	92	96%	91%	87%	100%
Beta Blocker at Discharge	297	99%	95%	90%	100%
Fibrinolytic Medication Timing	0	-	28%	31%	100%
PCI Within 90 Minutes of Arrival[1]	9	56%	60%	54%	95%
Smoking Cessation Advice	107	100%	85%	88%	100%
Heart Failure Care					
ACE Inhibitor or ARB for LVSD	128	91%	85%	82%	100%
Discharge Instructions	217	85%	53%	61%	93%
Evaluation of LVS Function	252	94%	85%	83%	99%
Smoking Cessation Advice	62	97%	75%	82%	100%
Pneumonia Care					
Appropriate Initial Antibiotic	91	87%	82%	83%	94%
Blood Culture Timing	76	89%	91%	90%	100%
Influenza Vaccine	31	71%	60%	70%	100%
Initial Antibiotic Timing	146	73%	77%	80%	93%
Oxygenation Assessment	186	100%	100%	99%	100%
Pneumococcal Vaccine	125	60%	68%	69%	94%
Smoking Cessation Advice	58	88%	79%	80%	100%
Surgical Infection Prevention					
Prophylactic Antibiotic Given[2,3]	351	90%	82%	77%	95%
Prophylactic Antibiotic Selection[2]	103	96%	91%	90%	100%
Prophylactic Antibiotic Stopped[2,3]	345	68%	75%	72%	95%
Pregnancy Care					
Inpatient Neonatal Mortality	-	-	-	-	-

NOTE: Hospital profiles are in alphabetical order by state, then city, then hospital within the city; Rankings are sorted by rate in descending order and exclude hospitals with less than 25 cases; (1) The number of cases is too small (n<25) for purposes of reliably predicting hospital performance; (2) Measure reflects the hospital's indication that its submission was based upon a sample of its relevant discharges; (3) Rate reflects fewer than the maximum possible quarters of data for the measure; (4) Inaccurate information submitted and suppressed for one or more quarters; (5) No data is available from the hospital for this measure; Please refer to the User's Guide for a full explanation of data

Third or Fourth Degree Laceration	-	-	3.98%	3.63%	3.27%

Holy Family Hospital

5633 North Lidgerwood
Spokane, WA 99208
Phone: 509-482-0111
Fax: 509-482-2587
E-mail: crabtrl@holy-family.org
URL: www.holy-family.org
Ownership: Voluntary non-profit - Church
Accredited: Yes
Emergency Services: Yes
Licensed Beds: 272

Key Personnel:

President/CEO. . . . . Thomas F Corley
Director Infection/Disease Control . . . . Kim Richardson
CCU Spvg. Nurse . . . . Kay Ely
OB/GYN Womens Health. . . . . Jane O'Hara
Director Radiology . . . . Al Wichtendahl
Director Respiratory Therapy . . . . June Davis

Measure	Cases	This Hospital	State Average	U.S. Average	Top Hospital
Heart Attack Care					
ACE Inhibitor or ARB for LVSD[1]	13	85%	84%	82%	100%
Aspirin at Arrival	97	99%	95%	92%	100%
Aspirin at Discharge	73	99%	95%	90%	100%
Beta Blocker at Arrival	86	99%	91%	87%	100%
Beta Blocker at Discharge	72	96%	95%	90%	100%
Fibrinolytic Medication Timing	0	-	28%	31%	100%
PCI Within 90 Minutes of Arrival[1]	12	42%	60%	54%	95%
Smoking Cessation Advice	29	97%	85%	88%	100%
Heart Failure Care					
ACE Inhibitor or ARB for LVSD	53	81%	85%	82%	100%
Discharge Instructions	129	66%	53%	61%	93%
Evaluation of LVS Function	165	86%	85%	83%	99%
Smoking Cessation Advice[1]	21	100%	75%	82%	100%
Pneumonia Care					
Appropriate Initial Antibiotic	280	87%	82%	83%	94%
Blood Culture Timing	240	95%	91%	90%	100%
Influenza Vaccine	64	88%	60%	70%	100%
Initial Antibiotic Timing	310	78%	77%	80%	93%
Oxygenation Assessment	393	100%	100%	99%	100%
Pneumococcal Vaccine	252	83%	68%	69%	94%
Smoking Cessation Advice	95	92%	79%	80%	100%
Surgical Infection Prevention					
Prophylactic Antibiotic Given[2,3]	151	87%	82%	77%	95%
Prophylactic Antibiotic Selection[2]	47	94%	91%	90%	100%
Prophylactic Antibiotic Stopped[2,3]	145	82%	75%	72%	95%
Pregnancy Care					
Inpatient Neonatal Mortality	1,150	0.00%	-	-	-
Third or Fourth Degree Laceration	876	2.63%	3.98%	3.63%	3.27%

Sacred Heart Medical Center

W 101 8th Avenue
Spokane, WA 99204
Phone: 509-474-3131
Fax: 509-474-3153
E-mail: pr@shmc.org
URL: www.shmc.org
Ownership: Voluntary non-profit - Church
Accredited: Yes
Emergency Services: Yes
Licensed Beds: 623

Key Personnel:

President/CEO. . . . . Ryland P Davis
President/COO. . . . . Michael Wilson
Chief Medical Staff. . . . . G Thomas Miller, MD
OB/GYN Womens Health. . . . . Sherry Maughan

Measure	Cases	This Hospital	State Average	U.S. Average	Top Hospital
Heart Attack Care					
ACE Inhibitor or ARB for LVSD	97	97%	84%	82%	100%
Aspirin at Arrival	193	100%	95%	92%	100%
Aspirin at Discharge	530	100%	95%	90%	100%
Beta Blocker at Arrival	168	99%	91%	87%	100%
Beta Blocker at Discharge	527	99%	95%	90%	100%
Fibrinolytic Medication Timing	0	-	28%	31%	100%
PCI Within 90 Minutes of Arrival[1]	13	85%	60%	54%	95%
Smoking Cessation Advice	196	100%	85%	88%	100%
Heart Failure Care					
ACE Inhibitor or ARB for LVSD	245	98%	85%	82%	100%
Discharge Instructions	414	96%	53%	61%	93%
Evaluation of LVS Function	457	99%	85%	83%	99%
Smoking Cessation Advice	70	100%	75%	82%	100%
Pneumonia Care					
Appropriate Initial Antibiotic	219	82%	82%	83%	94%
Blood Culture Timing	267	91%	91%	90%	100%
Influenza Vaccine	61	84%	60%	70%	100%
Initial Antibiotic Timing	391	75%	77%	80%	93%
Oxygenation Assessment	476	100%	100%	99%	100%
Pneumococcal Vaccine	285	80%	68%	69%	94%
Smoking Cessation Advice	112	100%	79%	80%	100%
Surgical Infection Prevention					
Prophylactic Antibiotic Given[2,3]	239	90%	82%	77%	95%
Prophylactic Antibiotic Selection[2]	84	96%	91%	90%	100%
Prophylactic Antibiotic Stopped[2,3]	233	90%	75%	72%	95%
Pregnancy Care					
Inpatient Neonatal Mortality	-	-	-	-	-
Third or Fourth Degree Laceration	-	-	3.98%	3.63%	3.27%

Valley Hospital & Medical Center

12606 E Mission Avenue
Spokane, WA 99216
Phone: 509-924-6650
Fax: 509-473-7684
URL: www.valleyhospital.org
Ownership: Voluntary non-profit - Private
Accredited: Yes
Emergency Services: Yes
Licensed Beds: 123

Key Personnel:

CEO. . . . . Jeff Nelson
Chief Medical Staff. . . . . Robert Hartman
Emergency Room Head. . . . . Wayne Tilson
Emergency Room . . . . T Brodie, MD
Director Infection/Disease Control . . . . Margaret Christian
Respiratory Care Head . . . . Dave Porter

Measure	Cases	This Hospital	State Average	U.S. Average	Top Hospital
Heart Attack Care					
ACE Inhibitor or ARB for LVSD[1]	1	0%	84%	82%	100%
Aspirin at Arrival[1]	14	79%	95%	92%	100%
Aspirin at Discharge[1]	9	100%	95%	90%	100%
Beta Blocker at Arrival[1]	15	93%	91%	87%	100%
Beta Blocker at Discharge[1]	9	89%	95%	90%	100%
Fibrinolytic Medication Timing[1]	1	100%	28%	31%	100%
PCI Within 90 Minutes of Arrival	0	-	60%	54%	95%
Smoking Cessation Advice	0	-	85%	88%	100%
Heart Failure Care					
ACE Inhibitor or ARB for LVSD[1]	23	78%	85%	82%	100%
Discharge Instructions	56	36%	53%	61%	93%
Evaluation of LVS Function	86	83%	85%	83%	99%
Smoking Cessation Advice[1]	13	85%	75%	82%	100%
Pneumonia Care					
Appropriate Initial Antibiotic	82	80%	82%	83%	94%
Blood Culture Timing	73	96%	91%	90%	100%
Influenza Vaccine[1]	19	68%	60%	70%	100%
Initial Antibiotic Timing	110	68%	77%	80%	93%
Oxygenation Assessment	152	100%	100%	99%	100%
Pneumococcal Vaccine	98	61%	68%	69%	94%
Smoking Cessation Advice	33	97%	79%	80%	100%
Surgical Infection Prevention					
Prophylactic Antibiotic Given[2,3]	227	89%	82%	77%	95%
Prophylactic Antibiotic Selection[2]	66	97%	91%	90%	100%
Prophylactic Antibiotic Stopped[2,3]	222	88%	75%	72%	95%
Pregnancy Care					
Inpatient Neonatal Mortality	-	-	-	-	-
Third or Fourth Degree Laceration	-	-	3.98%	3.63%	3.27%

Sunnyside Community Hospital

10th & Tacoma Avenue
Sunnyside, WA 98944
Phone: 509-837-1500
Fax: 509-837-1740
Ownership: Voluntary non-profit - Other
Accredited: Yes
Emergency Services: Yes
Licensed Beds: 38

Key Personnel:

CEO. . . . . Jon D Smiley
Chief Medical Staff. . . . . Coke R Smith, MD
Emergency Room . . . . David W Johnson, DO

NOTE: Hospital profiles are in alphabetical order by state, then city, then hospital within the city; Rankings are sorted by rate in descending order and exclude hospitals with less than 25 cases; (1) The number of cases is too small (n<25) for purposes of reliably predicting hospital performance; (2) Measure reflects the hospital's indication that its submission was based upon a sample of its relevant discharges; (3) Rate reflects fewer than the maximum possible quarters of data for the measure; (4) Inaccurate information submitted and suppressed for one or more quarters; (5) No data is available from the hospital for this measure; Please refer to the User's Guide for a full explanation of data

Director Infection/Disease Control . . . . S Robinson, RN
CCU Spvg. Nurse . . . . Kim Dokken, RN
Director Medical/Surgical Nursing . . . . Kim Dokken, RN
Chief Radiology . . . . Vivienne Kezuka, DO
Director Respiratory Therapy . . . . Dennis Criswell

Measure	Cases	This Hospital	State Average	U.S. Average	Top Hospital
Heart Attack Care					
ACE Inhibitor or ARB for LVSD[3]	0	-	84%	82%	100%
Aspirin at Arrival[1,3]	6	100%	95%	92%	100%
Aspirin at Discharge[1,3]	4	75%	95%	90%	100%
Beta Blocker at Arrival[1,3]	4	100%	91%	87%	100%
Beta Blocker at Discharge[1,3]	3	100%	95%	90%	100%
Fibrinolytic Medication Timing[1,3]	1	0%	28%	31%	100%
PCI Within 90 Minutes of Arrival[5]	-	-	60%	54%	95%
Smoking Cessation Advice[1,3]	1	0%	85%	88%	100%
Heart Failure Care					
ACE Inhibitor or ARB for LVSD[1,3]	9	89%	85%	82%	100%
Discharge Instructions[3]	27	19%	53%	61%	93%
Evaluation of LVS Function[3]	27	70%	85%	83%	99%
Smoking Cessation Advice[1,3]	4	25%	75%	82%	100%
Pneumonia Care					
Appropriate Initial Antibiotic[3]	33	82%	82%	83%	94%
Blood Culture Timing[1,3]	12	100%	91%	90%	100%
Influenza Vaccine[5]	-	-	60%	70%	100%
Initial Antibiotic Timing[3]	36	72%	77%	80%	93%
Oxygenation Assessment[3]	37	100%	100%	99%	100%
Pneumococcal Vaccine[1,3]	24	46%	68%	69%	94%
Smoking Cessation Advice[1,3]	7	43%	79%	80%	100%
Surgical Infection Prevention					
Prophylactic Antibiotic Given[1,3]	16	75%	82%	77%	95%
Prophylactic Antibiotic Selection[1]	6	100%	91%	90%	100%
Prophylactic Antibiotic Stopped[1,3]	12	92%	75%	72%	95%
Pregnancy Care					
Inpatient Neonatal Mortality	-	-	-	-	-
Third or Fourth Degree Laceration	-	-	3.98%	3.63%	3.27%

Saint Joseph Medical Center

1717 South J Street
PO Box 2197
Tacoma, WA 98405
URL: www.fhshealth.org
Phone: 253-627-4101
Fax: 253-426-6880
Ownership: Voluntary non-profit - Church
Emergency Services: Yes
Accredited: Yes
Licensed Beds: 320

Key Personnel:

President/CEO . . . . Joseph W Wilczek

Measure	Cases	This Hospital	State Average	U.S. Average	Top Hospital
Heart Attack Care					
ACE Inhibitor or ARB for LVSD	100	86%	84%	82%	100%
Aspirin at Arrival	296	99%	95%	92%	100%
Aspirin at Discharge	363	97%	95%	90%	100%
Beta Blocker at Arrival	157	96%	91%	87%	100%
Beta Blocker at Discharge	360	99%	95%	90%	100%
Fibrinolytic Medication Timing	0	-	28%	31%	100%
PCI Within 90 Minutes of Arrival[1]	13	62%	60%	54%	95%
Smoking Cessation Advice	135	94%	85%	88%	100%
Heart Failure Care					
ACE Inhibitor or ARB for LVSD	223	83%	85%	82%	100%
Discharge Instructions	471	42%	53%	61%	93%
Evaluation of LVS Function	559	94%	85%	83%	99%
Smoking Cessation Advice	95	72%	75%	82%	100%
Pneumonia Care					
Appropriate Initial Antibiotic	205	95%	82%	83%	94%
Blood Culture Timing	257	93%	91%	90%	100%
Influenza Vaccine	64	67%	60%	70%	100%
Initial Antibiotic Timing	320	84%	77%	80%	93%
Oxygenation Assessment	392	100%	100%	99%	100%
Pneumococcal Vaccine	209	74%	68%	69%	94%
Smoking Cessation Advice	112	82%	79%	80%	100%
Surgical Infection Prevention					
Prophylactic Antibiotic Given[3]	1,348	90%	82%	77%	95%
Prophylactic Antibiotic Selection	252	96%	91%	90%	100%
Prophylactic Antibiotic Stopped[3]	1,295	75%	75%	72%	95%
Pregnancy Care					
Inpatient Neonatal Mortality	5,174	0.02%	-	-	-
Third or Fourth Degree Laceration	3,741	3.07%	3.98%	3.63%	3.27%

Tacoma General Hospital

315 Martin Luther King Jr Way
Tacoma, WA 98405
E-mail: hrweb@multicare.org
URL: www.multicare.org
Phone: 253-403-1000
Fax: 253-403-1180
Ownership: Voluntary non-profit - Private
Emergency Services: Yes
Accredited: Yes
Licensed Beds: 593

Key Personnel:

Administrator . . . . John Folsom
President/CEO. . . . . Diane Cecchettini
Chief Medical Staff. . . . . Richard Stubbs, MD
Chief Catheterization Laboratory . . . . Eugene Lapin, MD
Emergency Room . . . . Harold Boyd, MD
Director Infection/Disease Control . . . . Christi McCarren
Director Medical/Surgical Nursing . . . . Linda DeCarlo
OB/GYN Womens Health. . . . . Claire Spain-Remy, MD
Director Radiology . . . . Nina Noldon
Director Respiratory Therapy . . . . Linda Nelson

Measure	Cases	This Hospital	State Average	U.S. Average	Top Hospital
Heart Attack Care					
ACE Inhibitor or ARB for LVSD[2]	71	85%	84%	82%	100%
Aspirin at Arrival[2]	210	96%	95%	92%	100%
Aspirin at Discharge[2]	251	99%	95%	90%	100%
Beta Blocker at Arrival[2]	163	98%	91%	87%	100%
Beta Blocker at Discharge[2]	279	96%	95%	90%	100%
Fibrinolytic Medication Timing[2]	0	-	28%	31%	100%
PCI Within 90 Minutes of Arrival[1,2]	12	83%	60%	54%	95%
Smoking Cessation Advice[2]	113	93%	85%	88%	100%
Heart Failure Care					
ACE Inhibitor or ARB for LVSD[2]	161	88%	85%	82%	100%
Discharge Instructions[2]	351	58%	53%	61%	93%
Evaluation of LVS Function[2]	454	95%	85%	83%	99%
Smoking Cessation Advice[2]	103	90%	75%	82%	100%
Pneumonia Care					
Appropriate Initial Antibiotic[2]	249	87%	82%	83%	94%
Blood Culture Timing[2]	214	94%	91%	90%	100%
Influenza Vaccine[4,5]	-	-	60%	70%	100%
Initial Antibiotic Timing[2]	311	83%	77%	80%	93%
Oxygenation Assessment[2]	405	100%	100%	99%	100%
Pneumococcal Vaccine[2]	224	27%	68%	69%	94%
Smoking Cessation Advice[2]	116	85%	79%	80%	100%
Surgical Infection Prevention					
Prophylactic Antibiotic Given[2]	539	78%	82%	77%	95%
Prophylactic Antibiotic Selection[2]	157	95%	91%	90%	100%
Prophylactic Antibiotic Stopped[2]	514	70%	75%	72%	95%
Pregnancy Care					
Inpatient Neonatal Mortality	3,316	0.72%	-	-	-
Third or Fourth Degree Laceration	2,113	3.79%	3.98%	3.63%	3.27%

Toppenish Community Hospital

502 W 4th Avenue
Toppenish, WA 98948
URL: www.hma-corp.com
Phone: 509-865-3105
Fax: 509-865-1519
Ownership: Proprietary
Emergency Services: Yes
Accredited: Yes
Licensed Beds: 63

Key Personnel:

Chief of Medical Staff. . . . . John Moran, MD
Emergency Room . . . . Linn Walker
Ob/Gyn . . . . Donna Howell

Measure	Cases	This Hospital	State Average	U.S. Average	Top Hospital
Heart Attack Care					
ACE Inhibitor or ARB for LVSD[1,3]	1	100%	84%	82%	100%
Aspirin at Arrival[1,3]	3	100%	95%	92%	100%
Aspirin at Discharge[1,3]	3	100%	95%	90%	100%
Beta Blocker at Arrival[1,3]	4	100%	91%	87%	100%

NOTE: Hospital profiles are in alphabetical order by state, then city, then hospital within the city; Rankings are sorted by rate in descending order and exclude hospitals with less than 25 cases; (1) The number of cases is too small (n<25) for purposes of reliably predicting hospital performance; (2) Measure reflects the hospital's indication that its submission was based upon a sample of its relevant discharges; (3) Rate reflects fewer than the maximum possible quarters of data for the measure; (4) Inaccurate information submitted and suppressed for one or more quarters; (5) No data is available from the hospital for this measure; Please refer to the User's Guide for a full explanation of data

Measure	Cases	This Hospital	State Average	U.S. Average	Top Hospital
Beta Blocker at Discharge[1,3]	3	100%	95%	90%	100%
Fibrinolytic Medication Timing[1,3]	2	0%	28%	31%	100%
PCI Within 90 Minutes of Arrival	0	-	60%	54%	95%
Smoking Cessation Advice[3]	0	-	85%	88%	100%
Heart Failure Care					
ACE Inhibitor or ARB for LVSD	34	91%	85%	82%	100%
Discharge Instructions	81	79%	53%	61%	93%
Evaluation of LVS Function	87	82%	85%	83%	99%
Smoking Cessation Advice[1]	23	74%	75%	82%	100%
Pneumonia Care					
Appropriate Initial Antibiotic	59	51%	82%	83%	94%
Blood Culture Timing	50	92%	91%	90%	100%
Influenza Vaccine[1]	12	58%	60%	70%	100%
Initial Antibiotic Timing	63	76%	77%	80%	93%
Oxygenation Assessment	94	100%	100%	99%	100%
Pneumococcal Vaccine	46	74%	68%	69%	94%
Smoking Cessation Advice[1]	24	54%	79%	80%	100%
Surgical Infection Prevention					
Prophylactic Antibiotic Given[2]	31	97%	82%	77%	95%
Prophylactic Antibiotic Selection[1,2]	6	67%	91%	90%	100%
Prophylactic Antibiotic Stopped[2]	31	81%	75%	72%	95%
Pregnancy Care					
Inpatient Neonatal Mortality	-	-	-	-	-
Third or Fourth Degree Laceration	-	-	3.98%	3.63%	3.27%

Legacy Salmon Creek Hospital

2211 Ne 139th Street
Vancouver, WA 98686
Phone: 360-487-1000
Ownership: Voluntary non-profit - Private
Accredited: No
Emergency Services: Yes

Measure	Cases	This Hospital	State Average	U.S. Average	Top Hospital
Heart Attack Care					
ACE Inhibitor or ARB for LVSD[1,2]	7	86%	84%	82%	100%
Aspirin at Arrival[2]	39	100%	95%	92%	100%
Aspirin at Discharge[2]	29	90%	95%	90%	100%
Beta Blocker at Arrival[1,2]	20	100%	91%	87%	100%
Beta Blocker at Discharge[1,2]	22	91%	95%	90%	100%
Fibrinolytic Medication Timing[1,2]	1	0%	28%	31%	100%
PCI Within 90 Minutes of Arrival[2]	0	-	60%	54%	95%
Smoking Cessation Advice[1,2]	3	100%	85%	88%	100%
Heart Failure Care					
ACE Inhibitor or ARB for LVSD[2]	62	66%	85%	82%	100%
Discharge Instructions[2]	147	31%	53%	61%	93%
Evaluation of LVS Function[2]	185	88%	85%	83%	99%
Smoking Cessation Advice[2]	41	78%	75%	82%	100%
Pneumonia Care					
Appropriate Initial Antibiotic[2]	88	91%	82%	83%	94%
Blood Culture Timing[2]	65	92%	91%	90%	100%
Influenza Vaccine[1]	24	50%	60%	70%	100%
Initial Antibiotic Timing[2]	142	84%	77%	80%	93%
Oxygenation Assessment[2]	161	100%	100%	99%	100%
Pneumococcal Vaccine[2]	112	59%	68%	69%	94%
Smoking Cessation Advice[2]	36	81%	79%	80%	100%
Surgical Infection Prevention					
Prophylactic Antibiotic Given[2,3]	93	67%	82%	77%	95%
Prophylactic Antibiotic Selection[2]	46	91%	91%	90%	100%
Prophylactic Antibiotic Stopped[2,3]	86	47%	75%	72%	95%
Pregnancy Care					
Inpatient Neonatal Mortality	-	-	-	-	-
Third or Fourth Degree Laceration	-	-	3.98%	3.63%	3.27%

Southwest Washington Medical Center

400 NE Mother Joseph Place
Vancouver, WA 98664
Phone: 360-256-2000
Fax: 360-514-2267
URL: www.swmedctr.com
Ownership: Voluntary non-profit - Private
Accredited: Yes
Emergency Services: Yes
Licensed Beds: 360

Key Personnel:

President/CEO. . . . . Joseph M Kortum
Executive VP/CFO. . . . . Eugene G Johnson
Chief Medical Officer . . . . Gilbert M Rodriguez, MD
Administrative Director Cardiovascular. . . . . John Capps
Emergency Room Director. . . . . Jackie Brown

Measure	Cases	This Hospital	State Average	U.S. Average	Top Hospital
Heart Attack Care					
ACE Inhibitor or ARB for LVSD	85	80%	84%	82%	100%
Aspirin at Arrival	415	100%	95%	92%	100%
Aspirin at Discharge	456	97%	95%	90%	100%
Beta Blocker at Arrival	369	98%	91%	87%	100%
Beta Blocker at Discharge	489	98%	95%	90%	100%
Fibrinolytic Medication Timing	0	-	28%	31%	100%
PCI Within 90 Minutes of Arrival[1]	17	76%	60%	54%	95%
Smoking Cessation Advice	173	90%	85%	88%	100%
Heart Failure Care					
ACE Inhibitor or ARB for LVSD	185	90%	85%	82%	100%
Discharge Instructions	481	58%	53%	61%	93%
Evaluation of LVS Function	551	90%	85%	83%	99%
Smoking Cessation Advice	97	64%	75%	82%	100%
Pneumonia Care					
Appropriate Initial Antibiotic[2]	119	39%	82%	83%	94%
Blood Culture Timing[2]	103	89%	91%	90%	100%
Influenza Vaccine	31	65%	60%	70%	100%
Initial Antibiotic Timing[2]	156	73%	77%	80%	93%
Oxygenation Assessment[2]	204	100%	100%	99%	100%
Pneumococcal Vaccine[2]	145	66%	68%	69%	94%
Smoking Cessation Advice[2]	52	77%	79%	80%	100%
Surgical Infection Prevention					
Prophylactic Antibiotic Given[2,3]	243	89%	82%	77%	95%
Prophylactic Antibiotic Selection[2]	77	97%	91%	90%	100%
Prophylactic Antibiotic Stopped[2,3]	232	77%	75%	72%	95%
Pregnancy Care					
Inpatient Neonatal Mortality	4,044	0.02%	-	-	-
Third or Fourth Degree Laceration	2,909	4.13%	3.98%	3.63%	3.27%

Saint Mary Medical Center

401 W Poplar
Walla Walla, WA 99362
Phone: 509-525-3320
Fax: 509-522-5950
E-mail: schima@smmc.com
URL: www.smmc.com
Ownership: Voluntary non-profit - Church
Accredited: Yes
Emergency Services: Yes
Licensed Beds: 142

Key Personnel:

President/CEO. . . . . John A Isely
Chief of Medical Staff. Lester Joseph Wojek
Emergency Room Director. . . . . Thomas Moroldo

Measure	Cases	This Hospital	State Average	U.S. Average	Top Hospital
Heart Attack Care					
ACE Inhibitor or ARB for LVSD[1]	2	50%	84%	82%	100%
Aspirin at Arrival	28	93%	95%	92%	100%
Aspirin at Discharge[1]	12	100%	95%	90%	100%
Beta Blocker at Arrival	27	100%	91%	87%	100%
Beta Blocker at Discharge[1]	16	94%	95%	90%	100%
Fibrinolytic Medication Timing[1]	2	50%	28%	31%	100%
PCI Within 90 Minutes of Arrival	0	-	60%	54%	95%
Smoking Cessation Advice[1]	1	100%	85%	88%	100%
Heart Failure Care					
ACE Inhibitor or ARB for LVSD	25	60%	85%	82%	100%
Discharge Instructions	68	53%	53%	61%	93%
Evaluation of LVS Function	98	95%	85%	83%	99%
Smoking Cessation Advice[1]	12	92%	75%	82%	100%
Pneumonia Care					
Appropriate Initial Antibiotic	79	86%	82%	83%	94%
Blood Culture Timing	77	92%	91%	90%	100%
Influenza Vaccine[1]	17	59%	60%	70%	100%
Initial Antibiotic Timing	98	86%	77%	80%	93%
Oxygenation Assessment	129	100%	100%	99%	100%
Pneumococcal Vaccine	77	78%	68%	69%	94%
Smoking Cessation Advice	34	71%	79%	80%	100%
Surgical Infection Prevention					
Prophylactic Antibiotic Given	341	91%	82%	77%	95%
Prophylactic Antibiotic Selection	64	97%	91%	90%	100%

NOTE: Hospital profiles are in alphabetical order by state, then city, then hospital within the city; Rankings are sorted by rate in descending order and exclude hospitals with less than 25 cases; (1) The number of cases is too small (n<25) for purposes of reliably predicting hospital performance; (2) Measure reflects the hospital's indication that its submission was based upon a sample of its relevant discharges; (3) Rate reflects fewer than the maximum possible quarters of data for the measure; (4) Inaccurate information submitted and suppressed for one or more quarters; (5) No data is available from the hospital for this measure; Please refer to the User's Guide for a full explanation of data

Prophylactic Antibiotic Stopped	329	84%	75%	72%	95%
Pregnancy Care					
Inpatient Neonatal Mortality	635	0.00%	-	-	-
Third or Fourth Degree Laceration	457	2.84%	3.98%	3.63%	3.27%

Walla Walla General Hospital

PO Box 1398
Walla Walla, WA 99362
Ownership: Voluntary non-profit - Church
Emergency Services: Yes
Phone: 509-525-0480
Fax: 509-527-8258
Accredited: Yes
Licensed Beds: 72

Key Personnel:

CEO. . . . . Moore Dean
Head of Emergency Room. . . . . Linda Givens
Emergency Room . . . . Adrian Selfa
Director Infection/Disease Control . . . . Doris Tucker

Measure	Cases	This Hospital	State Average	U.S. Average	Top Hospital
Heart Attack Care					
ACE Inhibitor or ARB for LVSD[1]	3	100%	84%	82%	100%
Aspirin at Arrival[1]	17	100%	95%	92%	100%
Aspirin at Discharge[1]	10	100%	95%	90%	100%
Beta Blocker at Arrival[1]	11	82%	91%	87%	100%
Beta Blocker at Discharge[1]	10	90%	95%	90%	100%
Fibrinolytic Medication Timing[1]	1	0%	28%	31%	100%
PCI Within 90 Minutes of Arrival	0	-	60%	54%	95%
Smoking Cessation Advice[1]	2	100%	85%	88%	100%
Heart Failure Care					
ACE Inhibitor or ARB for LVSD[1]	19	68%	85%	82%	100%
Discharge Instructions	30	43%	53%	61%	93%
Evaluation of LVS Function	47	96%	85%	83%	99%
Smoking Cessation Advice[1]	4	100%	75%	82%	100%
Pneumonia Care					
Appropriate Initial Antibiotic	47	89%	82%	83%	94%
Blood Culture Timing	47	96%	91%	90%	100%
Influenza Vaccine[1]	9	67%	60%	70%	100%
Initial Antibiotic Timing	52	85%	77%	80%	93%
Oxygenation Assessment	70	100%	100%	99%	100%
Pneumococcal Vaccine	48	67%	68%	69%	94%
Smoking Cessation Advice[1]	23	91%	79%	80%	100%
Surgical Infection Prevention					
Prophylactic Antibiotic Given[2,3]	110	87%	82%	77%	95%
Prophylactic Antibiotic Selection[2]	41	100%	91%	90%	100%
Prophylactic Antibiotic Stopped[2,3]	109	79%	75%	72%	95%
Pregnancy Care					
Inpatient Neonatal Mortality	323	0.31%	-	-	-
Third or Fourth Degree Laceration	233	3.00%	3.98%	3.63%	3.27%

Central Washington Hospital

1201 South Miller Street
PO Box 1887
Wenatchee, WA 98807
E-mail: contactus@cwhs.com
URL: www.cwhs.com
Ownership: Voluntary non-profit - Other
Emergency Services: Yes
Phone: 509-662-1511
Fax: 509-662-6770
Accredited: Yes
Licensed Beds: 210

Key Personnel:

President/CEO. . . . . Jack Evans
Chief of Medical Staff . . . . Russell Havlicek, MD
Director Emergency Room. . . . . Vickie Hammond
Director Respiratory Therapy . . . . Tom Gash

Measure	Cases	This Hospital	State Average	U.S. Average	Top Hospital
Heart Attack Care					
ACE Inhibitor or ARB for LVSD	33	82%	84%	82%	100%
Aspirin at Arrival	100	100%	95%	92%	100%
Aspirin at Discharge	161	99%	95%	90%	100%
Beta Blocker at Arrival	88	90%	91%	87%	100%
Beta Blocker at Discharge	172	95%	95%	90%	100%
Fibrinolytic Medication Timing	0	-	28%	31%	100%
PCI Within 90 Minutes of Arrival[1]	5	100%	60%	54%	95%
Smoking Cessation Advice	62	92%	85%	88%	100%
Heart Failure Care					
ACE Inhibitor or ARB for LVSD	72	88%	85%	82%	100%
Discharge Instructions	157	59%	53%	61%	93%
Evaluation of LVS Function	185	90%	85%	83%	99%
Smoking Cessation Advice	35	91%	75%	82%	100%
Pneumonia Care					
Appropriate Initial Antibiotic	99	89%	82%	83%	94%
Blood Culture Timing	116	89%	91%	90%	100%
Influenza Vaccine	35	77%	60%	70%	100%
Initial Antibiotic Timing	172	88%	77%	80%	93%
Oxygenation Assessment	206	100%	100%	99%	100%
Pneumococcal Vaccine	154	84%	68%	69%	94%
Smoking Cessation Advice	50	92%	79%	80%	100%
Surgical Infection Prevention					
Prophylactic Antibiotic Given[3]	285	86%	82%	77%	95%
Prophylactic Antibiotic Selection	104	98%	91%	90%	100%
Prophylactic Antibiotic Stopped[3]	282	77%	75%	72%	95%
Pregnancy Care					
Inpatient Neonatal Mortality	-	-	-	-	-
Third or Fourth Degree Laceration	-	-	3.98%	3.63%	3.27%

Wenatchee Valley Hospital

820 North Chelan Street
Wenatchee, WA 98801
Ownership: Government - Federal
Emergency Services: No
Phone: 509-663-8711
Accredited: No

Measure	Cases	This Hospital	State Average	U.S. Average	Top Hospital
Heart Attack Care					
ACE Inhibitor or ARB for LVSD[5]	-	-	84%	82%	100%
Aspirin at Arrival[5]	-	-	95%	92%	100%
Aspirin at Discharge[5]	-	-	95%	90%	100%
Beta Blocker at Arrival[5]	-	-	91%	87%	100%
Beta Blocker at Discharge[5]	-	-	95%	90%	100%
Fibrinolytic Medication Timing[5]	-	-	28%	31%	100%
PCI Within 90 Minutes of Arrival[5]	-	-	60%	54%	95%
Smoking Cessation Advice[5]	-	-	85%	88%	100%
Heart Failure Care					
ACE Inhibitor or ARB for LVSD[5]	-	-	85%	82%	100%
Discharge Instructions[5]	-	-	53%	61%	93%
Evaluation of LVS Function[5]	-	-	85%	83%	99%
Smoking Cessation Advice[5]	-	-	75%	82%	100%
Pneumonia Care					
Appropriate Initial Antibiotic[5]	-	-	82%	83%	94%
Blood Culture Timing[5]	-	-	91%	90%	100%
Influenza Vaccine[5]	-	-	60%	70%	100%
Initial Antibiotic Timing[5]	-	-	77%	80%	93%
Oxygenation Assessment[5]	-	-	100%	99%	100%
Pneumococcal Vaccine[5]	-	-	68%	69%	94%
Smoking Cessation Advice[5]	-	-	79%	80%	100%
Surgical Infection Prevention					
Prophylactic Antibiotic Given[3]	66	100%	82%	77%	95%
Prophylactic Antibiotic Selection[5]	-	-	91%	90%	100%
Prophylactic Antibiotic Stopped[3]	66	100%	75%	72%	95%
Pregnancy Care					
Inpatient Neonatal Mortality	-	-	-	-	-
Third or Fourth Degree Laceration	-	-	3.98%	3.63%	3.27%

Yakima Regional Medical & Cardiac Center

110 South 9th Avenue
Yakima, WA 98902
URL: www.yakimaregional.org
Ownership: Proprietary
Emergency Services: Yes
Phone: 509-575-5000
Fax: 509-454-6193
Accredited: Yes
Licensed Beds: 169

Key Personnel:

CEO. . . . . John R Finnegan
Chief Medical Staff. . . . . Ron Fought
Cardiac Lab . . . . Corinne Murphy-Hines
Chief Catheterization Laboratory . . . . Richard Spiegel, MD
Emergency Room . . . . Richard Plunkett, MD
ICU . . . . Maureen Ritter
Intensive Coronary Care . . . . Maureen Ritter
Respiratory Therapy. . . . . Dennis Criswell

NOTE: Hospital profiles are in alphabetical order by state, then city, then hospital within the city; Rankings are sorted by rate in descending order and exclude hospitals with less than 25 cases; (1) The number of cases is too small (n<25) for purposes of reliably predicting hospital performance; (2) Measure reflects the hospital's indication that its submission was based upon a sample of its relevant discharges; (3) Rate reflects fewer than the maximum possible quarters of data for the measure; (4) Inaccurate information submitted and suppressed for one or more quarters; (5) No data is available from the hospital for this measure; Please refer to the User's Guide for a full explanation of data

Measure	Cases	This Hospital	State Average	U.S. Average	Top Hospital
Heart Attack Care					
ACE Inhibitor or ARB for LVSD	56	98%	84%	82%	100%
Aspirin at Arrival	95	97%	95%	92%	100%
Aspirin at Discharge	180	99%	95%	90%	100%
Beta Blocker at Arrival	71	96%	91%	87%	100%
Beta Blocker at Discharge	177	99%	95%	90%	100%
Fibrinolytic Medication Timing	0	-	28%	31%	100%
PCI Within 90 Minutes of Arrival[1]	8	75%	60%	54%	95%
Smoking Cessation Advice	89	100%	85%	88%	100%
Heart Failure Care					
ACE Inhibitor or ARB for LVSD	67	93%	85%	82%	100%
Discharge Instructions	170	78%	53%	61%	93%
Evaluation of LVS Function	192	91%	85%	83%	99%
Smoking Cessation Advice	40	92%	75%	82%	100%
Pneumonia Care					
Appropriate Initial Antibiotic	87	90%	82%	83%	94%
Blood Culture Timing	88	82%	91%	90%	100%
Influenza Vaccine[1]	23	74%	60%	70%	100%
Initial Antibiotic Timing	117	84%	77%	80%	93%
Oxygenation Assessment	144	100%	100%	99%	100%
Pneumococcal Vaccine	79	73%	68%	69%	94%
Smoking Cessation Advice	56	98%	79%	80%	100%
Surgical Infection Prevention					
Prophylactic Antibiotic Given[2]	282	94%	82%	77%	95%
Prophylactic Antibiotic Selection[2]	50	98%	91%	90%	100%
Prophylactic Antibiotic Stopped[2]	280	59%	75%	72%	95%
Pregnancy Care					
Inpatient Neonatal Mortality	-	-	-	-	-
Third or Fourth Degree Laceration	-	-	3.98%	3.63%	3.27%

Yakima Valley Memorial Hospital

2811 Tieton Drive
Yakima, WA 98902
Phone: 509-575-8000
Fax: 509-576-5772
URL: www.yakimamemorialhospital.org
Ownership: Voluntary non-profit - Private
Accredited: Yes
Emergency Services: Yes
Licensed Beds: 218

Key Personnel:

President/CEO. . . . . Rick Linneweh, Jr
Infection Control. . . . . Gay Scott
Director Radiology . . . . Mike Klippert
Director Respiratory Therapy . . . . Jeanne Fasano

Measure	Cases	This Hospital	State Average	U.S. Average	Top Hospital
Heart Attack Care					
ACE Inhibitor or ARB for LVSD[1]	21	95%	84%	82%	100%
Aspirin at Arrival	161	97%	95%	92%	100%
Aspirin at Discharge	128	100%	95%	90%	100%
Beta Blocker at Arrival	121	98%	91%	87%	100%
Beta Blocker at Discharge	130	99%	95%	90%	100%
Fibrinolytic Medication Timing[1]	1	0%	28%	31%	100%
PCI Within 90 Minutes of Arrival[1]	7	100%	60%	54%	95%
Smoking Cessation Advice	47	100%	85%	88%	100%
Heart Failure Care					
ACE Inhibitor or ARB for LVSD	84	76%	85%	82%	100%
Discharge Instructions	220	36%	53%	61%	93%
Evaluation of LVS Function	261	86%	85%	83%	99%
Smoking Cessation Advice	28	96%	75%	82%	100%
Pneumonia Care					
Appropriate Initial Antibiotic	187	94%	82%	83%	94%
Blood Culture Timing	70	96%	91%	90%	100%
Influenza Vaccine	48	54%	60%	70%	100%
Initial Antibiotic Timing	275	85%	77%	80%	93%
Oxygenation Assessment	333	100%	100%	99%	100%
Pneumococcal Vaccine	221	71%	68%	69%	94%
Smoking Cessation Advice	78	97%	79%	80%	100%
Surgical Infection Prevention					
Prophylactic Antibiotic Given	819	99%	82%	77%	95%
Prophylactic Antibiotic Selection	192	97%	91%	90%	100%
Prophylactic Antibiotic Stopped	806	84%	75%	72%	95%
Pregnancy Care					
Inpatient Neonatal Mortality	-	-	-	-	-
Third or Fourth Degree Laceration	-	-	3.98%	3.63%	3.27%

NOTE: Hospital profiles are in alphabetical order by state, then city, then hospital within the city; Rankings are sorted by rate in descending order and exclude hospitals with less than 25 cases; (1) The number of cases is too small (n<25) for purposes of reliably predicting hospital performance; (2) Measure reflects the hospital's indication that its submission was based upon a sample of its relevant discharges; (3) Rate reflects fewer than the maximum possible quarters of data for the measure; (4) Inaccurate information submitted and suppressed for one or more quarters; (5) No data is available from the hospital for this measure; Please refer to the User's Guide for a full explanation of data

Heart Attack Care

1. ACE Inhibitor or ARB for LVSD

Hospital Name	City	Rate	Cases
Cheyenne Regional Medical Center-West	Cheyenne	92%	25
Wyoming Medical Center	Casper	89%	47

2. Aspirin at Arrival

Hospital Name	City	Rate	Cases
Wyoming Medical Center	Casper	98%	151
Cheyenne Regional Medical Center-West	Cheyenne	92%	133

3. Aspirin at Discharge

Hospital Name	City	Rate	Cases
Cheyenne Regional Medical Center-West	Cheyenne	98%	195
Wyoming Medical Center	Casper	96%	308

4. Beta Blocker at Arrival

Hospital Name	City	Rate	Cases
Wyoming Medical Center	Casper	93%	149
Cheyenne Regional Medical Center-West	Cheyenne	91%	129

5. Beta Blocker at Discharge

Hospital Name	City	Rate	Cases
Cheyenne Regional Medical Center-West	Cheyenne	95%	197
Wyoming Medical Center	Casper	93%	303

8. Smoking Cessation Advice

Hospital Name	City	Rate	Cases
Cheyenne Regional Medical Center-West	Cheyenne	96%	82
Wyoming Medical Center	Casper	88%	144

Heart Failure Care

9. ACE Inhibitor or ARB for LVSD

Hospital Name	City	Rate	Cases
Cheyenne Regional Medical Center-West	Cheyenne	89%	53
Wyoming Medical Center	Casper	89%	70

10. Discharge Instructions

Hospital Name	City	Rate	Cases
Saint John's Medical Center	Jackson	86%	36
Riverton Memorial Hospital	Riverton	79%	34
Cheyenne Regional Medical Center-West	Cheyenne	72%	138
Community Hospital	Torrington	68%	25
Lander Valley Medical Center	Lander	63%	30
Campbell County Memorial Hospital	Gillette	60%	35
Memorial Hospital of Sheridan County	Sheridan	59%	27
Wyoming Medical Center	Casper	58%	159
Memorial Hospital of Sweetwater County	Rock Springs	55%	53
Memorial Hospital of Carbon County	Rawlins	23%	48

11. Evaluation of LVS Function

Hospital Name	City	Rate	Cases
Ivinson Memorial Hospital	Laramie	90%	29
Wyoming Medical Center	Casper	86%	188
Cheyenne Regional Medical Center-West	Cheyenne	84%	176
Riverton Memorial Hospital	Riverton	83%	35
Washakie Medical Center	Worland	77%	26
Lander Valley Medical Center	Lander	75%	32
Community Hospital	Torrington	74%	31
Saint John's Medical Center	Jackson	64%	39
Campbell County Memorial Hospital	Gillette	62%	50
Memorial Hospital of Sweetwater County	Rock Springs	57%	65
Memorial Hospital of Sheridan County	Sheridan	42%	43
Memorial Hospital of Carbon County	Rawlins	41%	56

12. Smoking Cessation Advice

Hospital Name	City	Rate	Cases
Cheyenne Regional Medical Center-West	Cheyenne	84%	25
Wyoming Medical Center	Casper	62%	40

Pneumonia Care

13. Appropriate Initial Antibiotic

Hospital Name	City	Rate	Cases
Platte County Memorial Hospital	Wheatland	97%	33
Saint John's Medical Center	Jackson	92%	51
Evanston Regional Hospital	Evanston	89%	38
Wyoming Medical Center	Casper	85%	156
Lander Valley Medical Center	Lander	84%	56
Cheyenne Regional Medical Center-West	Cheyenne	81%	222
Community Hospital	Torrington	81%	36
Memorial Hospital of Sweetwater County	Rock Springs	81%	79
Memorial Hospital of Carbon County	Rawlins	78%	51
Memorial Hospital of Sheridan County	Sheridan	77%	82
Campbell County Memorial Hospital	Gillette	76%	71
Ivinson Memorial Hospital	Laramie	75%	71
Riverton Memorial Hospital	Riverton	74%	43

14. Blood Culture Timing

Hospital Name	City	Rate	Cases
Lander Valley Medical Center	Lander	100%	41
Memorial Hospital of Sheridan County	Sheridan	96%	52
Evanston Regional Hospital	Evanston	94%	33
Wyoming Medical Center	Casper	94%	135
Saint John's Medical Center	Jackson	89%	27
Campbell County Memorial Hospital	Gillette	85%	59
Ivinson Memorial Hospital	Laramie	84%	51
Riverton Memorial Hospital	Riverton	82%	28
Cheyenne Regional Medical Center-West	Cheyenne	81%	106
Memorial Hospital of Sweetwater County	Rock Springs	79%	58

15. Influenza Vaccine

Hospital Name	City	Rate	Cases
Wyoming Medical Center	Casper	100%	43
Cheyenne Regional Medical Center-West	Cheyenne	83%	41

16. Initial Antibiotic Timing

Hospital Name	City	Rate	Cases
Community Hospital	Torrington	97%	30
Evanston Regional Hospital	Evanston	96%	50
Platte County Memorial Hospital	Wheatland	94%	36
Riverton Memorial Hospital	Riverton	93%	45
Campbell County Memorial Hospital	Gillette	92%	86
Saint John's Medical Center	Jackson	89%	46
Hot Springs County Memorial Hospital	Thermopolis	88%	26
Memorial Hospital of Sheridan County	Sheridan	86%	97
Wyoming Medical Center	Casper	86%	208
Lander Valley Medical Center	Lander	85%	85
Memorial Hospital of Carbon County	Rawlins	85%	53
Memorial Hospital of Sweetwater County	Rock Springs	85%	96
Ivinson Memorial Hospital	Laramie	82%	98
Cheyenne Regional Medical Center-West	Cheyenne	71%	247

17. Oxygenation Assessment

Hospital Name	City	Rate	Cases
Campbell County Memorial Hospital	Gillette	100%	110
Cheyenne Regional Medical Center-West	Cheyenne	100%	285
Community Hospital	Torrington	100%	39
Evanston Regional Hospital	Evanston	100%	56
Hot Springs County Memorial Hospital	Thermopolis	100%	41
Ivinson Memorial Hospital	Laramie	100%	132
Lander Valley Medical Center	Lander	100%	98
Memorial Hospital of Carbon County	Rawlins	100%	66
Memorial Hospital of Converse County	Douglas	100%	25
Platte County Memorial Hospital	Wheatland	100%	43
Riverton Memorial Hospital	Riverton	100%	55
Washakie Medical Center	Worland	100%	31
Wyoming Medical Center	Casper	100%	244
Memorial Hospital of Sheridan County	Sheridan	99%	115
Memorial Hospital of Sweetwater County	Rock Springs	99%	110
Saint John's Medical Center	Jackson	97%	66

18. Pneumococcal Vaccine

Hospital Name	City	Rate	Cases
Hot Springs County Memorial Hospital	Thermopolis	100%	29
Evanston Regional Hospital	Evanston	96%	27
Platte County Memorial Hospital	Wheatland	96%	25
Wyoming Medical Center	Casper	88%	147
Cheyenne Regional Medical Center-West	Cheyenne	86%	161
Riverton Memorial Hospital	Riverton	85%	26
Ivinson Memorial Hospital	Laramie	84%	83
Community Hospital	Torrington	83%	29
Lander Valley Medical Center	Lander	82%	40
Campbell County Memorial Hospital	Gillette	76%	59
Memorial Hospital of Sweetwater County	Rock Springs	73%	59
Memorial Hospital of Carbon County	Rawlins	68%	37
Saint John's Medical Center	Jackson	65%	34
Memorial Hospital of Sheridan County	Sheridan	64%	85

NOTE: Hospital profiles are in alphabetical order by state, then city, then hospital within the city; Rankings are sorted by rate in descending order and exclude hospitals with less than 25 cases; (1) The number of cases is too small (n<25) for purposes of reliably predicting hospital performance; (2) Measure reflects the hospital's indication that its submission was based upon a sample of its relevant discharges; (3) Rate reflects fewer than the maximum possible quarters of data for the measure; (4) Inaccurate information submitted and suppressed for one or more quarters; (5) No data is available from the hospital for this measure; Please refer to the User's Guide for a full explanation of data

19. Smoking Cessation Advice

Hospital Name	City	Rate	Cases
Ivinson Memorial Hospital	Laramie	93%	30
Lander Valley Medical Center	Lander	92%	36
Memorial Hospital of Sweetwater County	Rock Springs	79%	33
Wyoming Medical Center	Casper	79%	89
Cheyenne Regional Medical Center-West	Cheyenne	77%	66
Campbell County Memorial Hospital	Gillette	63%	27
Memorial Hospital of Sheridan County	Sheridan	57%	28
Memorial Hospital of Carbon County	Rawlins	56%	25

Surgical Infection Prevention

20. Prophylactic Antibiotic Given

Hospital Name	City	Rate	Cases
Riverton Memorial Hospital	Riverton	95%	56
Memorial Hospital of Sheridan County	Sheridan	94%	182
Evanston Regional Hospital	Evanston	93%	30
Campbell County Memorial Hospital	Gillette	91%	126
Saint John's Medical Center	Jackson	83%	131
Lander Valley Medical Center	Lander	80%	128
Memorial Hospital of Converse County	Douglas	79%	75
Powell Vally Hospital	Powell	79%	38
Wyoming Medical Center	Casper	73%	394
Memorial Hospital of Sweetwater County	Rock Springs	70%	87
Ivinson Memorial Hospital	Laramie	67%	172
Cheyenne Regional Medical Center-West	Cheyenne	43%	510

21. Prophylactic Antibiotic Selection

Hospital Name	City	Rate	Cases
Lander Valley Medical Center	Lander	100%	61
Memorial Hospital of Converse County	Douglas	96%	28
Cheyenne Regional Medical Center-West	Cheyenne	95%	154
Saint John's Medical Center	Jackson	94%	47
Memorial Hospital of Sheridan County	Sheridan	92%	40
Ivinson Memorial Hospital	Laramie	89%	47
Wyoming Medical Center	Casper	86%	100
Memorial Hospital of Sweetwater County	Rock Springs	21%	28

22. Prophylactic Antibiotic Stopped

Hospital Name	City	Rate	Cases
Memorial Hospital of Sheridan County	Sheridan	95%	176
Memorial Hospital of Sweetwater County	Rock Springs	94%	77
Campbell County Memorial Hospital	Gillette	91%	121
Riverton Memorial Hospital	Riverton	89%	55
Lander Valley Medical Center	Lander	86%	125
Cheyenne Regional Medical Center-West	Cheyenne	78%	495
Powell Vally Hospital	Powell	78%	36
Saint John's Medical Center	Jackson	77%	124
Evanston Regional Hospital	Evanston	68%	28
Ivinson Memorial Hospital	Laramie	66%	169
Wyoming Medical Center	Casper	66%	372
Memorial Hospital of Converse County	Douglas	62%	74

Pregnancy Care

23. Inpatient Neonatal Mortality

Hospital Name	City	Rate	Cases
Saint John's Medical Center	Jackson	0.21%	487
Campbell County Memorial Hospital	Gillette	0.40%	752

24. Third or Fourth Degree Laceration

Hospital Name	City	Rate	Cases
Campbell County Memorial Hospital	Gillette	3.46%	549
Saint John's Medical Center	Jackson	3.83%	366

NOTE: Hospital profiles are in alphabetical order by state, then city, then hospital within the city; Rankings are sorted by rate in descending order and exclude hospitals with less than 25 cases; (1) The number of cases is too small (n<25) for purposes of reliably predicting hospital performance; (2) Measure reflects the hospital's indication that its submission was based upon a sample of its relevant discharges; (3) Rate reflects fewer than the maximum possible quarters of data for the measure; (4) Inaccurate information submitted and suppressed for one or more quarters; (5) No data is available from the hospital for this measure; Please refer to the User's Guide for a full explanation of data

Star Valley Medical Center

901 Adams Phone: 307-885-5800
Afton, WY 83110 Fax: 307-885-5889
E-mail: sperry@sv-mc.org
URL: svmcwy.org
Ownership: Govt - Hospital District or Authority Accredited: No
Emergency Services: Yes Licensed Beds: 39

Key Personnel:

CEO . . . . J Steve Perry
Chief Medical Staff . . . . Scott Bennett, DO
Emergency Room . . . . Marcia Bahr
Infection Control . . . . Amy Johnson
Medical Surgical Nursing . . . . Marta Heap, RN
OB/GYN/Womens Health . . . . Marta Heap
Respiratory . . . . Michael Ford

Measure	Cases	This Hospital	State Average	U.S. Average	Top Hospital
Heart Attack Care					
ACE Inhibitor or ARB for LVSD[3]	0	-	95%	82%	100%
Aspirin at Arrival[1,3]	1	0%	78%	92%	100%
Aspirin at Discharge[3]	0	-	78%	90%	100%
Beta Blocker at Arrival[1,3]	1	0%	77%	87%	100%
Beta Blocker at Discharge[3]	0	-	84%	90%	100%
Fibrinolytic Medication Timing[3]	0	-	36%	31%	100%
PCI Within 90 Minutes of Arrival	0	-	72%	54%	95%
Smoking Cessation Advice[3]	0	-	73%	88%	100%
Heart Failure Care					
ACE Inhibitor or ARB for LVSD[1]	1	100%	70%	82%	100%
Discharge Instructions[1]	4	0%	56%	61%	93%
Evaluation of LVS Function[1]	5	40%	60%	83%	99%
Smoking Cessation Advice[1]	1	0%	62%	82%	100%
Pneumonia Care					
Appropriate Initial Antibiotic[1]	14	71%	82%	83%	94%
Blood Culture Timing	0	-	92%	90%	100%
Influenza Vaccine[1]	2	50%	71%	70%	100%
Initial Antibiotic Timing[1]	15	100%	87%	80%	93%
Oxygenation Assessment[1]	17	100%	100%	99%	100%
Pneumococcal Vaccine[1]	13	23%	74%	69%	94%
Smoking Cessation Advice[1]	2	50%	73%	80%	100%
Surgical Infection Prevention					
Prophylactic Antibiotic Given[1]	20	50%	76%	77%	95%
Prophylactic Antibiotic Selection[1]	7	100%	90%	90%	100%
Prophylactic Antibiotic Stopped[1]	19	58%	78%	72%	95%
Pregnancy Care					
Inpatient Neonatal Mortality	-	-	-	-	-
Third or Fourth Degree Laceration	-	-	-	3.63%	3.27%

South Big Horn County Hospital

388 Us Highway 20 South Phone: 307-568-3311
Basin, WY 82410
Ownership: Govt - Hospital District or Authority Accredited: No
Emergency Services: Yes

Measure	Cases	This Hospital	State Average	U.S. Average	Top Hospital
Heart Attack Care					
ACE Inhibitor or ARB for LVSD[5]	-	-	95%	82%	100%
Aspirin at Arrival[5]	-	-	78%	92%	100%
Aspirin at Discharge[5]	-	-	78%	90%	100%
Beta Blocker at Arrival[5]	-	-	77%	87%	100%
Beta Blocker at Discharge[5]	-	-	84%	90%	100%
Fibrinolytic Medication Timing[5]	-	-	36%	31%	100%
PCI Within 90 Minutes of Arrival[5]	-	-	72%	54%	95%
Smoking Cessation Advice[5]	-	-	73%	88%	100%
Heart Failure Care					
ACE Inhibitor or ARB for LVSD[3]	0	-	70%	82%	100%
Discharge Instructions[1,3]	1	100%	56%	61%	93%
Evaluation of LVS Function[1,3]	1	100%	60%	83%	99%
Smoking Cessation Advice[3]	0	-	62%	82%	100%
Pneumonia Care					
Appropriate Initial Antibiotic[1,3]	1	100%	82%	83%	94%
Blood Culture Timing[3]	0	-	92%	90%	100%
Influenza Vaccine	0	-	71%	70%	100%
Initial Antibiotic Timing[3]	0	-	87%	80%	93%
Oxygenation Assessment[1,3]	2	100%	100%	99%	100%
Pneumococcal Vaccine[1,3]	1	100%	74%	69%	94%
Smoking Cessation Advice[1,3]	1	100%	73%	80%	100%
Surgical Infection Prevention					
Prophylactic Antibiotic Given[5]	-	-	76%	77%	95%
Prophylactic Antibiotic Selection[5]	-	-	90%	90%	100%
Prophylactic Antibiotic Stopped[5]	-	-	78%	72%	95%
Pregnancy Care					
Inpatient Neonatal Mortality	-	-	-	-	-
Third or Fourth Degree Laceration	-	-	-	3.63%	3.27%

Johnson County Healthcare Center

497 West Lott Phone: 307-684-5521
Buffalo, WY 82834
Ownership: Voluntary non-profit - Other Accredited: No
Emergency Services: Yes

Measure	Cases	This Hospital	State Average	U.S. Average	Top Hospital
Heart Attack Care					
ACE Inhibitor or ARB for LVSD[3]	0	-	95%	82%	100%
Aspirin at Arrival[1,3]	1	100%	78%	92%	100%
Aspirin at Discharge[1,3]	1	100%	78%	90%	100%
Beta Blocker at Arrival[1,3]	1	100%	77%	87%	100%
Beta Blocker at Discharge[1,3]	1	100%	84%	90%	100%
Fibrinolytic Medication Timing[1,3]	1	0%	36%	31%	100%
PCI Within 90 Minutes of Arrival[5]	-	-	72%	54%	95%
Smoking Cessation Advice[3]	0	-	73%	88%	100%
Heart Failure Care					
ACE Inhibitor or ARB for LVSD	0	-	70%	82%	100%
Discharge Instructions[1]	7	0%	56%	61%	93%
Evaluation of LVS Function[1]	6	17%	60%	83%	99%
Smoking Cessation Advice	0	-	62%	82%	100%
Pneumonia Care					
Appropriate Initial Antibiotic[1]	8	75%	82%	83%	94%
Blood Culture Timing[1]	2	100%	92%	90%	100%
Influenza Vaccine[1]	3	0%	71%	70%	100%
Initial Antibiotic Timing[1]	15	93%	87%	80%	93%
Oxygenation Assessment[1]	17	100%	100%	99%	100%
Pneumococcal Vaccine[1]	13	46%	74%	69%	94%
Smoking Cessation Advice[1]	1	100%	73%	80%	100%
Surgical Infection Prevention					
Prophylactic Antibiotic Given[5]	-	-	76%	77%	95%
Prophylactic Antibiotic Selection[5]	-	-	90%	90%	100%
Prophylactic Antibiotic Stopped[5]	-	-	78%	72%	95%
Pregnancy Care					
Inpatient Neonatal Mortality	-	-	-	-	-
Third or Fourth Degree Laceration	-	-	-	3.63%	3.27%

Wyoming Medical Center

1233 E Second Street Toll-Free: 800-822-7201
Casper, WY 82601 Phone: 307-577-7201
Fax: 307-237-1703
E-mail: info@wmcnet.org
URL: www.wmcnet.org
Ownership: Voluntary non-profit - Other Accredited: Yes
Emergency Services: Yes Licensed Beds: 282

Key Personnel:

President/CEO . . . . Pam Fulks
Chief Medical Staff . . . . John Barrasso, MD
Emergency Room . . . . Becky Hansen, RN
Director of Pulmonary . . . . Mark Neginley, MD

Measure	Cases	This Hospital	State Average	U.S. Average	Top Hospital
Heart Attack Care					
ACE Inhibitor or ARB for LVSD	47	89%	95%	82%	100%
Aspirin at Arrival	151	98%	78%	92%	100%
Aspirin at Discharge	308	96%	78%	90%	100%
Beta Blocker at Arrival	149	93%	77%	87%	100%
Beta Blocker at Discharge	303	93%	84%	90%	100%
Fibrinolytic Medication Timing	0	-	36%	31%	100%
PCI Within 90 Minutes of Arrival[1]	9	56%	72%	54%	95%
Smoking Cessation Advice	144	88%	73%	88%	100%

NOTE: Hospital profiles are in alphabetical order by state, then city, then hospital within the city; Rankings are sorted by rate in descending order and exclude hospitals with less than 25 cases; (1) The number of cases is too small (n<25) for purposes of reliably predicting hospital performance; (2) Measure reflects the hospital's indication that its submission was based upon a sample of its relevant discharges; (3) Rate reflects fewer than the maximum possible quarters of data for the measure; (4) Inaccurate information submitted and suppressed for one or more quarters; (5) No data is available from the hospital for this measure; Please refer to the User's Guide for a full explanation of data

Measure	Cases	This Hospital	State Average	U.S. Average	Top Hospital
Heart Failure Care					
ACE Inhibitor or ARB for LVSD	70	89%	70%	82%	100%
Discharge Instructions	159	58%	56%	61%	93%
Evaluation of LVS Function	188	86%	60%	83%	99%
Smoking Cessation Advice	40	62%	62%	82%	100%
Pneumonia Care					
Appropriate Initial Antibiotic[2]	156	85%	82%	83%	94%
Blood Culture Timing[2]	135	94%	92%	90%	100%
Influenza Vaccine[2]	43	100%	71%	70%	100%
Initial Antibiotic Timing[2]	208	86%	87%	80%	93%
Oxygenation Assessment[2]	244	100%	100%	99%	100%
Pneumococcal Vaccine[2]	147	88%	74%	69%	94%
Smoking Cessation Advice[2]	89	79%	73%	80%	100%
Surgical Infection Prevention					
Prophylactic Antibiotic Given[2,3]	394	73%	76%	77%	95%
Prophylactic Antibiotic Selection[2]	100	86%	90%	90%	100%
Prophylactic Antibiotic Stopped[2,3]	372	66%	78%	72%	95%
Pregnancy Care					
Inpatient Neonatal Mortality	-	-	-	-	-
Third or Fourth Degree Laceration	-	-	-	3.63%	3.27%

Cheyenne Regional Medical Center-West

214 E 23rd Street
Cheyenne, WY 82001
URL: www.umcwy.org
Ownership: Govt - Hospital District or Authority
Emergency Services: Yes
Phone: 307-634-2273
Fax: 307-633-7600
Accredited: No
Licensed Beds: 198

Key Personnel:

CEO.................................Jon M Gates
Chief Medical Staff.......................Bob Stuart, MD
Director Cardiac Services..................Heather Bagget
Director Infection/Disease Control ....Jay Jones
Director Cardiopulmonary ....Heather Baggett, RN

Measure	Cases	This Hospital	State Average	U.S. Average	Top Hospital
Heart Attack Care					
ACE Inhibitor or ARB for LVSD	25	92%	95%	82%	100%
Aspirin at Arrival	133	92%	78%	92%	100%
Aspirin at Discharge	195	98%	78%	90%	100%
Beta Blocker at Arrival	129	91%	77%	87%	100%
Beta Blocker at Discharge	197	95%	84%	90%	100%
Fibrinolytic Medication Timing	0	-	36%	31%	100%
PCI Within 90 Minutes of Arrival[1]	8	88%	72%	54%	95%
Smoking Cessation Advice	82	96%	73%	88%	100%
Heart Failure Care					
ACE Inhibitor or ARB for LVSD	53	89%	70%	82%	100%
Discharge Instructions	138	72%	56%	61%	93%
Evaluation of LVS Function	176	84%	60%	83%	99%
Smoking Cessation Advice	25	84%	62%	82%	100%
Pneumonia Care					
Appropriate Initial Antibiotic	222	81%	82%	83%	94%
Blood Culture Timing	106	81%	92%	90%	100%
Influenza Vaccine	41	83%	71%	70%	100%
Initial Antibiotic Timing	247	71%	87%	80%	93%
Oxygenation Assessment	285	100%	100%	99%	100%
Pneumococcal Vaccine	161	86%	74%	69%	94%
Smoking Cessation Advice	66	77%	73%	80%	100%
Surgical Infection Prevention					
Prophylactic Antibiotic Given[2,3]	510	43%	76%	77%	95%
Prophylactic Antibiotic Selection[2]	154	95%	90%	90%	100%
Prophylactic Antibiotic Stopped[2,3]	495	78%	78%	72%	95%
Pregnancy Care					
Inpatient Neonatal Mortality	-	-	-	-	-
Third or Fourth Degree Laceration	-	-	-	3.63%	3.27%

North Big Horn Hospital

1115 Lane 12
Lovell, WY 82431
URL: www.nbhh.com
Ownership: Govt - Hospital District or Authority
Emergency Services: Yes
Phone: 307-548-5200
Fax: 307-548-5205
Accredited: No
Licensed Beds: 15

Key Personnel:

President/CEO..........................Grant Wynnn
Chief Medical Staff.......................David Hoffman, MD
Cardiac Lab ....Jodi McLure
Infection Control.........................Jacqueline Bischoff, RN
Medical/Surgical Nursing ....Trish Mangus, RN, DON

Measure	Cases	This Hospital	State Average	U.S. Average	Top Hospital
Heart Attack Care					
ACE Inhibitor or ARB for LVSD[3]	0	-	95%	82%	100%
Aspirin at Arrival[1,3]	10	70%	78%	92%	100%
Aspirin at Discharge[1,3]	9	67%	78%	90%	100%
Beta Blocker at Arrival[1,3]	11	27%	77%	87%	100%
Beta Blocker at Discharge[1,3]	10	30%	84%	90%	100%
Fibrinolytic Medication Timing[3]	0	-	36%	31%	100%
PCI Within 90 Minutes of Arrival[5]	-	-	72%	54%	95%
Smoking Cessation Advice[1,3]	4	0%	73%	88%	100%
Heart Failure Care					
ACE Inhibitor or ARB for LVSD	0	-	70%	82%	100%
Discharge Instructions[1]	5	40%	56%	61%	93%
Evaluation of LVS Function[1]	13	8%	60%	83%	99%
Smoking Cessation Advice[1]	1	0%	62%	82%	100%
Pneumonia Care					
Appropriate Initial Antibiotic[1]	18	83%	82%	83%	94%
Blood Culture Timing[1]	4	100%	92%	90%	100%
Influenza Vaccine[1]	5	60%	71%	70%	100%
Initial Antibiotic Timing[1]	21	76%	87%	80%	93%
Oxygenation Assessment[1]	24	96%	100%	99%	100%
Pneumococcal Vaccine[1]	15	60%	74%	69%	94%
Smoking Cessation Advice[1]	3	33%	73%	80%	100%
Surgical Infection Prevention					
Prophylactic Antibiotic Given[5]	-	-	76%	77%	95%
Prophylactic Antibiotic Selection[5]	-	-	90%	90%	100%
Prophylactic Antibiotic Stopped[5]	-	-	78%	72%	95%
Pregnancy Care					
Inpatient Neonatal Mortality	-	-	-	-	-
Third or Fourth Degree Laceration	-	-	-	3.63%	3.27%

Memorial Hospital of Converse County

Alternate Name: Converse County Memorial Hospital
PO Box 1450
Douglas, WY 82633
E-mail: nprobert@wmcnet.org
Ownership: Government - Local
Emergency Services: Yes
Phone: 307-358-2122
Fax: 307-358-3630
Accredited: No
Licensed Beds: 34

Key Personnel:

Administrator ....Fred F Schroeder
Chief Medical Staff.......................Kirby C Kirkland, MD
Emergency Room ....Tracy Forward, RN
Director Infection/Disease Control ....Kirby C Kirkland, MD
Director Medical/Surgical Nursing ....Sharon Saunders, RN
OB/GYN Womens Health..................Beth C Robitaille, MD
Chief Radiology ....Sandy Thomas
Director Respiratory Therapy ....Kathy Summers

Measure	Cases	This Hospital	State Average	U.S. Average	Top Hospital
Heart Attack Care					
ACE Inhibitor or ARB for LVSD[3]	0	-	95%	82%	100%
Aspirin at Arrival[1,3]	1	100%	78%	92%	100%
Aspirin at Discharge[1,3]	1	100%	78%	90%	100%
Beta Blocker at Arrival[1,3]	1	100%	77%	87%	100%
Beta Blocker at Discharge[1,3]	1	100%	84%	90%	100%
Fibrinolytic Medication Timing[3]	0	-	36%	31%	100%
PCI Within 90 Minutes of Arrival[5]	-	-	72%	54%	95%
Smoking Cessation Advice[3]	0	-	73%	88%	100%
Heart Failure Care					
ACE Inhibitor or ARB for LVSD	0	-	70%	82%	100%
Discharge Instructions[1]	8	88%	56%	61%	93%
Evaluation of LVS Function[1]	9	78%	60%	83%	99%
Smoking Cessation Advice[1]	1	100%	62%	82%	100%
Pneumonia Care					
Appropriate Initial Antibiotic[1]	19	89%	82%	83%	94%
Blood Culture Timing[1]	7	86%	92%	90%	100%
Influenza Vaccine[1]	6	83%	71%	70%	100%

NOTE: Hospital profiles are in alphabetical order by state, then city, then hospital within the city; Rankings are sorted by rate in descending order and exclude hospitals with less than 25 cases; (1) The number of cases is too small (n<25) for purposes of reliably predicting hospital performance; (2) Measure reflects the hospital's indication that its submission was based upon a sample of its relevant discharges; (3) Rate reflects fewer than the maximum possible quarters of data for the measure; (4) Inaccurate information submitted and suppressed for one or more quarters; (5) No data is available from the hospital for this measure; Please refer to the User's Guide for a full explanation of data

Measure	Cases	This Hospital	State Average	U.S. Average	Top Hospital
Initial Antibiotic Timing[1]	20	90%	87%	80%	93%
Oxygenation Assessment	25	100%	100%	99%	100%
Pneumococcal Vaccine[1]	19	89%	74%	69%	94%
Smoking Cessation Advice[1]	4	100%	73%	80%	100%
Surgical Infection Prevention					
Prophylactic Antibiotic Given	75	79%	76%	77%	95%
Prophylactic Antibiotic Selection	28	96%	90%	90%	100%
Prophylactic Antibiotic Stopped	74	62%	78%	72%	95%
Pregnancy Care					
Inpatient Neonatal Mortality	-	-	-	-	-
Third or Fourth Degree Laceration	-	-	-	3.63%	3.27%

Evanston Regional Hospital

Alternate Name: IHC Evanston Regional Hospital
190 Arrowhead Drive
Evanston, WY 82930
Phone: 307-789-3636
Fax: 307-783-8237
Ownership: Proprietary
Accredited: Yes
Emergency Services: Yes
Licensed Beds: 42

Key Personnel:

CEO . . . . Chris Parj
Chief Medical Staff . . . . Gary Baldwan
Chief Medical Staff . . . . Mike Stellers
Emergency Room . . . . Kevin O'Meara
Respiratory Care . . . . Jamie Hunt

Measure	Cases	This Hospital	State Average	U.S. Average	Top Hospital
Heart Attack Care					
ACE Inhibitor or ARB for LVSD[3]	0	-	95%	82%	100%
Aspirin at Arrival[3]	0	-	78%	92%	100%
Aspirin at Discharge[3]	0	-	78%	90%	100%
Beta Blocker at Arrival[3]	0	-	77%	87%	100%
Beta Blocker at Discharge[3]	0	-	84%	90%	100%
Fibrinolytic Medication Timing[3]	0	-	36%	31%	100%
PCI Within 90 Minutes of Arrival[5]	-	-	72%	54%	95%
Smoking Cessation Advice[3]	0	-	73%	88%	100%
Heart Failure Care					
ACE Inhibitor or ARB for LVSD[1]	1	100%	70%	82%	100%
Discharge Instructions[1]	17	53%	56%	61%	93%
Evaluation of LVS Function[1]	19	74%	60%	83%	99%
Smoking Cessation Advice[1]	4	100%	62%	82%	100%
Pneumonia Care					
Appropriate Initial Antibiotic	38	89%	82%	83%	94%
Blood Culture Timing	33	94%	92%	90%	100%
Influenza Vaccine[1]	9	78%	71%	70%	100%
Initial Antibiotic Timing	50	96%	87%	80%	93%
Oxygenation Assessment	56	100%	100%	99%	100%
Pneumococcal Vaccine	27	96%	74%	69%	94%
Smoking Cessation Advice[1]	16	88%	73%	80%	100%
Surgical Infection Prevention					
Prophylactic Antibiotic Given[2,3]	30	93%	76%	77%	95%
Prophylactic Antibiotic Selection[1,2]	10	50%	90%	90%	100%
Prophylactic Antibiotic Stopped[2,3]	28	68%	78%	72%	95%
Pregnancy Care					
Inpatient Neonatal Mortality	-	-	-	-	-
Third or Fourth Degree Laceration	-	-	-	3.63%	3.27%

Campbell County Memorial Hospital

501 S Burma
Gillette, WY 82716
Phone: 307-682-8811
Fax: 307-688-1515
URL: www.ccmh.net
Ownership: Govt - Hospital District or Authority
Accredited: Yes
Emergency Services: Yes
Licensed Beds: 90

Key Personnel:

CEO . . . . Charles D Crow
Chief Medical Staff . . . . Larry Long, MD
Emergency Room . . . . Lorna Thomas
Emergency Room . . . . Stan Lawson
Infection Control . . . . Baerbel Merrill
ICU . . . . Bette Amith
Medical Surgical Nursing . . . . Anne Raga
Respiratory . . . . Linda Ducello

Measure	Cases	This Hospital	State Average	U.S. Average	Top Hospital
Heart Attack Care					
ACE Inhibitor or ARB for LVSD[1]	3	100%	95%	82%	100%
Aspirin at Arrival[1]	20	100%	78%	92%	100%
Aspirin at Discharge[1]	9	100%	78%	90%	100%
Beta Blocker at Arrival[1]	15	100%	77%	87%	100%
Beta Blocker at Discharge[1]	10	90%	84%	90%	100%
Fibrinolytic Medication Timing[1]	4	50%	36%	31%	100%
PCI Within 90 Minutes of Arrival	0	-	72%	54%	95%
Smoking Cessation Advice[1]	1	100%	73%	88%	100%
Heart Failure Care					
ACE Inhibitor or ARB for LVSD[1]	9	78%	70%	82%	100%
Discharge Instructions	35	60%	56%	61%	93%
Evaluation of LVS Function	50	62%	60%	83%	99%
Smoking Cessation Advice[1]	5	20%	62%	82%	100%
Pneumonia Care					
Appropriate Initial Antibiotic	71	76%	82%	83%	94%
Blood Culture Timing	59	85%	92%	90%	100%
Influenza Vaccine[1]	23	74%	71%	70%	100%
Initial Antibiotic Timing	86	92%	87%	80%	93%
Oxygenation Assessment	110	100%	100%	99%	100%
Pneumococcal Vaccine	59	76%	74%	69%	94%
Smoking Cessation Advice	27	63%	73%	80%	100%
Surgical Infection Prevention					
Prophylactic Antibiotic Given	126	91%	76%	77%	95%
Prophylactic Antibiotic Selection[1]	23	100%	90%	90%	100%
Prophylactic Antibiotic Stopped	121	91%	78%	72%	95%
Pregnancy Care					
Inpatient Neonatal Mortality	752	0.40%	-	-	-
Third or Fourth Degree Laceration	549	3.46%	-	3.63%	3.27%

Saint John's Medical Center

625 E Broadway
PO Box 425
Jackson, WY 83001
Phone: 307-733-3636
Fax: 307-739-7522
URL: www.tetonhospital.org
Ownership: Govt - Hospital District or Authority
Accredited: Yes
Emergency Services: Yes
Licensed Beds: 42

Key Personnel:

President . . . . Carol Lewis
Administrator/CEO . . . . John D Valiante
Chief Medical Staff . . . . William Neal, MD
Emergency Room . . . . Rick McKay, MD
Director Infection/Disease Control . . . . Janet Olsen, RN
ICU . . . . Kathy Martin, RN
Intensive Coronary . . . . Kathy Martin, RN
Medical & Surgical Nursing . . . . Pat Weber, RN
Director Respiratory Therapy . . . . Judy Bishop

Measure	Cases	This Hospital	State Average	U.S. Average	Top Hospital
Heart Attack Care					
ACE Inhibitor or ARB for LVSD[3]	0	-	95%	82%	100%
Aspirin at Arrival[1,3]	3	100%	78%	92%	100%
Aspirin at Discharge[1,3]	3	100%	78%	90%	100%
Beta Blocker at Arrival[1,3]	3	100%	77%	87%	100%
Beta Blocker at Discharge[1,3]	3	100%	84%	90%	100%
Fibrinolytic Medication Timing[3]	0	-	36%	31%	100%
PCI Within 90 Minutes of Arrival	0	-	72%	54%	95%
Smoking Cessation Advice[1,3]	1	100%	73%	88%	100%
Heart Failure Care					
ACE Inhibitor or ARB for LVSD[1]	18	61%	70%	82%	100%
Discharge Instructions	36	86%	56%	61%	93%
Evaluation of LVS Function	39	64%	60%	83%	99%
Smoking Cessation Advice[1]	5	100%	62%	82%	100%
Pneumonia Care					
Appropriate Initial Antibiotic	51	92%	82%	83%	94%
Blood Culture Timing	27	89%	92%	90%	100%
Influenza Vaccine[1]	6	67%	71%	70%	100%
Initial Antibiotic Timing	46	89%	87%	80%	93%
Oxygenation Assessment	66	97%	100%	99%	100%
Pneumococcal Vaccine	34	65%	74%	69%	94%
Smoking Cessation Advice[1]	11	45%	73%	80%	100%
Surgical Infection Prevention					
Prophylactic Antibiotic Given[3]	131	83%	76%	77%	95%

NOTE: Hospital profiles are in alphabetical order by state, then city, then hospital within the city; Rankings are sorted by rate in descending order and exclude hospitals with less than 25 cases; (1) The number of cases is too small (n<25) for purposes of reliably predicting hospital performance; (2) Measure reflects the hospital's indication that its submission was based upon a sample of its relevant discharges; (3) Rate reflects fewer than the maximum possible quarters of data for the measure; (4) Inaccurate information submitted and suppressed for one or more quarters; (5) No data is available from the hospital for this measure; Please refer to the User's Guide for a full explanation of data

Measure	Cases	This Hospital	State Average	U.S. Average	Top Hospital
Prophylactic Antibiotic Selection	47	94%	90%	90%	100%
Prophylactic Antibiotic Stopped[3]	124	77%	78%	72%	95%
Pregnancy Care					
Inpatient Neonatal Mortality	487	0.21%	-	-	-
Third or Fourth Degree Laceration	366	3.83%	-	3.63%	3.27%

South Lincoln Medical Center

711 Onyx Street
Kemmerer, WY 83101
E-mail: ms@allwest.net
Phone: 307-877-4401
Fax: 307-877-3236
Ownership: Govt - Hospital District or Authority
Emergency Services: No
Accredited: No
Licensed Beds: 16

Key Personnel:
CEO. . . . . Marla Shelby
Chief Medical Staff. . . . . G Cristopher Krell

Measure	Cases	This Hospital	State Average	U.S. Average	Top Hospital
Heart Attack Care					
ACE Inhibitor or ARB for LVSD[3]	0	-	95%	82%	100%
Aspirin at Arrival[3]	0	-	78%	92%	100%
Aspirin at Discharge[3]	0	-	78%	90%	100%
Beta Blocker at Arrival[3]	0	-	77%	87%	100%
Beta Blocker at Discharge[3]	0	-	84%	90%	100%
Fibrinolytic Medication Timing[3]	0	-	36%	31%	100%
PCI Within 90 Minutes of Arrival	0	-	72%	54%	95%
Smoking Cessation Advice[3]	0	-	73%	88%	100%
Heart Failure Care					
ACE Inhibitor or ARB for LVSD	0	-	70%	82%	100%
Discharge Instructions[1]	6	0%	56%	61%	93%
Evaluation of LVS Function[1]	8	0%	60%	83%	99%
Smoking Cessation Advice	0	-	62%	82%	100%
Pneumonia Care					
Appropriate Initial Antibiotic[1]	15	67%	82%	83%	94%
Blood Culture Timing[1]	4	100%	92%	90%	100%
Influenza Vaccine[1]	4	0%	71%	70%	100%
Initial Antibiotic Timing[1]	12	67%	87%	80%	93%
Oxygenation Assessment[1]	20	100%	100%	99%	100%
Pneumococcal Vaccine[1]	10	10%	74%	69%	94%
Smoking Cessation Advice[1]	7	71%	73%	80%	100%
Surgical Infection Prevention					
Prophylactic Antibiotic Given[1,3]	7	100%	76%	77%	95%
Prophylactic Antibiotic Selection[1]	2	100%	90%	90%	100%
Prophylactic Antibiotic Stopped[1,3]	6	100%	78%	72%	95%
Pregnancy Care					
Inpatient Neonatal Mortality	-	-	-	-	-
Third or Fourth Degree Laceration	-	-	-	3.63%	3.27%

Lander Valley Medical Center

1320 Bishop Randall Drive
Lander, WY 82520
E-mail: ccovert@landervalley.nahc.com
URL: www.landerhospital.com
Phone: 307-332-4420
Fax: 307-332-3548
Ownership: Proprietary
Emergency Services: Yes
Accredited: Yes
Licensed Beds: 107

Key Personnel:
President/CEO. . . . . Phil Paton
Chief of Medical Staff. . . . . Greg Clifford
Director of Pulmonary . . . . Tony Krvie

Measure	Cases	This Hospital	State Average	U.S. Average	Top Hospital
Heart Attack Care					
ACE Inhibitor or ARB for LVSD[1]	1	100%	95%	82%	100%
Aspirin at Arrival[1]	6	83%	78%	92%	100%
Aspirin at Discharge[1]	2	100%	78%	90%	100%
Beta Blocker at Arrival[1]	3	100%	77%	87%	100%
Beta Blocker at Discharge[1]	3	100%	84%	90%	100%
Fibrinolytic Medication Timing[1]	3	67%	36%	31%	100%
PCI Within 90 Minutes of Arrival	0	-	72%	54%	95%
Smoking Cessation Advice	0	-	73%	88%	100%
Heart Failure Care					
ACE Inhibitor or ARB for LVSD[1]	11	64%	70%	82%	100%
Discharge Instructions	30	63%	56%	61%	93%

Measure	Cases	This Hospital	State Average	U.S. Average	Top Hospital
Evaluation of LVS Function	32	75%	60%	83%	99%
Smoking Cessation Advice[1]	8	100%	62%	82%	100%
Pneumonia Care					
Appropriate Initial Antibiotic	56	84%	82%	83%	94%
Blood Culture Timing	41	100%	92%	90%	100%
Influenza Vaccine[1]	16	88%	71%	70%	100%
Initial Antibiotic Timing	85	85%	87%	80%	93%
Oxygenation Assessment	98	100%	100%	99%	100%
Pneumococcal Vaccine	40	82%	74%	69%	94%
Smoking Cessation Advice	36	92%	73%	80%	100%
Surgical Infection Prevention					
Prophylactic Antibiotic Given[2,3]	128	80%	76%	77%	95%
Prophylactic Antibiotic Selection[2]	61	100%	90%	90%	100%
Prophylactic Antibiotic Stopped[2,3]	125	86%	78%	72%	95%
Pregnancy Care					
Inpatient Neonatal Mortality	-	-	-	-	-
Third or Fourth Degree Laceration	-	-	-	3.63%	3.27%

Ivinson Memorial Hospital

255 North 30th Street
Laramie, WY 82072
URL: www.ivinsonhospital.org
Phone: 307-742-2141
Fax: 307-742-2150
Ownership: Govt - Hospital District or Authority
Emergency Services: Yes
Accredited: Yes
Licensed Beds: 99

Key Personnel:
CEO/President. . . . . Nelson Toebbe
Chief of Medical Staff . . . . Thomas Vienz
Emergency Room Director. . . . . Donald Swiatek, MD

Measure	Cases	This Hospital	State Average	U.S. Average	Top Hospital
Heart Attack Care					
ACE Inhibitor or ARB for LVSD[3]	0	-	95%	82%	100%
Aspirin at Arrival[1,3]	1	100%	78%	92%	100%
Aspirin at Discharge[1,3]	1	100%	78%	90%	100%
Beta Blocker at Arrival[1,3]	1	100%	77%	87%	100%
Beta Blocker at Discharge[1,3]	1	100%	84%	90%	100%
Fibrinolytic Medication Timing[3]	0	-	36%	31%	100%
PCI Within 90 Minutes of Arrival[5]	-	-	72%	54%	95%
Smoking Cessation Advice[3]	0	-	73%	88%	100%
Heart Failure Care					
ACE Inhibitor or ARB for LVSD[1]	10	100%	70%	82%	100%
Discharge Instructions[1]	17	65%	56%	61%	93%
Evaluation of LVS Function	29	90%	60%	83%	99%
Smoking Cessation Advice[1]	2	100%	62%	82%	100%
Pneumonia Care					
Appropriate Initial Antibiotic	71	75%	82%	83%	94%
Blood Culture Timing	51	84%	92%	90%	100%
Influenza Vaccine[1]	18	83%	71%	70%	100%
Initial Antibiotic Timing	98	82%	87%	80%	93%
Oxygenation Assessment	132	100%	100%	99%	100%
Pneumococcal Vaccine	83	84%	74%	69%	94%
Smoking Cessation Advice	30	93%	73%	80%	100%
Surgical Infection Prevention					
Prophylactic Antibiotic Given	172	67%	76%	77%	95%
Prophylactic Antibiotic Selection	47	89%	90%	90%	100%
Prophylactic Antibiotic Stopped	169	66%	78%	72%	95%
Pregnancy Care					
Inpatient Neonatal Mortality	-	-	-	-	-
Third or Fourth Degree Laceration	-	-	-	3.63%	3.27%

Niobrara County Memorial Hospital

PO Box 780
Lusk, WY 82225
Phone: 307-334-2711
Fax: 307-334-4059
Ownership: Govt - Hospital District or Authority
Emergency Services: Yes
Accredited: No
Licensed Beds: 51

Key Personnel:
Administrator . . . . Corolyn Gill
Director Infection/Disease Control . . . . Deana Sarr

Measure	Cases	This Hospital	State Average	U.S. Average	Top Hospital
Heart Attack Care					
ACE Inhibitor or ARB for LVSD[5]	-	-	95%	82%	100%

NOTE: Hospital profiles are in alphabetical order by state, then city, then hospital within the city; Rankings are sorted by rate in descending order and exclude hospitals with less than 25 cases; (1) The number of cases is too small (n<25) for purposes of reliably predicting hospital performance; (2) Measure reflects the hospital's indication that its submission was based upon a sample of its relevant discharges; (3) Rate reflects fewer than the maximum possible quarters of data for the measure; (4) Inaccurate information submitted and suppressed for one or more quarters; (5) No data is available from the hospital for this measure; Please refer to the User's Guide for a full explanation of data

Aspirin at Arrival[5]	-	-	78%	92%	100%
Aspirin at Discharge[5]	-	-	78%	90%	100%
Beta Blocker at Arrival[5]	-	-	77%	87%	100%
Beta Blocker at Discharge[5]	-	-	84%	90%	100%
Fibrinolytic Medication Timing[5]	-	-	36%	31%	100%
PCI Within 90 Minutes of Arrival[5]	-	-	72%	54%	95%
Smoking Cessation Advice[5]	-	-	73%	88%	100%
Heart Failure Care					
ACE Inhibitor or ARB for LVSD[3]	0	-	70%	82%	100%
Discharge Instructions[3]	0	-	56%	61%	93%
Evaluation of LVS Function[1,3]	1	0%	60%	83%	99%
Smoking Cessation Advice[3]	0	-	62%	82%	100%
Pneumonia Care					
Appropriate Initial Antibiotic[3]	0	-	82%	83%	94%
Blood Culture Timing[3]	0	-	92%	90%	100%
Influenza Vaccine[5]	-	-	71%	70%	100%
Initial Antibiotic Timing[3]	0	-	87%	80%	93%
Oxygenation Assessment[3]	0	-	100%	99%	100%
Pneumococcal Vaccine[3]	0	-	74%	69%	94%
Smoking Cessation Advice[3]	0	-	73%	80%	100%
Surgical Infection Prevention					
Prophylactic Antibiotic Given[5]	-	-	76%	77%	95%
Prophylactic Antibiotic Selection[5]	-	-	90%	90%	100%
Prophylactic Antibiotic Stopped[5]	-	-	78%	72%	95%
Pregnancy Care					
Inpatient Neonatal Mortality	-	-	-	-	-
Third or Fourth Degree Laceration	-	-	-	3.63%	3.27%

Weston County Health Services

1124 Washington Boulevard
Newcastle, WY 82701
Phone: 307-746-4491
Fax: 307-746-4579
Ownership: Govt - Hospital District or Authority
Accredited: No
Emergency Services: Yes
Licensed Beds: 25

Key Personnel:

CEO. . . . . George Minder
Chief Medical Staff. . . . . Cecellia Schlup, DON
CEO. . . . . Glenn Christian

Measure	Cases	This Hospital	State Average	U.S. Average	Top Hospital
Heart Attack Care					
ACE Inhibitor or ARB for LVSD[5]	-	-	95%	82%	100%
Aspirin at Arrival[5]	-	-	78%	92%	100%
Aspirin at Discharge[5]	-	-	78%	90%	100%
Beta Blocker at Arrival[5]	-	-	77%	87%	100%
Beta Blocker at Discharge[5]	-	-	84%	90%	100%
Fibrinolytic Medication Timing[5]	-	-	36%	31%	100%
PCI Within 90 Minutes of Arrival[5]	-	-	72%	54%	95%
Smoking Cessation Advice[5]	-	-	73%	88%	100%
Heart Failure Care					
ACE Inhibitor or ARB for LVSD[1]	1	0%	70%	82%	100%
Discharge Instructions[1]	4	0%	56%	61%	93%
Evaluation of LVS Function[1]	4	50%	60%	83%	99%
Smoking Cessation Advice[1]	1	100%	62%	82%	100%
Pneumonia Care					
Appropriate Initial Antibiotic[1]	11	73%	82%	83%	94%
Blood Culture Timing[1]	1	100%	92%	90%	100%
Influenza Vaccine[1]	5	60%	71%	70%	100%
Initial Antibiotic Timing[1]	12	92%	87%	80%	93%
Oxygenation Assessment[1]	13	100%	100%	99%	100%
Pneumococcal Vaccine[1]	9	89%	74%	69%	94%
Smoking Cessation Advice[1]	2	100%	73%	80%	100%
Surgical Infection Prevention					
Prophylactic Antibiotic Given[5]	-	-	76%	77%	95%
Prophylactic Antibiotic Selection[5]	-	-	90%	90%	100%
Prophylactic Antibiotic Stopped[5]	-	-	78%	72%	95%
Pregnancy Care					
Inpatient Neonatal Mortality	-	-	-	-	-
Third or Fourth Degree Laceration	-	-	-	3.63%	3.27%

Powell Vally Hospital

777 Avenue H
Powell, WY 82435
Phone: 307-754-2267
Fax: 307-754-3176
URL: www.pvhc.org
Ownership: Voluntary non-profit - Other
Accredited: No
Emergency Services: Yes
Licensed Beds: 25

Key Personnel:

CEO. . . . . Rod Barton
Chief Medical Staff. . . . . Mike Tracy, MD
Emergency Room . . . . Christine Winkleman, RN
Infection Control. . . . . Deb Kleinfeldt, RN
ICU . . . . Cathy Campbell, RN
OB/GYN/Women's Health . . . . Robert Ellis, MD
Respiratory/Cardiopulmonary. . . . . Diana Gorsuch

Measure	Cases	This Hospital	State Average	U.S. Average	Top Hospital
Heart Attack Care					
ACE Inhibitor or ARB for LVSD	0	-	95%	82%	100%
Aspirin at Arrival[1]	5	100%	78%	92%	100%
Aspirin at Discharge[1]	4	100%	78%	90%	100%
Beta Blocker at Arrival[1]	2	100%	77%	87%	100%
Beta Blocker at Discharge[1]	3	100%	84%	90%	100%
Fibrinolytic Medication Timing[1]	1	100%	36%	31%	100%
PCI Within 90 Minutes of Arrival	0	-	72%	54%	95%
Smoking Cessation Advice[1]	1	0%	73%	88%	100%
Heart Failure Care					
ACE Inhibitor or ARB for LVSD[1]	2	50%	70%	82%	100%
Discharge Instructions[1]	9	33%	56%	61%	93%
Evaluation of LVS Function[1]	21	38%	60%	83%	99%
Smoking Cessation Advice[1]	2	0%	62%	82%	100%
Pneumonia Care					
Appropriate Initial Antibiotic[1]	12	83%	82%	83%	94%
Blood Culture Timing[1]	4	100%	92%	90%	100%
Influenza Vaccine[1]	5	100%	71%	70%	100%
Initial Antibiotic Timing[1]	15	80%	87%	80%	93%
Oxygenation Assessment[1]	21	100%	100%	99%	100%
Pneumococcal Vaccine[1]	11	91%	74%	69%	94%
Smoking Cessation Advice[1]	4	50%	73%	80%	100%
Surgical Infection Prevention					
Prophylactic Antibiotic Given	38	79%	76%	77%	95%
Prophylactic Antibiotic Selection[1]	7	86%	90%	90%	100%
Prophylactic Antibiotic Stopped	36	78%	78%	72%	95%
Pregnancy Care					
Inpatient Neonatal Mortality	-	-	-	-	-
Third or Fourth Degree Laceration	-	-	-	3.63%	3.27%

Memorial Hospital of Carbon County

2221 W Elm
Rawlins, WY 82301
Phone: 307-324-2221
Fax: 307-324-8232
Ownership: Govt - Hospital District or Authority
Accredited: No
Emergency Services: Yes
Licensed Beds: 45

Key Personnel:

CEO. . . . . Cathy Carter
Chief Medical Staff. . . . . Duane Abell, DO
Emergency Room . . . . Duane Abell
Respiratory Care Chief. . . . . Tom Shrode

Measure	Cases	This Hospital	State Average	U.S. Average	Top Hospital
Heart Attack Care					
ACE Inhibitor or ARB for LVSD	0	-	95%	82%	100%
Aspirin at Arrival[1]	6	100%	78%	92%	100%
Aspirin at Discharge[1]	3	33%	78%	90%	100%
Beta Blocker at Arrival[1]	9	78%	77%	87%	100%
Beta Blocker at Discharge[1]	4	100%	84%	90%	100%
Fibrinolytic Medication Timing[1]	2	0%	36%	31%	100%
PCI Within 90 Minutes of Arrival	0	-	72%	54%	95%
Smoking Cessation Advice	0	-	73%	88%	100%
Heart Failure Care					
ACE Inhibitor or ARB for LVSD[1]	5	20%	70%	82%	100%
Discharge Instructions	48	23%	56%	61%	93%
Evaluation of LVS Function	56	41%	60%	83%	99%
Smoking Cessation Advice[1]	16	44%	62%	82%	100%
Pneumonia Care					

NOTE: Hospital profiles are in alphabetical order by state, then city, then hospital within the city; Rankings are sorted by rate in descending order and exclude hospitals with less than 25 cases; (1) The number of cases is too small (n<25) for purposes of reliably predicting hospital performance; (2) Measure reflects the hospital's indication that its submission was based upon a sample of its relevant discharges; (3) Rate reflects fewer than the maximum possible quarters of data for the measure; (4) Inaccurate information submitted and suppressed for one or more quarters; (5) No data is available from the hospital for this measure; Please refer to the User's Guide for a full explanation of data

Appropriate Initial Antibiotic	51	78%	82%	83%	94%
Blood Culture Timing[1]	17	82%	92%	90%	100%
Influenza Vaccine[1]	10	70%	71%	70%	100%
Initial Antibiotic Timing	53	85%	87%	80%	93%
Oxygenation Assessment	66	100%	100%	99%	100%
Pneumococcal Vaccine	37	68%	74%	69%	94%
Smoking Cessation Advice	25	56%	73%	80%	100%
Surgical Infection Prevention					
Prophylactic Antibiotic Given[1]	13	69%	76%	77%	95%
Prophylactic Antibiotic Selection[1]	2	100%	90%	90%	100%
Prophylactic Antibiotic Stopped[1]	13	0%	78%	72%	95%
Pregnancy Care					
Inpatient Neonatal Mortality	-	-	-	-	-
Third or Fourth Degree Laceration	-	-	-	3.63%	3.27%

Riverton Memorial Hospital

Alternate Name: Riverton Memorial Hospital
2100 W Sunset Drive
Riverton, WY 82501
Phone: 307-856-4161
Fax: 307-857-3571
E-mail: grant.scholes@lifepointhospitals.com
URL: www.riverton-hospital.com
Ownership: Government - State
Accredited: Yes
Emergency Services: Yes
Licensed Beds: 70

Key Personnel:

CEO . . . . William Russell
Chief Medical Staff . . . . John Reckling, MD
Emergency Room . . . . David Steger, MD
Director Infection/Disease Control . . . . Clare Miller
Director Medical/Surgical Nursing . . . . Vickie Bessey, RN
OB/GYN Womens Health . . . . N Cain, MD
Chief Radiology . . . . Thomas McCallum, MD
Director Respiratory Therapy . . . . Rick Kuhmley, RN

Measure	Cases	This Hospital	State Average	U.S. Average	Top Hospital
Heart Attack Care					
ACE Inhibitor or ARB for LVSD	0	-	95%	82%	100%
Aspirin at Arrival[1]	7	100%	78%	92%	100%
Aspirin at Discharge[1]	3	33%	78%	90%	100%
Beta Blocker at Arrival[1]	6	100%	77%	87%	100%
Beta Blocker at Discharge[1]	3	67%	84%	90%	100%
Fibrinolytic Medication Timing[1]	1	0%	36%	31%	100%
PCI Within 90 Minutes of Arrival	0	-	72%	54%	95%
Smoking Cessation Advice[1]	2	100%	73%	88%	100%
Heart Failure Care					
ACE Inhibitor or ARB for LVSD[1]	8	75%	70%	82%	100%
Discharge Instructions	34	79%	56%	61%	93%
Evaluation of LVS Function	35	83%	60%	83%	99%
Smoking Cessation Advice[1]	4	50%	62%	82%	100%
Pneumonia Care					
Appropriate Initial Antibiotic	43	74%	82%	83%	94%
Blood Culture Timing	28	82%	92%	90%	100%
Influenza Vaccine[1]	4	100%	71%	70%	100%
Initial Antibiotic Timing	45	93%	87%	80%	93%
Oxygenation Assessment	55	100%	100%	99%	100%
Pneumococcal Vaccine	26	85%	74%	69%	94%
Smoking Cessation Advice[1]	17	82%	73%	80%	100%
Surgical Infection Prevention					
Prophylactic Antibiotic Given[2,3]	56	95%	76%	77%	95%
Prophylactic Antibiotic Selection[1,2]	20	100%	90%	90%	100%
Prophylactic Antibiotic Stopped[2,3]	55	89%	78%	72%	95%
Pregnancy Care					
Inpatient Neonatal Mortality	-	-	-	-	-
Third or Fourth Degree Laceration	-	-	-	3.63%	3.27%

Memorial Hospital of Sweetwater County

1200 College Drive
Rock Springs, WY 82901
Phone: 307-362-3711
Fax: 307-362-8391
E-mail: mhschr@minershospital.com
URL: www.minershospital.com
Ownership: Government - Local
Accredited: Yes
Emergency Services: Yes
Licensed Beds: 99

Key Personnel:

CEO . . . . John Ferry
Chief Medical Staff . . . . Joseph Oliver, MD
Emergency Room . . . . Evelyn Normington
Infection Control . . . . Madlyna Rowland
ICU . . . . Barbara Walker
Medical/Surgical Nursing . . . . Brandy Sellers
Respiratory/Cardiopulmonary . . . . Janice Tripp

Measure	Cases	This Hospital	State Average	U.S. Average	Top Hospital
Heart Attack Care					
ACE Inhibitor or ARB for LVSD	0	-	95%	82%	100%
Aspirin at Arrival[1]	3	33%	78%	92%	100%
Aspirin at Discharge[1]	2	50%	78%	90%	100%
Beta Blocker at Arrival[1]	2	50%	77%	87%	100%
Beta Blocker at Discharge[1]	1	100%	84%	90%	100%
Fibrinolytic Medication Timing	0	-	36%	31%	100%
PCI Within 90 Minutes of Arrival	0	-	72%	54%	95%
Smoking Cessation Advice	0	-	73%	88%	100%
Heart Failure Care					
ACE Inhibitor or ARB for LVSD[1]	15	87%	70%	82%	100%
Discharge Instructions	53	55%	56%	61%	93%
Evaluation of LVS Function	65	57%	60%	83%	99%
Smoking Cessation Advice[1]	13	54%	62%	82%	100%
Pneumonia Care					
Appropriate Initial Antibiotic	79	81%	82%	83%	94%
Blood Culture Timing	58	79%	92%	90%	100%
Influenza Vaccine[1]	14	79%	71%	70%	100%
Initial Antibiotic Timing	96	85%	87%	80%	93%
Oxygenation Assessment	110	99%	100%	99%	100%
Pneumococcal Vaccine	59	73%	74%	69%	94%
Smoking Cessation Advice	33	79%	73%	80%	100%
Surgical Infection Prevention					
Prophylactic Antibiotic Given[3]	87	70%	76%	77%	95%
Prophylactic Antibiotic Selection	28	21%	90%	90%	100%
Prophylactic Antibiotic Stopped[3]	77	94%	78%	72%	95%
Pregnancy Care					
Inpatient Neonatal Mortality	-	-	-	-	-
Third or Fourth Degree Laceration	-	-	-	3.63%	3.27%

Memorial Hospital of Sheridan County

1401 W 5th Street
Sheridan, WY 82801
Phone: 307-672-1000
Fax: 307-674-8961
Ownership: Voluntary non-profit - Other
Accredited: Yes
Emergency Services: No
Licensed Beds: 88

Key Personnel:

CEO . . . . Ken Huey
Chief Medical Staff . . . . Lawrence Gill
Emergency Room . . . . Jane Scott
Director of Pulmonary . . . . Ken Bonnette

Measure	Cases	This Hospital	State Average	U.S. Average	Top Hospital
Heart Attack Care					
ACE Inhibitor or ARB for LVSD	0	-	95%	82%	100%
Aspirin at Arrival[1]	10	70%	78%	92%	100%
Aspirin at Discharge[1]	4	75%	78%	90%	100%
Beta Blocker at Arrival[1]	9	67%	77%	87%	100%
Beta Blocker at Discharge[1]	4	75%	84%	90%	100%
Fibrinolytic Medication Timing	0	-	36%	31%	100%
PCI Within 90 Minutes of Arrival	0	-	72%	54%	95%
Smoking Cessation Advice	0	-	73%	88%	100%
Heart Failure Care					
ACE Inhibitor or ARB for LVSD[1]	2	50%	70%	82%	100%
Discharge Instructions	27	59%	56%	61%	93%
Evaluation of LVS Function	43	42%	60%	83%	99%
Smoking Cessation Advice[1]	2	100%	62%	82%	100%
Pneumonia Care					
Appropriate Initial Antibiotic	82	77%	82%	83%	94%
Blood Culture Timing	52	96%	92%	90%	100%
Influenza Vaccine[1]	15	93%	71%	70%	100%
Initial Antibiotic Timing	97	86%	87%	80%	93%
Oxygenation Assessment	115	99%	100%	99%	100%
Pneumococcal Vaccine	85	64%	74%	69%	94%
Smoking Cessation Advice	28	57%	73%	80%	100%

NOTE: Hospital profiles are in alphabetical order by state, then city, then hospital within the city; Rankings are sorted by rate in descending order and exclude hospitals with less than 25 cases; (1) The number of cases is too small (n<25) for purposes of reliably predicting hospital performance; (2) Measure reflects the hospital's indication that its submission was based upon a sample of its relevant discharges; (3) Rate reflects fewer than the maximum possible quarters of data for the measure; (4) Inaccurate information submitted and suppressed for one or more quarters; (5) No data is available from the hospital for this measure; Please refer to the User's Guide for a full explanation of data

Surgical Infection Prevention					
Prophylactic Antibiotic Given	182	94%	76%	77%	95%
Prophylactic Antibiotic Selection	40	92%	90%	90%	100%
Prophylactic Antibiotic Stopped	176	95%	78%	72%	95%
Pregnancy Care					
Inpatient Neonatal Mortality	-	-	-	-	-
Third or Fourth Degree Laceration	-	-	-	3.63%	3.27%

Crook County Medical Services

PO Box 517
Sundance, WY 82729
Phone: 307-283-3501
Ownership: Govt - Hospital District or Authority
Accredited: No
Emergency Services: No

Measure	Cases	This Hospital	State Average	U.S. Average	Top Hospital
Heart Attack Care					
ACE Inhibitor or ARB for LVSD[5]	-	-	95%	82%	100%
Aspirin at Arrival[5]	-	-	78%	92%	100%
Aspirin at Discharge[5]	-	-	78%	90%	100%
Beta Blocker at Arrival[5]	-	-	77%	87%	100%
Beta Blocker at Discharge[5]	-	-	84%	90%	100%
Fibrinolytic Medication Timing[5]	-	-	36%	31%	100%
PCI Within 90 Minutes of Arrival[5]	-	-	72%	54%	95%
Smoking Cessation Advice[5]	-	-	73%	88%	100%
Heart Failure Care					
ACE Inhibitor or ARB for LVSD[1,3]	1	0%	70%	82%	100%
Discharge Instructions[1,3]	2	100%	56%	61%	93%
Evaluation of LVS Function[1,3]	2	50%	60%	83%	99%
Smoking Cessation Advice[3]	0	-	62%	82%	100%
Pneumonia Care					
Appropriate Initial Antibiotic[1]	12	92%	82%	83%	94%
Blood Culture Timing[1]	1	100%	92%	90%	100%
Influenza Vaccine[1]	1	0%	71%	70%	100%
Initial Antibiotic Timing[1]	12	83%	87%	80%	93%
Oxygenation Assessment[1]	14	100%	100%	99%	100%
Pneumococcal Vaccine[1]	7	43%	74%	69%	94%
Smoking Cessation Advice[1]	5	60%	73%	80%	100%
Surgical Infection Prevention					
Prophylactic Antibiotic Given[5]	-	-	76%	77%	95%
Prophylactic Antibiotic Selection[5]	-	-	90%	90%	100%
Prophylactic Antibiotic Stopped[5]	-	-	78%	72%	95%
Pregnancy Care					
Inpatient Neonatal Mortality	-	-	-	-	-
Third or Fourth Degree Laceration	-	-	-	3.63%	3.27%

Hot Springs County Memorial Hospital

Alternate Name: Hot Springs Memorial Hospital
150 East Arapahoe Street
Thermopolis, WY 82443
Toll-Free: 800-788-9459
Phone: 307-864-3121
Fax: 307-864-5050

E-mail: tim.knight@hscmh.org
URL: www.hscmh.org
Ownership: Govt - Hospital District or Authority
Accredited: No
Emergency Services: Yes
Licensed Beds: 25
Key Personnel:
CEO . . . . Trudy Chittick
Chief Staff . . . . Dr Miller
Surgical Services . . . . Robin Griffin
Respiratory/Cardiopulmonary . . . . Frank Hammond

Measure	Cases	This Hospital	State Average	U.S. Average	Top Hospital
Heart Attack Care					
ACE Inhibitor or ARB for LVSD[5]	-	-	95%	82%	100%
Aspirin at Arrival[5]	-	-	78%	92%	100%
Aspirin at Discharge[5]	-	-	78%	90%	100%
Beta Blocker at Arrival[5]	-	-	77%	87%	100%
Beta Blocker at Discharge[5]	-	-	84%	90%	100%
Fibrinolytic Medication Timing[5]	-	-	36%	31%	100%
PCI Within 90 Minutes of Arrival[5]	-	-	72%	54%	95%
Smoking Cessation Advice[5]	-	-	73%	88%	100%
Heart Failure Care					
ACE Inhibitor or ARB for LVSD[1,3]	1	100%	70%	82%	100%
Discharge Instructions[5]	-	-	56%	61%	93%
Evaluation of LVS Function[1,3]	3	100%	60%	83%	99%
Smoking Cessation Advice[1,3]	1	0%	62%	82%	100%
Pneumonia Care					
Appropriate Initial Antibiotic[1]	22	86%	82%	83%	94%
Blood Culture Timing[1]	9	100%	92%	90%	100%
Influenza Vaccine[1]	9	89%	71%	70%	100%
Initial Antibiotic Timing	26	88%	87%	80%	93%
Oxygenation Assessment	41	100%	100%	99%	100%
Pneumococcal Vaccine	29	100%	74%	69%	94%
Smoking Cessation Advice[1]	7	86%	73%	80%	100%
Surgical Infection Prevention					
Prophylactic Antibiotic Given[1]	17	88%	76%	77%	95%
Prophylactic Antibiotic Selection[1]	3	100%	90%	90%	100%
Prophylactic Antibiotic Stopped[1]	17	100%	78%	72%	95%
Pregnancy Care					
Inpatient Neonatal Mortality	-	-	-	-	-
Third or Fourth Degree Laceration	-	-	-	3.63%	3.27%

Community Hospital

2000 Campbell Drive
Torrington, WY 82240
Phone: 307-532-4181
Fax: 307-532-3783
Ownership: Voluntary non-profit - Private
Accredited: No
Emergency Services: Yes
Licensed Beds: 36
Key Personnel:
CEO/President . . . . Pardon Lewis
Chief of Medical Staff . . . . Richard Cambell
Director of Cardiology/Cardiac Lab. . . . . Diane Diane
Emergency Room Director . . . . Tedd Church
Director Infection/Disease Control . . . . Julia Kimsey
Director Respiratory Therapy . . . . Bill Bergstead

Measure	Cases	This Hospital	State Average	U.S. Average	Top Hospital
Heart Attack Care					
ACE Inhibitor or ARB for LVSD	0	-	95%	82%	100%
Aspirin at Arrival[1]	5	60%	78%	92%	100%
Aspirin at Discharge[1]	4	75%	78%	90%	100%
Beta Blocker at Arrival[1]	4	75%	77%	87%	100%
Beta Blocker at Discharge[1]	4	75%	84%	90%	100%
Fibrinolytic Medication Timing	0	-	36%	31%	100%
PCI Within 90 Minutes of Arrival	0	-	72%	54%	95%
Smoking Cessation Advice	0	-	73%	88%	100%
Heart Failure Care					
ACE Inhibitor or ARB for LVSD[1]	6	67%	70%	82%	100%
Discharge Instructions	25	68%	56%	61%	93%
Evaluation of LVS Function	31	74%	60%	83%	99%
Smoking Cessation Advice[1]	4	100%	62%	82%	100%
Pneumonia Care					
Appropriate Initial Antibiotic	36	81%	82%	83%	94%
Blood Culture Timing[1]	18	94%	92%	90%	100%
Influenza Vaccine[1]	12	92%	71%	70%	100%
Initial Antibiotic Timing	30	97%	87%	80%	93%
Oxygenation Assessment	39	100%	100%	99%	100%
Pneumococcal Vaccine	29	83%	74%	69%	94%
Smoking Cessation Advice[1]	3	67%	73%	80%	100%
Surgical Infection Prevention					
Prophylactic Antibiotic Given[1,3]	10	60%	76%	77%	95%
Prophylactic Antibiotic Selection[1]	10	100%	90%	90%	100%
Prophylactic Antibiotic Stopped[1,3]	9	89%	78%	72%	95%
Pregnancy Care					
Inpatient Neonatal Mortality	-	-	-	-	-
Third or Fourth Degree Laceration	-	-	-	3.63%	3.27%

Platte County Memorial Hospital

201 14th Street
Wheatland, WY 82201
Phone: 307-322-3636
Fax: 307-322-3690
URL: www.bannerhealth.com
Ownership: Voluntary non-profit - Other
Accredited: Yes
Emergency Services: Yes
Licensed Beds: 25
Key Personnel:
CEO . . . . Ken Leisher
Chief Medical Staff . . . . Jeremy Katzmann
Emergency Room . . . . Connie Marker, RN

NOTE: Hospital profiles are in alphabetical order by state, then city, then hospital within the city; Rankings are sorted by rate in descending order and exclude hospitals with less than 25 cases; (1) The number of cases is too small (n<25) for purposes of reliably predicting hospital performance; (2) Measure reflects the hospital's indication that its submission was based upon a sample of its relevant discharges; (3) Rate reflects fewer than the maximum possible quarters of data for the measure; (4) Inaccurate information submitted and suppressed for one or more quarters; (5) No data is available from the hospital for this measure; Please refer to the User's Guide for a full explanation of data

Infection Control . . . . Laurie Faber, RN
ICU Supervising Nurse. Marian Cole, RN
Coronary Care Unit Supervising Nurse . . . . Marian Cole, RN
Chief Radiology . . . . Randy Blackman
Director Respiratory Therapy . . . . Deborah Lockman, RN

Measure	Cases	This Hospital	State Average	U.S. Average	Top Hospital
Heart Attack Care					
ACE Inhibitor or ARB for LVSD[3]	0	-	95%	82%	100%
Aspirin at Arrival[1,3]	1	100%	78%	92%	100%
Aspirin at Discharge[1,3]	1	100%	78%	90%	100%
Beta Blocker at Arrival[1,3]	1	100%	77%	87%	100%
Beta Blocker at Discharge[1,3]	1	100%	84%	90%	100%
Fibrinolytic Medication Timing[3]	0	-	36%	31%	100%
PCI Within 90 Minutes of Arrival	0	-	72%	54%	95%
Smoking Cessation Advice[1,3]	1	100%	73%	88%	100%
Heart Failure Care					
ACE Inhibitor or ARB for LVSD[1]	4	100%	70%	82%	100%
Discharge Instructions[1]	6	100%	56%	61%	93%
Evaluation of LVS Function[1]	9	100%	60%	83%	99%
Smoking Cessation Advice[1]	2	100%	62%	82%	100%
Pneumonia Care					
Appropriate Initial Antibiotic	33	97%	82%	83%	94%
Blood Culture Timing[1]	13	85%	92%	90%	100%
Influenza Vaccine[1]	4	100%	71%	70%	100%
Initial Antibiotic Timing	36	94%	87%	80%	93%
Oxygenation Assessment	43	100%	100%	99%	100%
Pneumococcal Vaccine	25	96%	74%	69%	94%
Smoking Cessation Advice[1]	10	100%	73%	80%	100%
Surgical Infection Prevention					
Prophylactic Antibiotic Given[1,3]	5	80%	76%	77%	95%
Prophylactic Antibiotic Selection[1]	5	100%	90%	90%	100%
Prophylactic Antibiotic Stopped[1,3]	5	100%	78%	72%	95%
Pregnancy Care					
Inpatient Neonatal Mortality	-	-	-	-	-
Third or Fourth Degree Laceration	-	-	-	3.63%	3.27%

Washakie Medical Center

Alternate Name: Washakie County Memorial Hospital
400 S 15th
Worland, WY 82401
Phone: 307-347-3221
Fax: 307-347-6995
URL: www.washakiemedicalcenter.com
Ownership: Voluntary non-profit - Other
Accredited: No
Emergency Services: Yes
Licensed Beds: 30

Key Personnel:

President/CEO . . . . George Rohrich
Chief Medical Staff . . . . James Randolph
Cardiac Lab . . . . Juanita Noska
Emergency Room . . . . Evonne Charles
Infection Control . . . . Maryjo Hake
ICU . . . . Roy Peahoby
Medical/Surgical Nursing . . . . Robert Lindberg
OB/GYN Womens Health. . . . . Jody Costalez
Respiratory/Cardiopulmonary. . . . . Rob Lindberg

Measure	Cases	This Hospital	State Average	U.S. Average	Top Hospital
Heart Attack Care					
ACE Inhibitor or ARB for LVSD[3]	0	-	95%	82%	100%
Aspirin at Arrival[1,3]	1	0%	78%	92%	100%
Aspirin at Discharge[1,3]	1	0%	78%	90%	100%
Beta Blocker at Arrival[1,3]	1	0%	77%	87%	100%
Beta Blocker at Discharge[1,3]	1	0%	84%	90%	100%
Fibrinolytic Medication Timing[3]	0	-	36%	31%	100%
PCI Within 90 Minutes of Arrival[5]	-	-	72%	54%	95%
Smoking Cessation Advice[3]	0	-	73%	88%	100%
Heart Failure Care					
ACE Inhibitor or ARB for LVSD[1]	7	100%	70%	82%	100%
Discharge Instructions[1]	19	84%	56%	61%	93%
Evaluation of LVS Function	26	77%	60%	83%	99%
Smoking Cessation Advice[1]	3	33%	62%	82%	100%
Pneumonia Care					
Appropriate Initial Antibiotic[1]	23	74%	82%	83%	94%
Blood Culture Timing[1]	10	100%	92%	90%	100%
Influenza Vaccine[1]	6	83%	71%	70%	100%
Initial Antibiotic Timing[1]	21	100%	87%	80%	93%
Oxygenation Assessment	31	100%	100%	99%	100%
Pneumococcal Vaccine[1]	16	81%	74%	69%	94%
Smoking Cessation Advice[1]	4	25%	73%	80%	100%
Surgical Infection Prevention					
Prophylactic Antibiotic Given[1,3]	7	43%	76%	77%	95%
Prophylactic Antibiotic Selection[1]	8	100%	90%	90%	100%
Prophylactic Antibiotic Stopped[1,3]	5	80%	78%	72%	95%
Pregnancy Care					
Inpatient Neonatal Mortality	-	-	-	-	-
Third or Fourth Degree Laceration	-	-	-	3.63%	3.27%

NOTE: Hospital profiles are in alphabetical order by state, then city, then hospital within the city; Rankings are sorted by rate in descending order and exclude hospitals with less than 25 cases; (1) The number of cases is too small (n<25) for purposes of reliably predicting hospital performance; (2) Measure reflects the hospital's indication that its submission was based upon a sample of its relevant discharges; (3) Rate reflects fewer than the maximum possible quarters of data for the measure; (4) Inaccurate information submitted and suppressed for one or more quarters; (5) No data is available from the hospital for this measure; Please refer to the User's Guide for a full explanation of data

Hospital	Heart Attack Care								Heart Failure Care				Pneumonia Care							Surgical Infection Prevention			Pregnancy Care	
	1	2	3	4	5	6	7	8	9	10	11	12	13	14	15	16	17	18	19	20	21	22	23	24
ALASKA																								
Alaska Native Medical Center, Anchorage, AK	**100** 6	**100** 3	**91** 11	**100** 3	**92** 12	- 0	- 0	**57** 7	**100** 42	**5** 65	**97** 66	**57** 23	**91** 64	**90** 59	**54** 13	**77** 79	**99** 96	**94** 36	**65** 48	**84** 198	**93** 60	**81** 195	**0.40** 1501	**3.07** 1207
Alaska Regional Hospital, Anchorage, AK	**100** 21	**100** 67	**100** 117	**96** 69	**97** 115	- 0	**71** 7	**92** 49	**92** 36	**49** 75	**97** 78	**81** 16	**91** 34	**85** 20	**60** 5	**84** 37	**100** 50	**55** 22	**78** 18	**63** 273	**95** 133	**76** 271	- -	- -
Bartlett Regional Hospital, Juneau, AK	**100** 2	**100** 12	**100** 12	**93** 15	**100** 12	**14** 7	- 0	**33** 3	**85** 13	**51** 41	**89** 45	**50** 6	**70** 50	**96** 26	**75** 4	**83** 42	**100** 58	**47** 34	**78** 9	**37** 57	**56** 27	**63** 52	- -	- -
Central Peninsula Hospital, Soldotna, AK	**100** 1	**100** 3	**100** 1	**100** 3	**100** 1	**0** 1	- 0	- 0	**90** 10	**83** 35	**97** 38	**71** 7	**89** 35	**100** 30	**60** 5	**77** 39	**100** 52	**81** 32	**90** 10	**81** 75	**90** 21	**94** 78	- -	- -
Fairbanks Memorial Hospital, Fairbanks, AK	**75** 4	**90** 20	**100** 12	**94** 16	**100** 10	**50** 6	- 0	**100** 2	**90** 39	**66** 85	**99** 86	**95** 22	**80** 89	**97** 62	**95** 22	**80** 109	**100** 136	**88** 69	**95** 38	**71** 132	**85** 52	**82** 128	- -	- -
Ketchikan General Hospital, Ketchikan, AK	**100** 1	**100** 3	**100** 2	**67** 3	**100** 2	**0** 1	- 0	**100** 2	**100** 3	**33** 15	**81** 16	**100** 3	**77** 31	**89** 27	**57** 7	**72** 36	**100** 48	**76** 25	**100** 14	**84** 37	**100** 11	**76** 37	- -	- -
Mount Edgecumbe Hospital, Sitka, AK	- 0	**100** 2	**100** 2	**100** 2	**100** 2	- 0	- -	- 0	**100** 5	**33** 9	**100** 9	**100** 1	**100** 15	**100** 12	**100** 3	**79** 14	**100** 23	**100** 12	**73** 11	**80** 10	**100** 2	**50** 8	- -	- -
Providence Alaska Medical Center, Anchorage, AK	**85** 82	**98** 191	**95** 362	**95** 150	**97** 354	- 0	**54** 13	**90** 137	**90** 183	**43** 289	**96** 305	**55** 80	**76** 165	**89** 135	**63** 30	**72** 166	**100** 227	**48** 103	**66** 61	**87** 228	**95** 75	**71** 222	- -	- -
Samuel Simmonds Memorial Hospital, Barrow, AK	- -	- -	- -	- -	- -	- -	- -	- -	- 0	**0** 1	**50** 2	- 0	- -	- -	- -	**80** 5	**100** 5	**100** 2	- -	- -	- -	- -	- -	- -
Sitka Community Hospital, Sitka, AK	**0** 1	**100** 4	**100** 3	**100** 4	**67** 3	- 0	- 0	**0** 1	**50** 6	**0** 7	**73** 11	**100** 1	**100** 3	**100** 1	**0** 2	**100** 2	**100** 4	**25** 4	- 0	**100** 1	- 0	**100** 1	- -	- -
South Peninsula Hospital, Homer, AK	- 0	**50** 2	**100** 2	**0** 1	**0** 1	- 0	- 0	**100** 1	**67** 3	**93** 15	**62** 16	**50** 2	**73** 22	**100** 7	- -	**59** 17	**96** 25	**42** 19	**67** 3	**83** 6	**100** 4	**20** 5	- -	- -
Valley Hospital, Palmer, AK	**100** 3	**100** 37	**96** 23	**91** 32	**95** 22	**20** 5	- 0	**100** 11	**90** 20	**68** 56	**91** 57	**100** 14	**83** 75	**96** 48	**78** 9	**82** 80	**100** 91	**83** 54	**96** 24	**84** 141	**87** 38	**82** 136	- -	- -
Yukon-Kuskokwim Delta Regional Hospital, Bethel, AK	- 0	**100** 1	**100** 1	**100** 1	**100** 1	- -	- -	- -	**100** 1	**0** 5	**40** 15	**100** 1	**100** 15	**89** 18	- -	**64** 58	**100** 83	**63** 54	**67** 3	- -	- -	- -	- -	- -
ARIZONA																								
Arizona Heart Hospital, Phoenix, AZ	**88** 82	**100** 83	**99** 319	**100** 67	**97** 304	- 0	**80** 5	**96** 116	**90** 170	**85** 245	**97** 278	**93** 81	**84** 49	**89** 38	**42** 19	**74** 61	**100** 76	**62** 52	**79** 29	**81** 365	**97** 98	**67** 356	- -	- -
Arizona Orthopedic Surgical Hospital, Chandler, AZ	- -	- -	- -	- -	- -	- -	- -	- -	- -	- -	- -	- -	- -	- -	- -	- -	- -	- -	- -	**52** 25	- -	**64** 25	- -	- -
Arizona Spine and Joint Hospital, Mesa, AZ	- -	- -	- -	- -	- -	- -	- -	- -	- -	- -	- -	- -	- -	- -	- -	- -	- -	- -	- -	**94** 71	**100** 71	**66** 71	- -	- -
Arizona Surgical Hospital, Phoenix, AZ	- -	- -	- -	- -	- -	- -	- -	- -	- -	- -	- -	- -	- -	- -	- -	- -	- -	- -	- -	- 0	- -	- 0	- -	- -
Arrowhead Community Hospital, Glendale, AZ	**100** 14	**97** 101	**99** 78	**96** 81	**100** 82	- 0	**67** 3	**100** 22	**98** 51	**83** 101	**97** 124	**90** 20	**88** 312	**85** 170	**46** 80	**81** 342	**100** 382	**79** 210	**97** 86	**77** 485	**94** 155	**73** 496	- -	- -
Banner Baywood Heart Hospital, Mesa, AZ	**85** 60	**100** 7	**98** 248	**50** 4	**97** 247	- 0	- 0	**100** 99	**86** 145	**78** 260	**99** 283	**98** 44	**100** 1	- 0	**57** 14	**0** 1	**100** 2	**60** 20	**100** 4	**84** 182	**98** 61	**72** 161	- -	- -
Banner Baywood Medical Center, Mesa, AZ	**73** 11	**76** 51	**76** 25	**72** 43	**91** 34	- 0	- 0	**50** 4	**86** 76	**68** 206	**93** 264	**58** 24	**95** 118	**88** 82	**74** 23	**58** 134	**100** 163	**67** 99	**60** 30	**50** 121	**82** 39	**49** 109	- -	- -
Banner Estrella Medical Center, Phoenix, AZ	**83** 30	**98** 143	**97** 116	**93** 122	**97** 121	- 0	**12** 8	**94** 53	**85** 112	**70** 241	**92** 260	**87** 54	**86** 241	**57** 163	**44** 87	**75** 288	**100** 356	**55** 150	**72** 83	**74** 209	**89** 61	**87** 195	- -	- -
Banner Good Samaritan Medical Center, Phoenix, AZ	**77** 75	**98** 110	**98** 211	**94** 81	**95** 199	- 0	**14** 7	**95** 98	**75** 142	**54** 249	**97** 282	**89** 63	**86** 99	**93** 86	**37** 19	**67** 133	**100** 164	**49** 74	**40** 45	**71** 241	**92** 80	**64** 226	- -	- -
Banner Mesa Medical Center, Mesa, AZ	**50** 2	**95** 20	**80** 5	**80** 20	**100** 6	- 0	- 0	- 0	**77** 26	**67** 83	**90** 105	**89** 19	**97** 98	**87** 89	**38** 24	**76** 136	**100** 165	**59** 81	**51** 35	**83** 151	**94** 150	**69** 146	- -	- -
Banner Thunderbird Medical Center, Glendale, AZ	**81** 63	**94** 260	**95** 245	**81** 238	**96** 253	- 0	**50** 8	**90** 81	**78** 148	**49** 241	**96** 292	**63** 68	**89** 101	**91** 96	**40** 25	**57** 130	**100** 181	**39** 98	**57** 54	**73** 201	**80** 76	**63** 186	- -	- -
Benson Hospital, Benson, AZ	- 0	- 0	- 0	- 0	- 0	- 0	- -	- 0	**50** 4	**21** 14	**39** 18	**100** 3	**91** 35	**91** 22	**100** 4	**77** 39	**100** 47	**71** 28	**75** 16	- -	- -	- -	- -	- -
Carondelet Holy Cross Hospital, Nogales, AZ	- 0	**100** 1	**100** 1	**100** 1	**100** 1	- 0	- 0	- 0	**67** 3	**67** 12	**60** 10	- 0	**94** 36	**82** 17	**50** 12	**59** 29	**100** 51	**43** 30	**56** 9	**70** 54	**100** 13	**96** 49	- -	- -
Carondelet Saint Joseph's Hospital, Tucson, AZ	**89** 35	**98** 174	**98** 167	**96** 135	**98** 160	**0** 2	**77** 13	**100** 66	**88** 102	**94** 233	**96** 281	**92** 36	**89** 317	**82** 308	- -	**80** 388	**100** 499	**92** 305	**97** 102	**61** 183	**93** 60	**60** 167	**0.11** 2631	**6.07** 1795
Carondelet Saint Mary's Hospital, Tucson, AZ	**97** 66	**96** 311	**96** 280	**90** 253	**98** 291	- 0	**57** 7	**100** 76	**95** 133	**100** 350	**93** 382	**100** 58	**90** 319	**86** 288	**50** 114	**81** 396	**100** 483	**96** 249	**100** 145	**82** 144	**83** 48	**50** 145	- -	- -
Casa Grande Regional Medical Center, Casa Grande, AZ	**50** 14	**94** 80	**82** 28	**84** 67	**77** 30	**0** 1	- 0	**67** 6	**63** 54	**65** 163	**90** 182	**76** 33	**84** 334	**95** 187	**29** 112	**63** 400	**100** 449	**27** 254	**61** 108	**79** 224	**88** 73	**71** 220	- -	- -
Chandler Regional Hospital, Chandler, AZ	**88** 73	**97** 313	**98** 306	**97** 190	**96** 263	- 0	**41** 17	**100** 106	**80** 130	**67** 298	**95** 361	**100** 55	**91** 356	**87** 298	- -	**78** 418	**100** 549	**82** 310	**94** 89	**94** 208	**96** 68	**59** 194	**0.11** 5238	**3.93** 3434
Chinle Comprehensive Health Care Facility, Chinle, AZ	**100** 1	**100** 2	**100** 3	**100** 1	**100** 3	- 0	- 0	- 0	**82** 11	**42** 33	**51** 37	- 0	**76** 34	**75** 12	**14** 14	**72** 43	**100** 47	**21** 47	**0** 1	- 0	- 0	- 0	- -	- -
Copper Queen Community Hospital, Bisbee, AZ	- -	- -	- -	- -	- -	- -	- -	- -	- 0	**0** 4	**0** 3	**0** 1	**0** 6	**100** 6	- -	**75** 4	**100** 8	**100** 3	**33** 3	- -	- -	- -	- -	- -
Del E Webb Memorial Hospital, Sun City West, AZ	**86** 14	**98** 227	**96** 175	**98** 167	**98** 168	- 0	**100** 5	**97** 30	**69** 120	**23** 209	**88** 268	**70** 20	**90** 96	**94** 81	**43** 23	**77** 140	**100** 167	**60** 124	**76** 25	**79** 168	**88** 48	**42** 158	**0.10** 1951	**2.20** 1409
Desert Samaritan Medical Center, Mesa, AZ	**85** 62	**96** 227	**96** 221	**88** 146	**97** 237	- 0	**60** 15	**98** 98	**85** 130	**59** 234	**92** 273	**87** 52	**90** 139	**96** 119	**45** 20	**58** 154	**100** 198	**68** 87	**71** 56	**77** 233	**76** 83	**55** 223	**0.56** 9031	**3.84** 5599
Flagstaff Medical Center, Flagstaff, AZ	**79** 29	**98** 96	**97** 127	**91** 76	**93** 109	- 0	**33** 9	**97** 37	**97** 38	**85** 111	**91** 130	**86** 22	**89** 151	**95** 105	**56** 43	**70** 172	**100** 217	**58** 115	**76** 45	**89** 222	**92** 76	**61** 213	- -	- -
Fort Defiance Indian Hospital, Fort Defiance, AZ	- 0	**100** 1	**100** 1	**100** 1	**100** 1	- 0	- 0	- 0	**100** 3	**10** 10	**60** 10	- 0	**97** 39	**82** 22	**50** 8	**95** 42	**100** 45	**83** 29	**0** 3	- -	- -	- -	- -	- -
Gilbert Hospital, Higley, AZ	- -	- -	- -	- -	- -	- -	- -	- -	- -	- -	- -	- -	- -	- -	- -	- -	- -	- -	- -	- -	- -	- -	- -	- -
Havasu Regional Medical Center, Lake Havasu City, AZ	**89** 18	**85** 119	**83** 101	**78** 113	**87** 103	**0** 1	**50** 4	**74** 27	**85** 55	**58** 125	**80** 139	**82** 39	**90** 202	**85** 137	**75** 67	**50** 250	**99** 279	**69** 199	**77** 64	**50** 464	**78** 103	**46** 450	- -	- -
Hopi Health Care Center, Polacca, AZ	- -	- -	- -	- -	- -	- -	- -	- -	**100** 4	**0** 6	**88** 8	**100** 1	**45** 31	**94** 16	**83** 6	**94** 32	**100** 33	**60** 20	**0** 2	- -	- -	- -	- -	- -
John C Lincoln Hospital-Deer Valley, Phoenix, AZ	**90** 52	**98** 172	**99** 153	**90** 129	**99** 160	- 0	**17** 6	**100** 72	**91** 109	**57** 212	**97** 236	**100** 61	**90** 122	**95** 111	**84** 25	**59** 141	**100** 186	**78** 95	**98** 62	**84** 190	**97** 61	**64** 174	- -	- -
John C Lincoln Hospital-North Mountain, Phoenix, AZ	**84** 44	**94** 177	**99** 151	**93** 112	**97** 151	- 0	**30** 10	**97** 58	**88** 112	**66** 215	**98** 246	**92** 53	**87** 103	**92** 77	**96** 26	**77** 141	**100** 176	**80** 103	**87** 38	**85** 252	**87** 75	**60** 247	- -	- -
Kingman Regional Medical Center, Kingman, AZ	**73** 22	**88** 168	**82** 144	**82** 152	**86** 147	- 0	**14** 7	**88** 69	**81** 104	**41** 260	**70** 285	**67** 81	**90** 167	**81** 128	- -	**84** 187	**100** 214	**83** 96	**66** 86	**59** 190	**91** 46	**48** 183	- -	- -
La Paz Regional Hospital, Parker, AZ	- 0	**100** 2	**100** 2	**100** 2	**100** 2	- 0	- -	- 0	**100** 1	**37** 30	**61** 31	**86** 7	**96** 72	**68** 22	**79** 19	**84** 73	**99** 79	**80** 46	**64** 14	**67** 12	**0** 2	**9** 11	- -	- -
Maricopa Integrated Health, Phoenix, AZ	**69** 13	**100** 69	**84** 68	**89** 66	**81** 68	**0** 1	**50** 2	**50** 32	**86** 102	**9** 154	**94** 188	**56** 68	**83** 157	**79** 113	**23** 48	**67** 212	**100** 257	**21** 81	**63** 98	**50** 14	**89** 9	**100** 12	- -	- -
Maryvale Hospital Medical Center, Phoenix, AZ	**75** 24	**99** 148	**93** 121	**89** 143	**94** 123	- 0	**30** 10	**95** 59	**77** 83	**33** 170	**94** 190	**94** 71	**82** 176	**84** 121	**41** 41	**82** 196	**100** 229	**45** 87	**80** 82	**72** 76	**96** 26	**60** 72	- -	- -
Mayo Clinic Hospital, Phoenix, AZ	**88** 33	**98** 162	**98** 129	**98** 138	**99** 150	- 0	**78** 9	**100** 23	**97** 120	**81** 265	**100** 274	**100** 25	**96** 202	**94** 249	**91** 99	**87** 284	**100** 403	**96** 324	**100** 39	**92** 695	**97** 211	**90** 670	- -	- -

NOTE: The first number in each column (boldface) is the rate in percent, the second number is the number of patients; Please refer to the main entry for footnotes; ***Heart Attack Care:*** *1. ACE Inhibitor or ARB for LVSD; 2. Aspirin at Arrival; 3. Aspirin at Discharge; 4. Beta Blocker at Arrival; 5. Beta Blocker at Discharge; 6. Fibrinolytic Medication Timing; 7. PCI Within 90 Minutes of Arrival; 8. Smoking Cessation Advice;* ***Heart Failure Care:*** *9. ACE Inhibitor or ARB for LVSD; 10. Discharge Instructions; 11. Evaluation of LVS Function; 12. Smoking Cessation Advice;* ***Pneumonia Care:*** *13. Appropriate Initial Antibiotic; 14. Blood Culture Timing; 15. Influenza Vaccine; 16. Initial Antibiotic Timing; 17. Oxygenation Assessment; 18. Pneumococcal Vaccine; 19. Smoking Cessation Advice;* ***Surgical Infection Prevention:*** *20. Prophylactic Antibiotic Given; 21. Prophylactic Antibiotic Selection; 22. Prophylactic Antibiotic Stopped;* ***Pregnancy Care:*** *23. Inpatient Neonatal Mortality; 24. Third or Fourth Degree Laceration*

Hospital	Heart Attack Care								Heart Failure Care				Pneumonia Care							Surgical Infection Prevention			Pregnancy Care	
	1	2	3	4	5	6	7	8	9	10	11	12	13	14	15	16	17	18	19	20	21	22	23	24
Mercy Gilbert Medical Center, Gilbert, AZ	-	-	-	-	-	-	-	-	-	-	-	-	-	-	-	-	-	-	-	-	-	-	**0.00** 0	**0.00** 0
Mesa General Hospital, Mesa, AZ	**84** 25	**97** 59	**97** 73	**96** 45	**96** 76	- 0	**50** 2	**72** 36	**100** 61	**48** 112	**97** 144	**73** 33	**82** 85	**72** 60	-	**57** 109	**100** 123	**48** 66	**72** 36	**74** 121	**93** 29	**92** 108	**0.00** 1312	**8.76** 993
Mount Graham Regional Medical Center, Safford, AZ	- 0	**100** 1	- 0	- 0	- 0	- 0	- 0	- 0	**29** 7	**4** 24	**67** 24	**100** 3	**67** 92	**76** 38	-	**55** 94	**100** 125	**69** 77	**73** 26	**71** 114	**100** 21	**94** 112	-	-
Navapache Regional Medical Center, Show Low, AZ	**100** 4	**95** 41	**100** 34	**90** 20	**93** 30	**0** 6	**0** 1	**83** 18	**89** 18	**13** 68	**85** 73	**71** 14	**93** 128	**92** 83	**57** 23	**75** 152	**100** 168	**68** 78	**88** 33	**75** 159	**98** 41	**34** 158	-	-
Northern Cochise Community Hospital, Willcox, AZ	-	-	-	-	-	-	-	-	**86** 7	**29** 14	**69** 16	**33** 3	**98** 42	**100** 9	**40** 15	**77** 53	**100** 57	**70** 33	**56** 16	-	-	-	-	-
Northwest Medical Center, Tucson, AZ	**93** 44	**98** 174	**99** 202	**96** 120	**98** 199	**0** 1	**90** 10	**97** 70	**83** 117	**64** 286	**97** 352	**92** 48	**92** 358	**91** 331	**74** 119	**71** 479	**100** 604	**73** 361	**85** 119	**83** 1638	**96** 382	**65** 1523	-	-
Northwest Medical Center Oro Valley, Oro Valley, AZ	**94** 16	**98** 83	**99** 70	**90** 60	**93** 70	- 0	**100** 4	**95** 21	**76** 41	**51** 79	**91** 90	**79** 14	**91** 117	**94** 107	**58** 40	**79** 150	**100** 167	**81** 109	**90** 30	**91** 491	**96** 127	**47** 480	-	-
Page Hospital, Page, AZ	-	-	-	-	-	-	-	-	**100** 5	**91** 11	**100** 11	**100** 2	**100** 16	**67** 9	**100** 3	**93** 14	**100** 17	**100** 14	**50** 2	**100** 3	**100** 3	**100** 3	-	-
Paradise Valley Hospital, Phoenix, AZ	**80** 15	**96** 80	**97** 59	**88** 57	**94** 71	- 0	**40** 5	**100** 32	**81** 43	**34** 108	**96** 139	**92** 26	**90** 151	**90** 164	**41** 37	**86** 206	**100** 257	**56** 124	**91** 66	**84** 354	**94** 109	**63** 347	-	-
Payson Regional Medical Center, Payson, AZ	- 0	**67** 3	**50** 2	**57** 7	**100** 3	- 0	- 0	- 0	**71** 14	**61** 33	**87** 38	**71** 7	**92** 100	**88** 83	**78** 32	**89** 132	**100** 139	**82** 92	**88** 32	**72** 127	**84** 38	**70** 115	-	-
Phoenix Baptist Hospital and Medical Center, Phoenix, AZ	**93** 29	**99** 88	**99** 88	**91** 70	**96** 100	- 0	**33** 6	**100** 46	**94** 85	**48** 183	**91** 209	**91** 46	**81** 186	**85** 95	-	**76** 238	**100** 283	**66** 164	**82** 89	**86** 541	**79** 149	**100** 511	-	-
Phoenix Indian Medical Center, Phoenix, AZ	-	-	-	-	-	-	-	-	**67** 3	**83** 6	**100** 6	**100** 3	**84** 38	**90** 10	**50** 4	**78** 46	**100** 47	**75** 4	**41** 17	**72** 46	**64** 11	**95** 38	-	-
Phoenix Memorial Health System, Phoenix, AZ	**82** 33	**98** 96	**91** 128	**94** 87	**93** 124	**0** 1	**50** 6	**81** 64	**95** 59	**28** 109	**97** 120	**87** 52	**85** 151	**80** 104	-	**72** 184	**100** 195	**27** 73	**86** 84	**63** 76	**100** 14	**57** 72	-	-
PHS Indian Hospital-San Carlos, San Carlos, AZ	-	-	-	-	-	-	-	-	- 0	**0** 1	**100** 1	- 0	**88** 41	**70** 20	-	**85** 41	**100** 44	**87** 15	**0** 4	-	-	-	-	-
Sage Memorial Hospital, Ganado, AZ	-	-	-	-	-	-	-	-	- 0	**0** 8	**33** 9	- 0	**33** 33	**92** 13	**53** 19	**58** 36	**98** 47	**40** 40	**0** 2	-	-	-	-	-
Saint Joseph's Hospital & Medical Center, Phoenix, AZ	**100** 29	**97** 112	**100** 142	**97** 96	**100** 143	- 0	**71** 7	**100** 66	**96** 139	**81** 244	**99** 272	**98** 66	**94** 142	**88** 119	**82** 34	**84** 168	**100** 219	**80** 101	**68** 62	**70** 149	**92** 53	**66** 143	**1.01** 6028	**2.11** 4116
Saint Luke's Medical Center, Phoenix, AZ	**82** 17	**89** 44	**96** 48	**92** 26	**96** 52	- 0	**0** 1	**88** 26	**72** 69	**31** 113	**94** 129	**73** 41	**87** 90	**92** 79	**58** 19	**61** 117	**100** 139	**49** 70	**68** 47	**47** 145	**72** 50	**34** 139	-	-
Scottsdale Healthcare, Scottsdale, AZ	**78** 51	**97** 245	**97** 233	**92** 171	**98** 238	- 0	**83** 6	**100** 53	**69** 189	**61** 347	**93** 418	**95** 43	**91** 289	**88** 271	**64** 107	**84** 353	**100** 465	**78** 301	**95** 66	**59** 87	**79** 84	**66** 82	-	-
Scottsdale Healthcare-Osborn, Scottsdale, AZ	**81** 47	**95** 243	**98** 218	**93** 165	**98** 226	- 0	**25** 8	**100** 79	**82** 173	**55** 363	**95** 432	**100** 74	**89** 253	**90** 258	**57** 110	**84** 346	**100** 457	**79** 310	**98** 85	**89** 73	**75** 75	**41** 69	-	-
Sells Indian Hospital, Sells, AZ	-	-	-	-	-	-	-	-	- 0	- 0	**0** 7	- 0	**50** 4	**100** 4	-	**82** 22	**100** 32	**0** 11	- 0	-	-	-	-	-
Sierra Vista Regional Health Center, Sierra Vista, AZ	**83** 6	**94** 77	**66** 29	**88** 74	**79** 33	**50** 2	- 0	**56** 9	**75** 28	**16** 80	**85** 106	**71** 17	**86** 131	**91** 70	**70** 27	**70** 141	**99** 168	**65** 99	**71** 42	**82** 347	**95** 74	**61** 332	-	-
Southeast Arizona Medical Center, Douglas, AZ	- 0	**100** 1	- 0	**100** 1	- 0	**0** 2	-	- 0	**100** 2	**30** 10	**55** 11	**100** 3	**73** 41	**100** 6	**83** 6	**78** 37	**96** 47	**74** 31	**56** 9	-	-	-	-	-
Sun Health Boswell Hospital, Sun City, AZ	**64** 66	**94** 193	**95** 201	**88** 121	**96** 229	**50** 2	**20** 5	**89** 45	**65** 129	**24** 231	**92** 294	**66** 29	**94** 88	**97** 88	**48** 25	**65** 141	**100** 172	**58** 138	**74** 19	**86** 280	-	**46** 272	-	-
Tempe Saint Luke's Hospital, Tempe, AZ	**50** 4	**97** 33	**67** 12	**75** 32	**83** 12	**0** 1	- 0	**33** 3	**75** 32	**12** 112	**82** 127	**33** 30	**76** 149	**77** 47	**53** 19	**63** 148	**99** 163	**41** 69	**44** 48	**7** 30	**78** 9	**92** 24	-	-
Tuba City Indian Medical Center, Tuba City, AZ	- 0	- 0	**0** 1	- 0	**0** 1	- 0	- 0	- 0	**75** 28	**0** 36	**97** 36	**0** 2	**77** 79	**91** 54	**93** 27	**82** 85	**100** 98	**85** 71	- 0	**67** 9	**100** 3	**100** 8	**0.00** 498	**1.50** 399
Tucson Heart Hospital, Tucson, AZ	**100** 45	**100** 140	**98** 261	**100** 132	**100** 243	- 0	**100** 2	**100** 70	**100** 98	**92** 262	**95** 283	**95** 21	**96** 52	**88** 65	**100** 26	**85** 72	**100** 84	**97** 64	**100** 20	**99** 107	**100** 37	**100** 107	-	-
Tucson Medical Center, Tucson, AZ	**85** 66	**96** 224	**95** 270	**90** 202	**94** 271	- 0	**25** 4	**100** 85	**87** 95	**70** 197	**96** 256	**100** 42	**92** 72	**86** 74	-	**62** 108	**100** 151	**58** 86	**100** 32	**79** 266	**96** 96	**72** 249	-	-
University Medical Center, Tucson, AZ	**99** 70	**95** 192	**100** 267	**92** 169	**99** 260	- 0	**33** 6	**100** 91	**95** 183	**76** 295	**99** 318	**100** 59	**93** 73	**89** 45	**79** 19	**57** 142	**100** 188	**78** 74	**100** 48	**76** 66	**60** 72	**58** 65	-	-
UPH Hospital at Kino campus, Tucson, AZ	**71** 17	**97** 30	**96** 26	**91** 32	**85** 26	**9** 22	- 0	**73** 11	**94** 16	**73** 91	**92** 95	**32** 47	**89** 107	**77** 62	**53** 19	**55** 147	**99** 161	**40** 58	**47** 76	**98** 56	**100** 12	**96** 56	-	-
Valley View Medical Center, Fort Mohave, AZ	- 0	**100** 7	- 0	**100** 6	- 0	- 0	- 0	- 0	**75** 12	**53** 15	**86** 28	**80** 5	**62** 8	**100** 5	-	**66** 29	**100** 31	**71** 17	**60** 5	**60** 40	-	**65** 37	-	-
Verde Valley Medical Center, Cottonwood, AZ	**95** 41	**99** 133	**99** 186	**99** 113	**96** 167	- 0	**79** 14	**96** 55	**79** 34	**60** 86	**92** 84	**89** 19	**85** 158	**94** 127	**72** 50	**89** 183	**100** 216	**88** 164	**86** 51	**69** 90	**95** 64	**96** 69	-	-
West Valley Hospital, Goodyear, AZ	**81** 27	**98** 132	**95** 126	**95** 116	**95** 119	- 0	**10** 10	**86** 50	**88** 57	**60** 157	**90** 174	**91** 32	**82** 159	**76** 90	**58** 36	**75** 168	**100** 198	**44** 86	**77** 52	**69** 287	**97** 98	**66** 268	-	-
Western Arizona Regional Medical Center, Bullhead City, AZ	**95** 21	**98** 140	**99** 144	**98** 112	**98** 139	**26** 19	**50** 2	**100** 72	**80** 123	**67** 276	**94** 302	**94** 94	**76** 119	**88** 89	**65** 26	**85** 142	**100** 162	**66** 80	**85** 72	**44** 317	**68** 77	**98** 291	-	-
White Mountain Regional Medical Center, Springerville, AZ	- 0	**100** 2	**50** 2	**67** 3	**100** 2	-	-	-	**100** 3	**25** 4	**71** 28	**0** 2	**80** 5	**100** 2	-	**79** 33	**100** 38	**36** 22	**50** 2	-	-	-	-	-
Whiteriver Indian Hospital, Whiteriver, AZ	- 0	- 0	- 0	- 0	- 0	-	- 0	- 0	**67** 6	**57** 7	**100** 7	**0** 5	**79** 57	**79** 52	**100** 12	**83** 59	**99** 81	**97** 37	**57** 7	-	-	-	-	-
Wickenburg Regional Hospital, Wickenburg, AZ	-	-	-	-	-	-	-	-	**0** 3	**0** 3	**100** 5	- 0	**85** 33	**88** 16	**31** 13	**91** 33	**88** 33	**24** 25	**100** 2	-	-	-	-	-
Winslow Memorial Hospital, Winslow, AZ	- 0	**100** 1	**100** 1	**0** 1	- 0	**0** 2	- 0	- 0	**75** 4	**0** 14	**35** 17	**0** 2	**76** 21	**100** 5	-	**81** 27	**100** 30	**5** 21	**25** 4	- 0	- 0	- 0	-	-
Yavapai Regional Medical Center, Prescott, AZ	**83** 12	**97** 122	**95** 93	**92** 106	**86** 102	- 0	**67** 3	**96** 27	**84** 97	**61** 239	**87** 290	**85** 52	**86** 146	**90** 83	**70** 30	**76** 186	**100** 213	**78** 138	**87** 46	**91** 246	**98** 58	**69** 226	**0.22** 1378	**5.47** 896
Yavapai Regional Medical Center-East, Prescott Valley, AZ	- 0	- 0	- 0	- 0	**100** 1	- 0	- 0	- 0	**25** 4	**40** 10	**91** 11	**0** 1	**85** 26	**94** 17	-	**86** 28	**100** 33	**77** 22	**71** 7	**70** 23	-	**26** 23	-	-
Yuma Regional Medical Center, Yuma, AZ	**79** 68	**96** 277	**94** 236	**89** 227	**85** 275	**13** 30	**0** 6	**92** 74	**81** 221	**55** 425	**81** 488	**90** 78	**81** 354	**84** 370	**51** 172	**46** 721	**100** 848	**50** 545	**78** 131	**80** 898	**93** 182	**74** 886	**0.24** 3712	**3.02** 2580
CALIFORNIA																								
Alameda County Medical Center, Oakland, CA	**100** 10	**100** 50	**97** 30	**94** 49	**100** 29	**0** 1	- 0	**44** 9	**94** 140	**2** 266	**99** 279	**54** 136	**79** 141	**79** 119	-	**44** 156	**100** 220	**16** 58	**57** 86	**30** 27	**61** 23	**91** 23	-	-
Alameda Hospital, Alameda, CA	**71** 21	**98** 125	**97** 88	**99** 125	**99** 98	**15** 13	- 0	**87** 15	**80** 35	**12** 112	**87** 173	**95** 21	**71** 76	**86** 106	**16** 38	**85** 158	**100** 184	**23** 114	**96** 27	**79** 24	**100** 25	**83** 23	-	-
Alhambra Hospital Medical Center, Alhambra, CA	**75** 4	**89** 36	**59** 17	**68** 34	**60** 15	- 0	- 0	**25** 4	**48** 23	**10** 112	**76** 142	**33** 6	**70** 87	**87** 130	**8** 59	**74** 231	**100** 397	**13** 287	**26** 23	**69** 13	-	**8** 13	-	-
Alta Bates Summit Medical Center, Berkeley, CA	**85** 13	**98** 100	**100** 82	**95** 84	**98** 81	- 0	**100** 1	**100** 20	**83** 41	**82** 94	**94** 109	**100** 23	**91** 43	**96** 72	**67** 12	**68** 79	**100** 106	**63** 51	**100** 23	**92** 109	**100** 35	**70** 106	**0.32** 7706	**3.11** 5335
Alta Bates Summit Medical Center, Oakland, CA	**91** 109	**99** 238	**99** 777	**96** 198	**99** 799	- 0	**63** 19	**100** 206	**87** 85	**87** 159	**93** 203	**100** 33	**90** 60	**93** 105	**70** 20	**68** 125	**100** 146	**60** 96	**100** 35	**81** 169	**96** 56	**87** 157	-	-
Alvarado Hospital Medical Center, San Diego, CA	-	-	-	-	-	-	-	-	-	-	-	-	-	-	-	-	-	-	-	-	-	-	-	-
Anaheim General Hospital, Anaheim, CA	**0** 1	**100** 6	**43** 7	**67** 6	**0** 7	- 0	- 0	- 0	**70** 10	**0** 5	**77** 35	- 0	**50** 18	**73** 15	-	**83** 53	**95** 66	**0** 44	**0** 2	**25** 4	-	**100** 2	**0.00** 136	**2.08** 96

NOTE: The first number in each column (boldface) is the rate in percent, the second number is the number of patients; Please refer to the main entry for footnotes; ***Heart Attack Care:*** *1. ACE Inhibitor or ARB for LVSD; 2. Aspirin at Arrival; 3. Aspirin at Discharge; 4. Beta Blocker at Arrival; 5. Beta Blocker at Discharge; 6. Fibrinolytic Medication Timing; 7. PCI Within 90 Minutes of Arrival; 8. Smoking Cessation Advice;* ***Heart Failure Care:*** *9. ACE Inhibitor or ARB for LVSD; 10. Discharge Instructions; 11. Evaluation of LVS Function; 12. Smoking Cessation Advice;* ***Pneumonia Care:*** *13. Appropriate Initial Antibiotic; 14. Blood Culture Timing; 15. Influenza Vaccine; 16. Initial Antibiotic Timing; 17. Oxygenation Assessment; 18. Pneumococcal Vaccine; 19. Smoking Cessation Advice;* ***Surgical Infection Prevention:*** *20. Prophylactic Antibiotic Given; 21. Prophylactic Antibiotic Selection; 22. Prophylactic Antibiotic Stopped;* ***Pregnancy Care:*** *23. Inpatient Neonatal Mortality; 24. Third or Fourth Degree Laceration*

Hospital	Heart Attack Care								Heart Failure Care				Pneumonia Care							Surgical Infection Prevention			Pregnancy Care	
	1	2	3	4	5	6	7	8	9	10	11	12	13	14	15	16	17	18	19	20	21	22	23	24
Anaheim Memorial Medical Center, Anaheim, CA	100 49	99 204	99 396	100 162	100 384	50 2	73 15	100 108	96 207	89 495	98 576	99 82	78 286	95 281	63 93	87 437	100 524	79 377	98 83	84 418	69 64	53 408	0.39 2035	3.09 1457
Antelope Valley Hospital, Lancaster, CA	80 56	97 301	93 282	90 248	87 280	75 4	90 21	95 123	64 224	45 472	87 523	91 150	94 340	66 276	- -	80 476	100 539	67 263	82 149	45 413	91 134	67 347	- -	- -
Arrowhead Regional Medical Center, Colton, CA	94 31	98 87	100 71	95 65	98 65	12 17	0 3	61 28	90 207	4 322	94 337	34 124	93 138	76 129	- -	59 184	100 218	35 68	47 76	92 243	92 51	77 226	- -	- -
Arroyo Grande Community Hospital, Arroyo Grande, CA	100 6	97 32	90 21	94 31	90 21	- 0	- 0	100 2	92 24	93 90	89 103	100 12	88 128	90 92	88 24	88 132	99 160	71 112	88 24	90 116	100 37	99 115	- -	- -
Bakersfield Heart Hospital, Bakersfield, CA	90 80	99 193	98 264	96 141	92 262	- 0	27 11	98 103	80 135	64 251	94 277	95 42	92 89	92 75	78 27	82 112	100 161	81 112	95 43	95 185	93 69	80 159	- -	- -
Bakersfield Memorial Hospital, Bakersfield, CA	88 75	92 210	92 277	83 145	91 284	- 0	75 8	98 88	86 133	68 253	93 307	94 54	83 169	84 107	4 50	69 204	100 281	90 172	78 55	79 261	96 79	53 251	0.32 2854	1.71 2108
Banner Lassen Medical Center, Susanville, CA	100 2	100 4	100 2	75 4	100 3	0 1	- 0	100 1	100 12	100 15	100 20	100 2	87 45	100 6	100 7	100 11	100 46	95 22	100 12	50 10	100 1	67 9	- -	- -
Barstow Community Hospital, Barstow, CA	67 3	95 43	82 11	93 29	83 12	19 16	- 0	100 6	80 41	55 202	71 233	97 74	76 162	96 112	19 43	59 165	100 202	67 118	87 53	26 23	67 9	65 20	- -	- -
Barton Memorial Hospital, South Lake Tahoe, CA	100 1	86 7	100 3	83 6	100 3	- 0	- 0	- 0	94 18	14 65	80 64	65 20	73 83	71 48	57 14	74 61	100 90	60 47	46 24	90 124	100 34	15 121	0.00 560	3.59 390
Bear Valley Community Hospital, Big Bear Lake, CA	- 0	100 1	0 1	- 0	100 1	- -	- -	- -	- 0	100 5	10 10	- 0	100 4	100 2	- -	100 8	100 10	17 6	- 0	- -	- -	- -	- -	- -
Bellflower Medical Center, Bellflower, CA	33 3	82 11	40 5	75 8	33 6	0 1	- 0	- 0	64 28	50 14	87 94	100 4	73 11	84 32	- -	83 174	100 205	10 119	67 6	72 18	- -	56 18	- -	- -
Beverly Hospital, Montebello, CA	82 28	94 139	99 113	95 111	94 103	50 2	67 3	100 22	71 127	40 308	94 385	100 36	85 200	89 195	71 62	70 328	99 340	71 224	100 26	68 269	98 98	50 263	- -	- -
Brotman Medical Center, Culver City, CA	82 22	86 122	81 116	80 111	78 120	0 3	25 4	71 21	72 64	10 210	72 260	60 42	69 86	95 74	22 18	71 115	100 147	26 99	47 19	69 129	77 35	45 121	- -	- -
California Hospital Medical Center, Los Angeles, CA	100 12	100 75	100 40	100 43	100 44	33 3	- 0	100 9	100 218	100 378	100 433	100 128	91 113	93 98	100 19	76 143	100 181	96 83	100 42	85 152	83 54	42 147	0.27 4149	2.53 2841
California Pacific Medical Center, San Francisco, CA	91 56	99 147	99 179	96 108	99 181	- 0	75 8	93 46	92 177	47 384	98 457	88 57	85 84	97 106	29 21	78 133	100 178	72 119	74 23	92 244	98 82	80 242	0.40 1003	3.91 741
Catalina Island Medical Center, Avalon, CA	- -	- -	- -	- -	- -	- -	- -	- -	- -	- -	- -	- -	- -	- -	- -	- -	- -	- -	- -	- -	- -	- -	- -	- -
Cedars-Sinai Medical Center, Los Angeles, CA	98 54	100 352	100 347	100 234	100 312	0 1	85 13	100 72	99 336	44 777	100 880	100 96	94 334	98 480	66 122	94 519	100 720	88 455	100 86	96 2543	95 630	89 2442	- -	- -
Centinela Freeman Reg Med Ctr-Marina, Marina Del Rey, CA	- 0	96 28	100 11	86 22	89 9	0 2	- 0	100 1	93 27	32 102	86 123	91 11	93 83	87 39	56 16	73 88	98 98	67 60	100 11	88 72	95 19	54 69	- -	- -
Centinela Hospital Medical Center, Inglewood, CA	76 51	96 207	98 258	92 192	93 253	50 10	0 8	91 81	86 197	32 398	92 446	82 49	87 149	92 135	97 33	71 181	100 230	84 129	97 32	78 584	94 127	50 571	- -	- -
Central Valley General Hospital, Hanford, CA	- 0	100 2	0 1	100 2	100 1	- 0	- 0	- 0	75 8	40 35	30 40	92 12	84 67	90 20	78 9	72 65	100 71	46 39	86 14	35 34	67 3	91 23	0.29 2062	1.29 1319
Century City Doctors Hospital, Los Angeles, CA	100 2	100 6	100 4	100 9	80 5	100 1	- 0	- 0	80 5	28 25	83 35	33 3	64 22	100 28	38 8	50 40	98 53	20 44	33 3	89 206	97 65	96 202	- -	- -
Chapman Medical Center, Orange, CA	100 3	100 8	100 3	100 3	100 5	100 2	- 0	- 0	80 15	80 40	94 47	100 8	90 40	100 52	100 10	92 66	100 88	87 52	100 6	100 7	86 7	83 6	- -	- -
Chinese Hospital, San Francisco, CA	0 1	95 22	75 8	85 20	57 7	- 0	- 0	100 1	75 20	62 82	87 91	50 2	94 176	91 115	91 44	86 170	100 203	88 178	90 21	100 18	94 18	17 18	- -	- -
Chino Valley Medical Center, Chino, CA	100 9	100 54	100 19	100 46	100 21	100 3	- 0	100 3	97 31	100 49	98 127	100 21	100 8	89 54	- -	93 61	100 81	89 47	100 20	100 2	- 0	- 0	- -	- -
Chowchilla Memorial Hospital District, Chowchilla, CA	- -	- -	- -	- -	- -	- -	- -	- -	- -	- -	- -	- -	- -	- -	- -	- -	- -	- -	- -	- -	- -	- -	- -	- -
Citrus Valley Medical Center, Covina, CA	77 53	94 143	95 276	91 99	90 258	- 0	14 7	97 71	69 151	16 306	86 391	73 48	87 132	82 148	37 49	60 235	99 300	20 198	62 40	72 217	87 75	24 197	- -	- -
Citrus Valley Med Ctr Queen Valley Campus, West Covina, CA	67 12	90 62	78 32	95 41	72 43	0 1	- 0	83 6	78 154	19 317	88 388	72 50	84 207	67 205	23 64	62 300	99 378	11 207	67 51	73 314	63 105	41 296	- -	- -
City of Angels Medical Center, Los Angeles, CA	50 2	83 12	44 9	42 12	33 9	- 0	- 0	- 0	48 27	0 21	81 83	33 6	50 2	- 0	- -	60 42	97 86	5 56	100 1	- 0	- -	- 0	- -	- -
Coalinga Regional Medical Center, Coalinga, CA	- -	- -	- -	- -	- -	- -	- -	- -	- 0	0 2	0 1	- 0	79 19	14 7	- -	80 74	100 90	6 32	0 2	- -	- -	- -	- -	- -
Coast Plaza Doctors Hospital, Norwalk, CA	- 0	94 17	50 4	88 17	50 4	100 1	- 0	100 2	78 27	99 90	76 114	100 18	73 214	68 60	40 25	77 219	100 230	37 90	100 15	0 5	80 5	80 5	- -	- -
Coastal Communities Hospital, Santa Ana, CA	33 3	95 21	85 13	90 20	92 13	75 4	- 0	100 4	65 17	24 54	85 65	25 4	64 50	87 113	- -	87 105	100 142	43 69	89 9	79 101	96 26	69 99	- -	- -
College Hospital Costa Mesa, Costa Mesa, CA	- -	- -	- -	- -	- -	- -	- -	- -	- 0	- 0	100 1	- 0	- -	- -	- -	75 4	100 4	- 0	- -	- -	- -	- -	- -	- -
Colusa Regional Medical Center, Colusa, CA	- 0	100 3	50 2	50 2	100 1	- 0	- 0	- 0	50 6	3 36	66 41	50 4	78 32	70 10	33 3	74 31	100 35	93 27	25 4	- -	- -	- -	- -	- -
Community Hospital, Huntington Park, CA	100 4	93 28	69 13	71 28	46 13	- 0	- 0	- 0	74 27	48 142	54 156	43 7	61 127	78 50	24 29	62 113	89 142	10 78	23 13	39 31	75 4	95 22	- -	- -
Community Hospital of Gardena, Gardena, CA	- -	- -	- -	- -	- -	- -	- -	- -	100 2	- -	17 6	- -	- -	- -	- -	71 14	97 31	0 30	- -	- -	- -	- -	- -	- -
Community Hospital of Long Beach, Long Beach, CA	50 2	95 39	76 17	83 24	81 16	36 14	- 0	75 4	76 34	64 56	91 78	78 18	79 107	98 126	9 34	87 175	100 226	29 130	74 27	75 32	100 4	37 30	- -	- -
Community Hospital of Los Gatos, Los Gatos, CA	60 5	86 21	93 14	86 22	87 15	0 1	- 0	100 2	76 17	70 63	82 104	50 6	86 80	92 83	79 33	85 106	100 125	81 94	60 5	79 209	92 50	55 202	- -	- -
Community Hospital of San Bernardino, San Bernardino, CA	100 8	96 52	83 23	91 35	83 18	38 8	- 0	100 7	99 67	93 227	94 247	99 68	80 167	89 151	- -	74 212	100 289	85 134	95 65	65 68	94 18	39 64	0.16 2561	1.91 1570
Community Hospital of the Monterey Peninsula, Monterey, CA	83 24	96 138	84 85	95 93	96 74	- 0	60 5	100 3	70 91	70 56	92 282	100 11	76 21	100 24	- -	78 152	100 205	88 147	100 2	87 191	- -	73 188	- -	- -
Community Medical Center-Clovis, Clovis, CA	100 5	89 53	94 33	90 30	97 34	- 0	0 1	79 14	74 53	16 128	75 154	36 14	88 119	88 84	84 32	62 129	100 168	68 103	79 38	44 629	95 141	68 608	- -	- -
Community Memorial Hospital Ventura, Ventura, CA	92 37	97 181	100 226	92 165	94 220	- 0	62 8	91 53	97 73	33 206	95 253	62 24	83 181	87 231	57 60	82 292	100 375	29 266	69 58	34 127	96 114	50 124	- -	- -
Community Regional Medical Center, Fresno, CA	85 107	96 342	95 347	91 204	95 368	- 0	18 11	83 154	83 442	32 760	88 841	58 178	87 435	87 439	76 111	48 616	100 756	66 326	50 193	61 948	93 234	67 886	- -	- -
Contra Costa Regional Medical Center, Martinez, CA	- 0	100 26	100 25	88 25	92 25	50 2	- 0	80 5	96 70	0 25	99 151	18 11	84 19	78 23	- -	67 99	100 117	48 46	50 8	78 27	- -	68 25	- -	- -
Corcoran District Hospital, Corcoran, CA	- -	- -	- -	- -	- -	- -	- -	- -	33 3	12 8	10 40	- 0	100 1	- 0	- -	44 18	83 23	0 9	- 0	- -	- -	- -	- -	- -
Corona Regional Medical Center, Corona, CA	60 5	95 110	85 74	87 103	80 74	29 14	- 0	76 17	88 33	60 200	80 254	91 32	68 321	71 204	- -	71 315	99 375	66 214	71 49	70 238	86 76	47 226	- -	- -
Dameron Hospital, Stockton, CA	95 19	98 148	91 145	94 48	95 62	44 16	0 1	91 58	91 93	82 238	85 297	87 47	93 121	72 121	34 38	82 201	100 221	33 138	81 31	40 289	84 45	48 259	- -	- -
Davies Medical Center, San Francisco, CA	100 2	100 9	100 4	86 7	100 5	- 0	- -	0 1	90 20	58 53	97 63	86 14	82 50	92 62	20 15	77 75	100 101	67 51	79 29	90 21	100 4	100 20	- -	- -
Delano Regional Medical Center, Delano, CA	- 0	86 14	100 5	70 10	60 5	- 0	- -	- 0	70 27	54 124	58 146	45 22	74 69	80 44	12 26	69 124	99 157	11 104	29 17	69 13	77 13	46 13	- -	- -

NOTE: The first number in each column (boldface) is the rate in percent, the second number is the number of patients; Please refer to the main entry for footnotes; ***Heart Attack Care:*** *1. ACE Inhibitor or ARB for LVSD; 2. Aspirin at Arrival; 3. Aspirin at Discharge; 4. Beta Blocker at Arrival; 5. Beta Blocker at Discharge; 6. Fibrinolytic Medication Timing; 7. PCI Within 90 Minutes of Arrival; 8. Smoking Cessation Advice;* ***Heart Failure Care:*** *9. ACE Inhibitor or ARB for LVSD; 10. Discharge Instructions; 11. Evaluation of LVS Function; 12. Smoking Cessation Advice;* ***Pneumonia Care:*** *13. Appropriate Initial Antibiotic; 14. Blood Culture Timing; 15. Influenza Vaccine; 16. Initial Antibiotic Timing; 17. Oxygenation Assessment; 18. Pneumococcal Vaccine; 19. Smoking Cessation Advice;* ***Surgical Infection Prevention:*** *20. Prophylactic Antibiotic Given; 21. Prophylactic Antibiotic Selection; 22. Prophylactic Antibiotic Stopped;* ***Pregnancy Care:*** *23. Inpatient Neonatal Mortality; 24. Third or Fourth Degree Laceration*

Hospital	Heart Attack Care								Heart Failure Care				Pneumonia Care							Surgical Infection Prevention			Pregnancy Care	
	1	2	3	4	5	6	7	8	9	10	11	12	13	14	15	16	17	18	19	20	21	22	23	24
Desert Regional Medical Center, Palm Springs, CA	**83** 52	**97** 180	**97** 251	**96** 165	**94** 249	- 0	**80** 5	**94** 68	**88** 209	**87** 333	**92** 436	**96** 91	**93** 244	**94** 214	**83** 53	**91** 306	**100** 354	**86** 234	**89** 89	**86** 366	**93** 88	**43** 357	- -	- -
Desert Valley Hospital, Victorville, CA	**100** 10	**99** 106	**98** 86	**99** 102	**98** 90	**100** 3	- 0	**100** 29	**100** 64	**98** 118	**96** 257	**100** 54	**86** 14	**95** 134	- -	**90** 140	**100** 185	**91** 107	**100** 41	**65** 23	**100** 22	**56** 16	- -	- -
Doctor's Medical Center-San Pablo Campus, San Pablo, CA	**78** 63	**97** 147	**99** 171	**95** 123	**94** 160	**0** 2	**75** 8	**80** 56	**78** 213	**48** 366	**93** 441	**89** 114	**90** 205	**96** 224	**43** 65	**88** 295	**100** 344	**56** 213	**77** 73	**48** 225	**91** 53	**54** 216	- -	- -
Doctors Hospital of Manteca, Manteca, CA	**100** 1	**94** 36	**94** 16	**94** 33	**94** 17	**25** 4	- 0	**100** 3	**100** 30	**93** 90	**93** 105	**100** 23	**85** 108	**89** 96	**85** 34	**87** 141	**100** 161	**93** 95	**95** 38	**83** 115	**94** 32	**79** 113	- -	- -
Doctors Hospital of West Covina, West Covina, CA	- -	- -	- -	- -	- -	- -	- -	- -	- 0	**0** 4	**25** 4	- 0	**100** 2	- 0	**100** 1	**0** 2	**100** 3	**50** 2	**0** 1	**67** 12	**83** 12	**92** 12	- -	- -
Doctors Medical Center, Modesto, CA	**97** 75	**98** 192	**98** 364	**96** 163	**97** 348	**22** 9	**27** 11	**100** 119	**95** 165	**90** 350	**95** 422	**96** 105	**92** 299	**92** 360	**82** 102	**70** 436	**100** 560	**89** 292	**92** 157	**75** 607	**79** 192	**73** 578	- -	- -
Dominican Hospital, Santa Cruz, CA	**84** 50	**99** 157	**100** 160	**99** 142	**99** 153	- 0	**62** 8	**100** 39	**76** 96	**56** 259	**90** 342	**87** 47	**88** 185	**85** 168	**62** 55	**75** 242	**100** 292	**70** 194	**74** 39	**64** 214	**86** 69	**57** 207	- -	- -
Downey Regional Medical Center, Downey, CA	**74** 31	**98** 174	**97** 187	**89** 139	**97** 190	**38** 8	**0** 6	**100** 37	**83** 136	**67** 306	**92** 355	**100** 47	**84** 128	**86** 146	**53** 32	**71** 192	**100** 231	**72** 170	**70** 23	**90** 216	**97** 79	**52** 213	**0.25** 1574	**2.18** 1192
East Los Angeles Doctors Hospital, Los Angeles, CA	**75** 4	**86** 43	**73** 26	**86** 44	**70** 27	**33** 3	- 0	**88** 8	**85** 20	**99** 102	**53** 116	**100** 13	**69** 81	**71** 62	- -	**82** 96	**100** 120	**1** 73	**75** 4	**10** 10	**100** 1	**78** 9	- -	- -
East Valley Hospital Medical Center, Glendora, CA	**50** 6	**74** 43	**61** 31	**83** 41	**69** 32	- 0	- 0	**0** 1	**65** 20	**38** 8	**78** 67	- 0	**64** 36	**67** 18	- -	**83** 152	**99** 165	**26** 103	**100** 1	- 0	- -	- 0	**0.00** 398	**0.54** 184
Eastern Plumas Health Care, Portola, CA	- -	- -	- -	- -	- -	- -	- -	- -	- -	- -	- -	- -	**100** 1	**100** 1	- -	- 0	**100** 2	**0** 2	- 0	- -	- -	- -	- -	- -
Eden Medical Center, Castro Valley, CA	**78** 9	**90** 63	**86** 36	**92** 39	**97** 39	**0** 1	- 0	**75** 8	**76** 83	**63** 182	**89** 230	**94** 35	**85** 155	**95** 171	**43** 58	**64** 232	**100** 286	**52** 170	**80** 41	**87** 418	**98** 102	**79** 403	- -	- -
Eisenhower Medical Center, Rancho Mirage, CA	**80** 100	**92** 319	**91** 317	**85** 182	**92** 354	- 0	**82** 11	**96** 75	**86** 310	**56** 480	**90** 619	**95** 73	**77** 359	**79** 197	**71** 96	**67** 369	**100** 455	**64** 342	**92** 61	**86** 666	**96** 74	**75** 650	- -	- -
El Camino Hospital, Mountain View, CA	**95** 44	**100** 204	**99** 198	**96** 125	**98** 169	**0** 1	**29** 14	**100** 34	**93** 123	**46** 272	**85** 348	**98** 40	**77** 301	**92** 284	**56** 68	**67** 357	**100** 453	**61** 321	**93** 45	**81** 794	**93** 97	**79** 786	- -	- -
El Centro Regional Medical Center, El Centro, CA	**90** 10	**100** 85	**100** 28	**100** 76	**97** 31	**43** 7	- 0	**100** 5	**98** 60	**100** 206	**97** 222	**100** 8	**86** 135	**90** 96	**79** 39	**62** 139	**100** 167	**92** 108	**100** 16	**90** 244	**89** 71	**37** 71	- -	- -
Emanuel Medical Center, Turlock, CA	**80** 10	**94** 100	**93** 43	**90** 89	**74** 42	**27** 15	- 0	**75** 8	**92** 78	**80** 213	**90** 263	**70** 33	**91** 162	**86** 151	**75** 36	**77** 232	**100** 259	**78** 170	**68** 44	**83** 290	**89** 76	**51** 287	- -	- -
Encino-Tarzana Regional Medical Center, Encino, CA	**57** 7	**96** 47	**70** 30	**85** 46	**52** 23	- 0	- 0	- 0	**67** 15	**69** 75	**86** 106	**75** 4	**78** 86	**91** 123	**59** 44	**87** 154	**100** 225	**51** 173	**70** 10	**75** 121	**83** 24	**20** 120	- -	- -
Encino-Tarzana Regional Medical Center, Tarzana, CA	**89** 47	**94** 179	**88** 209	**86** 158	**85** 206	- 0	**36** 11	**93** 41	**82** 130	**68** 281	**93** 326	**75** 16	**88** 200	**81** 218	**55** 75	**83** 246	**100** 344	**55** 246	**57** 14	**73** 152	**80** 56	**56** 146	- -	- -
Enloe Medical Center, Chico, CA	**84** 83	**100** 118	**96** 233	**91** 75	**96** 270	**100** 1	**57** 7	**96** 95	**73** 112	**50** 233	**95** 296	**93** 41	**81** 232	**84** 223	- -	**79** 416	**100** 504	**50** 345	**92** 90	**87** 810	**97** 198	**66** 775	- -	- -
Fairchild Medical Center, Yreka, CA	- -	- -	- -	- -	- -	- -	- -	- -	- -	- -	- -	- -	- -	- -	- -	- -	- -	- -	- -	- -	- -	- -	- -	- -
Fallbrook Hospital, Fallbrook, CA	**100** 2	**94** 16	**75** 4	**91** 11	**80** 5	**0** 2	- 0	**100** 2	**92** 25	**26** 50	**88** 59	**100** 5	**73** 62	**91** 44	**37** 19	**75** 89	**99** 98	**45** 74	**100** 10	**67** 224	**88** 69	**83** 216	- -	- -
Feather River Hospital, Paradise, CA	**91** 11	**92** 62	**97** 35	**89** 61	**100** 42	**100** 1	- 0	**80** 5	**91** 22	**84** 64	**98** 84	**90** 10	**83** 119	**94** 128	**94** 36	**82** 164	**100** 203	**99** 138	**93** 46	**67** 119	**100** 38	**80** 116	- -	- -
Foothill Presbyterian Hospital, Glendora, CA	**71** 7	**94** 50	**81** 26	**89** 45	**76** 25	- 0	- 0	**100** 1	**60** 55	**68** 163	**97** 212	**96** 23	**78** 161	**89** 149	**51** 41	**76** 208	**100** 259	**53** 165	**42** 36	**62** 143	**87** 46	**61** 135	- -	- -
Fountain Valley Reg Hospital & Med Ctr, Fountain Valley, CA	**89** 35	**100** 174	**96** 218	**98** 152	**94** 226	- 0	**80** 10	**98** 58	**87** 150	**59** 328	**91** 397	**96** 48	**93** 179	**97** 249	**87** 52	**93** 281	**100** 360	**86** 229	**79** 39	**75** 328	**97** 100	**35** 304	- -	- -
Frank R Howard Memorial Hospital, Willits, CA	- 0	**100** 2	- 0	**100** 2	- 0	- 0	- 0	- 0	**100** 4	**50** 14	**94** 17	**33** 3	**80** 40	**90** 21	**88** 8	**91** 47	**100** 60	**68** 34	**95** 22	**100** 25	**96** 26	**84** 25	- -	- -
French Hospital Medical Center, San Luis Obispo, CA	**100** 12	**100** 47	**97** 117	**100** 42	**98** 123	- 0	- 0	**100** 35	**95** 42	**96** 110	**96** 131	**100** 16	**88** 103	**97** 91	**89** 19	**94** 109	**100** 129	**89** 98	**86** 7	**86** 224	**97** 75	**89** 217	- -	- -
Fresno Heart Hospital, Fresno, CA	**86** 22	**94** 33	**93** 101	**84** 32	**92** 108	- 0	- 0	**100** 23	**87** 52	**81** 123	**79** 133	**100** 9	**100** 1	**100** 1	- 0	**0** 1	**100** 2	**0** 1	**100** 1	**77** 303	**98** 163	**80** 276	- -	- -
Fresno Surgery Center, Fresno, CA	- -	- -	- -	- -	- -	- -	- -	- -	- -	- -	- -	- -	- -	- -	- -	- -	- -	- -	- -	**70** 27	- -	**67** 27	- -	- -
Garden Grove Hospital and Medical Center, Garden Grove, CA	**100** 7	**98** 54	**92** 24	**95** 39	**96** 23	**0** 2	- 0	**100** 3	**85** 26	**96** 71	**97** 103	**100** 17	**83** 162	**100** 143	**100** 32	**94** 178	**100** 225	**94** 144	**100** 17	**93** 163	**93** 41	**69** 162	- -	- -
Garfield Medical Center, Monterey Park, CA	**74** 23	**90** 123	**83** 126	**80** 85	**77** 115	**0** 1	**33** 3	**86** 21	**50** 64	**45** 260	**79** 295	**100** 9	**79** 103	**88** 95	**94** 18	**79** 149	**100** 177	**76** 124	**91** 11	**70** 198	**92** 52	**24** 190	- -	- -
George L Mee Memorial Hospital, King City, CA	- 0	**100** 4	**100** 3	**100** 3	**50** 2	- 0	- 0	- 0	**100** 4	**33** 6	**65** 20	- 0	**50** 6	- 0	- -	**63** 19	**100** 23	**31** 16	**100** 1	- 0	- -	- 0	**0.00** 590	**5.15** 408
Glendale Adventist Medical Center, Glendale, CA	**90** 81	**95** 236	**96** 249	**87** 174	**93** 257	- 0	**54** 13	**100** 83	**85** 176	**42** 330	**86** 430	**98** 53	**72** 188	**97** 199	**52** 60	**74** 260	**100** 334	**52** 231	**90** 51	**83** 481	**98** 156	**70** 462	- -	- -
Glendale Memorial Hospital and Health Center, Glendale, CA	**100** 54	**99** 175	**99** 201	**92** 123	**98** 205	- 0	**56** 9	**100** 61	**95** 256	**54** 478	**98** 578	**99** 80	**83** 206	**95** 182	**87** 68	**78** 285	**100** 367	**88** 252	**98** 50	**79** 238	**91** 80	**47** 230	- -	- -
Glenn Medical Center, Willows, CA	- -	- -	- -	- -	- -	- -	- -	- -	- -	- -	- -	- -	**75** 4	**100** 3	- -	**86** 7	**100** 7	**100** 2	**67** 3	- -	- -	- -	- -	- -
Goleta Valley Cottage Hospital, Santa Barbara, CA	- 0	**100** 3	**100** 1	**100** 3	**100** 1	- 0	- 0	- 0	**80** 5	**42** 19	**71** 24	**100** 2	**78** 36	**90** 21	**50** 4	**84** 38	**100** 48	**58** 36	**89** 9	**84** 108	**62** 40	**65** 102	**0.00** 296	**2.53** 237
Good Samaritan Hospital, Bakersfield, CA	- -	- -	- -	- -	- -	- -	- -	- -	- 0	**0** 15	**7** 69	**40** 5	**86** 7	**100** 2	- -	**37** 70	**97** 91	**44** 18	**50** 2	- -	- -	- -	- -	- -
Good Samaritan Hospital, San Jose, CA	**93** 56	**99** 166	**99** 638	**98** 131	**99** 625	**0** 1	**50** 6	**99** 133	**60** 113	**67** 273	**91** 368	**86** 29	**87** 227	**89** 215	**59** 71	**72** 253	**100** 322	**46** 237	**79** 42	**84** 274	**60** 129	**70** 259	- -	- -
Good Samaritan Hospital, Los Angeles, CA	**89** 55	**98** 137	**98** 264	**97** 106	**92** 250	**0** 13	**67** 6	**98** 65	**87** 197	**79** 391	**97** 463	**95** 74	**81** 165	**88** 148	- -	**77** 212	**99** 249	**65** 151	**78** 27	**83** 544	**80** 123	**74** 514	- -	- -
Greater El Monte Community Hospital, South El Monte, CA	**60** 5	**93** 41	**75** 12	**67** 36	**31** 13	**0** 1	- 0	- 0	**82** 22	**5** 75	**75** 95	**69** 13	**86** 98	**97** 134	**18** 33	**74** 206	**100** 247	**9** 150	**46** 24	**50** 14	**100** 1	**85** 13	- -	- -
Grossmont Hospital, La Mesa, CA	**98** 66	**97** 479	**100** 404	**95** 433	**99** 402	**0** 3	**53** 32	**99** 144	**89** 254	**71** 504	**97** 635	**98** 140	**91** 383	**84** 486	**27** 119	**85** 603	**100** 686	**47** 422	**85** 104	**83** 328	**74** 84	**71** 319	- -	- -
Hanford Community Medical Center, Hanford, CA	**20** 5	**93** 71	**69** 51	**88** 67	**73** 49	**17** 12	- 0	**82** 17	**77** 30	**37** 139	**40** 143	**90** 29	**77** 168	**87** 75	**53** 30	**61** 183	**99** 207	**54** 129	**83** 46	**39** 84	**88** 24	**40** 75	**0.14** 733	**2.35** 511
Hazel Hawkins Memorial Hospital, Hollister, CA	**0** 1	**88** 8	**100** 3	**75** 8	**83** 6	- 0	- 0	**100** 1	**100** 7	**51** 59	**59** 79	**50** 8	**81** 52	**60** 30	**70** 23	**83** 58	**96** 77	**53** 59	**33** 9	**54** 68	**92** 12	**80** 64	- -	- -
Healdsburg District Hospital, Healdsburg, CA	- 0	**50** 2	- 0	**0** 2	- 0	- 0	- -	- 0	**100** 1	**0** 17	**8** 25	**0** 1	**76** 29	**73** 11	**0** 10	**91** 32	**100** 38	**7** 29	**0** 7	**91** 53	**100** 4	**98** 52	- -	- -
Hemet Valley Medical Center, Hemet, CA	**77** 48	**93** 270	**79** 116	**88** 240	**81** 149	**81** 42	- 0	**43** 21	**66** 138	**49** 273	**89** 375	**69** 58	**65** 220	**88** 240	**32** 78	**58** 362	**100** 467	**39** 315	**63** 75	**53** 95	**52** 94	**9** 92	- -	- -
Henry Mayo Newhall Memorial Hospital, Valencia, CA	**83** 6	**98** 113	**89** 37	**96** 95	**93** 30	**50** 8	- 0	**33** 3	**75** 69	**36** 238	**89** 275	**47** 19	**75** 185	**84** 142	- -	**75** 234	**100** 287	**14** 182	**25** 32	**82** 147	**93** 68	**51** 145	- -	- -
Hi-Desert Medical Center, Joshua Tree, CA	**100** 1	**88** 25	**92** 13	**77** 31	**87** 15	- 0	- 0	**100** 7	**85** 33	**5** 65	**81** 106	**83** 23	**81** 118	**90** 142	**64** 45	**61** 241	**100** 290	**64** 182	**81** 77	**62** 61	**84** 25	**65** 57	- -	- -
Hoag Memorial Hospital Presbyterian, Newport Beach, CA	**96** 54	**99** 283	**100** 287	**98** 257	**99** 284	- 0	**93** 27	**93** 58	**87** 251	**73** 494	**95** 598	**84** 55	**89** 320	**91** 367	**81** 84	**87** 376	**100** 524	**75** 349	**85** 59	**90** 349	**94** 87	**83** 337	- -	- -
Hollywood Community Hospital, Hollywood, CA	**75** 4	**100** 3	**100** 5	**67** 3	**80** 5	- 0	- 0	**75** 4	**82** 11	**15** 27	**65** 34	**75** 16	**29** 35	**67** 3	**0** 12	**79** 48	**66** 50	**3** 37	**32** 34	**100** 6	**100** 6	**100** 6	- -	- -

NOTE: The first number in each column (boldface) is the rate in percent, the second number is the number of patients; Please refer to the main entry for footnotes; ***Heart Attack Care:*** *1. ACE Inhibitor or ARB for LVSD; 2. Aspirin at Arrival; 3. Aspirin at Discharge; 4. Beta Blocker at Arrival; 5. Beta Blocker at Discharge; 6. Fibrinolytic Medication Timing; 7. PCI Within 90 Minutes of Arrival; 8. Smoking Cessation Advice;* ***Heart Failure Care:*** *9. ACE Inhibitor or ARB for LVSD; 10. Discharge Instructions; 11. Evaluation of LVS Function; 12. Smoking Cessation Advice;* ***Pneumonia Care:*** *13. Appropriate Initial Antibiotic; 14. Blood Culture Timing; 15. Influenza Vaccine; 16. Initial Antibiotic Timing; 17. Oxygenation Assessment; 18. Pneumococcal Vaccine; 19. Smoking Cessation Advice;* ***Surgical Infection Prevention:*** *20. Prophylactic Antibiotic Given; 21. Prophylactic Antibiotic Selection; 22. Prophylactic Antibiotic Stopped;* ***Pregnancy Care:*** *23. Inpatient Neonatal Mortality; 24. Third or Fourth Degree Laceration*

Hospital	Heart Attack Care 1	2	3	4	5	6	7	8	Heart Failure Care 9	10	11	12	Pneumonia Care 13	14	15	16	17	18	19	Surgical Infection Prevention 20	21	22	Pregnancy Care 23	24
Hollywood Presbyterian Medical Center, Los Angeles, CA	100 19	98 129	100 89	97 126	98 89	22 9	- 0	89 19	100 115	42 352	95 409	80 56	61 354	94 278	- -	77 461	100 508	40 315	69 35	82 111	96 111	27 110	- -	- -
Huntington Beach Hospital, Huntington Beach, CA	43 7	93 41	94 16	83 36	78 23	33 3	- 0	20 5	88 26	56 97	91 128	63 27	72 107	96 99	70 20	92 132	100 156	86 96	64 25	56 68	94 16	42 60	- -	- -
Huntington Memorial Hospital, Pasadena, CA	90 51	94 249	98 235	93 170	96 224	- 0	64 11	93 60	75 178	33 418	87 493	86 72	83 289	90 391	14 132	71 462	100 630	9 443	79 84	85 319	96 313	30 315	- -	- -
Indian Valley Hospital, Greenville, CA	- -	- -	- -	- -	- -	- -	- -	- -	- -	- -	- -	- -	- -	- -	- -	- -	- -	- -	- -	- -	- -	- -	- -	- -
Irvine Regional Hospital, Irvine, CA	79 24	99 109	96 164	95 91	96 174	67 3	83 6	97 37	74 57	60 173	90 206	85 13	89 161	95 133	72 58	84 160	100 244	76 184	73 22	73 197	80 44	68 199	- -	- -
Jerold Phelps Community Hospital, Garberville, CA	- -	- -	- -	- -	- -	- -	- -	- -	- -	- -	- -	- -	100 1	100 1	- -	100 2	100 2	- 0	- 0	- -	- -	- -	- -	- -
John C Fremont Healthcare District, Mariposa, CA	- -	- -	- -	- -	- -	- -	- -	- -	- -	- -	- -	- -	- -	- -	- -	- -	- -	- -	- -	- -	- -	- -	- -	- -
John F Kennedy Memorial Hospital, Indio, CA	68 19	96 115	87 84	88 88	89 80	64 14	67 3	100 20	77 79	65 162	87 195	100 30	87 216	95 205	63 62	85 229	100 285	65 178	100 37	83 288	92 78	64 280	- -	- -
John Muir Medical Center, Walnut Creek, CA	88 26	100 157	100 133	97 123	100 126	- 0	33 9	100 25	98 88	92 225	96 272	100 22	92 121	99 132	96 28	78 162	100 207	80 152	95 21	81 181	62 55	53 171	0.16 620	6.19 679
John Muir Medical Center-Concord Campus, Concord, CA	96 45	99 183	98 281	97 155	100 276	100 1	40 5	100 78	93 106	84 257	96 317	100 46	89 116	95 122	52 29	81 152	100 195	77 123	100 36	77 231	67 79	76 218	- -	- -
Kaiser Foundation Hospital, Woodland Hills, CA	100 15	94 100	89 80	95 100	99 87	81 16	- 0	92 12	85 92	68 282	96 299	75 20	37 76	77 69	77 30	47 99	100 124	70 96	72 18	84 49	86 49	73 48	0.28 1761	3.77 1219
Kaiser Foundation Hospital, Baldwin Park, CA	83 12	99 104	93 68	99 80	96 72	71 17	- 0	91 11	84 122	58 346	96 382	94 50	81 85	89 97	- -	68 98	100 125	87 75	62 26	78 50	92 51	52 46	0.10 3158	2.80 2211
Kaiser Foundation Hospital, Hayward, CA	92 25	100 340	99 203	99 344	99 216	60 10	- 0	95 20	84 105	61 377	95 427	82 49	76 131	94 122	62 26	67 168	100 202	81 139	67 24	74 411	87 99	56 391	0.24 3342	5.23 2123
Kaiser Foundation Hospital-Fresno, Fresno, CA	88 34	97 183	94 140	91 176	96 152	43 14	- 0	85 27	83 103	54 206	98 244	92 38	91 105	89 100	60 30	63 121	100 163	82 123	100 21	87 161	93 42	74 159	0.00 1345	3.63 910
Kaiser Foundation Hospital-Manteca, Manteca, CA	89 9	96 49	97 37	87 39	97 35	67 3	- 0	78 9	93 56	16 152	94 181	86 22	81 113	83 100	44 34	72 119	100 164	59 106	72 46	62 114	100 14	66 113	- -	- -
Kaiser Foundation Hospital-Riverside, Riverside, CA	90 20	98 140	91 80	92 125	92 90	50 30	- 0	95 19	93 126	62 329	95 358	91 47	85 86	82 51	71 17	56 94	100 125	96 79	64 25	82 50	90 49	38 47	0.05 3785	2.38 2733
Kaiser Foundation Hospital-San Diego, San Diego, CA	93 27	92 235	93 95	95 215	96 101	14 7	- 0	53 19	86 242	53 575	94 625	82 67	36 94	85 71	69 29	66 112	100 144	81 86	65 17	58 31	100 30	57 28	0.40 3983	3.94 2640
Kaiser Foundation Hospital-Santa Rosa, Santa Rosa, CA	94 17	98 171	89 121	96 162	98 123	50 10	- 0	92 25	85 48	67 113	96 123	68 25	87 135	96 110	58 38	70 156	100 190	81 140	53 17	86 313	87 102	67 307	0.00 1458	5.01 959
Kaiser Foundation Hospital-South Sacramento, Sacramento, CA	100 30	100 246	97 152	97 207	99 166	42 12	- 0	90 30	98 101	83 255	99 285	96 46	89 202	92 179	81 47	80 210	100 285	89 189	98 50	90 735	93 177	71 730	0.03 3606	3.98 2866
Kaiser Foundation Hospital-Vallejo, Vallejo, CA	87 23	100 217	99 97	100 208	100 103	41 17	- 0	100 11	82 83	49 267	97 303	86 43	93 118	96 116	47 32	85 137	100 171	82 106	85 27	92 192	91 46	91 180	0.24 2510	3.71 1750
Kaiser Foundation Hospital-Walnut Creek, Walnut Creek, CA	100 17	96 225	97 86	99 197	100 97	41 22	- 0	89 9	93 41	60 188	98 216	94 16	88 108	73 113	66 29	66 115	100 168	86 124	79 19	90 322	91 53	81 313	0.24 4654	3.75 3228
Kaiser Permanente Anaheim Medical Center, Anaheim, CA	94 16	97 77	100 47	95 77	92 48	64 14	- 0	64 11	82 60	32 137	97 155	65 26	57 91	92 71	85 27	62 101	100 121	92 75	36 14	58 43	76 42	50 38	0.35 3398	2.30 2391
Kaiser Permanente Bellflower Medical Center, Bellflower, CA	80 30	99 155	96 112	98 149	99 118	46 24	- 0	82 17	87 212	67 478	89 525	72 82	72 95	96 75	54 24	69 108	100 122	83 76	69 13	88 42	98 42	62 42	0.58 3461	3.39 2447
Kaiser Permanente Fontana Medical Center, Fontana, CA	84 43	96 202	97 133	93 134	94 144	64 44	- 0	97 30	83 301	62 607	94 644	87 86	86 63	76 45	- -	78 74	100 102	87 70	77 22	73 48	91 47	49 47	0.46 4777	3.85 3321
Kaiser Permanente Los Angeles Medical Center, Los Angeles, CA	85 182	99 229	100 858	98 219	97 874	71 14	100 4	79 207	84 257	54 471	98 489	63 59	80 66	83 92	- -	72 95	100 127	59 81	53 15	60 68	90 72	80 65	0.61 2476	3.42 1520
Kaiser Permanente Panorama City Med Ctr, Panorama City, CA	82 17	94 98	95 63	95 100	93 71	71 17	- 0	90 10	75 134	60 340	83 371	82 45	36 67	75 51	64 25	66 94	99 118	60 91	67 15	71 41	98 41	52 40	0.06 1656	2.92 1026
Kaiser Permanente Sacramento Medical Center, Sacramento, CA	69 45	95 337	87 253	93 287	95 263	26 39	- 0	49 37	73 235	40 654	97 789	67 79	89 298	90 338	58 108	66 425	100 573	82 433	75 95	76 622	84 144	72 614	0.42 4283	2.85 2701
Kaiser Permanente San Francisco Med Ctr, San Francisco, CA	96 69	99 75	98 429	98 62	99 494	- 0	75 4	100 120	97 134	79 336	97 353	98 41	93 118	95 190	63 41	83 222	100 263	81 186	77 31	92 631	97 175	86 605	0.23 2612	6.87 1675
Kaiser Permanente Santa Clara Medical Center, Santa Clara, CA	72 29	99 149	97 90	100 114	100 94	33 21	- 0	86 14	60 115	69 397	99 467	78 27	86 90	92 106	69 26	71 132	100 173	91 128	78 18	79 197	84 45	74 193	0.14 725	5.73 489
Kaiser Permanente Santa Teresa Comm Med Ctr, San Jose, CA	93 28	99 204	99 120	98 171	100 135	50 4	70 10	100 39	90 138	76 346	99 373	100 49	90 105	92 101	57 28	72 130	100 160	78 111	100 15	41 197	76 49	74 183	0.00 510	4.19 382
Kaiser Permanente South Bay Medical Center, Harbor City, CA	77 26	97 137	94 102	94 132	97 109	29 14	- 0	100 13	87 120	54 382	93 414	88 43	46 103	92 101	52 21	54 115	100 138	92 79	64 22	76 51	98 50	63 51	0.16 1825	4.82 1223
Kaiser Permanente West Los Angeles Med Ctr, Los Angeles, CA	90 20	99 131	97 102	96 128	97 103	56 18	- 0	85 13	80 134	54 335	90 353	82 45	82 78	91 44	70 20	63 94	100 109	70 79	67 12	91 44	88 43	50 44	0.14 1461	2.34 1026
Kaiser Redwood City Medical Center, Redwood City, CA	100 6	100 104	96 50	100 98	100 53	58 12	- 0	100 4	97 37	40 112	98 124	78 9	89 96	89 114	65 31	84 137	100 168	81 119	73 26	82 367	95 82	85 367	0.42 1430	3.01 1131
Kaweah Delta Health Care District, Visalia, CA	96 57	98 231	96 310	93 196	91 304	0 1	58 12	96 91	77 160	46 329	87 399	86 59	87 446	82 247	- -	74 485	100 618	65 370	66 134	82 68	89 70	35 65	- -	- -
Kern Medical Center, Bakersfield, CA	67 3	100 15	100 8	85 13	100 8	- 0	- 0	- 0	95 76	0 23	98 129	25 8	100 12	81 16	- -	44 81	99 103	27 30	12 8	75 36	- -	66 35	0.43 932	3.50 742
Kern Valley Healthcare District, Lake Isabella, CA	- -	- -	- -	- -	- -	- -	- -	- -	- -	- -	- -	- -	100 20	78 32	- -	77 30	100 34	68 25	33 6	- -	- -	- -	- -	- -
Kingsburg District Hospital, Kingsburg, CA	- -	- -	- -	- -	- -	- -	- -	- -	- 0	0 3	0 5	100 1	0 1	100 1	- -	36 14	82 17	0 8	- 0	- -	- -	- -	- -	- -
La Palma Intercommunity Hospital, La Palma, CA	63 19	94 69	88 33	86 66	83 36	73 11	- 0	100 9	79 91	85 170	82 199	100 31	84 179	91 120	50 58	68 182	95 224	61 142	72 39	85 88	94 18	70 82	- -	- -
Laguna Honda Hospital and Rehab Center, San Francisco, CA	- 0	100 1	100 1	100 2	100 2	- -	- -	- -	100 1	- 0	100 1	- 0	- 0	100 1	- -	78 9	100 17	56 9	- 0	- -	- -	- -	- -	- -
Lakewood Regional Medical Center, Lakewood, CA	97 31	100 140	95 171	97 120	97 165	22 9	29 7	98 47	96 146	76 405	93 492	91 64	86 168	90 134	63 46	85 199	100 247	85 168	90 49	80 362	93 74	60 341	- -	- -
Lancaster Community Hospital, Lancaster, CA	88 34	92 129	83 112	81 122	80 123	- 0	75 4	97 37	77 105	11 282	72 321	74 58	90 163	75 96	34 41	63 159	99 222	46 121	63 60	76 371	88 110	50 360	- -	- -
Laurel Grove Hosp Acute Rehab Facility, Hayward, CA	- -	- -	- -	- -	- -	- -	- -	- -	- -	- -	- -	- -	- -	- -	- -	- -	- -	- -	- -	- -	- -	- -	- -	- -
Little Company of Mary Hospital, Torrance, CA	93 43	100 246	99 268	99 209	99 260	- 0	45 11	98 66	88 169	87 349	95 501	100 42	86 172	95 239	85 67	82 290	100 411	86 285	98 51	90 644	92 157	65 618	- -	- -
Little Company of Mary-San Pedro Hospital, San Pedro, CA	100 5	98 47	92 25	97 36	92 25	50 8	- 0	100 3	90 50	62 166	90 202	95 20	90 132	88 121	59 41	87 174	100 221	65 142	97 33	76 160	95 40	37 149	- -	- -
Lodi Memorial Hospital, Lodi, CA	77 13	98 80	100 32	98 55	94 35	70 20	- 0	78 9	71 55	59 139	84 193	92 38	91 77	90 77	75 24	69 123	100 158	71 109	82 33	73 214	85 52	35 202	- -	- -
Loma Linda University Medical Center, Loma Linda, CA	84 80	99 123	99 298	95 98	99 293	100 1	20 5	98 108	92 261	31 388	97 434	87 62	72 145	92 166	55 47	49 269	100 354	36 159	67 39	91 1147	98 343	52 1070	- -	- -
Lompoc Healthcare District Hospital, Lompoc, CA	100 3	100 4	100 2	0 1	67 3	- 0	- 0	100 1	97 29	69 49	88 58	77 13	92 63	95 43	7 14	85 82	100 94	13 52	50 22	75 142	89 35	68 142	0.00 473	3.23 341
Long Beach Memorial Medical Center, Long Beach, CA	97 60	99 292	99 310	96 235	97 309	- 0	40 5	100 87	84 330	81 599	92 717	84 119	86 287	92 399	30 118	75 485	100 619	60 373	95 105	70 332	74 92	67 316	- -	- -

NOTE: The first number in each column (boldface) is the rate in percent, the second number is the number of patients; Please refer to the main entry for footnotes; ***Heart Attack Care:*** *1. ACE Inhibitor or ARB for LVSD; 2. Aspirin at Arrival; 3. Aspirin at Discharge; 4. Beta Blocker at Arrival; 5. Beta Blocker at Discharge; 6. Fibrinolytic Medication Timing; 7. PCI Within 90 Minutes of Arrival; 8. Smoking Cessation Advice;* ***Heart Failure Care:*** *9. ACE Inhibitor or ARB for LVSD; 10. Discharge Instructions; 11. Evaluation of LVS Function; 12. Smoking Cessation Advice;* ***Pneumonia Care:*** *13. Appropriate Initial Antibiotic; 14. Blood Culture Timing; 15. Influenza Vaccine; 16. Initial Antibiotic Timing; 17. Oxygenation Assessment; 18. Pneumococcal Vaccine; 19. Smoking Cessation Advice;* ***Surgical Infection Prevention:*** *20. Prophylactic Antibiotic Given; 21. Prophylactic Antibiotic Selection; 22. Prophylactic Antibiotic Stopped;* ***Pregnancy Care:*** *23. Inpatient Neonatal Mortality; 24. Third or Fourth Degree Laceration*

Hospital	Heart Attack Care								Heart Failure Care				Pneumonia Care							Surgical Infection Prevention			Pregnancy Care	
	1	2	3	4	5	6	7	8	9	10	11	12	13	14	15	16	17	18	19	20	21	22	23	24
Los Alamitos Medical Center, Los Alamitos, CA	100 14	98 129	98 89	97 105	100 90	- 0	100 8	100 16	100 75	80 212	99 261	100 20	92 201	97 184	98 54	92 226	100 284	99 207	100 36	82 162	89 36	42 154	- -	- -
Los Angeles Community Hospital, Los Angeles, CA	67 3	100 8	100 7	78 9	75 8	20 5	- 0	0 1	61 41	59 115	80 136	96 23	64 72	75 16	0 16	57 93	98 104	0 53	44 78	64 25	96 25	96 25	- -	- -
Los Angeles County & USC Medical Center, Los Angeles, CA	83 66	97 178	97 193	86 142	90 187	- 0	0 13	69 83	90 307	20 579	86 617	47 211	83 281	84 122	58 66	38 341	99 368	56 87	32 137	15 995	92 211	73 960	1.09 1566	4.06 912
Los Angeles County Harbor-UCLA Medical Center, Torrance, CA	67 39	97 145	98 161	96 130	98 157	36 22	14 7	87 68	83 198	69 323	95 332	89 111	82 132	81 129	71 28	54 175	100 205	61 72	73 45	88 232	91 53	40 225	1.40 285	1.87 694
Los Angeles Metropolitan Med Ctr-LA Campus, Los Angeles, CA	- 0	0 1	0 1	0 1	0 1	- 0	- 0	- 0	25 8	4 51	56 72	7 29	40 40	100 4	0 20	26 53	95 62	9 33	0 25	- -	- -	- -	0.00 0	2.63 571
Los Robles Regional Medical Center, Thousand Oaks, CA	77 53	89 202	90 212	80 147	88 207	- 0	56 16	94 48	74 89	64 205	91 232	85 27	84 189	86 205	33 82	69 270	100 350	40 233	68 44	66 254	95 115	67 245	- -	- -
Mad River Community Hospital, Arcata, CA	50 2	95 19	85 13	100 15	94 17	- 0	- 0	100 2	88 24	60 10	72 78	100 3	67 3	100 6	- -	90 67	100 77	47 47	100 1	55 22	- -	57 21	- -	- -
Madera Community Hospital, Madera, CA	100 20	99 74	95 40	98 59	98 42	40 10	- 0	100 19	91 47	18 146	67 159	91 35	83 112	91 95	- -	80 160	100 193	44 90	90 52	53 207	89 63	74 205	- -	- -
Mammoth Hospital, Mammoth Lakes, CA	- -	- -	- -	- -	- -	- -	- -	- -	- 0	0 1	0 1	- 0	- -	- -	- -	- -	- -	- -	- -	- -	- -	- -	- -	- -
Marian Medical Center, Santa Maria, CA	100 6	99 141	99 127	100 88	100 102	81 21	100 1	100 35	96 78	97 223	100 254	100 22	93 185	93 172	72 69	86 234	100 307	75 225	100 44	96 493	91 172	62 481	- -	- -
Marin General Hospital, Greenbrae, CA	91 58	97 142	99 158	91 124	95 150	- 0	100 5	92 25	81 104	77 181	95 226	80 30	84 126	96 160	61 41	92 148	100 218	40 149	95 20	76 300	97 75	63 284	- -	- -
Mark Twain Saint Joseph's Hospital, San Andreas, CA	100 1	100 11	100 1	100 10	100 3	0 1	- 0	- 0	100 13	56 54	100 69	85 13	88 82	100 55	- -	76 89	100 122	72 79	100 25	84 32	100 32	94 31	- -	- -
Marshall Medical Center, Placerville, CA	62 8	94 35	94 18	94 32	92 24	40 5	- 0	75 4	73 55	37 137	89 171	100 16	84 111	95 120	- -	81 148	100 182	38 125	94 33	90 197	92 62	79 188	- -	- -
Martin Luther King Jr/Charles R Drew Med Ctr, Los Angeles, CA	83 6	94 108	90 59	66 102	79 61	0 10	- 0	10 10	92 50	1 310	72 308	11 128	72 134	47 74	0 25	62 164	99 202	9 44	11 61	45 77	62 16	90 68	- -	- -
Mayers Memorial Hospital District, Fall River Mills, CA	- -	- -	- -	- -	- -	- -	- -	- -	- -	- -	- -	- -	100 4	50 2	- -	100 3	100 5	50 4	100 2	- -	- -	- -	- -	- -
Memorial Hospital Los Banos, Los Banos, CA	- 0	75 8	80 5	50 8	40 5	- 0	- 0	100 1	62 8	67 43	45 55	90 10	78 92	78 41	18 17	81 98	100 112	61 71	85 26	28 36	90 10	97 34	- -	- -
Memorial Hospital of Gardena, Gardena, CA	86 7	100 59	87 30	88 51	71 31	0 15	- 0	67 12	91 82	26 161	86 200	42 36	54 209	93 196	0 56	64 299	100 323	1 170	48 29	40 48	57 14	63 30	- -	- -
Memorial Medical Center, Modesto, CA	77 52	94 224	98 264	90 170	99 287	50 6	71 7	98 118	82 153	55 331	91 388	92 76	88 104	78 110	74 35	67 163	99 197	67 120	84 51	58 351	90 78	56 344	- -	- -
Menifee Valley Medical Center, Sun City, CA	71 14	93 150	81 52	87 143	80 75	53 19	- 0	80 10	71 76	52 220	87 248	78 40	78 158	87 142	52 52	71 221	100 295	42 211	89 45	67 18	42 19	0 16	- -	- -
Mercy General Hospital, Sacramento, CA	85 165	99 233	99 966	96 190	98 997	82 11	71 14	99 329	89 269	91 511	96 562	99 127	83 166	97 214	81 79	89 365	100 409	83 286	98 64	82 299	90 104	69 285	0.12 2603	2.48 1897
Mercy Hospital, Bakersfield, CA	71 7	83 60	64 39	75 52	55 38	- 0	- 0	89 9	57 63	83 149	89 206	78 41	81 427	82 315	1 105	75 439	100 533	76 289	82 121	59 201	83 65	29 201	0.36 3587	6.66 2583
Mercy Hospital of Folsom, Folsom, CA	- 0	100 25	100 12	88 24	100 12	0 2	- 0	100 1	86 43	87 100	94 125	89 19	88 122	95 104	91 34	79 138	100 166	94 108	100 30	78 143	93 42	62 112	0.00 1084	5.18 830
Mercy Med Ctr Merced-Community Campus, Merced, CA	88 8	95 101	91 46	100 95	94 53	20 10	- 0	82 11	90 110	84 247	92 285	99 72	86 92	95 65	29 21	78 129	100 171	74 100	94 35	74 140	88 41	48 133	0.07 2764	3.38 2072
Mercy Medical Center-Mount Shasta, Mount Shasta, CA	67 3	100 8	86 7	100 9	83 6	0 1	- 0	- 0	92 24	90 40	93 44	100 8	89 70	96 49	70 10	84 73	99 85	91 58	100 15	89 97	92 38	100 94	- -	- -
Mercy Medical Center-Redding, Redding, CA	98 57	100 173	97 262	98 131	98 257	62 21	29 7	100 116	89 121	72 221	92 276	100 65	89 274	88 180	80 66	80 316	100 410	78 260	100 111	89 274	93 89	82 271	0.04 2239	2.09 1482
Mercy San Juan Hospital, Carmichael, CA	98 45	99 295	100 250	99 197	99 284	65 34	27 11	100 85	95 142	88 416	99 521	99 104	88 232	93 487	88 140	77 598	100 704	89 465	99 138	60 250	91 80	76 234	- -	- -
Methodist Hospital of Sacramento, Sacramento, CA	100 5	100 32	100 15	96 28	92 13	50 2	- 0	100 3	91 88	69 249	92 276	100 50	92 181	95 209	65 51	80 255	100 304	60 182	97 38	60 154	94 47	52 154	0.07 1473	2.60 960
Methodist Hospital of Southern California, Arcadia, CA	97 33	95 165	95 162	90 129	94 159	- 0	59 17	93 42	79 189	81 480	95 634	79 63	87 341	92 260	44 108	83 499	99 593	31 412	70 57	63 182	90 181	45 176	- -	- -
Mills-Peninsula Health Services, Burlingame, CA	90 29	98 108	98 131	98 88	96 121	- 0	11 9	100 40	92 76	68 217	97 305	86 37	87 113	96 110	58 31	76 152	100 186	72 155	93 27	80 296	100 58	49 283	- -	- -
Miracle Mile Medical Center, Los Angeles, CA	- -	- -	- -	- -	- -	- -	- -	- -	- -	- -	- -	- -	- -	- -	- -	- -	- -	- -	- -	- -	- -	- -	- -	- -
Mission Community Hospital, Panorama City, CA	53 15	92 37	82 34	89 36	72 32	0 2	- 0	0 3	71 68	48 25	82 171	57 7	57 21	81 37	- -	75 194	99 229	7 125	75 4	20 5	- -	25 4	- -	- -
Mission Hospital Regional Medical Center, Mission Viejo, CA	100 29	99 278	99 254	90 188	98 240	- 0	62 16	100 46	93 83	83 243	98 283	97 32	83 175	94 160	75 51	74 217	100 279	72 180	68 40	85 186	94 62	75 186	- -	- -
Modoc Medical Center, Alturas, CA	- 0	- 0	- 0	100 1	- 0	- -	- -	- -	- 0	0 1	20 5	0 1	100 2	- 0	- -	44 9	100 10	40 5	- 0	- -	- -	- -	- -	- -
Monterey Park Hospital, Monterey Park, CA	75 8	87 45	68 19	66 41	60 20	33 3	- 0	100 3	59 76	50 193	91 210	100 11	86 86	89 63	33 18	82 116	94 123	31 81	88 8	59 71	100 18	33 69	- -	- -
Moreno Valley Community Hospital, Moreno Valley, CA	33 3	81 42	46 13	79 29	54 13	25 4	- 0	0 1	70 50	41 153	70 158	54 26	82 127	90 88	- -	72 164	99 196	31 106	61 33	45 20	47 15	19 16	- -	- -
Motion Picture & Television Hospital, Woodland Hills, CA	- 0	100 5	- 0	67 3	- 0	- 0	- -	100 1	80 15	58 36	96 49	20 5	72 18	100 2	25 8	73 22	100 29	69 16	25 4	69 26	50 2	79 19	- -	- -
Mountain Community Medical Services, Weaverville, CA	- -	- -	- -	- -	- -	- -	- -	- -	- -	- -	- -	- -	100 7	100 4	- -	86 7	100 9	0 3	0 2	- -	- -	- -	- -	- -
Mountains Community Hospital, Lake Arrowhead, CA	- -	- -	- -	- -	- -	- -	- -	- -	- -	- -	- -	- -	- -	- -	- -	- -	- -	- -	- -	- -	- -	- -	- -	- -
Natividad Medical Center, Salinas, CA	- 0	100 10	100 5	100 5	100 3	- 0	- 0	0 1	100 28	15 65	97 73	38 16	85 86	90 69	36 11	76 89	100 118	39 36	38 32	74 50	100 17	100 54	0.31 2607	4.21 1853
NorthBay Medical Center, Fairfield, CA	83 6	94 50	96 25	92 48	93 27	44 16	- 0	40 5	71 92	28 163	94 181	84 50	96 159	89 184	50 34	78 223	100 265	46 140	84 44	83 179	90 52	63 163	- -	- -
Northridge Hospital Medical Center, Northridge, CA	98 41	98 196	99 169	99 124	98 177	25 4	33 3	100 42	94 125	76 293	99 354	100 48	87 199	94 221	79 70	73 296	100 396	82 262	97 62	69 211	78 73	44 198	- -	- -
Novato Community Hospital, Novato, CA	100 5	98 43	100 34	100 44	100 36	- 0	- 0	100 4	94 16	75 48	100 61	100 6	76 71	93 55	52 23	88 74	100 92	59 73	82 11	84 203	100 47	36 197	- -	- -
O'Connor Hospital, San Jose, CA	97 32	98 149	97 151	96 119	95 142	- 0	25 4	91 35	95 123	54 378	88 471	69 29	88 176	92 184	69 54	78 238	100 313	64 236	52 31	89 186	95 65	80 186	- -	- -
Oak Valley Hospital, Oakdale, CA	0 2	100 25	75 8	100 23	88 8	50 2	- 0	100 1	91 23	58 55	84 69	55 11	82 82	85 39	71 14	84 91	100 107	56 70	50 30	34 44	100 13	94 35	- -	- -
Oakland Medical Center, Oakland, CA	100 32	100 328	97 150	99 282	99 141	60 25	- 0	95 20	95 169	60 534	96 585	92 92	95 270	88 345	58 110	78 439	100 528	94 367	87 75	94 989	92 276	80 908	- -	- -
Ojai Valley Community Hospital, Ojai, CA	67 6	81 21	67 18	40 20	65 20	- 0	- 0	40 5	100 1	0 12	53 17	0 1	77 57	88 17	58 12	54 48	100 73	36 45	27 15	50 8	90 10	100 8	- -	- -
Olive View-UCLA Medical Center, San Fernando, CA	100 8	99 104	96 27	98 90	92 25	0 1	- 0	0 1	97 147	43 58	99 297	50 18	71 21	63 30	- -	61 158	100 178	33 70	57 7	82 22	- -	91 22	- -	- -
Olympia Medical Center, Los Angeles, CA	70 10	95 98	89 46	85 82	89 46	50 4	- 0	80 5	92 89	44 200	88 285	55 29	57 298	92 279	24 72	81 368	100 459	36 295	67 21	69 114	88 24	55 113	- -	- -

NOTE: The first number in each column (boldface) is the rate in percent, the second number is the number of patients; Please refer to the main entry for footnotes; ***Heart Attack Care:*** *1. ACE Inhibitor or ARB for LVSD; 2. Aspirin at Arrival; 3. Aspirin at Discharge; 4. Beta Blocker at Arrival; 5. Beta Blocker at Discharge; 6. Fibrinolytic Medication Timing; 7. PCI Within 90 Minutes of Arrival; 8. Smoking Cessation Advice;* ***Heart Failure Care:*** *9. ACE Inhibitor or ARB for LVSD; 10. Discharge Instructions; 11. Evaluation of LVS Function; 12. Smoking Cessation Advice;* ***Pneumonia Care:*** *13. Appropriate Initial Antibiotic; 14. Blood Culture Timing; 15. Influenza Vaccine; 16. Initial Antibiotic Timing; 17. Oxygenation Assessment; 18. Pneumococcal Vaccine; 19. Smoking Cessation Advice;* ***Surgical Infection Prevention:*** *20. Prophylactic Antibiotic Given; 21. Prophylactic Antibiotic Selection; 22. Prophylactic Antibiotic Stopped;* ***Pregnancy Care:*** *23. Inpatient Neonatal Mortality; 24. Third or Fourth Degree Laceration*

Hospital	Heart Attack Care								Heart Failure Care				Pneumonia Care							Surgical Infection Prevention			Pregnancy Care	
	1	2	3	4	5	6	7	8	9	10	11	12	13	14	15	16	17	18	19	20	21	22	23	24
Orange Coast Memorial Medical Center, Santa Ana, CA	**100** 15	**99** 92	**97** 70	**93** 55	**98** 83	- 0	**80** 5	**100** 9	**88** 103	**76** 297	**93** 364	**98** 53	**90** 200	**87** 157	**77** 61	**92** 253	**100** 310	**86** 260	**81** 36	**87** 445	**89** 105	**42** 424	**0.00** 1576	**1.98** 1059
Oroville Hospital, Oroville, CA	**75** 4	**83** 35	**91** 11	**81** 36	**73** 11	**0** 3	- 0	**0** 3	**84** 58	**11** 119	**77** 149	**17** 36	**80** 108	**85** 98	**24** 21	**74** 131	**100** 152	**12** 73	**41** 51	**63** 41	**92** 36	**100** 34	- -	- -
Pacific Alliance Medical Center, Los Angeles, CA	**67** 3	**66** 32	**52** 31	**43** 30	**43** 30	- 0	- 0	**100** 1	**36** 45	**67** 46	**79** 302	**50** 2	**0** 3	**100** 11	- -	**50** 149	**98** 162	**45** 114	**50** 2	**67** 12	- -	**67** 12	**0.00** 409	**0.71** 282
Pacific Hospital of Long Beach, Long Beach, CA	**50** 2	**100** 10	**100** 4	**90** 10	**83** 6	**50** 2	- 0	**100** 1	**92** 26	**82** 34	**89** 54	**67** 12	**67** 39	**91** 106	**50** 20	**91** 147	**99** 158	**80** 89	**80** 25	**91** 139	**97** 29	**52** 135	- -	- -
Pacifica Hospital of the Valley, Sun Valley, CA	**100** 2	**93** 42	**87** 15	**86** 36	**80** 15	**67** 3	- 0	**100** 1	**91** 11	**46** 13	**93** 83	**75** 4	**62** 8	**80** 10	- -	**73** 98	**100** 102	**28** 47	**33** 6	**89** 19	- -	**100** 18	- -	- -
Palm Drive Hospital, Sebastopol, CA	- 0	**100** 10	**80** 5	**86** 7	**25** 4	- -	- -	- -	**33** 9	**100** 4	**74** 31	- 0	**57** 7	**100** 5	- -	**77** 35	**100** 42	**52** 29	**50** 2	**95** 19	- -	**100** 19	- -	- -
Palo Verde Hospital, Blythe, CA	- 0	**0** 3	**100** 2	**40** 5	**100** 2	**100** 1	- -	**0** 1	- 0	**4** 25	**12** 25	**29** 7	**84** 49	**90** 20	**55** 11	**77** 44	**100** 64	**56** 39	**24** 17	**50** 10	**100** 2	**60** 5	- -	- -
Palomar Medical Center, Escondido, CA	**100** 48	**100** 278	**100** 313	**99** 253	**100** 313	- 0	**60** 25	**100** 96	**97** 162	**90** 365	**99** 434	**87** 54	**95** 279	**91** 264	**76** 80	**79** 374	**100** 398	**68** 290	**97** 60	**82** 221	**95** 65	**85** 214	- -	- -
Paradise Valley Hospital, National City, CA	**88** 17	**91** 88	**100** 40	**97** 61	**96** 46	**50** 4	- 0	**86** 14	**84** 161	**76** 326	**93** 370	**95** 96	**85** 174	**90** 126	**57** 58	**71** 259	**100** 289	**50** 175	**87** 53	**63** 126	**82** 38	**68** 109	- -	- -
Parkview Community Hospital, Riverside, CA	**80** 5	**97** 66	**91** 35	**100** 64	**95** 37	**22** 9	- 0	**89** 9	**90** 52	**49** 159	**78** 204	**90** 29	**83** 161	**91** 197	**43** 54	**82** 332	**100** 381	**30** 217	**94** 52	**59** 126	**94** 81	**97** 116	**0.34** 888	**3.25** 584
Patients' Hospital of Redding, Redding, CA	- -	- -	- -	- -	- -	- -	- -	- -	- -	- -	- -	- -	- -	- -	- -	- -	- -	- -	- -	**90** 79	**95** 20	**100** 78	- -	- -
Petaluma Valley Hospital, Petaluma, CA	**50** 4	**98** 51	**96** 27	**100** 40	**100** 25	**55** 11	- 0	**75** 4	**94** 16	**59** 56	**91** 82	**29** 14	**74** 95	**80** 45	**79** 28	**77** 101	**100** 139	**85** 87	**62** 24	**75** 81	**87** 30	**69** 81	- -	- -
Pioneers Memorial Healthcare District, Brawley, CA	**44** 18	**98** 42	**67** 33	**72** 39	**64** 33	**50** 6	- 0	**87** 15	**91** 66	**65** 110	**80** 122	**96** 26	**92** 158	**74** 92	- -	**81** 157	**100** 183	**57** 100	**80** 20	**78** 109	**82** 49	**41** 109	- -	- -
Placentia-Linda Hospital, Placentia, CA	**57** 7	**95** 37	**81** 16	**91** 23	**80** 20	**40** 5	- 0	- 0	**72** 36	**84** 74	**90** 110	**100** 3	**92** 146	**96** 145	**82** 40	**91** 187	**100** 229	**80** 164	**77** 30	**90** 145	**85** 41	**84** 139	- -	- -
Pomerado Hospital, Poway, CA	**100** 4	**100** 54	**96** 25	**100** 50	**100** 25	- 0	- 0	**60** 5	**100** 29	**81** 122	**98** 133	**100** 17	**90** 155	**89** 140	**49** 35	**80** 160	**100** 206	**64** 148	**77** 26	**76** 146	**87** 46	**81** 142	- -	- -
Pomona Valley Hospital Medical Center, Pomona, CA	**80** 98	**93** 259	**96** 265	**87** 164	**93** 254	**0** 1	**46** 13	**99** 78	**89** 261	**76** 484	**94** 604	**98** 123	**91** 180	**84** 198	**66** 68	**71** 311	**100** 406	**58** 226	**88** 69	**84** 712	**95** 173	**45** 683	**0.20** 1007	**2.51** 637
Presbyterian Intercommunity Hospital, Whittier, CA	**89** 28	**100** 204	**98** 196	**99** 194	**95** 188	**64** 22	**0** 2	**97** 37	**93** 76	**86** 218	**97** 255	**97** 33	**78** 96	**92** 101	**36** 22	**78** 125	**100** 156	**51** 100	**83** 12	**91** 237	**94** 64	**64** 225	- -	- -
Promise Hospital of San Diego, San Diego, CA	- -	- -	- -	- -	- -	- -	- -	- -	- 0	**50** 2	**50** 2	- 0	**50** 4	**100** 1	**33** 3	**80** 10	**100** 16	**33** 6	**75** 4	- -	- -	- -	- -	- -
Providence Holy Cross Medical Center, Mission Hills, CA	**92** 39	**100** 165	**98** 200	**97** 116	**97** 204	- 0	**69** 13	**94** 64	**87** 102	**45** 251	**98** 313	**94** 35	**90** 109	**96** 165	**62** 32	**86** 194	**100** 236	**81** 165	**85** 46	**94** 297	**96** 76	**54** 273	- -	- -
Providence Saint Joseph Medical Center, Burbank, CA	**97** 37	**99** 249	**98** 268	**95** 199	**98** 262	- 0	**75** 20	**96** 104	**97** 99	**63** 241	**99** 314	**96** 27	**72** 114	**91** 105	**81** 31	**77** 170	**100** 230	**69** 154	**91** 35	**92** 304	**81** 74	**47** 281	- -	- -
Queen of the Valley Hospital, Napa, CA	**76** 55	**94** 157	**95** 206	**85** 99	**96** 227	**100** 1	**100** 9	**98** 64	**75** 60	**46** 109	**93** 145	**100** 18	**98** 135	**92** 156	**87** 47	**89** 194	**100** 245	**98** 141	**100** 64	**77** 176	**95** 73	**57** 171	**0.56** 1062	**2.28** 745
Rancho Springs Medical Center, Murrieta, CA	**74** 23	**94** 222	**80** 84	**93** 167	**91** 90	**44** 39	- 0	**100** 18	**86** 146	**57** 391	**89** 389	**100** 54	**88** 259	**92** 182	**68** 68	**67** 321	**100** 384	**57** 247	**95** 65	**90** 798	**90** 175	**59** 744	- -	- -
Ranchos Los Amigos Nat'l Rehab Ctr, Downey, CA	- -	- -	- -	- -	- -	- -	- -	- -	**100** 6	**0** 3	**64** 22	- 0	- 0	- 0	- -	**100** 2	**100** 8	**0** 4	**0** 1	**50** 4	- -	**100** 4	- -	- -
Redbud Community Hospital, Clearlake, CA	- 0	**50** 4	**50** 2	**33** 3	**50** 2	- 0	- -	- 0	**69** 13	**24** 46	**71** 49	**56** 16	**83** 93	**91** 64	**27** 15	**69** 103	**100** 112	**17** 53	**54** 35	**63** 62	**100** 20	**59** 61	- -	- -
Redlands Community Hospital, Redlands, CA	**80** 30	**95** 163	**92** 88	**96** 114	**92** 91	**100** 1	- 0	**100** 1	**79** 110	**73** 45	**91** 265	**100** 7	**82** 22	**78** 49	- -	**75** 216	**100** 259	**67** 177	**100** 11	**84** 144	- -	**56** 140	**1.03** 583	**4.41** 431
Regional Medical Center of San Jose, San Jose, CA	**87** 23	**94** 169	**92** 138	**93** 89	**94** 124	**25** 4	**36** 14	**97** 36	**92** 113	**33** 353	**77** 429	**81** 54	**86** 292	**95** 346	**45** 100	**76** 417	**100** 483	**28** 349	**55** 53	**76** 127	**82** 56	**61** 114	- -	- -
Rideout Memorial Hospital, Marysville, CA	**64** 53	**99** 204	**94** 191	**90** 171	**86** 198	**33** 18	**0** 3	**83** 70	**84** 147	**13** 372	**84** 415	**61** 84	**73** 293	**86** 184	- -	**68** 353	**98** 400	**37** 279	**56** 126	**77** 269	**97** 68	**68** 237	- -	- -
Ridgecrest Regional Hospital, Ridgecrest, CA	**100** 1	**90** 21	**70** 10	**80** 15	**75** 8	**0** 3	- 0	**75** 4	**80** 25	**77** 74	**87** 82	**80** 15	**81** 97	**79** 24	- -	**68** 121	**100** 145	**59** 80	**63** 46	**47** 47	**61** 18	**76** 46	- -	- -
Riverside Community Hospital, Riverside, CA	**84** 85	**93** 245	**93** 358	**87** 218	**85** 346	**0** 1	**14** 14	**93** 116	**81** 193	**70** 439	**89** 542	**94** 107	**90** 261	**83** 308	**66** 90	**80** 523	**100** 618	**78** 321	**84** 116	**55** 284	**92** 136	**48** 255	- -	- -
Riverside County Regional Medical Center, Moreno Valley, CA	**80** 5	**97** 35	**67** 18	**81** 31	**82** 17	- 0	- 0	**100** 3	**91** 118	**55** 55	**91** 230	**63** 19	**90** 20	**78** 18	- -	**52** 109	**99** 138	**17** 36	**80** 5	**33** 52	- -	**84** 50	- -	- -
Saddleback Memorial Medical Center, Laguna Hills, CA	**96** 53	**95** 283	**96** 256	**93** 169	**97** 258	**40** 5	**46** 13	**100** 53	**94** 219	**82** 523	**96** 642	**96** 55	**90** 328	**95** 348	**92** 113	**90** 429	**100** 539	**84** 447	**97** 58	**90** 416	**93** 104	**75** 404	**0.21** 2890	**3.73** 1955
Saint Agnes Medical Center, Fresno, CA	**100** 71	**99** 299	**99** 352	**99** 198	**99** 365	- 0	**75** 12	**100** 84	**96** 158	**72** 357	**98** 430	**100** 54	**92** 159	**92** 213	**88** 56	**86** 318	**100** 378	**91** 253	**100** 55	**92** 477	**98** 151	**84** 458	- -	- -
Saint Bernardine Medical Center, San Bernardino, CA	**91** 45	**98** 101	**99** 273	**96** 50	**98** 248	**0** 2	**20** 5	**99** 76	**95** 91	**76** 275	**95** 310	**98** 55	**93** 85	**85** 72	**59** 17	**90** 115	**100** 147	**81** 77	**83** 29	**74** 239	**69** 80	**55** 235	- -	- -
Saint Elizabeth Community Hospital, Red Bluff, CA	**80** 5	**92** 40	**78** 23	**85** 39	**76** 25	**0** 1	- 0	**100** 7	**88** 17	**98** 65	**88** 67	**100** 13	**90** 152	**87** 89	**87** 30	**89** 168	**100** 200	**95** 121	**100** 48	**73** 168	**67** 54	**77** 164	**0.00** 721	**2.56** 507
Saint Francis Medical Center, Lynwood, CA	**93** 27	**98** 129	**96** 115	**95** 108	**96** 114	**39** 18	**0** 1	**97** 34	**91** 258	**62** 486	**97** 539	**98** 128	**94** 171	**96** 203	**70** 50	**59** 299	**100** 343	**64** 158	**91** 58	**87** 122	**76** 38	**57** 122	- -	- -
Saint Francis Memorial Hospital, San Francisco, CA	**100** 6	**100** 16	**82** 11	**100** 7	**100** 10	- 0	- 0	**100** 1	**100** 22	**84** 56	**97** 71	**100** 5	**82** 38	**95** 44	**75** 8	**91** 56	**100** 67	**89** 36	**100** 8	**97** 118	**85** 41	**72** 116	- -	- -
Saint Helena Hospital, Deer Park, CA	**94** 17	**100** 20	**100** 76	**100** 15	**97** 67	- 0	**50** 2	**100** 38	**83** 23	**90** 67	**98** 82	**95** 19	**96** 27	**100** 27	**36** 14	**93** 42	**100** 48	**50** 46	**100** 12	**95** 261	**97** 63	**80** 256	- -	- -
Saint John's Health Center, Santa Monica, CA	**84** 25	**99** 153	**94** 143	**91** 145	**94** 141	- 0	**33** 3	**93** 29	**91** 92	**44** 197	**81** 232	**38** 8	**78** 175	**90** 162	**2** 49	**72** 222	**100** 290	**29** 215	**71** 14	**71** 1293	**91** 355	**73** 1265	**0.22** 915	**6.13** 1288
Saint John's Pleasant Valley Hospital, Camarillo, CA	**62** 8	**94** 34	**86** 22	**96** 26	**100** 25	- 0	- 0	**75** 4	**94** 18	**67** 67	**100** 87	**100** 4	**86** 100	**90** 104	**66** 32	**72** 120	**99** 160	**56** 122	**53** 15	**72** 120	**100** 37	**36** 118	- -	- -
Saint John's Regional Medical Center, Oxnard, CA	**85** 40	**99** 203	**97** 222	**98** 189	**97** 227	- 0	**40** 5	**93** 46	**91** 92	**63** 299	**99** 342	**85** 26	**90** 187	**92** 207	**53** 43	**78** 268	**99** 326	**54** 227	**58** 43	**76** 207	**86** 65	**52** 203	- -	- -
Saint Joseph Hospital, Eureka, CA	**79** 24	**98** 54	**93** 105	**89** 53	**92** 102	- 0	**0** 2	**89** 37	**88** 41	**69** 101	**97** 106	**94** 33	**87** 93	**95** 96	**100** 25	**93** 115	**100** 147	**90** 81	**94** 49	**41** 256	**96** 128	**63** 252	- -	- -
Saint Joseph Hospital, Orange, CA	**93** 29	**100** 230	**96** 234	**98** 168	**98** 233	**100** 2	**83** 6	**100** 63	**93** 146	**63** 398	**97** 470	**97** 63	**81** 187	**96** 169	**85** 55	**88** 224	**100** 300	**79** 178	**95** 42	**82** 236	**97** 76	**81** 222	- -	- -
Saint Joseph's Medical Center of Stockton, Stockton, CA	**94** 48	**98** 185	**99** 270	**98** 122	**99** 261	**44** 9	**78** 9	**99** 106	**96** 119	**74** 216	**99** 296	**100** 43	**94** 126	**93** 114	**79** 24	**77** 154	**100** 186	**91** 118	**97** 35	**95** 189	**88** 64	**59** 185	- -	- -
Saint Jude Medical Center, Fullerton, CA	**81** 47	**98** 265	**97** 245	**96** 241	**97** 242	- 0	**71** 14	**97** 61	**88** 171	**95** 295	**98** 369	**100** 37	**85** 236	**92** 238	**96** 67	**81** 275	**100** 355	**86** 244	**82** 39	**93** 1253	**94** 302	**85** 1210	**0.13** 2255	**3.74** 1551
Saint Louisie Regional Hospital, Gilroy, CA	**75** 4	**98** 40	**69** 13	**89** 27	**92** 13	**50** 2	- 0	**100** 1	**66** 35	**98** 84	**76** 110	**92** 13	**88** 86	**86** 72	**80** 15	**84** 107	**100** 129	**53** 76	**83** 29	**86** 97	**84** 43	**69** 96	**0.14** 711	**3.89** 489
Saint Luke's Hospital, San Francisco, CA	**83** 6	**100** 43	**95** 22	**94** 34	**100** 25	- 0	- 0	**83** 6	**92** 75	**52** 160	**88** 191	**93** 44	**84** 116	**87** 108	**11** 27	**76** 148	**100** 169	**23** 102	**76** 46	**51** 136	**94** 33	**77** 128	**0.00** 255	**5.05** 376
Saint Mary Medical Center, Long Beach, CA	**86** 29	**96** 137	**97** 157	**96** 108	**94** 145	**0** 5	**50** 2	**94** 52	**84** 112	**91** 236	**91** 293	**92** 86	**84** 87	**90** 89	**33** 24	**80** 141	**100** 163	**36** 95	**96** 56	**67** 218	**90** 41	**57** 203	- -	- -
Saint Mary Medical Center, Apple Valley, CA	**72** 50	**98** 234	**91** 254	**93** 193	**76** 243	**29** 7	**60** 5	**98** 85	**76** 164	**60** 401	**75** 434	**95** 112	**87** 430	**90** 291	**44** 75	**78** 454	**99** 536	**72** 286	**82** 95	**82** 442	**90** 127	**59** 429	**0.49** 2855	**4.96** 2159

NOTE: The first number in each column (boldface) is the rate in percent, the second number is the number of patients; Please refer to the main entry for footnotes; ***Heart Attack Care:*** *1. ACE Inhibitor or ARB for LVSD; 2. Aspirin at Arrival; 3. Aspirin at Discharge; 4. Beta Blocker at Arrival; 5. Beta Blocker at Discharge; 6. Fibrinolytic Medication Timing; 7. PCI Within 90 Minutes of Arrival; 8. Smoking Cessation Advice;* ***Heart Failure Care:*** *9. ACE Inhibitor or ARB for LVSD; 10. Discharge Instructions; 11. Evaluation of LVS Function; 12. Smoking Cessation Advice;* ***Pneumonia Care:*** *13. Appropriate Initial Antibiotic; 14. Blood Culture Timing; 15. Influenza Vaccine; 16. Initial Antibiotic Timing; 17. Oxygenation Assessment; 18. Pneumococcal Vaccine; 19. Smoking Cessation Advice;* ***Surgical Infection Prevention:*** *20. Prophylactic Antibiotic Given; 21. Prophylactic Antibiotic Selection; 22. Prophylactic Antibiotic Stopped;* ***Pregnancy Care:*** *23. Inpatient Neonatal Mortality; 24. Third or Fourth Degree Laceration*

Hospital	Heart Attack Care								Heart Failure Care				Pneumonia Care							Surgical Infection Prevention			Pregnancy Care	
	1	2	3	4	5	6	7	8	9	10	11	12	13	14	15	16	17	18	19	20	21	22	23	24
Saint Mary's Medical Center, San Francisco, CA	**97** 32	**99** 88	**100** 133	**100** 73	**100** 141	- 0	**0** 3	**86** 29	**96** 78	**89** 151	**99** 199	**95** 22	**91** 116	**97** 147	**42** 36	**88** 184	**100** 229	**61** 162	**100** 31	**83** 173	**100** 55	**34** 166	- -	- -
Saint Rose Hospital, Hayward, CA	**90** 20	**97** 121	**91** 87	**90** 115	**93** 95	- 0	**47** 15	**92** 12	**81** 113	**70** 57	**86** 276	**100** 12	**72** 32	**82** 40	- -	**62** 200	**100** 216	**95** 130	**100** 5	**77** 39	- -	**100** 39	- -	- -
Saint Vincent Medical Center, Los Angeles, CA	**64** 25	**97** 79	**87** 113	**88** 74	**77** 118	- 0	- 0	**50** 20	**72** 109	**22** 289	**84** 361	**50** 36	**78** 159	**90** 184	**66** 59	**80** 306	**100** 357	**71** 256	**39** 31	**55** 289	**84** 57	**49** 269	- -	- -
Salinas Valley Memorial Health Care District, Salinas, CA	**92** 40	**95** 137	**100** 215	**97** 74	**99** 226	- 0	**100** 8	**94** 18	**88** 142	**86** 78	**92** 429	**100** 6	**85** 26	**89** 37	- -	**67** 280	**99** 296	**78** 206	**82** 11	**82** 221	- -	**72** 208	- -	- -
San Antonio Community Hospital, Upland, CA	**83** 54	**98** 227	**98** 219	**95** 153	**98** 209	**27** 11	**57** 7	**100** 70	**81** 207	**49** 380	**88** 487	**100** 70	**84** 338	**86** 306	**26** 92	**67** 427	**99** 551	**37** 331	**96** 89	**82** 694	**92** 241	**69** 680	**0.76** 2247	**3.46** 1302
San Diego Hospice & Palliative Care, San Diego, CA	- -	- -	- -	- -	- -	- -	- -	- -	- -	- -	- -	- -	- -	- -	- -	- -	- -	- -	- -	- -	- -	- -	- -	- -
San Dimas Community Hospital, San Dimas, CA	**100** 7	**100** 31	**100** 21	**78** 32	**82** 22	- 0	- 0	- 0	**74** 43	**78** 83	**92** 120	**92** 12	**87** 128	**90** 171	**96** 50	**90** 185	**100** 254	**92** 158	**100** 26	**90** 318	**96** 74	**44** 308	- -	- -
San Francisco General Medical Center, San Francisco, CA	**88** 16	**100** 101	**99** 67	**100** 87	**100** 63	**0** 1	**0** 4	**73** 26	**96** 200	**41** 280	**99** 294	**90** 122	**86** 174	**79** 176	**35** 26	**50** 244	**100** 271	**68** 62	**81** 128	**87** 121	**64** 36	**77** 113	- -	- -
San Gabriel Valley Medical Center, San Gabriel, CA	**95** 19	**98** 88	**89** 56	**95** 66	**98** 49	**0** 2	**25** 4	**86** 7	**87** 79	**73** 188	**94** 272	**94** 36	**82** 200	**90** 242	**44** 85	**78** 398	**100** 444	**68** 327	**95** 39	**59** 127	**82** 34	**40** 126	**0.33** 2142	**1.45** 1308
San Gorgonio Memorial Hospital, Banning, CA	**73** 15	**98** 81	**95** 44	**88** 80	**88** 50	- 0	- 0	**0** 1	**89** 37	**0** 23	**71** 164	**29** 7	**76** 41	**80** 44	- -	**85** 259	**99** 275	**2** 192	**62** 8	**11** 9	- -	**0** 7	**0.00** 415	**0.75** 266
San Joaquin Community Hospital, Bakersfield, CA	**69** 32	**99** 107	**91** 129	**89** 71	**89** 127	**100** 2	**75** 4	**94** 48	**92** 169	**71** 388	**90** 434	**97** 108	**89** 187	**96** 181	**100** 40	**79** 251	**100** 286	**84** 121	**97** 78	**63** 139	**94** 54	**52** 130	- -	- -
San Joaquin General Hospital, French Camp, CA	**100** 7	**99** 70	**100** 32	**96** 52	**100** 31	**67** 12	- 0	**77** 13	**98** 109	**74** 187	**100** 208	**83** 89	**91** 164	**77** 148	- -	**52** 221	**100** 241	**66** 82	**58** 101	**49** 136	**86** 29	**57** 120	**0.42** 3089	**3.04** 2139
San Leandro Hospital, San Leandro, CA	**88** 8	**98** 49	**97** 32	**100** 28	**95** 39	**0** 1	- 0	**100** 5	**87** 102	**62** 319	**89** 370	**100** 86	**94** 114	**92** 111	**69** 32	**74** 163	**100** 193	**77** 132	**94** 36	**86** 196	**100** 35	**75** 184	- -	- -
San Mateo Medical Center, San Mateo, CA	- 0	**100** 16	**100** 6	**100** 16	**100** 9	- 0	- 0	**100** 4	**100** 33	**100** 59	**100** 68	**100** 28	**77** 43	**85** 40	**89** 9	**87** 55	**100** 66	**92** 26	**100** 12	**85** 92	**91** 23	**79** 90	- -	- -
San Rafael Medical Center, San Rafael, CA	**90** 10	**99** 82	**93** 45	**99** 76	**100** 56	**67** 6	**40** 5	**100** 9	**98** 49	**75** 156	**97** 173	**82** 11	**97** 135	**91** 169	**92** 61	**82** 210	**100** 249	**96** 189	**89** 38	**85** 522	**95** 131	**82** 519	- -	- -
San Ramon Regional Medical Center, San Ramon, CA	**50** 6	**98** 60	**95** 60	**98** 58	**91** 55	- 0	**80** 5	**100** 16	**88** 33	**82** 80	**97** 106	**100** 8	**97** 118	**98** 54	**77** 35	**89** 115	**100** 143	**95** 112	**82** 17	**88** 325	**100** 79	**52** 313	- -	- -
Santa Barbara Cottage Hospital, Santa Barbara, CA	**70** 47	**94** 157	**96** 229	**89** 116	**90** 212	- 0	**71** 14	**98** 55	**77** 147	**47** 310	**88** 382	**73** 52	**82** 191	**92** 185	**54** 72	**80** 256	**100** 338	**59** 234	**54** 57	**52** 254	**96** 81	**29** 242	- -	- -
Santa Clara Valley Medical Center, San Jose, CA	**79** 14	**98** 131	**95** 134	**91** 122	**95** 137	**0** 1	**67** 9	**80** 50	**69** 172	**40** 308	**96** 329	**77** 112	**69** 245	**79** 201	- -	**56** 217	**99** 337	**18** 138	**47** 122	**85** 422	**72** 101	**86** 410	**0.43** 6066	**3.85** 4627
Santa Monica-UCLA Medical Center, Santa Monica, CA	**95** 21	**100** 109	**99** 103	**100** 97	**98** 103	- 0	**0** 3	**82** 17	**81** 68	**24** 176	**95** 247	**71** 24	**77** 74	**98** 109	**34** 32	**76** 160	**100** 186	**13** 134	**53** 19	**93** 285	**91** 46	**38** 276	**0.81** 369	**4.61** 781
Santa Rosa Memorial Hospital, Santa Rosa, CA	**83** 24	**97** 101	**99** 119	**94** 86	**97** 120	- 0	**100** 6	**95** 22	**89** 98	**75** 223	**96** 255	**97** 37	**72** 213	**87** 171	**63** 46	**82** 268	**98** 324	**65** 195	**84** 64	**58** 186	**82** 57	**54** 174	- -	- -
Santa Ynez Valley Cottage Hospital, Solvang, CA	- 0	- 0	- 0	- 0	- 0	- 0	- 0	- 0	**60** 5	**58** 19	**61** 23	**50** 2	**90** 20	**93** 15	**50** 6	**80** 25	**100** 32	**68** 25	**50** 2	- -	- -	- -	- -	- -
Scripps Green Hospital, La Jolla, CA	**100** 22	**100** 66	**99** 181	**100** 60	**98** 167	- 0	**33** 3	**91** 35	**92** 107	**83** 247	**100** 278	**93** 29	**94** 63	**100** 23	**86** 44	**84** 88	**100** 114	**84** 126	**94** 18	**93** 259	**88** 74	**79** 256	- -	- -
Scripps Memorial Hospital La Jolla, La Jolla, CA	**80** 49	**98** 101	**98** 286	**99** 73	**96** 280	**67** 3	**71** 7	**94** 71	**81** 119	**58** 224	**92** 270	**97** 31	**91** 91	**90** 107	**53** 34	**84** 140	**100** 176	**54** 122	**78** 27	**93** 241	**99** 78	**73** 232	**0.05** 3806	**6.04** 2534
Scripps Memorial Hospital-Encinitas, Encinitas, CA	**100** 16	**99** 116	**97** 99	**92** 71	**84** 93	**0** 2	**29** 7	**95** 21	**68** 59	**24** 120	**98** 170	**73** 11	**90** 126	**95** 144	**50** 40	**77** 145	**100** 205	**52** 130	**68** 28	**86** 94	**98** 50	**44** 91	**0.00** 1530	**3.42** 1228
Scripps Mercy Hospital, San Diego, CA	**95** 55	**100** 336	**98** 307	**99** 278	**97** 313	**0** 4	**77** 22	**95** 87	**86** 287	**69** 740	**89** 860	**92** 145	**70** 406	**88** 400	**11** 132	**63** 552	**100** 685	**22** 402	**77** 146	**79** 155	**91** 80	**57** 148	**0.07** 4352	**3.49** 2984
Seneca Hospital, Chester, CA	- -	- -	- -	- -	- -	- -	- -	- -	**100** 1	**0** 4	**0** 17	**0** 1	**67** 3	**50** 2	- -	**85** 20	**100** 32	**14** 21	**50** 2	- -	- -	- -	- -	- -
Sequoia Hospital, Redwood City, CA	**95** 21	**99** 82	**99** 79	**96** 51	**97** 73	- 0	**100** 4	**100** 13	**91** 95	**98** 262	**99** 285	**100** 17	**94** 67	**96** 71	**86** 29	**93** 92	**100** 119	**86** 98	**40** 10	**88** 248	**78** 86	**79** 244	**0.00** 1088	**3.30** 817
Seton Medical Center, Daly City, CA	**97** 30	**97** 127	**99** 130	**96** 107	**98** 122	- 0	**89** 9	**100** 8	**86** 151	**100** 71	**96** 431	**100** 6	**87** 23	**84** 32	- -	**86** 209	**100** 243	**41** 193	**100** 3	**77** 53	- -	**59** 51	- -	- -
Sharp Chula Vista Medical Center, Chula Vista, CA	**73** 66	**97** 279	**91** 284	**93** 243	**88** 280	**0** 2	**50** 10	**72** 57	**65** 179	**69** 478	**87** 574	**84** 56	**84** 270	**82** 283	**33** 67	**71** 390	**100** 468	**22** 278	**70** 54	**77** 222	**78** 64	**74** 208	- -	- -
Sharp Coronado Hospital, San Diego, CA	**100** 2	**100** 16	**100** 5	**100** 14	**100** 7	**33** 3	- 0	**100** 1	**100** 7	**54** 63	**74** 74	**75** 4	**81** 70	**92** 50	**55** 22	**93** 84	**100** 104	**52** 82	**95** 19	**94** 96	**89** 28	**87** 94	- -	- -
Sharp Mary Birch Hospital for Women, San Diego, CA	- -	- -	- -	- -	- -	- -	- -	- -	- -	- -	- -	- -	- -	- -	- -	- -	- -	- -	- -	**83** 35	- -	**94** 35	**0.46** 8388	**4.59** 5165
Sharp Memorial Hospital, San Diego, CA	**91** 56	**99** 275	**100** 298	**98** 196	**99** 307	**0** 2	**70** 10	**100** 61	**84** 161	**63** 365	**90** 454	**95** 42	**78** 235	**91** 216	**52** 69	**60** 308	**100** 366	**41** 237	**89** 55	**87** 461	**91** 172	**76** 449	- -	- -
Shasta Regional Medical Center, Redding, CA	**94** 32	**99** 94	**97** 114	**97** 69	**96** 111	**50** 4	**25** 4	**98** 47	**90** 98	**66** 176	**95** 216	**100** 61	**89** 232	**90** 229	**82** 65	**81** 313	**100** 381	**80** 241	**95** 153	**92** 736	**94** 189	**87** 714	- -	- -
Sherman Oaks Hospital, Sherman Oaks, CA	- 0	**100** 14	**100** 6	**100** 12	**100** 7	- 0	- 0	**100** 1	**100** 7	**100** 32	**99** 72	**100** 4	**100** 14	**92** 26	- -	**98** 43	**100** 56	**91** 32	**100** 3	**94** 17	- -	**82** 17	- -	- -
Sierra Kings District Hospital, Reedley, CA	- 0	**100** 1	**0** 1	**0** 1	**100** 1	- 0	- -	- -	**100** 1	**0** 1	**0** 25	- 0	**100** 8	**75** 8	- -	**83** 109	**100** 128	**53** 85	**100** 1	**100** 7	- -	**100** 7	**0.00** 1118	**2.61** 690
Sierra Nevada Memorial Hospital, Grass Valley, CA	**100** 2	**100** 45	**100** 26	**100** 42	**93** 28	**50** 2	- 0	**100** 3	**93** 73	**77** 112	**90** 157	**76** 21	**92** 251	**90** 191	**80** 56	**87** 276	**99** 333	**80** 254	**85** 74	**99** 174	**95** 57	**69** 170	- -	- -
Sierra View District Hospital, Porterville, CA	**91** 11	**95** 80	**93** 44	**73** 64	**95** 40	**50** 16	- 0	**100** 17	**94** 47	**73** 174	**67** 227	**92** 36	**79** 160	**84** 160	**65** 60	**63** 240	**100** 317	**66** 169	**93** 57	**53** 130	**98** 63	**39** 113	- -	- -
Sierra Vista Regional Medical Center, San Luis Obispo, CA	**95** 20	**97** 60	**96** 100	**98** 53	**95** 94	**0** 1	**40** 5	**97** 31	**90** 29	**91** 64	**91** 78	**92** 12	**85** 85	**96** 79	**85** 26	**86** 85	**100** 124	**70** 79	**84** 19	**75** 241	**98** 57	**71** 232	- -	- -
Simi Valley Hospital, Simi Valley, CA	**60** 5	**82** 49	**75** 8	**86** 36	**83** 12	**80** 5	- 0	**100** 2	**76** 38	**20** 90	**84** 133	**93** 15	**90** 105	**87** 107	**65** 34	**84** 122	**100** 185	**65** 106	**97** 35	**80** 193	**71** 38	**41** 187	- -	- -
Sonoma Developmental Center, Eldridge, CA	- -	- -	- -	- -	- -	- -	- -	- -	**0** 3	- 0	**100** 4	- 0	- 0	- 0	- -	**100** 4	**100** 9	**100** 2	- 0	- -	- -	- -	- -	- -
Sonoma Valley Hospital, Sonoma, CA	**100** 2	**88** 8	**83** 6	**25** 4	**100** 6	- 0	- 0	- 0	**71** 17	**25** 32	**92** 53	**89** 9	**94** 34	**97** 33	**47** 15	**82** 44	**100** 58	**24** 49	**80** 10	**86** 91	**95** 20	**58** 88	- -	- -
Sonora Regional Medical Center, Sonora, CA	**80** 5	**94** 47	**70** 20	**90** 29	**79** 24	**57** 7	- 0	**100** 9	**78** 23	**70** 80	**84** 93	**50** 4	**92** 113	**93** 74	**88** 24	**90** 149	**100** 172	**80** 140	**85** 39	**85** 271	**98** 85	**89** 262	- -	- -
South Coast Medical Center, Laguna Beach, CA	**75** 4	**100** 25	**100** 10	**93** 14	**100** 11	**0** 1	- 0	**100** 1	**87** 23	**79** 85	**97** 90	**80** 10	**82** 66	**87** 47	**64** 11	**88** 81	**100** 95	**70** 64	**65** 17	**79** 71	**89** 28	**69** 32	**0.00** 716	**3.36** 506
S San Francisco Medical Center, S San Francisco, CA	**86** 14	**98** 123	**97** 38	**100** 83	**100** 39	**88** 17	- 0	**100** 2	**90** 70	**64** 210	**99** 232	**77** 48	**81** 108	**94** 112	**64** 25	**84** 142	**100** 179	**90** 134	**45** 22	**97** 282	**95** 58	**89** 274	- -	- -
Southern Inyo Healthcare District, Lone Pine, CA	- -	- -	- -	- -	- -	- -	- -	- -	- -	- -	- -	- -	- -	- -	- -	- -	- -	- -	- -	- -	- -	- -	- -	- -
Stanford Hospital, Stanford, CA	**86** 37	**99** 158	**99** 215	**96** 115	**98** 185	- 0	**33** 6	**94** 33	**87** 150	**83** 288	**99** 339	**72** 25	**80** 178	**95** 199	**89** 47	**68** 259	**100** 351	**80** 223	**83** 29	**79** 110	**99** 68	**67** 102	- -	- -
Stanislaus Surgical Hospital, Modesto, CA	- -	- -	- -	- -	- -	- -	- -	- -	- -	- -	- -	- -	- -	- -	- -	- -	- -	- -	- -	**77** 35	- -	**74** 35	- -	- -
Surprise Valley Healthcare District, Cedarville, CA	- -	- -	- -	- -	- -	- -	- -	- -	- -	- -	- -	- -	- 0	**100** 1	- -	**100** 1	**100** 1	**100** 1	- 0	- -	- -	- -	- -	- -

NOTE: The first number in each column (boldface) is the rate in percent, the second number is the number of patients; Please refer to the main entry for footnotes; ***Heart Attack Care:*** *1. ACE Inhibitor or ARB for LVSD; 2. Aspirin at Arrival; 3. Aspirin at Discharge; 4. Beta Blocker at Arrival; 5. Beta Blocker at Discharge; 6. Fibrinolytic Medication Timing; 7. PCI Within 90 Minutes of Arrival; 8. Smoking Cessation Advice;* ***Heart Failure Care:*** *9. ACE Inhibitor or ARB for LVSD; 10. Discharge Instructions; 11. Evaluation of LVS Function; 12. Smoking Cessation Advice;* ***Pneumonia Care:*** *13. Appropriate Initial Antibiotic; 14. Blood Culture Timing; 15. Influenza Vaccine; 16. Initial Antibiotic Timing; 17. Oxygenation Assessment; 18. Pneumococcal Vaccine; 19. Smoking Cessation Advice;* ***Surgical Infection Prevention:*** *20. Prophylactic Antibiotic Given; 21. Prophylactic Antibiotic Selection; 22. Prophylactic Antibiotic Stopped;* ***Pregnancy Care:*** *23. Inpatient Neonatal Mortality; 24. Third or Fourth Degree Laceration*

Hospital	Heart Attack Care								Heart Failure Care				Pneumonia Care							Surgical Infection Prevention			Pregnancy Care	
	1	2	3	4	5	6	7	8	9	10	11	12	13	14	15	16	17	18	19	20	21	22	23	24
Sutter Amador Hospital, Jackson, CA	**40** 5	**80** 15	**86** 7	**100** 11	**100** 8	- 0	- 0	**100** 1	**68** 34	**30** 66	**63** 89	**80** 20	**76** 85	**90** 68	**0** 21	**96** 99	**100** 116	**31** 70	**75** 24	**71** 138	**100** 37	**57** 137	- -	- -
Sutter Auburn Faith Hospital, Auburn, CA	**100** 2	**100** 22	**90** 10	**100** 15	**100** 9	**75** 4	- 0	- 0	**98** 45	**89** 123	**99** 163	**100** 32	**94** 104	**99** 89	**74** 27	**90** 145	**100** 170	**93** 108	**100** 35	**83** 202	**88** 52	**81** 194	- -	- -
Sutter Coast Hospital, Crescent City, CA	- 0	**93** 14	**100** 6	**100** 7	**100** 6	**0** 1	- 0	**100** 2	**82** 34	**68** 91	**86** 86	**100** 21	**84** 76	**90** 78	**52** 21	**84** 105	**100** 124	**80** 69	**100** 47	**55** 62	**55** 11	**46** 61	**0.27** 376	**3.19** 282
Sutter Davis Hospital, Davis, CA	- 0	**100** 7	**100** 5	**100** 6	**100** 4	**100** 1	- 0	- 0	**87** 15	**74** 47	**94** 65	**89** 9	**95** 118	**90** 96	**93** 29	**90** 136	**100** 173	**96** 104	**88** 32	**84** 218	**87** 47	**84** 203	**0.13** 752	**2.47** 730
Sutter Delta Medical Center, Antioch, CA	**95** 19	**94** 154	**84** 73	**91** 148	**94** 81	**34** 32	- 0	**100** 22	**88** 78	**88** 253	**80** 300	**98** 61	**73** 134	**79** 111	**13** 23	**70** 162	**100** 195	**38** 94	**93** 41	**49** 150	**94** 34	**72** 131	- -	- -
Sutter General Hospital, Sacramento, CA	**91** 87	**98** 205	**98** 501	**93** 183	**98** 492	**50** 4	**0** 1	**99** 152	**94** 124	**85** 248	**99** 300	**100** 53	**90** 111	**90** 135	- -	**81** 180	**100** 207	**78** 130	**98** 50	**83** 370	**80** 88	**72** 356	- -	- -
Sutter Lakeside Hospital, Lakeport, CA	**100** 2	**95** 19	**89** 9	**89** 18	**88** 8	**0** 2	- 0	**67** 3	**80** 15	**81** 31	**95** 39	**73** 11	**76** 100	**93** 61	- -	**82** 107	**99** 131	**39** 89	**78** 27	**58** 189	**94** 53	**64** 182	- -	- -
Sutter Maternity and Surgery Center, Santa Cruz, CA	- -	- -	- -	- -	- -	- -	- -	- -	- 0	- 0	**0** 1	- 0	**80** 5	**100** 2	**100** 1	**25** 4	**100** 5	**50** 2	**100** 1	**68** 222	**89** 37	**84** 218	**0.00** 874	**5.81** 689
Sutter Medical Center of Santa Rosa, Santa Rosa, CA	**91** 53	**97** 70	**99** 177	**100** 65	**96** 171	- 0	**25** 4	**98** 58	**87** 97	**70** 183	**84** 208	**81** 43	**78** 126	**89** 89	**6** 32	**67** 120	**100** 156	**23** 75	**73** 56	**67** 507	**71** 122	**61** 473	**0.37** 818	**4.00** 826
Sutter Roseville Medical Center, Roseville, CA	**85** 33	**99** 201	**95** 129	**97** 159	**99** 139	**75** 20	**100** 1	**97** 31	**80** 94	**84** 222	**95** 279	**94** 32	**86** 119	**87** 97	**87** 31	**70** 159	**100** 200	**82** 142	**98** 43	**92** 228	**96** 52	**86** 224	**0.05** 2046	**1.74** 1554
Sutter Solano Medical Center, Vallejo, CA	**44** 9	**91** 69	**53** 34	**86** 63	**59** 32	**33** 12	- 0	**70** 10	**81** 80	**71** 313	**82** 328	**79** 106	**86** 96	**78** 55	**53** 30	**63** 131	**100** 167	**68** 73	**89** 53	**58** 182	**90** 10	**78** 169	- -	- -
Sutter Tracy Community Hospital, Tracy, CA	**100** 3	**96** 24	**100** 8	**95** 20	**100** 9	- 0	- 0	**100** 1	**100** 26	**72** 100	**93** 115	**91** 22	**81** 106	**93** 57	**63** 38	**82** 101	**100** 146	**61** 75	**84** 25	**82** 130	**100** 29	**60** 123	- -	- -
Tahoe Forest Hospital, Truckee, CA	- 0	**100** 3	**100** 1	**100** 3	**100** 1	**100** 1	- 0	- 0	**89** 9	**0** 6	**65** 26	- 0	**67** 6	**100** 3	- -	**91** 11	**97** 29	**21** 19	**0** 2	- -	- -	- -	- -	- -
Tehachapi Valley Healthcare District, Tehachapi, CA	- -	- -	- -	- -	- -	- -	- -	- -	- 0	**0** 1	**0** 1	- 0	**92** 12	**50** 2	- 0	**100** 9	**100** 13	**14** 7	**0** 1	- -	- -	- -	- -	- -
Temple Community Hospital, Los Angeles, CA	**100** 2	**100** 33	**100** 31	**100** 27	**100** 34	- 0	- 0	- 0	**100** 13	**100** 24	**98** 93	**100** 4	**100** 3	- 0	- -	**55** 53	**100** 75	**100** 48	**100** 4	**100** 4	- -	**25** 4	- -	- -
Thousand Oaks Surgical Hospital, Thousand Oaks, CA	- -	- -	- -	- -	- -	- -	- -	- -	- -	- -	- -	- -	- -	- -	- -	- -	- -	- -	- -	**56** 55	**91** 44	**87** 53	- -	- -
Torrance Memorial Medical Center, Torrance, CA	**76** 58	**98** 296	**93** 287	**88** 252	**92** 283	**0** 1	**82** 17	**91** 55	**83** 279	**76** 467	**97** 600	**89** 63	**86** 201	**93** 181	**5** 86	**83** 299	**100** 394	**37** 282	**67** 48	**91** 225	**93** 81	**75** 225	- -	- -
Tri-City Medical Center, Oceanside, CA	**81** 32	**97** 233	**95** 198	**97** 157	**97** 184	**25** 8	**50** 12	**100** 34	**79** 144	**81** 339	**93** 432	**98** 47	**91** 309	**86** 325	**78** 85	**83** 387	**100** 506	**70** 331	**95** 85	**86** 146	**94** 70	**85** 133	**0.26** 1948	**3.29** 1400
Tri-City Regional Medical Center, Hawaiian Gardens, CA	**75** 4	**80** 10	**86** 7	**57** 7	**67** 6	**100** 1	- 0	**50** 2	**62** 21	**58** 64	**87** 165	**92** 25	**66** 44	**84** 77	- -	**75** 145	**99** 178	**39** 116	**96** 25	**25** 16	**86** 7	**38** 8	- -	- -
Tulare District Hospital, Tulare, CA	**100** 4	**100** 55	**100** 19	**94** 50	**95** 21	**50** 2	- 0	**100** 10	**97** 59	**81** 124	**99** 144	**100** 21	**88** 128	**95** 74	**83** 36	**76** 158	**100** 197	**88** 113	**94** 35	**77** 35	**100** 35	**91** 35	**0.30** 1005	**3.27** 611
Tuolumne General Hospital, Sonora, CA	**100** 3	**90** 10	**100** 7	**70** 10	**75** 8	- 0	- 0	- 0	**92** 12	**0** 9	**56** 36	- 0	**62** 8	**100** 4	- -	**90** 72	**99** 80	**9** 47	**50** 2	- -	- -	- -	- -	- -
Tustin Hospital and Medical Center, Tustin, CA	- 0	**100** 1	- 0	**100** 1	- 0	- -	- -	- -	**100** 2	**0** 2	**40** 10	**100** 2	**33** 3	**100** 4	- -	**58** 26	**100** 41	**14** 7	**33** 3	- -	- -	- -	- -	- -
Twin Cities Community Hospital, Templeton, CA	**80** 5	**97** 35	**95** 19	**88** 33	**90** 20	- 0	- 0	- 0	**83** 41	**93** 123	**97** 142	**100** 10	**90** 100	**94** 100	**100** 30	**90** 153	**99** 176	**98** 130	**94** 35	**83** 375	**93** 86	**91** 351	- -	- -
UCLA Medical Center, Los Angeles, CA	**78** 36	**99** 103	**99** 77	**100** 57	**97** 108	- 0	**0** 2	**90** 20	**85** 194	**52** 314	**99** 326	**92** 50	**91** 77	**87** 85	**26** 23	**61** 115	**100** 201	**24** 105	**77** 26	**93** 387	**62** 55	**50** 367	- -	- -
UCSF Medical Center, San Francisco, CA	**72** 18	**99** 138	**99** 149	**96** 96	**98** 158	- 0	**50** 4	**85** 34	**82** 136	**63** 292	**99** 318	**69** 59	**94** 94	**90** 141	**52** 29	**65** 153	**100** 208	**81** 106	**82** 39	**83** 533	**99** 81	**86** 466	- -	- -
Ukiah Valley Medical Center, Ukiah, CA	- 0	**100** 24	**100** 8	**85** 20	**75** 8	**33** 3	- 0	**100** 3	**96** 26	**69** 70	**77** 84	**86** 14	**88** 102	**84** 32	**76** 25	**85** 128	**100** 150	**91** 91	**62** 37	**65** 173	**92** 40	**65** 170	- -	- -
University of California Davis Health System, Sacramento, CA	**75** 67	**98** 191	**99** 220	**95** 151	**98** 247	- 0	**44** 9	**96** 97	**77** 188	**46** 308	**99** 329	**95** 101	**85** 105	**86** 112	**74** 27	**55** 169	**100** 200	**69** 90	**92** 73	**94** 536	**87** 75	**73** 491	**1.29** 622	**3.70** 1893
University of California Irvine Med Ctr, Orange, CA	**84** 25	**100** 62	**94** 63	**98** 46	**97** 61	- 0	**50** 4	**96** 27	**88** 136	**68** 255	**98** 265	**100** 69	**71** 76	**93** 96	**36** 28	**59** 151	**100** 179	**41** 66	**100** 36	**75** 438	**91** 126	**68** 430	**2.64** 1667	**3.15** 1017
University of California San Diego Med Ctr, San Diego, CA	**63** 19	**100** 161	**100** 208	**100** 131	**99** 199	- 0	**67** 3	**98** 53	**88** 152	**60** 270	**96** 305	**96** 77	**68** 141	**95** 153	**34** 29	**65** 192	**100** 248	**56** 85	**97** 72	**81** 336	**89** 65	**53** 318	- -	- -
USC University Hospital, Los Angeles, CA	**80** 10	**100** 5	**100** 31	**100** 4	**85** 27	- 0	- 0	**80** 5	**91** 34	**45** 65	**100** 72	**67** 3	**75** 20	**100** 2	**75** 4	**67** 18	**97** 30	**79** 24	**33** 3	**53** 304	**91** 69	**26** 300	- -	- -
VacaValley Hospital, Vacaville, CA	**60** 5	**93** 55	**94** 17	**88** 42	**100** 18	**42** 12	- 0	**83** 6	**79** 39	**50** 107	**92** 120	**92** 25	**93** 138	**94** 160	**39** 31	**89** 186	**100** 221	**61** 141	**92** 50	**80** 86	**100** 18	**71** 85	- -	- -
Valley Presbyterian Hospital, Van Nuys, CA	**76** 34	**97** 119	**95** 138	**94** 79	**96** 142	- 0	**43** 7	**80** 15	**71** 52	**0** 43	**88** 214	**64** 11	**90** 10	**88** 32	- -	**59** 199	**100** 236	**15** 141	**50** 2	**35** 95	- -	**41** 94	- -	- -
Valleycare Medical Center, Livermore, CA	**83** 6	**98** 126	**95** 94	**96** 112	**97** 97	- 0	**83** 6	**94** 18	**86** 66	**58** 158	**84** 202	**83** 23	**81** 141	**91** 124	**79** 43	**82** 195	**100** 220	**90** 129	**30** 30	**87** 292	**97** 110	**62** 279	- -	- -
Ventura County Medical Center, Ventura, CA	**100** 7	**100** 25	**100** 19	**95** 19	**100** 17	- 0	- 0	**100** 6	**100** 39	**93** 88	**98** 102	**100** 17	**86** 87	**90** 71	**64** 14	**81** 73	**100** 105	**69** 39	**96** 28	**76** 17	**100** 16	**62** 16	**0.18** 3315	**2.82** 2412
Verdugo Hills Hospital, Glendale, CA	**50** 12	**92** 66	**84** 31	**79** 61	**79** 34	**0** 1	- 0	**75** 4	**63** 49	**34** 107	**76** 161	**29** 21	**68** 167	**83** 104	**7** 28	**66** 177	**93** 205	**9** 148	**60** 30	**78** 117	**60** 10	**47** 108	- -	- -
Veterans Home of California, Yountville, CA	- 0	**100** 1	**100** 1	**100** 1	**0** 1	- 0	- -	- 0	- 0	- 0	**0** 6	- 0	**92** 13	**100** 1	**75** 4	**94** 17	**100** 20	**94** 18	**75** 4	- -	- -	- -	- -	- -
Victor Valley Community Hospital, Victorville, CA	**67** 6	**81** 63	**55** 40	**64** 64	**49** 43	- 0	- 0	- 0	**66** 35	**35** 23	**57** 171	**56** 9	**100** 12	**77** 13	- -	**49** 168	**99** 201	**21** 107	**60** 5	**47** 38	- -	**66** 29	- -	- -
Washington Hospital, Fremont, CA	**88** 32	**97** 207	**94** 216	**87** 179	**86** 219	- 0	**93** 14	**96** 55	**73** 81	**54** 275	**83** 298	**88** 50	**85** 123	**87** 105	**72** 29	**76** 152	**100** 198	**66** 131	**88** 26	**81** 70	**84** 70	**80** 69	- -	- -
Watsonville Community Hospital, Watsonville, CA	**0** 2	**97** 30	**91** 22	**86** 21	**85** 20	**100** 2	- 0	**100** 3	**75** 36	**78** 156	**72** 177	**63** 27	**76** 110	**96** 92	**43** 30	**69** 151	**100** 163	**32** 100	**71** 24	**72** 126	**89** 35	**79** 112	- -	- -
West Anaheim Medical Center, Anaheim, CA	**79** 24	**93** 98	**84** 101	**86** 88	**83** 105	**30** 10	- 0	**89** 38	**77** 69	**79** 185	**89** 249	**97** 37	**65** 148	**93** 115	**0** 60	**81** 204	**98** 259	**13** 157	**100** 33	**79** 84	**81** 16	**87** 82	- -	- -
West Hills Hospital and Medical Center, West Hills, CA	**82** 17	**95** 92	**90** 91	**93** 75	**95** 88	**33** 6	**20** 5	**94** 17	**90** 49	**26** 138	**78** 201	**79** 14	**66** 210	**94** 264	**61** 80	**73** 339	**99** 446	**49** 292	**92** 36	**80** 211	**91** 95	**48** 204	- -	- -
Western Medical Center, Santa Ana, CA	**96** 26	**100** 86	**99** 176	**96** 79	**98** 170	- 0	**67** 6	**79** 47	**93** 101	**64** 222	**84** 283	**64** 47	**82** 101	**89** 89	**62** 29	**84** 129	**99** 168	**59** 111	**44** 18	**70** 33	**65** 34	**56** 32	- -	- -
Western Medical Center Hospital Anaheim, Anaheim, CA	**50** 14	**91** 34	**87** 132	**92** 26	**84** 126	**50** 2	- 0	**95** 39	**80** 20	**77** 35	**95** 59	**100** 13	**86** 36	**88** 57	**76** 17	**89** 85	**100** 99	**92** 59	**88** 17	**61** 18	**94** 18	**44** 18	- -	- -
White Memorial Medical Center, Los Angeles, CA	**54** 26	**94** 95	**92** 85	**85** 54	**93** 82	- 0	**100** 2	**94** 33	**76** 175	**71** 69	**94** 416	**100** 45	**94** 135	**92** 185	- -	**71** 284	**100** 325	**48** 220	**93** 57	**88** 50	- -	**78** 41	**0.50** 3828	**6.25** 2319
Whittier Hospital Medical Center, Whittier, CA	**67** 6	**98** 122	**89** 38	**91** 101	**90** 50	**38** 16	- 0	**100** 9	**92** 52	**95** 182	**96** 251	**96** 23	**88** 191	**93** 219	**79** 66	**77** 292	**100** 353	**78** 229	**96** 26	**88** 272	**83** 69	**38** 266	- -	- -
Woodland Healthcare, Woodland, CA	**100** 1	**100** 21	**71** 7	**100** 20	**100** 6	**40** 5	- 0	**0** 1	**94** 34	**81** 81	**97** 99	**100** 16	**81** 62	**97** 65	**62** 24	**91** 88	**100** 104	**91** 65	**76** 21	**82** 117	**96** 46	**91** 113	**0.13** 771	**1.41** 566
COLORADO																								
Animas Surgical Hospital, Durango, CO	- -	- -	- -	- -	- -	- -	- -	- -	- -	- -	- -	- -	- -	- -	- -	- -	- -	- -	- -	**92** 25	- -	**56** 25	- -	- -

NOTE: The first number in each column (boldface) is the rate in percent, the second number is the number of patients; Please refer to the main entry for footnotes; ***Heart Attack Care:*** *1. ACE Inhibitor or ARB for LVSD; 2. Aspirin at Arrival; 3. Aspirin at Discharge; 4. Beta Blocker at Arrival; 5. Beta Blocker at Discharge; 6. Fibrinolytic Medication Timing; 7. PCI Within 90 Minutes of Arrival; 8. Smoking Cessation Advice;* ***Heart Failure Care:*** *9. ACE Inhibitor or ARB for LVSD; 10. Discharge Instructions; 11. Evaluation of LVS Function; 12. Smoking Cessation Advice;* ***Pneumonia Care:*** *13. Appropriate Initial Antibiotic; 14. Blood Culture Timing; 15. Influenza Vaccine; 16. Initial Antibiotic Timing; 17. Oxygenation Assessment; 18. Pneumococcal Vaccine; 19. Smoking Cessation Advice;* ***Surgical Infection Prevention:*** *20. Prophylactic Antibiotic Given; 21. Prophylactic Antibiotic Selection; 22. Prophylactic Antibiotic Stopped;* ***Pregnancy Care:*** *23. Inpatient Neonatal Mortality; 24. Third or Fourth Degree Laceration*

Hospital	Heart Attack Care								Heart Failure Care				Pneumonia Care							Surgical Infection Prevention			Pregnancy Care	
	1	2	3	4	5	6	7	8	9	10	11	12	13	14	15	16	17	18	19	20	21	22	23	24
Arkansas Valley Regional Medical Center, La Junta, CO	- 0	100 14	100 3	82 17	71 7	33 3	- 0	100 1	86 14	49 51	69 70	64 11	86 117	92 74	64 44	84 146	99 175	69 116	86 37	62 13	67 3	91 11	- -	- -
Aspen Valley Hospital, Aspen, CO	100 2	100 6	100 5	100 5	100 4	- 0	- 0	0 1	- 0	9 11	100 12	0 1	100 19	94 16	- -	74 19	100 27	38 16	0 1	- -	- -	- -	- -	- -
Avista Adventist Hospital, Louisville, CO	100 6	100 26	96 23	95 21	86 22	- 0	0 2	100 4	43 7	26 23	77 26	50 2	81 58	91 45	70 20	88 66	100 88	75 48	79 19	85 158	100 48	88 155	0.00 2645	4.84 2003
Boulder Community Hospital, Boulder, CO	82 17	100 69	100 88	95 66	97 87	- 0	60 5	100 21	73 71	46 127	89 158	95 22	81 101	96 83	- -	77 145	100 191	68 114	94 31	80 246	94 65	47 231	- -	- -
Colorado Mental Health Institute-Pueblo, Pueblo, CO	- -	- -	- -	- -	- -	- -	- -	- -	- -	- -	- -	- -	- -	- -	- -	- -	- -	- -	- -	- -	- -	- -	- -	- -
Colorado Plains Medical Center, Fort Morgan, CO	- 0	88 8	67 3	75 4	0 1	0 1	- 0	100 1	86 14	62 26	76 41	86 7	87 61	88 60	- -	92 99	100 110	76 84	70 20	89 83	100 23	36 80	- -	- -
Community Hospital, Grand Junction, CO	100 1	85 13	100 7	91 11	86 7	- 0	- 0	50 2	89 9	82 34	81 48	88 8	90 39	84 31	92 13	79 48	100 55	92 36	86 14	87 134	91 46	77 133	- -	- -
Delta County Memorial Hospital, Delta, CO	100 4	89 38	85 26	95 39	86 29	33 3	- 0	100 4	87 15	49 47	83 63	100 7	90 90	89 73	90 30	89 114	100 140	75 91	82 33	87 143	98 55	81 140	- -	- -
Denver Health Medical Center, Denver, CO	80 15	97 79	97 59	95 62	97 59	- 0	- 0	90 41	89 159	64 247	98 259	79 117	87 127	90 79	87 23	72 162	100 184	83 53	80 104	84 200	85 48	70 191	- -	- -
East Morgan County Hospital, Brush, CO	- 0	0 1	100 1	100 1	100 2	- 0	- 0	- 0	100 1	67 6	86 14	100 2	96 28	87 15	- -	97 34	100 39	71 28	50 4	100 2	100 2	0 2	- -	- -
Estes Park Medical Center, Estes Park, CO	- -	- -	- -	- -	- -	- -	- -	- -	- 0	0 3	50 4	- 0	53 15	83 6	- -	75 16	100 20	79 14	33 6	92 12	100 1	100 11	- -	- -
Exempla Good Samaritan Medical Center, Lafayette, CO	95 22	98 126	97 110	98 95	98 133	- 0	88 8	97 38	76 62	87 201	94 232	91 33	88 101	85 75	81 21	70 109	100 148	83 109	83 36	94 171	95 42	59 168	- -	- -
Exempla Lutheran Medical Center, Wheat Ridge, CO	78 36	100 270	98 240	92 169	98 230	- 0	62 8	99 89	90 94	95 190	97 260	100 37	93 113	95 96	48 23	79 150	100 180	79 99	97 35	90 297	99 70	75 288	- -	- -
Exempla Saint Joseph Hospital, Denver, CO	85 34	99 182	100 204	96 133	100 255	- 0	79 14	97 74	84 92	91 223	95 278	97 31	87 83	92 87	83 23	85 115	100 146	65 97	84 37	94 307	97 72	73 300	- -	- -
Grand River Hospital District, Rifle, CO	- -	- -	- -	- -	- -	- -	- -	- -	100 1	29 14	63 19	67 3	90 29	94 18	80 5	71 41	100 43	87 23	20 10	- -	- -	- -	- -	- -
Gunnison Valley Hospital, Gunnison, CO	- 0	100 1	100 1	- 0	- 0	- 0	- -	- 0	100 1	0 11	25 12	0 1	44 16	100 2	100 1	79 14	95 19	70 10	67 3	71 21	100 4	90 21	- -	- -
Keefe Memorial Hospital, Cheyenne Wells, CO	- 0	100 1	- 0	0 1	- 0	0 1	- -	- 0	- -	- -	- -	- -	69 13	100 3	100 6	94 16	100 16	92 12	100 2	- -	- -	- -	- -	- -
Kit Carson County Memorial Hospital, Burlington, CO	- -	- -	- -	- -	- -	- -	- -	- -	- -	- -	- -	- -	- -	- -	- -	- -	- -	- -	- -	- -	- -	- -	- -	- -
Littleton Adventist Hospital, Littleton, CO	80 10	100 106	97 75	99 77	98 92	- 0	93 14	80 20	79 38	70 73	92 108	83 18	88 163	92 167	35 51	89 202	100 255	82 167	91 32	81 325	89 131	84 312	0.46 1737	4.27 1266
Longmont United Hospital, Longmont, CO	70 10	95 78	97 64	85 62	95 78	- 0	57 7	96 28	69 62	35 122	86 182	91 11	83 90	93 46	78 27	87 127	100 143	74 86	89 28	75 352	97 116	59 330	0.13 1505	3.77 1113
McKee Medical Center, Loveland, CO	93 14	97 62	100 46	98 48	98 48	- 0	- 0	90 10	93 29	87 63	96 90	100 8	91 88	97 68	91 32	83 119	100 142	82 107	70 30	93 45	42 45	52 44	- -	- -
Medical Center of Aurora, Aurora, CO	90 42	100 278	99 350	98 211	98 369	- 0	52 21	95 132	92 119	61 273	93 341	94 64	88 212	94 215	75 73	79 295	100 350	87 173	96 91	68 247	88 115	49 237	0.12 2570	3.34 1917
Melissa Memorial Hospital, Holyoke, CO	- 0	- 0	100 1	- 0	- 0	- 0	- -	- 0	100 1	62 8	92 12	100 1	100 5	50 2	100 2	100 5	100 9	67 6	- 0	- -	- -	- -	- -	- -
Memorial Hospital, Craig, CO	- 0	100 6	100 5	100 5	100 6	- 0	- 0	100 1	75 4	47 19	68 25	86 7	84 25	86 14	100 6	89 28	97 34	95 20	83 6	86 21	100 4	29 21	- -	- -
Memorial Hospital, Colorado Springs, CO	98 50	99 318	98 363	98 245	99 347	0 2	71 7	100 137	90 207	72 414	93 476	99 90	83 270	82 168	- -	65 309	100 363	66 214	100 113	93 412	98 135	84 399	- -	- -
Mercy Regional Medical Center, Durango, CO	100 7	98 49	100 66	100 36	95 63	- 0	50 2	100 16	92 25	73 56	100 61	86 7	97 58	94 71	83 23	91 88	100 103	66 73	100 26	96 247	97 69	82 243	- -	- -
Montrose Memorial Hospital, Montrose, CO	80 10	100 33	97 33	100 28	100 33	100 1	33 3	91 11	84 19	15 33	60 48	40 10	77 69	90 51	40 15	87 82	100 96	57 61	65 17	63 274	89 63	57 265	- -	- -
National Jewish Medical and Research Center, Denver, CO	- -	- -	- -	- -	- -	- -	- -	- -	- -	- -	- -	- -	- -	- -	- -	- -	- -	- -	- -	- -	- -	- -	- -	- -
North Colorado Medical Center, Greeley, CO	96 46	98 157	99 216	96 129	98 208	- 0	75 12	98 56	95 109	59 211	89 266	91 47	88 134	91 89	71 31	73 198	100 215	74 141	78 51	62 125	91 117	42 115	- -	- -
North Suburban Medical Center, Thornton, CO	100 6	100 106	100 89	100 74	99 74	100 1	100 5	100 50	100 26	92 61	100 87	100 11	93 97	92 120	97 29	88 157	100 205	90 89	100 74	81 129	94 49	45 121	0.15 1948	5.27 1461
Parker Adventist Hospital, Parker, CO	100 8	99 74	97 67	98 63	97 70	- 0	91 11	90 20	93 14	41 51	91 64	86 7	94 79	96 78	88 24	87 89	100 109	75 63	93 27	83 236	92 65	82 228	0.32 1262	4.15 891
Parkview Medical Center, Pueblo, CO	100 47	100 117	99 186	99 91	100 193	- 0	17 6	100 62	100 84	100 183	100 223	100 35	88 186	96 183	93 55	87 211	100 300	98 172	100 93	89 264	97 116	74 257	- -	- -
Penrose Saint Francis Health Services, Colorado Springs, CO	88 74	99 293	97 316	93 227	95 346	50 14	56 16	100 120	85 194	83 318	94 394	97 58	88 354	91 275	45 97	83 463	100 545	91 341	92 132	92 573	94 155	82 559	- -	- -
Pioneers Hospital of Rio Blanco County, Meeker, CO	- 0	100 2	100 1	100 2	100 1	- 0	- -	- 0	0 2	0 12	13 15	25 4	75 16	100 2	0 4	89 19	100 20	6 16	20 5	- -	- -	- -	- -	- -
Platte Valley Medical Center, Brighton, CO	100 1	94 18	88 8	94 16	71 7	- 0	- 0	0 1	85 20	68 40	82 50	100 11	86 65	90 31	64 14	84 74	100 94	79 47	83 18	90 197	100 41	72 188	- -	- -
Porter Adventist Hospital, Denver, CO	88 25	97 97	98 91	96 80	98 117	- 0	60 5	98 40	88 49	67 166	96 201	92 36	87 137	97 144	14 43	92 207	100 234	65 160	74 43	84 349	94 122	80 338	- -	- -
Poudre Valley Hospital, Fort Collins, CO	88 89	99 226	99 361	96 168	98 450	- 0	68 28	96 163	76 85	64 181	90 241	93 58	84 177	95 104	71 42	71 232	100 299	63 191	95 66	88 219	93 73	56 211	0.21 2818	5.01 1938
Presbyterian-Saint Luke's Medical Center, Denver, CO	100 13	100 39	100 115	100 25	99 135	- 0	- 0	100 40	95 66	84 142	98 165	97 31	80 55	95 59	57 21	76 94	100 115	64 64	62 32	72 218	73 90	61 203	3.62 1656	3.24 863
Prowers Medical Center, Lamar, CO	- 0	- 0	- 0	- 0	- 0	- 0	- -	- 0	50 2	0 25	50 28	- 0	73 45	100 27	0 12	55 47	100 62	10 41	7 14	- -	- -	- -	- -	- -
Rangely District Hospital, Rangely, CO	- -	- -	- -	- -	- -	- -	- -	- -	- 0	0 1	0 1	- 0	- -	- -	- -	- -	- -	- -	- -	- -	- -	- -	- -	- -
Rose Medical Center, Denver, CO	76 17	100 137	100 132	100 100	100 130	- 0	80 5	97 39	86 70	65 160	98 205	90 20	94 141	97 125	79 29	91 180	100 216	86 136	87 47	56 211	98 99	76 214	0.23 3846	4.85 2434
Saint Anthony Central Hospital, Denver, CO	100 58	100 182	100 270	97 154	100 252	- 0	100 12	100 102	89 76	59 150	95 187	100 40	84 103	90 124	84 31	78 194	100 213	95 135	100 61	84 363	97 115	81 341	- -	- -
Saint Anthony North Hospital, Westminster, CO	90 10	100 104	99 86	99 96	100 82	- 0	100 12	100 28	94 47	62 130	97 162	100 23	85 135	86 112	58 36	81 189	100 205	81 131	99 71	75 165	100 40	61 149	- -	- -
Saint Anthony Summit Medical Center, Frisco, CO	- -	- -	- -	- -	- -	- -	- -	- -	- 0	40 5	80 5	100 1	79 14	92 13	100 3	91 11	100 16	75 8	100 2	71 28	75 12	31 26	- -	- -
Saint Mary's Hospital & Medical Center, Grand Junction, CO	91 67	98 167	100 305	97 104	99 293	0 1	62 8	100 107	85 74	54 155	97 189	89 35	92 158	93 132	84 38	92 201	100 258	85 160	98 63	96 1047	94 235	92 1005	0.38 2338	1.97 1676
Saint Mary-Corwin Medical Center, Pueblo, CO	88 16	100 80	97 96	100 76	97 94	- 0	100 2	98 53	90 40	92 120	93 140	100 26	87 119	94 79	- -	89 131	100 167	86 118	95 44	86 315	93 76	74 303	- -	- -
Saint Thomas More Hospital, Canon City, CO	100 3	89 19	86 7	85 13	83 6	0 2	- 0	- 0	100 5	10 31	62 39	50 6	85 67	89 46	92 26	89 89	100 111	88 56	78 32	89 168	92 51	78 161	- -	- -
Saint Vincent General Hospital, Leadville, CO	- -	- -	- -	- -	- -	- -	- -	- -	- -	- -	- -	- -	- -	- -	- -	- -	- -	- -	- -	- -	- -	- -	- -	- -

*NOTE: The first number in each column (boldface) is the rate in percent, the second number is the number of patients; Please refer to the main entry for footnotes; **Heart Attack Care:** 1. ACE Inhibitor or ARB for LVSD; 2. Aspirin at Arrival; 3. Aspirin at Discharge; 4. Beta Blocker at Arrival; 5. Beta Blocker at Discharge; 6. Fibrinolytic Medication Timing; 7. PCI Within 90 Minutes of Arrival; 8. Smoking Cessation Advice; **Heart Failure Care:** 9. ACE Inhibitor or ARB for LVSD; 10. Discharge Instructions; 11. Evaluation of LVS Function; 12. Smoking Cessation Advice; **Pneumonia Care:** 13. Appropriate Initial Antibiotic; 14. Blood Culture Timing; 15. Influenza Vaccine; 16. Initial Antibiotic Timing; 17. Oxygenation Assessment; 18. Pneumococcal Vaccine; 19. Smoking Cessation Advice; **Surgical Infection Prevention:** 20. Prophylactic Antibiotic Given; 21. Prophylactic Antibiotic Selection; 22. Prophylactic Antibiotic Stopped; **Pregnancy Care:** 23. Inpatient Neonatal Mortality; 24. Third or Fourth Degree Laceration*

Hospital	Heart Attack Care								Heart Failure Care				Pneumonia Care							Surgical Infection Prevention			Pregnancy Care	
	1	2	3	4	5	6	7	8	9	10	11	12	13	14	15	16	17	18	19	20	21	22	23	24
San Luis Valley Regional Medical Center, Alamosa, CO	- 0	100 3	100 1	80 5	67 3	- 0	- 0	100 1	100 4	0 9	72 25	- 0	50 8	80 10	- -	87 53	100 58	48 40	100 3	68 41	- -	100 39	- -	- -
Sky Ridge Medical Center, Lone Tree, CO	90 10	100 63	100 54	95 41	98 61	- 0	88 8	95 21	79 29	29 70	98 92	75 8	83 78	85 60	57 14	86 93	100 115	67 52	100 26	85 176	92 74	70 174	0.07 3024	5.70 2105
Southwest Memorial Hospital, Cortez, CO	67 3	70 10	90 10	67 12	90 10	- 0	- 0	- 0	50 4	60 5	68 22	100 1	86 7	80 5	- -	83 66	100 87	54 54	100 4	76 33	- -	94 31	- -	- -
Spanish Peaks Regional Health Center, Walsenburg, CO	- -	- -	- -	- -	- -	- -	- -	- -	- 0	42 12	53 15	0 1	94 16	88 8	100 4	96 27	100 30	96 23	100 7	- -	- -	- -	- -	- -
Sterling Regional MedCenter, Sterling, CO	- 0	100 10	100 5	100 5	80 5	- 0	- 0	- 0	91 11	43 30	81 47	57 7	79 34	97 30	87 15	89 47	100 59	91 35	73 15	72 25	92 25	78 23	- -	- -
Swedish Medical Center, Englewood, CO	92 38	98 176	96 142	98 138	97 188	- 0	70 23	99 70	82 93	75 216	94 287	77 39	92 170	97 150	74 53	80 240	100 318	68 175	64 72	85 233	91 92	76 223	- -	- -
University of Colorado Hospital, Denver, CO	85 27	99 115	99 137	96 84	99 161	- 0	75 16	100 67	89 150	86 277	97 308	99 81	83 89	83 115	26 23	69 151	100 186	30 70	96 69	78 335	78 68	82 337	1.05 666	2.89 2280
Vail Valley Medical Center, Vail, CO	- 0	- 0	- 0	100 1	100 1	- 0	- 0	- 0	67 3	11 9	50 8	0 1	89 9	100 6	25 4	67 6	100 10	60 5	50 2	92 25	84 25	100 25	0.00 603	6.63 362
Valley View Hospital, Glenwood Springs, CO	100 2	100 18	82 11	100 13	100 10	50 2	- 0	100 3	90 10	82 28	97 33	100 7	68 40	97 34	58 12	68 41	100 55	78 32	89 9	93 208	88 51	86 206	- -	- -
Wray Community Hospital, Wray, CO	- 0	100 6	100 3	86 7	100 4	0 2	- 0	- 0	100 1	0 6	64 11	33 3	100 16	100 3	80 5	86 21	100 24	74 19	57 7	80 15	100 3	93 15	- -	- -
Yampa Valley Medical Center, Steamboat Springs, CO	100 1	100 1	100 1	100 1	100 1	33 3	- 0	- 0	100 7	100 11	100 12	100 1	89 46	100 9	33 6	87 52	100 55	40 25	45 11	98 46	100 47	54 46	- -	- -
HAWAII																								
Castle Medical Center, Kailua, HI	67 15	98 130	96 104	95 85	95 108	- 0	0 2	91 32	76 54	86 249	85 256	86 43	81 119	95 128	68 34	82 147	99 178	75 95	95 37	93 100	92 39	76 100	- -	- -
Hawaii Medical Center East, Honolulu, HI	66 32	95 86	95 169	84 75	95 171	50 2	- 0	59 58	86 71	24 211	86 234	44 45	77 94	85 96	75 40	77 158	100 204	49 136	53 30	79 261	86 50	42 239	- -	- -
Hawaii Medical Center West, Ewa Beach, HI	70 10	91 68	72 25	84 56	85 26	50 6	- 0	75 4	82 78	25 213	67 228	52 65	84 132	92 155	51 41	85 241	100 264	30 161	47 49	48 50	77 13	83 47	- -	- -
Hilo Medical Center, Hilo, HI	84 31	93 203	88 165	95 221	90 180	38 8	- 0	92 62	78 50	79 205	72 226	90 50	73 119	90 91	29 28	66 112	99 197	34 109	83 48	75 126	75 36	57 123	- -	- -
Kapiolani Health at Pali Momi, Aiea, HI	100 10	100 68	100 32	100 57	100 36	100 2	- 0	100 8	96 106	70 253	89 240	89 45	89 139	94 225	86 64	85 288	100 345	76 218	92 39	81 226	98 84	41 219	- -	- -
Kona Community Hospital, Kealakekua, HI	- 0	93 29	92 13	69 29	62 13	0 1	- 0	- 0	68 25	21 70	64 80	50 10	94 95	94 70	43 14	81 88	100 130	26 69	32 22	90 49	100 18	89 28	- -	- -
Kuakini Medical Center, Honolulu, HI	74 19	93 73	94 106	89 53	95 126	- 0	50 2	82 33	88 75	31 159	94 172	81 26	89 105	94 95	58 33	80 142	100 167	53 124	62 16	88 152	91 46	66 150	- -	- -
Kula Hospital, Kula, HI	- -	- -	- -	- -	- -	- -	- -	- -	- 0	0 1	0 1	- 0	- -	- -	- -	- -	- -	- -	- -	- -	- -	- -	- -	- -
Maui Memorial Hospital, Wailuku, HI	88 25	95 135	94 68	93 118	91 69	50 18	- 0	62 8	82 143	43 277	85 283	68 44	79 148	90 101	65 31	88 185	100 227	47 154	96 45	71 249	93 54	61 240	- -	- -
Moanalua Medical Center and Clinic, Honolulu, HI	85 68	97 173	97 293	96 160	97 292	- 0	100 4	92 65	88 114	38 270	96 275	95 41	83 269	93 193	64 56	77 266	100 362	89 251	60 47	80 537	99 147	49 521	0.67 1931	4.81 1435
North Hawaii Community Hospital, Kamuela, HI	50 2	88 25	73 11	85 26	83 12	40 5	- 0	0 2	100 16	23 61	77 53	50 10	52 56	91 35	28 18	72 50	100 65	24 41	45 11	84 38	89 18	69 35	- -	- -
Straub Clinic and Hospital, Honolulu, HI	62 69	97 158	94 277	97 137	94 267	67 6	50 4	84 73	72 107	36 207	91 229	58 24	61 131	91 152	82 38	71 182	100 223	62 156	30 20	88 125	96 77	87 119	- -	- -
The Queen's Medical Center, Honolulu, HI	86 88	95 242	96 400	98 173	98 390	25 4	23 13	92 131	88 293	78 482	93 515	94 113	83 245	83 262	53 75	73 319	100 413	58 234	77 81	88 1018	97 373	85 993	0.04 2275	5.45 1744
Wahiawa General Hospital, Wahiawa, HI	75 4	88 24	67 12	70 23	75 12	0 1	- 0	100 4	85 20	71 79	70 81	85 13	88 42	69 35	50 8	87 46	100 55	15 33	29 7	9 11	75 4	90 10	- -	- -
Wilcox Memorial Hospital, Lihue, HI	88 8	94 34	100 11	86 29	86 14	17 6	- 0	100 1	77 56	34 92	85 95	90 21	76 75	80 59	84 19	71 80	100 109	59 68	85 20	53 30	90 29	100 29	- -	- -
IDAHO																								
Bonner General Hospital, Sandpoint, ID	- 0	100 6	100 6	100 5	75 4	- 0	- 0	- 0	100 17	60 35	91 43	83 6	68 31	100 9	71 7	76 34	100 44	62 29	0 10	88 93	100 34	85 91	- -	- -
Cassia Regional Medical Center, Burley, ID	- 0	71 7	60 5	57 7	60 5	- 0	- 0	100 1	71 14	72 65	70 81	83 6	85 65	96 45	63 19	66 67	100 86	73 60	42 12	79 175	95 42	36 172	- -	- -
Eastern Idaho Regional Medical Center, Idaho Falls, ID	52 23	98 109	98 205	95 78	98 205	- 0	77 13	93 69	74 46	81 139	81 177	93 27	86 160	87 121	89 45	77 230	100 299	83 183	61 79	93 208	95 86	54 178	- -	- -
Healthsouth Treasure Valley Hospital, Boise, ID	- -	- -	- -	- -	- -	- -	- -	- -	- -	- -	- -	- -	- -	- -	- -	- -	- -	- -	- -	100 49	88 8	92 49	- -	- -
Idaho Doctors Hospital, Blackfoot, ID	- -	- -	- -	- -	- -	- -	- -	- -	- -	- -	- -	- -	- -	- -	- -	- -	- -	- -	- -	- -	- -	- -	- -	- -
Idaho Falls Recovery Center, Idaho Falls, ID	- -	- -	- -	- -	- -	- -	- -	- -	- -	- -	- -	- -	- -	- -	- -	- -	- -	- -	- -	- -	- -	- -	- -	- -
Kootenai Medical Center, Coeur d'Alene, ID	100 26	99 171	100 222	94 125	98 189	- 0	95 20	100 80	98 46	75 158	97 201	97 39	92 185	92 117	53 49	91 267	100 330	73 226	93 74	85 866	95 203	79 820	- -	- -
Madison Memorial Hospital, Rexburg, ID	100 1	100 6	100 1	100 5	50 2	0 1	- 0	- 0	0 3	36 25	55 33	33 3	89 54	83 6	89 9	98 49	100 62	83 36	85 13	76 177	84 50	67 174	- -	- -
Magic Valley Regional Medical Center, Twin Falls, ID	95 38	96 101	97 109	97 86	98 135	- 0	83 12	96 28	91 32	69 58	92 120	100 15	96 27	96 188	- -	93 282	100 333	76 210	91 64	66 53	91 54	80 54	- -	- -
Mercy Medical Center, Nampa, ID	94 18	100 95	100 87	100 85	100 81	- 0	80 10	100 32	95 20	94 72	96 96	86 14	91 151	96 114	97 38	83 183	100 215	92 122	98 52	93 190	98 57	60 191	0.34 1478	3.34 1257
Mountain View Hospital, Idaho Falls, ID	- -	- -	- -	- -	- -	- -	- -	- -	- -	- -	- -	- -	- -	- -	- -	- -	- -	- -	- -	52 33	97 33	33 33	- -	- -
Northwest Specialty Hospital, Post Falls, ID	- -	- -	- -	- -	- -	- -	- -	- -	- -	- -	- -	- -	- -	- -	- -	- -	- -	- -	- -	89 103	89 18	24 102	- -	- -
Portneuf Medical Center, Pocatello, ID	65 26	97 98	98 120	93 69	94 109	33 12	50 4	92 38	71 58	12 150	76 169	76 29	85 136	94 145	66 32	59 212	100 246	60 150	88 73	83 510	93 123	51 485	- -	- -
Saint Alphonsus Regional Medical Center, Boise, ID	100 31	99 151	99 285	99 137	99 276	0 1	45 11	99 92	95 87	85 184	98 228	88 25	91 108	88 116	- -	91 187	100 237	91 153	92 76	91 358	92 113	81 350	- -	- -
Saint Joseph Regional Medical Center, Lewiston, ID	80 5	100 11	100 10	88 8	70 10	- 0	- 0	75 4	78 32	67 55	86 81	73 22	89 66	95 83	75 28	78 92	99 148	43 95	67 27	86 429	95 101	78 418	- -	- -
Saint Luke's Medical Center, Ketchum, ID	- 0	100 2	100 1	100 2	100 1	- 0	- -	- 0	0 1	54 13	86 14	- 0	92 25	100 10	75 4	74 23	100 32	83 24	50 4	- -	- -	- -	- -	- -
Saint Luke's Regional Medical Center, Boise, ID	95 58	99 144	100 387	100 136	100 373	- 0	100 14	100 141	88 148	90 284	96 345	94 52	91 270	91 245	54 74	88 328	100 403	67 280	85 102	91 518	96 522	92 505	- -	- -
West Valley Medical Center, Caldwell, ID	60 5	89 27	83 12	75 28	100 20	- 0	- 0	100 1	76 25	62 80	92 98	76 29	84 103	89 55	57 28	87 128	100 145	85 104	60 48	80 117	95 41	67 112	- -	- -
MONTANA																								
Barrett Hospital, Dillon, MT	- 0	100 3	100 1	67 3	100 1	50 4	- 0	- 0	100 6	92 13	93 14	- 0	100 42	94 18	100 13	86 43	100 47	100 32	100 5	73 26	100 4	88 25	- -	- -

NOTE: The first number in each column (boldface) is the rate in percent, the second number is the number of patients; Please refer to the main entry for footnotes; ***Heart Attack Care:*** *1. ACE Inhibitor or ARB for LVSD; 2. Aspirin at Arrival; 3. Aspirin at Discharge; 4. Beta Blocker at Arrival; 5. Beta Blocker at Discharge; 6. Fibrinolytic Medication Timing; 7. PCI Within 90 Minutes of Arrival; 8. Smoking Cessation Advice;* ***Heart Failure Care:*** *9. ACE Inhibitor or ARB for LVSD; 10. Discharge Instructions; 11. Evaluation of LVS Function; 12. Smoking Cessation Advice;* ***Pneumonia Care:*** *13. Appropriate Initial Antibiotic; 14. Blood Culture Timing; 15. Influenza Vaccine; 16. Initial Antibiotic Timing; 17. Oxygenation Assessment; 18. Pneumococcal Vaccine; 19. Smoking Cessation Advice;* ***Surgical Infection Prevention:*** *20. Prophylactic Antibiotic Given; 21. Prophylactic Antibiotic Selection; 22. Prophylactic Antibiotic Stopped;* ***Pregnancy Care:*** *23. Inpatient Neonatal Mortality; 24. Third or Fourth Degree Laceration*

Hospital	Heart Attack Care								Heart Failure Care				Pneumonia Care							Surgical Infection Prevention			Pregnancy Care	
	1	2	3	4	5	6	7	8	9	10	11	12	13	14	15	16	17	18	19	20	21	22	23	24
Benefis Healthcare, Great Falls, MT	77 22	99 94	99 136	95 77	99 136	0 1	88 8	98 45	92 78	82 175	97 221	100 30	93 179	93 125	60 43	82 231	99 309	87 199	91 87	98 200	99 68	67 189	- -	- -
Billings Clinic, Billings, MT	98 53	99 157	98 311	96 130	99 302	- 0	75 8	100 114	96 121	90 215	99 249	100 27	88 109	88 132	100 32	89 154	100 207	98 128	100 59	96 1171	99 278	94 1150	- -	- -
Bozeman Deaconess Hospital, Bozeman, MT	100 9	100 82	96 68	97 68	97 71	- 0	88 8	100 16	81 36	42 131	93 143	67 15	80 76	96 57	100 13	90 93	100 119	89 71	73 11	94 241	90 49	92 230	- -	- -
Central Montana Medical Center, Lewistown, MT	0 1	83 6	75 4	67 3	0 4	- 0	- 0	- 0	100 3	100 6	46 13	100 1	82 34	100 18	100 7	92 39	100 42	84 31	83 6	67 48	94 17	90 48	- -	- -
Central Montana Surgical Hospital, Great Falls, MT	- -	- -	- -	- -	- -	- -	- -	- -	- 0	- 0	- 0	- 0	- -	- -	- -	- -	- -	- -	- -	90 10	- -	100 10	- -	- -
Community Hosp and Nursing Home of Anaconda, Anaconda, MT	- 0	100 11	100 3	100 7	100 3	100 1	- 0	100 1	100 2	92 13	95 20	100 3	94 34	94 17	100 10	96 50	100 56	100 37	100 11	100 15	100 5	100 15	- -	- -
Community Medical Center, Missoula, MT	100 22	100 49	97 87	98 45	99 85	- 0	75 4	92 37	90 20	75 68	94 89	100 13	90 68	90 59	82 11	78 82	100 98	90 58	92 39	93 621	92 50	87 612	- -	- -
Crow/Northern Cheyenne Hospital, Crow Agency, MT	- 0	- 0	- 0	- 0	- 0	- 0	- -	- 0	100 5	25 8	88 16	50 2	71 21	83 12	67 6	100 19	100 24	100 15	40 5	50 8	100 2	100 6	- -	- -
Daniels Memorial Hospital & Nursing Home, Scobey, MT	- -	- -	- -	- -	- -	- -	- -	- -	- 0	0 1	40 5	- 0	100 5	100 4	100 1	80 10	100 10	57 7	- 0	- -	- -	- -	- -	- -
Frances Mahon Deaconess Hospital, Glasgow, MT	- 0	100 1	- 0	100 1	100 1	0 1	- 0	- 0	100 3	61 18	67 18	100 8	89 19	- 0	100 10	83 23	100 26	89 19	100 6	93 14	100 3	100 14	- -	- -
Garfield County Health Center, Jordan, MT	- -	- -	- -	- -	- -	- -	- -	- -	- -	- -	- -	- -	- -	- -	- -	- -	- -	- -	- -	- -	- -	- -	- -	- -
Glendive Medical Center, Glendive, MT	100 1	78 9	40 5	88 8	100 4	- 0	- 0	- 0	83 6	57 14	60 20	80 5	78 40	96 26	89 9	84 56	100 60	88 40	67 9	81 73	92 13	91 70	- -	- -
Health Center Northwest, Kalispell, MT	- 0	- 0	- 0	0 1	0 1	- 0	- 0	- 0	- 0	0 2	67 3	- 0	100 5	100 1	50 2	100 3	100 6	38 16	71 7	73 239	96 25	80 232	- -	- -
Holy Rosary Health Care, Miles City, MT	100 1	100 6	100 5	100 4	75 4	0 1	- 0	0 1	100 11	82 34	64 50	60 5	88 81	97 38	100 11	95 76	100 95	94 72	82 11	89 56	96 23	89 56	- -	- -
Kalispell Regional Medical Center, Kalispell, MT	92 24	99 151	98 198	99 134	96 191	- 0	83 12	88 69	89 47	66 105	91 139	89 18	82 121	90 119	57 23	93 155	100 195	58 126	69 55	77 502	92 108	53 491	0.00 572	4.88 430
Livingston Memorial Hospital, Livingston, MT	50 2	100 7	100 4	100 7	80 5	67 9	- 0	- 0	100 5	63 27	88 33	0 1	78 50	90 30	100 8	89 57	100 67	94 47	93 14	81 74	100 20	96 72	- -	- -
Marcus Daly Memorial Hospital, Hamilton, MT	- 0	75 4	50 2	50 4	0 2	- 0	- 0	- 0	50 2	20 15	65 17	0 1	82 28	80 10	- -	84 38	100 44	100 28	22 9	96 47	69 13	72 46	- -	- -
Marias Medical Center, Shelby, MT	- 0	100 2	100 1	100 2	100 2	0 1	- -	- 0	0 1	50 6	38 8	0 1	80 20	100 1	100 7	96 24	100 29	95 22	57 7	- -	- -	- -	- -	- -
Mccone County Health Center, Circle, MT	- -	- -	- -	- -	- -	- -	- -	- -	- 0	0 2	0 5	0 1	50 2	- 0	- 0	50 2	100 2	50 2	- 0	- -	- -	- -	- -	- -
Missouri River Medical Center, Fort Benton, MT	- -	- -	- -	- -	- -	- -	- -	- -	- -	0 4	- -	- 0	60 5	100 1	50 2	100 4	100 6	43 7	100 1	- -	- -	- -	- -	- -
Mountainview Medical Center, White Sulphur Springs, MT	- -	- -	- -	- -	- -	- -	- -	- -	- 0	100 1	100 2	- 0	33 3	- 0	- -	100 4	25 4	33 3	- 0	- -	- -	- -	- -	- -
North Valley Hospital, Whitefish, MT	- 0	- 0	- 0	- 0	- 0	- 0	- -	- 0	80 5	0 13	100 15	100 1	72 43	90 31	25 4	94 51	100 60	88 40	69 16	74 95	83 12	98 80	- -	- -
Northeast Montana Healthcare Poplar Hospital, Poplar, MT	- -	- -	- -	- -	- -	- -	- -	- -	67 3	8 12	50 14	50 2	76 21	100 3	43 7	77 31	100 32	67 9	47 15	- -	- -	- -	- -	- -
Northern Montana Hospital, Havre, MT	100 2	100 2	100 1	75 4	100 2	50 2	- 0	- 0	83 6	41 39	87 45	88 8	86 57	95 43	57 14	77 69	100 85	59 51	83 23	90 89	100 15	84 87	- -	- -
PHS Indian Hospital-Browning, Browning, MT	- -	- -	- -	- -	- -	- -	- -	- -	100 2	60 5	41 27	100 1	0 2	60 5	- -	85 47	100 57	88 34	75 4	- -	- -	- -	- -	- -
Pioneer Medical Center, Big Timber, MT	100 1	100 1	0 1	100 1	100 1	- 0	- 0	- 0	100 4	0 4	56 9	100 1	92 13	100 2	100 5	95 22	100 24	94 16	0 1	- -	- -	- -	- -	- -
Pondera Medical Center, Conrad, MT	- -	- -	- -	- -	- -	- -	- -	- -	100 2	86 7	100 8	100 1	80 5	100 1	100 1	67 6	83 6	80 5	- 0	- -	- -	- -	- -	- -
Prairie Community Hospital, Terry, MT	- -	- -	- -	- -	- -	- -	- -	- -	- -	- -	- -	- -	- -	- -	- -	- -	- -	- -	- -	- -	- -	- -	- -	- -
Roundup Memorial Hospital & Nursing Home, Roundup, MT	- 0	- 0	- 0	- 0	- 0	- -	- -	- -	80 5	0 1	44 27	- 0	100 3	100 1	- -	88 34	100 38	9 23	0 1	- -	- -	- -	- -	- -
Saint James Community Hospital, Butte, MT	69 13	96 67	94 50	90 50	81 54	50 2	100 2	94 34	65 20	48 75	85 102	100 15	85 91	97 72	95 20	89 105	100 130	74 72	78 36	97 346	79 72	75 334	0.00 525	3.82 393
Saint John's Lutheran Hospital, Libby, MT	- -	- -	- -	- -	- -	- -	- -	- -	- -	- -	- -	- -	88 17	100 9	- -	85 20	100 19	73 15	12 8	- -	- -	- -	- -	- -
Saint Joseph Hospital, Polson, MT	- -	- -	- -	- -	- -	- -	- -	- -	57 7	12 16	73 22	50 2	75 32	100 13	33 3	93 27	100 33	64 22	50 10	81 36	100 9	88 34	- -	- -
Saint Luke Community Hospital, Ronan, MT	- -	- -	- -	- -	- -	- -	- -	- -	50 4	11 19	64 25	17 6	95 43	80 30	100 7	83 53	100 61	79 28	50 22	- -	- -	- -	- -	- -
Saint Patrick Hosp and Health Sci Ctr, Missoula, MT	96 50	99 125	100 284	99 111	99 273	- 0	90 10	100 85	97 115	69 189	100 220	100 35	79 92	94 93	96 24	88 131	100 159	91 105	95 41	93 402	98 152	92 391	- -	- -
Saint Peter's Hospital, Helena, MT	100 14	99 75	96 71	100 59	98 66	- 0	0 2	86 22	88 16	66 56	94 71	100 11	94 95	96 74	96 27	89 122	100 159	96 102	84 32	95 237	100 59	91 229	0.00 875	3.54 594
Saint Vincent Healthcare, Billings, MT	69 81	95 151	98 302	90 145	90 294	- 0	62 8	99 94	92 86	78 200	89 242	88 43	87 209	90 132	100 39	83 215	100 260	81 154	85 86	94 1334	93 295	89 1317	- -	- -
Sheridan Memorial Hospital, Plentywood, MT	- 0	100 2	100 1	50 2	- 0	- 0	- 0	- 0	- 0	17 6	50 10	100 1	100 10	100 2	100 2	94 18	100 22	89 19	- 0	- -	- -	- -	- -	- -
Sidney Health Center, Sidney, MT	0 1	80 5	50 4	80 5	50 4	0 2	- 0	- 0	40 5	50 28	78 37	100 7	69 13	86 7	100 1	100 15	100 23	92 13	67 3	96 53	100 11	81 53	- -	- -
Stillwater Community Hospital, Columbus, MT	- -	- -	- -	- -	- -	- -	- -	- -	- -	- -	- -	- -	- -	- -	- -	- -	- -	- -	- -	- -	- -	- -	- -	- -
Teton Medical Center, Choteau, MT	- -	- -	- -	- -	- -	- -	- -	- -	- -	- -	- -	- -	- -	- -	- -	- -	- -	- -	- -	- -	- -	- -	- -	- -
Trinity Hospital, Wolf Point, MT	- 0	100 1	- 0	0 1	- 0	- 0	- -	- 0	100 4	41 32	63 35	75 4	85 20	- 0	86 7	70 27	100 31	100 18	78 9	- 0	- 0	- 0	- -	- -
NEVADA																								
Banner Churchill Community Hospital, Fallon, NV	50 2	80 10	80 5	75 12	100 8	33 3	- 0	100 2	83 12	81 36	90 39	83 6	79 89	91 55	84 19	84 88	100 112	68 72	56 32	67 45	100 12	74 42	- -	- -
Carson Valley Medical Center, Gardnerville, NV	- 0	100 4	67 3	25 4	33 3	- 0	- 0	- 0	86 7	55 11	64 11	0 2	88 34	83 29	43 7	82 39	100 44	79 29	33 3	- -	- -	- -	- -	- -
Carson-Tahoe Hospital, Carson City, NV	96 27	96 143	92 144	96 127	97 150	- 0	0 2	100 12	88 88	54 50	95 245	90 10	84 49	96 55	- -	77 315	100 399	45 283	73 22	75 77	- -	83 65	- -	- -
Desert Springs Hospital, Las Vegas, NV	72 40	95 243	90 276	87 174	87 259	67 12	36 14	93 122	70 83	41 229	85 291	93 54	90 100	68 87	28 25	54 117	100 167	43 100	74 43	74 243	92 61	42 238	- -	- -
Grover C Dils Medical Center, Caliente, NV	- -	- -	- -	- -	- -	- -	- -	- -	100 1	0 1	11 9	0 1	100 4	- 0	- -	58 12	100 13	0 7	0 1	- -	- -	- -	- -	- -
Humboldt General Hospital, Winnemucca, NV	- 0	100 2	100 2	100 2	100 2	- 0	- -	- 0	- 0	0 2	50 2	100 2	75 20	100 7	50 2	77 22	100 26	65 17	25 12	- -	- -	- -	- -	- -

NOTE: The first number in each column (boldface) is the rate in percent, the second number is the number of patients; Please refer to the main entry for footnotes; ***Heart Attack Care:*** *1. ACE Inhibitor or ARB for LVSD; 2. Aspirin at Arrival; 3. Aspirin at Discharge; 4. Beta Blocker at Arrival; 5. Beta Blocker at Discharge; 6. Fibrinolytic Medication Timing; 7. PCI Within 90 Minutes of Arrival; 8. Smoking Cessation Advice;* ***Heart Failure Care:*** *9. ACE Inhibitor or ARB for LVSD; 10. Discharge Instructions; 11. Evaluation of LVS Function; 12. Smoking Cessation Advice;* ***Pneumonia Care:*** *13. Appropriate Initial Antibiotic; 14. Blood Culture Timing; 15. Influenza Vaccine; 16. Initial Antibiotic Timing; 17. Oxygenation Assessment; 18. Pneumococcal Vaccine; 19. Smoking Cessation Advice;* ***Surgical Infection Prevention:*** *20. Prophylactic Antibiotic Given; 21. Prophylactic Antibiotic Selection; 22. Prophylactic Antibiotic Stopped;* ***Pregnancy Care:*** *23. Inpatient Neonatal Mortality; 24. Third or Fourth Degree Laceration*

Hospital	Heart Attack Care								Heart Failure Care				Pneumonia Care							Surgical Infection Prevention			Pregnancy Care	
	1	2	3	4	5	6	7	8	9	10	11	12	13	14	15	16	17	18	19	20	21	22	23	24
Mesa View Regional Hospital, Mesquite, NV	- -	- -	- -	- -	- -	- -	- -	- -	- -	- -	- -	- -	- -	- -	- -	- -	- -	- -	- -	- -	- -	- -	- -	- -
MountainView Hospital, Las Vegas, NV	**90** 50	**98** 272	**98** 246	**92** 203	**96** 236	**23** 13	**27** 11	**99** 97	**83** 158	**62** 402	**95** 482	**85** 92	**92** 222	**94** 212	**46** 96	**51** 301	**100** 398	**75** 244	**70** 105	**70** 269	**91** 118	**57** 249	- -	- -
North Vista Hospital, North Las Vegas, NV	**75** 8	**96** 89	**78** 36	**89** 73	**68** 34	**19** 21	- 0	**90** 10	**67** 99	**63** 244	**87** 306	**99** 105	**87** 172	**90** 151	**24** 41	**66** 209	**100** 252	**18** 95	**91** 100	**77** 216	**96** 46	**36** 201	- -	- -
Northeasetern Nevada Regional Hospital, Elko, NV	**100** 3	**100** 38	**85** 13	**94** 31	**100** 11	**47** 15	- 0	**40** 5	**100** 20	**49** 69	**82** 76	**67** 21	**96** 72	**83** 41	**75** 12	**88** 78	**100** 102	**69** 52	**79** 28	**60** 83	**96** 27	**26** 81	- -	- -
Northern Nevada Medical Center, Sparks, NV	**67** 3	**92** 38	**55** 20	**61** 38	**52** 21	**0** 1	- 0	**100** 5	**75** 52	**33** 93	**88** 122	**76** 34	**74** 76	**86** 57	**67** 12	**84** 81	**100** 96	**60** 58	**88** 34	**92** 212	**97** 39	**26** 208	- -	- -
Nye Regional Medical Center, Tonopah, NV	**0** 1	**100** 1	**100** 1	**100** 1	**100** 1	**0** 1	- -	**100** 1	- 0	**17** 24	**67** 15	**88** 8	**22** 23	**33** 3	**50** 2	**70** 23	**100** 24	**31** 13	**100** 10	- -	- -	- -	- -	- -
Renown Regional Medical Center, Reno, NV	**88** 84	**97** 173	**97** 362	**99** 144	**99** 338	**50** 2	**53** 15	**85** 162	**87** 157	**37** 315	**95** 354	**77** 107	**82** 161	**84** 127	- -	**81** 204	**100** 242	**78** 120	**78** 76	**71** 494	**90** 169	**56** 481	**0.81** 992	**3.79** 712
Renown South Meadows Medical Center, Reno, NV	- 0	**100** 3	**100** 4	**100** 2	**100** 3	**50** 2	- 0	**100** 1	**88** 16	**44** 45	**95** 56	**91** 11	**91** 68	**98** 52	**89** 18	**87** 67	**100** 86	**86** 51	**79** 24	**81** 70	**94** 32	**32** 68	- -	- -
Saint Mary's Regional Medical Center, Reno, NV	**87** 47	**100** 210	**97** 291	**98** 186	**98** 307	**0** 1	**29** 14	**90** 118	**90** 105	**31** 239	**97** 282	**96** 50	**91** 87	**72** 101	**50** 22	**80** 131	**100** 165	**65** 101	**81** 48	**85** 350	**98** 82	**72** 326	- -	- -
Saint Rose Dominican Hospital, Henderson, NV	**88** 16	**99** 165	**95** 119	**96** 133	**93** 124	**67** 9	**0** 2	**96** 57	**71** 56	**69** 162	**93** 231	**89** 61	**79** 108	**86** 71	- -	**80** 131	**100** 169	**75** 97	**84** 45	**86** 140	**90** 51	**45** 132	**0.16** 3704	**5.19** 2504
Saint Rose Dominican Hospital-Siena, Henderson, NV	**81** 36	**100** 253	**97** 261	**94** 186	**95** 241	**38** 13	**100** 3	**94** 103	**77** 115	**65** 275	**97** 334	**90** 63	**78** 122	**86** 77	**48** 27	**66** 140	**100** 187	**75** 113	**86** 49	**78** 251	**93** 90	**44** 229	- -	- -
Sierra Surgery & Imaging, Carson City, NV	- -	- -	- -	- -	- -	- -	- -	- -	- -	- -	- -	- -	- -	- -	- -	- -	- -	- -	- -	**93** 94	- -	**80** 94	- -	- -
South Lyon Medical Center, Yerington, NV	- 0	**100** 1	**0** 1	**0** 1	**0** 1	- -	- -	- -	**100** 1	- 0	**46** 13	- 0	**67** 3	**100** 1	- -	**84** 25	**100** 28	**15** 20	**100** 1	- -	- -	- -	- -	- -
Southern Hills Hospital and Medical Center, Las Vegas, NV	**83** 6	**98** 53	**87** 31	**98** 41	**90** 29	**0** 3	**0** 3	**100** 9	**80** 65	**40** 147	**99** 166	**97** 30	**94** 96	**92** 99	**57** 35	**69** 112	**100** 166	**57** 91	**98** 45	**53** 164	**96** 98	**39** 153	- -	- -
Spring Valley Hospital, Las Vegas, NM	**77** 13	**96** 183	**91** 80	**86** 134	**81** 80	**65** 17	**33** 3	**98** 40	**92** 77	**99** 183	**98** 234	**99** 69	**90** 125	**80** 70	**90** 20	**75** 139	**100** 145	**85** 72	**96** 48	**71** 208	**88** 50	**54** 200	- -	- -
Summerlin Hospital Medical Center, Las Vegas, NV	**96** 23	**99** 220	**95** 182	**94** 177	**95** 167	**25** 4	**20** 5	**85** 66	**83** 78	**72** 187	**95** 243	**81** 32	**80** 124	**63** 105	**100** 28	**70** 142	**100** 194	**71** 109	**79** 38	**67** 304	**87** 68	**59** 286	- -	- -
Sunrise Hospital & Medical Center, Las Vegas, NV	**86** 56	**97** 271	**96** 278	**86** 171	**93** 295	**0** 4	**21** 14	**99** 153	**76** 334	**36** 610	**92** 710	**87** 213	**86** 403	**79** 331	**36** 118	**65** 506	**100** 655	**50** 333	**86** 208	**59** 319	**88** 162	**71** 295	- -	- -
University Medical Center, Las Vegas, NV	**95** 39	**99** 206	**97** 209	**96** 158	**93** 191	**25** 4	**0** 4	**96** 97	**93** 180	**75** 296	**97** 326	**87** 142	**78** 165	**66** 76	**12** 32	**52** 206	**100** 244	**38** 64	**86** 101	**37** 294	**91** 57	**75** 271	- -	- -
Valley Hospital Medical Center, Las Vegas, NV	**72** 57	**98** 250	**92** 293	**90** 189	**89** 277	**33** 24	**0** 5	**95** 130	**73** 154	**72** 284	**92** 338	**96** 95	**93** 96	**62** 104	**30** 23	**63** 138	**100** 164	**26** 88	**93** 46	**76** 401	**93** 94	**41** 380	- -	- -
NEW MEXICO																								
ACL-IHS Hospital, San Fidel, NM	- -	- -	- -	- -	- -	- -	- -	- -	**50** 2	- -	**100** 3	- -	**100** 3	**75** 4	- -	**76** 49	**98** 50	**90** 31	- 0	- -	- -	- -	- -	- -
Alta Vista Regional Hospital, Las Vegas, NM	- 0	**100** 8	**100** 6	**75** 8	**100** 4	- 0	- -	**50** 2	**76** 25	**2** 63	**77** 75	**37** 19	**77** 87	**79** 72	**33** 21	**73** 122	**100** 136	**53** 73	**62** 47	**62** 52	**88** 16	**76** 46	- -	- -
Artesia General Hospital, Artesia, NM	- 0	**60** 5	**80** 5	**75** 4	**80** 5	- 0	- 0	- 0	**100** 2	**25** 16	**17** 18	**50** 4	**79** 48	**95** 21	**82** 11	**60** 52	**95** 60	**64** 36	**32** 19	**33** 6	**75** 4	**83** 6	- -	- -
Carlsbad Medical Center, Carlsbad, NM	**100** 13	**97** 78	**98** 60	**96** 70	**100** 61	**44** 9	**0** 1	**100** 26	**93** 28	**77** 56	**93** 69	**100** 16	**93** 100	**95** 107	**88** 52	**88** 137	**100** 168	**92** 100	**98** 43	**97** 224	**100** 59	**85** 220	- -	- -
Cibola General Hospital, Grants, NM	- 0	**100** 3	**100** 3	**67** 3	**100** 3	- 0	- 0	**100** 1	**0** 1	**20** 15	**24** 17	**100** 1	**88** 40	**100** 30	**40** 10	**61** 36	**100** 45	**42** 26	**62** 8	**50** 20	**83** 6	**100** 19	- -	- -
Doctor Dan C Trigg Memorial Hospital, Tucumcari, NM	- 0	**100** 2	**83** 6	**100** 2	**67** 6	**0** 1	- 0	**0** 1	- 0	**0** 12	**0** 17	**0** 2	**77** 26	**100** 10	**0** 9	**72** 36	**100** 40	**8** 26	**33** 6	- -	- -	- -	- -	- -
Eastern New Mexico Medical Center, Roswell, NM	**83** 6	**98** 62	**94** 36	**89** 54	**93** 29	**0** 1	- 0	**92** 13	**89** 47	**41** 155	**86** 173	**85** 33	**76** 181	**97** 127	**94** 69	**66** 271	**100** 298	**87** 175	**83** 75	**77** 309	**89** 74	**90** 301	- -	- -
Espanola Hospital, Espanola, NM	- 0	**100** 5	**100** 1	**60** 5	**100** 1	- 0	- 0	- 0	**82** 17	**74** 50	**74** 54	**100** 8	**80** 87	**85** 62	**76** 21	**92** 100	**100** 111	**66** 70	**96** 25	**77** 44	**100** 16	**95** 42	**0.32** 310	**3.29** 243
Gallup Indian Medical Center, Gallup, NM	**0** 1	**100** 2	**100** 1	**100** 1	**100** 1	- 0	- 0	- 0	**82** 22	**11** 37	**98** 40	**0** 1	**85** 97	**93** 59	**71** 21	**73** 112	**99** 136	**81** 67	**17** 6	**67** 33	**88** 8	**78** 32	- -	- -
Gerald Champion Memorial Hospital, Alamogordo, NM	**100** 1	**88** 17	**82** 17	**75** 20	**80** 15	- 0	- 0	**14** 7	**71** 45	**63** 153	**61** 179	**67** 36	**85** 96	**74** 47	**45** 51	**72** 162	**100** 197	**46** 118	**37** 49	**62** 143	**96** 76	**58** 137	- -	- -
Gila Regional Medical Center, Silver City, NM	- 0	**100** 9	**83** 6	**100** 9	**100** 6	**45** 11	- 0	**100** 1	**70** 20	**16** 95	**50** 117	**27** 11	**93** 103	**96** 74	**60** 20	**91** 141	**100** 144	**48** 90	**48** 25	**52** 223	**93** 71	**44** 208	- -	- -
Guadalupe County Hospital, Santa Rosa, NM	- 0	**100** 1	**100** 1	- 0	**100** 1	- 0	- 0	**100** 1	**100** 2	**100** 1	**90** 10	- 0	- 0	- 0	- -	**89** 9	**100** 19	**71** 7	**100** 1	- -	- -	- -	- -	- -
Heart Hospital of New Mexico, Albuquerque, NM	**91** 192	**99** 158	**99** 644	**99** 152	**98** 646	- 0	**77** 13	**86** 256	**84** 154	**65** 254	**98** 277	**81** 31	**83** 6	**100** 11	**20** 5	**69** 16	**100** 18	**61** 18	**71** 7	**95** 309	**100** 89	**91** 293	- -	- -
Holy Cross Hospital, Taos, NM	**100** 1	**80** 5	**100** 1	**50** 4	**100** 1	- 0	- 0	- 0	**79** 14	**18** 39	**90** 49	**86** 7	**84** 88	**81** 91	- -	**81** 134	**100** 163	**44** 105	**95** 19	**73** 15	**100** 15	**100** 14	- -	- -
Lea Regional Medical Center, Hobbs, NM	- 0	**100** 11	**100** 6	**82** 11	**100** 6	**0** 1	- 0	**80** 5	**92** 13	**59** 29	**88** 49	**92** 13	**90** 84	**91** 75	**48** 21	**73** 104	**100** 116	**78** 69	**85** 33	**94** 220	**99** 73	**88** 209	**0.09** 1072	**3.18** 785
Lincoln County Medical Center, Ruidoso, NM	- 0	**100** 5	**80** 5	**50** 4	**80** 5	**0** 4	- -	- 0	- 0	**0** 37	**5** 44	**38** 8	**74** 39	**100** 20	**80** 10	**82** 40	**100** 44	**93** 27	**71** 14	**55** 49	**87** 15	**81** 43	- -	- -
Los Alamos Medical Center, Los Alamos, NM	- 0	**50** 2	**100** 1	**100** 2	**100** 1	- 0	- 0	- 0	**100** 6	**15** 20	**64** 22	**33** 6	**83** 47	**84** 32	- -	**79** 58	**100** 63	**40** 35	**43** 7	**78** 79	**96** 24	**62** 79	- -	- -
Lovelace Health Systems, Albuquerque, NM	**94** 53	**99** 201	**97** 250	**93** 182	**92** 250	- 0	**73** 11	**90** 60	**93** 122	**89** 249	**99** 279	**68** 37	**87** 252	**96** 185	- -	**70** 284	**100** 349	**68** 237	**77** 64	**87** 164	**93** 27	**78** 152	- -	- -
Lovelace Westside Hospital, Albuquerque, NM	**100** 1	**75** 4	**75** 4	**67** 6	**100** 4	- 0	- -	**100** 1	**73** 15	**22** 45	**92** 51	**78** 9	**81** 108	**88** 68	**77** 26	**70** 107	**100** 150	**71** 78	**65** 34	**100** 14	**100** 14	**93** 14	- -	- -
Loveless Medical Center-Downtown, Albuquerque, NM	**100** 3	**100** 6	**89** 9	**50** 8	**78** 9	- 0	- 0	**100** 1	**85** 13	**14** 36	**89** 45	**25** 8	**80** 121	**93** 110	**46** 41	**71** 141	**100** 193	**49** 127	**68** 50	**81** 36	**89** 35	**80** 35	- -	- -
Memorial Medical Center, Las Cruces, NM	**58** 48	**91** 70	**97** 137	**70** 63	**92** 167	- 0	**43** 7	**79** 67	**73** 102	**10** 209	**81** 239	**59** 32	**82** 261	**91** 193	**57** 69	**57** 337	**96** 369	**49** 219	**79** 66	**69** 227	**93** 118	**68** 223	- -	- -
Mescalero PHS Indian Hospital, Mescalero, NM	- -	- -	- -	- -	- -	- -	- -	- -	- -	- -	- -	- -	**100** 2	- 0	- -	**0** 1	**100** 2	**0** 1	- 0	- -	- -	- -	- -	- -
Mimbres Memorial Hospital, Deming, NM	**0** 1	**80** 15	**100** 12	**85** 13	**75** 12	- 0	- 0	**50** 4	**50** 8	**0** 67	**32** 80	**27** 15	**93** 81	**96** 26	- -	**75** 100	**100** 107	**8** 65	**33** 30	**39** 18	**10** 10	**100** 17	- -	- -
Miners' Colfax Medical Center, Raton, NM	- 0	**100** 8	**86** 7	**83** 6	**62** 8	**50** 2	- 0	**100** 1	**75** 4	**6** 18	**47** 30	**0** 1	**76** 21	**100** 20	**67** 3	**76** 49	**100** 57	**65** 37	**38** 8	**22** 9	**0** 5	**89** 9	- -	- -
Mountain View Regional Medical Center, Las Cruces, NM	**65** 54	**91** 85	**95** 145	**85** 62	**91** 159	- 0	**25** 4	**97** 63	**79** 73	**50** 141	**91** 163	**91** 22	**87** 127	**95** 126	**81** 42	**70** 152	**100** 193	**89** 128	**95** 38	**82** 536	**98** 124	**85** 520	- -	- -
Nor-Lea General Hospital, Lovington, NM	- 0	**0** 1	**0** 1	**0** 1	**0** 1	- 0	- -	- 0	**75** 4	**8** 13	**54** 13	**0** 2	**85** 27	**100** 11	**0** 13	**61** 31	**100** 38	**55** 20	**60** 10	**20** 5	- -	**100** 4	- -	- -
Northern Navajo Medical Center, Shiprock, NM	- 0	**100** 4	**100** 1	**75** 4	**100** 1	- 0	- 0	- 0	**75** 16	**0** 9	**60** 42	**0** 2	**95** 19	**86** 7	- -	**78** 95	**98** 120	**40** 84	**0** 1	- -	- -	- -	- -	- -
PHS Indian Hospital, Santa Fe, NM	- 0	**0** 2	**0** 1	**0** 2	**0** 1	- -	- -	- -	- 0	**0** 2	**0** 5	- 0	- -	- -	- -	**83** 6	**100** 18	**92** 12	- -	- -	- -	- -	- -	- -

NOTE: The first number in each column (boldface) is the rate in percent, the second number is the number of patients; Please refer to the main entry for footnotes; ***Heart Attack Care:*** *1. ACE Inhibitor or ARB for LVSD; 2. Aspirin at Arrival; 3. Aspirin at Discharge; 4. Beta Blocker at Arrival; 5. Beta Blocker at Discharge; 6. Fibrinolytic Medication Timing; 7. PCI Within 90 Minutes of Arrival; 8. Smoking Cessation Advice;* ***Heart Failure Care:*** *9. ACE Inhibitor or ARB for LVSD; 10. Discharge Instructions; 11. Evaluation of LVS Function; 12. Smoking Cessation Advice;* ***Pneumonia Care:*** *13. Appropriate Initial Antibiotic; 14. Blood Culture Timing; 15. Influenza Vaccine; 16. Initial Antibiotic Timing; 17. Oxygenation Assessment; 18. Pneumococcal Vaccine; 19. Smoking Cessation Advice;* ***Surgical Infection Prevention:*** *20. Prophylactic Antibiotic Given; 21. Prophylactic Antibiotic Selection; 22. Prophylactic Antibiotic Stopped;* ***Pregnancy Care:*** *23. Inpatient Neonatal Mortality; 24. Third or Fourth Degree Laceration*

Hospital	Heart Attack Care								Heart Failure Care				Pneumonia Care							Surgical Infection Prevention			Pregnancy Care	
	1	2	3	4	5	6	7	8	9	10	11	12	13	14	15	16	17	18	19	20	21	22	23	24
Plains Regional Medical Center, Clovis, NM	**37** 19	**75** 28	**43** 30	**63** 27	**42** 31	**0** 3	- 0	**60** 5	**66** 92	**58** 109	**75** 128	**34** 29	**89** 101	**98** 63	**60** 30	**80** 138	**99** 154	**45** 101	**44** 34	**84** 321	**86** 72	**78** 318	**0.07** 1435	**2.80** 1036
Presbyterian Hospital, Albuquerque, NM	**72** 50	**99** 219	**98** 285	**94** 176	**97** 290	- 0	**84** 19	**98** 112	**76** 132	**48** 248	**94** 292	**93** 54	**93** 55	**90** 90	**56** 25	**74** 129	**100** 158	**48** 115	**82** 49	**95** 436	**98** 104	**80** 424	**0.40** 1005	**1.74** 749
Presbyterian Kaseman Hospital, Albuquerque, NM	**0** 1	**100** 6	**100** 5	**50** 6	**100** 4	- 0	- 0	- 0	**90** 10	**5** 22	**84** 31	**50** 4	**95** 42	**92** 66	**57** 23	**75** 91	**100** 112	**42** 89	**73** 22	**96** 105	**82** 28	**80** 105	- -	- -
Rehoboth McKinley Christian Health Care Svcs, Gallup, NM	- 0	**100** 4	- 0	**75** 4	**100** 1	- 0	- 0	- 0	**77** 13	**27** 66	**40** 73	**73** 11	**80** 108	**82** 80	**48** 33	**82** 125	**100** 161	**40** 91	**79** 29	**86** 63	**89** 18	**80** 61	- -	- -
Roosevelt General Hospital, Portales, NM	**100** 1	**50** 2	**67** 3	**50** 2	**0** 3	- 0	- 0	**0** 1	**100** 6	**10** 48	**25** 60	**20** 10	**79** 84	**92** 40	**15** 20	**80** 100	**100** 113	**14** 77	**22** 37	**0** 1	- 0	**100** 1	- -	- -
Saint Joseph's North East Heights Hospital, Albuquerque, NM	**50** 2	**100** 7	**100** 6	**78** 9	**83** 6	- 0	- 0	- 0	**60** 5	**18** 17	**96** 23	**40** 5	**84** 105	**87** 71	**75** 28	**75** 109	**100** 133	**71** 92	**79** 34	**87** 30	**96** 28	**52** 29	**0.00** 0	**0.00** 0
Saint Vincent Regional Medical Center, Santa Fe, NM	**100** 27	**97** 120	**93** 170	**94** 97	**96** 168	- 0	**29** 7	**90** 63	**91** 69	**5** 152	**95** 169	**54** 24	**83** 160	**73** 130	- -	**74** 184	**99** 232	**51** 134	**57** 42	**71** 732	**92** 165	**74** 658	- -	- -
San Juan Regional Medical Center, Farmington, NM	**100** 14	**99** 85	**91** 45	**97** 70	**95** 44	**53** 15	- 0	**82** 11	**97** 98	**52** 165	**96** 198	**76** 21	**87** 157	**87** 156	**66** 76	**82** 261	**100** 317	**62** 226	**80** 45	**82** 249	**98** 64	**70** 241	- -	- -
Sierra Vista Hospital, Truth or Consequences, NM	- 0	- 0	- 0	- 0	- 0	- 0	- -	- 0	- 0	**6** 16	**15** 20	**0** 3	**74** 23	**80** 15	**40** 5	**77** 39	**96** 45	**66** 29	**31** 13	- -	- -	- -	- -	- -
Socorro General Hospital, Socorro, NM	- 0	**100** 1	**100** 1	**100** 1	**100** 1	- 0	- -	**100** 1	**64** 11	**26** 19	**48** 31	**80** 5	**79** 42	**76** 17	**83** 12	**76** 41	**100** 46	**59** 29	**72** 18	**100** 1	- -	**100** 1	**0.00** 222	**0.62** 161
Union County General Hospital, Clayton, NM	- 0	**100** 1	- 0	**100** 1	- 0	- 0	- 0	- 0	**50** 2	**20** 5	**60** 5	**0** 1	**60** 10	- 0	**67** 6	**82** 17	**100** 19	**80** 15	**0** 3	**75** 8	**100** 1	**62** 8	- -	- -
University of New Mexico Hospital, Albuquerque, NM	**71** 28	**96** 135	**97** 146	**95** 128	**97** 143	- 0	**83** 6	**93** 69	**86** 96	**15** 163	**99** 182	**81** 58	**80** 121	**82** 115	**50** 26	**37** 161	**100** 197	**33** 73	**38** 52	**84** 390	**97** 67	**69** 383	- -	- -
US Public Health Service Indian Hospital, Crownpoint, NM	- 0	- 0	- 0	- 0	- 0	- 0	- 0	- 0	**50** 2	**0** 5	**60** 10	- 0	**78** 18	**100** 12	- -	**81** 43	**96** 57	**93** 41	**0** 1	- -	- -	- -	- -	- -
Zuni Hospital, Zuni, NM	- -	- -	- -	- -	- -	- -	- -	- -	- 0	**0** 2	**50** 2	- 0	**100** 2	**100** 5	- -	**89** 18	**94** 33	**5** 22	- 0	- -	- -	- -	- -	- -
OREGON																								
Albany General Hospital, Albany, OR	**88** 8	**88** 24	**100** 15	**90** 20	**100** 20	- 0	- 0	**100** 3	**85** 40	**69** 97	**95** 123	**77** 26	**84** 142	**92** 118	**90** 39	**90** 176	**100** 210	**84** 136	**69** 55	**89** 266	**98** 56	**93** 263	**0.28** 715	**1.76** 510
Ashland Community Hospital, Ashland, OR	**100** 1	**57** 7	**86** 7	**83** 6	**86** 7	- 0	- 0	**100** 1	**67** 6	**77** 22	**79** 24	**67** 3	**82** 33	**87** 23	**78** 9	**82** 34	**100** 48	**77** 31	**60** 10	**76** 181	**100** 59	**29** 175	**0.32** 312	**1.25** 240
Bay Area Hospital, Coos Bay, OR	- 0	**94** 16	**100** 2	**88** 16	**100** 2	**17** 6	- 0	- 0	**90** 80	**69** 106	**76** 200	**78** 18	**91** 93	**86** 111	**67** 33	**89** 173	**100** 211	**69** 144	**74** 46	**72** 299	**91** 98	**59** 275	**0.15** 649	**2.39** 460
Blue Mountain Hospital District, John Day, OR	**100** 1	**100** 4	**100** 2	**75** 4	**100** 2	**0** 1	- -	- 0	**0** 1	**14** 7	**22** 9	**0** 1	**93** 15	**91** 11	**100** 2	**82** 11	**100** 18	**67** 12	**0** 3	- -	- -	- -	- -	- -
Columbia Memorial Hospital, Astoria, OR	**100** 1	**100** 17	**80** 5	**92** 12	**100** 6	**50** 2	- 0	**100** 1	**79** 14	**41** 44	**47** 53	**50** 10	**83** 99	**90** 21	**69** 16	**85** 100	**100** 116	**66** 65	**58** 19	**87** 70	**100** 13	**85** 65	- -	- -
Coquille Valley Hospital, Coquille, OR	**100** 1	**75** 8	**83** 6	**75** 8	**83** 6	**50** 2	- 0	**50** 2	**100** 1	**0** 14	**12** 16	**33** 3	**57** 21	**71** 7	**0** 5	**75** 24	**100** 28	**0** 16	**33** 12	**0** 3	**100** 1	**0** 1	- -	- -
Cottage Grove Community Hospital, Cottage Grove, OR	- -	- -	- -	- -	- -	- -	- -	- -	- -	- -	- -	- -	**77** 44	**100** 18	**94** 17	**61** 49	**100** 60	**88** 43	**73** 11	- -	- -	- -	- -	- -
Good Samaritan Regional Medical Center, Corvallis, OR	**90** 30	**99** 96	**100** 206	**96** 69	**99** 221	- 0	**88** 8	**93** 86	**87** 63	**51** 123	**84** 149	**90** 21	**90** 84	**90** 67	**75** 24	**91** 127	**100** 163	**63** 123	**66** 35	**78** 1049	**89** 182	**79** 1034	- -	- -
Good Shepherd Health Care System, Hermiston, OR	**100** 1	**100** 3	**100** 2	**100** 2	**100** 1	- 0	- -	**0** 1	**100** 8	**85** 20	**75** 24	**67** 3	**83** 42	**90** 20	**67** 3	**70** 37	**96** 45	**45** 31	**50** 12	**72** 58	**88** 24	**32** 53	- -	- -
Grande Ronde Hospital, La Grande, OR	**50** 2	**100** 19	**80** 10	**100** 17	**100** 11	**0** 4	- 0	**100** 1	**87** 15	**82** 45	**93** 56	**60** 5	**76** 89	**80** 41	**89** 28	**76** 103	**99** 128	**68** 87	**42** 12	- -	- -	- -	- -	- -
Holy Rosary Medical Center, Ontario, OR	**80** 5	**100** 14	**70** 10	**92** 12	**100** 10	- 0	- 0	**100** 1	**71** 14	**29** 51	**82** 60	**100** 9	**67** 83	**77** 30	**31** 16	**76** 84	**99** 106	**34** 79	**74** 19	**50** 133	**63** 43	**34** 131	**0.15** 663	**1.04** 479
Kaiser Sunnyside Medical Center, Clackamas, OR	**83** 18	**98** 137	**100** 98	**100** 132	**100** 112	**0** 2	- 0	**78** 32	**91** 85	**79** 246	**97** 274	**80** 41	**79** 90	**92** 86	**58** 24	**71** 122	**100** 150	**85** 88	**82** 34	**79** 47	**96** 48	**64** 47	- -	- -
Lake District Hospital, Lakeview, OR	- -	- 0	- 0	- 0	- 0	- 0	- -	- 0	- -	**20** 5	- -	- -	- 0	- 0	- -	- -	**100** 1	- 0	- 0	- -	- -	- -	- -	- -
Legacy Emanuel Hospital/Health Center, Portland, OR	**83** 35	**97** 73	**98** 129	**90** 42	**99** 122	**100** 1	**75** 4	**89** 46	**77** 64	**33** 107	**98** 126	**79** 34	**84** 69	**86** 65	**45** 20	**68** 102	**99** 110	**56** 50	**70** 47	**67** 124	**95** 58	**77** 114	- -	- -
Legacy Good Samaritan Hospital, Portland, OR	**66** 76	**99** 122	**98** 272	**97** 76	**94** 259	- 0	**27** 11	**91** 108	**66** 177	**30** 270	**95** 332	**63** 62	**87** 78	**96** 67	**60** 20	**71** 134	**100** 152	**56** 95	**72** 54	**51** 138	**97** 71	**90** 128	- -	- -
Legacy Meridian Park Hospital, Tualatin, OR	**82** 34	**94** 108	**92** 75	**93** 75	**96** 83	**33** 3	**33** 3	**94** 18	**75** 93	**30** 173	**93** 216	**82** 11	**79** 89	**96** 72	**36** 22	**91** 172	**100** 186	**53** 133	**68** 25	**77** 98	**98** 50	**74** 92	- -	- -
Legacy Mount Hood Medical Center, Gresham, OR	**71** 7	**97** 36	**88** 16	**100** 20	**83** 18	**33** 3	- 0	**40** 5	**72** 36	**11** 84	**93** 95	**50** 16	**90** 89	**97** 61	**41** 27	**86** 140	**100** 159	**44** 86	**66** 47	**79** 73	**95** 40	**44** 70	- -	- -
McKenzie-Willamette Medical Center, Springfield, OR	**100** 8	**97** 74	**90** 39	**97** 65	**88** 42	- 0	- 0	**100** 7	**74** 35	**76** 91	**94** 131	**96** 25	**87** 150	**92** 142	**97** 30	**85** 206	**100** 249	**83** 149	**92** 78	**72** 196	**91** 74	**87** 192	**0.00** 799	**3.42** 555
Mercy Medical Center, Roseburg, OR	**100** 9	**97** 76	**90** 41	**95** 81	**94** 48	**63** 19	- 0	**100** 14	**77** 61	**4** 215	**75** 240	**67** 27	**88** 139	**88** 82	**8** 37	**80** 132	**100** 182	**35** 108	**75** 48	**68** 240	**70** 60	**49** 231	**0.19** 1042	**3.31** 756
Merle West Medical Center, Klamath Falls, OR	**64** 11	**96** 73	**97** 65	**89** 57	**92** 63	**0** 1	**44** 9	**89** 18	**89** 46	**51** 131	**92** 155	**73** 22	**90** 139	**88** 105	**66** 35	**83** 167	**100** 199	**80** 125	**62** 56	**80** 97	**62** 97	**41** 95	**0.23** 870	**5.25** 591
Mid-Columbia Medical Center, The Dalles, OR	**100** 1	**100** 18	**100** 6	**94** 16	**100** 8	**50** 4	- 0	**100** 2	**93** 15	**98** 50	**98** 59	**100** 17	**79** 70	**96** 71	**58** 19	**89** 83	**100** 103	**82** 65	**100** 22	**93** 163	**100** 58	**81** 164	- -	- -
Mountain View Hospital District, Madras, OR	- 0	**67** 3	**100** 3	**67** 3	**67** 3	- 0	- -	- 0	**100** 2	**25** 16	**30** 20	**62** 8	**100** 28	**95** 20	**80** 5	**84** 37	**100** 42	**87** 23	**75** 12	**45** 22	**89** 9	**82** 22	- -	- -
Oregon Health Sciences University, Portland, OR	**86** 28	**99** 73	**99** 93	**98** 62	**99** 93	- 0	**100** 1	**77** 26	**94** 108	**41** 199	**98** 216	**49** 45	**72** 68	**95** 84	**26** 23	**64** 135	**100** 167	**67** 51	**63** 62	**74** 373	**93** 83	**80** 373	- -	- -
Peace Harbor Hospital, Florence, OR	**100** 1	**80** 5	**100** 3	**71** 7	**100** 6	- 0	- 0	**0** 1	**92** 12	**24** 38	**90** 39	**80** 5	**82** 34	**88** 26	**100** 3	**82** 38	**100** 51	**91** 35	**82** 11	**78** 18	**100** 17	**81** 16	- -	- -
Pioneer Memorial Hospital, Prineville, OR	- 0	**50** 4	**100** 2	**100** 1	**100** 1	- 0	- 0	- 0	**100** 5	- -	**65** 34	**33** 3	**84** 25	**96** 23	- -	**85** 34	**100** 40	**45** 20	**22** 9	**92** 37	**89** 9	**73** 37	- -	- -
Pioneer Memorial Hospital, Heppner, OR	- -	- -	- -	- -	- -	- -	- -	- -	- -	- -	- -	- -	- -	- -	- -	- -	- -	- -	- -	- -	- -	- -	- -	- -
Portland Adventist Medical Center, Portland, OR	**87** 15	**96** 96	**98** 88	**94** 50	**98** 95	- 0	**50** 10	**100** 32	**93** 44	**75** 133	**95** 153	**98** 45	**90** 164	**97** 167	**93** 42	**81** 236	**100** 304	**84** 204	**83** 76	**84** 158	**90** 52	**68** 153	- -	- -
Providence Hood River Memorial Hospital, Hood River, OR	**100** 3	**100** 16	**100** 9	**100** 14	**100** 9	**0** 2	- 0	**0** 2	**100** 9	**10** 20	**74** 23	**50** 2	**91** 43	**91** 11	**86** 7	**90** 48	**100** 61	**90** 49	**25** 4	**96** 125	**100** 44	**74** 125	- -	- -
Providence Medford Medical Center, Medford, OR	**91** 11	**98** 64	**100** 45	**97** 60	**96** 52	- 0	- 0	**82** 11	**74** 39	**10** 136	**85** 162	**65** 40	**83** 107	**82** 68	**83** 24	**70** 132	**100** 166	**45** 115	**80** 50	**65** 108	**85** 27	**78** 108	- -	- -
Providence Milwaukie Hospital, Portland, OR	**100** 5	**100** 41	**92** 25	**97** 37	**96** 27	- 0	- 0	**75** 4	**92** 37	**27** 86	**93** 105	**73** 26	**76** 98	**86** 79	**74** 27	**84** 129	**100** 156	**74** 99	**79** 43	**69** 113	**95** 39	**55** 105	- -	- -
Providence Newberg Hospital, Newberg, OR	**100** 1	**100** 15	**100** 9	**93** 15	**100** 11	**50** 2	- 0	- 0	**57** 14	**22** 41	**91** 55	**25** 8	**74** 50	**92** 36	**57** 7	**82** 62	**100** 78	**37** 49	**62** 13	**93** 99	**95** 37	**89** 96	- -	- -
Providence Portland Medical Center, Portland, OR	**98** 106	**98** 389	**99** 545	**98** 336	**99** 500	**0** 2	**70** 23	**96** 154	**89** 132	**61** 280	**94** 323	**98** 59	**86** 125	**94** 123	**92** 25	**78** 179	**100** 215	**77** 123	**98** 56	**84** 222	**95** 79	**55** 215	- -	- -
Providence Saint Vincent Medical Center, Portland, OR	**90** 136	**99** 716	**98** 1008	**96** 648	**96** 923	**100** 1	**78** 23	**86** 297	**80** 131	**57** 308	**90** 346	**78** 41	**89** 157	**90** 147	**57** 28	**78** 185	**100** 230	**82** 164	**72** 47	**92** 263	**99** 94	**83** 259	- -	- -

NOTE: The first number in each column (boldface) is the rate in percent, the second number is the number of patients; Please refer to the main entry for footnotes; ***Heart Attack Care:*** *1. ACE Inhibitor or ARB for LVSD; 2. Aspirin at Arrival; 3. Aspirin at Discharge; 4. Beta Blocker at Arrival; 5. Beta Blocker at Discharge; 6. Fibrinolytic Medication Timing; 7. PCI Within 90 Minutes of Arrival; 8. Smoking Cessation Advice;* ***Heart Failure Care:*** *9. ACE Inhibitor or ARB for LVSD; 10. Discharge Instructions; 11. Evaluation of LVS Function; 12. Smoking Cessation Advice;* ***Pneumonia Care:*** *13. Appropriate Initial Antibiotic; 14. Blood Culture Timing; 15. Influenza Vaccine; 16. Initial Antibiotic Timing; 17. Oxygenation Assessment; 18. Pneumococcal Vaccine; 19. Smoking Cessation Advice;* ***Surgical Infection Prevention:*** *20. Prophylactic Antibiotic Given; 21. Prophylactic Antibiotic Selection; 22. Prophylactic Antibiotic Stopped;* ***Pregnancy Care:*** *23. Inpatient Neonatal Mortality; 24. Third or Fourth Degree Laceration*

Hospital	Heart Attack Care								Heart Failure Care				Pneumonia Care							Surgical Infection Prevention			Pregnancy Care	
	1	2	3	4	5	6	7	8	9	10	11	12	13	14	15	16	17	18	19	20	21	22	23	24
Providence Seaside Hospital, Seaside, OR	100 2	100 17	89 9	89 18	100 10	- 0	- 0	50 2	88 8	10 39	64 45	78 9	83 41	75 20	79 14	80 45	100 56	91 33	75 8	38 8	100 1	75 8	- -	- -
Rogue Valley Medical Center, Medford, OR	95 58	99 219	99 421	98 162	97 448	- 0	53 19	95 142	91 221	73 402	94 428	85 68	91 188	96 176	69 62	76 259	100 325	67 230	94 77	82 590	99 78	84 574	- -	- -
Sacred Heart Medical Center, Eugene, OR	89 149	98 302	99 606	96 285	99 665	- 0	71 21	99 239	90 246	93 408	99 476	94 79	92 295	94 345	83 112	81 526	100 624	76 388	97 215	83 148	93 150	70 142	- -	- -
Saint Charles Medical Center-Bend-Redmond, Bend, OR	94 48	98 244	98 339	95 195	95 293	- 0	73 15	98 88	92 84	49 167	93 178	87 38	90 136	85 124	20 41	76 184	100 226	24 137	62 45	79 1197	98 308	68 1149	0.10 1998	2.02 1487
Saint Charles Medical Center-Redmond, Redmond, OR	100 6	92 40	80 25	82 34	85 26	- 0	- 0	0 1	88 16	40 40	87 45	88 8	81 53	80 45	15 13	78 69	100 81	20 50	68 19	88 204	91 45	56 194	0.00 255	3.55 197
Saint Elizabeth Health Services, Baker City, OR	- -	- -	- -	- -	- -	- -	- -	- -	- -	- -	- -	- -	- -	- -	- -	- -	- -	- -	- -	- -	- -	- -	- -	- -
Salem Hospital, Salem, OR	73 67	99 343	98 387	97 296	99 345	57 7	73 15	95 119	77 156	59 303	95 388	92 64	90 254	91 245	95 78	78 371	100 478	87 303	88 112	82 1171	62 277	89 1109	- -	- -
Samaritan Lebanon Community Hospital, Lebanon, OR	50 2	96 23	93 15	83 23	95 19	- 0	- 0	100 2	85 26	46 70	77 96	100 17	86 95	92 61	74 23	92 118	100 139	70 105	94 36	83 88	100 17	92 85	- -	- -
Samaritan North Lincoln Hospital, Lincoln City, OR	100 2	100 10	80 10	80 5	83 6	- 0	- 0	100 1	82 11	24 29	74 43	40 10	72 39	91 22	44 9	77 48	100 59	44 41	43 23	59 64	44 9	35 60	- -	- -
Samaritan Pacific Community Hospital, Newport, OR	100 2	80 15	77 13	100 11	100 11	- 0	- 0	33 3	78 9	23 39	76 37	70 10	80 49	83 23	33 9	86 42	100 58	52 31	81 16	80 54	100 10	82 51	- -	- -
Santiam Memorial Hospital, Stayton, OR	- 0	67 6	60 5	100 4	100 3	- 0	- 0	100 1	100 3	67 24	76 29	50 2	76 42	72 18	78 9	63 43	100 61	47 36	100 12	0 2	50 2	0 2	- -	- -
Silverton Hospital, Silverton, OR	75 4	83 23	100 14	93 14	82 11	- 0	- 0	100 1	100 8	75 24	87 30	100 2	94 51	91 34	73 11	91 53	100 67	68 44	45 11	78 110	72 29	81 101	- -	- -
Southern Coos Hospital & Health Center, Bandon, OR	- 0	100 1	- 0	100 1	- 0	0 1	- 0	- 0	- -	- -	- -	- -	79 34	100 9	29 7	85 39	100 45	31 32	90 10	50 20	50 2	30 20	- -	- -
Three Rivers Community Hospital/Health Center, Grants Pass, OR	91 11	93 83	88 52	89 72	95 43	- 0	- 0	56 9	91 65	6 174	82 213	57 35	88 232	98 80	49 59	85 275	100 323	56 229	65 84	75 231	97 35	72 214	- -	- -
Tillamook County General Hospital, Tillamook, OR	100 1	100 14	100 9	100 13	100 10	0 4	- 0	100 3	100 5	84 38	79 38	90 10	82 50	86 28	83 12	93 45	100 59	80 35	100 12	57 75	89 19	34 77	- -	- -
Tuality Community Hospital, Hillsboro, OR	20 10	95 131	94 125	85 105	89 130	0 1	40 5	41 37	60 47	25 134	78 156	41 22	90 128	94 112	62 39	84 172	100 209	52 156	50 48	69 288	91 110	49 284	- -	- -
West Valley Hospital, Dallas, OR	- -	- -	- -	- -	- -	- -	- -	- -	- -	- -	- -	- -	- -	- -	- -	- -	- -	- -	- -	- -	- -	- -	- -	- -
Willamette Falls Hospital, Oregon City, OR	100 3	92 52	100 18	90 41	82 22	- 0	- 0	60 5	94 33	75 16	87 118	50 2	83 92	93 56	- -	90 104	100 129	75 79	71 7	40 45	93 43	98 40	0.09 1125	4.05 839
Willamette Valley Medical Center, McMinnville, OR	100 4	94 36	100 21	96 23	90 21	0 3	- 0	100 7	79 38	85 96	100 122	96 25	88 132	97 147	96 45	78 180	100 224	88 155	96 55	96 230	96 51	86 222	- -	- -
UTAH																								
Alta View Hospital, Sandy, UT	- 0	100 7	40 5	75 8	67 6	- 0	- 0	- 0	83 18	69 45	95 65	67 3	84 110	96 100	- -	85 160	100 194	82 119	91 33	95 261	100 81	77 260	0.09 2234	3.65 1780
American Fork Hospital, American Fork, UT	- 0	100 3	100 1	67 3	50 2	- 0	- 0	- 0	67 12	88 65	94 87	86 7	81 112	94 65	84 19	89 126	100 156	83 92	48 21	92 219	97 60	77 216	0.00 2845	3.09 2397
Ashley Valley Medical Center, Vernal, UT	- 0	100 1	100 1	0 1	0 1	- 0	- 0	- 0	100 4	86 14	100 18	100 6	84 45	100 23	100 6	93 54	100 56	100 31	100 21	78 32	100 9	38 32	0.28 352	3.80 263
Bear River Valley Hospital, Tremonton, UT	- 0	- 0	- 0	0 1	0 1	- 0	- -	- 0	- 0	80 10	89 9	- 0	88 26	100 2	75 4	86 22	100 28	72 18	83 6	47 19	50 4	84 19	- -	- -
Beaver Valley Hospital, Beaver, UT	0 1	100 2	50 2	33 3	33 3	- 0	- -	- 0	- 0	13 15	15 20	33 3	96 53	100 5	27 15	98 54	100 70	57 54	14 7	0 1	- 0	100 1	- -	- -
Brigham City Community Hospital, Brigham City, UT	- 0	- 0	- 0	- 0	- 0	- 0	- 0	- 0	100 1	0 4	75 8	100 1	83 23	80 5	88 8	91 23	100 31	90 21	60 5	40 70	80 25	100 68	0.28 358	1.46 274
Cache Valley Speciality Hospital, North Logan, UT	- -	- -	- -	- -	- -	- -	- -	- -	- 0	0 2	50 2	- 0	100 1	- 0	- -	0 1	100 1	0 1	- 0	16 64	91 64	17 64	- -	- -
Castleview Hospital, Price, UT	- 0	100 1	100 1	100 2	100 1	- 0	- 0	- 0	100 5	58 19	67 33	71 7	72 101	99 88	73 33	90 123	100 151	70 87	92 37	85 129	100 57	84 121	- -	- -
Central Valley Medical Center, Nephi, UT	- -	- -	- -	- -	- -	- -	- -	- -	100 3	11 18	64 25	100 1	81 27	100 4	8 12	85 34	100 42	18 22	60 5	90 50	100 17	96 48	- -	- -
Cottonwood Hospital, Murray, UT	77 13	92 127	93 106	93 104	94 117	- 0	43 7	94 31	77 30	88 91	92 105	85 20	84 257	94 163	84 67	73 329	99 382	79 212	85 74	81 260	92 78	62 254	0.00 3852	3.51 2992
Davis Hospital and Medical Center, Layton, UT	94 17	93 107	97 100	89 93	97 98	- 0	75 8	93 29	90 29	53 72	89 89	94 16	90 125	87 79	74 35	81 134	100 178	68 107	79 34	84 476	94 111	77 463	0.00 753	2.14 562
Delta Community Medical Center, Delta, UT	- 0	0 2	0 1	50 2	0 1	- 0	- -	- 0	- 0	86 7	67 9	- 0	81 21	80 5	80 5	87 23	100 26	65 17	0 3	- 0	- 0	- 0	- -	- -
Dixie Regional Medical Center, Saint George, UT	100 32	98 170	99 216	96 145	100 244	- 0	58 12	98 57	100 79	93 147	99 187	100 22	83 202	89 178	90 83	82 288	100 364	77 269	94 50	93 518	95 172	83 496	0.21 2875	3.40 2296
Fillmore Community Medical Center, Fillmore, UT	- 0	100 1	- 0	100 1	- 0	- 0	- 0	- 0	- -	- -	- -	- -	73 11	0 1	100 1	67 12	100 15	80 10	50 2	- 0	- 0	- 0	- -	- -
Garfield Memorial Hospital & Clinics, Panguitch, UT	- 0	- 0	- 0	- 0	- 0	- 0	- 0	- 0	0 1	25 8	42 12	100 1	94 34	100 2	50 4	100 34	100 40	58 26	78 9	- 0	- 0	- 0	- -	- -
Gunnison Valley Hospital, Gunnison, UT	- -	- -	- -	- -	- -	- -	- -	- -	- 0	27 11	44 16	100 2	78 40	100 5	50 4	83 36	100 47	77 26	57 7	- 0	- 0	- 0	- -	- -
Heber Valley Medical Center, Heber City, UT	- 0	100 1	0 1	0 1	0 1	- 0	- -	- 0	- 0	40 5	38 8	0 1	84 37	100 8	73 11	85 34	98 42	65 20	29 7	38 76	89 18	71 77	- -	- -
Jordan Valley Hospital, West Jordan, UT	100 3	100 25	89 18	91 23	87 15	67 3	33 6	100 6	87 15	57 67	87 79	100 14	89 151	95 112	100 35	84 177	100 211	97 98	100 49	70 341	98 92	63 329	0.07 1502	3.05 1213
Kane County Hospital, Kanab, UT	- 0	100 1	0 1	100 1	100 1	- 0	- 0	- 0	- 0	0 10	0 12	- 0	72 47	100 2	0 9	81 47	100 53	8 36	0 7	40 5	100 2	100 5	- -	- -
Lakeview Hospital, Bountiful, UT	100 7	100 66	100 60	95 55	100 56	0 2	100 7	100 7	88 16	55 38	94 52	- 0	84 115	91 100	81 36	81 134	100 184	73 127	62 21	91 218	99 134	24 215	- -	- -
LDS Hospital, Salt Lake City, UT	80 70	96 178	99 393	93 148	93 387	- 0	72 18	99 95	78 190	89 337	100 369	86 58	85 169	89 132	65 60	79 225	100 314	58 170	76 70	84 549	92 196	67 548	0.55 4215	3.34 3169
Logan Regional Hospital, Logan, UT	- 0	100 14	100 5	100 11	100 4	- 0	- 0	- 0	67 6	89 38	85 47	100 7	78 83	85 62	86 28	90 116	100 159	87 109	67 9	79 242	97 69	70 235	0.00 2645	2.89 2147
McKay-Dee Hospital Center, Ogden, UT	96 25	99 177	97 248	88 144	95 229	- 0	75 8	97 68	93 116	83 221	98 256	96 27	92 292	84 231	82 62	90 323	100 444	71 268	86 101	88 508	92 173	69 498	0.20 3920	2.14 2849
Mountain View Hospital, Payson, UT	100 4	95 39	95 39	85 26	89 35	- 0	50 4	100 6	92 13	53 45	98 57	100 6	83 72	95 60	88 33	80 99	100 124	85 79	100 20	94 138	89 61	89 133	- -	- -
Mountain West Medical Center, Tooele, UT	- 0	100 4	100 4	100 2	75 4	- 0	- 0	- 0	67 12	18 28	87 39	60 10	86 43	91 32	62 8	76 55	100 63	51 37	77 13	32 75	43 23	21 62	- -	- -
Ogden Regional Medical Center, Ogden, UT	100 10	99 81	97 105	94 62	98 104	0 1	25 8	92 38	89 38	54 78	92 109	100 13	89 129	84 75	90 40	90 145	100 174	86 119	85 39	64 199	93 94	72 198	0.12 2431	0.79 1768
Orem Community Hospital, Orem, UT	- -	- -	- -	- -	- -	- -	- -	- -	- -	- -	- -	- -	- -	- -	- -	- -	- -	- -	- -	100 18	100 3	100 18	- -	- -
Pioneer Valley Hospital, West Valley City, UT	76 17	98 89	99 113	91 66	91 101	25 8	38 16	95 55	90 31	29 78	94 88	87 23	81 183	93 135	98 44	79 202	100 226	84 128	88 59	71 190	98 54	72 179	0.00 287	1.86 215

NOTE: The first number in each column (boldface) is the rate in percent, the second number is the number of patients; Please refer to the main entry for footnotes; ***Heart Attack Care:*** *1. ACE Inhibitor or ARB for LVSD; 2. Aspirin at Arrival; 3. Aspirin at Discharge; 4. Beta Blocker at Arrival; 5. Beta Blocker at Discharge; 6. Fibrinolytic Medication Timing; 7. PCI Within 90 Minutes of Arrival; 8. Smoking Cessation Advice;* ***Heart Failure Care:*** *9. ACE Inhibitor or ARB for LVSD; 10. Discharge Instructions; 11. Evaluation of LVS Function; 12. Smoking Cessation Advice;* ***Pneumonia Care:*** *13. Appropriate Initial Antibiotic; 14. Blood Culture Timing; 15. Influenza Vaccine; 16. Initial Antibiotic Timing; 17. Oxygenation Assessment; 18. Pneumococcal Vaccine; 19. Smoking Cessation Advice;* ***Surgical Infection Prevention:*** *20. Prophylactic Antibiotic Given; 21. Prophylactic Antibiotic Selection; 22. Prophylactic Antibiotic Stopped;* ***Pregnancy Care:*** *23. Inpatient Neonatal Mortality; 24. Third or Fourth Degree Laceration*

Hospital	Heart Attack Care								Heart Failure Care				Pneumonia Care							Surgical Infection Prevention			Pregnancy Care	
	1	2	3	4	5	6	7	8	9	10	11	12	13	14	15	16	17	18	19	20	21	22	23	24
Saint Mark's Hospital, Salt Lake City, UT	79 28	98 132	98 174	95 106	86 169	0 1	56 16	86 49	85 100	56 186	96 222	89 36	93 269	97 261	78 94	78 361	100 472	73 311	68 85	91 290	95 134	81 283	- -	- -
Salt Lake Regional Medical Center, Salt Lake City, UT	71 7	75 20	90 52	69 16	73 44	- 0	100 2	75 20	75 32	35 66	87 86	44 18	85 68	61 54	89 19	77 78	100 93	84 44	62 29	78 211	100 52	83 193	0.00 814	2.20 682
Sanpete Valley Hospital, Mount Pleasant, UT	- 0	- 0	- 0	0 1	0 1	- 0	- 0	- 0	- 0	33 3	0 3	- 0	82 44	88 8	82 11	74 47	100 49	58 33	14 7	33 9	100 3	44 9	- -	- -
Sevier Valley Hospital, Richfield, UT	- 0	100 1	- 0	0 1	- 0	- 0	- -	- 0	50 2	30 20	43 23	50 2	80 61	100 17	89 9	78 68	100 79	52 42	47 17	83 29	83 6	56 27	0.38 265	4.35 207
The Orthopedic Specialty Hospital, Murray, UT	- -	- -	- -	- -	- -	- -	- -	- -	- -	- -	- -	- -	- -	- -	- -	- -	- -	- -	- -	87 194	99 71	34 194	- -	- -
Timpanogos Regional Hospital, Orem, UT	50 8	88 26	92 26	85 27	90 31	- 0	- 0	80 5	75 20	61 36	91 46	100 2	71 63	87 53	82 17	79 82	100 111	80 56	80 15	85 152	97 65	88 146	0.11 1852	2.11 1471
Uintah Basin Medical Center, Roosevelt, UT	100 1	50 4	50 4	75 4	75 4	- 0	- 0	- 0	100 4	0 16	67 21	0 4	86 21	82 11	33 3	81 26	100 33	12 17	43 7	36 36	100 14	56 34	- -	- -
University Health Care/Univ of Utah Hosp, Salt Lake City, UT	90 42	96 85	98 165	95 78	92 172	0 1	22 9	95 74	88 121	57 153	98 183	53 34	81 52	94 72	50 18	55 103	100 208	66 74	39 46	79 385	96 83	85 382	1.03 679	3.87 2349
Utah Valley Regional Medical Center, Provo, UT	89 37	98 157	98 334	94 135	96 305	- 0	70 10	100 82	80 82	86 187	98 236	93 29	90 149	87 119	75 51	78 211	100 272	78 155	57 35	79 534	95 169	77 520	0.34 5901	3.39 4579
Valley View Medical Center, Cedar City, UT	- 0	75 4	100 1	50 4	50 2	- 0	- 0	100 1	78 9	65 20	96 23	57 7	85 79	81 42	100 16	86 83	100 111	90 58	70 20	78 228	92 50	30 224	0.34 885	2.51 718
WASHINGTON																								
Auburn Regional Medical Center, Auburn, WA	62 55	93 142	97 118	95 147	89 119	52 27	20 10	81 42	76 79	56 124	70 156	85 33	79 159	86 97	53 32	82 163	100 201	61 111	57 44	88 388	96 98	81 388	- -	- -
Capital Medical Center, Olympia, WA	92 12	90 29	95 42	88 25	92 39	- 0	0 4	82 17	79 19	19 42	84 68	75 4	89 53	97 35	56 16	73 52	100 67	65 43	31 13	93 91	96 93	67 90	- -	- -
Cascade Valley Hosp/N Snohomish Co Sys, Arlington, WA	50 2	89 19	100 16	85 13	88 17	- 0	- 0	75 4	67 12	44 43	75 61	36 11	50 58	87 54	14 14	85 72	100 93	49 65	85 34	56 63	90 30	68 60	- -	- -
Central Washington Hospital, Wenatchee, WA	82 33	100 100	99 161	90 88	95 172	- 0	100 5	92 62	88 72	59 157	90 185	91 35	89 99	89 116	77 35	88 172	100 206	84 154	92 50	86 285	98 104	77 282	- -	- -
Coulee Community Hospital, Grand Coulee, WA	- -	- -	- -	- -	- -	- -	- -	- -	- -	- -	- -	- -	- -	- -	- -	- -	- -	- -	- -	- -	- -	- -	- -	- -
Deaconess Medical Center, Spokane, WA	89 70	99 105	100 270	96 92	99 297	- 0	56 9	100 107	91 128	85 217	94 252	97 62	87 91	89 76	71 31	73 146	100 186	60 125	88 58	90 351	96 103	68 345	- -	- -
Deer Park Health Center & Hospital, Deer Park, WA	- -	- -	- -	- -	- -	- -	- -	- -	- 0	0 1	100 1	- 0	100 2	- 0	- -	0 1	100 2	100 2	- 0	- -	- -	- -	- -	- -
Enumclaw Regional Hospital, Enumclaw, WA	50 2	100 4	100 3	75 4	100 3	- 0	- -	- 0	75 4	21 19	81 26	67 3	85 26	79 14	50 6	67 33	100 42	58 26	62 8	- -	- -	- -	- -	- -
Evergreen Hospital Medical Center, Kirkland, WA	98 46	99 205	97 191	94 136	98 181	- 0	47 15	82 56	89 80	63 175	95 223	74 19	86 146	94 166	89 44	75 207	100 254	88 146	81 43	83 128	95 39	79 123	- -	- -
Good Samaritan Hospital & Rehab Center, Puyallup, WA	91 33	99 225	91 188	99 206	95 190	- 0	33 15	96 68	85 82	35 211	90 292	75 40	76 147	89 120	68 28	73 176	99 229	45 140	61 44	55 247	96 90	87 222	- -	- -
Grays Harbor Community Hospital-West Campus, Aberdeen, WA	100 2	78 50	82 22	86 43	83 24	22 9	- 0	67 9	90 41	32 192	72 224	72 43	74 189	95 116	38 45	80 231	100 254	44 153	64 72	77 146	92 53	75 138	- -	- -
Group Health Eastside Hospital, Redmond, WA	100 8	97 31	100 17	100 22	100 23	- 0	- 0	- 0	89 54	46 35	99 149	100 2	90 20	93 27	- -	81 125	100 177	92 163	80 5	90 199	- -	83 192	- -	- -
Harborview Medical Center, Seattle, WA	96 24	100 98	100 63	100 61	100 80	- 0	67 9	91 54	90 113	59 176	98 199	74 102	83 121	80 119	21 24	68 177	100 214	46 68	66 119	76 133	83 36	78 131	- -	- -
Harrison Medical Center, Bremerton, WA	91 47	95 239	98 288	96 209	98 304	- 0	58 12	86 85	86 151	53 300	91 439	67 60	80 246	93 251	- -	70 371	100 448	79 325	56 114	86 792	74 297	65 761	- -	- -
Highline Community Hospital, Burien, WA	80 10	99 85	94 79	99 70	92 78	- 0	100 4	100 30	74 57	48 157	87 186	90 41	83 177	92 188	79 53	88 269	100 318	85 199	97 74	93 293	99 99	94 283	0.00 1252	1.90 843
Holy Family Hospital, Spokane, WA	85 13	99 97	99 73	99 86	96 72	- 0	42 12	97 29	81 53	66 129	86 165	100 21	87 280	95 240	88 64	78 310	100 393	83 252	92 95	87 151	94 47	82 145	0.00 1150	2.63 876
Hospice Care Center Hospital, Longview, WA	- -	- -	- -	- -	- -	- -	- -	- -	- -	- -	- -	- -	- -	- -	- -	- -	- -	- -	- -	- -	- -	- -	- -	- -
Island Hospital, Anacortes, WA	100 4	84 19	100 13	88 16	100 17	- 0	- 0	0 1	75 12	47 38	84 44	100 4	81 63	88 64	83 23	74 84	100 114	96 85	100 21	69 35	92 36	85 33	- -	- -
Jefferson General Hospital, Port Townsend, WA	- 0	83 6	75 4	100 5	100 3	- 0	- 0	- 0	81 16	25 36	83 46	40 10	83 48	92 36	58 12	87 63	100 77	62 50	70 10	89 152	76 46	65 151	- -	- -
Kadlec Medical Center, Richland, WA	84 55	90 115	96 298	82 106	92 275	- 0	80 15	63 19	67 67	41 32	89 161	75 4	76 25	93 30	- -	78 156	100 211	86 123	100 4	70 60	- -	74 57	- -	- -
Kennewick General Hospital, Kennewick, WA	89 9	82 33	70 23	73 33	77 26	- 0	- 0	100 4	69 35	62 92	83 118	91 22	75 76	92 86	- -	90 119	100 157	88 109	96 25	79 162	92 59	47 152	- -	- -
Kittitas Valley Community Hospital, Ellensburg, WA	100 2	100 7	100 8	100 5	100 5	- 0	- 0	- 0	100 4	67 24	90 31	100 3	93 29	95 21	83 6	88 32	100 36	65 23	88 8	94 65	100 12	85 62	- -	- -
Lake Chelan Community Hospital, Chelan, WA	- 0	- 0	- 0	- 0	- 0	0 1	- 0	- 0	- 0	100 1	0 2	- 0	67 3	100 1	0 1	100 3	100 3	0 2	- 0	- -	- -	- -	- -	- -
Legacy Salmon Creek Hospital, Vancouver, WA	86 7	100 39	90 29	100 20	91 22	0 1	- 0	100 3	66 62	31 147	88 185	78 41	91 88	92 65	50 24	84 142	100 161	59 112	81 36	67 93	91 46	47 86	- -	- -
Lincoln Hospital, Davenport, WA	- -	- -	- -	- -	- -	- -	- -	- -	100 2	100 1	100 2	50 2	100 6	- 0	- -	50 6	100 7	50 4	100 1	100 7	- -	100 7	- -	- -
Lourdes Medical Center, Pasco, WA	60 5	75 12	71 7	75 8	78 9	- 0	- 0	67 3	57 7	67 30	73 37	29 7	74 54	87 38	0 12	75 55	99 83	44 54	73 15	- -	- -	- -	- -	- -
Mark Reed Hospital, McCleary, WA	- -	- -	- -	- -	- -	- -	- -	- -	- -	- -	- -	- -	92 12	100 4	100 4	91 11	100 12	100 6	75 4	- -	- -	- -	- -	- -
Mason General Hospital, Shelton, WA	67 3	100 18	86 7	83 18	71 7	- 0	- 0	- 0	90 29	62 45	74 68	89 19	58 12	88 40	- -	88 83	100 99	83 58	94 16	- -	- -	- -	- -	- -
Mount Carmel Hospital, Colville, WA	100 1	100 7	100 8	100 10	100 8	0 1	- 0	- 0	100 14	97 34	93 41	100 5	80 82	98 63	100 18	88 95	100 112	99 80	91 23	88 25	100 9	68 25	- -	- -
Northwest Hospital and Medical Center, Seattle, WA	93 29	95 114	99 101	96 89	100 114	- 0	50 10	97 32	86 85	69 158	89 218	92 26	72 119	91 125	- -	73 145	100 188	92 125	78 41	76 363	83 60	56 349	0.00 999	6.75 696
Ocean Beach Hospital, Ilwaco, WA	- -	- -	- -	- -	- -	- -	- -	- -	100 1	67 3	100 3	- 0	- -	- -	- -	- -	- -	- -	- -	- -	- -	- -	- -	- -
Olympic Medical Center, Port Angeles, WA	100 7	91 35	85 20	96 27	95 19	60 5	- 0	60 5	89 62	84 128	98 172	67 15	89 150	93 155	65 60	79 225	100 269	69 199	79 52	80 319	81 70	91 306	- -	- -
Othello Community Hospital, Othello, WA	- 0	100 1	- 0	0 1	- 0	- 0	- -	- 0	100 8	79 19	80 20	71 7	- -	100 4	67 3	64 11	100 16	100 11	- 0	- -	- -	- -	- -	- -
Overlake Hospital Medical Center, Bellevue, WA	78 77	94 213	98 253	86 149	97 265	0 2	46 13	92 59	77 134	16 269	97 344	68 22	82 130	98 142	19 53	76 197	100 245	23 175	70 40	63 220	85 79	80 210	0.02 4155	5.66 2703
Prosser Memorial Hospital, Prosser, WA	- -	- -	- -	- -	- -	- -	- -	- -	100 1	0 7	18 11	0 4	73 15	89 9	40 5	69 13	100 15	58 12	0 2	58 19	88 8	83 18	- -	- -
Providence Centralia Hospital, Centralia, WA	80 5	98 43	94 33	85 34	97 32	- 0	- 0	100 6	92 50	80 133	92 157	80 25	88 154	78 109	67 24	80 180	100 226	85 145	84 49	67 203	96 72	85 184	- -	- -
Providence Everett Medical Center, Everett, WA	76 62	99 406	98 453	98 394	99 450	- 0	70 30	93 142	95 115	51 255	89 331	93 46	77 104	92 95	29 31	57 152	100 189	77 125	92 60	90 225	95 82	82 214	0.13 1516	3.16 1013

NOTE: The first number in each column (boldface) is the rate in percent, the second number is the number of patients; Please refer to the main entry for footnotes; ***Heart Attack Care:*** *1. ACE Inhibitor or ARB for LVSD; 2. Aspirin at Arrival; 3. Aspirin at Discharge; 4. Beta Blocker at Arrival; 5. Beta Blocker at Discharge; 6. Fibrinolytic Medication Timing; 7. PCI Within 90 Minutes of Arrival; 8. Smoking Cessation Advice;* ***Heart Failure Care:*** *9. ACE Inhibitor or ARB for LVSD; 10. Discharge Instructions; 11. Evaluation of LVS Function; 12. Smoking Cessation Advice;* ***Pneumonia Care:*** *13. Appropriate Initial Antibiotic; 14. Blood Culture Timing; 15. Influenza Vaccine; 16. Initial Antibiotic Timing; 17. Oxygenation Assessment; 18. Pneumococcal Vaccine; 19. Smoking Cessation Advice;* ***Surgical Infection Prevention:*** *20. Prophylactic Antibiotic Given; 21. Prophylactic Antibiotic Selection; 22. Prophylactic Antibiotic Stopped;* ***Pregnancy Care:*** *23. Inpatient Neonatal Mortality; 24. Third or Fourth Degree Laceration*

Hospital	Heart Attack Care								Heart Failure Care				Pneumonia Care							Surgical Infection Prevention			Pregnancy Care	
	1	2	3	4	5	6	7	8	9	10	11	12	13	14	15	16	17	18	19	20	21	22	23	24
Providence St Peter Chemical Dependency Ctr, Lacey, WA	- -	- -	- -	- -	- -	- -	- -	- -	- -	- -	- -	- -	- -	- -	- -	- -	- -	- -	- -	- -	- -	- -	- -	- -
Providence Saint Peter Hospital, Olympia, WA	**80** 103	**97** 377	**97** 570	**93** 338	**90** 540	- 0	**50** 22	**81** 213	**92** 161	**41** 355	**87** 431	**78** 79	**76** 242	**91** 225	**48** 52	**82** 311	**99** 401	**62** 261	**52** 118	**86** 310	**92** 132	**60** 305	- -	- -
Pullman Memorial Hospital, Pullman, WA	**100** 1	**100** 4	**100** 4	**75** 4	**100** 4	**0** 2	- 0	- 0	**100** 1	**20** 5	**33** 9	**0** 1	**43** 7	**77** 22	- -	**75** 32	**100** 42	**34** 32	**0** 3	- -	- -	- -	- -	- -
Sacred Heart Medical Center, Spokane, WA	**97** 97	**100** 193	**100** 530	**99** 168	**99** 527	- 0	**85** 13	**100** 196	**98** 245	**96** 414	**99** 457	**100** 70	**82** 219	**91** 267	**84** 61	**75** 391	**100** 476	**80** 285	**100** 112	**90** 239	**96** 84	**90** 233	- -	- -
Saint Clare Hospital, Lakewood, WA	**100** 7	**98** 47	**100** 26	**95** 21	**100** 28	**0** 1	- 0	**100** 3	**96** 77	**60** 203	**98** 263	**86** 56	**94** 197	**89** 191	**54** 56	**83** 254	**100** 327	**79** 205	**83** 94	**94** 314	**96** 46	**91** 303	- -	- -
Saint Francis Hospital, Federal Way, WA	**94** 31	**98** 145	**100** 109	**95** 61	**100** 111	- 0	**90** 10	**93** 28	**95** 57	**39** 145	**99** 194	**91** 34	**96** 110	**90** 121	**61** 28	**84** 153	**100** 181	**82** 105	**86** 44	**86** 251	**96** 56	**77** 248	- -	- -
Saint John Medical Center, Longview, WA	**82** 22	**100** 115	**97** 64	**99** 90	**99** 69	**18** 11	- 0	**100** 13	**82** 93	**76** 172	**91** 209	**94** 50	**82** 140	**93** 125	**100** 62	**85** 335	**100** 428	**62** 227	**98** 102	**80** 152	**88** 155	**80** 146	- -	- -
Saint Joseph Hospital, Bellingham, WA	**95** 59	**100** 283	**98** 306	**98** 237	**99** 318	**100** 1	**71** 14	**90** 82	**95** 174	**71** 268	**99** 337	**92** 49	**89** 172	**97** 180	**82** 61	**81** 318	**100** 372	**89** 267	**97** 73	**97** 804	**98** 261	**93** 782	- -	- -
Saint Joseph Medical Center, Tacoma, WA	**86** 100	**99** 296	**97** 363	**96** 157	**99** 360	- 0	**62** 13	**94** 135	**83** 223	**42** 471	**94** 559	**72** 95	**95** 205	**93** 257	**67** 64	**84** 320	**100** 392	**74** 209	**82** 112	**90** 1348	**96** 252	**75** 1295	**0.02** 5174	**3.07** 3741
Saint Joseph's Hospital, Chewelah, WA	- 0	**100** 5	**86** 7	**67** 6	**60** 5	- 0	- 0	- 0	**75** 4	**90** 21	**91** 23	**100** 1	**92** 59	**97** 29	**100** 10	**91** 86	**100** 100	**86** 57	**93** 27	**50** 2	**100** 1	**50** 2	- -	- -
Saint Mary Medical Center, Walla Walla, WA	**50** 2	**93** 28	**100** 12	**100** 27	**94** 16	**50** 2	- 0	**100** 1	**60** 25	**53** 68	**95** 98	**92** 12	**86** 79	**92** 77	**59** 17	**86** 98	**100** 129	**78** 77	**71** 34	**91** 341	**97** 64	**84** 329	**0.00** 635	**2.84** 457
Samaritan Healthcare, Moses Lake, WA	**100** 1	**79** 24	**100** 14	**89** 18	**92** 12	- 0	- 0	**100** 2	**83** 12	**35** 51	**63** 73	**50** 8	**78** 54	**97** 38	**18** 17	**74** 85	**100** 103	**41** 61	**94** 16	**64** 213	**98** 47	**48** 207	- -	- -
Schick-Shadel Hospital, Seattle, WA	- -	- -	- -	- -	- -	- -	- -	- -	- -	- -	- -	- -	- -	- -	- -	- -	- -	- -	- -	- -	- -	- -	- -	- -
Skagit Valley Hospital, Mount Vernon, WA	**81** 26	**100** 88	**96** 91	**96** 79	**98** 113	- 0	**80** 5	**94** 31	**72** 54	**54** 127	**96** 172	**68** 22	**92** 108	**81** 121	**68** 34	**82** 147	**100** 195	**81** 135	**92** 38	**79** 355	**83** 54	**86** 341	- -	- -
Snoqualmie Valley Hospital, Snoqualmie, WA	- -	- -	- -	- -	- -	- -	- -	- -	**100** 1	**0** 5	**62** 8	- 0	**67** 9	**75** 4	**50** 2	**70** 10	**100** 12	**50** 6	**100** 1	- -	- -	- -	- -	- -
Southwest Washington Medical Center, Vancouver, WA	**80** 85	**100** 415	**97** 456	**98** 369	**98** 489	- 0	**76** 17	**90** 173	**90** 185	**58** 481	**90** 551	**64** 97	**39** 119	**89** 103	**65** 31	**73** 156	**100** 204	**66** 145	**77** 52	**89** 243	**97** 77	**77** 232	**0.02** 4044	**4.13** 2909
Stevens Hospital, Edmonds, WA	**95** 22	**93** 115	**99** 88	**97** 63	**97** 73	- 0	**20** 5	**94** 33	**79** 47	**40** 112	**89** 137	**70** 23	**83** 186	**93** 170	**70** 37	**78** 245	**100** 272	**73** 174	**72** 57	**79** 490	**88** 111	**73** 478	**0.08** 1208	**4.50** 866
Sunnyside Community Hospital, Sunnyside, WA	- 0	**100** 6	**75** 4	**100** 4	**100** 3	**0** 1	- -	**0** 1	**89** 9	**19** 27	**70** 27	**25** 4	**82** 33	**100** 12	- -	**72** 36	**100** 37	**46** 24	**43** 7	**75** 16	**100** 6	**92** 12	- -	- -
Swedish Medical Center, Seattle, WA	**76** 42	**98** 152	**96** 196	**92** 145	**94** 216	- 0	**0** 2	**79** 53	**81** 150	**22** 361	**91** 453	**48** 61	**79** 261	**88** 249	**63** 92	**78** 399	**100** 506	**71** 329	**86** 116	**79** 270	**98** 93	**52** 263	- -	- -
Swedish Medical Center/Providence, Seattle, WA	**78** 36	**98** 99	**99** 168	**97** 88	**93** 176	- 0	**43** 7	**80** 49	**85** 124	**27** 222	**94** 271	**54** 63	**84** 88	**93** 74	**61** 23	**76** 114	**100** 142	**60** 90	**87** 45	**73** 149	**100** 60	**69** 145	- -	- -
Tacoma General Hospital, Tacoma, WA	**85** 71	**96** 210	**99** 251	**98** 163	**96** 279	- 0	**83** 12	**93** 113	**88** 161	**58** 351	**95** 454	**90** 103	**87** 249	**94** 214	- -	**83** 311	**100** 405	**27** 224	**85** 116	**78** 539	**95** 157	**70** 514	**0.72** 3316	**3.79** 2113
Toppenish Community Hospital, Toppenish, WA	**100** 1	**100** 3	**100** 3	**100** 4	**100** 3	**0** 2	- 0	- 0	**91** 34	**79** 81	**82** 87	**74** 23	**51** 59	**92** 50	**58** 12	**76** 63	**100** 94	**74** 46	**54** 24	**97** 31	**67** 6	**81** 31	- -	- -
Tri-State Memorial Hospital, Clarkston, WA	**0** 2	**82** 11	**67** 6	**67** 12	**80** 5	- 0	- 0	- 0	**78** 9	**58** 26	**52** 56	**57** 7	**100** 4	**89** 36	- -	**75** 36	**100** 63	**71** 49	**33** 9	- -	- -	- -	- -	- -
United General Hospital, Sedro Woolley, WA	**100** 1	**100** 6	**100** 5	**100** 3	**100** 3	- 0	- 0	- 0	**100** 14	**88** 24	**91** 34	**100** 3	**94** 107	**96** 50	**62** 16	**82** 92	**100** 113	**96** 79	**100** 24	**100** 1	**0** 1	**0** 1	- -	- -
University of Washington Medical Center, Seattle, WA	**91** 22	**100** 51	**99** 82	**95** 42	**99** 105	- 0	**50** 4	**100** 36	**97** 231	**51** 333	**99** 352	**100** 63	**86** 83	**97** 97	**33** 30	**47** 173	**100** 200	**38** 87	**100** 51	**81** 343	**92** 74	**56** 331	- -	- -
Valley General Hospital, Monroe, WA	**100** 2	**100** 7	**100** 5	**100** 6	**100** 7	- 0	- 0	**100** 1	**100** 13	**90** 39	**98** 49	**83** 12	**74** 54	**87** 53	- -	**76** 79	**100** 83	**82** 49	**76** 17	**83** 75	**81** 31	**81** 73	**0.50** 401	**1.76** 284
Valley Hospital & Medical Center, Spokane, WA	**0** 1	**79** 14	**100** 9	**93** 15	**89** 9	**100** 1	- 0	- 0	**78** 23	**36** 56	**83** 86	**85** 13	**80** 82	**96** 73	**68** 19	**68** 110	**100** 152	**61** 98	**97** 33	**89** 227	**97** 66	**88** 222	- -	- -
Valley Medical Center, Renton, WA	**85** 40	**97** 261	**97** 209	**96** 223	**96** 200	- 0	**88** 17	**85** 20	**88** 113	**71** 55	**84** 303	**67** 9	**90** 20	**90** 30	- -	**61** 239	**100** 284	**57** 169	**88** 8	**67** 64	**91** 66	**84** 64	**0.14** 3571	**4.19** 2243
Virginia Mason Medical Center, Seattle, WA	**88** 48	**98** 139	**99** 244	**100** 125	**98** 240	- 0	**50** 8	**98** 47	**77** 123	**59** 288	**97** 375	**100** 15	**96** 177	**87** 202	**74** 78	**81** 235	**100** 352	**61** 266	**98** 61	**70** 524	**94** 134	**91** 496	- -	- -
Walla Walla General Hospital, Walla Walla, WA	**100** 3	**100** 17	**100** 10	**82** 11	**90** 10	**0** 1	- 0	**100** 2	**68** 19	**43** 30	**96** 47	**100** 4	**89** 47	**96** 47	**67** 9	**85** 52	**100** 70	**67** 48	**91** 23	**87** 110	**100** 41	**79** 109	**0.31** 323	**3.00** 233
Wenatchee Valley Hospital, Wenatchee, WA	- -	- -	- -	- -	- -	- -	- -	- -	- -	- -	- -	- -	- -	- -	- -	- -	- -	- -	- -	**100** 66	- -	**100** 66	- -	- -
Whidbey General Hospital, Coupeville, WA	**100** 2	**95** 22	**100** 9	**89** 18	**100** 10	**100** 1	- 0	**0** 2	**77** 13	**41** 27	**70** 37	**33** 3	**70** 82	**90** 49	**58** 19	**81** 83	**100** 101	**44** 79	**67** 9	**84** 62	**90** 20	**81** 59	- -	- -
Yakima Regional Medical & Cardiac Center, Yakima, WA	**98** 56	**97** 95	**99** 180	**96** 71	**99** 177	- 0	**75** 8	**100** 89	**93** 67	**78** 170	**91** 192	**92** 40	**90** 87	**82** 88	**74** 23	**84** 117	**100** 144	**73** 79	**98** 56	**94** 282	**98** 50	**59** 280	- -	- -
Yakima Valley Memorial Hospital, Yakima, WA	**95** 21	**97** 161	**100** 128	**98** 121	**99** 130	**0** 1	**100** 7	**100** 47	**76** 84	**36** 220	**86** 261	**96** 28	**94** 187	**96** 70	**54** 48	**85** 275	**100** 333	**71** 221	**97** 78	**99** 819	**97** 192	**84** 806	- -	- -
WYOMING																								
Campbell County Memorial Hospital, Gillette, WY	**100** 3	**100** 20	**100** 9	**100** 15	**90** 10	**50** 4	- 0	**100** 1	**78** 9	**60** 35	**62** 50	**20** 5	**76** 71	**85** 59	**74** 23	**92** 86	**100** 110	**76** 59	**63** 27	**91** 126	**100** 23	**91** 121	**0.40** 752	**3.46** 549
Cheyenne Regional Medical Center-West, Cheyenne, WY	**92** 25	**92** 133	**98** 195	**91** 129	**95** 197	- 0	**88** 8	**96** 82	**89** 53	**72** 138	**84** 176	**84** 25	**81** 222	**81** 106	**83** 41	**71** 247	**100** 285	**86** 161	**77** 66	**43** 510	**95** 154	**78** 495	- -	- -
Community Hospital, Torrington, WY	- 0	**60** 5	**75** 4	**75** 4	**75** 4	- 0	- 0	- 0	**67** 6	**68** 25	**74** 31	**100** 4	**81** 36	**94** 18	**92** 12	**97** 30	**100** 39	**83** 29	**67** 3	**60** 10	**100** 10	**89** 9	- -	- -
Crook County Medical Services, Sundance, WY	- -	- -	- -	- -	- -	- -	- -	- -	**0** 1	**100** 2	**50** 2	- 0	**92** 12	**100** 1	**0** 1	**83** 12	**100** 14	**43** 7	**60** 5	- -	- -	- -	- -	- -
Evanston Regional Hospital, Evanston, WY	- 0	- 0	- 0	- 0	- 0	- 0	- -	- 0	**100** 1	**53** 17	**74** 19	**100** 4	**89** 38	**94** 33	**78** 9	**96** 50	**100** 56	**96** 27	**88** 16	**93** 30	**50** 10	**68** 28	- -	- -
Hot Springs County Memorial Hospital, Thermopolis, WY	- -	- -	- -	- -	- -	- -	- -	- -	**100** 1	- -	**100** 3	**0** 1	**86** 22	**100** 9	**89** 9	**88** 26	**100** 41	**100** 29	**86** 7	**88** 17	**100** 3	**100** 17	- -	- -
Ivinson Memorial Hospital, Laramie, WY	- 0	**100** 1	**100** 1	**100** 1	**100** 1	- 0	- -	- 0	**100** 10	**65** 17	**90** 29	**100** 2	**75** 71	**84** 51	**83** 18	**82** 98	**100** 132	**84** 83	**93** 30	**67** 172	**89** 47	**66** 169	- -	- -
Johnson County Healthcare Center, Buffalo, WY	- 0	**100** 1	**100** 1	**100** 1	**100** 1	**0** 1	- -	- 0	- 0	**0** 7	**17** 6	- 0	**75** 8	**100** 2	**0** 3	**93** 15	**100** 17	**46** 13	**100** 1	- -	- -	- -	- -	- -
Lander Valley Medical Center, Lander, WY	**100** 1	**83** 6	**100** 2	**100** 3	**100** 3	**67** 3	- 0	- 0	**64** 11	**63** 30	**75** 32	**100** 8	**84** 56	**100** 41	**88** 16	**85** 85	**100** 98	**82** 40	**92** 36	**80** 128	**100** 61	**86** 125	- -	- -
Memorial Hospital of Carbon County, Rawlins, WY	- 0	**100** 6	**33** 3	**78** 9	**100** 4	**0** 2	- 0	- 0	**20** 5	**23** 48	**41** 56	**44** 16	**78** 51	**82** 17	**70** 10	**85** 53	**100** 66	**68** 37	**56** 25	**69** 13	**100** 2	**0** 13	- -	- -
Memorial Hospital of Converse County, Douglas, WY	- 0	**100** 1	**100** 1	**100** 1	**100** 1	- 0	- -	- 0	- 0	**88** 8	**78** 9	**100** 1	**89** 19	**86** 7	**83** 6	**90** 20	**100** 25	**89** 19	**100** 4	**79** 75	**96** 28	**62** 74	- -	- -
Memorial Hospital of Sheridan County, Sheridan, WY	- 0	**70** 10	**75** 4	**67** 9	**75** 4	- 0	- 0	- 0	**50** 2	**59** 27	**42** 43	**100** 2	**77** 82	**96** 52	**93** 15	**86** 97	**99** 115	**64** 85	**57** 28	**94** 182	**92** 40	**95** 176	- -	- -
Memorial Hospital of Sweetwater County, Rock Springs, WY	- 0	**33** 3	**50** 2	**50** 2	**100** 1	- 0	- 0	- 0	**87** 15	**55** 53	**57** 65	**54** 13	**81** 79	**79** 58	**79** 14	**85** 96	**99** 110	**73** 59	**79** 33	**70** 87	**21** 28	**94** 77	- -	- -

NOTE: The first number in each column (boldface) is the rate in percent, the second number is the number of patients; Please refer to the main entry for footnotes; ***Heart Attack Care:*** *1. ACE Inhibitor or ARB for LVSD; 2. Aspirin at Arrival; 3. Aspirin at Discharge; 4. Beta Blocker at Arrival; 5. Beta Blocker at Discharge; 6. Fibrinolytic Medication Timing; 7. PCI Within 90 Minutes of Arrival; 8. Smoking Cessation Advice;* ***Heart Failure Care:*** *9. ACE Inhibitor or ARB for LVSD; 10. Discharge Instructions; 11. Evaluation of LVS Function; 12. Smoking Cessation Advice;* ***Pneumonia Care:*** *13. Appropriate Initial Antibiotic; 14. Blood Culture Timing; 15. Influenza Vaccine; 16. Initial Antibiotic Timing; 17. Oxygenation Assessment; 18. Pneumococcal Vaccine; 19. Smoking Cessation Advice;* ***Surgical Infection Prevention:*** *20. Prophylactic Antibiotic Given; 21. Prophylactic Antibiotic Selection; 22. Prophylactic Antibiotic Stopped;* ***Pregnancy Care:*** *23. Inpatient Neonatal Mortality; 24. Third or Fourth Degree Laceration*

Hospital	Heart Attack Care								Heart Failure Care				Pneumonia Care							Surgical Infection Prevention			Pregnancy Care	
	1	2	3	4	5	6	7	8	9	10	11	12	13	14	15	16	17	18	19	20	21	22	23	24
Niobrara County Memorial Hospital, Lusk, WY	- -	- -	- -	- -	- -	- -	- -	- -	- 0	- 0	0 1	- 0	- 0	- 0	- -	- 0	- 0	- 0	- 0	- -	- -	- -	- -	- -
North Big Horn Hospital, Lovell, WY	- 0	70 10	67 9	27 11	30 10	- 0	- -	0 4	- 0	40 5	8 13	0 1	83 18	100 4	60 5	76 21	96 24	60 15	33 3	- -	- -	- -	- -	- -
Platte County Memorial Hospital, Wheatland, WY	- 0	100 1	100 1	100 1	100 1	- 0	- 0	100 1	100 4	100 6	100 9	100 2	97 33	85 13	100 4	94 36	100 43	96 25	100 10	80 5	100 5	100 5	- -	- -
Powell Vally Hospital, Powell, WY	- 0	100 5	100 4	100 2	100 3	100 1	- 0	0 1	50 2	33 9	38 21	0 2	83 12	100 4	100 5	80 15	100 21	91 11	50 4	79 38	86 7	78 36	- -	- -
Riverton Memorial Hospital, Riverton, WY	- 0	100 7	33 3	100 6	67 3	0 1	- 0	100 2	75 8	79 34	83 35	50 4	74 43	82 28	100 4	93 45	100 55	85 26	82 17	95 56	100 20	89 55	- -	- -
Saint John's Medical Center, Jackson, WY	- 0	100 3	100 3	100 3	100 3	- 0	- 0	100 1	61 18	86 36	64 39	100 5	92 51	89 27	67 6	89 46	97 66	65 34	45 11	83 131	94 47	77 124	0.21 487	3.83 366
South Big Horn County Hospital, Basin, WY	- -	- -	- -	- -	- -	- -	- -	- -	- 0	100 1	100 1	- 0	100 1	- 0	- 0	- 0	100 2	100 1	100 1	- -	- -	- -	- -	- -
South Lincoln Medical Center, Kemmerer, WY	- 0	- 0	- 0	- 0	- 0	- 0	- 0	- 0	- 0	0 6	0 8	- 0	67 15	100 4	0 4	67 12	100 20	10 10	71 7	100 7	100 2	100 6	- -	- -
Star Valley Medical Center, Afton, WY	- 0	0 1	- 0	0 1	- 0	- 0	- 0	- 0	100 1	0 4	40 5	0 1	71 14	- 0	50 2	100 15	100 17	23 13	50 2	50 20	100 7	58 19	- -	- -
Washakie Medical Center, Worland, WY	- 0	0 1	0 1	0 1	0 1	- 0	- -	- 0	100 7	84 19	77 26	33 3	74 23	100 10	83 6	100 21	100 31	81 16	25 4	43 7	100 8	80 5	- -	- -
Weston County Health Services, Newcastle, WY	- -	- -	- -	- -	- -	- -	- -	- -	0 1	0 4	50 4	100 1	73 11	100 1	60 5	92 12	100 13	89 9	100 2	- -	- -	- -	- -	- -
Wyoming Medical Center, Casper, WY	89 47	98 151	96 308	93 149	93 303	- 0	56 9	88 144	89 70	58 159	86 188	62 40	85 156	94 135	100 43	86 208	100 244	88 147	79 89	73 394	86 100	66 372	- -	- -

NOTE: The first number in each column (boldface) is the rate in percent, the second number is the number of patients; Please refer to the main entry for footnotes; ***Heart Attack Care:*** *1. ACE Inhibitor or ARB for LVSD; 2. Aspirin at Arrival; 3. Aspirin at Discharge; 4. Beta Blocker at Arrival; 5. Beta Blocker at Discharge; 6. Fibrinolytic Medication Timing; 7. PCI Within 90 Minutes of Arrival; 8. Smoking Cessation Advice;* ***Heart Failure Care:*** *9. ACE Inhibitor or ARB for LVSD; 10. Discharge Instructions; 11. Evaluation of LVS Function; 12. Smoking Cessation Advice;* ***Pneumonia Care:*** *13. Appropriate Initial Antibiotic; 14. Blood Culture Timing; 15. Influenza Vaccine; 16. Initial Antibiotic Timing; 17. Oxygenation Assessment; 18. Pneumococcal Vaccine; 19. Smoking Cessation Advice;* ***Surgical Infection Prevention:*** *20. Prophylactic Antibiotic Given; 21. Prophylactic Antibiotic Selection; 22. Prophylactic Antibiotic Stopped;* ***Pregnancy Care:*** *23. Inpatient Neonatal Mortality; 24. Third or Fourth Degree Laceration*

Hospitals whose Mortality Rate is Better than the U.S. National Rate

Heart Attack

Hospital	City	State	Phone	Web Site
Abbott-Northwestern Hospital	Minneapolis	Minnesota	612-863-4000	www.abbottnorthwestern.com
Advocate Lutheran General Hospital	Park Ridge	Illinois	847-723-2210	www.advocatehealth.com
Aurora Saint Lukes Medical Center	Milwaukee	Wisconsin	414-649-6000	www.aurorahealthcare.org
Avera Heart Hospital of South Dakota	Sioux Falls	South Dakota	605-977-7000	www.southdakotaheart.com
Barnes Jewish Hospital	Saint Louis	Missouri	314-747-3000	www.barnesjewish.org
Cape Cod Hospital	Hyannis	Massachusetts	508-771-1800	www.capecodhealth.org/
Evergreen Hospital Medical Center	Kirkland	Washington	425-899-1000	www.evergreenhealthcare.org
Hartford Hospital	Hartford	Connecticut	860-545-5000	www.harthosp.org
Hillcrest Hospital	Mayfield Heights	Ohio	440-312-4500	www.hillcresthospital.org
Maimonides Medical Center	Brooklyn	New York	718-283-6000	www.maimonidesmed.org
Maine Medical Center	Portland	Maine	207-871-0111	www.mmc.org
New York-Presbyterian Hospital	New York	New York	212-746-5454	www.nyp.org
Rex Hospital	Raleigh	North Carolina	919-784-3100	www.rexhealth.com
Saint Vincent Heart Center of Indiana	Indianapolis	Indiana	317-583-5000	www.theheartcenter.com
Saint Vincent's Medical Center	Bridgeport	Connecticut	203-576-6000	www.stvincents.org
Suburban Hospital Association	Bethesda	Maryland	301-896-3100	www.suburbanhospital.org
Trumbull Memorial Hospital	Warren	Ohio	330-841-9011	www.trumhosp.org

Note: Table shows hospitals whose 30-day risk-adjusted death (mortality) rate from heart attack is lower than the U.S. national rate of 16%

Heart Failure

Hospital	City	State	Phone	Web Site
Aventura Hospital & Medical Center	Aventura	Florida	305-682-7000	www.aventurahospital.com
Bay Medical Center	Panama City	Florida	850-769-1511	www.baymedical.org
Bayonne Medical Center	Bayonne	New Jersey	201-858-5000	www.bayonnemedicalcenter.org
Beth Israel Deaconess Medical Center	Boston	Massachusetts	617-667-7000	www.bidmc.harvard.edu
Beth Israel Medical Center	New York	New York	212-420-2000	www.bethisraelny.com
Brigham and Women's Hosptial	Boston	Massachusetts	617-732-5500	www.brighamandwomens.org
Christiana Hospital	Newark	Delaware	302-733-1000	www.christianacare.org
Community Hospital	Munster	Indiana	219-836-1600	www.comhs.org/community
Genesys Regional Medical Center	Grand Blanc	Michigan	810-606-5000	www.genesys.org
Glendale Memorial Hospital & Health Center	Glendale	California	818-502-1900	www.glendalememorial.com
Good Samaritan Hospital	Baltimore	Maryland	410-532-8000	www.goodsam-md.org
Hackensack University Medical Center	Hackensack	New Jersey	201-996-3760	www.humed.com
Harper University Hospital	Detroit	Michigan	313-745-8040	www.harperhospital.org
Healtheast Saint John's Hospital	Maplewood	Minnesota	651-232-7000	www.stjohnshospital-mn.org
Hillcrest Hospital	Mayfield Heights	Ohio	440-312-4500	www.hillcresthospital.org
Liberty Hospital	Liberty	Missouri	816-781-7200	www.libertyhospital.org
Loyola University Medical Center	Maywood	Illinois	708-216-9000	www.luhs.org
Maimonides Medical Center	Brooklyn	New York	718-283-6000	www.maimonidesmed.org
Marymount Hospital	Garfield Heights	Ohio	216-581-0500	www.marymount.org
Mclaren Regional Medical Center	Flint	Michigan	810-342-2000	www.mclaren.org
Memorial Hermann Healthcare System	Houston	Texas	281-929-6100	www.mhhs.org
Mercy Hospital	Miami	Florida	305-854-4400	www.mercymiami.com
Methodist Hospitals	Gary	Indiana	219-886-4000	www.methodisthospital.org
Miami Valley Hospital	Dayton	Ohio	937-208-8000	www.miamivalleyhospital.com
Mount Sinai Medical Center	Miami Beach	Florida	305-674-2121	www.msmc.com
New York-Presbyterian Hospital	New York	New York	212-746-5454	www.nyp.org
Northwestern Memorial Hospital	Chicago	Illinois	312-926-2000	www.nmh.org
Olympia Medical Center	Los Angeles	California	310-657-5900	www.olympiamedicalcenter.com
Providence Hospital	Southfield	Michigan	248-849-3000	www.stjohn.org/Providence/
Saint Agnes Hospital	Baltimore	Maryland	410-368-6000	www.stagnes.org
Sinai-Grace Hospital	Detroit	Michigan	313-966-3300	www.sinaigrace.org
Southcoast Hospital Group	Fall River	Massachusetts	508-679-3131	www.southcoast.org/charlton/
Southwest General Health Center	Middleburg Heights	Ohio	440-816-8000	www.swgeneral.com
Saint Catherine Hospital	East Chicago	Indiana	219-392-1700	www.comhs.org/stcatherine/
Western Pennsylvania Hospital Forbes Reg Campus	Monroeville	Pennsylvania	412-858-2000	www.wpahs.org
White Plains Hospital Center	White Plains	New York	914-681-0600	www.wphospital.org
William Beaumont Hospital	Royal Oak	Michigan	248-898-5000	www.beaumonthospitals.com
Willis Knighton Medical Center	Shreveport	Louisiana	318-212-4000	www.wkmc.com

Note: Table shows hospitals whose 30-day risk-adjusted death (mortality) rate from heart failure is lower than the U.S. national rate of 11%

Hospitals whose Mortality Rate is Worse than the U.S. National Rate

Heart Attack

Hospital	City	State	Phone	Web Site
Christus Saint Michael Health System	Texarkana	Texas	903-614-1000	www.christusstmichael.org/
Danville Regional Medical Center	Danville	Virginia	434-799-2100	www.danvilleregional.org
Kingman Regional Medical Center	Kingman	Arizona	928-757-2101	www.azkrmc.com
Southern Ohio Medical Center	Portsmouth	Ohio	740-356-5000	www.somc.org
Sparks Regional Medical Center	Fort Smith	Arkansas	479-441-4000	www.sparks.org
SVCMC-Catholic Medical Center of Brooklyn Queens	Jamaica	New York		
Yuma Regional Medical Center	Yuma	Arizona	928-344-2000	www.yumaregional.org

Note: Table shows hospitals whose 30-day risk-adjusted death (mortality) rate from heart attack is lower than the U.S. national rate of 16%

Heart Failure

Hospital	City	State	Phone	Web Site
Advocate Christ Hospital & Medical Center	Oak Lawn	Illinois	708-684-8000	www.advocatehealth.com
Athens Regional Medical Center	Athens	Tennessee	423-745-1411	www.athensrmc.com
Banner Thunderbird Medical Center	Glendale	Arizona	602-865-5555	www.bannerhealth.com
Baptist Memorial Hospital	Memphis	Tennessee	901-226-5000	www.baptistonline.org
Baylor All Saints Medical Center at Fort Worth	Fort Worth	Texas	817-926-2544	www.baylorhealth.com/locations/allsaints
Bromenn Healthcare	Normal	Illinois	309-454-1400	www.bromenn.org
Christus Saint Francis Cabrini Hospital	Alexandria	Louisiana	318-448-6760	www.cabrini.org
Claremore Regional Hospital	Claremore	Oklahoma	918-341-2556	www.claremorereghospital.com
Conway Regional Medical Center	Conway	Arkansas	501-329-3831	www.conwayregional.org
Corona Regional Medical Center	Corona	California	951-737-4343	www.coronaregional.com
Danville Regional Medical Center	Danville	Virginia	434-799-2100	www.danvilleregional.org
Faith Regional Health Services	Norfolk	Nebraska	402-371-3402	www.frhs.org
Forrest General Hospital	Hattiesburg	Mississippi	601-288-7000	www.forrestgeneral.com
Gnaden Huetten Memorial Hospital	Lehighton	Pennsylvania	610-377-1300	www.bluemountainhealthsystem.org
Hardin Medical Center	Savannah	Tennessee	731-926-8000	www.hardinmedicacenter.org
Hendrick Medical Center	Abilene	Texas	325-670-2000	www.hendrickhealth.org
Huguley Health System	Fort Worth	Texas	817-293-9110	www.huguley.org
Jackson Hospital & Clinic	Montgomery	Alabama	334-293-8000	www.jackson.org
Kenmore Mercy Hospital	Kenmore	New York	716-447-6100	www.chsbuffalo.org
Lodi Memorial Hospital	Lodi	California	209-334-3411	www.lodihealth.org
Manatee Memorial Hospital	Bradenton	Florida	941-745-6862	www.manateememorial.com
Massena Memorial Hospital	Massena	New York	315-769-4233	www.massenahospital.org
Medical Center of Central Georgia	Macon	Georgia	478-633-1000	www.mccg.org
Mercy Medical Center	Redding	California	530-225-6000	www.redding.mercy.org
Olympic Medical Center	Port Angeles	Washington	360-417-7000	www.olympicmedical.org
Plainview Hospital	Plainview	New York	516-719-3000	www.northshorelij.com
Port Huron Hospital	Port Huron	Michigan	810-987-5000	www.porthuronhospital.org
Providence Hospital	Mobile	Alabama	251-633-1000	www.providencehospital.org
Providence Saint Vincent Medical Center	Portland	Oregon	503-216-1234	www.providence.org
Sacred Heart Medical Center	Eugene	Oregon	541-686-7300	www.peacehealth.org
Samaritan Hospital	Troy	New York	518-271-3300	www.nehealth.com
Saint Josephs Medical Center of Stockton	Stockton	California	209-943-2000	www.stjospehscares.org
Saint Marys Hospital Medical Center	Green Bay	Wisconsin	920-498-4200	www.stmgb.org
Sutter General Hospital	Sacramento	California	916-454-2222	www.suttermedicalcenter.org
Tri-City Medical Center	Oceanside	California	760-940-5780	www.tricitymed.org

Note: Table shows hospitals whose 30-day risk-adjusted death (mortality) rate from heart failure is lower than the U.S. national rate of 11%

Hospital Mortality from Heart Attack and Heart Failure: State Summary

State	Number of Hospitals					
	Heart Attack			Heart Failure		
	Better than U.S. National Rate[1]	No Different than U.S. National Rate[2]	Worse than U.S. National Rate[3]	Better than U.S. National Rate[4]	No Different than U.S. National Rate[5]	Worse than U.S. National Rate[6]
Alabama	0	93	0	0	99	2
Alaska	0	13	0	0	20	0
Arizona	0	62	2	0	71	1
Arkansas	0	81	1	0	82	1
California	0	316	0	2	323	6
Colorado	0	61	0	0	68	0
Connecticut	2	29	0	0	32	0
Delaware	0	5	0	1	4	0
District of Columbia	0	7	0	0	7	0
Florida	0	182	0	4	180	1
Georgia	0	134	0	0	141	1
Guam	0	1	0	0	1	0
Hawaii	0	15	0	0	18	0
Idaho	0	33	0	0	37	0
Illinois	1	184	0	2	184	2
Indiana	1	117	0	3	119	0
Iowa	0	112	0	0	125	0
Kansas	0	114	0	0	132	0
Kentucky	0	100	0	0	103	0
Louisiana	0	108	0	1	117	1
Maine	1	37	0	0	39	0
Maryland	1	44	0	2	43	0
Massachusetts	1	63	0	3	62	0
Michigan	0	132	0	6	131	1
Minnesota	1	131	0	1	137	0
Mississippi	0	80	0	0	98	1
Missouri	1	117	0	1	123	0
Montana	0	41	0	0	60	0
N. Mariana Islands	0	1	0	0	1	0
Nebraska	0	74	0	0	87	1
Nevada	0	28	0	0	31	0
New Hampshire	0	26	0	0	26	0
New Jersey	0	75	0	2	73	0
New Mexico	0	38	0	0	42	0
New York	2	185	1	4	187	4
North Carolina	1	108	0	0	114	0
North Dakota	0	33	0	0	43	0
Ohio	2	155	1	4	159	0
Oklahoma	0	100	0	0	115	1
Oregon	0	57	0	0	56	2
Pennsylvania	0	170	0	1	170	1
Puerto Rico	0	47	0	0	49	0
Rhode Island	0	10	0	0	11	0
South Carolina	0	57	0	0	58	0
South Dakota	1	44	0	0	54	0
Tennessee	0	116	0	0	116	3
Texas	0	320	1	1	357	3
Utah	0	31	0	0	39	0
Vermont	0	15	0	0	16	0
Virgin Islands	0	2	0	0	2	0
Virginia	0	79	1	0	83	1
Washington	1	75	0	0	85	1
West Virginia	0	53	0	0	53	0
Wisconsin	1	118	0	0	124	1
Wyoming	0	23	0	0	26	0
U.S. and Territories	17	4453	7	38	4734	35

Note: (1) 30-day risk-adjusted death rate is lower than U.S. rate of 16%; (2) 30-day risk-adjusted death rate is about the same as U.S. rate of 16% or difference is uncertain; (3) 30-day risk-adjusted death rate is higher than U.S. rate of 16%; (4) 30-day risk-adjusted death rate is lower than U.S. rate of 11%; (2) 30-day risk-adjusted death rate is about the same as U.S. rate of 11% or difference is uncertain; (3) 30-day risk-adjusted death rate is higher than U.S. rate of 11%

What Do These Mortality Categories Show?

These categories show how hospitals' risk-adjusted 30-Day Death (mortality) rates compare to the rate across the U.S., after making adjustments for how sick patients were before they were admitted to the hospital and taking into account differences in death rates that might be due to chance.

Hospitals are shown to be Better or Worse Than U.S. National Rate only if we can be 95% certain that the difference between their risk-adjusted death (mortality) rates and the U.S. National rate is not due to chance. All others are shown in the No Different Than U.S. National Rate category.

Better than U.S. National Rate. Hospitals in the Better Than U.S. National Rate category have risk-adjusted 30-day death (mortality) rates that are lower than the U.S. National rate, and we can be 95% certain that this difference is not due to chance.

No Different than U.S. National Rate. Many hospitals in the No Different Than U.S. National Rate category have risk-adjusted 30-day death (mortality) rates that are about the same as the U.S. National rate. Other hospitals in this category have rates that are higher or lower than the U.S. National rate, but we cannot be 95% certain that these differences are not due to chance. One cannot be certain about differences when a hospital has very few relevant patients.

Worse than U.S. National Rate. Hospitals in the Worse Than U.S. National Rate category have risk-adjusted 30-day death (mortality) rates that are higher than the U.S. National rate, and we can be 95% certain that this difference is not due to chance.

Why are Death Rates for Individual Hospitals Not Shown?

Comparisons based on estimated death (mortality) rates alone can be misleading. Risk-adjusted death (mortality) rates are estimated for individual hospitals based on information taken from a particular time period (in this case, July 1, 2005 - June 30, 2006). If a slightly different time period had been chosen, chances are that each hospital's results would have been somewhat different.

Researchers almost always report a range ("confidence interval" or in this case an "interval estimate") around their estimates, to show how much variation might be due to this kind of chance. A confidence interval or interval estimate tells us we can be reasonably "confident" (in this case, 95% confident) that a hospital's death (mortality) rate fell somewhere within this specified range. The smaller the range, the more precise the estimate.

When hospitals treat a very large number of patients, chance differences will not have much effect on the overall rates. The range will be small, and the estimated death (mortality) rates will be more precise. In hospitals that treat smaller numbers of patients, however, even small chance differences could have a big impact on death (mortality) rates. The 95% confidence interval, or range, will be large, and the estimated death (mortality) rates will be much less precise.

Because the number of patients treated at U.S. hospitals varies widely, the precision of hospitals' estimated death (mortality) rates also varies.

Calculation of 30-Day Risk-Adjusted Mortality Rates

CMS calculates 30-day death (mortality) rates for heart attack and heart failure. The rates are "risk-adjusted" using Medicare claims and enrollment data in a complex statistical model. The model predicts how many patients will die within 30 days of being admitted to each hospital for heart attack or heart failure. It includes deaths whether the patients die in the hospital or after leaving, and whether or not they die for heart attack/heart failure or something else. By "risk-adjusted", we mean that the model calculates a death (mortality) rate that adjusts for the kinds of patients who go to that hospital so that hospitals that take care of sicker patients won't have a worse rate just because their patients were sicker before they arrived at the hospital.

For each hospital's rate, the model also calculates an "interval estimate" (which is like a confidence interval), which describes how much uncertainty there is around the rate-how much bigger or smaller the rate might really be. A hospital with many relevant patients will have a rate that is more precise or certain; that is, the "interval estimate" will be relatively narrow. A hospital with few relevant patients will have a rate that is less precise or certain; that is, will have a wide "interval estimate." The "risk-adjusted" hospital rate with its "interval estimate" can be compared to the U.S. National death (mortality) rate (the "national crude mortality rate"). If the interval estimate includes (overlaps with) the national crude mortality rate, the hospital's performance is considered to be "no different than U.S. National rate" and so is placed in that category. If the entire interval estimate is below the national crude mortality rate, then the hospital's performance is "worse than U.S. National rate." If the entire interval estimate is above the national crude mortality rate, the hospital's performance is "better than U.S. National rate."

Data Collection Methods

Cases Included in the Model. All Medicare beneficiaries aged 65 or older who were enrolled in Original Medicare (traditional fee-for-service Medicare) for the entire 12 months prior to their hospital admission for heart attack or heart failure, and for whom complete administrative data for that 12-month period are available, are included in the model. The model identifies (1) all short-stay acute-care hospital discharges for heart attack or heart failure in the reference year based on a principal discharge diagnosis on the Medicare beneficiary's inpatient claim, and (2) all deaths (for all causes) within 30 days of admission. Hospital stays that lasted one day or less are excluded, provided the patient was discharged alive and not against medical advice. (For the initial publication of the rates in June 2007, the reference year used for calculating mortality rates is July 2005 through June 2006. Subsequent updates to the rates are expected to use the same July/June reference year.)

Hospital mortality rates for heart attack are calculated based on all admissions for heart attack, even if an individual Medicare beneficiary was hospitalized more than once for this condition during the 12-month period. However, for purposes of calculating heart failure mortality rates, if a beneficiary had multiple admissions during the 12-month period, one admission is chosen randomly for inclusion in the model.

Use of a 30-Day Period to Assess Mortality

The model tracks deaths that occur within 30 days of a hospital admission, rather than inpatient mortality only, or mortality over some other post-discharge period. Thirty-day mortality was chosen over inpatient mortality because variability across hospitals in lengths of stay can make differences in inpatient mortality hard to interpret. For example, a heart attack patient hospitalized for 12 days may have a higher chance of dying during the hospital stay than a patient hospitalized for only 7 days, merely because the first patient's outcome is tracked for 5 days longer than the second patient's. Thirty-day mortality was chosen over longer windows (such as 90 days or one year), because mortality over longer periods may have less to do with the care received in the hospital and more to do with other complicating illnesses, patients' own behavior, or the care they received after discharge.

Use of Administrative Claims Data

Administrative claims data, rather than medical records data, are used to predict 30-day mortality. These data are widely available for Original Medicare (traditional fee-for-service) beneficiaries, are relatively inexpensive to acquire, and are timely. Using administrative data makes it possible to calculate mortality without having to do chart reviews or requiring hospitals to report additional data. Research conducted when the measures were being developed demonstrated that the administrative claims-based models perform well in predicting mortality compared with models based on chart reviews.

Risk-Adjustment and Covariates Included in the Model

Risk-Adjustment. The model adjusts for differences in patients' risks unrelated to their hospital care (risk-adjustment). The characteristics that Medicare patients bring with them when they arrive at a hospital with a heart attack or heart failure are not under the control of the hospital. However, some patient characteristics may make death more likely (increase the "risk" of death), no matter where the patient is treated or how good the care is. Moreover, some hospitals may treat people with a history of more severe disease. Therefore, when mortality rates are calculated for each hospital for a 12-month period, they are adjusted based on the unique mix of patients that hospital treated during that period. Factors included in the risk-adjustment model include age, gender, past medical history, and other diseases or conditions (comorbidities) that patients had when they arrived at the hospital that are known to increase their risk.

Past medical history and comorbidities are included in the model using CMS's hierarchical condition categories (HCCs) and a history of certain procedures. Medicare patients are assigned to one or more HCCs based on diagnoses (ICD-9 codes) obtained from the patient's discharge claim, and from the hospital inpatient, hospital outpatient, and physician Medicare claims submitted for the patient one year prior to the admission. Secondary diagnoses from the patient's hospital discharge claim that might represent complications that occurred while the patient was in the hospital, rather than conditions that were present on admission, are not included in assigning the patient's HCC. Research has shown that coding differences among providers affect HCCs only slightly. Diagnoses from unreliable sources (such as laboratory or other claims that were not based on face-to-face encounters) are not included when assigning the HCCs in the model.

To "risk-adjust" mortality rates for patient characteristics, the statistical model estimates the independent effects of age, gender, comorbidities, and a hospital-specific component of quality on mortality of patients within 30 days of hospital admission (the dependent variable). Using these estimates, the model calculates an adjusted mortality rate for each hospital that can be compared with those of other hospitals with different case mixes.

Covariates in 30-Day Mortality Risk-Adjustment Models	
Heart Attack	Heart Failure
Age-65	Age-65
Gender (male)	Gender (male)
History of PTCA	History of PTCA
History of CABG	History of CABG
History of heart failure	History of heart failure
History of MI	History of MI
AMI location (Group 1): anterior, anterolateral	
AMI location (Group 2): inferolateral, inferoposterior, inferior, other lateral, and true posterior	
Unstable angina	Unstable angina
Chronic atherosclerosis	Chronic atherosclerosis
Cardiopulmonary-respiratory failure and shock	Cardiopulmonary-respiratory failure and shock
Valvular heart disease	Valvular heart disease
Hypertension	Hypertension
Stroke	Stroke
Cerebrovascular disease	
Renal failure	Renal failure
COPD	COPD
Pneumonia	Pneumonia
Diabetes	Diabetes
Protein-calorie malnutrition	Protein-calorie malnutrition
Dementia	Dementia
Functional disability	Functional disability
Peripheral vascular disease	Peripheral vascular disease
Metastatic cancer	Metastatic cancer
Trauma in last year	Trauma in last year
Major psych disorder	Major psych disorder
Chronic liver disease	Chronic liver disease

Statistical Methods Used to Calculate Mortality Rates

Hierarchical Regression Model. The statistical model for computing 30-day risk-adjusted mortality rate measures is a "hierarchical regression model." This type of model is based on the assumption that any heart attack or heart failure patients treated at a particular hospital will experience a level of quality of care that applies to all patients treated for the same condition in that hospital. In other words, the expected risk of death for two similar heart attack or heart failure patients treated in the same hospital would be more alike than the risk of death for the same two patients treated in two different hospitals.

The likelihood that an individual patient will die is therefore a combination of (1) his or her individual risk characteristics (for example, gender, comorbidities, and past medical history) and 2) the hospital's unique quality of care for all patients treated for that condition in that hospital. The model estimates the effects of both of these components on mortality.

Calculating Mortality Rates. Each hospital's "30-day risk-adjusted mortality rate" (also called the "Risk Standardized Mortality Rate" or RSMR) is computed in several steps. First, the predicted 30-day mortality for a particular hospital obtained from the hierarchical regression model is divided by the expected mortality for that hospital, which is also obtained from the regression model. Predicted mortality is the rate of deaths from heart attack or heart failure that would be anticipated in the particular hospital during the 12-month period, given the patient case mix and the hospital's unique quality of care effect on mortality. Expected mortality is the rate of deaths from heart attack or heart failure that would be expected if the same patients with the same characteristics had instead been treated at an "average" hospital, given the "average" hospital's quality of care effect on mortality for patients with that condition. This ratio is then multiplied by the national unadjusted mortality rate for the condition for all hospitals to compute a "risk-adjusted mortality rate" for the hospital. So, the higher a hospital's predicted 30-day mortality rate, relative to expected mortality for the hospital's particular case mix of patients, the higher its adjusted mortality rate will be. Hospitals with better quality will have lower rates.

(Predicted 30-day mortality/Expected mortality) * U.S. National mortality rate = RSMR

For example, suppose the model predicts that 10 percent of Hospital A's heart attack patients would die within 30 days of admission in a given year, based on their ages, gender mix, and pre-existing health conditions, and based on the estimate of the hospital's specific quality of care. Then, suppose that the expected rate of 30-day deaths for those same patients were higher – say, 15 percent – if they had instead been treated at an "average" U.S. hospital. If the actual mortality rate for the 12-month period for all heart attack patients in all hospitals in the U.S. is 12 percent, then the hospital's risk-adjusted 30-day mortality rate would be 8 percent.

(10%/15%)* 12% = RSMR for Hospital A 8%

If, instead, 9 percent of these patients would be expected to have died if treated at the average hospital, then the hospital's mortality rate would be 13.3 percent.

(10%/9%)* 12% = RSMR for Hospital A 13.3%

In the first case, the hospital performed better than the average hospital and had a relatively low risk-adjusted mortality rate (8 percent); in the second case it performed worse and had a relatively high rate (13.3 percent).

Hospitals with relatively low-risk patients whose predicted mortality rate is the same as the expected mortality rate for the average hospital for the same group of low-risk patients would have an adjusted mortality rate equal to the national rate (12 percent in this example). Similarly, hospitals with high-risk patients whose predicted mortality rate is the same as the expected mortality rate for the average hospital for the same group of high-risk patients would also have an adjusted mortality rate equal to the national rate of 12 percent. Thus, each hospital's case mix should not affect the adjusted mortality rates used to compare hospitals.

Adjusting for Small Hospitals or a Small Number of Cases. The hierarchical regression model also adjusts mortality rates results for small hospitals or hospitals with few heart attack or heart failure cases in a given year. This reduces the chance that such hospitals' performance will fluctuate wildly from year to year or that they will be wrongly classified as either a worse or better performer. For these hospitals, the model not only considers deaths among patients treated for the condition in the small sample size of cases, but pools together patients from all hospitals treated for the given condition, to make the result more reliable. In essence, the predicted mortality rate for a hospital with a small number of cases is moved toward the overall U.S. National mortality rate for all hospitals. The estimates of mortality for hospitals with few patients will rely considerably on the pooled data for all hospitals, making it less likely that small hospitals will fall into either of the outlier categories. This pooling affords a "borrowing of statistical strength" that provides more confidence in the results.

Significance Testing, Interval Estimates, and Comparing Rates Among Hospitals

Significance Testing and Interval Estimates. The model also calculates how precise the estimates of the adjusted mortality rate are, and determines upper and lower bounds (Interval Estimates) for each hospital's risk-adjusted rate. Interval estimates, which are like confidence intervals, describe how much uncertainty there is around the rate—how much bigger or smaller the rate might really be. Larger hospitals typically have more precise estimates and smaller interval estimates, since more data are available to estimate mortality. The smaller the sample size, the greater the difference in mortality rates between a hospital and the national rate must be in order for that difference to be statistically meaningful.

Comparing Mortality Rates Among Hospitals. The risk-adjusted hospital rate with its interval estimate can be compared to the U.S. National crude mortality rate. If the interval estimate includes (overlaps with) the national crude mortality rate, the hospital's performance is in the "no different than U.S. National rate" category. If the entire interval estimate is below the national crude mortality rate, then the hospital is performing "worse than U.S. National rate." If the entire interval estimate is above the national crude mortality rate, it is "better than U.S. National rate."

Glossary of Terms

Accreditation
An evaluative process in which a healthcare organization undergoes an examination of its policies, procedures and performance by an external private sector organization ("accrediting body") to ensure that it is meeting predetermined criteria. It usually involves both on- and off-site surveys. Also see the terms AOA, The Joint Commission, and Medicare-Certified Hospitals.

Acute Care Hospital
A hospital that provides inpatient medical care and other related services for surgery, acute medical conditions or injuries (usually for a short term illness or condition).

Acute Myocardial Infarction (AMI)
A condition (also called a heart attack) that occurs when the arteries leading to the heart become blocked and the blood supply is slowed or stopped. When the heart muscle can't get the oxygen and nutrients it needs, the part of the heart tissue that is affected may die.

Additional Measures
Measures included in the Hospital Quality Alliance measure set, reflecting care for discharges occurring on or after April 1, 2004 (Collection period varies by measure).

Acute Myocardial Infarction

- Fibrinolytic agent received within 30 minutes of hospital arrival
- Percutaneous Coronary Intervention (PCI) received within 90 minutes of hospital arrival (previously PCI received within 120 minutes of hospital arrival, as well as, Percutaneous Transluminal Coronary Angioplasty (PTCA) received within 90 minutes of hospital arrival)
- Smoking cessation advice/counseling
- 30-Day Risk Adjusted Heart Attack Mortality

Heart Failure

- Discharge instructions
- Smoking cessation advice/counseling
- 30-Day Risk Adjusted Heart Failure Mortality

Pneumonia

- Blood culture performed in the emergency department prior to initial antibiotic received in hospital (previously Blood culture performed prior to first antibiotic received in hospital)
- Smoking cessation advice/counseling
- Appropriate initial antibiotic selection
- Influenza vaccination status

Surgical Care Improvement/Surgical Infection Prevention

- Prophylactic antibiotic received within 1 hour prior to surgical incision
- Prophylactic antibiotic selection
- Prophylactic antibiotic discontinued within 24 hours after surgery end time

American Hospital Association (AHA)
The national organization that represents and serves all types of hospitals, health care networks, and their patients and communities. AHA takes part in national health policy development, legislative and regulatory debates, and legal matters. AHA provides education for health care leaders and is a source of information on health care issues and trends.

American Osteopathic Association (AOA)
A member association representing approximately 52,000 osteopathic physicians (D.O.s). The AOA serves as the primary certifying body for D.O.s, and is the accrediting agency for all osteopathic medical colleges and health care facilities.

The AOA writes a performance report on each hospital that it checks. You can call or write to AOA to find out a hospital's level of accreditation.

Angioplasty
In angioplasty, a catheter is used to insert a balloon that is inflated to open a blocked blood vessel. Percutaneous transluminal coronary angioplasty (PTCA) is one of several procedures used to open a blocked blood vessel, known collectively as a percutaneous coronary intervention or PCI.

Angiotensin Converting Enzyme (ACE) Inhibitor
A medicine used to treat heart attacks, heart failure, or a decreased function of the left heart. They stop production of a hormone that can narrow blood vessels. This helps reduce the pressure in the heart and lower blood pressure.

Angiotensin Receptor Blocker (ARB)
A medicine used to treat patients with heart failure and a decreased function of the left heart. ARBs block the action of a hormone that can narrow blood vessels. This helps reduce the pressure in the heart and lower blood pressure.

Antibiotic
Medicine used to fight bacteria in the body.

Atherectomy
A procedure where a blade or laser on a catheter cuts through and removes blockages in blood vessels. It is one of several procedures used to open a blocked blood vessel (known as a Percutaneous Coronary Intervention or PCI).

Beta Blocker
A type of medicine that is used to lower blood pressure, treat chest pain (angina) and heart failure, and to help prevent a heart attack. Beta blockers relieve the stress on the heart by slowing the heart rate and reducing the force with which the heart muscles contract to pump blood. They also help keep blood vessels from constricting in the heart, brain, and body.

Blood Culture
A blood test that shows if there are bacteria in the blood, and what type of bacteria it is. It helps your doctor decide which antibiotic to use to treat a bacterial infection.

Centers for Medicare & Medicaid Services (CMS)
The federal agency that runs the Medicare program for the elderly aged and disabled. In addition, CMS works with the states to run the Medicaid program for low-income individuals. CMS works to make sure that the people in these programs are able to get high quality health care. Also see the term DHHS.

Certification (Medicare-Certified)
State government agencies inspect health care providers, including hospitals, nursing homes, dialysis facilities and home health agencies, as well as other health care providers. These providers are certified if they pass inspection. Being certified is not the same as being accredited. Medicare or Medicaid only pays for care provided by certified or accredited providers.

Critical Access Hospital (CAH)
A small, generally geographically remote facility that provides outpatient and inpatient hospital services to people in rural areas. The designation was established by law, for special payments under the Medicare program. To be designated as a CAH, a hospital must be located in a rural area, provide 24-hour emergency services; have an average length-of-stay for its patients of 96 hours or less; be located more than 35 miles (or more than 15 miles in areas with mountainous terrain) from the nearest hospital or be designated by its State as a "necessary provider". Hospitals may have no more than 25 beds.

Department of Health and Human Services (DHHS)
A division of the U.S. government that administers many of the social programs at the Federal level dealing with the health and welfare of the citizens of the United States. CMS is an agency within DHHS.

Diastolic Pressure
The lowest pressure in the artery when the heart is filling with blood. In a blood pressure reading, the diastolic pressure is the second number recorded.

Do hospitals that treat sicker patients have worse death rates? (Risk-adjustment)
Hospitals that treat sicker patients do not necessarily have worse death rates. The hospital-specific 30-day death (mortality) rates used in this report have been adjusted to account for differences in patients' health before their hospital admission.

Sicker patients or patients with more health-related risks may be more likely to die than healthier patients. Moreover, patients who are sicker may be more likely to be treated at particular hospitals while patients who are healthier may be more likely to be treated at other hospitals.

To compare hospitals fairly (and to avoid penalizing those that treat sicker patients) it is therefore important to consider differences in patients' health before they were admitted to the hospital. The statistical process of accounting for differences in patients' sickness before they were admitted to the hospital is called risk-adjustment. This statistical process aims to 'level the playing field' by accounting for health risks that patients have before they enter the hospital.

Fibrinolysis, Fibrinolytic Drugs
Fibrinolytic drugs are "clot-busting" medicines that can help dissolve blood clots in blood vessels and improve blood flow to your heart. They are important for treating heart attacks. If you have a heart attack, your doctor may give you a fibrinolytic drug, perform a percutaneous coronary intervention (PCI), or both.

Hospital Quality Alliance (HQA): Improving Care Through Information
In December 2002, the American Hospital Association (AHA), Federation of American Hospitals (FAH), and Association of American Medical Colleges (AAMC) launched the Hospital Quality Alliance (HQA), a national public-private collaboration to encourage hospitals to voluntarily collect and report hospital quality performance information. This effort is intended to make important information about hospital performance accessible to the public and to inform and invigorate efforts to improve quality. CMS and the Joint Commission participate in the HQA, along with the AHA, the FAH, the AAMC, the American Medical Association, the American Nurses Association, the National Association of Children's Hospitals and Related Organizations, American Association of Retired People, American Federation of Labor and Council of Industrial Organizations, the Consumer-Purchaser Disclosure Project, the Agency for Healthcare Research and Quality, the National Quality Forum, the Blue Cross and Blue Shield Association, the National Business Coalition on Health, General Electric, and the U.S. Chamber of Commerce.

Influenza
Influenza is a serious and sometimes deadly lung infection that can spread quickly in a community. Symptoms include fever-often a high temperature of more than 102° Fahrenheit (38.9° Celsius), headache, muscle aches and pains, chills, cough and chest pain when you take a breath ("pleuritic chest pain"). Although most people recover from the illness, the Centers for Disease Control and Prevention (the CDC) estimates that in the United States more than 200,000 people are hospitalized and about 36,000 people die from the flu and its complications every year.

Influenza Vaccination ("Flu Shot")
The main way to keep from getting flu is to get a yearly flu vaccination. Scientists make a different vaccine every year because the strains of flu viruses change from year to year. Nine to 10 months before the flu season begins, they prepare a new vaccine made from inactivated (killed) flu viruses. Because the viruses have been killed, they cannot cause infection. The vaccine preparation is based on the strains of the flu viruses that are in circulation at the time.

Hospitals should check to make sure that pneumonia patients get a flu shot during flu season to protect them from another lung infection and to help prevent the spread of influenza in the community. You can also get the vaccine at your doctor's office or a local clinic, and in many communities at workplaces, supermarkets, and drugstores. You must get the vaccine every year because it changes.

Inpatient Hospital Services
Services provided to patients admitted to a hospital that include bed and board, nursing services, diagnostic or therapeutic services, and medical or surgical services.

Left Ventricular Function Assessment
A test to check how well the heart is pumping.

Long-term Care Hospital
A facility, like a nursing home, that provides a variety of services that help people with health or personal needs and activities of daily living (like walking, eating, and going to the bathroom) over a period of time. Most long-term care is custodial care, for which Medicare does not pay.

Measurement
The process of collecting data to assess performance conducted at a single point in time or repeated over time.

Medicaid
A joint federal and state program that helps with medical costs for some people with low incomes and limited resources. Medicaid programs vary from state to state, but most health care costs are covered if you qualify for both Medicare and Medicaid.

Medicare-Certified Hospital
In order to receive any payment from either the Medicare or Medicaid programs, a hospital must meet a set of basic standards for quality of care, called "conditions of participation". Medicare-certified hospitals are reviewed periodically (every three years) to assure that they are continuing to provide services of acceptable quality.

Medicare also considers or "deems" hospitals as Medicare-certified that meet the accreditation requirements of the The Joint Commission or the American Osteopathic Association. Most short-term acute care hospitals in the United States choose to be Medicare-certified, either directly or through accreditation.

Medicare Provider Number
Medicare identifies the hospitals with which it works using a unique number. These numbers were used to identify the facilities that reported data for Hospital Compare. If hospitals share a Medicare Provider Number (for example, they bill Medicare for services as a single legal entity), the performance data for those hospitals are, in effect, combined into an aggregate rate representing all of the hospitals represented by the Medicare Provider Number. If you are interested in a hospital that is part of a system or network, you may not be able to find your specific hospital.

Medigap Policy
A Medicare supplement insurance policy sold by private insurance companies to fill "gaps" in Original Medicare Plan coverage. Except in Massachusetts, Minnesota and Wisconsin, there are 10 standardized plans labeled Plan A through Plan J. Medigap policies only work with the Original Medicare Plan.

Original Medicare Plan
A pay-per-visit health plan that lets you go to any doctor, hospital, or other health care supplier who accepts Medicare and is accepting new Medicare patients. You must pay the deductible. Medicare pays its share of the Medicare-approved amount, and you pay your share (coinsurance). In some cases you may be charged more than the Medicare-approved amount. The Original Medicare Plan has two parts: Part A (Hospital Insurance) and Part B (Medical Insurance).

Osteopathic Doctor
A licensed physician who can do surgery and prescribe drugs who has training in manipulative therapy. Also called a Doctor of Osteopathy or DO.

Outcome Measures
Measures designed to reflect the results of care, rather than how frequently a specific treatment or intervention was performed.

Oxygenation Assessment
Test that measures the amount of oxygen in your blood to see if you need oxygen therapy.

Percutaneous Coronary Interventions (PCI)
The procedures called Percutaneous Coronary Interventions (PCI), such as angioplasty and atherectomy are among those that are the most effective for opening blocked blood vessels that cause heart attacks. Doctors may perform a PCI, or give medicine to open the blockage, and in some cases, may do both.

Plan of Care
A written plan of care created with your physician and hospital staff. It tells what services you will get to reach and keep your best physical, mental, and social well being. The hospital staff keeps your doctor up-to-date on how you are doing and updates your care plan as needed.

Pneumonia
An inflammation of the lungs caused by a viral or bacterial infection. This fills your lungs with mucus and lowers the oxygen level in your blood. Symptoms can include fever, fatigue, difficulty breathing, chills, a "wet" cough, and chest pain.

Pneumonia (pneumococcal) Vaccination
Vaccine given to prevent pneumonia, estimated to protect against 80% of bacteria causing pneumonia.

Process of Care Measures
Measures that show, in percentage form or as a rate, how often a health care provider gives recommended care; that is, the treatment known to give the best results for most patients with a particular condition.

Provider
A doctor, hospital, health care professional, or health care facility.

Psychiatric Hospital
A facility that provides inpatient psychiatric services for the diagnosis and treatment of mental illness on a 24-hour basis, by or under the supervision of a physician.

Quality
Quality health care is how well a doctor, hospital, health plan, or other provider of health care, keeps its members healthy or treats them when they are sick. Good quality health care means doing the right thing at the right time, in the right way, for the right person and getting the best possible results.

Quality Assurance
The process of looking at how well a medical service is provided. The process may include formally reviewing health care given to a person, or group of persons, locating the problem, correcting the problem, and then checking to see if what you did worked.

Quality Improvement Organizations (QIOs)
Groups of practicing doctors and other health care experts who are paid by the federal government to check and improve the care given to Medicare patients. They must review your complaints about the quality of care given by: inpatient hospitals, hospital outpatient departments, hospital emergency rooms, skilled nursing facilities, home health agencies, Private Fee-for-Service plans, and ambulatory surgical centers.

Rehabilitation Hospital
A hospital that specializes in improving or restoring a patient's functional ability through therapies. Sometimes called a post-acute hospital.

Risk-Adjusted 30-Day Death (Mortality) Rates
The 30-day Risk-Adjusted Death (Mortality) Rates are produced using a complex statistical model, that relies on Medicare claims and enrollment information. The model predicts patient deaths for any cause within 30 days of hospital admission for heart attack or heart failure, whether the patients die while still in the hospital or after discharge. Thirty-day mortality is used because this is the time period when deaths are most likely to be related to the care patients received in the hospital. Deaths that occur outside the hospital within 30 days are included along with deaths that occur in the hospital, because some hospitals discharge patients sooner than others.

"Starter Set" Measures

Heart Attack
- Aspirin at arrival
- Aspirin at discharge
- ACE Inhibitor or ARB for Left Ventricular Systolic Dysfunction*
- Beta Blocker at arrival
- Beta Blocker at discharge

Heart Failure
- Evaluation of Left Ventricular Systolic (LVS) Function**
- ACE Inhibitor or ARB for Left Ventricular Systolic Dysfunction*

Pneumonia
- Oxygenation Assessment
- Initial Antibiotic Timing
- Pneumococcal Vaccination Status

*Modified, effective 1Q2005 discharges. For more information, see http://www.cms.hhs.gov/HospitalQualityInits/downloads/HospitalSummaryOfMeeting1.pdf.

**Modified, effective 1Q2006 discharges.

Stent
A small wire tube inserted in a blood vessel by a catheter to hold open a blocked blood vessel. One of several procedures to open a blocked blood vessel called a percutaneous coronary intervention (PCI).

The Joint Commission
An organization that evaluates and accredits health care organizations and programs in the United States. The Joint Commission is an independent, not-for-profit organization. The Joint Commission looks at how well a hospital treats patients and how good a hospital's staff and equipment are. A hospital is accredited by The Joint Commission if it meets certain quality standards. These checks are done at least every 3 years. Most hospitals take part in these accreditations.

The Joint Commission writes a "performance report" on each hospital that it checks. You can order these reports free of charge.

Thirty-Day Mortality Model Information
See Krumholtz, H., et al. "An Administrative Claims Model Suitable for Profiling Hospital Performance Based on 30-Day Mortality Rates Among Patients with an Acute Myocardial Infarction." Circulation. Vol. 113: 1683-1692, 2006, for details on the development of the AMI model. An accompanying article in the same volume discusses the heart failure model.

Treatment
Something done to help with a health problem. For example, medicine and surgery are treatments.

Treatment Options
The choices you have when there is more than one way to treat your health problem.

Sedgwick Press
Hospital & Health Plan Directories

'he Directory of Hospital Personnel, 2007

'*he Directory of Hospital Personnel* is the best resource you can have at your fingertips when researching or marketing a product or ervice to the hospital market. A "Who's Who" of the hospital universe, this directory puts you in touch with over 150,000 key ecision-makers. With 100% verification of data you can rest assured that you will reach the right person with just one call. Every ospital in the U.S. is profiled, listed alphabetically by city within state. Plus, three easy-to-use, cross-referenced indexes put the facts t your fingertips faster and more easily than any other directory: Hospital Name Index, Bed Size Index and Personnel Index. *The)irectory of Hospital Personnel* is the only complete source for key hospital decision-makers by name. Whether you want to define or estructure sales territories... locate hospitals with the purchasing power to accept your proposals... keep track of important contacts r colleagues... or find information on which insurance plans are accepted, *The Directory of Hospital Personnel* gives you the information ou need – easily, efficiently, effectively and accurately.

"Recommended for college, university and medical libraries." -ARBA

,500 pages; Softcover ISBN 1-59237-178-7 $325.00 ◆ Online Database $545.00 ◆ Online Database & Directory Combo, $650.00

'he Directory of Health Care Group Purchasing Organizations, 2006

'his comprehensive directory provides the important data you need to get in touch with over 800 Group Purchasing Organizations. y providing in-depth information on this growing market and its members, *The Directory of Health Care Group Purchasing Organizations* ills a major need for the most accurate and comprehensive information on over 800 GPOs – Mailing Address, Phone & Fax Numbers, -mail Addresses, Key Contacts, Purchasing Agents, Group Descriptions, Membership Categorization, Standard Vendor Proposal equirements, Membership Fees & Terms, Expanded Services, Total Member Beds & Outpatient Visits represented and more. Five ndexes provide a number of ways to locate the right GPO: Alphabetical Index, Expanded Services Index, Organization Type Index, ;eographic Index and Member Institution Index. With its comprehensive and detailed information on each purchasing organization, '*he Directory of Health Care Group Purchasing Organizations* is the go-to source for anyone looking to target this market.

"The information is clearly arranged and easy to access...recommended for those needing this very specialized information." –ARBA

,000 pages; Softcover ISBN 1-59237-0091-8, $325.00 ◆ Online Database, $650.00 ◆ Online Database & Directory Combo, $750.00

'he HMO/PPO Directory, 2007

'*he HMO/PPO Directory* is a comprehensive source that provides detailed information about Health Maintenance Organizations and 'referred Provider Organizations nationwide. This comprehensive directory details more information about more managed health care rganizations than ever before. Over 1,100 HMOs, PPOs, Medicare Advantage Plans and affiliated companies are listed, arranged lphabetically by state. Detailed listings include Key Contact Information, Prescription Drug Benefits, Enrollment, Geographical Areas erved, Affiliated Physicians & Hospitals, Federal Qualifications, Status, Year Founded, Managed Care Partners, Employer References, 'ees & Payment Information and more. Plus, five years of historical information is included related to Revenues, Net Income, Medical ,oss Ratios, Membership Enrollment and Number of Patient Complaints. Five easy-to-use, cross-referenced indexes will put this vast rray of information at your fingertips immediately: HMO Index, PPO Index, Other Providers Index, Personnel Index and Enrollment ndex. *The HMO/PPO Directory* provides the most comprehensive data on the most companies available on the market place today.

"Helpful to individuals requesting certain HMO/PPO issues such as co-payment costs, subscription costs and patient complaints. Individuals concerned (or those with questions) about their insurance may find this text to be of use to them." -ARBA

;00 pages; Softcover ISBN 1-59237-158-2, $325.00 ◆ Online Database, $495.00 ◆ Online Database & Directory Combo, $600.00

To preview any of our Directories Risk-Free for 30 days, call (800) 562-2139 or fax to (518) 789-0556

Medical Device Register, 2007

The only one-stop resource of every medical supplier licensed to sell products in the US. This award-winning directory offers immediate access to over 13,000 companies - and more than 65,000 products – in two information-packed volumes. This comprehensive resource saves hours of time and trouble when searching for medical equipment and supplies and the manufacturers who provide them. Volume I: The Product Directory, provides essential information for purchasing or specifying medical supplies for every medical device supply, and diagnostic available in the US. Listings provide FDA codes & Federal Procurement Eligibility, Contact information for every manufacturer of the product along with Prices and Product Specifications. Volume 2 - Supplier Profiles, offers the most complete and important data about Suppliers, Manufacturers and Distributors. Company Profiles detail the number of employees, ownership, method of distribution, sales volume, net income, key executives detailed contact information medical products the company supplies, plus the medical specialties they cover. Four indexes provide immediate access to this wealth of information: Keyword Index, Trade Name Index, Supplier Geographical Index and OEM (Original Equipment Manufacturer) Index. Medical Device Register, 2007 is the only one-stop source for locating suppliers and products; looking for new manufacturers or hard-to-find medical devices; comparing products and companies; know who's selling what and who to buy from cost effectively. This directory has become the standard in its field and will be a welcome addition to the reference collection of any medical library, large public library, university library along with the collections that serve the medical community.

"A wealth of information on medical devices, medical device companies… and key personnel in the industry is provide in this comprehensive reference work... A valuable reference work, one of the best hardcopy compilations available." -Doody Publishing

3,000 pages Two Volumes; Hardcover ISBN 1-59237-181-7; $325.00

The Directory of Independent Ambulatory Care Centers

This first edition of *The Directory of Independent Ambulatory Care Centers* provides access to detailed information that, before now, could only be found scattered in hundreds of different sources. This comprehensive and up-to-date directory pulls together a vast array of contact information for over 7,200 Ambulatory Surgery Centers, Ambulatory General and Urgent Care Clinics, and Diagnostic Imaging Centers that are not affiliated with a hospital or major medical center. Detailed listings include Mailing Address, Phone & Fax Numbers, E-mail and Web Site addresses, Contact Name and Phone Numbers of the Medical Director and other Key Executives and Purchasing Agents, Specialties & Services Offered, Year Founded, Numbers of Employees and Surgeons, Number of Operating Rooms, Number of Cases seen per year, Overnight Options, Contracted Services and much more. Listings are arranged by State, by Center Category and then alphabetically by Organization Name. Two indexes provide quick and easy access to this wealth of information: Entry Name Index and Specialty/Service Index. *The Directory of Independent Ambulatory Care Centers* is a must-have resource for anyone marketing a product or service to this important industry and will be an invaluable tool for those searching for a local care center that will meet their specific needs.

"Among the numerous hospital directories, no other provides information on independent ambulatory centers. A handy, well-organized resource that would be useful in medical center libraries and public libraries." –Choice

986 pages; Softcover ISBN 1-930956-90-8, $185.00 • Online Database, $365.00 • Online Database & Directory Combo, $450.00

Sedgwick Press
Health Directories

The Complete Directory for People with Disabilities, 2007

A wealth of information, now in one comprehensive sourcebook. Completely updated, this edition contains more information than ever before, including thousands of new entries and enhancements to existing entries and thousands of additional web sites and e-mail addresses. This up-to-date directory is the most comprehensive resource available for people with disabilities, detailing Independent Living Centers, Rehabilitation Facilities, State & Federal Agencies, Associations, Support Groups, Periodicals & Books, Assistive Devices, Employment & Education Programs, Camps and Travel Groups. Each year, more libraries, schools, colleges, hospitals, rehabilitation centers and individuals add *The Complete Directory for People with Disabilities* to their collections, making sure that this information is readily available to the families, individuals and professionals who can benefit most from the amazing wealth of resources cataloged here.

"No other reference tool exists to meet the special needs of the disabled in one convenient resource for information." –Library Journal

1,200 pages; Softcover ISBN 1-59237-147-7, $165.00 ◆ Online Database $215.00 ◆ Online Database & Directory Combo $300.00

The Complete Directory for People with Chronic Illness, 2007/08

Thousands of hours of research have gone into this completely updated 2005/06 edition – several new chapters have been added along with thousands of new entries and enhancements to existing entries. Plus, each chronic illness chapter has been reviewed by an medical expert in the field. This widely-hailed directory is structured around the 90 most prevalent chronic illnesses – from Asthma to Cancer to Wilson's Disease – and provides a comprehensive overview of the support services and information resources available for people diagnosed with a chronic illness. Each chronic illness has its own chapter and contains a brief description in layman's language, followed by important resources for National & Local Organizations, State Agencies, Newsletters, Books & Periodicals, Libraries & Research Centers, Support Groups & Hotlines, Web Sites and much more. This directory is an important resource for health care professionals, the collections of hospital and health care libraries, as well as an invaluable tool for people with a chronic illness and their support network.

"A must purchase for all hospital and health care libraries and is strongly recommended for all public library reference departments." –ARBA

1,200 pages; Softcover ISBN 1-59237-183-3, $165.00 ◆ Online Database $215.00 ◆ Online Database & Directory Combo $300.00

The Complete Learning Disabilities Directory, 2007

The Complete Learning Disabilities Directory is the most comprehensive database of Programs, Services, Curriculum Materials, Professional Meetings & Resources, Camps, Newsletters and Support Groups for teachers, students and families concerned with learning disabilities. This information-packed directory includes information about Associations & Organizations, Schools, Colleges & Testing Materials, Government Agencies, Legal Resources and much more. For quick, easy access to information, this directory contains four indexes: Entry Name Index, Subject Index and Geographic Index. With every passing year, the field of learning disabilities attracts more attention and the network of caring, committed and knowledgeable professionals grows every day. This directory is an invaluable research tool for these parents, students and professionals.

"Due to its wealth and depth of coverage, parents, teachers and others... should find this an invaluable resource." -Booklist

900 pages; Softcover ISBN 1-59237-122-1, $145.00 ◆ Online Database $195.00 ◆ Online Database & Directory Combo $280.00

The Complete Mental Health Directory, 2006/07

This is the most comprehensive resource covering the field of behavioral health, with critical information for both the layman and the mental health professional. For the layman, this directory offers understandable descriptions of 25 Mental Health Disorders as well as detailed information on Associations, Media, Support Groups and Mental Health Facilities. For the professional, *The Complete Mental Health Directory* offers critical and comprehensive information on Managed Care Organizations, Information Systems, Government Agencies and Provider Organizations. This comprehensive volume of needed information will be widely used in any reference collection.

"... the strength of this directory is that it consolidates widely dispersed information into a single volume." –Booklist

800 pages; Softcover ISBN 1-59237-124-8, $165.00 ◆ Online Database $215.00 ◆ Online & Directory Combo $300.00

To preview any of our Directories Risk-Free for 30 days, call (800) 562-2139 or fax to (518) 789-0556

Older Americans Information Directory, 2006/07

Completely updated for 2006/07, this sixth edition has been completely revised and now contains 1,000 new listings, over 8,000 updates to existing listings and over 3,000 brand new e-mail addresses and web sites. You'll find important resources for Older Americans including National, Regional, State & Local Organizations, Government Agencies, Research Centers, Libraries & Information Centers, Legal Resources, Discount Travel Information, Continuing Education Programs, Disability Aids & Assistive Devices, Health, Print Media and Electronic Media. Three indexes: Entry Index, Subject Index and Geographic Index make it easy to find just the right source of information. This comprehensive guide to resources for Older Americans will be a welcome addition to any reference collection.

"Highly recommended for academic, public, health science and consumer libraries…" –Choice

1,200 pages; Softcover ISBN 1-59237-136-1, $165.00 ◆ Online Database $215.00 ◆ Online Database & Directory Combo $300.00

The Complete Directory for Pediatric Disorders, 2007

This important directory provides parents and caregivers with information about Pediatric Conditions, Disorders, Diseases and Disabilities, including Blood Disorders, Bone & Spinal Disorders, Brain Defects & Abnormalities, Chromosomal Disorders, Congenital Heart Defects, Movement Disorders, Neuromuscular Disorders and Pediatric Tumors & Cancers. This carefully written directory offers: understandable Descriptions of 15 major bodily systems; Descriptions of more than 200 Disorders and a Resources Section, detailing National Agencies & Associations, State Associations, Online Services, Libraries & Resource Centers, Research Centers, Support Groups & Hotlines, Camps, Books and Periodicals. This resource will provide immediate access to information crucial to families and caregivers when coping with children's illnesses.

"Recommended for public and consumer health libraries." –Library Journal

1,200 pages; Softcover ISBN 1-59237-150-7 $165.00 ◆ Online Database $215.00 ◆ Online Database & Directory Combo $300.00

The Directory of Drug & Alcohol Residential Rehabilitation Facilities

This brand new directory is the first-ever resource to bring together, all in one place, data on the thousands of drug and alcohol residential rehabilitation facilities in the United States. *The Directory of Drug & Alcohol Residential Rehabilitation Facilities* covers over 1,000 facilities, with detailed contact information for each one, including mailing address, phone and fax numbers, email addresses and web sites, mission statement, type of treatment programs, cost, average length of stay, numbers of residents and counselors, accreditation, insurance plans accepted, type of environment, religious affiliation, education components and much more. It also contains a helpful chapter on General Resources that provides contact information for Associations, Print & Electronic Media, Support Groups and Conferences. Multiple indexes allow the user to pinpoint the facilities that meet very specific criteria. This time-saving tool is what so many counselors, parents and medical professionals have been asking for. *The Directory of Drug & Alcohol Residential Rehabilitation Facilities* will be a helpful tool in locating the right source for treatment for a wide range of individuals. This comprehensive directory will be an important acquisition for all reference collections: public and academic libraries, case managers, social workers, state agencies and many more.

"This is an excellent, much needed directory that fills an important gap…" –Booklist

300 pages; Softcover ISBN 1-59237-031-4, $135.00

Sedgwick Press
Education Directories

'he Comparative Guide to American Elementary & Secondary Schools, 2007

'he only guide of its kind, this award winning compilation offers a snapshot profile of every public school district in the United States erving 1,500 or more students – more than 5,900 districts are covered. Organized alphabetically by district within state, each chapter egins with a Statistical Overview of the state. Each district listing includes contact information (name, address, phone number and veb site) plus Grades Served, the Numbers of Students and Teachers and the Number of Regular, Special Education, Alternative and 'ocational Schools in the district along with statistics on Student/Classroom Teacher Ratios, Drop Out Rates, Ethnicity, the Numbers f Librarians and Guidance Counselors and District Expenditures per student. As an added bonus, *The Comparative Guide to American Elementary and Secondary Schools* provides important ranking tables, both by state and nationally, for each data element. For easy avigation through this wealth of information, this handbook contains a useful City Index that lists all districts that operate schools vithin a city. These important comparative statistics are necessary for anyone considering relocation or doing comparative research on heir own district and would be a perfect acquisition for any public library or school district library.

"This straightforward guide is an easy way to find general information. Valuable for academic and large public library collections." –ARBA

,400 pages; Softcover ISBN 1-59237-223-6, $125.00

Educators Resource Directory, 2007/08

Educators Resource Directory is a comprehensive resource that provides the educational professional with thousands of resources and tatistical data for professional development. This directory saves hours of research time by providing immediate access to Associations & Organizations, Conferences & Trade Shows, Educational Research Centers, Employment Opportunities & Teaching Abroad, School Library Services, Scholarships, Financial Resources, Professional Consultants, Computer Software & Testing Resources and much more. Plus, this comprehensive directory also includes a section on Statistics and Rankings with over 100 tables, including statistics on Average Teacher Salaries, SAT/ACT scores, Revenues & Expenditures and more. These important statistics will allow the user to see how their school rates among others, make relocation decisions and so much more. For quick access to information, this directory contains four indexes: Entry & Publisher Index, Geographic Index, a Subject & Grade Index and Web Sites Index. *Educators Resource Directory* will be a well-used addition to the reference collection of any school district, education department or public library.

"Recommended for all collections that serve elementary and secondary school professionals." –Choice

,000 pages; Softcover ISBN 1-59237-179-5, $145.00 ◆ Online Database $195.00 ◆ Online Database & Directory Combo $280.00

To preview any of our Directories Risk-Free for 30 days, call (800) 562-2139 or fax to (518) 789-0556

Grey House Publishing
Business Directories

The Directory of Business Information Resources, 2007

With 100% verification, over 1,000 new listings and more than 12,000 updates, this 2007 edition of *The Directory of Business Information Resources* is the most up-to-date source for contacts in over 98 business areas – from advertising and agriculture to utilities and wholesalers. This carefully researched volume details: the Associations representing each industry; the Newsletters that keep members current; the Magazines and Journals - with their "Special Issues" - that are important to the trade, the Conventions that are "must attends," Databases, Directories and Industry Web Sites that provide access to must-have marketing resources. Includes contact names, phone & fax numbers, web sites and e-mail addresses. This one-volume resource is a gold mine of information and would be a welcome addition to any reference collection.

"This is a most useful and easy-to-use addition to any researcher's library." –The Information Professionals Institut

2,500 pages; Softcover ISBN 1-59237-146-9, $195.00 ◆ Online Database $495.00

Nations of the World, 2007/08 A Political, Economic and Business Handbook

This completely revised edition covers all the nations of the world in an easy-to-use, single volume. Each nation is profiled in a single chapter that includes Key Facts, Political & Economic Issues, a Country Profile and Business Information. In this fast-changing world, it is extremely important to make sure that the most up-to-date information is included in your reference collection. This edition is just the answer. Each of the 200+ country chapters have been carefully reviewed by a political expert to make sure that the text reflects the most current information on Politics, Travel Advisories, Economics and more. You'll find such vital information as a Country Map, Population Characteristics, Inflation, Agricultural Production, Foreign Debt, Political History, Foreign Policy, Regional Insecurity, Economics, Trade & Tourism, Historical Profile, Political Systems, Ethnicity, Languages, Media, Climate, Hotels, Chambers of Commerce, Banking, Travel Information and more. Five Regional Chapters follow the main text and include a Regional Map, an Introductory Article, Key Indicators and Currencies for the Region. As an added bonus, an all-inclusive CD-ROM is available as a companion to the printed text. Noted for its sophisticated, up-to-date and reliable compilation of political, economic and business information, this brand new edition will be an important acquisition to any public, academic or special library reference collection.

"A useful addition to both general reference collections and business collections." –RUSQ

1,700 pages; Print Version Only Softcover ISBN 1-59237-177-9, $155.00

The Directory of Venture Capital & Private Equity Firms, 2007

This edition has been extensively updated and broadly expanded to offer direct access to over 2,800 Domestic and International Venture Capital Firms, including address, phone & fax numbers, e-mail addresses and web sites for both primary and branch locations. Entries include details on the firm's Mission Statement, Industry Group Preferences, Geographic Preferences, Average and Minimum Investments and Investment Criteria. You'll also find details that are available nowhere else, including the Firm's Portfolio Companies and extensive information on each of the firm's Managing Partners, such as Education, Professional Background and Directorships held, along with the Partner's E-mail Address. *The Directory of Venture Capital & Private Equity Firms* offers five important indexes: Geographic Index, Executive Name Index, Portfolio Company Index, Industry Preference Index and College & University Index. With its comprehensive coverage and detailed, extensive information on each company, *The Directory of Venture Capital & Private Equity Firms* is an important addition to any finance collection.

"The sheer number of listings, the descriptive information provided and the outstanding indexing make this directory a better value than its principa competitor, Pratt's Guide to Venture Capital Sources. Recommended for business collections in large public, academic and business libraries." –Choic

1,300 pages; Softcover ISBN 1-59237-176-0, $565.00/$450.00 Library ◆ Online Database (includes a free copy of the directory) $889.0C

To preview any of our Directories Risk-Free for 30 days, call (800) 562-2139 or fax to (518) 789-0556

The Directory of Mail Order Catalogs, 2007

Published since 1981, the *Directory of Mail Order Catalogs* is the premier source of information on the mail order catalog industry. It is the source that business professionals and librarians have come to rely on for the thousands of catalog companies in the US. New for 2007, The Directory of Mail Order Catalogs has been combined with its companion volume, *The Directory of Business to Business Catalogs,* to offer all 13,000 catalog companies in one easy-to-use volume. Section I: Consumer Catalogs, covers over 9,000 consumer catalog companies in 44 different product chapters from Animals to Toys & Games. Section II: Business to Business Catalogs, details 5,000 business catalogs, everything from computers to laboratory supplies, building construction and much more. Listings contain detailed contact information including mailing address, phone & fax numbers, web sites, e-mail addresses and key contacts along with important business details such as product descriptions, employee size, years in business, sales volume, catalog size, number of catalogs mailed and more. Three indexes are included for easy access to information: Catalog & Company Name Index, Geographic Index and Product Index. *The Directory of Mail Order Catalogs,* now with its expanded business to business catalogs, is the largest and most comprehensive resource covering this billion-dollar industry. It is the standard in its field. This important resource is a useful tool for entrepreneurs searching for catalogs to pick up their product, vendors looking to expand their customer base in the catalog industry, market researchers, small businesses investigating new supply vendors, along with the library patron who is exploring the available catalogs in their areas of interest.

"This is a godsend for those looking for information." –Reference Book Review

1,700 pages; Softcover ISBN 1-59237-156-6 $350.00/$250.00 Library ◆ Online Database (includes a free copy of the directory) $495.00

Sports Market Place Directory, 2007

For over 20 years, this comprehensive, up-to-date directory has offered direct access to the Who, What, When & Where of the Sports Industry. With over 20,000 updates and enhancements, the *Sports Market Place Directory* is the most detailed, comprehensive and current sports business reference source available. In 1,800 information-packed pages, *Sports Market Place Directory* profiles contact information and key executives for: Single Sport Organizations, Professional Leagues, Multi-Sport Organizations, Disabled Sports, High School & Youth Sports, Military Sports, Olympic Organizations, Media, Sponsors, Sponsorship & Marketing Event Agencies, Event & Meeting Calendars, Professional Services, College Sports, Manufacturers & Retailers, Facilities and much more. *The Sports Market Place Directory* provides organization's contact information with detailed descriptions including: Key Contacts, physical, mailing, email and web addresses plus phone and fax numbers. Plus, nine important indexes make sure that you can find the information you're looking for quickly and easily: Entry Index, Single Sport Index, Media Index, Sponsor Index, Agency Index, Manufacturers Index, Brand Name Index, Facilities Index and Executive/Geographic Index. For over twenty years, *The Sports Market Place Directory* has assisted thousands of individuals in their pursuit of a career in the sports industry. Why not use "THE SOURCE" that top recruiters, headhunters and career placement centers use to find information on or about sports organizations and key hiring contacts.

1,800 pages; Softcover ISBN 1-59237-189-2, $225.00 ◆ Online Database $479.00

Food and Beverage Market Place, 2007

Food and Beverage Market Place is bigger and better than ever with thousands of new companies, thousands of updates to existing companies and two revised and enhanced product category indexes. This comprehensive directory profiles over 18,000 Food & Beverage Manufacturers, 12,000 Equipment & Supply Companies, 2,200 Transportation & Warehouse Companies, 2,000 Brokers & Wholesalers, 8,000 Importers & Exporters, 900 Industry Resources and hundreds of Mail Order Catalogs. Listings include detailed Contact Information, Sales Volumes, Key Contacts, Brand & Product Information, Packaging Details and much more. *Thomas Food and Beverage Market Place* is available as a three-volume printed set, a subscription-based Online Database via the Internet, on CD-ROM, as well as mailing lists and a licensable database.

"An essential purchase for those in the food industry but will also be useful in public libraries where needed. Much of the information will be difficult and time consuming to locate without this handy three-volume ready-reference source." –ARBA

8,500 pages, 3 Volume Set; Softcover ISBN 1-59237-152-3, $595.00 ◆ Online Database $795.00 ◆ Online Database & 3 Volume Set Combo, $995.00

The Grey House Homeland Security Directory, 2007

This updated edition features the latest contact information for government and private organizations involved with Homeland Security along with the latest product information and provides detailed profiles of nearly 1,000 Federal & State Organizations & Agencies and over 3,000 Officials and Key Executives involved with Homeland Security. These listings are incredibly detailed and include Mailing Address, Phone & Fax Numbers, Email Addresses & Web Sites, a complete Description of the Agency and a complete list of the Officials and Key Executives associated with the Agency. Next, *The Grey House Homeland Security Directory* provides the go-to source for Homeland Security Products & Services. This section features over 2,000 Companies that provide Consulting, Products or Services. With this Buyer's Guide at their fingertips, users can locate suppliers of everything from Training Materials to Access Controls, from Perimeter Security to BioTerrorism Countermeasures and everything in between – complete with contact information and product descriptions. A handy Product Locator Index is provided to quickly and easily locate suppliers of a particular product. Lastly, an Information Resources Section provides immediate access to contact information for hundreds of Associations, Newsletters, Magazines, Trade Shows, Databases and Directories that focus on Homeland Security. This comprehensive, information-packed resource will be a welcome tool for any company or agency that is in need of Homeland Security information and will be a necessary acquisition for the reference collection of all public libraries and large school districts.

"Compiles this information in one place and is discerning in content. A useful purchase for public and academic libraries." –Booklis

800 pages; Softcover ISBN 1-59237-151-5, $195.00 ◆ Online Database (includes a free copy of the directory) $385.00

The Grey House Transportation Security Directory & Handbook

This brand new title is the only reference of its kind that brings together current data on Transportation Security. With information on everything from Regulatory Authorities to Security Equipment, this top-flight database brings together the relevant information necessary for creating and maintaining a security plan for a wide range of transportation facilities. With this current, comprehensive directory at the ready you'll have immediate access to: Regulatory Authorities & Legislation; Information Resources; Sample Security Plans & Checklists; Contact Data for Major Airports, Seaports, Railroads, Trucking Companies and Oil Pipelines; Security Service Providers; Recommended Equipment & Product Information and more. Using the *Grey House Transportation Security Directory & Handbook*, managers will be able to quickly and easily assess their current security plans; develop contacts to create and maintain new security procedures; and source the products and services necessary to adequately maintain a secure environment. This valuable resource is a must for all Security Managers at Airports, Seaports, Railroads, Trucking Companies and Oil Pipelines.

800 pages; Softcover ISBN 1-59237-075-6, $195

The Grey House Safety & Security Directory, 2007

The Grey House Safety & Security Directory is the most comprehensive reference tool and buyer's guide for the safety and security industry. Arranged by safety topic, each chapter begins with OSHA regulations for the topic, followed by Training Articles written by top professionals in the field and Self-Inspection Checklists. Next, each topic contains Buyer's Guide sections that feature related products and services. Topics include Administration, Insurance, Loss Control & Consulting, Protective Equipment & Apparel, Noise & Vibration, Facilities Monitoring & Maintenance, Employee Health Maintenance & Ergonomics, Retail Food Services, Machine Guards, Process Guidelines & Tool Handling, Ordinary Materials Handling, Hazardous Materials Handling, Workplace Preparation & Maintenance, Electrical Lighting & Safety, Fire & Rescue and Security. The Buyer's Guide sections are carefully indexed within each topic area to ensure that you can find the supplies needed to meet OSHA's regulations. Six important indexes make finding information and product manufacturers quick and easy: Geographical Index of Manufacturers and Distributors, Company Profile Index, Brand Name Index, Product Index, Index of Web Sites and Index of Advertisers. This comprehensive, up-to-date reference will provide every tool necessary to make sure a business is in compliance with OSHA regulations and locate the products and services needed to meet those regulations.

"Presents industrial safety information for engineers, plant managers, risk managers, and construction site supervisors…" –Choic

1,500 pages, 2 Volume Set; Softcover ISBN 1-59237-160-4, $225.00

˜he Grey House Biometric Information Directory

˜*he Biometric Information Directory* is the only comprehensive source for current biometric industry information. This 2006 edition is the ırst published by Grey House. With 100% updated information, this latest edition offers a complete, current look, in both print and nline form, of biometric companies and products – one of the fastest growing industries in today's economy. Detailed profiles of nanufacturers of the latest biometric technology, including Finger, Voice, Face, Hand, Signature, Iris, Vein and Palm Identification ystems. Data on the companies include key executives, company size and a detailed, indexed description of their product line. Plus, he Directory also includes valuable business resources, and current editorial make this edition the easiest way for the business ommunity and consumers alike to access the largest, most current compilation of biometric industry information available on the narket today. The new edition boasts increased numbers of companies, contact names and company data, with over 700 manufacturers nd service providers. Information in the directory includes: Editorial on Advancements in Biometrics; Profiles of 700+ companies isted with contact information; Organizations, Trade & Educational Associations, Publications, Conferences, Trade Shows and Expositions Worldwide; Web Site Index; Biometric & Vendors Services Index by Types of Biometrics; and a Glossary of Biometric Terms. This resource will be an important source for anyone who is considering the use of a biometric product, investing in the levelopment of biometric technology, support existing marketing and sales efforts and will be an important acquisition for the business eference collection for large public and business libraries.

ı00 pages; Softcover ISBN 1-59237-121-3, $225

The Rauch Guide to the US Adhesives & Sealants, Cosmetics & Toiletries, Ink, Paint, lastics, Pulp & Paper and Rubber Industries

The Rauch Guides are known worldwide for their comprehensive marketing information. Acquired by Grey House Publishing in 2005, ıew updated and revised editions will be published throughout 2005 and 2006. Each Guide provides market facts and figures in a ighly organized format, ideal for today's busy personnel, serving as ready-references for top executives as well as the industry ıewcomer. *The Rauch Guides* save time and money by organizing widely scattered information and providing estimates for important ɔusiness decisions, some of which are available nowhere else. Each Guide is organized into several information-packed chapters. After a brief introduction, the ECONOMICS section provides data on industry shipments; long-term growth and forecasts; prices; company performance; employment, expenditures, and productivity; transportation and geographical patterns; packaging; foreign trade; ınd government regulations. Next, TECHNOLOGY & RAW MATERIALS provide market, technical, and raw material information for chemicals, equipment and related materials, including market size and leading suppliers, prices, end uses, and trends. PRODUCTS & MARKETS provide information for each major industry product, including market size and historical trends, leading suppliers, five-year forecasts, industry structure, and major end uses. For easy access, each *Guide* contains a chapter on INDUSTRY ACTIVITIES, ORGANIZATIONS & SOURCES OF INFORMATION with detailed information on meetings, exhibits, and trade shows, sources of statistical information, trade associations, technical and professional societies, and trade and technical periodicals. Next, the COMPANY DIRECTORY profiles major industry companies, both public and private. Generally several hundred companies are analyzed. Information includes complete contact information, web address, estimated total and domestic sales, product description, and recent mergers and acquisitions. Each Guide also contains several APPENDICES that provide a cross-reference of suppliers, subsidiaries and divisions. The Rauch Guides will prove to be an invaluable source of market information, company data, trends and forecasts that anyone in these fast-paced industries.

The Rauch Guide to the U.S. Paint Industry Softcover ISBN 1-59237-127-2 $595 ♦ The Rauch Guide to the U.S. Plastics Industry Softcover ISBN 1-59237-128-0 $595 ♦ The Rauch Guide to the U.S. Adhesives and Sealants Industry Softcover ISBN 1-59237-129-9 $595 ♦ The Rauch Guide to the U.S. Ink Industry Softcover ISBN 1-59237-126-4 $595 ♦ The Rauch Guide to the U.S. Rubber Industry Softcover ISBN 1-59237-130-2 $595 ♦ The Rauch Guide to the U.S. Pulp and Paper Industry Softcover ISBN 1-59237-131-0 $595 ♦ The Rauch Guide to the U.S. Cosmetic and Toiletries Industry Softcover ISBN 1-59237-132-9 $895

The Grey House Performing Arts Directory, 2007

The Grey House Performing Arts Directory is the most comprehensive resource covering the Performing Arts. This important directory provides current information on over 8,500 Dance Companies, Instrumental Music Programs, Opera Companies, Choral Groups, Theater Companies, Performing Arts Series and Performing Arts Facilities. Plus, this edition now contains a brand new section on Artist Management Groups. In addition to mailing address, phone & fax numbers, e-mail addresses and web sites, dozens of other fields of available information include mission statement, key contacts, facilities, seating capacity, season, attendance and more. This directory also provides an important Information Resources section that covers hundreds of Performing Arts Associations, Magazines, Newsletters, Trade Shows, Directories, Databases and Industry Web Sites. Five indexes provide immediate access to this wealth of information: Entry Name, Executive Name, Performance Facilities, Geographic and Information Resources. *The Grey House Performing Arts Directory* pulls together thousands of Performing Arts Organizations, Facilities and Information Resources into an easy-to-use source – this kind of comprehensiveness and extensive detail is not available in any resource on the market place today.

"Immensely useful and user-friendly … recommended for public, academic and certain special library reference collections." –Booklist

1,500 pages; Softcover ISBN 1-59237-138-8, $185.00 ♦ Online Database $335.00

New York State Directory, 2007/08

The New York State Directory, published annually since 1983, is a comprehensive and easy-to-use guide to accessing public officials and private sector organizations and individuals who influence public policy in the state of New York. *The New York State Directory* include important information on all New York state legislators and congressional representatives, including biographies and key committee assignments. It also includes staff rosters for all branches of New York state government and for federal agencies and departments that impact the state policy process. Following the state government section are 25 chapters covering policy areas from agriculture through veterans' affairs. Each chapter identifies the state, local and federal agencies and officials that formulate or implement policy. In addition, each chapter contains a roster of private sector experts and advocates who influence the policy process. The directory also offers appendices that include statewide party officials; chambers of commerce; lobbying organizations; public and private universities and colleges; television, radio and print media; and local government agencies and officials.

New York State Directory - 800 pages; Softcover ISBN 1-59237-190-6; $145.00
New York State Directory with Profiles of New York – 2 volumes; 1,600 pages; Softcover ISBN 1-59237-191-4; $225

Profiles of New York ♦ Profiles of Florida ♦ Profiles of Texas ♦ Profiles of Illinois ♦ Profiles of Michigan ♦ Profiles of Ohio ♦ Profiles of New Jersey ♦ Profiles of Massachusetts ♦ Profiles of Pennsylvania ♦ Profiles of Wisconsin ♦ Profiles of Connecticut ♦ Profiles of Indiana ♦ Profiles of North Carolina ♦ Profiles of Virginia ♦ Profiles of California

Packed with over 50 pieces of data that make up a complete, user-friendly profile of each state, these directories go even further by then pulling selected data and providing it in ranking list form for even easier comparisons between the 100 largest towns and cities! The careful layout gives the user an easy-to-read snapshot of every single place and county in the state, from the biggest metropolis to the smallest unincorporated hamlet. The richness of each place or county profile is astounding in its depth, from history to weather, all packed in an easy-to-navigate, compact format. No need for piles of multiple sources with this volume on your desk. Here is a look at just a few of the data sets you'll find in each profile: History, Geography, Climate, Population, Vital Statistics, Economy, Income, Taxes, Education, Housing, Health & Environment, Public Safety, Newspapers, Transportation, Presidential Election Results, Information Contacts and Chambers of Commerce. As an added bonus, there is a section on Selected Statistics, where data from the 100 largest towns and cities is arranged into easy-to-use charts. Each of 22 different data points has its own two-page spread with the cities listed in alpha order so researchers can easily compare and rank cities. A remarkable compilation that offers overviews and insights into each corner of the state, *Profiles of New York, Profiles of Florida* and *Profiles of Texas* go beyond Census statistics, beyond metro area coverage, beyond the 100 best places to live. Drawn from official census information, other government statistics and original research, you will have at your fingertips data that's available nowhere else in one single source. Data will be published on additional states in 2006 and 2007.

Each Profiles of... title ranges from 400-800 pages, priced at $149.00 each

Research Services Directory: Commercial & Corporate Research Centers

This Ninth Edition provides access to well over 8,000 independent Commercial Research Firms, Corporate Research Centers and Laboratories offering contract services for hands-on, basic or applied research. *Research Services Directory* covers the thousands of types of research companies, including Biotechnology & Pharmaceutical Developers, Consumer Product Research, Defense Contractors, Electronics & Software Engineers, Think Tanks, Forensic Investigators, Independent Commercial Laboratories, Information Brokers, Market & Survey Research Companies, Medical Diagnostic Facilities, Product Research & Development Firms and more. Each entry provides the company's name, mailing address, phone & fax numbers, key contacts, web site, e-mail address, as well as a company description and research and technical fields served. Four indexes provide immediate access to this wealth of information: Research Firms Index, Geographic Index, Personnel Name Index and Subject Index.

"An important source for organizations in need of information about laboratories, individuals and other facilities." –ARBA

1,400 pages; Softcover ISBN 1-59237-003-9, $395.00 ♦ Online Database (includes a free copy of the directory) $850.00

International Business and Trade Directories

Completely updated, the Third Edition of *International Business and Trade Directories* now contains more than 10,000 entries, over 2,000 more than the last edition, making this directory the most comprehensive resource of the worlds business and trade directories. Entries include content descriptions, price, publisher's name and address, web site and e-mail addresses, phone and fax numbers and editorial staff. Organized by industry group, and then by region, this resource puts over 10,000 industry-specific business and trade directories at the reader's fingertips. Three indexes are included for quick access to information: Geographic Index, Publisher Index and Title Index. Public, college and corporate libraries, as well as individuals and corporations seeking critical market information will want to add this directory to their marketing collection.

"Reasonably priced for a work of this type, this directory should appeal to larger academic, public and corporate libraries with an international focus." –Library Journal

1,800 pages; Softcover ISBN 1-930956-63-0, $225.00 ♦ Online Database (includes a free copy of the directory) $450.00

To preview any of our Directories Risk-Free for 30 days, call (800) 562-2139 or fax to (518) 789-0556

Grey House Publishing Canada
Canadian Information Resources

Canadian Almanac & Directory, 2007

The Canadian Almanac & Directory contains ten directories in one – giving you all the facts and figures you will ever need about Canada. No other single source provides users with the quality and depth of up-to-date information for all types of research. This national directory and guide gives you access to statistics, images and over 45,000 names and addresses for everything from Airlines to Zoos - updated every year. It's Ten Directories in One! Each section is a directory in itself, providing robust information on business and finance, communications, government, associations, arts and culture (museums, zoos, libraries, etc.), health, transportation, law, education, and more. Government information includes federal, provincial and territorial - and includes an easy-to-use quick index to find key information. A separate municipal government section includes every municipality in Canada, with full profiles of Canada's largest urban centers. A complete legal directory lists judges and judicial officials, court locations and law firms across the country. A wealth of general information, the Canadian Almanac & Directory also includes national statistics on population, employment, imports and exports, and more. National awards and honors are presented, along with forms of address, Commonwealth information and full color photos of Canadian symbols. Postal information, weights, measures, distances and other useful charts are also incorporated. Complete almanac information includes perpetual calendars, five-year holiday planners and astronomical information. Published continuously for 160 years, The Canadian Almanac & Directory is the best single reference source for business executives, managers and assistants; government and public affairs executives; lawyers; marketing, sales and advertising executives; researchers, editors and journalists.

Hardcover ISBN 978-1-89502-149-3; 1,600 pages; $315.00

Associations Canada, 2007

The Most Powerful Fact-Finder to Business, Trade, Professional and Consumer Organizations

Associations Canada covers Canadian organizations and international groups including industry, commercial and professional associations, registered charities, special interest and common interest organizations. This annually revised compendium provides detailed listings and abstracts for nearly 20,000 regional, national and international organizations. This popular volume provides the most comprehensive picture of Canada's non-profit sector. Detailed listings enable users to identify an organization's budget, founding date, scope of activity, licensing body, sources of funding, executive information, full address and complete contact information, just to name a few. Powerful indexes help researchers find information quickly and easily. The following indexes are included: subject, acronym, geographic, budget, executive name, conferences & conventions, mailing list, defunct and unreachable associations and registered charitable organizations. In addition to annual spending of over $1 billion on transportation and conventions alone, Canadian associations account for many millions more in pursuit of membership interests. Associations Canada provides complete access to this highly lucrative market. Associations Canada is a strong source of prospects for sales and marketing executives, tourism and convention officials, researchers, government officials - anyone who wants to locate non-profit interest groups and trade associations.

Hardcover ISBN 978-1-59237-219-5; 1,600 pages; $315.00

Financial Services Canada, 2007/08

Financial Services Canada is the only master file of current contacts and information that serves the needs of the entire financial services industry in Canada. With over 18,000 organizations and hard-to-find business information, Financial Services Canada is the most up-to-date source for names and contact numbers of industry professionals, senior executives, portfolio managers, financial advisors, agency bureaucrats and elected representatives. Financial Services Canada incorporates the latest changes in the industry to provide you with the most current details on each company, including: name, title, organization, telephone and fax numbers, e-mail and web addresses. Financial Services Canada also includes private company listings never before compiled, government agencies, association and consultant services - to ensure that you'll never miss a client or a contact. Current listings include: banks and branches, non-depository institutions, stock exchanges and brokers, investment management firms, insurance companies, major accounting and law firms, government agencies and financial associations. Powerful indexes assist researchers with locating the vital financial information they need. The following indexes are included: alphabetic, geographic, executive name, corporate web site/e-mail, government quick reference and subject. Financial Services Canada is a valuable resource for financial executives, bankers, financial planners, sales and marketing professionals, lawyers and chartered accountants, government officials, investment dealers, journalists, librarians and reference specialists.

900 pages; Hardcover ISBN 978-1-59237-221-8 $315.00

To preview any of our Directories Risk-Free for 30 days, call (800) 562-2139 or fax to (518) 789-0556

Directory of Libraries in Canada, 2007/08

The Directory of Libraries in Canada brings together almost 7,000 listings including libraries and their branches, information resource centers, archives and library associations and learning centers. The directory offers complete and comprehensive information on Canadian libraries, resource centers, business information centers, professional associations, regional library systems, archives, library schools and library technical programs. The Directory of Libraries in Canada includes important features of each library and service, including library information; personnel details, including contact names and e-mail addresses; collection information; services available to users; acquisitions budgets; and computers and automated systems. Useful information on each library's electronic access is also included, such as Internet browser, connectivity and public Internet/CD-ROM/subscription database access. The directory also provides powerful indexes for subject, location, personal name and Web site/e-mail to assist researchers with locating the crucial information they need. The Directory of Libraries in Canada is a vital reference tool for publishers, advocacy groups, students, research institutions, computer hardware suppliers, and other diverse groups that provide products and services to this unique market.

850 pages; Hardcover ISBN 978-1-59237-222-5; $315.00

Canadian Environmental Directory, 2007/08

The Canadian Environmental Directory is Canada's most complete and only national listing of environmental associations and organizations, government regulators and purchasing groups, product and service companies, special libraries, and more! The extensive Products and Services section provides detailed listings enabling users to identify the company name, address, phone, fax, e-mail, Web address, firm type, contact names (and titles), product and service information, affiliations, trade information, branch and affiliate data. The Government section gives you all the contact information you need at every government level – federal, provincial and municipal. We also include descriptions of current environmental initiatives, programs and agreements, names of environment-related acts administered by each ministry or department PLUS information and tips on who to contact and how to sell to governments in Canada. The Associations section provides complete contact information and a brief description of activities. Included are Canadian environmental organizations and international groups including industry, commercial and professional associations, registered charities, special interest and common interest organizations. All the Information you need about the Canadian environmental industry: directory of products and services, special libraries and resource, conferences, seminars and tradeshows, chronology of environmental events, law firms and major Canadian companies, The Canadian Environmental Directory is ideal for business, government, engineers and anyone conducting research on the environment.

Hardcover ISBN 978-1-59237-218-8; 900 pages; $315.00

Grey House Publishing
General Reference Titles

The Value of a Dollar 1600-1859, The Colonial Era to The Civil War

Following the format of the widely acclaimed, *The Value of a Dollar, 1860-2004*, *The Value of a Dollar 1600-1859, The Colonial Era to The Civil War* records the actual prices of thousands of items that consumers purchased from the Colonial Era to the Civil War. Our editorial department had been flooded with requests from users of our Value of a Dollar for the same type of information, just from an earlier time period. This new volume is just the answer – with pricing data from 1600 to 1859. Arranged into five-year chapters, each 5-year chapter includes a Historical Snapshot, Consumer Expenditures, Investments, Selected Income, Income/Standard Jobs, Food Basket, Standard Prices and Miscellany. There is also a section on Trends. This informative section charts the change in price over time and provides added detail on the reasons prices changed within the time period, including industry developments, changes in consumer attitudes and important historical facts. This fascinating survey will serve a wide range of research needs and will be useful in all high school, public and academic library reference collections.

600 pages; Hardcover ISBN 1-59237-094-2, $135.00

The Value of a Dollar 1860-2004, Third Edition

A guide to practical economy, *The Value of a Dollar* records the actual prices of thousands of items that consumers purchased from the Civil War to the present, along with facts about investment options and income opportunities. This brand new Third Edition boasts a brand new addition to each five-year chapter, a section on Trends. This informative section charts the change in price over time and provides added detail on the reasons prices changed within the time period, including industry developments, changes in consumer attitudes and important historical facts. Plus, a brand new chapter for 2000-2004 has been added. Each 5-year chapter includes a Historical Snapshot, Consumer Expenditures, Investments, Selected Income, Income/Standard Jobs, Food Basket, Standard Prices and Miscellany. This interesting and useful publication will be widely used in any reference collection.

"Recommended for high school, college and public libraries." –ARBA

600 pages; Hardcover ISBN 1-59237-074-8, $135.00

Working Americans 1880-1999
Volume I: The Working Class, Volume II: The Middle Class, Volume III: The Upper Class

Each of the volumes in the *Working Americans 1880-1999* series focuses on a particular class of Americans, The Working Class, The Middle Class and The Upper Class over the last 120 years. Chapters in each volume focus on one decade and profile three to five families. Family Profiles include real data on Income & Job Descriptions, Selected Prices of the Times, Annual Income, Annual Budgets, Family Finances, Life at Work, Life at Home, Life in the Community, Working Conditions, Cost of Living, Amusements and much more. Each chapter also contains an Economic Profile with Average Wages of other Professions, a selection of Typical Pricing, Key Events & Inventions, News Profiles, Articles from Local Media and Illustrations. The *Working Americans* series captures the lifestyles of each of the classes from the last twelve decades, covers a vast array of occupations and ethnic backgrounds and travels the entire nation. These interesting and useful compilations of portraits of the American Working, Middle and Upper Classes during the last 120 years will be an important addition to any high school, public or academic library reference collection.

"These interesting, unique compilations of economic and social facts, figures and graphs will support multiple research needs. They will engage and enlighten patrons in high school, public and academic library collections." –Booklist

Volume I: The Working Class ◆ 558 pages; Hardcover ISBN 1-891482-81-5, $145.00 ◆ Volume II: The Middle Class ◆ 591 pages; Hardcover ISBN 1-891482-72-6; $145.00 ◆ Volume III: The Upper Class ◆ 567 pages; Hardcover ISBN 1-930956-38-X, $145.00

Working Americans 1880-1999 Volume IV: Their Children

This Fourth Volume in the highly successful *Working Americans 1880-1999* series focuses on American children, decade by decade from 1880 to 1999. This interesting and useful volume introduces the reader to three children in each decade, one from each of the Working, Middle and Upper classes. Like the first three volumes in the series, the individual profiles are created from interviews, diaries, statistical studies, biographies and news reports. Profiles cover a broad range of ethnic backgrounds, geographic area and lifestyles – everything from an orphan in Memphis in 1882, following the Yellow Fever epidemic of 1878 to an eleven-year-old nephew of a beer baron and owner of the New York Yankees in New York City in 1921. Chapters also contain important supplementary materials including News Features as well as information on everything from Schools to Parks, Infectious Diseases to Childhood Fears along with Entertainment, Family Life and much more to provide an informative overview of the lifestyles of children from each decade. This interesting account of what life was like for Children in the Working, Middle and Upper Classes will be a welcome addition to the reference collection of any high school, public or academic library.

600 pages; Hardcover ISBN 1-930956-35-5, $145.00

To preview any of our Directories Risk-Free for 30 days, call (800) 562-2139 or fax to (518) 789-0556

Working Americans 1880-2003 Volume V: Americans At War

Working Americans 1880-2003 Volume V: Americans At War is divided into 11 chapters, each covering a decade from 1880-2003 and examines the lives of Americans during the time of war, including declared conflicts, one-time military actions, protests, and preparations for war. Each decade includes several personal profiles, whether on the battlefield or on the homefront, that tell the stories of civilians, soldiers, and officers during the decade. The profiles examine: Life at Home; Life at Work; and Life in the Community. Each decade also includes an Economic Profile with statistical comparisons, a Historical Snapshot, News Profiles, local News Articles, and Illustrations that provide a solid historical background to the decade being examined. Profiles range widely not only geographically, but also emotionally, from that of a girl whose leg was torn off in a blast during WWI, to the boredom of being stationed in the Dakotas as the Indian Wars were drawing to a close. As in previous volumes of the *Working Americans* series, information is presented in narrative form, but hard facts and real-life situations back up each story. The basis of the profiles come from diaries, private print books, personal interviews, family histories, estate documents and magazine articles. For easy reference, *Working Americans 1880-2003 Volume V: Americans At War* includes an in-depth Subject Index. The *Working Americans* series has become an important reference for public libraries, academic libraries and high school libraries. This fifth volume will be a welcome addition to all of these types of reference collections.

600 pages; Hardcover ISBN 1-59237-024-1; $145.00
Five Volume Set (Volumes I-V), Hardcover ISBN 1-59237-034-9, $675.00

Working Americans 1880-2005 Volume VI: Women at Work

Unlike any other volume in the *Working Americans* series, this Sixth Volume, is the first to focus on a particular gender of Americans. *Volume VI: Women at Work*, traces what life was like for working women from the 1860's to the present time. Beginning with the life of a maid in 1890 and a store clerk in 1900 and ending with the life and times of the modern working women, this text captures the struggle, strengths and changing perception of the American woman at work. Each chapter focuses on one decade and profiles three to five women with real data on Income & Job Descriptions, Selected Prices of the Times, Annual Income, Annual Budgets, Family Finances, Life at Work, Life at Home, Life in the Community, Working Conditions, Cost of Living, Amusements and much more. For even broader access to the events, economics and attitude towards women throughout the past 130 years, each chapter is supplemented with News Profiles, Articles from Local Media, Illustrations, Economic Profiles, Typical Pricing, Key Events, Inventions and more. This important volume illustrates what life was like for working women over time and allows the reader to develop an understanding of the changing role of women at work. These interesting and useful compilations of portraits of women at work will be an important addition to any high school, public or academic library reference collection.

600 pages; Hardcover ISBN 1-59237-063-2; $145.00

Working Americans 1880-2005 Volume VII: Social Movements

The newest addition to the widely-successful *Working Americans* series, *Volume VII: Social Movements* explores how Americans sought and fought for change from the 1880s to the present time. Following the format of previous volumes in the Working Americans series, the text examines the lives of 34 individuals who have worked – often behind the scenes — to bring about change. Issues include topics as diverse as the Anti-smoking movement of 1901 to efforts by Native Americans to reassert their long lost rights. Along the way, the book will profile individuals brave enough to demand suffrage for Kansas women in 1912 or demand an end to lynching during a March on Washington in 1923. Each profile is enriched with real data on Income & Job Descriptions, Selected Prices of the Times, Annual Incomes & Budgets, Life at Work, Life at Home, Life in the Community, along with News Features, Key Events, and Illustrations. The depth of information contained in each profile allow the user to explore the private, financial and public lives of these subjects, deepening our understanding of how calls for change took place in our society. A must-purchase for the reference collections of high school libraries, public libraries and academic libraries.

600 pages; Hardcover ISBN 1-59237-101-9; $145.00
Seven Volume Set (Volumes I-VII), Hardcover ISBN 1-59237-133-7, $945.00

The Encyclopedia of Warrior Peoples & Fighting Groups

Many military groups throughout the world have excelled in their craft either by fortuitous circumstances, outstanding leadership, or intense training. This new second edition of The Encyclopedia of Warrior Peoples and Fighting Groups explores the origins and leadership of these outstanding combat forces, chronicles their conquests and accomplishments, examines the circumstances surrounding their decline or disbanding, and assesses their influence on the groups and methods of warfare that followed. This edition has been completely updated with information through 2005 and contains over 20 new entries. Readers will encounter ferocious tribes, charismatic leaders, and daring militias, from ancient times to the present, including Amazons, Buffalo Soldiers, Green Berets, Iron Brigade, Kamikazes, Peoples of the Sea, Polish Winged Hussars, Sacred Band of Thebes, Teutonic Knights, and Texas Rangers. With over 100 alphabetical entries, numerous cross-references and illustrations, a comprehensive bibliography, and index, the Encyclopedia of Warrior Peoples and Fighting Groups is a valuable resource for readers seeking insight into the bold history of distinguished fighting forces.

"This work is especially useful for high school students, undergraduates, and general readers with an interest in military history." –Library Journal

Pub. Date: May 2006; Hardcover ISBN 1-59237-116-7; $135.00

To preview any of our Directories Risk-Free for 30 days, call (800) 562-2139 or fax to (518) 789-0556

he Encyclopedia of Invasions & Conquests, From the Ancient Times to the Present

Throughout history, invasions and conquests have played a remarkable role in shaping our world and defining our boundaries, both hysically and culturally. This second edition of the popular Encyclopedia of Invasions & Conquests, a comprehensive guide to over 50 invasions, conquests, battles and occupations from ancient times to the present, takes readers on a journey that includes the Roman onquest of Britain, the Portuguese colonization of Brazil, and the Iraqi invasion of Kuwait, to name a few. New articles will explore he late 20th and 21st centuries, with a specific focus on recent conflicts in Afghanistan, Kuwait, Iraq, Yugoslavia, Grenada and Chechnya. Categories of entries include countries, invasions and conquests, and individuals. In addition to covering the military spects of invasions and conquests, entries cover some of the political, economic, and cultural aspects, for example, the effects of a onquest on the invade country's political and monetary system and in its language and religion. The entries on leaders – among them Sargon, Alexander the Great, William the Conqueror, and Adolf Hitler – deal with the people who sought to gain control, expand power, or exert religious or political influence over others through military means. Revised and updated for this second edition, entries re arranged alphabetically within historical periods. Each chapter provides a map to help readers locate key areas and geographical eatures, and bibliographical references appear at the end of each entry. Other useful features include cross-references, a cumulative bibliography and a comprehensive subject index. This authoritative, well-organized, lucidly written volume will prove invaluable for a variety of readers, including high school students, military historians, members of the armed forces, history buffs and hobbyists.

"Engaging writing, sensible organization, nice illustrations, interesting and obscure facts, and useful maps make this book a pleasure to read." –ARBA

Pub. Date: March 2006; Hardcover ISBN 1-59237-114-0; $135.00

Encyclopedia of Prisoners of War & Internment

This authoritative second edition provides a valuable overview of the history of prisoners of war and interned civilians, from earliest imes to the present. Written by an international team of experts in the field of POW studies, this fascinating and thought-provoking volume includes entries on a wide range of subjects including the Crusades, Plains Indian Warfare, concentration camps, the two world wars, and famous POWs throughout history, as well as atrocities, escapes, and much more. Written in a clear and easily understandable style, this informative reference details over 350 entries, 30% larger than the first edition, that survey the history of prisoners of war and interned civilians from the earliest times to the present, with emphasis on the 19th and 20th centuries. Medical conditions, international law, exchanges of prisoners, organizations working on behalf of POWs, and trials associated with the treatment of captives are just some of the themes explored. Entries range from the Ardeatine Caves Massacre to Kurt Vonnegut. Entries are arranged alphabetically, plus illustrations and maps are provided for easy reference. The text also includes an introduction, bibliography, appendix of selected documents, and end-of-entry reading suggestions. This one-of-a-kind reference will be a helpful addition to the reference collections of all public libraries, high schools, and university libraries and will prove invaluable to historians and military enthusiasts.

"Thorough and detailed yet accessible to the lay reader. Of special interest to subject specialists and historians; recommended for public and academic libraries." - Library Journal

Pub. Date: March 2006; Hardcover ISBN 1-59237-120-5; $135.00

The Religious Right, A Reference Handbook

Timely and unbiased, this third edition updates and expands its examination of the religious right and its influence on our government, citizens, society, and politics. From the fight to outlaw the teaching of Darwin's theory of evolution to the struggle to outlaw abortion, the religious right is continually exerting an influence on public policy. This text explores the influence of religion on legislation and society, while examining the alignment of the religious right with the political right. A historical survey of the movement highlights the shift to "hands-on" approach to politics and the struggle to present a unified front. The coverage offers a critical historical survey of the religious right movement, focusing on its increased involvement in the political arena, attempts to forge coalitions, and notable successes and failures. The text offers complete coverage of biographies of the men and women who have advanced the cause and an up to date chronology illuminate the movement's goals, including their accomplishments and failures. This edition offers an extensive update to all sections along with several brand new entries. Two new sections complement this third edition, a chapter on legal issues and court decisions and a chapter on demographic statistics and electoral patterns. To aid in further research, The Religious Right, offers an entire section of annotated listings of print and non-print resources, as well as of organizations affiliated with the religious right, and those opposing it. Comprehensive in its scope, this work offers easy-to-read, pertinent information for those seeking to understand the religious right and its evolving role in American society. A must for libraries of all sizes, university religion departments, activists, high schools and for those interested in the evolving role of the religious right.

" Recommended for all public and academic libraries." - Library Journal

Pub. Date: November 2006; Hardcover ISBN 1-59237-113-2; $135.00

From Suffrage to the Senate, America's Political Women

From Suffrage to the Senate is a comprehensive and valuable compendium of biographies of leading women in U.S. politics, past and present, and an examination of the wide range of women's movements. Up to date through 2006, this dynamically illustrated reference work explores American women's path to political power and social equality from the struggle for the right to vote and the abolition of slavery to the first African American woman in the U.S. Senate and beyond. This new edition includes over 150 new entries and a branc new section on trends and demographics of women in politics. The in-depth coverage also traces the political heritage of the abolition, labor, suffrage, temperance, and reproductive rights movements. The alphabetically arranged entries include biographies of every woman from across the political spectrum who has served in the U.S. House and Senate, along with women in the Judiciary and the U.S Cabinet and, new to this edition, biographies of activists and political consultants. Bibliographical references follow each entry. For easy reference, a handy chronology is provided detailing 150 years of women's history. This up-to-date reference will be a must-purchase for women's studies departments, high schools and public libraries and will be a handy resource for those researching the key players in women's politics, past and present.

"An engaging tool that would be useful in high school, public, and academic libraries looking for an overview of the political history of women in the US." –Booklis

Pub. Date: October 2006; Two Volume Set; Hardcover ISBN 1-59237-117-5; $195.00

An African Biographical Dictionary

This landmark second edition is the only biographical dictionary to bring together, in one volume, cultural, social and political leaders – both historical and contemporary – of the sub-Saharan region. Over 800 biographical sketches of prominent Africans, as well as foreigners who have affected the continent's history, are featured, 150 more than the previous edition. The wide spectrum of leaders includes religious figures, writers, politicians, scientists, entertainers, sports personalities and more. Access to these fascinating individuals is provided in a user-friendly format. The biographies are arranged alphabetically, cross-referenced and indexed. Entries include the country or countries in which the person was significant and the commonly accepted dates of birth and death. Each biographical sketch is chronologically written; entries for cultural personalities add an evaluation of their work. This information is followed by a selection of references often found in university and public libraries, including autobiographies and principal biographical works. Appendixes list each individual by country and by field of accomplishment – rulers, musicians, explorers, missionaries, businessmen, physicists – nearly thirty categories in all. Another convenient appendix lists heads of state since independence by country. Up-to-date and representative of African societies as a whole, An African Biographical Dictionary provides a wealth of vital information for students of African culture and is an indispensable reference guide for anyone interested in African affairs.

"An unquestionable convenience to have these concise, informative biographies gathered into one source, indexed, and analyzed by appendixes listing entrants by nation and occupational field." –Wilson Library Bulletir

Pub. Date: July 2006; Hardcover ISBN 1-59237-112-4; $125.00

American Environmental Leaders, From Colonial Times to the Present

A comprehensive and diverse award winning collection of biographies of the most important figures in American environmentalism. Few subjects arouse the passions the way the environment does. How will we feed an ever-increasing population and how can that food be made safe for consumption? Who decides how land is developed? How can environmental policies be made fair for everyone, including multiethnic groups, women, children, and the poor? American Environmental Leaders presents more than 350 biographies of men and women who have devoted their lives to studying, debating, and organizing these and other controversial issues over the last 200 years. In addition to the scientists who have analyzed how human actions affect nature, we are introduced to poets, landscape architects, presidents, painters, activists, even sanitation engineers, and others who have forever altered how we think about the environment. The easy to use A–Z format provides instant access to these fascinating individuals, and frequent cross references indicate others with whom individuals worked (and sometimes clashed). End of entry references provide users with a starting point for further research.

"Highly recommended for high school, academic, and public libraries needing environmental biographical information." –Library Journal/Starred Review

Two Volume Set; Hardcover ISBN 1-57607-385-8 $175.00

World Cultural Leaders of the Twentieth Century

An expansive two volume set that covers 450 worldwide cultural icons, World Cultural Leaders of the Twentieth Century includes each person's works, achievements, and professional careers in a thorough essay. Who was the originator of the term "documentary"? Which poet married the daughter of the famed novelist Thomas Mann in order to help her escape Nazi Germany? Which British writer served as an agent in Russia against the Bolsheviks before the 1917 revolution? These and many more questions are answered in this illuminating text. A handy two volume set that makes it easy to look up 450 worldwide cultural icons: novelists, poets, playwrights, painters, sculptors, architects, dancers, choreographers, actors, directors, filmmakers, singers, composers, and musicians. World Cultural Leaders of the Twentieth Century provides entries (many of them illustrated) covering the person's works, achievements, and professional career in a thorough essay and offers interesting facts and statistics. Entries are fully cross-referenced so that readers can learn how various individuals influenced others. A thorough general index completes the coverage.

"Fills a need for handy, concise information on a wide array of international cultural figures."-ARBA

Two Volume Set; Hardcover ISBN 1-57607-038-7 $175.00

To preview any of our Directories Risk-Free for 30 days, call (800) 562-2139 or fax to (518) 789-0556

The Asian Databook: Statistics for all US Counties & Cities with Over 10,000 Population

This is the first-ever resource that compiles statistics and rankings on the US Asian population. *The Asian Databook* presents over 20 statistical data points for each city and county, arranged alphabetically by state, then alphabetically by place name. Data reported for each place includes Population, Languages Spoken at Home, Foreign-Born, Educational Attainment, Income Figures, Poverty Status, Homeownership, Home Values & Rent, and more. Next, in the Rankings Section, the top 75 places are listed for each data element. These easy-to-access ranking tables allow the user to quickly determine trends and population characteristics. This kind of comparative data can not be found elsewhere, in print or on the web, in a format that's as easy-to-use or more concise. A useful resource for those searching for demographics data, career search and relocation information and also for market research. With data ranging from Ancestry to Education, *The Asian Databook* presents a useful compilation of information that will be a much-needed resource in the reference collection of any public or academic library along with the marketing collection of any company whose primary focus in on the Asian population.

1,000 pages; Softcover ISBN 1-59237-044-6 $150.00

The Hispanic Databook: Statistics for all US Counties & Cities with Over 10,000 Population

Previously published by Toucan Valley Publications, this second edition has been completely updated with figures from the latest census and has been broadly expanded to include dozens of new data elements and a brand new Rankings section. The Hispanic population in the United States has increased over 42% in the last 10 years and accounts for 12.5% of the total US population. For ease-of-use, *The Hispanic Databook* presents over 20 statistical data points for each city and county, arranged alphabetically by state, then alphabetically by place name. Data reported for each place includes Population, Languages Spoken at Home, Foreign-Born, Educational Attainment, Income Figures, Poverty Status, Homeownership, Home Values & Rent, and more. Next, in the Rankings Section, the top 75 places are listed for each data element. These easy-to-access ranking tables allow the user to quickly determine trends and population characteristics. This kind of comparative data can not be found elsewhere, in print or on the web, in a format that's as easy-to-use or more concise. A useful resource for those searching for demographics data, career search and relocation information and also for market research. With data ranging from Ancestry to Education, *The Hispanic Databook* presents a useful compilation of information that will be a much-needed resource in the reference collection of any public or academic library along with the marketing collection of any company whose primary focus in on the Hispanic population.

"This accurate, clearly presented volume of selected Hispanic demographics is recommended for large public libraries and research collections."-Library Journa

1,000 pages; Softcover ISBN 1-59237-008-X, $150.00

Ancestry in America: A Comparative Guide to Over 200 Ethnic Backgrounds

This brand new reference work pulls together thousands of comparative statistics on the Ethnic Backgrounds of all populated places in the United States with populations over 10,000. Never before has this kind of information been reported in a single volume. Section One, Statistics by Place, is made up of a list of over 200 ancestry and race categories arranged alphabetically by each of the 5,000 different places with populations over 10,000. The population number of the ancestry group in that city or town is provided along with the percent that group represents of the total population. This informative city-by-city section allows the user to quickly and easily explore the ethnic makeup of all major population bases in the United States. Section Two, Comparative Rankings, contains three tables for each ethnicity and race. In the first table, the top 150 populated places are ranked by population number for that particular ancestry group, regardless of population. In the second table, the top 150 populated places are ranked by the percent of the total population for that ancestry group. In the third table, those top 150 populated places with 10,000 population are ranked by population number for each ancestry group. These easy-to-navigate tables allow users to see ancestry population patterns and make city-by-city comparisons as well. Plus, as an added bonus with the purchase of *Ancestry in America*, a free companion CD-ROM is available that lists statistics and rankings for all of the 35,000 populated places in the United States. This brand new, information-packed resource will serve a wide-range or research requests for demographics, population characteristics, relocation information and much more. *Ancestry in America: A Comparative Guide to Over 200 Ethnic Backgrounds* will be an important acquisition to all reference collections.

"This compilation will serve a wide range of research requests for population characteristic ... it offers much more detail than other sources." –Booklis

1,500 pages; Softcover ISBN 1-59237-029-2, $225.00

'he American Tally: Statistics & Comparative Rankings for U.S. Cities with Populations over 10,000

'his important statistical handbook compiles, all in one place, comparative statistics on all U.S. cities and towns with a 10,000+ opulation. *The American Tally* provides statistical details on over 4,000 cities and towns and profiles how they compare with one nother in Population Characteristics, Education, Language & Immigration, Income & Employment and Housing. Each section begins vith an alphabetical listing of cities by state, allowing for quick access to both the statistics and relative rankings of any city. Next, the ighest and lowest cities are listed in each statistic. These important, informative lists provide quick reference to which cities are at oth extremes of the spectrum for each statistic. Unlike any other reference, *The American Tally* provides quick, easy access to omparative statistics – a must-have for any reference collection.

"A solid library reference." -Bookwatch

00 pages; Softcover ISBN 1-930956-29-0, $125.00

'he Environmental Resource Handbook, 2007/08

'he Environmental Resource Handbook is the most up-to-date and comprehensive source for Environmental Resources and Statistics. ection I: Resources provides detailed contact information for thousands of information sources, including Associations &)rganizations, Awards & Honors, Conferences, Foundations & Grants, Environmental Health, Government Agencies, National Parks x Wildlife Refuges, Publications, Research Centers, Educational Programs, Green Product Catalogs, Consultants and much more. ection II: Statistics, provides statistics and rankings on hundreds of important topics, including Children's Environmental Index, Aunicipal Finances, Toxic Chemicals, Recycling, Climate, Air & Water Quality and more. This kind of up-to-date environmental data, ll in one place, is not available anywhere else on the market place today. This vast compilation of resources and statistics is a must-ave for all public and academic libraries as well as any organization with a primary focus on the environment.

"...the intrinsic value of the information make it worth consideration by libraries with environmental collections and environmentally concerned users." –Booklist

,000 pages; Softcover ISBN 1-59237-195-7, $155.00 ◆ Online Database $300.00

Weather America, A Thirty-Year Summary of Statistical Weather Data and Rankings

This valuable resource provides extensive climatological data for over 4,000 National and Cooperative Weather Stations throughout he United States. *Weather America* begins with a new Major Storms section that details major storm events of the nation and a National Rankings section that details rankings for several data elements, such as Maximum Temperature and Precipitation. The main ody of *Weather America* is organized into 50 state sections. Each section provides a Data Table on each Weather Station, organized lphabetically, that provides statistics on Maximum and Minimum Temperatures, Precipitation, Snowfall, Extreme Temperatures, 'oggy Days, Humidity and more. State sections contain two brand new features in this edition – a City Index and a narrative)escription of the climatic conditions of the state. Each section also includes a revised Map of the State that includes not only weather tations, but cities and towns.

"Best Reference Book of the Year." –Library Journal

2,013 pages; Softcover ISBN 1-891482-29-7, $175.00

Crime in America's Top-Rated Cities

This volume includes over 20 years of crime statistics in all major crime categories: violent crimes, property crimes and total crime. *Crime in America's Top-Rated Cities* is conveniently arranged by city and covers 76 top-rated cities. *Crime in America's Top-Rated Cities* offers details that compare the number of crimes and crime rates for the city, suburbs and metro area along with national crime trends for violent, property and total crimes. Also, this handbook contains important information and statistics on Anti-Crime Programs, Crime Risk, Hate Crimes, Illegal Drugs, Law Enforcement, Correctional Facilities, Death Penalty Laws and much more. A much-needed resource for people who are relocating, business professionals, general researchers, the press, law enforcement officials and students of criminal justice.

"Data is easy to access and will save hours of searching." –Global Enforcement Review

832 pages; Softcover ISBN 1-891482-84-X, $155.00